Diagnostic
Pathology of
NERVOUS SYSTEM
TUMOURS

We dedicate this book to patients and their families, in the hope that better knowledge of the diagnostic features of nervous system tumours will improve care and lead to a cure.

Commissioning Editor: Michael J. Houston
Project Development Manager: Aoibhe O'Shea
Project Manager: Helen MacDonald at Prepress Projects Ltd
Designer: Sarah Russell
Illustrator: Robin Dean

Diagnostic Pathology of NERVOUS SYSTEM TUMOURS

James W. Ironside BMSc MBChB FRCPEdin FRCPath
Professor of Clinical Neuropathology, Honorary Consultant Neuropathologist,
Department of Pathology, University of Edinburgh,
Edinburgh, UK

Tim H. Moss MBChB PhD FRCPath
Consultant Neuropathologist, Honorary Senior Clinical Lecturer in Neuropathology,
Department of Neuropathology, Frenchay Hospital,
Bristol, UK

David N. Louis MD
Professor of Pathology,
Department of Pathology
Massachusetts General Hospital and Harvard Medical School,
Boston, MA, USA

James S. Lowe BMedSci BMBS DM FRCPath
Professor of Neuropathology,
Division of Pathology, School of Clinical Laboratory Sciences,
University of Nottingham Medical School, Queen's Medical Centre,
Nottingham, UK

Roy O. Weller BSc MD PhD FRCPath
Professor of Neuropathology,
Department of Pathology and Division of Clinical Neuroscience,
University of Southampton School of Medicine,
Southampton General Hospital,
Southampton, UK

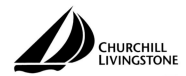

CHURCHILL
LIVINGSTONE

LONDON   EDINBURGH   NEW YORK   PHILADELPHIA   ST LOUIS   SYDNEY   TORONTO   2002

CHURCHILL LIVINGSTONE
An imprint of Elsevier Science Limited

First published 2002

ISBN 0 44304 5585

British Library Cataloguing in Publication Data
A catalogue record for this book is available from the British Library

Library of Congress Cataloging in Publication Data
A catalog record for this book is available from the Library of Congress

Note
Medical knowledge is constantly changing. As new information becomes
available, changes in treatment, procedures, equipment and the use of
drugs become necessary. The editors and the publishers have taken care
to ensure that the information given in this text is accurate and up to date.
However, readers are strongly advised to confirm that the information,
especially with regard to drug usage, complies with the latest legislation
and standards of practice.

The
publisher's
policy is to use
**paper manufactured
from sustainable forests**

Printed in China by RDC Group Limited

Contents

Preface

Our understanding of tumours arising in the tissues of the human nervous system has grown beyond measure in the last decade, and continues to do so with seemingly unceasing momentum. Fundamental research into the cell biology and genetics of these neoplasms is yielding a wealth of information about their predisposing factors, pathogenetic mechanisms, cells of origin, growth kinetics and many other exciting insights. The emergence of new tumour entities, increasing complexities of classification and the identification of features governing both treatment susceptibility and prognosis have all increased the need for a greater precision in pathological diagnosis.

This book is aimed primarily at practising clinical pathologists, but it has been written in the firm belief that pathological information in isolation is no longer sufficient for proper assessment and diagnosis in such a complex and rapidly evolving field of oncology. A multidisciplinary approach is required in clinical practice, and pathologists need not only to interact closely with their clinical neuroscience colleagues, but to understand for themselves the relevant clinical information, features of radiological scans, anatomical sites, current treatment options and prognostic issues. In addition, assessment of the pathology of nervous system tumours requires a thorough knowledge of their background genetics and biology, which are becoming increasingly relevant in classification, growth prediction and potential for treatment. Tumour genetics have been given particular attention in this volume, including detailed description of inherited tumour syndromes. Finally, there is the pathology itself, the core of this book and still the mainstay of diagnosis of nervous system tumours. Carefully chosen illustrations are important for any pathology book and are to be found here, but, as every pathologist knows, diagnosis is much more than matching gross and microscopic images. Emphasis has also been placed on providing textual information that encourages a structured approach to pathological assessment, including choice of stains or other diagnostic techniques and careful consideration of differential diagnosis. For those needing to research a tumour entity in more detail, the book has been referenced throughout, while for the less experienced there are introductory chapters providing more basic advice on the art of pathological diagnosis. Attention has been paid not just to neoplasms of the brain, spinal cord and peripheral nerves, but to any mass lesions that may involve the neuraxis and its coverings, including tumour extensions from local structures and tumour-like lesions such as cysts and vascular malformations. These, after all, are just as likely to be encountered in clinical practice.

You may put this book on your bookshelf, to take down and consult from time to time as a reference volume, and it will not let you down. But we suspect that its practical value will be such that it will rapidly find a permanent home out there on the bench next to the microscope. Those are our intentions, together with the hope that it will become well thumbed and that you will enjoy using it.

James W. Ironside   February 2002
Tim H. Moss
David N. Louis
James S. Lowe
Roy O. Weller

Acknowledgements

We extend heartfelt thanks to our families, friends and mentors for their support during this project. We also wish to thank our colleagues and our technical and secretarial staff for their for their invaluable contributions.

1 An introduction to tumours of the nervous system

Introduction

Tumours of the nervous system are the second most common form of cancer in children and the sixth most common in adults. Affecting the brain and spinal cord with the onset of focal neurological signs, changes in personality or raised intracranial pressure, these tumours can be very distressing for patients and for carers. Although successful treatments are offered for certain types of tumour of the nervous system, some of the most common tumours, such as glioblastoma, have a poor prognosis and treatment is only marginally successful. With the increasing use of imaging by computerised tomography (CT) and magnetic resonance imaging (MRI) worldwide, there is a rising demand for the biopsy diagnosis of intracranial and intraspinal tumours. This demand has been met by the introduction of highly sophisticated CT or MRI guided stereotactic biopsies in which small but well targeted samples of tissue are taken for pathological analysis. Although most biopsies and the histological diagnosis of intracranial and intraspinal tumours are performed in specialised centres, there is a need for a general awareness of the pathology of these tumours among all pathologists, radiologists and clinicians if the management of patients is to be effective and appropriate. This is also true for the autopsy investigation of central nervous system (CNS) tumours, which continues to supply vital information for the audit of biopsy diagnoses and for the control of clinical trials.

An understanding of the pathology of CNS tumours plays a vital role in the management of patients and in clinical and biological research. Although CT and MRI allow accurate localisation of intracranial and spinal lesions, and often serve as a very good guide to the nature of the lesion, the final diagnosis of a tumour relies almost exclusively on histological evaluation of tissue taken at biopsy or autopsy. Pathology, radiology and clinical evaluation all play key roles in the diagnosis of tumours of the nervous system.

In parallel with the advances in imaging and surgical techniques, histological and molecular genetic methodologies for the study of CNS tumours continue to devleop. The widespread use of immunocytochemistry has replaced the older tinctorial and silver stains for tissue diagnoses but the constant need for clinico-pathological and radiological correlation in the diagnosis of CNS tumours remains. Tissue samples taken at biopsy form a valuable resource for molecular research in the quest for new data to improve therapeutic strategies and for investigating the biological properties of CNS tumour cells in vitro, including their response to chemotherapeutic agents. Pathological diagnoses also play a key role in clinical trials of therapeutic agents.

The effective use of pathology in the management of patients with CNS tumours requires firm diagnostic criteria and an agreed classification; these are essential for accurate communication between pathologists and clinicians. But flexibility of approach is also desirable so that new ideas and concepts can be incorporated into clinical and research activity.

Histological basis of CNS tumours

The CNS is composed of a number of cell types, which are depicted diagrammatically in Fig. 1.1. The incidence of primary brain tumours appears to be increasing, although it has been suggested that this finding may be an artefact of improvements in diagnosis.[1,2] The cells of origin for most brain tumours remain a subject for debate. Molecular enquiries are beginning to shed light on the issue and have suggested that the most likely cells of origin are multipotential stem cells that reside in both the developing and adult brain.[3,4] Astrocytic tumours are the most common primary CNS tumours; they occur at all ages, but the most aggressive tumour, glioblastoma, occurs predominantly in subjects over the age of 50 years. Other tumours, such as ependymomas and choroid plexus papillomas, also occur at all ages but are more commonly encountered in children or young adults (Fig. 1.2). Neurons are stable cells that undergo little if any proliferation postnatally, and the majority of tumours

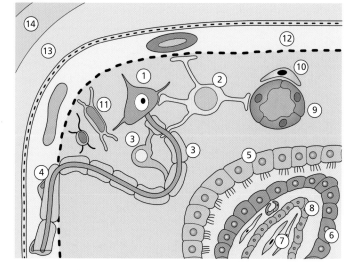

Fig. 1.1 **Histological basis of nervous system tumours.** This is a diagrammatic representation of the major cell components in the normal cortex and white matter of the brain. The meningeal and bony coverings are also shown. Key: 1, neuron; 2, astrocyte; 3, oligodendrocyte and myelin sheath; 4, Schwann cells myelinating cranial and spinal nerves; 5, ependyma lining the ventricles; 6, Choroid plexus epithelium; 7, meningeal cells in the stroma of the choroid plexus; 8, blood vessels of the choroid plexus; 9, blood vessels of the cortex and white matter; 10, perivascular cells – resident macrophages in the perivascular spaces; 11, microglia – resident histiocytes of the CNS; 12, subarachnoid space lined on the inner (brain) aspect by pia mater and on the outer aspect by arachnoid mater (the subarachnoid space houses arteries, veins and nerves); 13, dura mater; 14, skull.

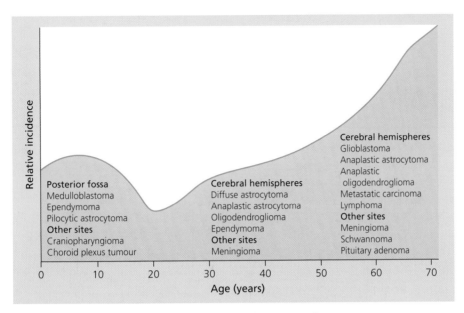

Fig. 1.2 **Overview of the age distribution of the major intracranial tumours.**

with a neuronal phenotype in the CNS occur in children or young adults. Although oligodendrogliomas were so named by Bailey and Cushing[5] because of their histomorphological resemblance to oligodendrocytes, it is difficult to demonstrate phenotypic markers for oligodendrocytes in most of these tumours. Nevertheless, the name persists, and oligodendrogliomas occur at all ages with anaplastic oligodendrogliomas arising mainly in older age groups. True tumours of blood vessels are rare in the CNS, although malformations of blood vessels are relatively common. Although microglia are widespread as resident histiocytes throughout the CNS, tumours related to these cells rarely, if ever, occur. The original 'microglioma' is, in fact, a misnomer as reactive microglia were mistakenly identified as the tumour cells in lymphomas before the introduction of immunocytochemistry. A variety of cell types is seen in the coverings of the brain, but arachnoid cells predominate and are the cells of origin for meningiomas. Schwannomas and neurofibromas arise from Schwann cells associated with intracranial and spinal peripheral nerves. Primary tumours of bone arising from skull or spine may compress and damage the brain and spinal cord. Although distant metastases of primary intracranial and intraspinal tumours are uncommon, the CNS and its coverings are frequent sites of metastases from tumours elsewhere in the body.

Classification of nervous system tumours

Although tumours affecting the brain and spinal cord were well described in the nineteenth century and the first recorded operation for the removal of a primary brain tumour took place in the 1890s, the widely accepted classification of brain tumours upon which all subsequent classifications have been based was formulated by Bailey and Cushing in 1926.[5] Their classification was based upon the cytological and histological similarity of tumour cells to cells in the adult or developing nervous system. Tumours arising outside the brain or spinal cord from meninges, pituitary, spinal cord and other tissues surrounding the nervous system were also recognised but perhaps the most lasting contribution of Bailey and Cushing[5] was the histological classification of *primary neuroepithelial (neuroectodermal) tumours* arising from nervous tissue itself. Loosely called gliomas in the nineteenth century, because of their 'glue-like' consistency or their derivation from the 'glue-like' glial cells of the nervous system, it was Bailey and Cushing who introduced a logical classification of primary neuroepithelial tumours, based on cell type and embryonic cell patterns.

In the years that followed the introduction of Bailey and Cushing's classification, the diversity of histological appearance in primary neuroepithelial tumours, even within one diagnostic category, was widely recognised. Such a feature is well demonstrated by the names given in the past to the numerous histological variations seen in glioblastomas. Different subgroups of tumours were inserted into classifications during the 1930s and 1940s and, in an attempt to rationalise the description of neuroepithelial tumours, Kernohan and Sayre introduced a system of grading in 1949.[6] Their system was based mainly upon autopsy material and related histological features to clinical prognosis.

The current system of classification is based on the World Health Organisation (WHO) series of international

Table 1.1 Histological classification of brain tumours – WHO (2000)

Tumours of neuroepithelial tissue

Astrocytic tumours
Diffuse astrocytoma
   Fibrillary astrocytoma
   Protoplasmic astrocytoma
   Gemistocytic astrocytoma
Anaplastic astrocytoma
Glioblastoma
   Giant cell glioblastoma
   Gliosarcoma
Pilocytic astrocytoma
Pleomorphic xanthoastrocytoma
Subependymal giant cell astrocytoma (tuberous sclerosis)

Oligodendroglial tumours
Oligodendroglioma
Anaplastic oligodendroglioma

Mixed gliomas
Oligoastrocytoma
Anaplastic oligoastrocytoma

Ependymal tumours
Ependymomas
   Cellular
   Papillary
   Clear cell
   Tanycytic
Anaplastic ependymoma
Myxopapillary ependymoma
Subependymoma

Choroid plexus tumours
Choroid plexus papilloma
Choroid plexus carcinoma

Glial tumours of uncertain origin
Astroblastoma
Gliomatosis cerebri
Chordoid glioma of the third ventricle

Neuronal and mixed neuronal-glial tumours
Gangliocytoma
Dysplastic gangliocytoma of cerebellum (Lhermitte-Duclos)
Desmoplastic infantile astrocytoma/ganglioglioma
Dysembryoplastic neuroepithelial tumour
Ganglioglioma
Anaplastic ganglioglioma
Central neurocytoma
Cerebellar liponeurocytoma
Paraganglioma of the filum terminale

Neuroblastic tumours
Olfactory neuroblastoma (aesthesioneuroblastoma)
Olfactory neuroepithelioma
Neuroblastomas of the adrenal gland and sympathetic nervous system

Pineal parenchymal tumours
Pineocytoma
Pineoblastoma
Pineal parenchymal tumour of intermediate differentiation

Embryonal tumours
Medulloepithelioma
Ependymoblastoma
Medulloblastoma
   Desmoplastic medulloblastoma
   Large cell medulloblastoma
   Medullomyoblastoma
   Melanotic medulloblastoma
Supratentorial primitive neuroectodermal tumour (PNET)
   Neuroblastoma
   Ganglioneuroblastoma
(Polar spongioblastoma)
Atypical teratoid-rhabdoid tumour

Tumours of peripheral nerve

Schwannoma
(Neurilemmoma, Neurinoma)
   Cellular
   Plexiform
   Melanotic

Neurofibroma
Plexiform

Perineurioma
Intraneural perineurioma
Soft tissue perineurioma

Malignant peripheral nerve sheath tumour (MPNST)
Epithelioid
MPNST with divergent mesenchymal and/or epithelial differentiation
Melanotic
Melanotic psammomatous

Tumours of the meninges

Tumours of meningothelial cells
Meningioma
   Meningothelial
   Fibrous (fibroblastic)
   Transitional (mixed)
   Psammomatous
   Angiomatous
   Microcystic
   Secretory
   Lymphoplasmacyte-rich
   Metaplastic
   Clear cell
   Chordoid
   Atypical
   Papillary
   Rhabdoid
   Anaplastic meningioma

Mesenchymal, non-meningothelial tumours
Lipoma
Angiolipoma
Hibernoma
Liposarcoma (intracranial)
Solitary fibrous tumour

Table 1.1 (*Cont'd*)

Fibrosarcoma	**Tumours of the sellar region**
Malignant fibrous histiocytoma	Pituitary adenoma
Leiomyoma	Pituitary carcinoma
Leiomyosarcoma	Craniopharyngioma
Rhabdomyoma	Adamantionomatous
Rhabdomyosarcoma	Papillary
Chondroma	Granular cell tumour
Chondrosarcoma	(Choristoma, Pituicytoma)
Osteoma	Hypothalamic neuronal hamartoma
Osteosarcoma	
Osteochondroma	**Local extensions from regional tumours**
Haemangioma	Paraganglioma
Epithelial haemangioendothelioma	Chordoma
Haemangiopericytoma	Chondroma
Angiosarcoma	Chondrosarcoma
Kaposi's sarcoma	Adenoid cystic carcinoma
	(Cylindroma)
Primary melanocytic lesions	
Diffuse melancytosis	**Cysts and tumour-like lesions**
Melanocytoma	Rathke's cleft cyst
Malignant melanoma	Epidermoid cyst
Meningeal melanomatosis	Dermoid cyst
	Colloid cyst of the third ventricle
Tumour of uncertain histogenesis	Enterogenous cyst
Haemangioblastoma	Neuroglial cyst
	Arachnoid cyst
Lymphomas and haematopoietic neoplasms	Other cysts
Malignant lymphomas	Lipoma
Plasmacytoma	Nasal glial heterotopia
Granulocytic sarcoma	
	Metastatic tumours
Germ cell tumours	
Germinoma	**Unclassified tumours**
Embryonal carcinoma	
Yolk sac tumour	
Choriocarcinoma	
Teratoma	
Mature	
Immature	
Teratoma with malignant transformation	
Mixed germ cell tumours	

Note: For the purposes of this book, certain categories of neoplastic and non-neoplastic lesions that are not included in the WHO classification of tumours of the nervous system have been included. These categories are seen in neurosurgical and neuropathological practice and are described in the text. They are *Pituitary adenoma and carcinoma; Local extensions from regional tumours; Cysts and tumour-like lesions.*

histological classifications of tumours. Zülch and an international team published the first WHO classification of tumours of the CNS in 1979. This classification was subsequently revised in 1990 by an international team of neuropathologists and published under the editorship of Kleihues et al. in 1993[7] and a subsequent modification in 2000 by Kleihues and Cavanee and their international team.[8] As set out in Table 1.1, the 2000 WHO classification forms the basis for a logical approach to tumours of the nervous system. Inevitably, in such a vibrant field of histological, molecular genetic and clinical research, the 2000 WHO classification is likely to be modified in the future as new tumour entities and new relationships between tumours emerge.

Grading of CNS tumours

In addition to the 2000 WHO classification, a number of systems have been introduced to grade tumours of the nervous system according to their biological behaviour. A modification of the Kernohan system of grading has been adopted by the WHO classification with grade I tumours having the most favourable prognosis and grade IV tumours the least favourable prognosis; such grading systems have been most widely applied to astrocytic tumours (see Chapter 4).

Grading systems are very useful in certain respects and, in particular, in the analysis of large clinical trials but they should be used with caution. Numerical grading does not surplant the need for a firm understanding of the histological criteria for diagnosis of specific types of tumour and grading is probably best used once a firm name has been applied to the tumour. It is also essential that there is a firm understanding among pathologists, radiologists and clinicians of the significance of names and grades, particularly since the criteria used for assigning diagnoses and grades differ between the various systems in use.

In this volume, the nomenclature of the 2000 WHO classification will be used, although a brief explanation of grading will be given for each type of tumour where appropriate.

Age incidence and sites of nervous system tumours

There is a distinct pattern in the incidence of nervous system tumours in relation to the ages and sites at which they occur. An overview of the age distribution of major intracranial tumours is depicted in Fig. 1.2. The majority of CNS tumours in childhood arise in the posterior fossa in relation to the brain stem and cerebellum. Intracranial tumours are relatively uncommon in adolescents and young adults but the incidence of diffuse astrocytomas, in particular, starts to rise in the third and fourth decades; these tumours are located mainly in the cerebral hemispheres and they frequently progress to anaplastic astrocytomas or glioblastomas. The majority of intracranial tumours occur over the age of 50 years; glioblastoma, metastatic carcinoma, meningioma, and Schwannoma are the most common types of tumour in this older age group.

Although the relative incidence of the various types of tumour is difficult to estimate with a high degree of accuracy, the figures shown in Fig. 1.3 for intracranial tumours, neuroepithelial tumours in childhood and adults and for spinal tumours are derived from analyses over the last 20 or 30 years.[9]

Aetiology of tumours of the nervous system

Few definite aetiologies and risk factors have been identified for tumours of the nervous system in humans. Among these, the most definitive is the hereditary predisposition to nervous system tumours found in particular genetic syndromes. These include neurofibromatosis 1, neurofibromatosis 2, tuberous sclerosis, von Hippel–Lindau syndrome, Li–Fraumeni syndrome, Turcot syndrome, Gorlin syndrome and Cowden syndrome, among others. Each is caused by a mutation in a growth regulatory gene, the study of which has already shed light on the genetic basis of specific brain tumours, including the sporadic counterparts to the familial lesions.[10,11] Thus, the genes mutated in the germline in familial syndromes which lead to specific tumour types (e.g. the NF2 gene in neurofibromatosis 2 patients leading to meningiomas) are also mutated in sporadic tumours (e.g. somatic mutations in the NF2 gene in sporadic meningiomas). The specific syndromes and the genes involved are discussed in detail in Chapter 19.

Epidemiological studies[12–17] have revealed a number of factors that could be associated with an increase in nervous system tumours and have defined how improvements in treatment have influenced the patterns of diagnosis and survival.[13,18,19] Anaplastic astrocytomas and glioblastomas are increasing in the elderly population[14,16] and factors such as birth weight may play a role in the induction of childhood tumours.[15] Although some studies have suggested that farmers, coal miners and industrial workers exposed to chemicals show an increased risk of developing tumours in the CNS, the associations remain weak and no environmental factors inducing brain tumours have been definitely established.[1,16,18,20] Similarly, the suggestion that electrical fields are important in the aetiology of brain tumours has not been established conclusively.[9]

A clear association between therapeutic X-irradiation and intracranial[21,22] and spinal tumours[23] has been established, but long term, low dose, X-ray exposure and exposure to irradiation for workers in nuclear plants has not been firmly related to an increase in nervous system tumours.[11] The most frequent use of X-irradiation therapeutically, in the past, has been for treating fungal disease of the scalp and such low dose irradiation is associated with an increase in meningiomas which are often multiple and anaplastic.[9] A similar increase in meningiomas has been observed following high dose irradiation for intracranial tumours with a mean period of 8–10 years between exposure and the development of the second tumour.[9] Treatment of acute lymphoblastic leukaemia by irradiation is associated with an increase in astrocytomas and glioblastomas and primitive neuroectodermal tumours.[9] Estimates for the increased incidence of brain tumours, postirradiation, range from 1.9 to 2.5%;[9] they are especially high in children under 5 years of age.

Immmunosuppression with an increased incidence of Epstein–Barr virus infection is associated with primary lymphomas of the brain,[8,9] but not with an increase in primary neuroepithelial tumours with the possible exception of astrocytomas.[24] An increased incidence of childhood brain tumours has been reported in rural communities.[20] Other factors, such as smoking and trauma do not have a firm association with an increased incidence of brain tumours.[9] Despite the potency of N-nitroso compounds in inducing brain tumours in rodents,[25] particularly when administered prenatally, a role for these compounds in the diet in the induction of brain tumours in man has yet to be established.[8]

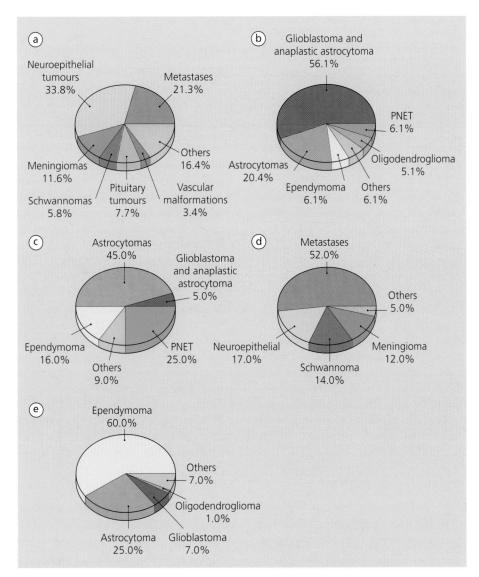

Fig. 1.3 **Comparative incidence of intracranial tumours. (a)** All intracranial tumours. **(b)** Intracranial neuroepithelial tumours, all ages. **(c)** Primary neuroepithelial tumours of childhood. **(d)** Spinal tumours, overall. **(e)** Spinal tumours, neuroepithelial.

Oncogenic viruses such as SV40 and other animal viruses have been implicated in brain tumours in experimental animals and transformation of cells following infection with oncogenic papovaviruses implicated in progressive multifocal leucoencephalopathy have been shown in culture in human material. Despite these associations, there is no firm evidence of a constant association of viruses with human brain tumours.[8]

Molecular genetics of nervous system tumours

General concepts

Cancer is a genetic disease: most human tumours arise when alterations occur in key growth regulatory genes. In familial tumour syndromes (see Chapter 19), critical genes are inherited in mutant forms, predisposing such patients to the development of tumours. The majority of human neoplasms, however, arise sporadically as a result of somatic insults to growth regulatory genes, in the absence of familial syndromes. Such changes may occur due to environmental insults, for example, cigarette smoke for lung cancer or sunlight for skin cancer; alternatively, they can be random genetic changes that are not adequately corrected by DNA repair mechanisms. Far less commonly, tumours may develop when the function of protein products of key growth regulatory genes are affected; for example, human papillomaviruses interfere with the function of cell cycle regulatory molecules in the genesis of cervical cancer. Regardless of an aetiology, alteration of growth regulatory genes or their protein products results in uncontrolled growth, hence tumorigenesis.[8]

Two major classes of genes are targeted in human cancers:

1. growth promoting genes, known as *oncogenes*, which are abnormally activated in cancer; and
2. growth suppressing genes, termed *tumour suppressor genes*, which are inactivated in cancer.

Oncogenes are typically activated by mechanisms that increase the expression levels (e.g. gene amplification or overexpression) or activity (e.g. mutations) of these growth promoting genes. Tumour suppressor genes, on the other hand, are inactivated by events that delete genes (e.g. chromosomal loss, gene deletion) and/or inactivate gene products (gene mutations or binding proteins). Other families of regulatory genes also exist, such as genes that encode regulators of cell death or facilitators of DNA repair. Preventing the normal control pathways of cell death and DNA repair may contribute to tumorigenesis, by immortalising cells and by facilitating mutagenesis, respectively.

Various combinations of alterations of these gene types have now been demonstrated in a wide variety of human tumours; some genetic abnormalities are common to many lesions and others are fairly specific to a few cancers. A major goal of neuro-oncology research has been to identify the genetic culprits that underlie the formation of brain tumours. The genes involved in specific types of nervous system tumours are discussed in the individual chapters.

Clinical use of molecular genetic analyses

Analysis of the genetic alterations in human tumours may provide important clinical information. This has been most strikingly shown for childhood systemic neuroblastoma, in which amplification of the *NMYC* gene is closely correlated with clinical course. In the management of childhood neuroblastoma, therefore, molecular analysis of *NMYC* copy number is an important diagnostic test. For brain tumours, molecular genetic analysis has clarified the classification of some lesions and suggested new ways for diagnosing others. The impact of molecular genetic investigations is discussed within each of the following chapters, particularly in relation to the astrocytomas, oligodendrogliomas, medulloblastoma and meningioma.[11] It is likely that molecular analyses will prove to be useful in the evaluation of many kinds of nervous system tumours over the next decade, and the molecular assays will become routine in neuro-oncology.[26–29]

Molecular approaches to detect common types of gene alterations

A number of techniques exist for the analysis of genetic changes and the resultant alterations in expression of gene products.[11] As these approaches become common-place and find diagnostic utility, it will be necessary to incorporate oncogene and tumour suppressor gene analysis into diagnostic pathology. The major techniques for molecular assays are catalogued in Table 1.2.

Briefly, oncogene activation can be detected by assessing either the gene itself or the gene product. Often oncogenes are present in greatly increased numbers, so-called gene amplification, and this can be determined by a variety of techniques, such as Southern blotting, polymerase chain reaction (PCR), fluorescence in situ hybridisation (FISH) or comparative genomic hybridisation (CGH). Alternatively, oncogene amplification is typically accompanied by overexpression at both the mRNA and protein levels. mRNA overexpression can be measured using Northern blots or in situ hybridisation, while protein expression can be assayed by Western blotting or immunohistochemistry. On the other hand, tumour suppressor gene inactivation is most often accomplished via mutations and/or deletions that affect both chromosomal (or allelic) copies of the gene. Typically, one allele is affected by a point mutation whereas the second allele is lost through deletion of a chromosomal arm. Point mutations must be detected using detailed PCR-based screening assays such as single strand conformation polymorphism (SSCP) and DNA sequencing. Allelic loss of a chromosomal arm is more easily assessed, using approaches such as loss of heterozygosity (LOH) studies or FISH.

Clinical presentation of nervous system tumours

Tumours affecting the brain and spinal cord produce clinical signs and symptoms due to various combinations of local tissue destruction, oedema, distortion and shift of intracranial contents, raised intracranial pressure and the onset of epilepsy.[30] In general, the signs and symptoms are progressive and the speed of progression depends upon the rate of enlargement of the tumour. This pattern contrasts with the sudden onset of signs and symptoms in stroke due to cerebral infarction or intracerebral haemorrhage but confusion can occur when there is infarction or haemorrhage into a tumour and the onset of signs and symptoms mimics a stroke. Alternatively, subacute evolution of a cerebral infarct can mimic a tumour, so an infarct should always be considered in the differential diagnosis of a brain tumour.

Signs and symptoms related to the site of the tumour

Most intracranial and intraspinal tumours enlarge as focal masses so the pattern of clinical presentation depends largely upon the site of the tumour.[30–32] In the brain, enlargement of a tumour may result in focal neurological deficit, in a less well defined neurological syndrome, or in raised intracranial pressure. Thus,

Table 1.2 Molecular assays commonly used in cancer diagnosis

DNA analyses: structural changes in genes and chromosomes

Southern blot
DNA is separated by size using an electrophoretic gel and then transferred to a membrane. The DNA is then detected using complementary DNA probes to the gene of interest. This method is most often used for detecting gene amplification or rearrangements, or chromosomal loss

Polymerase chain reaction (PCR)
Small fragments of DNA are amplified exponentially using oligonucleotide primers specific to the gene of interest. This powerful technique has found a myriad of uses in cancer genetics, and forms the basis of most diagnostic assays. For instance, PCR is used to detect gene amplification, mutation and loss

Fluorescence in situ hybridisation (FISH)
Complementary DNA probes can be labelled fluorescently and hybridised to intact nuclei, thereby providing a means of detecting increases or losses of chromosomes in whole cells

Single strand conformation polymorphism (SSCP) analysis
One of the more popular DNA mutation detection techniques, SSCP is based on PCR amplification of the gene of interest, followed by separation of the single stranded products in a non-denaturing electrophoretic gel. Mutant fragments migrate in an aberrant manner

Loss of heterozygosity (LOH) analysis
Chromosomal loss, reflecting inactivation of tumour suppressor genes, can be detected by LOH. The two chromosomes, or alleles, are visualised by either Southern blot or PCR techniques; the normal state, with two alleles, is termed 'heterozygous'. Loss of the 'heterozygous' state occurs when the tumour loses one chromosome when compared with DNA from normal cells

Comparative genomic hybridisation (CGH)
A screening technique for detecting large genomic gains or losses, CGH competitively cohybridises tumour and normal DNA onto metaphase chromosomes, with tumour and normal DNA each labelled with a different colour. Chromosomal gains appear as an excess of the tumour DNA-labelled colour (i.e. there is more of a particular chromosomal region in the tumour when compared to the blood), whereas chromosomal losses appear as an excess of the normal DNA-labelled colour (i.e. the tumour DNA contains fewer copies of the chromosomal region than does normal blood DNA)

RNA analyses: changes in levels of mRNA expression

Northern blot
RNA is separated by size using an electrophoretic gel and then transferred to a membrane. The RNA is then detected using a complementary DNA probe to the gene of interest

In situ hybridisation (ISH)
RNA is detected in tissue sections, usually frozen sections, when the RNA is hybridised with labelled DNA or RNA probes. ISH provides a means of determining which cells express which genes

Protein analyses: changes in levels of protein expression; structural and functional protein changes

Western blot
Protein extracts are separated by size using an electrophoretic gel and then transferred to a membrane. The protein of interest is then detected using antibodies to the protein. Truncated, mutant proteins can be visualised, as can increases or decrease in protein expression

Immunohistochemistry
Antibodies are used to detect proteins in intact cells or tissue sections

involvement of the motor or sensory cortex, the internal capsules and corticospinal tracts in the brain stem and spinal cord will result in focal motor or sensory deficit or complete hemiparesis or quadriparesis. Tumours that affect 'silent areas' such as the non-dominant temporal lobe, the corpus callosum, the frontal lobe and the thalamus, produce less specific symptomatology. Lesions arising in the temporal lobe may produce signs and symptoms due to transtentorial herniation and compression of the brain stem whereas thalamic tumours may present with hydrocephalus due to obstruction of the third ventricle and the upper aqueduct. Tumours at other sites may also obstruct the ventricular system and present with raised intracranial pressure due to hydrocephalus. Lesions in the pineal region, third ventricle, and in the vermis of the cerebellum characteristically present with hydrocephalus due to obstruction of cerebrospinal fluid (CSF) flow in the ventricular system.

Tumours of the frontal lobe may present with progressive dementia, characterised by alteration in personality, loss of intellectual capability and of memory. Features of parkinsonism may occur when tumours invade the basal ganglia or there is a combination of tissue destruction in the frontal lobes and distortion of the premotor cortex and its connections with the basal ganglia. The less specific signs of frontal lobe tumours may be confused with the onset of dementia in the elderly. Tumours in the pons and medulla may result in damage to the corticospinal tracts with quadriplegia or in destruction of cranial nerve nuclei causing cranial nerve palsies. Lesions of the cerebellum may produce ataxia.

Intrinsic tumours of the spinal cord, such as astrocytomas and ependymomas often result in damage to long descending corticospinal tracts or the ascending sensory tracts. Tumours in the cervical region may result in quadriparesis, sensory signs and ataxia in all four limbs; those in the thoracic and lumbar regions result in paraparesis with sensory signs confined to the lower limbs. In addition to long tract signs, there may be muscle wasting, particularly if a tumour affects the anterior horn cells in the cervical or lumbar regions. Extrinsic tumours of the spine, be they meningiomas arising from the arachnoid coating of the cord, or Schwannomas and neurofibromas arising from peripheral nerve roots, result mainly in cord compression with long tract signs. Tethering of peripheral nerves may result in back pain and pain on leg or arm movement. Metastatic tumours and lymphomas frequently involve the extradural fatty tissue or bone and, again, the symptomatology is due to spinal cord compression.

Raised intracranial pressure

A progressively enlarging intracranial mass will eventually result in raised intracranial pressure. As seen in Fig. 1.4, the pressure–volume curve allows for some increase in the volume of intracranial content as CSF and blood are expelled from inside the skull to accommodate the enlarging mass. Eventually, however, the tolerance of the system is exceeded and pressure rises rapidly, producing headache, nausea, decline in the level of consciousness, visual failure and eventually death. Once the pressure has risen above that of arterial pressure, no blood enters the skull and brain death occurs.[33]

It is least difficult to diagnose raised intracranial pressure when it occurs suddenly. However, chronically raised pressure with insidious onset may produce visual failure, without other signs, and this may go unrecognised by the patient and clinician unless specifically sought.

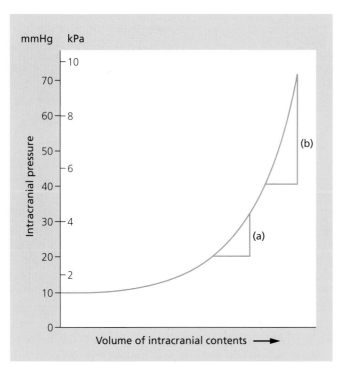

Fig. 1.4 **Theoretical intracranial pressure–volume curve.** This diagram illustrates how the volume of intracranial contents may increase, initially, with little change in intracranial pressure. Once a certain threshold has been reached following expulsion of blood and CSF from the intracranial compartment, the pressure rises exponentially and, as the curve steepens, a small rise in volume results in a significant increase in intracranial pressure. **(a)** and **(b)** illustrate the relationship between rise in intracranial volume and the theoretical rise in intracranial pressure at two parts of the curve (modified from Ref. 33).

Enlargement of the physiological blind spot, with or without reduced visual acuity, is a much more reliable sign of raised intracranial pressure than papilloedema. Although it is a helpful sign when present, papilloedema is absent in two-thirds of patients with intracranial tumours at the time of surgery. Headache, on the whole, is an unhelpful symptom, although it may be a reliable feature when it is a new symptom for that patient.

The age of the patient has some effect on the onset of raised intracranial pressure, as does the speed with which the tumour grows. In elderly patients, cerebral atrophy may allow a larger tumour mass to develop before the onset of raised intracranial pressure, and in young children separation of the skull sutures may allow an expanding mass to develop within the skull without an accompanying rise in intracranial pressure. Some tumours grow very slowly, for example meningiomas, and they may reach a considerable size with slow compression and displacement of the brain before the onset of raised intracranial pressure. Rapidly growing glioblastomas, on the other hand, may result in raised intracranial pressure within a few weeks of the onset of other neurological signs and symptoms.

Epilepsy

Approximately, one-third of patients with brain tumours suffer from epilepsy.[34] The seizures may be focal or generalised in nature although the focus can usually be detected by electroencephalography if the epilepsy is due to a tumour in a cerebral hemisphere. When it occurs, epilepsy tends to present early in the growth of the tumour. Epilepsy is a presenting symptom in approximately 50% of those parietal tumours which cause epilepsy, 80% of those frontal tumours and 90% of those temporal tumours which cause epilepsy. Overall, epilepsy occurs four times more frequently in slowly growing tumours, such as oligodendrogliomas (81% of cases) than in rapidly growing tumours such as metastases (19% of cases). Tumours are the cause in a significant number of patients with temporal lobe epilepsy.

Imaging of nervous system tumours

There are now a number of techniques that are used to detect the location and physiological properties of intracranial and intraspinal tumours. They include CT, MRI, positron emission tomography (PET) and the use of cerebral and spinal angiography for the localisation of arteriovenous malformations and other lesions of vascular tissue.[35–38] Apart from the angiographic demonstration of lesions of vascular tissue, none of the other techniques allows a specific diagnosis to be made with absolute certainty and biopsy is still the gold standard in establishing the diagnosis in the majority of intracranial and intraspinal tumours.

CT scanning

Based on computerised integration of tomographic X-ray data, CT scans are visualised as horizontal or coronal sections of the skull, the brain and its surrounding structures or as horizontal sections of the spinal column. Distortion of brain or spinal cord anatomy and variation in atenuation of the X-rays allows localisation of intracranial and intraspinal lesions and an assessment of their pathological nature. Lesions may appear less dense (black), e.g. astrocytoma or oedema around a glioblastoma, or hyperdense (white), in the case of fresh haemorrhage or calcification. Intravenous injection of iodine-containing contrast media, which do not cross the normal blood–brain barrier, can be used to locate regions of blood–brain barrier breakdown. Such areas appear as white contrast-enhancing regions, e.g. those seen in glioblastoma, metastatic carcinoma and meningiomas. Some contrast enhancement occurs normally in the choroid plexus and in the pineal as these regions lack a blood–brain barrier.

MRI

Based on images derived from the magnetically induced changes in the orientation of water molecules, MRI offers a variety of modes and is used either alone or in various combinations with CT scanning to localise cerebral tumours and to investigate their physiology. High resolution anatomical images of brain, spinal cord, the eye and orbit can be obtained from MRI and intravenous injection of gadolinium containing compounds allows contrast enhancement of lesions in a similar way to the contrast enhancement of CT scans. By the use of T1- and T2-weighted images, different characteristics of pathological lesions and normal structures can be depicted.

CT and MRI guided stereotactic biopsies

By the use of a fixed frame on the patient's skull, co-ordinates can be established by both CT and MRI for accurate targeting of stereotactic tumour biopsies.

PET

PET imaging relies upon the intravenous injection of radioisotopes and detection of their differential uptake by different regions of the brain. Used mainly for the investigation of glucose uptake capacity in different regions of the brain in stroke and dementia patients, this technique has also been used for the investigation of physiological functions of brain tumour tissue and for the differential diagnosis of recurrent tumour versus radiation necrosis.

Strategies for the diagnosis of nervous system tumours

The relative inaccessibility of intracranial and intraspinal tumours in particular, combined with the risk of biopsy or open operation on a tumour, has led to the widespread use of frozen sections and smears for the intraoperative diagnosis of nervous system tumours.[39,40] At craniotomy, an intraoperative diagnosis may need to be established by frozen section and smear or the resection margins of the tumour examined so that the appropriate surgery can be performed. In many cases, however, particularly those involving stereotactic biopsy, the major role of the frozen section and smear may be just to establish that there is adequate tumour tissue in the biopsy so that a definitive diagnosis can be made later in paraffin sections, with or without immunocytochemistry (see Chapter 2).

Diagnosis and classification of a tumour in frozen section and smear preparations are, overall, less reliable than diagnoses made on paraffin sections. This is largely due to the greater amount of tissue that can be assessed in paraffin sections, the better cytology, more time to assess the sections and the application of immuno-cytochemistry to paraffin sections. In many cases, such as glioblastoma and other astrocytic tumours, a firm diagnosis can be given on frozen section but the limitations for identification of less common lesions should be recognised. In general, cryostat sections are more informative for firm tumours such as meningiomas, Schwannomas and for determining the epithelial pattern of metastatic carcinomas, whereas smears are frequently more valuable in soft neuroepithelial tumours, as the morphology of individual cells or groups of cells can be assessed as can the blood vessels (e.g. microvascular proliferation in glioblastoma).

Detailed features upon which the diagnosis of individual tumour types depend are reviewed in individual chapters, but there are some general principles which can be applied to nervous system tumours in general which may be helpful in formulating an approach to diagnosis.

The age of the patient, site of the tumour and imaging characteristics

There are a number of essential pieces of clinical information that are required for the diagnosis of nervous system tumours and should accompany the biopsy request. They include: the age of the patient, the site of the tumour, whether it is enhancing on CT or MRI and whether there is evidence of a primary tumour in another organ. It may be dangerous to attempt a diagnosis on a tumour biopsy in the absence of these clinical data.

The age and site distributions of CNS tumours are depicted in Figs 1.2 and 1.3 which show that primitive neuroectodermal tumours, pilocytic astrocytomas and ependymomas occur mainly in the posterior fossa in children whereas cerebral diffuse astrocytomas and anaplastic astrocytomas are more common in young adults; glioblastoma is most frequently seen in the cerebral hemispheres of older adults. Meningiomas and

Schwannomas are more common in older adults. Glioblastoma is rare in the spinal cord, and oligodendroglioma is almost unknown at this site. Ependymomas are much more common than astrocytomas or anaplastic astrocytomas in the spinal cord. The majority of spinal tumours encountered in clinical practice are ependymomas, Schwannomas, meningiomas and metastases.

Details of the CT and MRI appearances should always accompany a request for histological diagnosis as a guide to the most probable nature of the tumour. Such information is most valuable for the diagnosis of primary neuroepithelial tumours. Diffuse astrocytomas do not enhance following the injection of contrast; anaplastic astrocytomas characteristically show patchy diffuse enhancement whereas glioblastoma has a ring enhancing pattern due to the presence of a central area of necrosis. Pilocytic astrocytomas, central neurocytomas and ependymomas usually enhance as do primitive neuroectodermal tumours such as medulloblastoma. Virtually all the tumours arising from tissues other than brain or spinal cord show enhancement as would be expected for tissues that do not normally possess a blood–brain barrier. Such tumours include meningiomas, Schwannomas, pituitary tumours, haemangioblastomas and metastatic tumours in the brain, cord and their coverings. Cysts, which are often large, occur in a number of primary brain and spinal cord tumours, most notably pilocytic astrocytomas, diffuse astrocytomas and glioblastomas. In the cerebellum, pilocytic astrocytomas may be difficult to distinguish from haemangioblastoma as both enhance and both may be cystic.

Behaviour of nervous system tumours – benign or malignant

The terms 'benign and malignant' in relation to primary neuroepithelial tumours must be used with caution as they do not have the same connotation as the same terms used for tumours derived from other tissues and organs. Diffuse invasion of surrounding brain or spinal cord tissue and involvement of vital structures in the brain often preclude excision as a therapeutic option even in the most slowly growing primary neurepithelial tumours, such that patients develop severe neurological deficit and die from the effects of the expanding tumour. The term 'malignant' is often applied to tumours such as glioblastoma which enlarge rapidly and have a very poor prognosis. But, malignancy in the normal sense of the word, whereby there is metastatic spread to distant organs of the body, is very rare with glioblastoma. Spread of primitive neuroectodermal tumours such as medulloblastoma to bone or lung is more common but still rare.

There are obvious examples of intracranial and intraspinal tumours that can be classified as 'benign'. Easily accessible intracranial or intraspinal meningiomas or Schwannomas that are well demarcated from the adjacent brain or spinal cord may be excised with no recurrence and few sequelae for the patient. However, similar tumours in inaccessible sites involving delicate structures that are essential for the preservation of neurological function may be inoperable and continued growth of the tumour frequently results in disability or death of the patient. Other examples in which complicated, but otherwise 'benign', slowly growing tumours such as craniopharyngioma and pituitary adenomas result in neurological deficit due to the progressive destruction of adjacent neurological tissue are well documented. Anaplastic change in meningiomas and nerve sheath tumours may result in local invasion of brain tissue and very occasionally metastatic spread outside the CNS as truly malignant tumours.

Intraoperative diagnosis of intracranial and intraspinal tumours

The diagnosis of a tumour may be straightforward if adequate tissue is available, and there is sufficient time to prepare paraffin sections and complete the appropriate immunocytochemical profiles. In practice, however, there may be a clinical need for an immediate diagnosis to be made on the frozen section or smear preparation. This is particularly so if the surgeon requires advice during the operation on the nature of the tumour in order to determine appropriate management. There are a number of features that can be used to distinguish between certain types of tumour that present difficulties in frozen sections and smears. These issues are discussed in detail in Chapter 3, but are highlighted here.

Primary neuroepithelial tumours can usually be distinguished from other types of tumour by the fibrillary nature of the cytoplasm and the indistinct cell borders. Often there is an indication of the astrocytic nature of a tumour by the presence of a small amount of paranuclear eosinophilic cytoplasm; the long processes of astrocytic tumour cells are well demonstrated in smear preparations. Diffuse invasion of brain tissue is a characteristic of primary neuroepithelial tumours; this can be detected in frozen sections by the presence of myelin sheaths or normal neurons incorporated into the tumour. Absence of collagen or reticulin, except around blood vessels, is another valuable feature in most neuroepithelial tumours which may help to identify them in cryostat or paraffin sections. In some cases, however, the fibrous tissue element is high, especially in gliosarcomas, pleomorphic xanthoastrocytomas and desmoplastic medulloblastomas. In these cases, the presence of reticulin-free glial elements in the tumour may be a useful guide to the nature of the tumour.

Immunocytochemistry using antibodies to gliofibrillary acidic protein (GFAP) for astrocytes, synaptophysin and neurofilament protein for neuronal cells and axons can be performed on either cryostat or paraffin sections. These techniques will help to define the neuroepithelial histogenesis of the tumour and the intercellular relationships, both within the tumour and in the surrounding tissue. Futher details regarding the immunocytochemical identification of individual tumours are found in the relevant chapters.

Meningiomas may be confused with astrocytic tumours, particularly in small biopsies both in frozen sections and in smears. As meningiomas are often treated successfully by excision, it is very important to distinguish these tumours from astrocytic tumours at biopsy. Confusion may occur because the meningioma cells often have long processes in smear preparations and in cryostat sections the cell borders are indistinct. However, the nuclear characteristics in meningiomas with regular round or oval nuclei and small but prominent nucleoli may aid diagnosis. Bands of fibrous tissue are usually found in meningiomas and can be stained by the haematoxylin van Giesen technique on frozen sections and may offer a further clue to the diagnosis of meningioma. Immunocytochemistry on the cryostat sections will, in general, reveal GFAP expression in primary neuroepithelial tumours and epithelial membrane antigen in meningiomas.

Lymphomas diffusely spread through brain tissue and may, therefore, be confused with primary neuroepithelial tumours and, in particular, oligodendrogliomas, medulloblastoma and other primitive neuroectodermal tumours or glioblastoma. In frozen sections, a diagnosis of lymphoma can be made by recognising the perivascular accumulation of lymphoma cells, particularly at the infiltrating edge of the tumour, by the relative uniformity of the nuclear shape and the prominent nucleoli compared with astrocytic tumours; the nuclei differ from the more bizarre or rod shaped morphology of the nuclei in glioblastoma. A reticulin stain on a frozen section is useful for identifying the complex proliferation of fibrous tissue in the perivascular spaces associated with lymphomas. Immunocytochemistry on cryostat sections will reveal expression of leucocyte common antigen in the lymphoma cells. Lastly, touch or dab preparations stained with Giemsa-based techniques are very valuable for the rapid diagnosis of lymphomas, as the lymphoma cytology is usually distinctive. The tumour cells become detached from the tissue and adhere to the slide in a way that is uncommon for astrocytic tumours or primitive neuroectodermal tumours.

Schwannomas may occur at very similar sites to meningiomas, particularly in the posterior fossa around the internal auditory meatus and in the spinal column as intradural tumours. The majority of meningiomas can be distinguished on their cell morphology from Schwannomas. Meningioma nuclei are oval, pale, with small but prominent nucleoli and occasional cytoplasmic inclusions whereas the Schwannoma nuclei are spindle shaped, densely stained and rarely show prominent nucleoli. Nevertheless, in frozen sections such features may not be immediately apparent and the firmness of the tissue may not allow cytological characteristics to be assessed in smear preparations. One very useful feature for distinguishing between Schwannomas and meningiomas is the presence of an intimate reticulin network in Schwannomas which stains the basement membrane and small collagen fibres between the neoplastic Schwann cells. In the majority of meningiomas, reticulin is only seen around blood vessels and as broad fibrous bands within the tumour, reticulin is not seen between individual cells. The only major exception is in fibroblastic meningiomas in which the tumour cells are not only spindle shaped but there may also be an abundance of reticulin. Immunocytochemistry on the cryostat sections will, in general, reveal S-100 protein expression in the Schwannomas and epithelial membrane antigen expression in the meningiomas.

Prognostic indicators in the histology of tumours of the nervous system

There are certain criteria which can help to determine whether a particular tumour will behave aggressively. The cytoplasmic features of tumour cells, the expression of proteins detectable by immunocytochemistry and organoid arrangements of the cells in some tumours may be useful in determining the diagnosis of a tumour. However, it is the nuclear characteristics of the tumour cells, the mitotic and proliferative activity; the presence of necrosis and microvascular proliferation, and the pattern of spread of the tumour cells that are the most important guides to prognosis.

Nuclear hyperchromasia and nuclear : cytoplasmic ratio
Nuclear hyperchromasia and an increase in nuclear : cytoplasmic ratio are clear indicators of neoplasia, particularly in the primary neuroepithelial tumours. Large, densely staining nuclei identify neoplastic astrocytes both within the main bulk of the tumour and infiltrating adjacent normal brain tissue. Recognition of enlarged hyperchromatic nuclei is a major step in confirming the presence of diffuse astrocytoma cells in a biopsy. Detection of anaplastic change in an astrocytic tumour also depends largely on the detection of nuclear changes. Anaplasia in a diffuse astrocytoma is accompanied by an increase in the nuclear : cytoplasmic ratio (often loosely referred to as increased cellularity) and the presence of rod shaped tumour nuclei. In oligodendrogliomas, on the other hand, even the most slowly growing tumours may have a relatively high nuclear : cytoplasmic ratio and factors such as necrosis and mitotic

rate or Ki-67/MIB-1 labelling index are more reliable indicators of anaplasia.

Enlarged nuclei showing hyperchromasia and pleomorphism are prominent features of highly aggressive tumours such as glioblastoma and metastatic carcinoma. But such features may also be seen in slowly growing Schwannomas and (pleomorphic) meningiomas. In these tumours the nuclear changes have no adverse prognostic significance unless there is a high mitotic or Ki-67/MIB-1 labelling index. In Schwannomas, the presence of large hyperchromatic nuclei in the absence of mitoses is referred to as 'ancient change.'

Mitotic and proliferation indices Although the presence of mitoses in tumours such as meningiomas and primitive neuroectodermal tumours may be a useful diagnostic feature, most particularly in the assessment of the growth potential of the tumour, the search for mitoses in astrocytic tumours may be less fruitful. Mitoses are usually absent in diffuse astrocytomas, infrequent but present in anaplastic astrocytomas, and seen in varying numbers in glioblastoma. With very small biopsies, mitoses may be missed. The use of immunocytochemistry for proliferation antigens such as Ki-67/MIB-1 has, therefore, improved the analysis of small biopsies of astrocytic tumours. A number of studies have illustrated the correlation between Ki-67/MIB-1 labelling indices and prognosis for diffuse astrocytic tumours and ependymomas but there is wide variation and the labelling index should be only one of the features used to decide upon the well differentiated or anaplastic nature of such tumours. In oligodendrogliomas, the well differentiated tumours have low labelling indices whereas both mitotic rates and the labelling indices are high in anaplastic oligodendrogliomas. Ki-67/MIB-1 labelling may be variable in primitive neuroectodermal tumours, it may be higher in the areas showing few features of differentiation than in areas where there is morphological evidence of ganglion cell differentiation.

Necrosis Areas of necrosis in are usually an indication of poor prognosis. Typically seen in glioblastoma, primitive neuroectodermal tumours, anaplastic oligodendrogliomas, atypical meningiomas (microinfarction) and metastatic tumours in the brain. The presence of thrombosed arteries, commonly associated with areas of necrosis in glioblastomas, suggest that the necrosis is due to ischaemic infarction. Large areas of infarction in glioblastoma, with associated swelling of the tumour and an increased intracranial pressure, may explain the sudden deterioration of neurological status in some patients with this tumour.

Blood vessels, blood–brain barrier and oedema Functional features of the vascular supply of intracranial tumours and the presence of associated oedema are key factors in the CT and MRI diagnosis of intracranial and spinal tumours. Metastatic tumours and those derived from tissues other than the CNS within the skull or spinal column show enhancement on CT and MRI as they do not posses a blood–brain barrier. Thus, meningiomas, Schwannomas, pituitary tumours and pineal germinomas typically enhance.

Histological features of blood vessels are particularly valuable in the pathological diagnosis and in the evaluation of the prognosis of primary neuroepithelial tumours. In diffuse astrocytic tumours, there is a change in the morphology of blood vessels, the blood–brain barrier and the degree of peritumoral oedema as astrocytomas evolve into anaplastic astrocytomas or glioblastoma. In diffuse astrocytomas, the blood vessels are well formed and resemble those in normal brain. On CT and MRI, there is no enhancement as the blood–brain barrier is intact and peritumoral oedema is minimal. With the onset of anaplastic change in a diffuse astrocytoma, the blood–brain barrier becomes more permeable and enhancement is seen on CT scan and MRI. In glioblastoma, there are substantial changes in the blood vessels, probably associated with the production of abnormal growth factors and the presence of growth factor receptors. The glomeruloid disordered structure of blood vessels showing microvascular proliferation in glioblastomas is accompanied by a breakdown of the blood–brain barrier and bright contrast enhancement on CT and MRI. Coincident with the breakdown of the blood–brain barrier is peritumoral oedema around glioblastomas. Radiologically, a region of central necrosis, a rim of enhancing tumour and the presence of peritumoral oedema on CT and MRI are good indicators of glioblastoma. Microvascular proliferation and the presence of necrosis in an anaplastic glial tumour are the histological indicators of glioblastoma.

Invasion, spread and metastasis Metastatic spread of tumours to the CNS is very common but metastasis outside the CNS from intracranial tumours is rare. Carcinomas from lung, breast, kidney and other organs spread to the CNS in two major forms; most commonly as single or multiple well circumscribed deposits, or less commonly by diffusely spreading over the surface of the brain in the subarachnoid space as carcinomatous meningitis.

Tumours arising from the meninges occasionally directly invade the brain; but more frequently they compress adjacent structures during growth. Similarly, Schwannomas associated with the vestibular nerve and other cranial or spinal nerves grow as localised masses and compress or displace adjacent structures. Neurofibromas, on the other hand, may invade both peripheral nerves and nearby structures such as bone. Pituitary adenomas tend to compress neural structures, such as the optic chiasm. Craniopharyngiomas arising from the pituitary region may also spread into the brain by budding in a similar way to some meningiomas; this makes complete excision of the tumour sometimes very difficult.

Primary neuroepithelial tumours spread by directly invading surrounding brain but they also seed through the subarachnoid space. Diffuse astrocytomas and anaplastic astrocytoma are typical examples of tumours that spread diffusely through the brain so that the limits of the tumour are difficult, if not impossible, to define by radiology, at surgery and even by histological examination. Characteristically, astrocytic tumour cells spread along fibre tracts within the brain and cord and may be so diffuse that no localised tumour mass is recognised, as in gliomatosis cerebri. Glioblastomas show a similar spread into surrounding tissues, although histologically the margin of invasion in these tumours and in some oligodendrogliomas is more sharply defined; this may be because the tumour cells destroy the tissue as they invade. Primitive neuroectodermal tumours typically invade surrounding brain structures and also seed through the CSF; the recognition of such seeding is key to the therapy of such tumours. Ependymomas may also spread diffusely through the cranial and spinal subarachnoid spaces.

Virtually the only non-neural tumours to spread diffusely through brain or spinal cord tissue are lymphomas, and, occasionally, small cell carcinoma of the lung.

REFERENCES

1. Davis FG, Preston-Martin S. Epidemiology: incidence and survival. In: Bigner DD, McLendon RE, Bruner JM (eds). Russell and Rubinstein's pathology of tumors of the nervous system. London: Arnold, 1998, pp 5–45
2. Jukich PJ, McCarthy BJ, Surawicz TS, Freels S, Davis FG. Trends in the incidence of primary brain tumors in the United States, 1985–1994. Neuro-oncol 2001; 3:141–151
3. Louis DN, Holland EC, Cairncross JG. Glioma classification: a molecular reappraisal. Am J Pathol 2001; 159:779–786
4. Maher EA, Furnari FB, Bachoo RM, Rowitch DH, Louis DN, Cavanee WK, DePinho RA. Malignant glioma: genetics and biology of a grave matter. Genes Dev 2001; 15:1311–1333
5. Bailey P, Cushing H. A classification of the tumours of the glioma group on a histogenetic basis with a correlated study of prognosis. Philadelphia: JB Lippincott, 1926
6. Kernohan JW, Sayre GP. Tumors of the central nervous system. Atlas of tumor pathology, section x, fascicle 35. Washington D C: Armed Forces Institute of Pathology, 1952
7. Kleihues P, Burger PC, Scheithauer BW. Histological typing of tumours of the central nervous system. Berlin: Springer-Verlag, 1993
8. Kleihues P, Cavenee WK. Pathology and genetics of tumours of the nervous system. Lyon: IARC, 2000
9. Russell DS, Rubinstein LJ. Pathology of tumours of the nervous system, 5th edn. Baltimore: Williams & Wilkins, 1989
10. McLendon RE, Tien RD. Tumors and tumor-like lesions of maldevelopmental origin. In: Bigner DD, McLendon RE, Brunner JM, eds. Russell and Rubinstein's pathology of tumors of the nervous system II. London: Edward Arnold, 1998, pp 295–370
11. Louis DN, Cavanee WK. Molecular biology of central nervous system tumours. In DeVita VT, Hellman S, Rosenberg SA, eds. Cancer: principles and practice of oncology, 6th edn. Philadelphia: Lippincott-Raven, 2001
12. Barker DJ, Weller RO, Garfield JS. Epidemiology of primary tumours of the brain and spinal cord: a regional survey in southern England. J Neurol Neurosurg Psych 1976; 39:290–296
13. McKinney PA, Parslow RC, Lane SA et al. Epidemiology of childhood brain tumours in Yorkshire, UK, 1974–95: geographical distribution and changing patterns of occurrence. Br J Cancer 1998; 78:974–979
14. Davis FG, Freels S, Grutsch J, Barlas S, Brem S. Survival rates in patients with primary malignant brain tumors stratified by patient age and tumor histological type: an analysis based on Surveillance, Epidemiology, and End Results (SEER) data, 1973–1991. J Neurosurg 1998; 88:1–10
15. Heuch JM, Heuch I, Akslen LA, Kvale G. Risk of primary childhood brain tumors related to birth characteristics: a Norwegian prospective study. Int J Cancer 1998; 77:498–503
16. Fleury A, Menegoz F, Grosclaude P et al. Descriptive epidemiology of cerebral gliomas in France. Cancer 1997; 79:1195–1202
17. Pobereskin LH, Chadduck JB. Incidence of brain tumours in two English counties: a population based study. J Neurol Neurosurg Psych 2001; 69:464–471
18. Polednak AP. Interpretation of secular increases in incidence rates for primary brain cancer in Connecticut adults, 1965–1988. Neuroepidemiology 1996; 15:51–56
19. Rickert CH, Probst Cousin S, Gullotta F. Primary intracranial neoplasms of infancy and early childhood. Childs Nerv Syst 1997; 13:507–513
20. Yeni-Komshian H, Holly EA. Childhood brain tumours and exposure to animals and farm life: a review. Paediatr Perinat Epidemiol 2000; 14:248–256
21. Furuta T, Sugiu K, Tamiya T, Matsumoto K, Ohmoto T. Malignant cerebellar astrocytoma developing 15 years after radiation therapy for a medulloblastoma. Clin Neurol Neurosurg 1998; 100:56–59
22. Saiki S, Kinouchi T, Usami M, Nakagawa H, Kotake T. Glioblastoma multiforme after radiotherapy for metastatic brain tumor of testicular cancer. Int J Urol 1997; 4:527–529
23. Grabb PA, Kelly DR, Fulmer BB, Palmer C. Radiation-induced glioma of the spinal cord. Pediatr Neurosurg 1996; 25:214–219
24. Neal JW, Llewelyn MB, Morrison HL, Jasani B, Borysiewicz LK. A malignant astrocytoma in a patient with AIDS: a possible association between astrocytomas and HIV infection. J Infect 1996; 33:159–162
25. Zook BC, Simmens SJ, Jones RV. Evaluation of ENU-induced gliomas in rats: nomenclature, immunochemistry, and malignancy. Toxicol Pathol 2000; 28:193–201
26. Simmons ML, Lamborn KR, Takahashi M et al. Analysis of complex relationships between age, TP53, epidermal growth factor receptor, and survival in glioblastoma patients. Cancer Res 2001; 61:1122–1128
27. Pomeroy SL, Tamayo P, Gaasenbeek M et al. Gene expression-based classification and outcome prediction of central nervous system embryonal tumours. Nature 2002; 415:436–442
28. Nozaki M, Tada M, Kobayashi H et al. Roles of the functional loss of p53 and other genes in astrocytoma tumorigenesis and progression. Neuro-oncol 1999; 1:124–137
29. Ino Y, Betensky RA, Zlatescu MC et al. Molecular subtypes of anaplastic oligodendroglioma: implications for patient management at diagnosis. Clin Cancer Res 2001; 7:839–845
30. Cher LM. Cancer and the nervous system. Med J Aust 2001; 175:277–282
31. Akinwunmi J, Powell M. Understanding cerebral tumours. Practitioner 2001; 245:498–502
32. Bouffet E. Common brain tumours in children: diagnosis and treatment. Paediatr Drugs 2000; 2:57–66
33. Ironside JW, Pickard J. Raised intracranial pressure, oedema and hydrocephalus. In: Graham DI, Lantos PL, eds. Greenfield's neuropathology, 7th edn. London: Arnold (in press)
34. Berger MS, Keles E. Epilepsy associated with brain tumors. In Kaye AH, Laws ER, eds. Brain tumors. An encyclopedic approach. Edinburgh: Churchill Livingstone, 1995, pp 239–246

35. Black P, Wen PY. Clinical, imaging and laboratory diagnosis of brain tumors. In: Kaye AH, Laws ER, eds. Brain Tumors. An Encyclopedic Approach. Edinburgh: Churchill Livingstone, 1995, pp 191–214

36. Brunelle F. Noninvasive diagnosis of brain tumours in children. Childs Nerv Syst 2000; 16:731–734

37. Goldman S, Wikler D, Damhaut P et al. Positron emission tomography and brain tumours. Acta Neurol Belg 1997; 97:183–186

38. Plowman PN, Saunders CA, Maisey M. On the usefulness of brain

PET scanning to the paediatric neuro-oncologist Br J Neurosurg 1997; 11:525–532

39. Firlik KS, Martinez AJ, Lunsford LD. Use of cytological preparations for the intraoperative diagnosis of stereotactically obtained brain biopsies: a 19-year experience and survey of neuropathologists. J Neurosurg 2000; 91:454–458

40. Moss TH, Nicoll JAR, Ironside JW. Intra-operative diagnosis of nervous system tumours. London: Arnold, 1997

2 A practical approach to the diagnosis of neurosurgical biopsies

The diagnosis of brain tumours is a multidisciplinary exercise, which requires close communication between neurologists, neurosurgeons, neuroradiologists and neuropathologists. It is therefore particularly important that when tissue samples are submitted for pathological diagnosis, clinical and neuroradiological information on the case should be clearly provided on the request form which is sent with the specimen to the neuropathology laboratory. Experience has taught us that by no means all request forms are ideally completed, but it is essential to have a concise summary of the clinical, neuroradiological and surgical findings in each case in order to facilitate pathological diagnosis. The approach to the diagnosis of brain tumours is discussed below mainly in terms of paraffin section histology (see Chapter 3 for intraoperative techniques), but although the vast majority of definitive brain tumour diagnoses are made on surgical biopsy specimens, the role of the autopsy and cerebrospinal fluid (CSF) cytology in the investigation and diagnosis of central nervous system (CNS) tumours should not be overlooked. Finally, in order to maintain a high standard of diagnostic practice it is essential to undertake regular audit and external quality assessment programmes. All these issues are included towards the end of this chapter.

Clinical diagnosis: essential parameters

Basic patient data

It is critically important that the pathologist should be aware of the age and sex of the patient at the time of diagnosis. Both parameters play a major role in influencing differential diagnosis and this important information should be readily available. Although it is accepted that neither age nor sex is seldom an absolute contraindication to any diagnosis, the characteristic spectrum of brain tumours, particularly in relation to age, is clearly documented. Further important information is the relevant family history, which is paramount in establishing whether or not an underlying genetic disorder may be responsible for the patient's neurological abnormalities; conversely, the presence of an established family history of a tumour associated syndrome will clearly direct the neuropathologist at the time of diagnosis. Additional relevant information on medical history is also important, and in particular details of previous neurological illnesses (especially any previous neurosurgical procedures) along with the relevant neuropathological diagnosis (and if possible the associated laboratory reference numbers for specimen retrieval) and details of treatment. The importance of knowing the nature of previous treatment for brain tumours is discussed at greater length in Chapter 20, and familial tumour associated syndromes are described in detail in Chapter 19.

Clinical history

The nature and duration of the neurological symptoms is also important in helping establish diagnosis. Most patients with brain tumours present with non-specific signs and symptoms associated with raised intracranial pressure including headaches, visual disturbances, nausea and vomiting, seizures or focal neurological signs. Over the past decade, as the sophistication and availability of sensitive neurological investigative techniques has increased, there is an increasing awareness of the need to consider brain and spinal cord tumours as the underlying cause for a more subtle range of neurological abnormalities than was hitherto suspected clinically, allowing earlier diagnosis in many cases, e.g. complex partial seizures in children.

Neuroradiology

Information on the neuroradiological findings in patients with suspected brain or spinal cord tumours is essential in allowing the neuropathologist the opportunity to formulate a differential diagnosis before even looking down the microscope. Neuroradiology also allows the accurate recognition of tissue changes occurring adjacent to and within CNS tumours including haemorrhage, calcification, cyst formation and the space occupying effect of an expanding intracranial mass. It is also possible to recognise individual tissue constituents, for example adipose tissue within CNS tumours. However, even these sophisticated techniques are not always capable of reliably establishing the infiltrating margin of most tumours, and this is of particular importance when biopsy sites are being considered. Apart from giving important information on the anatomical localisation of a brain or spinal cord tumour, modern magnetic resonance imaging (MRI) techniques also allow a much more accurate assessment of tumour margins, tumour associated oedema and in particular enhancement following the administration of intravenous contrast material. Contrast enhancement in a diffuse intracerebral lesion is a strong indication that this is likely to be a malignant lesion and a clinical diagnosis of benign tumours must always be questioned by the pathologist in the face of this information. A summary of the patterns of contrast enhancement in common CNS tumours is listed in Table 2.1. Although it is ideal under many circumstances to have the opportunity to inspect the neuroradiological images oneself prior to making a diagnosis, this is not practicable in all centres and can be resolved by adequate communication with the neuroradiologist.

The widespread use of stereotaxy as an investigative tool for diagnosis has had a major impact on the practice of surgical neuropathology. The design of most stereotactic frames allows multiple biopsies to be sampled by the biopsy needle at various sites within and around a

Table 2.1 Summary of MRI/CT enhancement patterns in common CNS neoplasms

Neoplasm	Pattern of contrast enhancement
Astrocytoma	Non-enhancing
Anaplastic astrocytoma	Non-homogeneous, variable
Glioblastoma	Ring enhancement around areas of necrosis
Pilocytic astrocytoma	Diffuse; ring enhancement around large cysts
Metastases	Multiple, non-homogeneous with ring enhancement around necrotic foci
Meningioma	Homogeneous, with variable patterns following embolism
Oligodendroglioma	Non-enhancing, small areas of calcification
Ependymoma	Homogeneous enhancement; cystic change may produce a ring-like effect
Medulloblastoma	Non-homogeneous, intense enhancement around foci of necrosis
Lymphoma	Strong enhancement, with ring-like areas of intensity around necrotic foci

suspected brain tumour. Whenever possible, it is advisable for the neuropathologist to be involved in the discussion of biopsy targets using the stereotactic approach, in order to ensure that representative tumour material is included in at least one of the targets, and not just tissue showing reactive changes or tissue which has undergone extensive necrosis. If this is not practical, it is essential to establish whether a series of stereotactic biopsies has been taken from the centre of the tumour, the infiltrating edge, the area of necrosis or haemorrhage. It is therefore important to ensure the accurate identification of biopsy specimens taken from various tumour co-ordinates, in order that an accurate assessment of the histological and cytological features may be made following biopsy. This is of particular relevance when subsequent neurosurgical excision of an intracerebral tumour is being considered.

Neurosurgical operative findings

The increasing use of stereotaxy to obtain tissue for the diagnosis of intrinsic CNS tumours obviates a need for a detailed description of the operative findings in such cases; however, a brief summary of the neurosurgical findings in patients undergoing craniotomy and biopsy, subtotal or complete excision of intracranial tumours is helpful to the neuropathologist. Particularly useful is information on the relationship of the lesion to adjacent structures and changes in the character and nature of the tissue including the presence of necrosis, haemorrhage and cystic change. Calcification is often appreciated at the time of biopsy, even when it is not readily demonstrable

using MRI techniques. The neuropathologist should be informed of any changes in the tissue specimen that have occurred as a result of neurosurgery, in particular haemorrhage occurring during the biopsy procedure or collapse of a cystic structure following incision. In meningiomas, a history of therapeutic embolism should be given when appropriate; this can result in tumour infarction and necrosis, and may make intraoperative diagnosis particularly difficult.

It is also important to have information on the precise location of different portions of a biopsy, and to record whether or not certain key areas were sampled, for example a mural nodule within a cystic lesion. Other factors, including the presence of apparent multiple lesions, should be recorded, as should the extent of the resection. This is particularly important in lobectomy or other larger resection specimens when total excision of the lesion has been attempted. In such cases, it is important to identify the resection margins to allow proper orientation of the specimen prior to histological sampling (see below). Finally, an experienced neuro-surgeon will be able to provide additional information or other parameters including the relationship to blood vessels, other associated lesions (particularly those not identified prior to surgery) and reactive changes in adjacent tissues which should not be confused with the lesion at the time of sampling of histology. Adequate specimen documentation and a record of tissue samples from the neurosurgeon will help avoid confusion between the lesion which is under investigation and any secondary reactive or associated changes in the surrounding tissue.

Tissue handling and sampling

Tissue fixation

There is much to be said for receiving all CNS tumour specimens unfixed from the neurosurgical theatre, since this allows tissue to be sampled and stored for a number of techniques including microbiology, virology and (more commonly) molecular genetic analysis, or cell culture.[1] It also allows the use of a greater range of tissue fixatives; optimal fixation in glutaraldehyde for electron microscopy can easily be achieved. Most neuropathology laboratories fix biopsy specimens in 10% formalin, usually buffered at a neutral pH. Once brain tumour biopsy specimens are placed in fixative, sampling for paraffin section processing can be carried out within 6–24 h depending on size and volume of the specimens. As with unfixed tissue, the dimensions of the specimen should be recorded (and the specimen weight if large tumours are resected) and a careful description made with respect to the relationship of the tumour with any adjacent brain tissue, the appearance and consistency of the tumour tissue with particular attention to the presence of necrosis, haemorrhage, cystic change and infiltration of the surrounding tissue, particularly at the margins of the specimen.

Specimen sampling

Once the material from the brain tumour biopsy resection specimen has been adequately fixed, examined macroscopically (and photographed if necessary) then it should be sampled for histological examination. In the case of stereotactic biopsies the entire material must be examined and the specimen should be labelled in order to allow comparison with the corresponding MRI target site of the tumour. Any specimens taken for cryostat section examination should also be processed separately and given a separate identification number or subheading in order that a direct comparison can be made between the cryostat sections and the corresponding paraffin embedded sections. Sampling of other specimens depends on the volume and nature of the tumour material and the relevant clinical association. For example, most biopsies of intrinsic tumours should be sampled in their entirety for histological examination in order to allow full assessment of tumour heterogeneity, which is of major prognostic significance in gliomas.

When resection or lobectomy specimens are received in the laboratory then it is important that the specimens should be examined and sampled in a way that a meaningful comment can be made on the adequacy of the excision, and precise anatomical correlates identified. This is often best achieved by serial sectioning of the lobectomy specimen after appropriate orientation, which allows a large number of surfaces throughout the lesion to be inspected, photographed and sampled for histology.[1] This is particularly important in the case of lobectomy specimens when a tumour cannot be identified on macroscopic examination (a protocol for lobectomy specimens is listed in Table 2.2). The tumour resection margins should always be studied with particular care and should be sampled histologically, trying to ensure that the orientation of the specimen is appropriate for the size of the lesion and the relationship of the excision margin to adjacent structures. Familiarity with the neuroradiological features in such cases is helpful when the orientation and resection margins sampling procedures are under consideration.

With other tumours, for example metastatic carcinoma, the need for extensive sampling is not so great as tumour heterogeneity is of lesser clinical significance. With extrinsic tumours, particularly meningiomas, there is a need to sample adequately the interface between the tumour and the brain to investigate the possibility of cortical infiltration, which is of prognostic significance, and to examine the relationship of the tumour to adjacent structures including the dura mater, blood vessels and skull if this is submitted for examination.

Table 2.2 Protocol for handling a lobectomy specimen[1]

1. The specimen should be received fresh and orientated prior to dissection
2. The specimen should be described carefully, paying particular attention to the presence of any tumour on the external surface, and its relationship to specialised structures (e.g. the hippocampus) and the resection margins
3. Fresh tissue should be sampled as appropriate for microbiology, virology or molecular genetic studies
4. The specimen may then be fixed overnight for further dissection, or dissected fresh (the former procedure usually facilitates identification and orientation of small lesions)
5. After fixation, the specimen should be sectioned serially in the coronal plane at 5 mm intervals
6. The cut surfaces should be carefully inspected and photographed as necessary. Any lesions should be recorded, and the hippocampus identified
7. The entire specimen should be blocked out on non-adjacent faces; the hippocampus may be examined separately
8. All tissues should be processed for histology, with the use of special stains and immunocytochemistry as appropriate

Calcified specimens

Tumours involving the skull and the vertebral column are frequently biopsied and submitted for examination in neuropathology laboratories. These inevitably cause problems in sampling; the presence of bone, cartilage and other calcified material will hinder processing of the specimen, since microtome sections cannot readily be cut until the specimen is decalcified. Under these circumstances it is obviously advisable to sample as extensively as possible from areas where there is only a limited component of bone; surface decalcification can be employed on the tissue blocks to allow sections to be obtained much sooner than conventional decalcification, which can take up to several weeks. It should also be borne in mind that prolonged decalcification (by whatever method) does interfere with tissue morphology and particularly with antigen preservation should immunocytochemistry be required for subsequent diagnosis.

Section preparation and staining

The accuracy of histological diagnosis is dependent on the provision of adequate material for interpretation. This is influenced by the nature and duration of tissue fixation, processing, section cutting and staining. In most neuropathology laboratories neurosurgical biopsies are cut at a reduced thickness in relation to brain autopsy tissues. In surgical practice, $5 \mu m$ biopsy sections are adequate and it is occasionally necessary to obtain thinner ($2–3 \mu m$) sections to study nuclear morphology, e.g. in lymphoid neoplasms.

Tinctorial staining

Sections are stained conventionally with haematoxylin and eosin (H & E) in neuropathology laboratories across the world. The widespread use of haematoxylin and eosin is testimony to the remarkable extent to which it allows visualisation of many critical morphological features. Other tinctorial stains may be helpful, for example a reticulin stain in lymphomas or haemangiopericytomas, or a periodic acid–Schiff (PAS) stain for mucins in metastatic carcinomas. Tinctorial stains which are commonly used in neurosurgical tumour diagnosis are listed in Table 2.3.

Basic immunocytochemical staining

Diagnosis of brain tumours requires use of immunocytochemistry in the context of an experienced laboratory where familiarity with the many antibodies which are not used in general histological diagnosis is readily available. Most immunocytochemistry is used to investigate cellular differentiation in tumours and many of the most frequently used antibodies recognise different classes of intermediate filaments, including glial fibrillary acidic protein (GFAP), neurofilament protein, cytokeratins and desmin. Other antibodies recognise epitopes which are frequently encountered in certain categories of tumour for example epithelial membrane antigen in carcinomas, synaptophysin in tumours showing neuronal differentiation and the leucocyte common antigen (CD45) in the lymphoid tumours. These antibodies are supplemented by other groups of antibodies which recognise specific tumour products including placental alkaline phosphatase, alpha-fetoprotein and beta-human chorionic gonadotropin in germ cell tumours. Diagnostic immunocytochemistry is best performed using a panel of antibodies, particularly for tumours which are difficult to classify using standard tinctorial methods.[2–4] The use of one single antibody to confirm or refute diagnosis of a particular category of tumour is generally not a helpful approach, although in practice the use of GFAP for the diagnosis of astrocytic tumours frequently does not require an extensive panel of other antibodies for its successful use. However, this instance represents the exception rather than the rule and most tumours which are difficult to interpret on routine histology should be investigated with a panel of antibodies. (See below under General principles of histological diagnosis.)[5,6] Details of antibodies commonly used in diagnostic surgical neuropathology are listed in Table 2.4.

An important issue in the interpretation of immunocytochemistry concerns artefacts and unsuspected technical difficulties. Control tissue should be carefully selected for each antibody and the results examined on every staining run. Even then, unexpected negative results on the test section may still be caused by accidental omission of a reagent layer on that particular slide but not on the control section. Where the staining is very faint in the control tissue, a naturally limited expression of the epitope in the tumour may result in a false negative result, and the expiry dates of the primary antibody and other reagents should be carefully scrutinised. Uneven staining over the area of a section is another trap, especially if diagnostic tumour tissue is only visible in one area of the section. As a general rule, if the result of an immunocytochemical stain is very unexpected and there is any doubt about technical aspects, it is wise to repeat the procedure, if necessary replacing suspect reagents.

Cell proliferation indices

In addition to antibodies employed to define cellular differentiation, there is a wider range of antibodies which have been employed to study cell biology in human brain tumours. This includes antibodies used to detect proliferating cells, and there is increasing evidence to suggest that these may be helpful in both diagnostic and prognostic terms particularly for astrocytic gliomas. These include the Ki-67 antigen. In practice Ki-67/MIB-1 is probably the most frequently employed and is of considerable use on paraffin sections including archival material.[7–11]

Oncogene and tumour suppressor products

Antibodies to oncogene and tumour suppressor gene products are generally still used for research purposes only in neuropathology. We believe that these will play an increasing role in tumour diagnosis and categorisation in future years since there is increasing evidence to suggest that the expression of certain gene products (or the absence of others) may be characteristic of certain tumours and of prognostic value, for example the expression of EGFR, p16 or p53 mutant protein in malignant astrocytic gliomas.[12,13]

Table 2.3 Tinctorial stains commonly used in the diagnosis of CNS tumours

Stain	Demonstration
Haematoxylin and eosin	General histological features
Toluidine blue	Useful for rapid staining of smears for intraoperative diagnosis
Reticulin	Reticulin framework around blood vessels in gliomas and lymphomas; soft tissue tumours
van Gieson	Dural infiltration in meningiomas
Periodic acid–Schiff	Glycogen (diastase sensitive) Mucins (intra- and extracellular)
Alcian blue	Mucins (intra- and extracellular)
Mucicarmine	Mucins (intracellular)
Singh, Masson–Fontana	Melanin
Luxol fast blue	Myelin
Solochrome cyanin	Myelin

Table 2.4 Antibodies commonly used in the diagnosis of CNS tumours* [3–6]

Tumour type	Antibodies used
Astrocytic tumours	Glial fibrillary acidic protein
Oligodendrogliomas	Glial fibrillary acidic protein Leu7
Ependymomas	S-100 protein Glial fibrillary acidic protein Epithelial membrane antigen
Choroid plexus tumours	Transthyretin Carbonic anhydrase C Cathepsin D Glial fibrillary acidic protein Epithelial membrane antigen Cytokeratins
Medulloblastoma	Glial fibrillary acidic protein Synaptophysin Neuron specific enolase Neurofilament protein
Neuronal tumours	Synaptophysin Neuron specific enolase Neurofilament protein MAP-2 NeuN
Germ cell tumours	Placental alkaline phosphatase Alpha-fetoprotein Beta-human chorionic gonadotrophin Carcinoembryonic antigen
Lymphomas	CD3, 20, 45, 68, 79a Immunoglobulins Epstein–Barr virus latent proteins
Meningiomas	Epithelial membrane antigen Vimentin Cytokeratins Progesterone receptor
Melanoma	S-100 protein Neuron specific enolase HMB45 MART-1
Nerve sheath tumours	S-100 protein Neurofilament protein (for axons)
Pituitary tumours	GH, PRL, ACTH, FSH, LH, TSH Alpha-glycoprotein subunit
Metastatic tumours	Cytokeratins (pan- and mono-, e.g. CK7, CK20) Epithelial membrane antigen Chromogranin Neuron specific enolase As above for melanoma, lymphoma, germ cell tumours Cell specific markers, e.g. ER, PSA, prostatic acid phosphatase, thyroglobulin

*See subsequent chapters for more information on individual tumours.
ACTH, adrenocorticotropic hormone; FSH, follicle stimulating hormone;
GH growth hormone; LH luteinising hormone; PRL, prolactin; TSH, thyroid
stimulating hormone; PSA, prostate specific antigen
[1] ER, oestrogen receptor;
[2] MAP-2 microtubule associated protein-2;

In addition, expression of these molecules at the messenger RNA level (as determined by expression profiling using microassays) holds promise to improve the classification of brain tumours.[14]

Antigen retrieval techniques

The use of immunocytochemistry in recent years has been greatly facilitated by the development of antigen retrieval techniques, particularly the use of microwave ovens and pressure cookers which have allowed antibodies previously used only in cryostat sections to be employed routinely on paraffin sections for diagnosis.[15] The use of antigen retrieval techniques also allows the investigation of archival material using techniques which were not available for use on paraffin sections at the time of initial diagnosis. However, the use of these techniques is not without complications and the sensitivity and specificity of the antibodies employed within a particular diagnostic setting should always be borne in mind. There is a great need to ensure adequate quality control of immunocytochemistry and it is the diagnostic pathologist's responsibility to ensure that technical staff are given appropriate support to maintain high standards and consistency in immunocytochemistry and to participate in relevant quality assurance programmes.

Molecular genetics

In recent years there has been an explosion of interest in molecular genetic techniques to investigate neoplasms including brain tumours.[16,17] While some of these techniques require unfixed tissue, the acquisition and storage of appropriate material is the province of the diagnostic neuropathologist and this should be borne in mind whenever a tumour specimen is received in the laboratory.[1] The increasing information on specific genetic abnormalities in individual tumours is included in subsequent chapters but it is important to emphasise the need to store appropriately sampled material in order that these investigations can be employed. There is already evidence to indicate that in some tumours, for example anaplastic oligodendrogliomas, the recognition of certain molecular abnormalities may be of major clinical and prognostic significance in determining response to therapy[18,19] (see Chapter 5).

General principles of histological diagnosis

Histological assessment of a presumptive tumour biopsy requires the pathologist to go through a series of mental steps in a disciplined fashion, avoiding hasty conclusions and their ensuing mistakes (Fig. 2.1). The first stage is to decide whether the tissue being examined is from a neoplasm at all. For example it may be that the surgeon has biopsied only the reactive edges of a tumour, or that

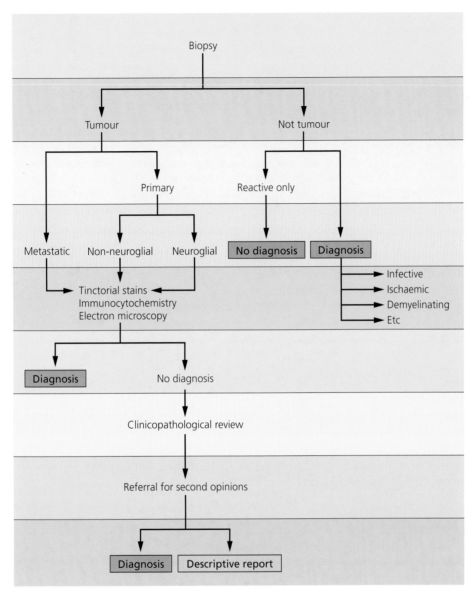

Fig. 2.1 **An outline approach to histological diagnosis of tumour biopsies.**

the lesion is not neoplastic at all but of some other aetiology. Only after it has been established that the biopsy does indeed contain tumour, can its nature be progressively refined. The aim is to consider all possibilities in the light of the observed features, work through the range of available diagnostic techniques as required and eventually arrive at a definitive diagnosis, including relevant grading and prognostic information.

Is it a neoplastic or reactive process?

Reactive brain is present around the margins of a variety of primary pathologies, including neoplastic, infective, ischaemic and demyelinating lesions. It may also occur without an adjacent primary lesion, as for example in the case of delayed radiation change. Care must always be taken not to interpret florid astrocytic reaction as diffusely infiltrating astrocytic tumour, although this distinction can be impossible if the biopsy is from the margins of an astrocytoma and shows both changes intermingled (see below). Reactive astrocytes usually have distinctive cytological features, showing both hypertrophied perinuclear cytoplasm and prominent radiating cell processes. Their nuclei are relatively uniform in size and shape, but binucleate forms are not uncommon in florid reaction and there may even be occasional mitoses. The background stroma has a characteristic loose, coarse, fibrillar appearance, usually accompanied by oedema vacuoles. In biopsies showing reactive changes only, it is most important to remember that the appearances are not specific and do not imply any particular underlying pathology, tumour or otherwise. Such a situation should ideally be avoided by the process of careful intraoperative diagnosis (see Chapter 3) but in practice will inevitably occur from time to time. All the material should be embedded and sectioned, and further levels cut through the block to look for diagnostic areas, but failing this, the biopsy has to be reported as non-diagnostic.

Ischaemic lesions may sometimes mimic neoplasms clinically and radiologically, especially where the differential diagnosis lies between an evolving infarct and a malignant astrocytic tumour. Hypertrophied reactive astrocytes and proliferating capillaries in the early stages of infarction may confuse the unwary, although if the lesion is in grey matter, the presence of neurones showing acute ischaemic change can be helpful. Macrophages may occur in either instance, but they are particularly numerous in the later stages of infarction, whereas in gliomas they are usually confined to areas of necrosis within obvious solid tumour tissue. As ever, careful review of the clinical history and radiology in conjunction with the biopsy findings will usually resolve the issue.

Demyelination is another trap for the unwary pathologist expecting a biopsy from a brain tumour. An initial presentation of unsuspected multiple sclerosis, especially where only a single large cavitating lesion is visible radiologically, may be sufficiently persuasive of tumour to prompt referral for a surgical biopsy. Such solitary giant demyelinating plaques are usually very acute, and the biopsy will show florid reactive changes (see above) together with abundant foamy macrophages. The latter are typically cuffed around blood vessels in demyelination and there may also be foci of lymphocytic infiltration. Special stains showing loss of myelin but relative sparing of axons, at least in the less destructive areas, are also a helpful feature.

Infective lesions also need to be kept in mind as a differential diagnosis of brain tumour. The commonest problem lies in the clinical and radiological distinction between a maturing bacterial abscess and a circumscribed glioblastoma. Both appear as ring enhancing mass lesions on radiological scans and they may be associated with very similar clinical presentations. Surgical biopsy of an abscess usually produces acutely reactive brain with prominent mononuclear cell infiltration, sheets of necrotic polymorphs (i.e. pus) or a mixture of the two. If there was any doubt at the time of surgery, some fresh tissue should have been sent for microbiological assessment, which can offer timely help for a neuropathologist examining the paraffin sections. Other, atypical, infective lesions also need to be considered, including the bewildering array of infective intracranial masses which may present in individuals who are immunosuppressed. These are often multiple, although that does not exclude multifocal tumours, including the lymphomas which also occur in immune deficiency. In biopsies of such infective lesions, florid astrocytic reaction and destructive changes again

need to be distinguished from glial tumour, often helped in this instance by the abundance of causative organism, such as *Toxoplasma* for example.

Is the tumour intrinsic or extrinsic to brain parenchyma?

If tumour tissue is present but the precise diagnosis is not immediately apparent, it can be helpful in the first instance to try and identify the basic tissue of origin. A major division in the diagnostic process lies between tumours derived from brain tissue and those arising from non-neuroglial elements such as meningeal or other connective tissues, bone, cartilage, etc. The site of the lesion is very important here, but such 'extrinsic' tumours may sometimes arise within the brain or cord itself, as in the case of intraventricular meningiomas. The converse is also true, with myxopapillary ependymomas and ectopic gliomas as examples of tumours derived from intrinsic brain elements but sited entirely outside the neuraxis. A list of the more common extrinsic tumours which may involve the neuraxis is given in Table 2.5. The nature of such lesions may be immediately apparent if they show characteristic histological features, but otherwise they can be separated from glial and other intrinsic brain tumours by using a variety of special stains. In addition to using immunocytochemistry for epitopes such as GFAP, simple connective tissue stains such as a reticulin preparation can be very helpful here, since most primary brain tumours lack a

Table 2.5 Tumours of non-neuroglial origin affecting the craniospinal axis

1. *Primary tumours*
   Nerve sheath tumours
   Meningeal tumours
      Meningiomas
      Haemangiopericytoma
      Sarcomas
      Melanomas
   Choroid plexus tumours
   Haemangioblastoma
   Germ cell tumours
      Germinoma
      Teratomas
   Haemopoetic tumours
      Lymphomas
      Histiocytic tumours
   Craniopharyngioma
   Pituitary gland tumours
   Osteocartilaginous tumours
   Chordoma

2. *Metastatic tumours*
   Carcinomas
   Melanomas
   Lymphomas
   Germ cell tumours
   Sarcomas

systematic connective tissue framework. There are exceptions to this of course, and in particular desmoplasia in intrinsic tumours such as gliomas and medulloblastomas needs to be kept in mind. It is also worth remembering that gliomas can be good mimics of extrinsic tumours, as for example with spindle cell and chordoid glioma variants. Again, stains for reticulin and GFAP soon unmask these as being of primary glial origin. A particular difficulty lies with genuinely sarcomatous lesions involving the brain, since these may be pure lesions, as with meningeal sarcomas and angiosarcomas, but are more commonly part of a mixed gliosarcoma with an unsuspected intrinsic component (see below).

Is the tumour primary or metastatic?

Patients with intracranial metastases referred to a neurosurgical centre for biopsy are mostly from a clinically preselected group in whom there is no known systemic primary tumour, with no metastatic disease apparent elsewhere and often only a solitary intracranial lesion. Such cases constitute more of a diagnostic challenge to the clinicians, which usually explains the referral for biopsy. Even where the intracranial lesions are multiple, a multicentric glioma cannot always be ruled out purely on radiological grounds. Solitary metastases may be radiologically indistinguishable from hemispheric glioblastomas, cerebellopontine angle Schwannomas or meningiomas, spinal haemangioblastomas and cauda equina ependymomas, to name but a few.

For the pathologist, examination of an adequate biopsy usually allows identification of a metastatic tumour without too much difficulty. The overwhelming majority of craniospinal metastases are carcinomas or melanomas, where the histological diagnosis is immediately apparent, sometimes even without the need to immunostain for cytokeratin or S-100 protein. Primitive and poorly differentiated lesions may present more of a problem, however, and require more extensive immunocytochemistry. More detailed diagnostic information relating to metastatic tumours will be found in Chapter 12. The important thing at this early stage of diagnostic thought is for the pathologist to keep in mind the possibility of a metastatic lesion, even if this has not been the clinical impression before biopsy.

Towards a specific diagnosis

Assuming that diagnostic tumour tissue is present in the biopsy, and having considered the possibility of non-neuroglial or metastatic origin, the next stage is to try and reach a specific diagnosis. The specific microscopic features of individual nervous system tumours are described in the chapters that follow, together with details about the differential diagnosis in each case, but there are some basic steps relating to this stage of diagnostic microscopy which are worth outlining here.

Specific cellular and architectural features are displayed by many nervous system tumours, especially when better differentiated, and may usually be assessed with routine stains. Without being exhaustive, the following features are of particular diagnostic relevance:

- *Rosettes* take many forms (Fig. 2.2 and Table 2.6). They are particularly helpful in the identification of tumours such as ependymomas, pineocytomas, ependymoblastomas and retinoblastomas. Less specific rosettes such as the solid Homer Wright type are found in a wide variety of primitive neuroectodermal tumours, but can still be useful. True rosettes need in turn to be distinguished from perivascular pseudorosettes, which are less specific still, but characteristically prominent in ependymomas.
- *Papillary formations* (Fig. 2.3 and Table 2.7) are a constant feature of tumours such as choroid plexus papillomas and myxopapillary ependymomas, and may also be prominent in metastatic adenocarcinomas. In addition, there are uncommon papillary tumour variants to consider, such as papillary ependymomas and meningiomas.
- *Clear cell change* (Fig. 2.4 and Table 2.8) may again be integral to a tumour type, such as haemangioblastomas, oligodendrogliomas and germinomas, or represent a tumour variant, as with clear cell ependymomas and meningiomas. Xanthomatous change has a slightly different appearance, with foamy rather than 'empty' or optically clear cytoplasm. It may be a focal phenomenon in tumours such as meningiomas and glioblastomas, or a more constant feature, as in pleomorphic xanthoastrocytoma.
- *Pigment* is mostly melanin or iron pigment, which may be distinguished using Perl's and Masson–Fontana stains or simply a bleached H & E. Iron pigment is very non-specific and usually derives from old haemorrhage into the tumour. Tumour melanin, however, is more useful in diagnosis (Table 2.9). It may be intrinsic to the tumour type, as in the case of melanocytic tumours, or signify unusual tumour variants such as melanotic Schwannomas, medulloblastomas and ependymomas. It is therefore important to remember that not all melanin containing tumours are melanomas. A particular trap lies in the common expression of S-100 protein by both primary melanocytic tumours and melanocytic Schwannomas.

Special stains have already been alluded to earlier in this chapter (Table 2.3). Since the introduction of immunocytochemistry, they have had a rather limited role in nervous system tumour diagnosis, but there are some notable exceptions.[19] In particular, reticulin staining remains helpful in assessing whether a connective tissue stroma is present in tumours (see above under Extrinsic

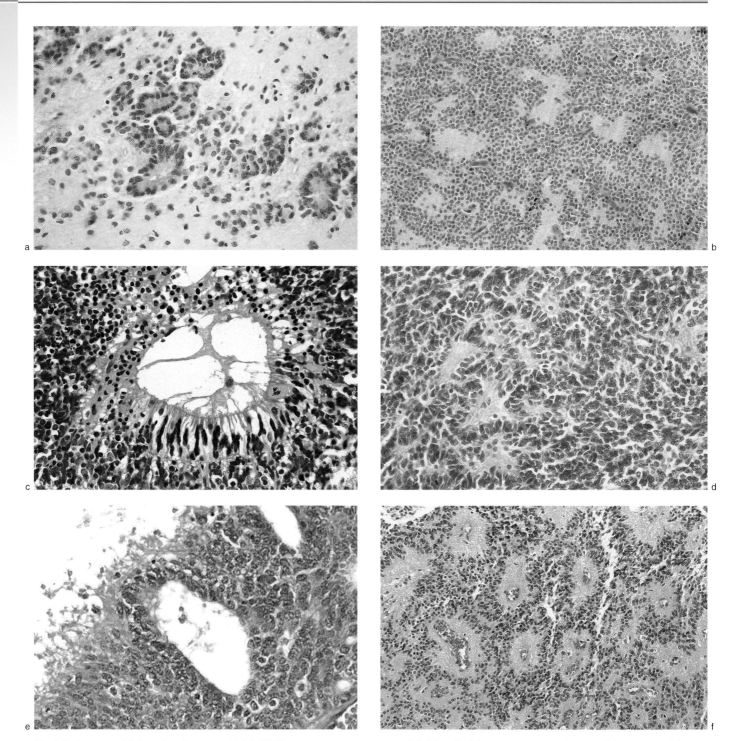

Fig. 2.2 **Rosettes. (a)** Ependymal rosettes. H & E. **(b)** Pineocytomatous rosettes. H & E. **(c)** Retinoblastoma rosette. H & E × 40. **(d)** Homer Wright rosettes from a medulloblastoma. H & E × 40. **(e)** Ependymoblastoma rosette. H & E. **(f)** Perivascular pseudorosettes from an ependymoma. H & E. (See also Chapter 7, Fig. 7.9)

tumours) and in demonstrating their vascular architecture. Mucin stains are still used to identify a glandular primary origin in poorly differentiated metastatic carcinomas and tumour pigments can be investigated using stains such as Masson–Fontana and Perl's (see above). It has to be admitted, however, that in many cases, special tinctorial stains do no more than illustrate the features of lesions which can be diagnosed using just H & E staining, as in the case of PAS/Alcian blue staining of chordomas and myxopapillary ependymomas. In a similar way, a van Gieson stain rarely helps in tumour identification but is recommended to demonstrate infiltration of pre-existing connective tissue structures, for example where meningiomas are invading dural venous sinuses.

Table 2.6 Rosettes in nervous system tumours

Rosette	Structure	Tumours
True rosettes		
Homer Wright	Nuclei around a round, solid central fibrillary zone	Primitive neuroectodermal tumours
Flexner–Wintersteiner	Nuclei around a central tubule EM: cilia, no microvilli	Retinoblastoma
Fleurette	Nuclei around a central tubule EM: projecting bulbous processes	Retinoblastoma
Ependymal	Nuclei around a central tubule EM: microvilli and cilia	Ependymoma
Pineocytomatous	Nuclei around irregular fibrillary areas. Club ended argyrophilic processes	Pineocytoma (adult type)
Medulloepithelial	Pseudostratified cells around ovoid lumen. External limiting membrane. Mitoses	Medulloepithelioma
Ependymoblastic	Multilayered cells around central lumen. Mitoses	Ependymoblastoma
Perivascular pseudorosettes		
Ependymal	Anucleate, radiating fibrillar zone around central vessel	Ependymoma
Astroblastic	Nuclei separated from central vessel by broad radiating processes	Astroblastoma

EM, electron microscopy

Table 2.7 Papillary architecture in nervous system tumours

1. *Integral to the tumour type*
   Choroid plexus tumours
   Myxopapillary ependymoma
   Metastatic adenocarcinoma
   Germ cell tumours
     Yolk sac
     Embryonal carcinoma

2. *Tumour variants*
   Meningioma
   Ependymoma
   Pituitary adenoma

Table 2.8 Clear cell change in nervous system tumours[25]

1. *True clear cell change*
   Integral to the tumour type
     Oligodendroglioma
     Haemangioblastoma
     Germinoma
     Central neurocytoma
     Paraganglioma

   Tumour variants
     Meningioma
     Ependymoma

2. *Xanthomatous change*
   Glioblastoma
   Pleomorphic xanthoastrocytoma
   Meningioma
   Xanthogranuloma
     Sellar region
     Choroid plexus

Immunocytochemistry has been discussed earlier in this chapter and a list of the more common antibodies available for nervous system tumour diagnosis is given in Table 2.4. Used correctly, immunocytochemistry is a very powerful diagnostic aid, *but only in intelligent and experienced hands*.

- The first question to ask is whether immunostaining is really necessary or likely to prove useful. Tumours showing typical features, diagnostic using tinctorial stains, really do not need to be subjected to the time and expense of immunocytochemistry just for the 'sake of completeness'. Conversely, in non-diagnostic situations such as biopsies consisting entirely of reactive brain tissue, no amount of immunocytochemical staining is likely to help matters.
- The next issue concerns the number of stains to perform and how to select them. Panels of reagents are usually recommended, but this does not simply mean using large numbers of antibody stains in an indiscriminate fashion when confronted by a difficult tumour biopsy. Antibodies which are totally inappropriate to the basic type of tumour tissue can produce confusing and unhelpful results, such as with GFAP immunostaining in some systemic tumours, for example. In addition, antibodies to some epitopes, such as S-100 protein, will stain a wide range of normal tissues and tumours, and such lack of specificity needs careful interpretation, exactly as with tinctorial stains. Ideally, interpretation of the results should rely on prior knowledge of the staining pattern expected for each antibody in all the possible tumour diagnoses being considered.

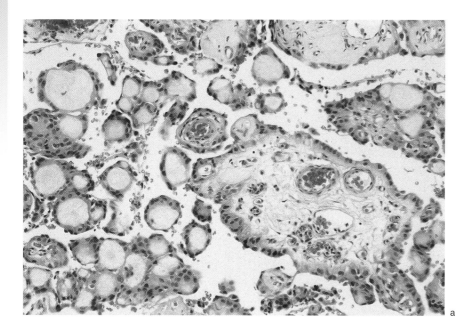

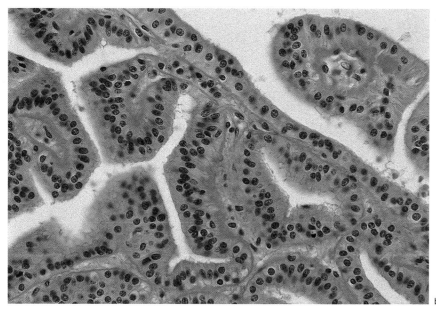

Fig. 2.3 **Papillary architecture. (a)** Myxopapillary ependymoma. H & E × 10. **(b)** Choroid plexus papilloma. H & E.

- The best approach is to arrive at a differential of two or more possible tumour types, whittled down by the diagnostic sequence outlined in the preceding sections, and then customise a panel of antibodies which would positively identify or exclude each possibility. Inevitably, there are going to be occasions where the results appear to exclude all the diagnoses considered, but this can then trigger further thought and a second round of immunostaining to investigate other possibilities. Where the amount of tissue is very sparse, thus limiting the number of sections available, there needs to be even greater discipline in selecting antibody stains, with careful consideration of the usefulness or otherwise of each reagent in relation to the diagnoses being considered.

Table 2.9 Melanin pigment in nervous system tumours

Integral to the tumour type
Melanoma
Melanocytoma

Tumour variants
Melanotic Schwannoma
Pigmented ependymoma
Pigmented medulloblastoma

Electron microscopy has a rather limited role to play in the practical diagnosis of nervous system tumours and is hampered by the constraints of time, expense, specialised fixation and the expertise required for ultrathin section preparation. Despite these practical considerations,

Fig. 2.3 (*Cont'd*) **Papillary architecture.**
(c) Papillary variant of meningioma. H & E.
(d) Papillary variant of ependymoma. H & E.

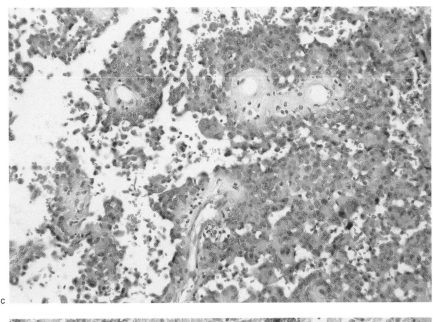

c

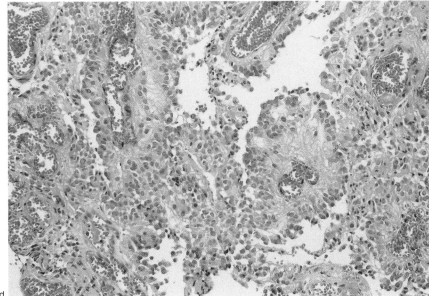

d

however, there are situations where ultrastructural examination can be of diagnostic help. Even where fresh biopsy tissue has not been selected for primary glutaraldehyde fixation, postfixing reserve formalin fixed tissue can produce surprisingly good results. In general, electron microscopy is most useful in primitive or poorly differentiated tumours where tinctorial and immunocytochemical staining have failed to elucidate the diagnosis. There are a number of ultrastructural features which may indicate tumour differentiation in such cases, and the most important of these are illustrated in Fig. 2.5 and listed in Table 2.10. Some of the more useful ones include microrosettes in ependymal tumours, basement membrane, cilia and microvilli in choroid plexus tumours, photoreceptor structures in pineal tumours,

and dense core or synaptic vesicles in neuroblastic tumours. Desmosomes and intercellular junction complexes are less specific but can also be very helpful in poorly differentiated tumours of meningeal or choroid plexus origin. For non-neural tumours involving the nervous system, special mention should be made of periodic filamentous densities in leiomyosarcoma and Birbeck granules in Langerhans cell tumours, since these are quite specific and notoriously robust structures. It should go without saying that the results of ultrastructural examination must always be interpreted in the context of all the other findings and will prove most helpful if conducted in a goal orientated fashion, i.e. with specific diagnostic possibilities and corresponding ultrastructural features in mind before commencing.

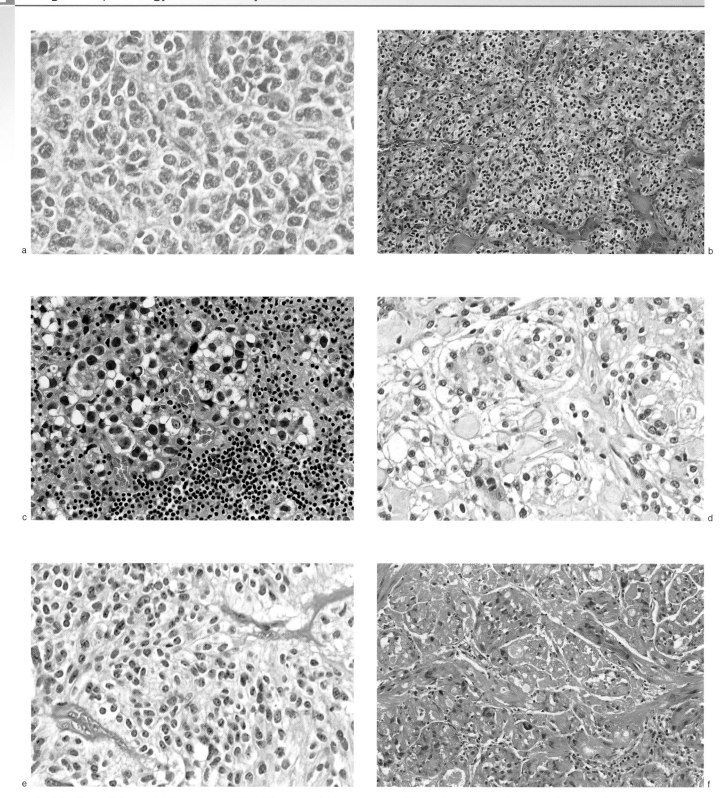

Fig. 2.4 **Clear cell change. (a)** Neurocytoma. H & E. **(b)** Haemangioblastoma. H & E. **(c)** Germinoma. H & E. **(d)** Clear cell variant of meningioma. H & E. **(e)** Clear cell variant of ependymoma. H & E. **(f)** Xanthomatous change in a pleomorphic xanthoastrocytoma. H & E.

Is it a mixed tumour?

There is a time honoured maxim that aims to dissuade pathologists from considering two diagnoses where one will suffice, which still has much to commend it. For nervous system tumours, however, this principle should be tempered with the knowledge that mixed lesions are not uncommon and may have both prognostic and management implications. Some of the more frequently encountered combinations (also see Table 2.11) are as follows:

- *Gliosarcomas*. These may be mistaken surgically for meningeal tumours, with a false plane at their deep margins which results in the pathologist receiving only the superficial, predominantly sarcomatous, part of the lesion. A careful search using reticulin stains and GFAP immunocytochemistry will usually reveal incorporated foci of glioma and may prompt the surgeon to review the scans and consider a debulking of the deeper, predominantly gliomatous part of the lesion.
- *Mixed gliomas*. Oligoastrocytomas and their anaplastic counterpart are the most commonly encountered mixed glial tumours and may consist of segregated areas of each tumour type of more diffusely intermingled elements. Mixed ependymoma and subependymoma is prognostically important because the ependymoma element confers a poorer prognosis than with subependymoma alone.
- *Glioneuronal tumours*. There is a wide range of these lesions, including gangliogliomas, desmoplastic infantile gangliogliomas and dysembryoplastic neuroepithelial tumours, all fully described in Chapter 8. Immunocytochemistry for GFAP and neuronal epitopes such as neurone specific enolase and synaptophysin is invaluable in the evaluation of such lesions. The same applies to the assessment of glial and neuronal differentiation in primitive neuroectodermal tumours, although strictly speaking this situation does not constitute a true mixed tumour.

Grading and malignancy

Assessment of malignancy is one of the most important steps in the histological diagnosis of any tumour, in the nervous system no less than elsewhere. Information about the biological potential of a tumour gives guidance for prognosis and the subsequent management of the patient, and is frequently as important as trying to arrive at a specific diagnosis. Even when particularly unusual or poorly differentiated tumours cannot be assigned a specific diagnostic label, some comment about the malignant potential of the lesion is usually still possible and gives invaluable information to the clinician. For some tumour entities, such as myxopapillary ependymoma (low grade) or medulloblastoma (highly malignant), a precise diagnosis will itself imply the biological potential of a lesion. In many instances, however, the diagnosis needs to be qualified by an assessment of malignancy, whether this is a formal numerical grade, as for astrocytic gliomas, or a descriptive qualification such as 'atypical' or 'anaplastic' meningioma. The World Health Organisation (WHO) classification[20] is a useful basis for standardising this process (see also under Formulating a report, below), but like any grading system it needs intelligent interpretation on the part of the pathologist. Clear distinction between benign and malignant is sometimes difficult in tumours of the nervous system, and lesions which are borderline between numeric grades or descriptive categories are by no means uncommon. Furthermore, gliomas in particular are often non-uniform in their malignant potential and a small biopsy from a large lesion can lead to serious sampling error unless the radiology, history and other information are taken into account. Samples showing only diffusely infiltrated brain from the margins of a high grade glioma are a particular trap in this respect. In addition to assessing the usual histological features of malignant potential, such as tumour necrosis, mitoses, cellularity, cytological atypia etc., it is also necessary to consider the actual behaviour of the lesion, as it presents in any particular case. For example, frank invasion of adjacent bone and other adjacent structures is of vital importance in pituitary adenomas and meningiomas, even when these tumours are apparently entirely benign using intrinsic histological parameters. In the same way, a tumour which has recurred in a short space of time after adequate primary treatment has clearly declared its biological potential, regardless of the interpretation of the initial biopsy.

Finally, immunocytochemical stains for markers of proliferation (e.g. Ki-67/MIB-1; see above under Preparation and staining of sections) are finding increasing favour in the assessment of biological potential in nervous system tumours, and are likely to become a powerful and more objective tool, particularly for gliomas. It should be noted, however, that their use in routine diagnosis is still in its relative infancy and the results can easily give a misleading impression of tumour grade unless used with sufficient experience or automated numerical analysis technology.

Problem cases

From time to time it is inevitable that all pathologists will encounter adequate tumour biopsies which prove diagnostically elusive, despite following all the steps outlined above. There are no hard and fast rules here, but one or more of the following courses of action may prove helpful, not necessarily in the order given:

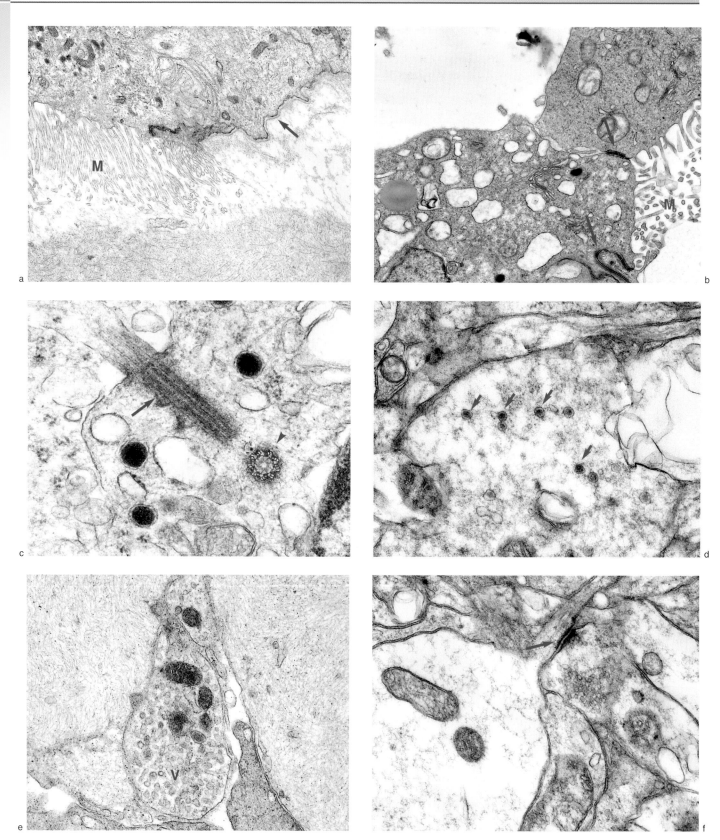

Fig. 2.5 **Ultrastructural features useful in tumour diagnosis. (a)** Microvilli (M) and tumour cell basement membrane (arrow) from a myxopapillary ependymoma. **(b)** Desmosomes (arrows) and microvilli (M) from a metastatic carcinoma. **(c)** Cilia from a pineoblastoma (arrow). The cross-section (arrowhead) shows a 9 + 0 axial structure. **(d)** Dense core vesicles (arrows) from a central neuroblastoma. **(e)** Synaptic vesicles (V) from a ganglioglioma. **(f)** Synapse (arrow) from a central neuroblastoma.

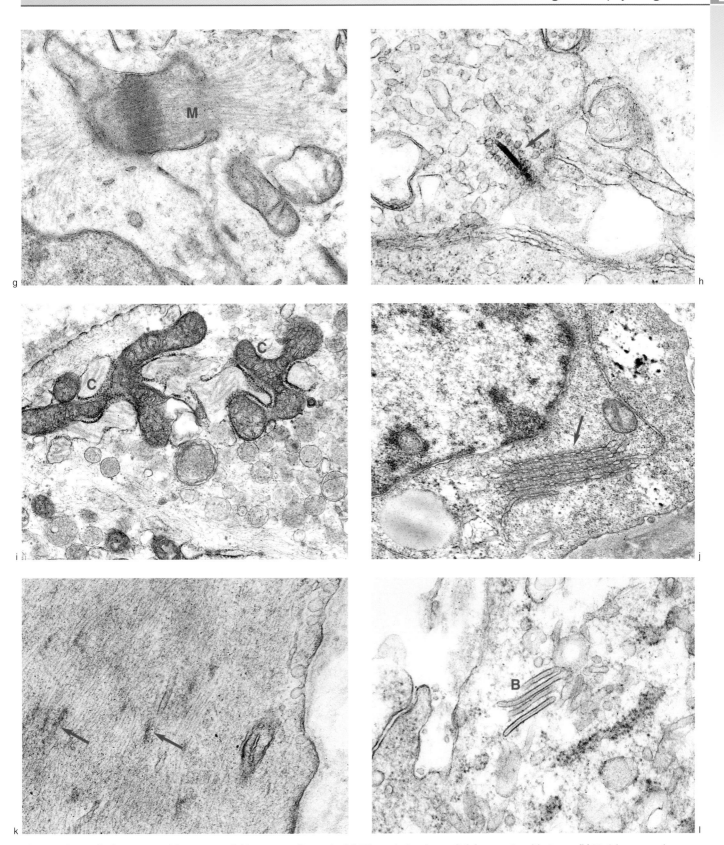

Fig. 2.5 *(Cont'd)* **Ultrastructural features useful in tumour diagnosis. (g)** Microtubular sheave (M) from a pineoblastoma. **(h)** Vesicle crowned lamellus (arrow) from a pineoblastoma. **(i)** Mitochondria/rough endoplasmic reticulum organelle complexes from a chordoma. **(j)** Annulate lamellae (arrow) from a germinoma. **(k)** Filamentous densities (arrows) from a sellar leiomyosarcoma. **(l)** Birbeck granules (B) from a Langerhans cell tumour of the skull vault.

Table 2.10 Useful ultrastructural features in nervous system tumours[19,20]

Structure	Tumour	Notes
Basement membrane (non-vascular)	Choroid plexus tumours	Basal epithelial surfaces
	Myxopapillary ependymoma	Basal, expanded
	Craniopharyngioma	Basal epithelial surfaces
	Schwannoma	Pericellular
	Neurofibroma	Schwann cell related
	Muscle sarcomas	Pericellular
Cilia	Ependymoma	In microrosettes 9 + 2
	Choroid plexus tumours	Apical 9 + 2
	Retinoblastoma	In rosettes 9 + 0
	Pineoblastoma	Photoreceptor diff. 9 + 0
Microvilli	Ependymoma	In microrosettes
	Myxopapillary ependymoma	Apical surfaces
	Subependymoma	Sparse tufts
	Choroid plexus tumours	Apical surfaces
	Chordoma	Between adjacent cells
	Adenocarcinoma	Intracytoplasmic lumina
	Craniopharyngioma	Intracytoplasmic lumina
Desmosomes	Ependymoma	In microrosettes
	Meningioma	Especially meningothelial
	Choroid plexus tumours	At apical surfaces
	Craniopharyngioma	Between cell processes
	Metastatic carcinoma	Especially squamous
	Chordoma	Infrequent
Dense core vesicles	PNETs	Neuroblastic differentiation
	Ganglionic tumours	Neuroblastic differentiation
	Pineocytoma	Neuroblastic differentiation
	Pituitary adenomas	Neurosecretory granules
Synapses/synaptic vesicles	PNETs	Neuroblastic differentiation
	Ganglionic tumours	Neuroblastic differentiation
	Pineocytomas	Neuroblastic differentiation
Annulate lamellae	Retinoblastoma	Photoreceptor differentiation
	Germinoma	Not specific
Vesicle crowned lamellae	Retinoblastoma	Photoreceptor differentiation
	Pineoblastoma	Photoreceptor differentiation
Microtubular sheaves	Retinoblastoma	Photoreceptor differentiation
	Pineoblastoma	Photoreceptor differentiation
Organelle complexes	Chordoma	Mitochondria and RER
Birbeck granules	Langerhans histiocytosis	Constant, specific feature
Filamentous densities	Leiomyosarcoma	Thin filaments, multiple

PNETs, primary neuroectodermal tumours; RER, rough endoplasmic reticulum

Table 2.11 Mixed tumours of the nervous system

Gliosarcoma

Mixed gliomas
Oligoastrocytoma
Anaplastic oligoastrocytoma
Subependymoma/ependymoma
Rarities e.g. ependymoastrocytoma

Ganglioneuronal tumours
Ganglioglioma
Desmoplastic infantile ganglioglioma
Dysembryoplastic neuroepithelial tumour

- Return to the original H & E stained sections and examine them again with no preconceptions. This is especially recommended if subsequent staining with numerous antibody reagents has produced conflicting or confusing results.
- Re-examine the differential diagnosis list and check that no possibilities have been overlooked.
- Show the biopsy informally to a local pathology colleague with some experience of nervous system tumour diagnosis.

- Discuss the clinical, radiological and surgical aspects of the case thoroughly in the light of the biopsy findings. In particular, ascertain how precise or otherwise your diagnostic comment needs to be in order for the clinicians to plan their further management. This is best achieved at a multidisciplinary biopsy review meeting, bringing together the surgeons, radiologists, scans and projected histological images.
- Send the case away for a second opinion by one or more experts in the field. This is the most time consuming option and also carries the risk of receiving conflicting opinions if more than one is sought. However it can be a useful course of action as a last resort or in specialised areas, such as osteoarticular or sarcomatous tumours.

In the end, with some biopsies it may still prove difficult to come to a single, conclusive diagnosis. When this happens, the only course of action is to present the clinicians with as much information as possible, including any second opinions received. Even in the most difficult cases, it is usually possible to conclude with a generic diagnosis and some indication as to the likely behaviour of the tumour, for example 'unusual glial tumour with features suggesting that it is growing rapidly and likely to recur'.

Quality assessment in diagnostic neuropathology

In addition to appropriate quality control measures for immunocytochemistry and other technical considerations there is a recognised need for quality control in diagnostic neuropathology and this is achievable under a number of systems operating in various countries. In the UK there is a National External Quality Assessment Scheme in neuropathology which allows participants to assess their performance in routine diagnosis, based on H & E stained sections in relation to a peer group. This scheme has been operating successfully for a number of years and serves to draw the participants' attention to areas of diagnostic practice which require further interpretation and study. In cases of poor performance a remedial arm has been identified which will allow individuals who have been deemed to perform at a substandard level to undergo further training before re-entering the scheme.

Clinical audit continues to play a major role in hospital practice across the world and it is important that diagnostic surgical neuropathology is involved in audit processes. This can be achieved by stand alone exercises including the investigation of parameters readily identifiable in relation to diagnosis, such as turnaround time, accuracy of intraoperative diagnosis, use of immuno-cytochemistry and ancillary investigative techniques, and the clarity and accuracy of the final report. It is also important to participate in multigroup projects with relevant clinicians in order to ensure that the best quality of diagnostic care is delivered to patients with brain tumours. This is probably best achieved in the setting of a neuro-oncology group comprising neurologists, neuro-radiologists, neurosurgeons, neuropathologists, radio-therapists, oncologists and related staff. Such groups can review and discuss individual cases at particular intervals as well as participate in larger audit projects and clinical trials, in which the importance of adequate neuro-pathological input cannot be overemphasised.

Formulating a diagnostic report

The surgical neuropathology report is the final written document conveying the diagnosis to the clinician and the patient. As such, it should be a carefully constructed and accurate account of what is known and, equally important, what is not known about the submitted specimen. Surgical pathology reports vary in format from institution to institution, but nearly all include:

- patient and specimen identification;
- brief clinical summary;
- macroscopic description;
- microscopic description;
- diagnosis (and comments as appropriate).

From a neuropathological point of view, a few issues deserve special mention in relation to the diagnosis of CNS tumours:

1. *Site*. Because the nervous system is a complex structure, with different subdivisions that have differing functions and different susceptibility to particular neoplasms, it is important not only to designate the overall site of a tumour (brain, spinal cord, meninges, cranial nerve, spinal nerve, peripheral nerve) but also to specify a region, e.g. 'brain (right frontal)' or 'meninges (left frontal convexity)' or 'peripheral nerve (right sciatic)'. Such designations are of great value for future studies, since the behaviour of CNS tumours varies by site, e.g. the different prognosis of a frontal convexity meningioma in comparison to one growing along the sphenoid ridge.
2. *Classification*. This book presents a detailed diagnostic approach to brain tumour classification, that is, assigning an understood name to a tumour biopsy; in this regard, we have been primarily following the most recent WHO consensus. Such classification allows the clinician to predict a certain behaviour and response to therapy for a given lesion. While most pathologists attempt to assign one of the conventional names to a biopsy specimen, it must be stressed that not all tumours fit in well to the WHO classification. It is not uncommon for a lesion, particularly a poorly differentiated neoplasm, to defy exact classification. In such a situation, it makes little sense to attempt to force a lesion into one of the existing entities, because the behaviour of the tumour

may not correspond to that entity. For tumours that do not correspond to the WHO definitions, we encourage a descriptive diagnosis, followed by a note elaborating the findings and the differential diagnosis, accompanied by a dialogue with the neurosurgeon or oncologist caring for the patient. For instance, some malignant gliomas do not fit neatly into the categories of either glioblastoma, anaplastic oligodendroglioma or anaplastic oligoastrocytoma. Such cases may be designated simply as 'malignant glioma (see note)' along with a note describing the differential diagnostic issues and the difficulties of recognising oligodendroglial components in malignant glial tumours.

3. *Tumour grade.* A variety of systems exist for grading CNS tumours,[19] the most widely used of which is the WHO classification. This book has followed, to a large extent, the 2000 WHO recommendations,[20] which incorporate a four-tier grading system (in Roman numerals I to IV) that can be applied to all tumours. Grade I tumours are considered benign in the sense that if they can be resected, they can be cured. As discussed in Chapter 1, not all biologically benign tumours can be resected, particularly those arising deep within the brain, or in the brain stem. Grade IV tumours, at the other end of the spectrum, are highly malignant tumours with a generally poor prognosis. However, some effective therapies exist for some WHO grade IV tumours, for example irradiation and chemotherapy for medulloblastoma.

In practical terms, while all tumours can be assigned a WHO grade, most clinicians only utilise this information in the management of glial tumours, particularly for the astrocytic group of tumours. The vast majority of CNS neoplasms do not strictly require a grade to be appended within a report, since the tumour name in the WHO classification conveys adequate information about the biological behaviour. In practice, most neuropathologists will assign a WHO grade to astrocytomas and other glial neoplasms, but not to most other CNS neoplasms.

In some situations, however, it may be prudent not to grade even astrocytic tumours. Such a situation arises occasionally in the setting of a stereotactic biopsy of a diffuse astrocytic glioma that may not appear representative of what is expected (based on neuroimaging studies). For instance, a biopsy may show scattered infiltrating astrocytoma cells or solid WHO grade II diffuse astrocytoma, whereas the neuroimaging studies demonstrate a ring enhancing mass that strongly suggests a glioblastoma. In such situations, one can omit assigning a definite grade in the diagnosis, and simply discuss some of the issues of sample bias and tumour grading in the accompanying note, using phrases such as 'the histological features described above may not be representative of the tumour as a whole' or 'there is an apparent discrepancy between the neuroradiological and histopathological features in this case, which suggests that the prognosis should remain guarded'.

Other approaches to diagnosis: cytology and autopsy

CSF cytology in brain tumour diagnosis

Cytological examination of CSF is an important tool in the investigation of patients with suspected brain tumours, and can be used for the following purposes:

1. Primary cytopathological diagnosis of a CNS tumour.
2. Staging and the assessment of CSF involvement by a known primary tumour, e.g. medulloblastoma.
3. To monitor the possibility of tumour responses to treatment, or recurrence.
4. Biochemical investigations on the CSF tumour cell 'markers' particularly in germ cell tumours.

The specialised techniques required for CSF diagnosis of CNS tumours are not the primary concern of this book; more detailed information is readily available,[21–23] but the importance of CSF cytology diagnosis is reinforced by the increasing use of immunocytochemical and molecular genetic techniques on CSF samples which are relevant to tumour diagnosis and the investigation of responses to therapy. Descriptions of CSF cytology for the diagnosis of CNS tumours can be found under individual tumour headings in subsequent chapters.

The autopsy in brain tumour diagnosis

Although the emphasis in this volume is appropriately centred on biopsy based diagnosis, the importance of the autopsy in patients with brain tumours should be reinforced, since it allows a unique opportunity to investigate the changes occurring in brain tumours as they spread throughout the CNS and to determine the complications arising from such spread; also to investigate the effects of surgery, irradiation and other forms of treatment, to investigate unexpected clinical complications in individual cases and to study the growth and dissemination of tumours in the CNS and elsewhere in the body.[1,24] When undertaking an autopsy in a patient with a brain tumour, the neuropathologist should particularly bear in mind the need for a thorough investigation of the CNS, including the brain and spinal cord with cranial and peripheral nerves as appropriate. In patients with tumours arising adjacent to the brain and spinal cord, other tissues may be required for diagnosis and the dissection technique should be modified to reflect these needs.[24] The autopsy also allows (where appropriate consent has been obtained) tissue to be obtained for teaching and research purposes and macroscopic examination of the tumour in the CNS permits a particularly informative comparison with neuroimaging studies. Acquisition of relatively large volumes of tumour tissue allows more extensive pathological, immunocytochemical and molecular genetic studies to be performed and the pathologist should also be reminded that it is entirely possible to establish cell cultures from autopsy tissues including the brain and spinal cord tumours.

The autopsy is a particularly important investigation in patients with recurrent tumours, tumours which have pursued an unexpected clinical course and in particular where there has been an unexpected or adverse response to therapy. Autopsy can provide the pathologists, clinicians and relatives with important information which will enable all concerned to widen their understanding of the disease mechanisms operating in individual patients and to place this information in the wider perspective of clinical practice. The autopsy is an important tool for clinical audit and the declining autopsy rates in many countries is an unfortunate reflection on the current resource restrictions which appear to operate in many centres. A detailed protocol for autopsy brain and spinal cord fixation, processing and dissection is beyond the scope of this book; readers are referred to other detailed sources.[1,24]

REFERENCES

1. Esiri MM. Oppenheimer's diagnostic neuropathology. A practical manual. Oxford: Blackwell Science, 1996
2. Morrison CD, Prayson RA. Immunohistochemsitry in the diagnosis of neoplasms of the central nervous system. Semin Diagn Pathol, 2000; 17:204–215
3. McKeever PE, Blaivas M, Nelson JS. Tumors: applications of light microscopic methods. In: Garcia JH, Budka H, McKeever PE et al., eds. Neuropathology: the diagnostic approach. Philadelphia: Mosby, 1997, pp 31–95
4. McKeever PE. Insights about brain tumours gained through immunohistochemical and in situ hybridisation of nuclear and phenotypic markers. J Histochem Cytochem, 1998; 46:585–594
5. Cáccamo DV, Rubinstein LJ. Tumors: applications of immunocytochemical methods. In Garcia JH, Budka H, McKeever PE et al., eds. Neuropathology: the diagnostic approach. Philadelphia: Mosby, 1997, pp 193–218
6. Kleinman GM, Zagzag D, Miller DC. Diagnostic use of immunohistochemistry in neuropathology. Neurosurg Clin N Am, 1994; 5:97–126
7. Hoyt JW, Gown AM, Kim DK et al. Analysis of proliferative grade in glial neoplasms using antibodies to the Ki-67 defined antigen and PCNA in formalin fixed, deparaffinized tissues. J Neurooncol, 1995; 24:163–169
8. Mikhail AA, Yamini B, McKeever PE et al. MIB-1 proliferation index predicts survival among patients with low grade astrocytoma. Lab Invest, 1996; 74:141A
9. Montine TJ, Vandersteenhoven JJ, Aguzzi A et al. Prognostic significance of Ki-67 proliferation index in supratentorial fibrillary astrocytic neoplasms. Neurosurgery, 1994; 34:674–678
10. Raghavan R, Steart P, Weller RO. Cell proliferation patterns in the diagnosis of astrocytomas, anaplastic astrocytomas, and glioblastoma multiforme: a Ki-67 study. Neuropathol Appl Neurobiol, 1990; 16:123–133
11. Revesz T, Alsanjari N, Darling JL et al. Proliferating cell nuclear antigen (PCNA): expression in samples of human astrocytic gliomas. Neuropathol Appl Neurobiol, 1993; 19:152–158
12. Burns KL, Ueki K, Jhung SL, Koh J, Louis DN. Molecular genetic correlates of p16, cdk4 and pRb immunohistochemistry in glioblastomas. J Neuropathol Exp Neurol 1998; 57:122–130
13. Simmons ML, Lamborn KR, Takahashi M et al. Analysis of complex relationships between age, p53, epidermal growth factor receptor, and survival in glioblastoma patients. Cancer Res 2001; 61:1122–1128
14. Pomeroy SL, Tamayo P, Gaasenbeek M et al. Gene expression-based classification and outcome prediction of central nervous system embryonal tumours. Nature 2002; 415:436–442
15. Shri S-R, Cote RJ, Taylor CR. Antigen retrieval immunohistochemistry: past, present, and future. J Histochem Cytochem, 1997; 45:327–343
16. Louis DN, Cavanee WK. Molecular biology of central nervous system tumours. In DeVita VT, Hellman S, Rosenberg SA, eds. Cancer: principles and practice of oncology, 6th edn. Philadelphia: Lippincott-Raven, 2001
17. Louis DN, Holland EC, Cairncross JG. Glioma classification: a molecular reappraisal. Am J Pathol 2001; 159:779–786
18. Cairncross JG, Ueki K, Zlatescu MC et al. Specific genetic predictors of chemotherapeutic response and survival in patients with anaplastic oligodendrogliomas. J Natl Cancer Inst, 1998; 7:1473–1479
19. Ino Y, Betensky RA, Zlatescu MC et al. Molecular subtypes of anaplastic oligodendroglioma: implications for patient management at diagnosis. Clin Cancer Res 2001; 7:839–845
20. Kleihues P, Cavenee WK (eds). World Health Organisation classification of tumours. Tumours of the nervous system. Pathology & genetics. Lyons: IARC Press, 2000
21. MacKenzie JM. Malignant meningitis: a rational approach to cerebrospinal fluid cytology. J Clin Pathol, 1996; 49:497–499
22. Oschmann P, Kaps M, Volker J et al. Meningeal carcinomatosis: CSF cytology, imunohistochemistry and biochemical tumor markers. Acta Neurol Scand, 1994; 89:395–399
23. Bigner SH, Johnston WW. Cytopathology of the central nervous system. Chicago: ASCP Press, 1994
24. Adams JH, Graham DI. An introduction to neuropathology, 2nd edn. Edinburgh: Churchill Livingstone, 1994

3   Intraoperative diagnosis

Intraoperative diagnosis in general pathology is dependent primarily on the use of cryostat section histology and touch imprint cytology preparations, but in the investigation of central nervous system (CNS) neoplasms, smear cytology has been used in numerous centres for many years with great success for intraoperative diagnosis.[1–4] Its use reflects the generally soft consistency and texture of most intrinsic CNS tumours, which facilitates the preparation of smears. Cryostat sections are also used for the intraoperative diagnosis of CNS tumours, and are particularly useful for firm or rubbery lesions which are unsuitable for smear cytology preparations.[1–5] This chapter gives an overview of the techniques and principles used in the intraoperative diagnosis of CNS tumours. It will therefore be of interest primarily to trainees, general histopathologists and cytologists, and neurosurgeons. This general guidance is supplemented by detailed descriptions relating to intraoperative diagnosis of individual tumour entities in subsequent chapters. A general approach to the histological diagnosis of nervous system tumours is outlined in Chapter 2.

Criteria for requesting an intraoperative diagnosis

The intraoperative diagnosis of CNS tumours forms a large part of the workload in most neuropathology laboratories. Whilst individual working arrangements between neurosurgeons and neuropathologists will inevitably vary from one centre to another, it is possible to identify major criteria for requesting an intraoperative neuropathological diagnosis:

1. Definitive neurosurgical management will be influenced by the diagnosis during the neurosurgical procedure.
2. When an unexpected lesion is encountered during surgery, or when the appearances of the lesion visualised during surgery suggest an alternative to the clinical and/or neuroradiological diagnosis.
3. The main aim of the neurosurgical procedure is to obtain a tissue-based diagnosis.
4. The neurosurgeon aims to perform a radical excision of the tumour, which requires intraoperative assessment of the resection margins.

These criteria are not exclusive, but it is not uncommon for a request for intraoperative diagnosis to be made in other circumstances where the benefits to the patient or neurosurgeon of a precise diagnosis during the surgical procedure are not immediately apparent. This can be avoided by a clear discussion between the neurosurgeon and the neuropathologist in advance of the surgical procedure, when all the relevant information is available on the case in question.

Ideally, it should be possible for the neurosurgeon to discuss the cases in which intraoperative diagnosis may be requested with the neuropathologist in advance of the procedure. This cannot always be achieved, but there is a need to discuss particularly difficult or complicated cases, especially if previous surgery has been performed or if the patient has received chemotherapy or radiation therapy for a previous tumour. This advance warning is particularly helpful when an earlier biopsy has been examined, since it allows review of the relevant sections prior to the day of the neurosurgical procedure. It is also helpful for the neuropathologist to have a full knowledge of the neuroradiological features of the case in question; an informed discussion on the suitability of targets for stereotactic biopsy may then be possible.

Laboratory facilities for intraoperative diagnosis

The laboratory used for the intraoperative diagnosis of neurosurgical specimens should be located as close to the operating theatre as possible, since this facilitates rapid transport of specimens and allows clear communication between the neuropathologist and the neurosurgeon. This is particularly helpful if there is difficulty in interpreting the specimens, so the scans can be reviewed or additional tissue specimens submitted. In some departments, there is a satellite laboratory situated adjacent to the neurosurgical operating theatre; such a laboratory need not be full of expensive equipment, since the smear technique is cheap, fast and not dependent on apparatus other than a safety hood in which to examine the unfixed tissue. When unfixed material has been submitted for examination, it is necessary to use appropriate facilities to ensure that existing health and safety measures are fulfilled. In the UK, unfixed tissue should be examined in a Class 1 hood with protective clothing and gloves employed by anyone handling the material. This is particularly important in brain tumour biopsies, since non-neoplastic infective lesions are occasionally biopsied with an initial clinical diagnosis of the tumour. Furthermore, under certain circumstances brain tumours may be accompanied by infective processes, e.g. cerebral lymphomas arising in immunocompromised patients.[6]

The laboratory equipment therefore required is:

1. A ventilated safety hood which fulfils local health and safety guidelines, with adequate space for tissue handling, fixation and staining.
2. A microscope, preferably with a teaching head.
3. A cryostat, if cryostat microtomy is to be performed (otherwise this can be performed in the main neuropathology laboratory).
4. Benchspace and sink for slide staining and mounting.

Macroscopic inspection and tissue sampling

On receipt of a biopsy or resection specimen in the neuropathology laboratory, the details on the laboratory request form and specimen container should be checked to ensure that they correspond. The specimen should then undergo careful macroscopic examination in order to select appropriate tissue for intraoperative diagnosis. Specimens which arrive in multiple containers (for example stereotactic biopsies) should be consecutively numbered and checked in order that they correspond to the stated details on the request form, particularly with respect to the biopsy sites or targets. Each specimen should be examined and the dimensions of the tissue specimen recorded along with any distinguishing macroscopic features. The small amount of tissue available in stereotactic biopsy specimens places a high priority on the efficient use of this material, particularly if intraoperative diagnosis is requested or if material is to be stored for molecular biological studies.

If intraoperative diagnosis is requested on a stereotactic biopsy specimen, it is suggested that the smear technique is used in the first instance. This has the advantage over cryostat section examination in that less material is used (1–2 mm² of tissue is sufficient for an adequate smear preparation); the relative advantages and drawbacks of smear preparations and cryostat sections for intraoperative diagnosis are listed in Table 3.1. Tissue samples for smear preparations may be taken from either end of the stereotactic biopsy core, provided that viable tissue is present. For intraoperative diagnosis it is recommended that frankly necrotic tissue is avoided; diagnostic yield is greater when tissue adjacent to an area

Table 3.1 Comparison of smear preparations and cryostat sections[1]

Smears	Cryostat sections
Advantages	
No special equipment needed	Applicable to soft and firm lesions
Quick and easy to prepare	Tissue architecture readily apparent
Use very little tissue	Widely used for non-CNS lesions
Multiple areas can readily be sampled	More tissue is sampled than in a smear
A range of stains can be used	A range of stains can be used
Good quality cytology	Multiple levels can be cut and examined
Disadvantages	
Only applicable to soft lesions	Require special equipment
Tissue architecture not apparent	Take time to prepare
Not widely used for non-CNS lesions	Dependent on technical expertise

of necrosis is inspected rather than the necrotic tissue itself. Similarly, tissue that is excessively haemorrhagic should if at all possible be avoided, since widespread haemorrhage can mask the cytological features of tumour cells, particularly in smear preparations.

With larger resection specimens, multiple regions of the lesion can be examined. Cerebral tissue infiltrated by a glial neoplasm may be abnormally tough or rubbery in consistency and this can occasionally produce difficulties in the preparation of satisfactory smears. With experience, it is usually possible to identify other softer areas of the tumour which are more amenable to the process of smear preparation; alternatively, if the lesion is excessively firm in consistency then cryostat sections can be used for intraoperative diagnosis. If the material is largely calcified (for example in a spinal cord meningioma) then neither smear preparations nor cryostat sections may be possible and imprint preparations can be made which will often allow a diagnosis based on tumour cell cytology.

Smear preparations

Making and staining the smears

After inspection of the specimen for intraoperative diagnosis, a 1–2 mm² portion of tissue is dissected with a scalpel and placed at one end of a clean glass slide which is labelled appropriately (Fig. 3.1). The smear preparation is made by compressing the tissue with a second slide (Fig. 3.2) and drawing the second slide quickly along the surface of the first slide in order to produce a relatively uniform tissue layer (Fig. 3.3). Care is required in gauging the amount of pressure required to do this for most tumours; undue pressure will cause one or both slides to break, and can result in crush artefact in the cytology (Fig. 3.4). Insufficient pressure will not allow the tumour cells to form an adequate monolayer for cytological inspection and the resulting preparation will be too thick to be diagnostically useful (Fig 3.5).

In making the smear preparations, the neuropathologist should study the distribution of tissue in the smear before fixation as this can often give an indication as to whether or not tumour tissue is present, since normal brain tends to spread out in a uniform monolayer. Some tumours, particularly pituitary adenomas, also spread out readily, but most intrinsic neoplasms, metastases and meningiomas spread out in an irregular aggregated pattern. Other tumours, such as Schwannomas and haemangioblastomas may be difficult to smear at all; these are best investigated by cryostat section histology. Calcification can be detected as a gritty sensation between the slides whilst the smear is being prepared.

The smear preparations should be rapidly fixed without the need to air dry the specimen. A range of fixatives can be used for smear prepartions (Table 3.2). Two

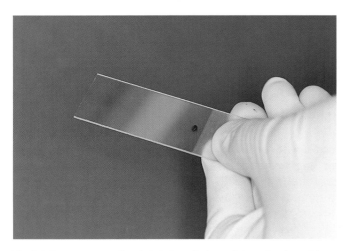

Fig. 3.1 **Smear preparation 1**. A 1–2 mm² piece of tissue is selected for a smear preparation and placed on one end of a clean glass slide.

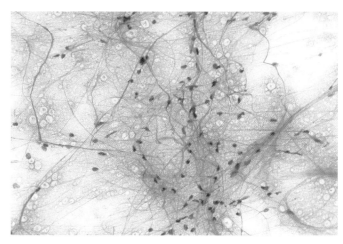

Fig. 3.4 **Crush artefact**. Excess pressure during the production of a smear preparation results in crush artefact, where nuclear detail is obscured, staining is impaired and cytoplasm is distorted and elongated into thread-like structures. H & E.

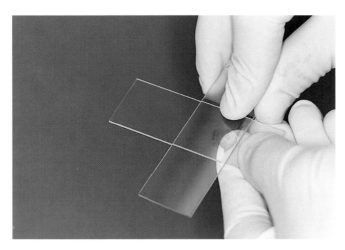

Fig. 3.2 **Smear preparation 2**. The smear preparation is made by compressing the tissue sample by a second slide, ensuring that the smeared tissue spreads across the base of the slide.

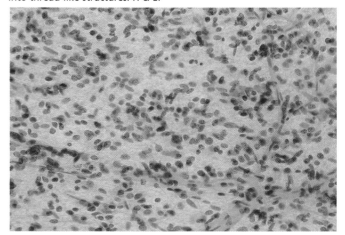

Fig. 3.5 **Unsatisfactory smear**. Insufficient pressure in the production of a smear will result in a tissue layer which is too thick, with nuclei present at multiple levels and both nuclear and cytological detail obscured. H & E.

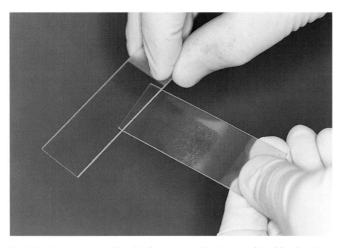

Fig. 3.3 **Smear preparation 3**. The preparation is completed by drawing the second slide across the surface of the first slide with uniform pressure, taking care to produce an even layer of tissue.

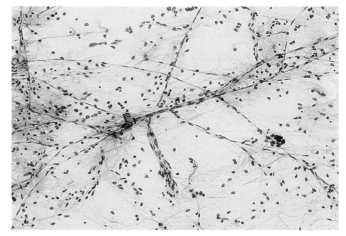

Fig. 3.6 **Satisfactory smear**. A good smear preparation will contain blood vessels and cells which have spread out in a monolayer, to facilitate analysis of cytological and nuclear detail, without excess crush artefact. Toluidine blue.

Table 3.2 Fixation and staining techniques for smear preparations

Smear preparations are best fixed immediately after preparation in:
a. 95% alcohol for 1 min, or
b. 95% alcohol with a small quantity of acetic acid for 1 min is advantageous if a haematoxylin and eosin stain is to be used, or
c. 50% alcohol/50% ether (this mixture is potentially explosive on storage)

A variety of staining techniques may be used, including methylene blue, Papanicolaou, and haematoxylin/toluidine blue. The two most popular methods are:

1. Toluidine blue:
a. After fixation, rinse slides gently in water
b. Stain with 1% aqueous toluidine blue for 60–90 s
c. Rinse slides gently in water
d. Dehydrate rapidly through graded alcohols
e. Clear in xylene (or alternative)
f. Mount in DPX or another synthetic medium

2. Haematoxylin and eosin
a. Rinse slides gently in water
b. Stain in haematoxylin (e.g. Harris's haematoxylin) for 60 s
c. Rinse slides gently in water
d. Differentiate in acid alcohol (1% hydrochloric acid in 70% alcohol) for 10–15 s
e. Rinse slides gently in tap water
f. Blue in Scott's tap water substitute for 10–15 s
g. Rinse slides gently in water
h. Counterstain with 5% eosion for 30 s
i. Rinse slides gently in water
j. Fix eosin in tap water with 5–10 ml of potassium alum added for 10 s
k. Dehydrate rapidly through graded alcohols
l. Clear in xylene (or alternative)
m. Mount in DPX or another synthetic medium.

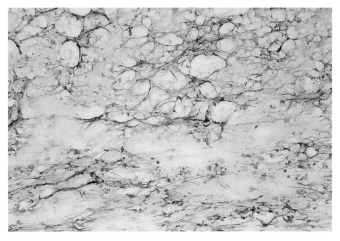

Fig. 3.7 **Smear immunocytochemistry**. Immunocytochemistry for glial fibrillary acidic protein in an astrocytoma gives strong staining of the cytoplasm of the tumour cells and their cell processes.

staining methods have been found to be particularly useful for smear preparations: toluidine blue and haematoxylin and eosin (H & E). The former is easier and quicker to produce and shows excellent nuclear detail (Fig. 3.6); the latter is slightly more complex and takes longer to produce adequate differentiation, but has the advantages of allowing a direct comparison with cryostat sections and providing better cytological detail than toluidine blue. It is also possible to employ a much wider range of stains on smear preparations, including immunocytochemistry (Fig. 3.7)[7–9] and even molecular genetic techniques such as fluorescent in situ hybridisation.[4–11] However, these techniques are more suited towards research purposes rather than intraoperative diagnosis.

During the staining procedure it is important to handle the specimens gently, particularly those with a relatively thick smear on the glass slide, as these tend to fragment and dislodge from the specimen when the slide is being rinsed in water. After staining, the specimen should be dehydrated, cleared and mounted using a suitable synthetic medium. The entire process of smear preparation, staining and mounting can be accomplished within 5–10 min depending on the numbers of specimens to be stained and the staining techniques employed. After

inspection of the smears, the diagnosis should be conveyed to the neurosurgeon as soon as possible, preferably in the form of a written record, a copy of which should be kept within the laboratory for comparison with the final paraffin section diagnosis.

Interpretation of smear preparations

The use of the smear technique for intraoperative diagnosis provides a rapid and efficient means of pathological assessment which, in experienced hands, is capable of obtaining a high degree of diagnostic accuracy.[2,5,12–19] Its use is therefore strongly commended for this purpose; the increasing use of stereotaxy for brain tumour diagnosis will ensure the continuing need for this technique. Before attempting to use the smear technique for intraoperative diagnosis it is essential to become acquainted with the normal cytology of the CNS and smear preparations. The best way of doing this is to use unfixed autopsy tissue to allow a widespread sampling of different anatomical regions which are likely to be encountered in surgical neuropathology. In practice, this should comprise the cerebral cortex, white matter, subcortical grey matter regions, cerebellar cortex, brain stem and spinal cord. Specialised tissues, including choroid plexus and arachnoid granulations should also be studied since these can be misinterpreted by the inexperienced as neoplastic tissue (Table 3.3). The importance of this familiarity cannot be overemphasised, as it is all too common to encounter the diagnosis of lymphoma or metastatic small cell carcinoma by the inexperienced when confronted with a smear preparation that contains normal cerebellar granular neurons, or the diagnosis of choroid plexus papilloma when a portion of the normal choroid plexus has been included in the smear preparations. The descriptions of smear preparations listed below are not

Table 3.3 Common errors in the interpretation of normal cytological features in smears[1,2]

Normal feature	Mistaken interpretation
Cerebral cortex	Ganglion cell tumour
Cerebellar cortex	Metastatic small cell carcinoma
	Lymphoma
	Medulloblastoma
Choroid plexus	Choroid plexus papilloma
	Metastatic papillary carcinoma
Ependymal cells	Metastatic carcinoma
Anterior pituitary cells	Pituitary adenoma
Arachnoidal cells	Meningioma
Pineocytes	Pineocytoma

comprehensive, and for further information and illustrations on this important topic, specialised texts should be consulted[1,2] in addition to subsequent chapters.

Normal cytological appearances

1. Cerebral cortex – most cerebral cortical biopsies contain large neurons, with pyramidal cells easily identified by their distinctive size and abundant dendritic branches. However, small compact neurons are usually included and these should be distinguished from small glial cells (including oligodendrocytes) which lack dendritic branches (Fig. 3.8). In elderly patients the larger neurons can contain lipofuscin, which appears as a green/blue pigment in toluidine blue stained smears. Glial cells are represented by oligodendrocytes with small uniform darkly staining nuclei and scanty cytoplasm, whilst astrocytes tend to have a larger ovoid nucleus with speckled chromatin and variable cytoplasm. Microglial cells are often inconspicuous but thin walled branching capillaries are usually present.
2. White matter – the cytological features of normal white matter in smear preparations comprise nuclei of oligodendrocytes and astrocytes with occasional microglia and thin walled branching capillaries. The background neuropil tends to stain more intensely than in the grey matter because of the more abundant myelinated fibres.
3. Deep cerebral grey matter – smears taken from the basal ganglia, thalamus and hypothalamus show similar appearances to the cerebral cortex but with a much more pronounced variability in the size and shape of neurons which can include characteristic cell populations, e.g. from the substantia nigra. The larger neurons in the basal ganglia also contain abundant lipofuscin in elderly patients and there can be an admixture of white matter elements with a more prominent staining of the neuropil.
4. Cerebellar cortex – smear preparations of the cerebellar cortex show a characteristic population of small rounded uniform intensely staining nuclei of normal granule cells with the much larger Purkinje cells being a prominent and readily identifiable feature with their unique shape and branching dendritic tree (Fig. 3.9). Molecular layer constituents, comprising small neurons with relatively few oligodendrocyte and astrocyte nuclei, may also be identified; molecular layer capillaries are thin walled and usually less conspicuous than in the cerebral cortex.
5. Brain stem and spinal cord – depending on the area sampled, the smear preparations from these sites will contain white matter and grey matter elements in an admixture which sometimes resembles smears taken from the region of the basal ganglia.
6. Choroid plexus – this tissue is occasionally included in smear preparations of lesions in the vicinity of the ventricular system. The epithelial cells in normal choroid plexus are relatively uniform in size and shape, often densely cohesive around a core of thick fibrovascular tissue which does not easily smear. The cohesive nature of the epithelial cells in smear preparations often give the appearance of the epithelial layer being greater than one cell in thickness; this should not be misinterpreted as indicative of a choroid plexus neoplasm.
7. Ependymal cells – these are also encountered in biopsies from lesions in the vicinity of the ventricular system. Unlike choroid plexus, ependymal cells tend to smear out in a sheet of cells which bear no relationship to a fibrovascular stroma. These cells often appear epithelial in nature with compact rounded uniform nuclei.
8. Arachnoidal cells – in biopsies of superficially sited lesions, or if in the trajectory path of a needle passing into the underlying brain, arachnoidal cells can be incorporated into the smear preparations and appear as rounded or whorled collections of polygonal cells which have ill-defined cytoplasmic boundaries and uniform rounded nuclei. These may be mistaken for fragments of a meningioma, particularly if psammoma bodies are present.

Basic diagnostic principles

The differential diagnosis of smear cytology can be reduced to the consideration of the following simple questions:

1. Is the cytology normal?
2. If the cytology is abnormal, does it show:
   a. reactive changes only?; or
   b. tumour cells (and if so, which type)?

It is not uncommon for both reactive changes and tumour cells to be present in a single smear preparation, e.g. in a

Fig. 3.8 **Cerebral cortex**. A smear preparation containing cerebral cortical tissue shows small finely branching capillaries with the large nuclei of pyramidal neurons (centre). Smaller neuronal and glial cell nuclei are also present. H & E.

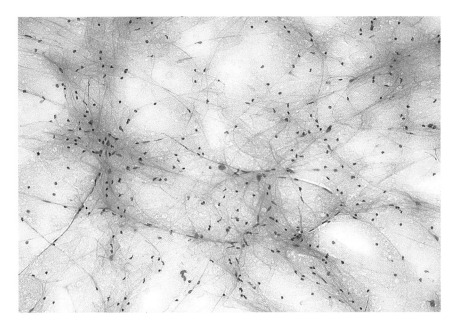

Fig. 3.9 **Cerebellar cortex**. A smear preparation from the cerebellar cortex contains occasional large Purkinje cells (centre) with the nuclei of small granule layer neurones, which are sometimes aggregated in clusters. H & E.

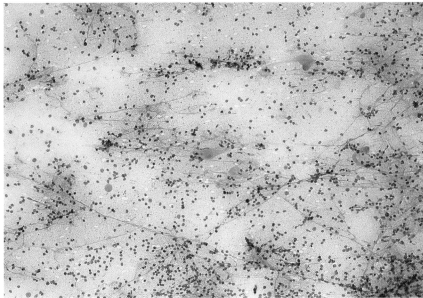

necrotic neoplasm, or at the infiltrating edge of a glioma. There is no substitute for personal experience of the wide range of reactive and neoplastic conditions that may be identified on smear cytology. The commoner of these are considered in brief detail below.

Reactive changes in smear preparations

The CNS exhibits only a limited number of reactions to a wide variety of insults and consequently the cytological features of reactive changes can be identified under a wide variety of circumstances and sites. The severity of these changes is obviously extremely variable, but at their most pronounced can be mistaken even by experienced pathologists for neoplastic lesions[1,13] (Table 3.4).

The most common reactive change occurring in the CNS is *astrocytosis*, which is evident in smear preparations as increased numbers of hypertrophied astrocytes containing abundant cytoplasm (Fig. 3.10), usually with an eccentric nucleus and a finely stippled chromatin pattern. The cytoplasm characteristically extends into fine fibrillary processes (Fig. 3.11). *Reactive microglia* can be identified as rod cells in smear preparations, with characteristically elongated nuclei and relatively scanty cytoplasm, but under conditions of established tissue damage they can assume the features of *phagocytic macrophages* with abundant cytoplasm and an eccentric nucleus (Fig. 3.12). Occasional *mitotic figures* may be identified in reactive astrocytes and microglia and should not be taken as evidence of malignancy.

Table 3.4 Common errors in the interpretation of reactive changes in smears[1,2]

Reactive change	Mistaken interpretation
Astrocytosis	Astrocytoma
Infarction	Glioblastoma
Perivascular lymphocytic cuffing	Lymphoma
Acute inflammation, abscess	Glioblastoma
Capillary proliferation	Haemangioblastoma Glioblastoma
Arachnoiditis	Meningioma
Recent haemorrhage	Glioblastoma Vascular malformation
Haemosiderin in macrophages	Malignant melanoma

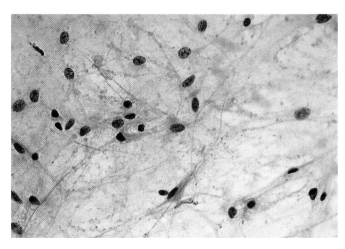

Fig. 3.11 **Astrocytes**. Reactive astrocytes contain relatively uniform oval nuclei with finely stippled chromatin. The pale staining cytoplasm has numerous fine branches. H & E.

Reactive conditions in the CNS are often associated with *oedema*, which alters the staining of the neuropil, imparting a faint metachromatic property in a toluidine blue stain. Capillary proliferation is a feature of *cerebral infarction*, which can be accompanied by polymorph infiltration into the area of tissue damage, later followed by macrophages, which will exhibit a characteristic foamy cytology once myelin has been broken down into neutral lipids and phagocytosed in a maturing infarct (Fig. 3.12). Rod shaped microglial nuclei are often present in cerebral infarcts and the overall cytology is quite markedly heterogenous, since reactive astrocytes are also present in established lesions.

Glomeruloid capillary loops, characteristic of malignant gliomas are not a characteristic feature in reactive conditions, although the vascular changes occurring in *vascular malformations* can occasionally be mistaken for neoplastic vascular proliferation. Evidence of previous haemorrhage in these lesions can be detected by the presence of haemoglobin breakdown products (haemosiderin, haematoidin) in macrophages.

Inflammatory conditions affecting the CNS are characterised by acute or chronic inflammatory cells as one would expect. Acute inflammatory cells (mainly neutrophil polymorphs) are most often seen in cerebral abscesses or cerebritis, but can occur in the early stages of cerebral infarction and in tumour necrosis.

Cerebral abscesses are accompanied by a characteristic fibrovascular reaction and the firm abscess capsule can be difficult to smear. A marked astrocytic response occurs in the oedematous brain around cerebral abscesses and this can occasionally mimic tumour, particularly if an area of vascular proliferation is included in the smear preparations. Acute abscesses are seldom resected (as they lack a well formed capsule), but evidence of cerebritis can

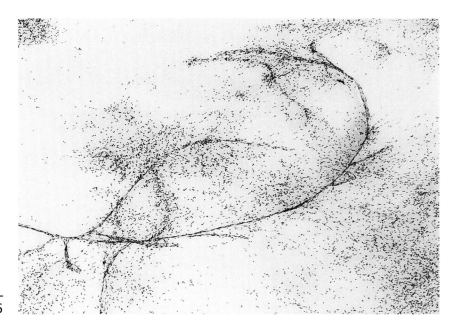

Fig. 3.10 **Astrocytosis**. Astrocytosis in smear preparations comprises increased numbers of astrocytic cell nuclei, often aggregated around capillaries but spreading in a monolayer with a faintly-staining gliofibrillary matrix adjacent to the blood vessel. Toluidine blue.

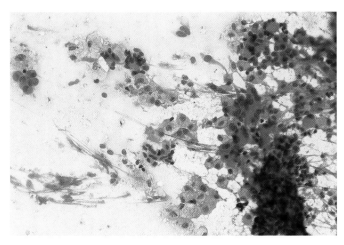

Fig. 3.12 **Macrophages**. Macrophages identified at the edge of an infarct contain abundant foamy cytoplasm, with a uniform rounded nucleus. Reactive astrocytes (with more intensely eosinophilic cytoplasm) are also present. H & E.

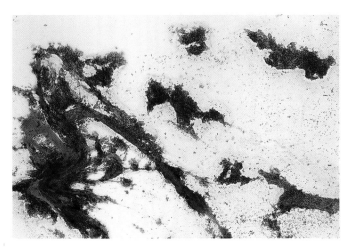

Fig. 3.13 **Necrosis.** Necrosis in a metastatic carcinoma, with intensely eosinophilic necrotic blood vessels and cells (left) adjacent to which are clusters of viable tumour cells. H & E.

Table 3.5 Common errors in the interpretation of artefacts in smears[1,2]

Artefact	Mistaken interpretation
Crush artefact	Fibrillary astrocytoma
Thick smear	Malignant glioma
Bone dust	Calcospherites
Starch powder	Psammoma bodies
Drying artefact (cellular)	Necrosis
Drying artefact (nuclear)	Mitotic or apoptotic figures
Haemostatic sponge	Calcification

detected. The tissue surrounding the abscess capsule is gliotic and in smears contains numerous hypertrophied astrocytes, microglia and chronic inflammatory cells; the last-mentioned may be particularly conspicuous around blood vessels.

Chronic inflammatory conditions in the CNS, including multiple sclerosis, are characterised by perivascular lymphocytic cuffing, which is well demonstrated using the smear technique. The perivascular cells are small T-lymphocytes which exhibit a uniform nuclear profile and scanty cytoplasm. These cells usually extend into the neuropil, which is usually hypercellular and contains reactive astrocytes and microglia. In certain infective conditions, numerous macrophages may also be present; these can occasionally contain organisms (as in cryptococcal infections) or fuse to form multinucleate giant cells, for example in human immunodeficiency virus (HIV) infection or tuberculosis (neither of which should normally be subject to smear examination if the diagnosis is suspected in advance).

Haemorrhage is a common finding in neurosurgical biopsies often relating to the biopsy procedure itself but is often a characteristic feature of malignant gliomas, metastatic tumours and a wide range of vascular malformations and vasculitic conditions affecting the CNS. Acute haemorrhage is readily identified but chronic haemorrhage can also be recognised by the presence of numerous haemosiderin-laden macrophages.

Necrosis is a characteristic feature of many pathological conditions, the most relevant of which is tumour associated necrosis in glioblastomas, metastatic carcinoma and other malignant brain tumours. Occasionally, stereotactic biopsies will contain tissue which is totally necrotic. Such material is unsuitable for a definitive diagnosis but it should be recalled that the 'ghost' cytological features will depend on the underlying lesion; in particular, the gliofibrillary background of malignant glial tumours and the extensive network of hyperplastic endothelium is usually identifiable and careful inspection can occasionally identify small clusters of viable tumour cells adjacent to the larger blood vessels (Fig. 3.13). However, under these circumstances diagnosis should be reserved until all the available material has been subjected to examination on paraffin sections.

Artefacts can arise at several stages in the preparation and staining of smears, most of which are easily recognised. If severe, however, they can hinder diagnosis by producing distortions in the cytological features. The commonest artefacts and their causes are listed in Table 3.5.

CNS neoplasms

The smear cytology of individual CNS tumours is described in detail in subsequent chapters, but the following approach will help identify key features of diagnostic significance:

be identified in smears by the presence of numerous neutrophil polymorphs. Chronic abscesses contain pus, which appears as necrotic material containing numerous degenerate polymorphs and in which bacteria may be

1. *Check the clinical details,* particularly the site of the lesion and the neuroradiological findings.
2. *Inspect the pattern of the smear preparation* on the glass slide. Most primary and secondary CNS tumours have an irregular pattern of aggregation, but some tumours, including oligodendrogliomas and pituitary adenomas, will form a smooth uniform layer on the slide.
3. *Study the pattern of the blood vessels* in the tumour at low magnification. Malignant glial tumours have numerous large thick walled vessels, with glomeruloid loops present in glioblastomas (Fig. 3.14). Astrocytomas have much finer vessels, while oligodendrogliomas have delicately branching capillaries.
4. *Study the relationship of the cells to the blood vessels* at medium magnification. Most gliomas contain tumour cells which are closely cohesive to blood vessels, sometimes with a marked perivascular orientation, as in ependymomas (Fig. 3.15). Non-glial tumours often lack this feature.
5. *Study the relationships of the cells to each other.* Metastatic carcinomas contain irregular clusters of cells (Fig. 3.16), whereas in glial tumours (Fig. 3.17) and lymphomas (Fig. 3.18) a monolayer of non-cohesive tumour cells is usually present.
6. *Study the nuclear and cytological features of the cells* at high magnification. Is the population of cells uniform, or is there evidence of nuclear pleomorphism and cellular atypia (Fig. 3.19)? The presence of specialised features, e.g. astrocytic processes, a gliofibrillary matrix in glioma, cellular whorls and psammoma bodies in meningiomas, papillary structures in a choroid plexus papilloma, are key diagnostic features (Fig. 3.20).
7. *Is there any evidence of necrosis or mitotic activity?* Necrosis is common in glioblastomas and metastatic carcinomas (Fig. 3.21), but should not be confused with cerebral infarction or active demyelination. Mitotic activity is not confined to CNS neoplasms, but may also be encountered in populations of reactive astrocytes and microglia, and in proliferating capillary endothelium at the edge of an infarct.
8. *Review the morphological features in relation to the clinical diagnosis.* Convey the diagnosis in writing and preferably also in person to the neurosurgeon. Check that you are speaking about the correct patient before giving a verbal report through the operating theatre door, and also that the patient is anaesthetised, not just sedated. If necessary discuss the need for additional material or specialised investigations. In difficult cases do not be tempted to guess at specific diagnoses where you are not sure, simply give as much information as you can, i.e. 'tumour, probably of glial origin'. Consider the need for a cryostat section if

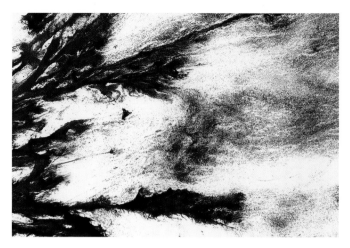

Fig. 3.14 **Endothelium.** Vascular endothelial proliferation is a prominent feature in glioblastomas (left), with numerous thick walled blood vessels which stain intensely and a population of tumour cells which spreads away from the abnormal vessel. Toluidine blue.

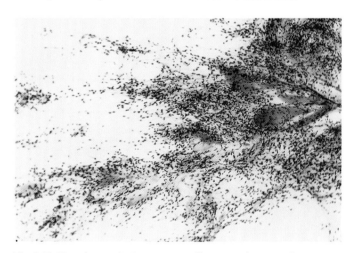

Fig. 3.15 **Metachromasia.** In a myxopapillary ependymoma, the tumour cells are closely adherent to blood vessels which contain large quantities of metachromatic mucinous material (purple). Toluidine blue.

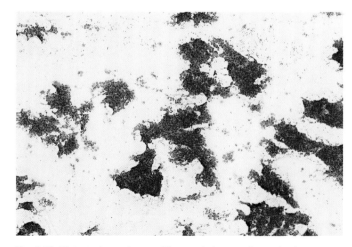

Fig. 3.16 **Metastatic carcinoma.** Metastatic large cell anaplastic bronchial carcinoma, with large aggregates of densely cohesive tumour cells. There is little relationship to blood vessels. H & E.

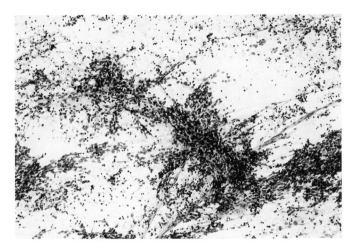

Fig. 3.17 **Anaplastic astrocytoma.** In an anaplastic astrocytoma, the tumour cells surround finely branching capillaries, and spread out in a monolayer, which exhibits a layer of pleomorphic nuclei. Toluidine blue.

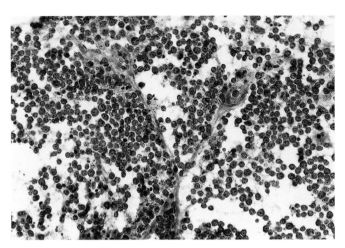

Fig. 3.18 **Primary CNS lymphoma.** A population of small non-cohesive tumour cells which form a monolayer around the irregularly thickened capillaries, and spread out in a uniform sheet of cells. Toluidine blue.

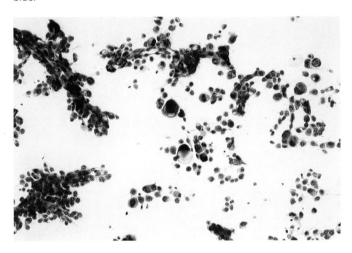

Fig. 3.19 **Cytological atypia.** Marked cytological atypia in a smear preparation from a metastatic adenocarcinoma, which contains large vacuolated cells with marked nuclear pleomorphism. Toluidine blue.

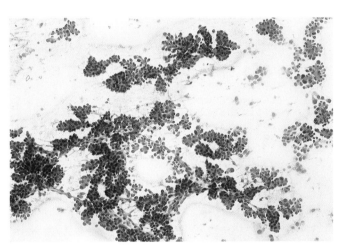

Fig. 3.20 **Choroid plexus papilloma.** A choroid plexus papilloma exhibits a characteristic papillary structure, with rounded aggregates of relatively uniform cells with a prominent apical nucleus. H & E.

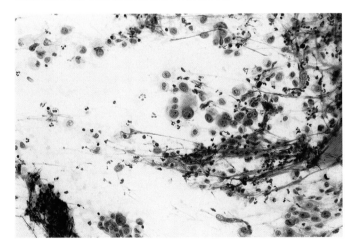

Fig. 3.21 **Incipient necrosis.** Incipient necrosis in a metastatic carcinoma, characterised by a neutrophil polymorph infiltrate. The nuclei of polymorphs are scattered throughout the smear preparation, and the blood vessels appear necrotic. Toluidine blue.

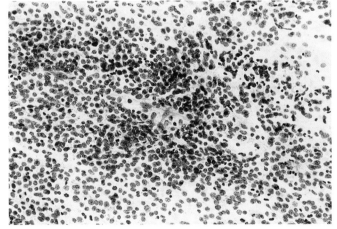

Fig. 3.22 **Medulloblastoma.** A smear preparation from a medulloblastoma shows a population of small malignant cells with pleomorphic neuclei and occasional mitotic figures. Occasional larger cells are present (centre), suggestive of neuronal differentiation. Toluidine blue.

this has not already been performed; comparison of the histological and cytological features of a tumour can often be constructive (Figs 3.22 and 3.23). It is also important to be aware of the kind of information the surgeon requires at the time of surgery. For example, in some biopsy procedures intraoperative knowledge of a specific tumour identity may not be necessary, merely the knowledge that the biopsied material is likely to prove diagnostic when paraffin histology is examined later on.

Cryostat sections

In the selection of tissue for cryostat section examination it is also important to avoid tissue which is necrotic or excessively haemorrhagic. Many intrinsic tumours are soft and there is usually marked oedema in the surrounding brain. This can cause problems when the tissue is frozen, resulting in ice crystal artefact if a rapid freezing technique is not employed (Fig. 3.24). With care it is usually possible to select suitable blocks of tissue for this purpose which should be generally no more than 10 mm^2 in area and up to 5 mm in thickness. The specimen should be carefully orientated (in order to ensure that the appropriate face of the tissue is sectioned) and then rapidly frozen. This can be achieved in a number of ways, but direct immersion in liquid nitrogen or in isopentane chilled with liquid nitrogen will provide satisfactory results with minimal ice crystal artefact. After sectioning on the cryostat at around 10 μm, the sections are fixed (for example in 95% alcohol or 10% buffered formalin) and stained. The sections can be briefly microwaved in order to enhance nuclear and cytological detail and to improve section adhesion to the slides (Fig. 3.25).[20] H & E is the stain of choice for cryostat sections (Figs 3.26 and 3.27),

but other stains, including the van Gieson and reticulin techniques can also be performed,[1,21] and of course additional sections can be cut for specialised techniques including immunocytochemistry and molecular biological techniques.[9] After staining, the specimens should then be dehydrated and mounted in a suitable synthetic medium.

After sampling and the preparation of smears for cryostat sections it is important to ensure that the residual unfixed tissue does not dry out prior to fixation. The tissue should not be fixed until a diagnosis has been made and discussed with the surgeon and the need for ancillary investigations including molecular genetic techniques, virological and bacteriological culture etc. have been considered. Once the intraoperative diagnosis has been made and discussed with the surgeon the cryostat block can be thawed, fixed as for routine specimens and processed into

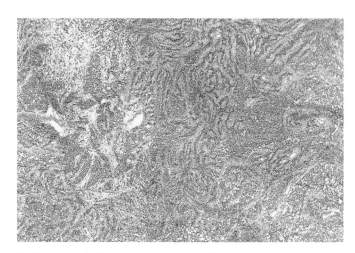

Fig. 3.24 **Medulloblastoma.** Ice crystal artefact is present in this cryostat section from a medulloblastoma. This has resulted from uneven freezing of a large tissue fragment. The characteristic architecture of this tumour can, however, still be identified. H & E.

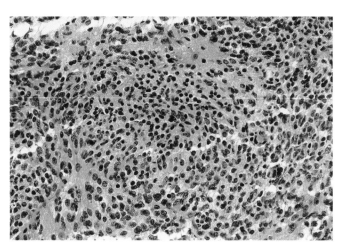

Fig. 3.23 **Medulloblastoma.** Cryostat section from a medulloblastoma (same case as Fig. 2.22) showing small tumour cells with a variable quantity of eosinophilic cytoplasm, also suggestive of neuronal differentiation. H & E.

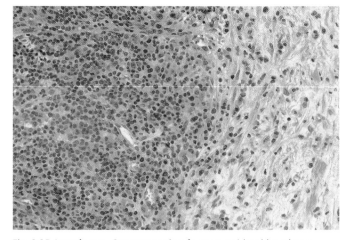

Fig. 3.25 **Lymphoma.** Cryostat section from an epidural lymphoma, showing infiltration of the dura mater (right) by the tumour cells. This section was microwaved prior to staining, with good morphological preservation and little evidence of ice crystal artefact. H & E.

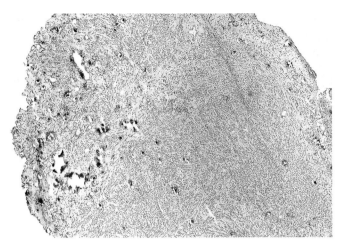

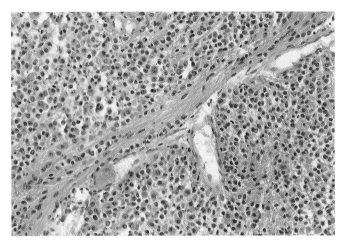

Fig. 3.26 **Oligodendroglioma.** A cryostat section from an oligodendroglioma, which shows some scoring and chattering as a result of calcification within the tumour. The characteristic tumour architecture, however, is well preserved. H & E.

Fig. 3.27 **Anaplastic oligoendroglioma.** Cryostat section from an anaplastic oligodendroglioma showing a population of small pleomorphic cells, many of which contain abundant eosinophilic cytoplasm, situated around thick walled blood vessels. Occasional apoptotic nuclei are identifiable. H & E.

paraffin wax. It is recommended that the block of tissue used for cryostat section diagnosis is identified and processed separately to allow comparison with the original cryostat sections and audit of the intraoperative diagnosis.

Diagnostic accuracy of smear preparations and cryostat sections

In most published series, these techniques appear to be highly reliable in experienced hands.[5,12–19,22–35] A recent survey found that most centres in the USA used a combination of smear cytology and cryostat sections for intra-

operative diagnosis.[12] Most reviews of the diagnostic accuracy of these techniques report a correlation rate of around 90% in relation to the final diagnosis made on paraffin sections, with a high sensitivity (greater than 95%) in the detection of diagnostic specimens.[2,12] These reviews have also highlighted areas of diagnostic difficulty, which include accurate tumour typing and grading, and the distinction between reactive and neoplastic astrocytic proliferations;[12,13,15,16,19] particularly difficult problems are listed in Table 3.6. Clinical audit has shown that there is a clear need for an intraoperative neuropathological diagnostic service as a prerequisite for neurosurgical patient care, particularly in relation to stereotactic biopsy procedures.[36] As advances in neurosurgery and neuroimaging allow 'neuronavigation' in the surgery of intracranial and spinal tumours in both adults and children,[37–39] this need is likely to increase.

Table 3.6 Common problems in differentiating between CNS tumours at intraoperative diagnosis[1,2,5,12,15,19]

CNS tumour	Misdiagnosis
Pilocytic astrocytoma	Fibrillary astrocytoma Glioblastoma
Diffuse astrocytoma	Anaplastic astrocytoma
Anaplastic astrocytoma	Glioblastoma
Pleomorphic xanthoastrocytoma	Glioblastoma
Subependymal giant cell astrocytoma	Glioblastoma
Cerebral cortical infiltration by glioma	Ganglion cell tumour
Ependymoma	Fibrillary astrocytoma
Central neurocytoma	Oligodendroglioma
Desmoplastic neuroepithelial tumour	Oligodendroglioma Ganglion cell tumour
Craniopharyngioma	Epidermoid cyst Dermoid cyst
Haemangioblastoma	Metastatic renal carcinoma

REFERENCES

1. Moss TH, Nicoll JAR, Ironside JW. Intra-operative diagnosis of nervous system tumours. London: Arnold, 1997
2. Adams HJ, Graham DI, Doyle D. The smear technique for surgical biopsies. London: Chapman & Hall, 1981
3. Eisenhardt L, Cushing H. Diagnosis of intracranial tumours by supravital technique. Am J Pathol, 1930; 6:541–552
4. Russell DS, Krayenbuhl H, Cairns H. The wet film technique in histological diagnosis of intracranial tumours. A rapid method. J Pathol Bacteriol, 1937; 45:501–505
5. Folkerth RD. Smears and frozen sections in the intraoperative diagnosis of central nervous system lesions. Neurosurg Clin N Am, 1994; 5:1–18
6. Miller DC, Najjar S, Budzilovich GN. Neuropathology of AIDS in surgical biopsy specimens. Neurosurg Clin N Am, 1994; 5:57–70
7. Ng HK, Lo ST. Immunohistochemical diagnosis of central nervous system tumours on smear preparations. Eur Neurol, 1988; 28:142–145
8. Ironside JW. Update on central nervous system cytopathology. II. Brain smear technique. J Clin Pathol, 1994; 47:683–688

9. McKeever PE. Insights about brain tumours gained through immunohistochemical and in situ hybridisation of nuclear and phenotypic markers. J Histochem Cytochem, 1998; 46:585–594

10. Low M, Feiden W, Moringlane JR et al. Detection of numerical chromosome aberrations in brain tumours by fluorescence in situ hybridisation on smear preparations of small tumour biopsies. Neuropathol Appl Neurobiol, 1994; 20:432–438

11. Amalfitano G, Chatel M, Paquis P et al. Fluorescence in situ hybridisation study of aneuploidy of chromosomes 7, 10, X, and Y in primary and secondary glioblastomas. Cancer Genet Cytogenet, 2000; 116:6–9

12. Firlik KS, Martinez AJ, Lunsford LD. Use of cytological preparations for the intraoperative diagnosis of stereotactically obtained brain biopsies: a 19-year experience and survey of neuropathologists. J Neurosurg, 1999; 91:454–458

13. Slowinski J, Harabin-Slowinska M, Mrowka R. Smear technique in the intra-operative brain tumour diagnosis: its advantages and limitations. Neurol Res, 1999; 21:121–124

14. Robbins PD, Yu LL, Lee M et al. Stereotactic biopsy of 100 intracerebral lesions at Sir Charles Gairdner Hospital. Pathology, 1994; 26:410–413

15. Kitchen ND, Bradford R, McLaughlin JE. The value of per-operative smear examination during stereotactic biopsy. Acta Neurochir, 1993; 121:196–198

16. Mennel HD, Rossberg C, Lorenz H et al. Reliability of simple cytological methods in brain tumour biopsy diagnosis. Neurochirurgia, 1989; 32:129–134

17. Ferracini R, Poletti V, Manetto V et al. Smear biopsy for on-the-spot diagnosis in stereotactic surgery of CNS tumours. Experience of 101 cases. Ital J Neurol Sci, 1987; 8:347–349

18. Burger PC. Use of cytological preparations in frozen section diagnosis of central nervous system neoplasia. Am J Surg Pathol, 1985; 9:344–354

19. Kleihues P, Volk B, Anagnostopoulos J et al. Morphologic evaluation of stereotactic brain tumour biopsies. Acta Neurochir (Suppl), 1984; 33:171–181

20. Ainley C, Ironside JW. Microwave technology in diagnostic neuropathology. J Neurosci Methods, 1994; 55:183–190

21. Velasco ME, Sindely SO, Roessmann U. Reticulum stain for frozen-section diagnosis of pituitary adenomas. Technical note. J Neurosurg, 1977; 46:548–550

22. Wober G, Jellinger K. The value of imprint cytology in neurosurgical diagnosis. Wien Klin Wochenschr, 1977; 89:122–126

23. Tashiro K, Tsuru M. The rapid microscopical diagnosis of brain and spinal cord tumours by cryostat-cut frozen section. No Shinkei Geka, 1975; 3:323–327

24. Monabati A, Kumar PV, Kamkarpour A. Intraoperative cytodiagnosis of metastatic brain tumours confused clinically with brain abscess. A report of three cases. Acta Cytol, 2000; 44:437–441

25. Smith AR, Elsheikh TM, Silverman JF. Intraoperative cytologic diagnosis of suprasellar and sellar cystic lesions. Diagn Cytopathol, 1999; 20:137–147

26. Brainard JA, Prayson RA, Barnett GH. Frozen section evaluation of stereotactic brain biopsies: diagnostic yield at the stereotactic target position in 188 cases. Arch Pathol Lab Med, 1997; 121:481–484

27. Reyes MG, Homsi MF, McDonald LW et al. Imprints, smears and frozen sections of brain tumours. Neurosurgery, 1991; 29:575–579

28. Patt S, Weigel K, Zimmer C et al. Experience with the intraoperative frozen section technique for stereotaxic brain tumour biopsies. Zentralbl Pathol, 1991; 137:35–40

29. Nguyen GK, Johnson ES, Mielke BW. Cytology of neuroectodermal tumours of the brain in crush preparations. A review of 56 cases of deep-seated tumours sampled by CT-guided stereotactic needle biopsy. Acta Cytol, 1989; 33:67–73

30. Colbassani HJ, Nishio S, Sweeney KM et al. CT-assisted stereotactic brain biopsy: value of intraoperative frozen section diagnosis. J Neurol Neurosurg Psychiatry 1988; 51:332–341

31. Silverman JF. Cytopathology of fine-needle aspiration biopsy of the brain and spinal cord. Diagn Cytopathol, 1986; 2:312–319

32. Cahill EM, Hidvegi DF. Crush preparations of lesions of the central nervous system. A useful adjunct to the frozen section. Acta Cytol, 1985; 29:279–285

33. Frederiksen P, Knudsen V, Reske-Nielsen E. Diagnostic aid of aspiration biopsy cytology in brain lesions. Neurochirurgie, 1979; 22:229–235

34. Adelman LS, Post KD. Intra-operative frozen section technique for pituitary adenomas. Am J Surg Pathol, 1979; 3:173–175

35. Meyermann R, Kletter G. Comparative evaluation of various histological techniques for the rapid diagnosis of brain tumours. Acta Neurochir 1976; 35:171–180

36. O'Neill KS, Dyer PV, Bell BA et al. Is peroperative smear cytology necessary for CT-guided stereotaxic biopsy? Br J Neurosurg 1992; 6:421–427

37. Haberland L, Ebmeirer K, Hilscs R et al. Neuronavigation in surgery of intracranial and spinal tumours. J Cancer Res Clin Oncol, 2000; 126:529–541

38. Wirtz CR, Albert FK, Schwaderer M et al. The benefit of neuronavigation for neurosurgery analyzed by its impact on glioblastoma surgery. Neurol Res, 2000; 22:354–360

39. Wagner W, Gaab MR, Schroeder HW et al. Experiences with cranial neuronavigation in pediatric neurosurgery. Pediatr Neurosurg, 1999; 31:231–236

4 Astrocytic tumours

Astrocytic tumours can arise in almost any part of the brain or spinal cord; in adults they have a predilection for the cerebral hemispheres and in children for the cerebellum and brain stem. The major characteristic by which astrocytic tumours are grouped together is the histological resemblance of the tumour cells to either normal or reactive astrocytes. In most cases, therefore, the presence of cells with fine fibrillary processes, expressing glial fibrillary acidic protein (GFAP), is a major diagnostic feature.

The majority of astrocytic tumours diffusely infiltrate the brain and are thus termed 'diffuse' astrocytomas. These tumours range from well differentiated diffuse astrocytomas, through anaplastic astrocytomas to glioblastoma. Genetic studies suggest that diffuse astrocytomas frequently, if not inevitably, progress to anaplastic astrocytoma or glioblastoma, although a proportion of glioblastomas arise de novo. A number of slowly growing astrocytic tumours, such as pilocytic astrocytomas and others described in this chapter, also occur and should be distinguished from the diffuse, infiltrating astrocytomas as, in general, they have a more favourable prognosis.

The importance of astrocytic tumours to neuro-oncology lies in their relatively high frequency compared with other types of central nervous system (CNS) tumour, the very poor prognosis of anaplastic astrocytomas and glioblastoma, and the problems that may arise in diagnosis clinically, radiologically and from biopsy material.

In the present chapter, there is first a brief outline of the morphological and functional aspects of astrocytes followed by an account of the clinical, radiological and pathological features of astrocytic tumours concentrating upon those aspects that are of value in their diagnosis. The biological characteristics of astrocytic tumours and their molecular biology are considered towards the end of the chapter.

Astrocytes

The histological diagnosis of astrocytic tumours depends upon distinguishing tumour astrocytes from normal and reactive astrocytes and from other types of tumour cells. It is therefore appropriate that some of the histological and physiological features of normal astrocytes and of reactive astrocytes are reviewed before embarking upon a description of astrocytic tumours.

Embryologically, astrocytes are derived from neuro-ectoderm and, in the developing nervous system, form several distinct types of radial glia along which neuroblasts from germinal zones migrate.[1] Remnants of such glia can be seen in the adult cerebellum as processes of Bergmann glia in the Purkinje cell layer extend radially across the molecular layer to the surface of the cerebellar cortex. During development, astrocytes and oligodendrocytes appear to arise from common progenitor cells. In tissue culture, a distinct pattern of development[1] as type I and type 2 astrocytes is seen with further differentiation of grey matter astrocytes from type I cells and of oligodendrocytes and fibrous astrocytes in the white matter from type 2 cells. Attempts have been made to relate such developmental characteristics to tumour cell migration and invasion in astrocytic tumours, but no clear correlation has been established.

In the adult nervous system, there are a number of specialised types of astrocyte, such as tanycytes and Bergmann glia but the majority of astrocytes can be divided into protoplasmic astrocytes in grey matter and fibrous astrocytes in the white matter. Protoplasmic astrocytes contain few GFAP intermediate filaments in their processes or cell bodies, whereas the fibrous astrocytes in the white matter have stainable GFAP filaments in their delicate stellate processes. Astrocytes perform a variety of functions in the normal nervous system; they form a layer of compacted cell processes at the glia limitans on the surface of the brain and around blood vessels and play a major role in the induction and maintenance of the blood–brain barrier in CNS microvessels. In addition, astrocytes play a key role in the metabolic support of neurons. Positioned as they are with processes surrounding the cell bodies and synapses of neurons, astrocytes maintain intimate metabolic exchanges with neurons. Glucose is taken up by astrocytes and converted to glycogen; the release of glutamate from neuronal synapses induces glycolysis in the astrocytes and the formation of lactate, which is then utilised through pyruvate by neuronal mitochondria.[2] In addition, astrocytes play a role in the maintenance of electrolyte and fluid balance within the extracellular space of the brain; following tissue damage, astrocytes swell and take up protein and fluid from the extracellular space.[3]

Astrocytes, together with microglia, are the major cell elements that react to injury in the CNS and such reactions are accompanied by hypertrophy and proliferation of astrocytes and by the production of increased amounts of GFAP, both in protoplasmic astrocytes and in fibrous astrocytes. Typical reactive astrocytes are seen after 2 or 3 days around infarcts; there is an increase in the size of the nuclei which lie eccentrically in the enlarged cell bodies. Perhaps most striking, however, is the increase in size of the processes which contain large numbers of GFAP filaments. As inflammation and brain damage subside, reactive astrocytes become smaller and the processes more compacted to form dense gliotic scar tissue as, for example, in chronic gliotic multiple sclerosis plaques. In such longstanding gliosis, binucleate astrocytes may be seen and some cells may have large, hyperchromatic nuclei which may be confused with neoplastic cells. Another feature of longstanding gliosis is the presence of Rosenthal fibres which are swollen astrocytic processes containing ubiquitin, GFAP and alpha-B crystallin. Rosenthal fibres are a feature of pilocytic astrocytomas and sometimes ependymomas, in addition to being present in longstanding gliotic scar tissue.[3]

The role of astrocytes in forming the glia limitans at the surface of the brain and around blood vessels is connected also with their capacity to form basement membrane. This feature is reflected in reactive brain, particularly around abscesses in which there is formation of fibrous tissue. Extensive basement membrane formation can be seen in reticulin stains of a number of astrocytic tumours, in particular pleomorphic xanthoastrocytomas and gliosarcomas (see below).

Astrocytic tumours

Astrocytic tumours are composed of cells which morphologically resemble astrocytes and express GFAP. In the more undifferentiated and anaplastic tumours, only a proportion of the cells show astrocytic features and GFAP staining is very important for identifying such cells.

There are many classifications of astrocytic tumours. In this chapter the World Health Organisation (WHO) classification (see Chapter 1) will be followed, as set out in Table 4.1a and b.

Age, incidence and site

Astrocytic tumours show a wide spectrum of clinical presentation, radiological characteristics, macroscopic appearance, histological structure and molecular genetic features, age and site of occurrence and a wide variation in response to therapy and in prognosis. The age distribution of the major astrocytic tumours is illustrated graphically in Fig. 4.1 and in Table 4.2.

The majority of astrocytic tumours in the first two decades of life are slow growing and fall into the defined histological categories of *pilocytic astrocytoma, diffuse astrocytoma, pleomorphic xanthoastrocytoma* and *subependymal giant cell astrocytoma*. The number of reported cases and the incidence in routine surgical practice of *pleomorphic xanthoastrocytoma* and *subependymal giant cell astrocytoma* is too low to construct a meaningful graph showing the age and sex incidence. *Pilocytic astrocytoma* is more common and has its major incidence in both sexes in the first two decades; it rarely undergoes anaplastic change and differs from *diffuse astrocytomas, anaplastic astrocytoma* and *glioblastoma* in its molecular genetic profile (see below). *Subependymal giant cell astrocytoma* is associated with the hereditary condition of tuberous sclerosis and is most frequently found in the central grey matter areas of the brain related to the lateral and third ventricles.

The majority of astrocytic tumours in the first two decades of life are infratentorial, involving the brain stem, cerebellum and spinal cord, whereas from the third decade onwards, most astrocytic tumours arise in the cerebral hemispheres (Fig. 4.2) and show progression from *diffuse astrocytoma* to *anaplastic astrocytoma* and *glioblastoma*. *Glioblastoma* and *gliosarcoma* occur mainly in the cerebral hemispheres and are uncommon in the spinal cord, brain stem and cerebellum. *Giant cell glioblastoma* arises at a younger age than *glioblastoma* and diffuse invasion of the brain by astrocytoma cells (*gliomatosis cerebri*) may be seen in childhood and in adults but this tumour is very much less common than the more focal astrocytoma and glioblastoma.

Familial aspects of astrocytic tumours

Astrocytic tumours occurring in a familial setting are uncommon but well described. Hereditary predisposition to astrocytic tumours may occur in the presence or the absence of a distinct tumour syndrome (see Chapter 19 and below). Those families that have multiple astrocytic tumours in the absence of defined syndromes typically have just a few affected members, often just enough to raise suspicion of 'cancer family'[4] and to elicit a case report in the literature.[5] Usually, such families have two or three affected members in subsequent generations

Table 4.1 (a)   Astrocytic tumours – classification based on WHO 2000

Pilocytic astrocytoma	*Diffuse astrocytoma*
Pleomorphic xanthoastrocytoma	Fibrillary
Subependymal giant cell astrocytoma	Protoplasmic
Chordoid glioma of the third ventricle	Gemistocytic
Astroblastoma	*Anaplastic astrocytoma*
Gliomatosis cerebri	*Glioblastoma*
	Giant cell glioblastoma
	Gliosarcoma

Table 4.1 (b)   Terminology used for the major astrocytic tumours in the present chapter

Terminology based on WHO 2000	Other commonly used terms
Pilocytic astrocytoma	Low grade astrocytoma/glioma Astrocytoma grade I
Diffuse astrocytoma Fibrillary Protoplasmic Gemistocytic	Low grade astrocytoma/glioma Astrocytoma grade II
Anaplastic astrocytoma	High grade astrocytoma/glioma Malignant astrocytoma Malignant glioma Diffuse astrocytoma grade III Astrocytoma grade III
Glioblastoma	Glioblastoma multiforme High grade astrocytoma/glioma Malignant glioma Diffuse astrocytoma grade IV Astrocytoma grade IV

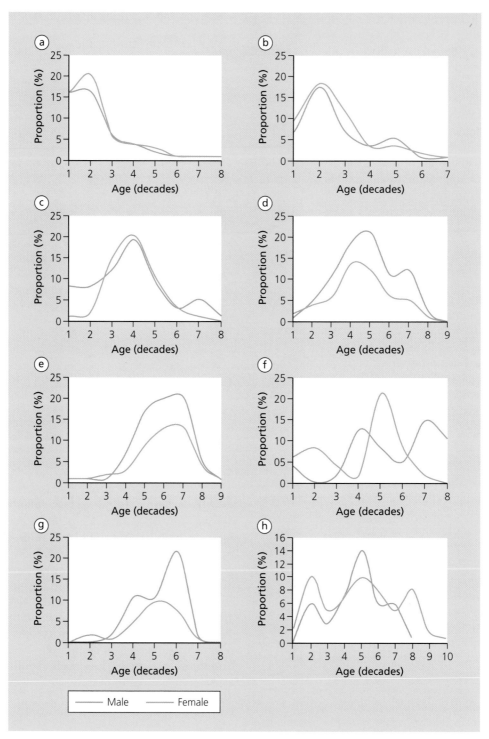

Fig. 4.1 Relative age and sex incidence of astrocytic tumours. (Data derived from Ref. 17) **(a)** Pilocytic astrocytoma. **(b)** Pleomorphic xanthoastrocytoma. **(c)** Diffuse astrocytoma. **(d)** Anaplastic astrocytoma. **(e)** Glioblastoma. **(f)** Giant cell glioblastoma. **(g)** Gliosarcoma. **(h)** Gliomatosis cerebri.

(parent–child) or two siblings. It is important to emphasise that it is currently unclear whether the aetiologies for isolated familial clustering of occasional astrocytic tumours are genetic or environmental. As discussed elsewhere, with the exception of radiation, definite enviromental aetiologies of astrocytic tumours have not been identified. Therefore, although such astrocytic tumour families may arise from common environmental carcinogen exposure, this cannot be proven at the present time. As a result, most of the studies on such families

Table 4.2 Age distribution of the major astrocytic tumours

Decade of peak incidence		Type of astrocytic tumour
Seventh decade	60–69 years	Glioblastoma Gliosarcoma
Sixth decade	50–59 years	Glioblastoma Gliosarcoma
Fifth decade	40–49 years	Anaplastic astrocytoma Giant cell glioblastoma
Fourth decade	30–39 years	Diffuse astrocytoma
Third decade	20–29 years	Diffuse astrocytoma
Second decade	10–19 years	Pilocytic astrocytoma Subependymal giant cell astrocytoma
First decade	0–9 years	Pilocytic astrocytoma Pleomorphic xanthoastrocytoma

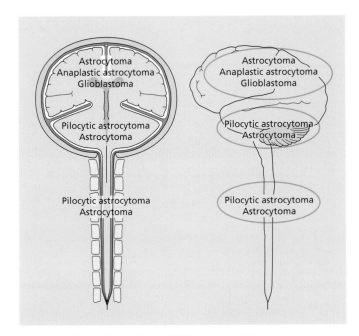

Fig. 4.2 **Preferential sites in the CNS for astrocytic tumours.**

have focussed on excluding mutation of genes responsible for known syndromes that may predispose to astrocytic tumours (see below). Thus, mutations in genes such as *TP53* or *NF1* are unlikely to be responsible for isolated astrocytic tumour families;[6] nonetheless, alternative methods of inactivating these genes have not been conclusively excluded. At the same time, a few astrocytic tumour families have been reported with germline *TP53* gene mutations;[7] in essentially all of these families, other tumour types have been reported, suggesting that these families are more likely formes frustes of Li–Fraumeni syndrome.[8]

Among the defined syndromes that predispose patients to astrocytic tumours, Li–Fraumeni syndrome, neurofibromatosis 1 (NF1), tuberous sclerosis and Turcot

syndrome stand out as the most prominent. Patients with Li–Fraumeni syndrome develop breast carcinomas, soft tissue sarcomas, adrenal tumours, lymphoid tumours, amongst other less common lesions. Brain tumours represent the third most common tumour type in patients with Li–Fraumeni syndrome, with anaplastic astrocytoma and glioblastoma by far the most predominant tumour types. There are no described histological differences between sporadic astrocytic tumours and those that occur in Li–Fraumeni syndrome. Most of these families can be shown to have germline mutations in the *TP53* tumour suppressor gene.[8] As a corollary (see below), sporadic astrocytic tumours frequently have *TP53* gene mutations as well, even in diffuse astrocytic tumours.[9] The fact that Li–Fraumeni patients are at great risk for developing astrocytic tumours has been cited as evidence that alterations of *TP53* are important early in astrocytic tumorigenesis.

NF1 also predisposes affected patients to the development of a variety of astrocytic tumours, including both pilocytic and diffuse astrocytomas, and to focal subarachnoid and subependymal astrocytic proliferations that fall short of being frank tumours. As mentioned above, pilocytic astrocytomas are highly characteristic of NF1; in fact, NF1 remains unique as the only tumour syndrome that specifically predisposes to pilocytic tumours. Pilocytic astrocytomas in NF1 are particularly common in the optic nerves, with symptomatic optic nerve gliomas occurring in about 1.5–7.5% of NF1 patients, and bilateral optic nerve gliomas being virtually pathognomonic of NF1.[10] The optic nerve pilocytic astrocytomas in NF1 appear particularly indolent, and many resolve without treatment.[10] Pilocytic astrocytomas, however, may occur throughout the neuraxis in NF1 patients, with some patients developing multiple tumours. Studies of sporadic pilocytic astrocytomas have shown allelic loss affecting the NF1 region of chromosome 17q in some cases,[11] but (perhaps because of the large size of the *NF1* gene) *NF1* gene mutations have not been documented in sporadic pilocytic astrocytomas. Those diffuse astrocytic tumours that arise in NF1 patients are typically anaplastic astrocytomas and glioblastomas that often lead to the patient's death; they occur throughout the neuraxis but most commonly affect the cerebral hemispheres. Interestingly, rare *NF1* gene mutations have been demonstrated in sporadic anaplastic astrocytomas.[12] The exception to diffuse astrocytic tumours in NF1 resembling their sporadic counterparts is the diffuse brain stem enlargement that is sometimes seen on neuroimaging of NF1 patients. While on neuroimaging these may resemble brain stem astrocytic tumours, they may resolve spontaneously.

Patients with Turcot syndrome may be affected by a variety of brain tumours in addition to their colonic tumours. Turcot syndrome has been divided phenotypically and genetically; most patients have mutations of the *APC* gene and suffer from colonic polyposis, and are therefore phenotypically and genetically similar to familial adenomatous polyposis; other patients harbour mutations of the mismatch repair genes such as *hMLH1* and have hereditary non-polyposis colorectal carcinoma (HNPCC).[13] While there is an association between the HNPCC phenotype and glioblastoma, and the colonic polyposis phenotype and medulloblastoma, the correlation is not exact. Furthermore, mutations in mismatch repair genes in sporadic glioblastomas are rare and microsatellite instability is rare in sporadic glioblastomas.[14]

Tuberous sclerosis patients are predisposed to the unique subependymal giant cell astrocytomas (see below and Chapter 19). Indeed, some authors consider the occurrence of a subependymal giant cell astrocytoma as pathognomonic of tuberous sclerosis. There is no increased incidence of anaplastic astrocytoma or glioblastoma in tuberous sclerosis patients nor have alterations of the *TSC1* or *TSC2* genes been detected in diffuse astrocytic tumours.

A number of other rare syndromes are also associated with predisposition to neuroepithelial tumours including astrocytic tumours. Rare families have been described with melanoma and other nervous system tumours, including diffuse astrocytomas. Two of these families have been reported to have germline deletions of the *CDKN2A/p16* gene,[15] and deletions of this gene are common in melanomas and astrocytic tumours. Other syndromes that include a predisposition to diffuse gliomas such as astrocytic tumours include Ollier and Maffuci syndromes (enchondromatoses).

Pilocytic astrocytoma

Pilocytic astrocytomas are slow growing, often well defined, tumours that occur mainly under the age of 20 years, at any site in the brain and spinal cord but particularly in the optic nerves and cerebellum. They have a relatively good prognosis as they rarely undergo malignant change to anaplastic pilocytic astrocytoma and may be effectively treated by surgical excision. The 10-year survival rate in patients under 20 years for pilocytic astrocytomas is 81%, whereas it is only 15% for other astrocytic tumours.[16] Optic nerve pilocytic astrocytomas are associated with NF1.

Incidence

Comprising some 6% of surgically biopsied or excised astrocytic tumours,[17] 70% of pilocytic astrocytomas occur under the age of 20 (Fig. 4.3). They are rare over the age of 50 but may occur in older patients particularly in the cerebral hemispheres where they may be confused clinically with metastatic carcinomas as they enhance on

computerised tomography (CT) scanning. There is little difference in incidence between males and females.[17]

Site

Pilocytic astrocytomas in children occur in such widely dispersed sites as the optic nerve, optic chiasm, cerebral hemispheres, brain stem, cerebellum and spinal cord (Fig. 4.4).

The cerebellum is one of the most common sites for pilocytic astrocytoma; in effect, most cerebellar astrocytomas are pilocytic, particularly under the age of 18 years.[16] Cerebellar pilocytic astrocytomas are frequently

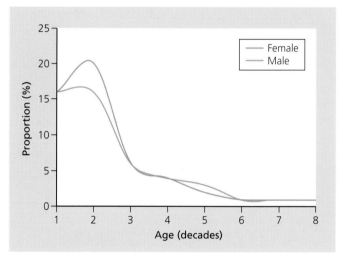

Fig. 4.3 **Relative age and sex incidence of pilocytic astrocytomas.** (Data derived from Ref. 17).

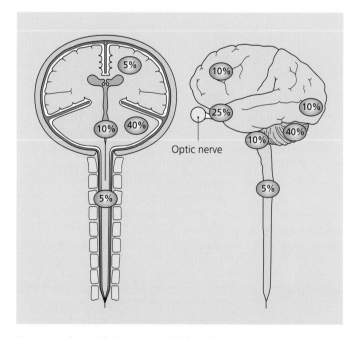

Fig. 4.4 **Preferential sites in the CNS for pilocytic astrocytomas**.

Table 4.3 Differential diagnosis of 'brain stem glioma' in children and adults.

Children	Adults
Pilocytic astrocytoma	Anaplastic astrocytoma
Diffuse astrocytoma	Glioblastoma
Anaplastic astrocytoma	Lymphoma
Medulloblastoma	Oligodenroglioma
Ependymoma	Demyelination
Glioblastoma	

cystic and have an excellect prognosis.[18] In the brain stem, pilocytic astrocytomas may be exophytic and amenable to excision;[19] there is a subgroup confined to the tectum or tegmentum that has a favourable outcome.[16] Pilocytic astrocytoma is an important member of the various lesions that may be diagnosed radiologically as 'brain stem gliomas' (Table 4.3). Pilocytic astrocytomas occur in the spinal cord in children; they grow slowly and have a much better prognosis than diffuse astrocytomas.

A high proportion of the astrocytic tumours affecting the optic nerve, optic chiasm and hypothalamus are pilocytic astrocytomas;[16] anaplastic astrocytoma and glioblastoma are uncommon at this site. Some 55% of optic pathway astrocytomas (optic chiasmatic-hypothalamic gliomas) occur in children under 5 years and 50–85% involve the chiasm and hypothalamus.[20] Most of the astrocytomas confined to the optic nerve are pilocytic astrocytomas and they are less aggressive than those involving the chiasm and hypothalamus. The majority of patients with optic nerve gliomas have NF1, and tumours of the posterior part of the optic tract tend to be more aggressive than those confined to the optic nerve; they are also more aggressive in children under the age of 5 years.[20] Anaplastic change is occasionally seen in optic nerve astrocytomas in adults, but this very rarely occurs in children. Sixty per cent of optic chiasmatic, hypothalamic gliomas are pilocytic astrocytomas and 40% are diffuse fibrillary astrocytomas.[20]

Pilocytic astrocytomas also occur in the thalamus from which there is frequently intraventricular extension.[16] Such tumours at this site are difficult to excise and thus the prognosis may be poor, particularly if bilateral thalamic involvement is present.[21] Within the cerebral hemispheres, diffuse astrocytomas are much more common than pilocytic astrocytomas but it is important to recognise pilocytic astrocytomas as they may be amenable to surgical excision and, unlike diffuse astrocytomas, rarely undergo anaplastic change.

Clinical features

Pilocytic astrocytomas produce signs and symptoms due to raised intracranial pressure with headache, vomiting and eventually drowsiness and unconsciousness. Haemorrhage into a pilocytic astrocytoma may cause a sudden rise in intracranial pressure or the sudden onset of focal neurological signs. Tumours growing in the thalamus or extending into the lateral ventricles may obstruct the flow of cerebrospinal fluid (CSF) through the ventricular system and cause hydrocephalus. Similar obstruction to CSF may occur with cystic or solid cerebellar tumours compressing the fourth ventricle. Optic nerve pilocytic astrocytomas result in loss of visual acuity and may result in proptosis due to the bulk of the tumour. Those tumours involving the chiasm and hypothalamus may produce not only loss of visual acuity but also interference with hypothalamic function, resulting in sexual precosity, obesity and diabetes insipidus.[17] Cerebral pilocytic astrocytomas rarely cause seizures and more frequently result in raised intracranial pressure either from the bulk of the tumour, haemorrhage into the tumour, or obstruction of CSF flow. Involvement of the corticospinal tracts at the internal capsule may result in hemiparesis. Ataxia and clumsiness may occur in cerebellar pilocytic astrocytomas or patients may present with raised intracranial pressure due to compression of the fourth ventricle and the resulting hydrocephalus. In the brain stem, pilocytic astrocytomas are usually associated with hydrocephalus due to the exophytic growth into the fourth ventricle, whereas in the spinal cord, such tumours interfere with motor and sensory long tract function and may cause local damage to anterior horn cells and thus muscle wasting.

Radiology

Pilocytic astrocytomas characteristically enhance on CT and magnetic resonance imaging (MRI) (Fig. 4.5) and may, therefore, be confused with medulloblastomas or with haemangioblastomas, particularly when associated with a cyst. Other sites such as the optic nerve and hypothalamus cause fewer problems with neuroradiological diagnosis. Both cerebral and cerebellar pilocytic astrocytomas frequently have an associated cyst and this feature, together with their enhancing nature, may be of value in distinguishing pilocytic astrocytomas from diffuse astrocytomas in which contrast enhancement is not a feature. CT and MRI may also delineate the extent of pilocytic astrocytomas which are frequently well circumscribed and the enhancing border may define the tumour. This is not totally reliable as invasion of pilocytic astrocytoma cells into the brain away from the main enhancing edge of the tumour is also seen.[16] Haemorrhage associated with pilocytic astrocytoma will also be visible on CT scans. Imaging of the spinal cord reveals pilocytic astrocytomas as enhancing fusiform lesions causing expansion of the cord; as they are slowly growing, they may result in expansion of the spinal canal.

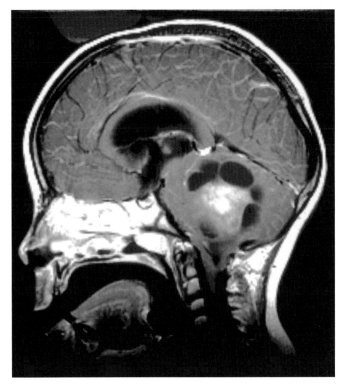

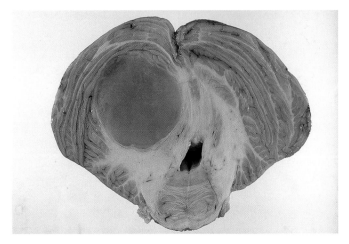

Fig. 4.6 **Pilocytic astrocytoma**. A large cyst filled with proteinaceous material is present in one cerebellar hemisphere. The pilocytic astrocytoma is a small mural nodule. There is distortion of the fourth ventricle.

Fig. 4.5 **Pilocytic astrocytoma**. A contrast-enhanced MRI scan shows a large cerebellar pilocytic astrocytoma with irregular enhancement, surrounded by satellite cysts. There is obstructive hydrocephalus and lateral ventricular dilation. (Courtesy of Dr D Collie, Edinburgh.)

Familial aspects

The major familial and genetic associations of pilocytic astrocytomas are with NF1 (see Chapter 19). NF1 patients may develop pilocytic astrocytomas in the optic nerve, third ventricular region, cerebellum or spinal cord, but optic nerve tumours are most common and most characteristic. Bilateral optic nerve pilocytic astrocytomas are virtually pathognomonic of NF1. On the other hand, pilocytic astrocytomas are not as common in NF1 as previously reported, with more recent estimates suggesting an incidence between 1.5 and 7.5% of cases.[10] In addition, many of the optic nerve pilocytic astrocytomas in NF1 patients follow an extremely indolent course, with spontaneous regression occurring in some cases.[10] Pilocytic astrocytomas of the cerebellum do not have the same association with NF1.

Pathology

Macroscopic features

Pilocytic astrocytomas vary in their macroscopic appearance and texture. They may be firm, greyish-pink, well defined tumours, particularly in the occipital lobes or cerebellum, but soft, opalescent and poorly defined in the optic nerve, hypothalamus and pons. Focal mucoid and cystic change occurs, and large cysts form in some

cerebellar pilocytic astrocytomas (Fig. 4.6). In the spinal cord, pilocytic astrocytomas usually have well defined borders with a central cyst or a number of cysts extending over several segments. Haemorrhage is a recognised complication in pilocytic astrocytoma; thus tumours may appear brown or rust coloured due to haemosiderin deposition or they may be associated with fresh haemorrhage.

Intraoperative diagnosis

Pilocytic astrocytomas are usually suspected preoperatively from the clinical history of slow onset of visual disturbance due to an optic nerve tumour, long tract signs from a spinal cord tumour or from raised intracranial pressure, hydrocephalus and ataxia from a cerebellar pilocytic astrocytoma. Cerebellar, cerebral and brain stem pilocytic astrocytomas may be cystic or uniformly enhancing, well circumscribed tumours on CT and MRI. Occasionally, however, the diagnosis may not be clear and pilocytic astrocytomas may be confused on imaging with medulloblastomas in the cerebellum, ependymomas in the fourth ventricle or, rarely, with haemangioblastoma or metastastic carcinoma. Intraoperative diagnosis is, therefore, desirable, as the ideal management for many pilocytic astrocytomas is total excision.

Some pilocytic astrocytomas are firm and do not smear well so these tumours are often best examined by cryostat sectioning. The cytological features of softer tumours are well demonstrated, both in smears and cryostat sections. Key features for rapid diagnosis are the presence of elongated pilocytic cells, well demontrated in smear preparations, (Fig. 4.7) and Rosenthal fibres which are best demonstrated in cryostat sections stained with haematoxylin and eosin (H & E) (Fig. 4.8). Granular eosinophilic droplets are also well visualised in cryostat sections. If there is confusion between the pilocytic cells and fibroblasts, reticulin stains or haematoxylin van Gieson are useful for excluding the presence of fibrous tissue. In highly vascular, poorly cellular, pilocytic astrocytomas, the hyaline blood vessels may be a very confusing feature but the pilocytic cells may be identified in smear preparations and by the presence of elongated cells in reticulin-free regions of cryostat sections.

Histological features

Despite the name 'pilocytic' meaning hair-like cells, there is wide variation of cytological appearance in pilocytic astrocytomas. The diagnosis, therefore, in some cases may depend upon a combination of clinical, radiological and pathological data. A tumour occurring at a typical site for pilocytic astrocytoma, showing enhancement on CT scan, with a well defined border may exhibit a mixture of the cytological features described below, perhaps with one pattern predominating. Rosenthal fibres and eosinophilic granular bodies (protein droplets) are particularly valuable in establishing the diagnosis of pilocytic astrocytoma, although they are also found in longstanding gliosis and are, therefore, not specific for pilocytic astrocytoma without the other histological and clinical features.

Cytologically, pilocytic cells are long, bipolar cells with fine terminal processes (Figs 4.7 and 4.9); arranged in densely packed sheaths or more dispersed and randomly orientated. Most pilocytic astrocytomas have a *biphasic* histological pattern (Fig. 4.10) with areas of pilocytic cells and microcystic areas containing stellate cells with defined processes; both types of cell contain glial fibrils (Fig. 4.11). Stellate cells may predominate in some cerebral pilocytic astrocytomas (Fig. 4.12). For the most part,

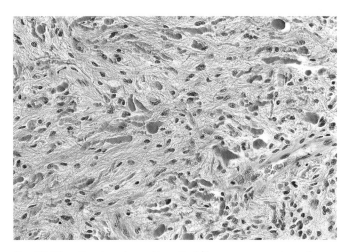

Fig. 4.8 **Pilocytic astrocytoma**. Rosenthal fibres are seen as irregular brightly eosinophilic structures abundant within this part of the tumour. Occasional granular protein droplets are also seen (far left). H & E.

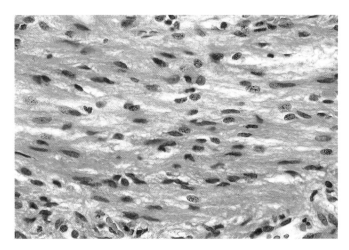

Fig. 4.9 **Pilocytic astrocytoma.** This solid area is composed of elongated cells with regular round or oval nuclei. H & E.

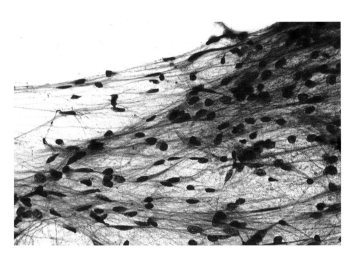

Fig. 4.7 **Pilocytic astrocytoma**. Smear of a pilocytic astrocytoma showing cells with regular round or oval nuclei and fine pilocytic processes. Toluidine blue.

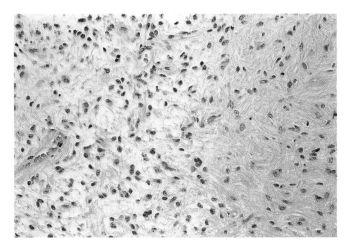

Fig. 4.10 **Pilocytic astrocytoma**. A biphasic histological pattern is present. In one area (right) the pilocytic cells are fibrillary and compacted, whereas on the left the cells are more loosely packed. H & E.

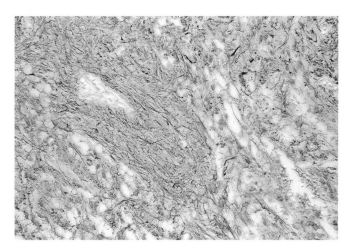

Fig. 4.11 **Pilocytic astrocytoma.** Compacted pilocytic cells are seen around an unstained blood vessel, whereas in other fields the tumour cells are more loosely packed. Immunocytochemistry for GFAP.

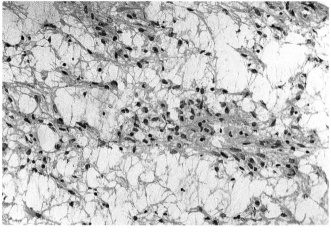

Fig. 4.12 **Pilocytic astrocytoma**. This optic nerve tumour shows wide dispersion of pilocytic cells. There is some concentration around the blood vessels in the tumour. H & E.

pilocytic astrocytoma cells have bland, regular, ovoid nuclei with some hyperchromasia; a significant fraction of pilocytic astrocytomas is aneuploid.[23] Mitoses are rarely seen and the proliferation index with Ki-67/MIB-1 is generally little greater than 1%;[24] in some cases, Ki-67/MIB-1 labelling indices are up to 5% but this has little predictive value for prognosis,[25] unless accompanied by other signs of anaplasia. Hyperchromatic nuclei may be present, but should not cause concern unless there are mitoses in the tumour or a high Ki-67/MIB-1 proliferation index. Multinucleated giant cells, with peripherally arranged nuclei may be seen but the nuclei are usually not hyperchromatic or mitotically active.

Rosenthal fibres are characteristic of most, but not all, pilocytic astrocytomas; they are rare in other astrocytic tumours but are seen sometimes in ependymomas. Typically, Rosenthal fibres are elongated, irregularly swollen, refractile, eosinophilic hyaline structures 20 μm or more in diameter (Fig. 4.8). They occur either singly or in groups in the fibrillary regions of pilocytic astrocytomas. Rosenthal fibres have roughly the same degree of eosinophilia as erythrocytes with which they should not be confused. Immunocytochemistry reveals a core of alpha-B crystallin[17] and varying amounts of GFAP, often arranged as a skein around the periphery of the Rosenthal fibre. By electron microscopy, Rosenthal fibres have dense, osmiophilic cores, with associated glial intermediate filaments (GFAP). Although typical of pilocytic astrocytoma, Rosenthal fibres occur in areas of long-standing gliosis especially around craniopharyngiomas. Care is required in interpreting small biopsies of cyst walls, particularly in the cerebellum, as Rosenthal fibres also occur in the walls of cysts associated with haemangioblastomas.

Granular bodies (protein droplets) are also characteristic of pilocytic astrocytomas but occur more frequently in the loosely packed areas of the tumour. In conjunction with other histological features, the presence of these bodies is a valuable diagnostic feature. They are brightly eosinophilic, spherical, granular structures up to 20 μm in diameter. Immunocytochemistry has demonstrated that they contain alpha-B crystallin and ubiquitin and, in addition, alpha-1 antitrypsin, alpha-1 antichymotrypsin and beta-amyloid precursor protein. Ultrastructurally, granular eosinophilic bodies are membrane bound acretions of osmiophilic material.[17]

Blood vessels in pilocytic astrocytomas show some unexpected features for a slowly growing astrocytic tumour. Pilocytic astrocytomas enhance on CT and MRI[26,27] and in the cerebellum may be confused radiologically in children with medulloblastomas or ependymomas, and in older patients with haemangioblastomas or metastases. Histology shows many multichannelled blood vessel complexes which are not the typical glomeruloid form seen in glioblastoma but appear as groups of distinct thin walled vessels encompassed by basement membrane of the glia limitans and a perivascular space (Fig. 4.13). It is presumably the perivascular space along which fluid drains from the tumour as in normal grey matter.[28] Even when the vessel walls are thicker, there is a distinct lumen (Fig. 4.14) which distinguishes these vessels from the glomeruloid form of microvascular (capillary endothelial) proliferation in glioblastomas (see Fig. 4.51) Expression of vascular endothelial growth factor (VEGF)[29] by tumour cells may account for the vascular proliferation. In most pilocytic astrocytomas blood vessels with thick, hyaline walls are seen. Such vessels may be so numerous that they obscure the astrocytic tumour cells and the lesion may be mistaken for a cavernous haemangioma. However, the presence of elongated GFAP positive pilocytic astrocytoma cells, rather than stellate reactive astrocytes,

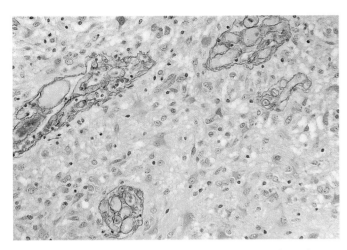

Fig. 4.13 **Pilocytic astrocytoma.** Multiple thin walled blood vessels are encompassed by the black stained basement membrane of the perivascular glia limitans. Reticulin stain.

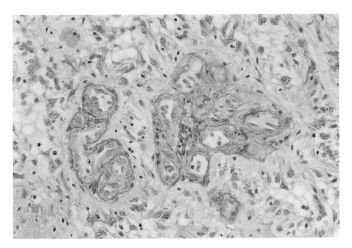

Fig. 4.14 **Pilocytic astrocytoma.** Aggregations of blood vessels with hypertrophic endothelium and some hyalinisation of the walls are present. Distinct channels distinguish them from the glomeruloid structures of microvascular (capillary endothelial) proliferation in glioblastomas. Reticulin stain.

between the blood vessels should allow the distinction to be made. Such vascular pilocytic astrocytomas have been referred to as 'angiogliomas' but there is no particular reason to separate them from other pilocytic astrocytomas.

Macrophages containing haemosiderin may be present in the tumour, reflecting old haemorrhage and, although calcification is uncommon,[17] it may be seen in association with hyalinised blood vessel walls. Occasionally, groups of lymphocytes are present in the tumour and there may be areas of necrosis. However, individual cell necrosis and apoptosis are not usually a feature of pilocytic astrocytomas. Necrosis does not necessarily mean that anaplastic or malignant change has occurred within a pilocytic astrocytoma as it would in a diffuse astrocytic tumour.

At surgery, the firm consistency of pilocytic astrocytomas may allow total excision to be achieved from accessible sites such as the cerebellum or occipital lobes.[30,31] However, examination of the margins of pilocytic astrocytomas frequently shows a narrow edge of 1–2 mm, where tumour cells infiltrate normal tissue and incorporate normal cell elements, such as neurons, into the tumour. Extensive diffuse spread into surrounding tissue is only usually seen in optic nerve pilocytic astrocytomas. Growth of tumour into the subarachnoid space may occur, often exciting a desmoplastic reaction with the formation of reticulin and collagen bands.[17] Subarachnoid invasion is quite common in pilocytic astrocytomas associated with NF1. Distant spread through the subarachnoid space also occurs but it is uncommon[22] and, as with the tumour at the primary site, seedlings grow slowly.[32]

Variations of pilocytic astrocytoma

Diffuse pilocytic astrocytoma

Diffuse pilocytic astrocytoma is very rare. It presents clinically in a similar way to a diffuse astrocytoma with enlargement of the affected region of the brain. Histologically, the major feature is Rosenthal fibres diffusely spread through the tissue and gathered as collars around blood vessels. The appearances resemble Alexander's disease but the lesion is focal and the age and clinical history are not those of Alexander's disease. Identification of the genetic defect in Alexander's disease as a *GFAP* mutation will further allow a firm distinction between these two conditions. Few cases of diffuse pilocytic astrocytoma have been described and the prognosis is unclear;[17] care must be taken not to interpret the edge of a nodular pilocytic astrocytoma as a diffuse tumour.

Anaplastic pilocytic astrocytoma

Anaplastic change in pilocytic astrocytomas is uncommon and there is no good correlation between malignant histology and malignant behaviour.[33] They are recognised by the presence of a mitotically active small cell component with necrosis and vascular proliferation within a pre-existing pilocytic astrocytoma.[16] Such tumours may progress to glioblastoma.[34] Some cases may arise following irradiation of a pilocytic astrocytoma.[16] An aggressive, infantile pilocytic astrocytoma has also been described in the suprasellar region in children under the age of 3 years[17] with extensive mucoid change and high mitotic activity. Invasion of the base of the skull and spenid sinus has been reported.[35]

Monomorphous pilomyxoid astrocytoma

A recent study of paediatric astrocytomas has reported a group of 18 supatentorial tumours (occurring in the hypothalamus, optic chiasm, thalamus and temporal lobe) (Fig. 4.15) with a distinctive monomorphous pilomyxoid histological pattern.[36] These tumours affected young children (median age 10 months) and presented with failure to thrive, developmental delay and features of raised intracranial pressure. Histologically, the tumours were characterised by small spindle bipolar cells in a loose fibrillar and strikingly myxoid background. The classical biphasic pattern of pilocytic astrocytomas was absent, no Rosenthal fibres were identified, and eosinophilic bodies were present in only one case. A marked angiocentric pattern was common (Fig. 4.16) and vascular proliferation was widespread, often in association with cyst formation. The tumour cells exhibited immunoreactivity for GFAP, with negative results for synaptophysin and chromogranin. Ki-67/MIB-1 labelling indices were around 4%, and a moderate degree of nuclear pleomorphism was present. Foci of necrosis were identified in 4/18 cases, and there was infiltration of the adjacent brain in 3/18 of cases. Similar histological features were seen in repeat biopsies from two cases. At the end of the (variable) follow-up period, 6/18 patients were dead and 12/18 were alive with evidence of disease. Progression-free survival at 1 year was 38.7%. The authors suggest that the monomorphous pilomyxoid tumour is a more aggressive entity than pilocytic astrocytoma; further studies are required to define the clinical and pathological spectrum of these lesions, and their relationship to conventional pilocytic astrocytomas.

Differential diagnosis

Pilocytic astrocytomas may occur in the cerebellar or cerebral hemispheres, in the brain stem or in the spinal cord in children and in adults. They enhance on CT and MRI and they are prone to bleed. Although there is obvious overlap, the differential diagnosis of this tumour from other intracranial or spinal lesions depends upon the site and the age of the patient. The main differential diagnoses for pilocytic astrocytoma in children are medulloblastoma, ependymoma, cavernous haemangioma, and, if haemorrhage has occurred, arteriovenous malformation. In adults, cerebellar haemangioblastoma, metastatic carcinoma, vestibular Schwannoma, arteriovenous malformation and diffuse astrocytic tumour are the main lesions to be considered. The differential diagnosis of 'brain stem glioma' in adults and children is summarised in Table 4.3.

In the majority of cases, the typical histological features of elongated pilocytic GFAP positive tumour cells with little nuclear pleomorphism, few if any mitoses and the presence of Rosenthal fibres and granular protein droplets will be a strong indication of pilocytic astrocytoma. However, the biopsy may be small, some of the histological features may not be present and the clinical and radiological picture may suggest one of the lesions described below.

Medulloblastoma

Medulloblastoma is a primitive neuroectodermal tumour arising in the midline of the cerebellum in children and more laterally in the cerebellum in adults. The main confusion clinically between this tumour and pilocytic astrocytomas arises due to the position of both tumours in the cerebellum and the fact that they both enhance on CT and MRI. Histologically, however, medulloblastomas consist of cells with hyperchromatic nuclei that are more irregular than those of pilocytic astrocytoma and very sparse amounts of cytoplasm. Thus in smears, medulloblastoma cells do not have the long astrocytic processes of the pilocytic cells and in cryostat sections their high nuclear cytoplasmic ratio can be appreciated. In paraffin sections, mitoses and apoptotic cells will be present in the medulloblastoma and not in the pilocytic astrocytoma.

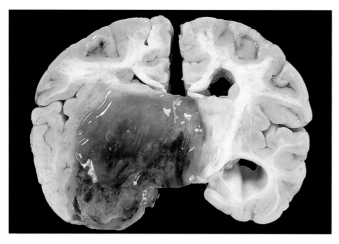

Fig. 4.15 **Pilomyxoid astrocytoma**. A large gelatinous tumour with areas of haemorrhage occupies most of the left temporal lobe in the brain of a 12-month-old infant.

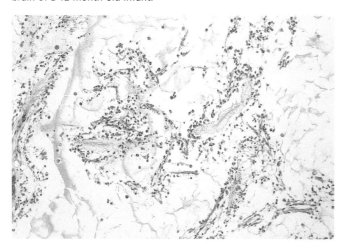

Fig. 4.16 **Pilomyxoid astrocytoma**. Bipolar tumour cells exhibit a perivascular arrangement within a gelatinous matrix. No solid areas are present and Rosenthal fibres and eosinophilic bodies are both absent. H & E.

Immunocytochemistry usually reveals patchy expression of GFAP and synaptophysin in medulloblastoma cells but more widespread strong expression of GFAP in the pilocytic astrocytoma cells.

Ependymomas

Ependymomas present as enhancing tumours in the fourth ventricle and may invade the brain stem and cerebellum, particularly in children. For this reason, there may be confusion clinically and radiologically with pilocytic astrocytoma. Histologically, confusion between ependymoma and pilocytic astrocytoma may occur as they are both glial tumours and both express GFAP. Furthermore, Rosenthal fibres may occur in ependymomas and there may be long processes extending from ependymoma cells. In well differentiated ependymomas, the nuclei are round and show little pleomorphism and few mitoses. The main points of differentiation between ependymomas and pilocytic astrocytomas lie in the histological organisation of ependymomas with the presence of pseudorosettes around blood vessels and, occasionally, true rosettes of cuboidal ependymal cells. In a cryostat or paraffin section stained with H & E, pseudo-rosettes in ependymomas appear as pink eosinophilic halos of fine, GFAP positive fibrillary processes around blood vessels. A further point of distinction between the two tumours is the structure of the blood vessels. Although both tumours may show hyalinisation of blood vessel walls, the complex multichannelled blood vessels seen in pilocytic astrocytomas (Figs 4.13 and 4.14) are not usually seen in ependymomas. It is important to make the distinction between pilocytic astrocytoma and ependymoma, as the prognosis and treatment for each tumour differ. Surgical excision of pilocytic astrocytoma is frequently successful, whereas ependymomas may spread more readily through the subarachnoid space and thus the prognosis is not as favourable. Furthermore, radiotherapy or chemotherapy is more likely to be considered for ependymoma than for pilocytic astrocytoma.

Ganglioglioma

Ganglioglioma (see Chapter 8) is often entertained in the differential diagnosis of pilocytic astrocytoma. Gangliogliomas also affect children and young adults and are well-demarcated, often cystic, neoplasms. Both may present as large cysts with mural nodules. The cyst walls and glial component of gangliogliomas can closely resemble pilocytic astrocytoma. For instance, granular bodies may be numerous, Rosenthal fibres may be present (particularly in cyst walls) and nuclear cytological features tend to be bland. The main diagnostic finding to support a diagnosis of ganglioglioma is the presence of large neoplastic neuronal cells that resemble ganglion cells. These often have a decidedly neuronal appearance, with large nuclei and prominent, large nucleoli, as well as granular, basophilic cytoplasmic material that resembles Nissl substance. These cells can be distinguished from trapped normal neurons by their variable appearance from cell to cell and their irregular distribution, as normal groups of neurons appear relatively homogeneous in appearance and distribution. Binucleate neuronal cells as well as ganglion cells abutting one another should raise the suspicion of neoplastic ganglion cells. Immunohistochemistry for markers such as synaptophysin and Neu N may be of great help in establishing the neuronal nature of these cells. In addition to the ganglion cells, the glial component of gangliogliomas often has other features that may help distinguish it from pilocytic astrocytoma – although no one of these is diagnostic by itself. The glial component of ganglioglioma, in comparison with pilocytic astrocytoma, usually has plumper, less elongated cells, fewer Rosenthal fibers, more lymphocytic cuffs around blood vessels and more irregular, vascular malformation-like blood vessels.

Cavernous haemangioma

Cavernous haemangioma may occur in the cerebellum and pilocytic astrocytoma may be confused with this lesion, particularly if there is a prominent hyalinised vascular component to the pilocytic astrocytoma. Both lesions enhance and both are prone to haemorrhage. Distinction between the two lesions lies in the identification of pilocytic astrocytoma cells. Reliance should not be placed upon the presence of Rosenthal fibres, as these may occur in the gliotic tissue around cavernous haemangiomas. Detection of elongated pilocytic astrocytoma cells is a more reliable index for the presence of the tumour. Using immunocytochemistry for GFAP as a guide, groups of pilocytic astrocytoma cells can be identified and their nature confirmed by the presence of nuclei which are usually oval and frequently possess small nucleoli which are unlike the smaller darker nuclei present in chronic gliosis, which do not exhibit the same small, but prominent, nucleoli.

Arteriovenous malformation

Arteriovenous malformation also shares the propensity for haemorrhage shown by pilocytic astrocytomas and such lesions occur in the cerebellum. The presence of large, irregular, poorly formed arterial and venous vessels with collagenous walls in the arteriovenous malformation will help to distinguish it from pilocytic astrocytoma. Nevertheless, care must be taken to ensure that the gliotic tissue between the vessels does not have the cytological appearances of the pilocytic astrocytoma cells described in the section on cavernous haemangioma.

Cerebellar haemangioblastoma

Cerebellar haemangioblastoma may be confused with cerebellar pilocytic astrocytoma both clinically and pathologically. Both lesions may be cystic and, although the enhancing characteristics of cerebellar haemangioblastoma may differ from that of pilocytic astrocytoma, both may present as nodules in the wall of the cyst. However, the most confusing feature of cerebellar haemangioblastoma is that the cyst wall, away from the main tumour nodule, may show extensive gliosis with prominent Rosenthal fibre formation, which may be confused with pilocytic astrocytoma. Discussion with the surgeon with regard to the site of the biopsy is an obvious first step to avoid confusion between these two lesions; if the main nodule of haemangioblastoma is biopsied, the diagnosis should be immediately apparent as the tumour tissue is often yellow and red in colour due to the presence of lipid and on cryostat section, the haemangioblastoma cells are gathered in small packets and contain sudanophilic lipid. On paraffin sections, the groups of cells in haemangioblastoma are surrounded by reticulin and the blood vessels have thin walls with fine branches, quite distinct from the more hyalinised vessels of the pilocytic astrocytoma. Astrocytic elements are rarely seen in the centre of the haemangioblastoma. If the main nodule of the tumour is not available and distinction between pilocytic astrocytoma and haemangioblastoma must be made on the wall of the cyst, the cytological characteristics of the glial cells and Rosenthal fibres will be the main guide to the identity of the lesion. As described above with cavernous haemangioma, the nuclear characteristics of pilocytic astrocytoma cells differ from those of chronic longstanding gliosis. Furthermore, large sheets of Rosenthal fibres suggest longstanding gliosis rather than pilocytic astrocytoma, as the Rosenthal fibres are more widely separated within the tumour.

Metastatic carcinoma

Metastatic carcinoma may enter the differential diagnosis, particularly with enhancing cerebellar lesions and, more rarely, with single enhancing cerebral lesions in adults. Histologically, the cytological features of pilocytic astrocytoma, with its elongated GFAP positive cells should be clearly distinguished from the epithelial or anaplastic carcinomatous elements of the metastasis. Although metastatic sarcomas may superficially resemble pilocytic astrocytoma, the presence of reticulin within the sarcoma and the presence of GFAP expression in the pilocytic astrocytoma will help to distinguish these two lesions even on very small biopsies.

Vestibular Schwannoma

Vestibular Schwannoma presents as an enhancing lesion in the cerebellar pontine angle in adults. There is usually a clear history of deafness and the consistency of the tumour at surgery is usually much firmer than that of pilocytic astrocytoma. However, a small biopsy from a vestibular Schwannoma adjacent to the cerebellum may be confused histologically with a pilocytic astrocytoma, due to the spindle cell nature of both tumours. However, the presence of an intimate reticulin network in the Schwannoma and the presence of GFAP expression in pilocytic astrocytoma should allow distinction between the two tumours despite the shared expression of S-100 protein by both tumours.

Other astrocytic tumours

Other astrocytic tumours should also be included in the differential diagnosis of pilocytic astrocytoma. Although in most cases the pilocytic nature of the tumour would be obvious from the presence of Rosenthal fibres, such structures are not always present in pilocytic astrocytomas. The main distinction between diffuse astrocytoma and pilocytic astrocytoma lies in a careful analysis of the clinical history, radiological appearances and the histology. Diffuse astrocytomas do not enhance, are poorly circumscribed radiologically and show nuclear hyperchromasia and fine astrocytic processes. Pilocytic astrocytomas, on the other hand, enhance, are usually well defined, and, although nuclear hyperchromasia may be seen within pilocytic astrocytomas, the pilocytic cells in smears and paraffin sections are unlike the more stellate cells in diffuse astrocytomas. A further distinction can be seen in the blood vessels with the multichannelled and often hyaline blood vessels of pilocytic astrocytoma contrasting with the delicate thin walled vessels of a diffuse astrocytoma. For distinguishing pilocytic astrocytoma from anaplastic astrocytoma, Ki-67/MIB-1 immunocytochemistry will show a proliferation rate in anaplastic astrocytoma which is much higher than in pilocytic astrocytoma unless anaplastic change has occurred.

Genetics

Pilocytic astrocytomas differ clinically and histopathologically from the diffuse, fibrillary astrocytoma that arise in adults; accordingly, they differ genetically as well. Because pilocytic astrocytomas frequently affect patients with NF1 and the *NF1* gene maps to chromosome 17q11.2, pilocytic astrocytomas show allelic loss of chromosome 17q in about one-quarter of cases.[11] These data suggest the presence of a tumour suppressor gene on 17q that is associated with pilocytic astrocytomas. While the logical candidate for this gene is the NF1 tumour suppressor gene, analysis of the *NF1* gene in sporadic pilocytic astrocytomas has shown paradoxical up-regulation.[37] The other genetic changes that are so common in diffuse, fibrillary astrocytomas, however, including *TP53* mutations, *CDKN2A/p16* deletions and *EGFR* amplification, are rare in pilocytic astrocytomas.

Therapy and prognosis

Pilocytic astrocytomas are among the most benign of the astrocytic tumours. They grow slowly and rarely undergo anaplastic change; unlike diffuse astrocytomas, the prognosis of pilocytic astrocytomas does not relate to the Ki-67/MIB-1 or the p53 labelling indices.[38] Nevertheless, a significant proportion of pilocytic astrocytomas are associated with intracranial haemorrhage and, if incompletely excised, these tumours do recur. The treatment of choice is surgical excision and, particularly for cerebellar astrocytomas, the overall 25-year survival rate has been estimated at 75%. Repeated excision may be required. Similar treatment may be successful in occipital lobe pilocytic astrocytomas. Treatment is more complicated for optic nerve and hypothalamic pilocytic astrocytomas. Complete surgical excision is often impractical and radiotherapy may be employed to slow the growth of these tumours. Radiotherapy may have long term consequences with the induction of second tumours of the CNS. Chemotherapy has also been employed for surgically inaccessible pilocytic astrocytomas.

Subependymal giant cell astrocytoma

Incidence and site

This tumour occurs as part of the tuberous sclerosis complex which is an autosomal dominantly inherited multisystem disorder characterised by hamartomas and benign tumours (see Chapter 19). Patients with tuberous sclerosis are predisposed to develop cortical hamartomas (tubers), which are associated with extensive gliosis (sclerosis); they also develop subependymal giant cell astrocytomas and a number of extraneural manifestations.[39]

Clinical features

Patients with tuberous sclerosis mainly present with epilepsy and autistic withdrawal or with mild mental retardation and behavioural disorders.[40] Fully developed cases present before the age of 10 years and the incidence is between 1 in 5000 and 1 in 10 000 of the population. Formes frustes of the disease are such that relatives of patients who present with this disease may have a number of minor lesions, which include the cerebral lesions, adenoma sebaceum, shagreen patches and peri- and subungual fibromata. A number of patients also develop angiomyolipomas of the kidney or cardiac rhabdomyomas which may grow in atria and obstruct blood flow. A variety of other lesions is also described.[39]

Subependymal giant cell astrocytoma most commonly occurs in the brain but can arise in the retina. The cerebral tumours have an incidence of 6% in confirmed cases of tuberous sclerosis complex but isolated tumours are often considered a forme fruste of the disease.[40,41] It usually presents under the age of 20 with worsening of epilepsy or raised intracranial pressure.

Radiology

Tumours can be identified radiologically as nodules arising in the walls of the lateral ventricles and extending into the third ventricle with obstruction of the foramina of Munro. Calcification may be seen and spontaneous haemorrhage may occur in these lesions.

Pathology

Macroscopic features

The brain of a patient with tuberous sclerosis complex shows firm nodules of gliotic hamartomatous tissue in the cortex or in the central grey matter of the brain. Subependymal giant cell astrocytomas appear as irregular nodules or streaks on the ventricular aspect of the central grey matter, often referred to as 'candle guttering' because of the drip-like appearance of the nodules.

Intraoperative diagnosis

Rapid intraoperative diagnosis of these tumours relies upon the recognition of the large giant astrocytes, both in cryostat sections and in smears. It is often not possible to reach a definitive diagnosis until there has been a thorough examination of the paraffin sections.

Histological features

Paraffin sections of subependymal giant cell astrocytomas reveal a heterogeneous population of cells. These cells include both astrocytic and neuronal elements. The large cells include polygonal cells with eosinophilic cytoplasm and granular nuclei with distinct nucleoli, giving the appearance of ganglion cells (Fig. 4.17). Other large cells have more hypochromatic nuclei and eosinophilic glassy cytoplasm, more resembling atypical astrocytes as seen elsewhere in the brain of patients with tuberous sclerosis (see Chapter 19). Admixed with the giant cells is a population of smaller and spindled astrocytic cells. These smaller cells may form the dominant population of the tumour; indeed, some subependymal giant cell astrocytomas are nearly exclusively composed of spindled cells. Calcification may be prominent in these lesions, with some tumours having extensive central cores of course mineralised debris. Some mineral deposits have the appearance of psammoma bodies, but most are ill-defined and not concentrically laminated. The border with normal brain is sharp, and is well demonstrated in post-mortem samples from tuberous sclerosis patients,

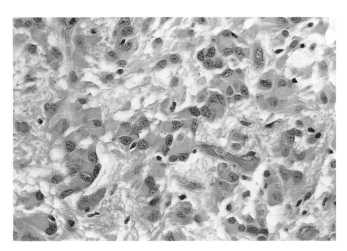

Fig. 4.17 **Subependymal giant cell astrocytoma**. Large cells with copious eosinophilic cytoplasm and nuclei with prominent nucleoli; some resemble neurons, others are binucleate. A dense fibrillary background of processes is present. H & E.

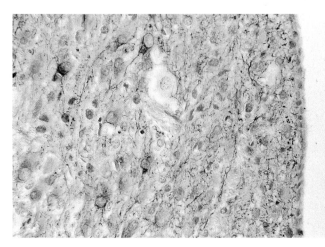

Fig. 4.18 **Subependymal giant cell astrocytoma**. The ependyma is on the right. The tumour cells show variable expression of GFAP with some positive and some negative cells. Immunocytochemistry for GFAP.

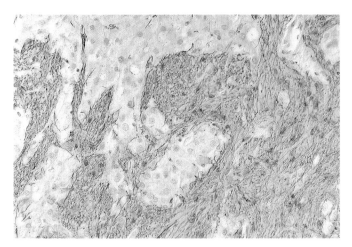

Fig. 4.19 **Subependymal giant cell astrocytoma**. This tumour exhibits variability of GFAP expression. Islands of completely negative cells are surrounded by more fibrillary GFAP positive areas. Immunocytochemistry for GFAP.

although the adjacent brain may contain scattered atypical cells as well as gliosis and other reactive changes. However, in the setting of tuberous sclerosis, atypical cells in the adjacent brain do not necessarily represent tumour infiltraion and more likely are the result of the underlying dysgenetic condition (see Chapter 19). Immunohistochemistry shows variable expression of GFAP (Figs 4.18 and 4.19) and S-100 protein but neuro-filament protein and beta tubulin are also seen in cell processes.[17] Microtubules and dense core vesicles have also been described by electron microscopy in these tumours.[17] Although cells in other lesions associated with tuberous sclerosis express a protein detected by the monoclonal antibody HMB45, subependymal giant cell astrocytomas are negative.[41]

A certain degree of nuclear pleomorphism may be seen histologically but Ki-67/MIB-1 shows low labelling indices.[41] Tumours that recur following excision do not undergo malignant transformation.

The histogenesis of the giant cells in the tubers them-selves appears to be mixed. Immunocytochemistry reveals expression of synaptophysin in many of the neuronal giant cells and GFAP or synaptophysin in the inter-mediate cells.[42,43] Subependymal giant cell astrocytomas show a similar mixture of cell types with expression of glial and neuronal proteins as outlined above. It seems therefore that although these tumours are designated astrocytomas, they are of mixed histogenesis which may be related to the histogenesis of cortical tubers.

Differential diagnosis

The major differential diagnosis of subependymal giant cell astrocytoma is from other tumours arising in the region of the basal ganglia and within the lateral and third ventricles. In patients with an obvious syndrome of tuberous sclerosis, diagnosis of subependymal giant cell astrocytoma may be reasonably certain before biopsy is performed. However, in about one-third of cases, the tumour may be the first manifestation of tuberous sclerosis, or tumour may arise in patients with a forme fruste of the disease. The major differential diagnosis is with other primary tumours occurring in the region of the basal ganglia and ventricles, and these include diffuse astrocytoma, central neurocytoma, ependymoma and choroid plexus papilloma. The young age of the patients (mean age 13 years, with a range of 1–30 years) makes metastatic carcinoma as a differential diagnosis less likely.

Diffuse astrocytoma

Diffuse astrocytoma may arise in central grey matter regions of the brain in young people, but can usually be distinguished from subependymal giant cell astrocytoma by its low density appearance on CT scan and its uniform appearance on MRI. This contrasts with the nodular appearance of subependymal giant cell astrocytoma on imaging and its variable density. Histologically, diffuse astrocytoma lacks the heterogeneity of cell population of subependymal giant cell astrocytoma and on immunocytochemistry, the only cells that express the neuronal markers of neurofilament protein and synaptophysin are normal neurons in tissue infiltrated by astrocytoma cells. Furthermore, the large vesicular nuclei associated with subependymal giant cell astrocytoma are not a feature of diffuse astrocytoma.

Central neurocytoma

Central neurocytoma presents mainly as an intraventricular lesion with enhancement on MRI and CT scan and histologically presents a picture of sheets of uniform cells with small round nuclei and fine fibrillary cytoplasm showing expression of synaptophysin. GFAP expression is only seen in the stromal astrocytes. This picture contrasts with subependymal giant cell astrocytoma which shows considerable cytological heterogeneity and tumour cells expressing GFAP as well as neurofilament protein. It is important to distinguish between these two tumours, as central neurocytoma is largely located in the ventricles and, therefore, more amenable to extirpation and does not carry the same risk of tuberous sclerosis as subependymal giant cell astrocytoma.

Ependymomas

Ependymomas arise within the lateral and third ventricles; they enhance on CT and MRI and present a histological appearance characterised by perivascular pseudorosettes of glial filaments and a moderately uniform nuclear population. These tumours lack the expression of neurofilament protein and the cytological heterogeneity typical of subependymal giant cell astrocytomas. Whereas ependymomas are liable to spread through the ventricular system, dissemination of subependymal giant cell astrocytoma is not usually a significant feature.

Choroid plexus papilloma

Choroid plexus papilloma may arise in the lateral or third ventricles as an enhancing tumour on CT and MRI, usually resulting in obstruction of CSF flow and hydrocephalus. A clear distinction can usually be made between this tumour and subependymal giant cell astrocytoma as choroid plexus papillomas have an epithelial and papillary structure with connective tissue stroma. Such an appearance is quite distinct from the hetero-

geneous glial and neuronal tumour cell population of subependymal giant cell astrocytoma. Choroid plexus papillomas are not associated with tuberous sclerosis and, if excised, have a relatively favourable prognosis.

Genetics

Subependymal giant cell astrocytomas, because of their close association with tuberous sclerosis, have been studied genetically for alterations at the tuberous sclerosis gene loci, *TSC1* on chromosome 9q and *TSC2* on chromosome 16p. Although few tumours have been studied, allelic loss of chromosome 16p in the *TSC2* region has been noted in TS patients who harbour *TSC2* gene mutations, suggesting that the *TSC2* gene functions as a tumour suppressor in these tumours.[44] The situation with *TSC1* is less clear, although some reports have noted chromosome 9q loss in subependymal giant cell astrocytomas.[45] Since there is disagreement as to whether subependymal giant cell astrocytomas are ever truly sporadic tumours or sometimes represent formes frustes of tuberous sclerosis, the role of the *TSC1* and *TSC2* genes in sporadic astrocytoma tumorigenesis remains unclear.

Therapy and prognosis

The prognosis of patients with tuberous sclerosis depends upon a combination of factors within the tuberous sclerosis complex, of which the subependymal giant cell astrocytoma is one factor.[46] These are slow-growing tumours that do not undergo malignant progression. Prognosis is typically related to the location of the tumour and the attendant hydrocephalus. Debulking of the tumour mass may be possible especially if it is mainly within the ventricle, but as these tumours arise from central grey matter regions of the brain, wide excision is for the most part not possible.

Pleomorphic xanthoastrocytoma

Pleomorphic xanthoastrocytoma (PXA) is an astrocytic tumour that most often affects children and young adults, and is distinguished by its superficial meningocerebral location, striking histological appearance and usually benign behaviour.[47–50]

Incidence

PXAs are uncommon tumours, accounting for less than 1% of astrocytic tumours. They usually present in children and young adults, (Fig. 4.20) but occasional cases have been reported in older adults as well. The aetiology of PXA remains unclear and there are no known risk factors, although rare PXAs have been reported in the setting of NF1.[51,52]

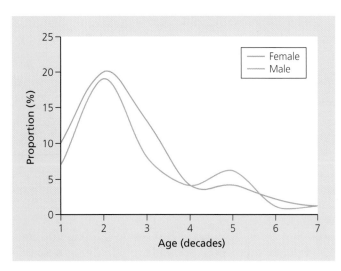

Fig. 4.20 Relative age and sex incidence of pleomorphic xanthoastrocytomas. (Data derived from Ref. 17).

Site

PXAs almost invariably occur as superficial cerebral masses.[48,51] While any of the lobes may be affected, the most common location is the temporal lobe. The tumours often appear as primarily subarachnoid masses. At the same time, they demonstrate attachment to and involvement of the underlying superficial cerebral cortex as well as sometimes conspicuous attachment to the overlying dura mater. Indeed, PXAs may sometimes be confused with primary meningeal tumours on neuroimaging and at surgery. Nonetheless, rare tumours with the histological features of PXA may occur as deep seated cerebral lesions, and PXAs have also been reported in the cerebellum and spinal cord.[53] Thus, an 'atypical' location does not preclude a diagnosis of PXA; however, it is unclear whether PXAs in such anomalous locations have the same good prognosis as the meningocerebral forms.

Clinical features

Patients with PXAs usually present with seizures, with some patients having longstanding seizure disorders.[47–50] The type of seizure varies, but given the propensity for PXAs to arise in the temporal lobe, complex partial seizures may occur. PXAs may also present with symptoms and signs of mass effect, most often with headache. Those rare PXAs that affect infratentorial sites usually present with localising signs to suggest a cerebellar or spinal lesion.

Radiology

Neuroimaging often demonstrates PXAs as superficial masses that are typically, but not always, associated with a cyst. PXAs may enhance with contrast, particularly the mural nodule if the tumour is associated with a cyst.

The cyst contents are fluid and do not enhance, although there may be some highlighting of the tumour periphery. Peritumoral oedema is not prominent, in keeping with the slow growth of these lesions. In some patients with longstanding superficial tumours, overlying skull thinning may be noted. Calcification of the mass may also be present.

Pathology

Macroscopic features

Macroscopically, PXAs vary from being soft to rubbery tan masses. Particularly collagen rich components involving the subarachnoid space are firmer than intra-parenchymal portions. Despite the presence of a xanthomatous component, this is usually not extensive enough to impart a yellowish colour to the mass. Most lesions are nodular, although plaque-like growth may also occur. The tumour commonly forms a nodule in the wall of a smooth walled cyst ('mural nodule'), filled with proteinaceous fluid. PXAs are usually well demarcated from the surrounding brain; in particular, the cyst wall is sharply demarcated. On the other hand, infiltration of the superficial cerebral cortex may make the tumour–cerebrum margin less well defined. However, except in rare cases, this infiltration is not as extensive as that of diffuse, fibrillary astrocytomas.

Intraoperative diagnosis

It may be difficult to make a definitive diagnosis of PXA on smear or cryostat section and the bizarre nature of the cells in the tumour may at first suggest a diagnosis of glioblastoma.[54] However, an oil red O stain for lipid on the cryostat section should reveal the fine lipid droplets within the tumour cells and a reticulin stain will demontrate the fine reticulin stroma of the tumour. In addition, PXAs typically lack the other features of glioblastoma, such as brisk mitotic activity, microvascular proliferation and necrosis with pseudopalisading.

Histological features

In their most classical form, PXAs demonstrate three rather distinctive histological features: marked cytological pleomorphism, xanthomatous changes and prominent reticulin deposition.[47] Nonetheless, many tumours do not display all of these characteristics, and the presence of any of the above features in the setting of a superficial, well demarcated astrocytoma in a young patient should prompt the histopathologist to consider a diagnosis of PXA.

Cellular pleomorphism is the most constant histological feature of these tumours, but may be only focal within any individual lesion. The typical tumour cells are markedly enlarged, with both large nuclei and copious cytoplasm (Fig. 4.21). The nuclei may be bizarre, often

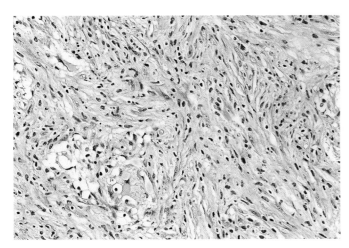

Fig. 4.21 **Pleomorphic xanthoastrocytoma.** There are large cells with multiple nuclei and lipid vacuoles within the cytoplasm. Fascicles of spindle shaped cells are also seen. H & E.

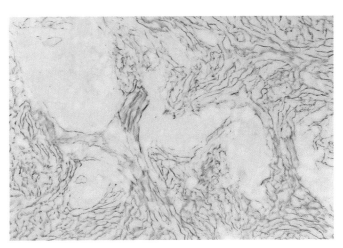

Fig. 4.22 **Pleomorphic xanthoastrocytoma.** A characteristic dense intercellular reticulin network. Reticulin stain.

gigantic and multilobated, sometimes multinucleated, and usually irregularly hyperchromatic. The cytoplasm of these cells tends to be eosinophilic, having an 'astrocytic' appearance, although tapering cell processes, when present, are often short and stubby. This eosinophilic cytoplasm can be demonstrated immunohistochemically to contain GFAP, and ultrastructurally intermediate filaments are apparent. Indeed, it was the demonstration of these astrocytic features that first allowed Kepes and colleagues to separate PXA from xanthomatous mesenchymal lesions of the meninges.[47,49,55]

The cytoplasm of some large cells may be distorted by lipid droplets (Fig. 4.21). Usually, these are multiple and moderate in size; sometimes single droplets may be present in cells, but 'adipocyte-like' cells are rare. These xanthomatous cells can sometimes be highlighted by GFAP staining, since the lipids will appear as negative vacuoles against the silhouette of the GFAP positive cytoplasm. It is important to emphasise, however, that xanthomatous cells may be rare in PXAs, and the diagnosis does not depend on the presence of these cells. Furthermore, as discussed below (see Differential diagnosis), lipidised cells are not specific for PXA among astrocytic tumours. Some glioblastomas may be heavily lipidised (see below) and occasional lipidised cells may be seen in other diffuse astrocytomas as well.

A conspicuous reticulin network is also characteristic of PXA (Fig. 4.22). As with other 'reticulin rich' astrocytic tumours, the reticulin surrounds individual tumour cells, but primarily when the tumour is present in the subarachnoid space. The infiltrating component, which is typically minor and restricted to the superficial cerebrum, does not display much desmoplasia. The reticulin network can be demonstrated by immunocytochemistry for type IV collagen in addition to a standard reticulin stain, and can be seen as extensive pericellular basal lamina by

electron microscopy. Again, a prominent reticulin network does not imply that the tumour is a PXA, as this may be seen in other superficial astrocytic tumours, such as *desmoplastic infantile gangliogliomas*, *desmoplastic cerebral astrocytomas of infancy*, and in *giant cell glioblastomas* and *gliofibromas*.

The combination of pleomorphism, xanthomatous change and reticulin deposition in a superficial meningocerebral astrocytoma is virtually pathognomonic of PXA. Nonetheless, some PXAs show a predominantly spindled pattern to their cells, with only scattered pleomorphic cells. Sometimes these spindle cells may form fascicles or even structures reminiscent of a storiform pattern. For this reason, the diagnosis of PXA should be entertained even in a predominantly spindle cell astrocytic lesion if it is occurring in a superficial location in a young person.

Eosinophilic granular bodies and Rosenthal fibres, histological findings characteristic of pilocytic astrocytomas, may also be found in PXAs. Indeed, eosinophilic granular bodies are quite common and may be numerous. Rosenthal fibres tend to be less plentiful than in pilocytic astrocytomas. Lymphocytic infiltrates, typically composed of perivascular cuffs of reactive T cells, may be conspicuous in PXAs and constitute a classic feature of these lesions.

PXAs have also been reported as components of mixed lesions, particularly in combination with gangliogliomas. In addition, some studies have suggested that typical PXAs may also show immunohistochemical positivity with neuronal markers. Thus, the presence of neuronal cells or immunopositivity for neuronal markers in an otherwise typical PXA should not detract from the diagnosis of PXA.

Immunocytochemistry and electron microscopy

PXAs are GFAP-positive tumours, although the number of GFAP-positive cells varies markedly between tumours. In the absence of extensive GFAP immuno-positivity, S-100 staining may be useful, since most tumours will be S-100 positive. Recent reports have suggested that focal positivity for neuronal markers may be characteristic of PXAs.[48] Other immunohistochemical markers are not of practical help in establishing the diagnosis, but may help in excluding other lesions (see below). In most cases, electron microscopy is not necessary for diagnosis. Ultrastructural findings include typical astrocytic features (see elsewhere in this chapter) with the noted difference of finding discrete basal lamina around many individual cells. While characteristic of PXAs, the presence of discrete basal lamina around astrocytoma cells is not specific and is a feature shared by other astrocytic tumours that either elaborate reticulin from the tumour cells or from involvement of the leptomeninges (e.g. desmoplastic cerebral astrocytoma of infancy).

Spread of PXA

The infiltrative portion of PXA may display single cell invasion, and individual high power fields at the infiltrating margin may look disturbingly like a diffuse, fibrillary astrocytoma. As mentioned above, the cells do not spread as far afield as in diffuse astrocytomas, but this may be little comfort to the histopathologist confronted with a small biopsy of the infiltrative edge of a PXA. Fortunately, most PXAs are surgically accessible lesions and inspection of resected specimens will usually reveal typical PXA in other regions.

Anaplastic PXA

Histological features of malignancy are uncommon in PXAs[56] and, if present, should prompt consideration of other diagnostic possibilities.[57] For instance, mitotic figures should not be plentiful in typical PXAs,[58] nor should proliferative activity as measured immunohisto-chemically (e.g. Ki-67/MIB-1 indices) be high. Necrosis is also not common[59] and, when present, appears infarctive in nature, without pseudopalisading. Endothelial proliferation, particularly glomeruloid vascular proliferation, is uncommon. The presence of these findings (substantial mitotic activity, necrosis and vascular proliferation) should call the diagnosis of PXA into doubt and prompt consideration of glioblastoma. Nonetheless, some tumours with convincing, classical features of PXA display such microscopic features of malignancy. The terminology for such lesions is confusing, with some authors endorsing the term 'anaplastic PXA'[60] and others preferring the term 'pleomorphic xanthoastrocytoma with anaplastic features'.[48] Some of these lesions may be glioblastomas arising in the setting of a PXA; such tumours may have a somewhat better prognosis than standard glioblastomas, but large series of similar tumours are not available to address this question.

Differential diagnosis

The differential diagnosis of PXA centres on two issues: establishing that the lesion is astrocytic and excluding histological features of malignancy. In the characteristic clinical setting of a superficial meningocerebral, cystic tumour in a young person with seizures, consideration of PXA in the differential diagnosis will prompt obtaining GFAP immunocytochemistry if the tumour has bizarre cytological features. If the tumour is GFAP positive and has other features of PXA (e.g. lipidised cells, reticulin deposition, inflammation), the diagnosis is relatively straightforward. Notably, GFAP immunoreactivity may be relatively focal, in which case staining for S-100 protein may be more extensive. If histological features of malignancy are conspicuous, a diagnosis of anaplastic or malignant PXA may be suggested if the tumour otherwise resembles a PXA.

Glioblastoma

Glioblastoma and a number of glioblastoma variants have pathological features that may mimic PXA. For instance, giant cell glioblastomas display huge, monstrous giant cells and may be superficial, well demarcated tumours. The giant cells of giant cell glioblastoma, however, are often mitotically active, with highly atypical mitotic figures, and feature larger, more multinucleated and hyperchromatic bizarre nuclei, without the glassy, eosinophilic cytoplasm typical of PXA. Similarly, some glioblastoma may be heavily lipidised.[61] Thus, the presence of markedly pleomorphic or lipidised cells is not sufficient to diagnose PXA, and it may be impossible to distinguish such giant cell or heavily lipidised glioblastomas from PXAs transforming into glioblastomas.

Ganglioglioma

Ganglioglioma is usually a superficial, often temporal lobe tumour that is cystic and well demarcated and which may be associated with a long history of seizures. It may thus be confused with PXA. Gangliogliomas also feature large cells with prominent nucleoli and commonly have eosinophilic granular bodies and prominent inflammation. A careful search for ganglion cells is therefore required to distinguish gangliogliomas from PXA. In addition, the astrocytic component in ganglioglioma is composed of small, bland-appearing astrocytic cells, often in a coarsely fibrillary background; this appearance differs markedly from the bizarre astrocytic cells of PXA with their inconspicuous background fibrillarity. However, gangliogliomas and PXAs may rarely coexist;[62,63] thus, the presence of one does not exclude the possibility of a second lesion existing as well in the same overall tumour.

Subependymal giant cell astrocytoma

Subependymal giant cell astrocytoma is the other type of astrocytoma that consistently features large cells, often with a spindle cell component as well. Usually, the periventricular location and association with tuberous sclerosis clarifies any possible confusion with PXA. In rare cases of deep seated PXAs, however, the bizarre pleomorphic PXA cells should be readily distinguishable from the rather uniform 'ganglioid' subependymal giant cell astrocytoma cells. The remaining entities in the differential diagnosis of PXA involve the differential diagnosis of astrocytomas in general and are discussed elsewhere in this chapter.

Genetics

While pleomorphic xanthoastrocytomas are typically slowly growing astrocytic tumours that predominantly affect young adults and are sometimes amenable to surgical cure, some PXAs recur as glioblastomas. However, the genetic events that underlie PXA formation and progression appear to differ from those involved in diffuse astrocytoma tumorigenesis.[64] While PXAs may have *TP53* mutations, the mutations are somewhat different from those usually found in diffuse, astrocytic tumours.[64] In addition, although *EGFR* gene amplification has not been noted in PXAs, glioblastomas that arise from PXAs can display *EGFR* gene amplification. Furthermore, allelic losses of chromosomes 9, 10 and 19q have not been noted in PXA.[64]

Therapy and prognosis

Most PXAs are superficial and well demarcated, making their surgical extirpation practicable. Thus, surgery remains the mainstay of treatment for PXAs, effecting apparent cures in a large percentage of cases and recorded survival of 40 years.[65] Unfortunately, a small number of PXAs display a propensity for recurrence and for transformation to anaplastic astrocytomas and glioblastomas.[57,66] Clearly, those tumours that have histological features of malignancy at the time of initial diagnosis have a greater chance for aggressive behaviour and such tumours may be candidates for other treatments such as radiation therapy. Some tumours, however, appear histologically benign at first diagnosis but recur years after resection as malignant lesions. At the time of recurrence, such tumours are treated in a similar way to anaplastic astrocytomas and glioblastomas, with radiation and chemotherapy.

Chordoid glioma of the third ventricle

Chordoid gliomas are rare tumours and have only been reported in the anterior third ventricle of adults, primarily in women.[67,68] They are well demarcated tumours that compress the adjacent brain, resulting in extensive gliosis and Rosenthal fibre deposition, as well as reactive inflammatory changes in the brain. While chordoid gliomas of the third ventricle are slow growing lesions, their deep seated location makes complete resection problematic.

Chordoid glioma of the third ventricle[65] is characterised microscopically by cords and aggregates of epithelioid cells in a prominent myxoid background, giving these tumours a distinctly 'chordoid' appearance (Fig. 4.23). The cells are glial, and often stain strongly for GFAP on immunohistochemical analysis (Fig. 4.24).[67,69] Cytologically, some of the tumour cells have glial features, with astrocytic nuclei and glassy, eosinophilic cytoplasm that sometimes forms processes – 'epithelioid gemistocytes'. Recent ultrastructural studies have shown evidence of ependymal differentiation.[70] Mitotic activity is absent or

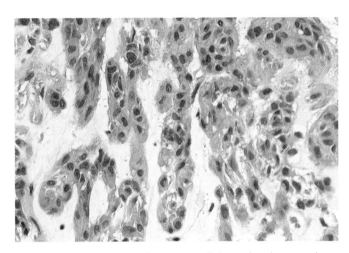

Fig. 4.23 Chordoid glioma. The tumour cells have abundant cytoplasm with irregular processes and are arranged in cords and clusters within a myxoid matrix. H & E.

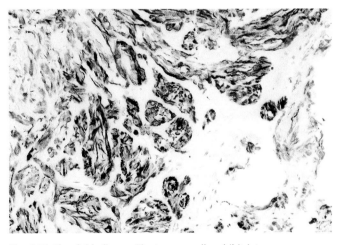

Fig. 4.24 Chordoid glioma. The tumour cells exhibit intense immunoreactivity for GFAP, which also demonstrates the irregular cell processes. The myxoid matrix is unstained.

rare and proliferation indices are low. Inflammation is typically prominent, with numerous lymphocytes and plasma cells. The plasma cell infiltrate may be accompanied by Russell bodies. Fibrosis is also common, often with broad collagen rich zones. Proliferation rates appear to be low with Ki-67/MIB-1 labelling of up to 5%.[66,71] No chromosomal imbalances have been detected by comparative genomic hybridisation; molecular genetic analyses have shown no abnormalities in *TP53* or *CDKN2A* and no amplification of *EGFR*, *CDK4* or *MDM2*.[71]

The major differential diagnostic entities are pituitary adenoma and meningioma; knowledge of chordoid gliomas and their expression of GFAP on immunocytochemistry should help to exclude these other possibilities. As more cases of this rare neoplasm are reported, the clinico-pathological entity of chordoid glioma will no doubt become better defined and diagnostic issues and approaches refined.

Astroblastoma

Astroblastomas were originally described by Bailey and Bucy in 1930. They are rare, but may occur as a pure form in young adults or children;[72,73] although astroblastomas have been recorded at 70 years of age.[74] Most common in the cerebral hemispheres, they also occur in the cerebellum, optic nerves, brain stem and cauda equina as well defined lesions which often enhance on CT or MRI.

Macroscopically, astroblastomas are well circumscribed with a homogeneous cut surface, with or without cyst formation or necrosis.

Histologically, astroblastomas have a varied appearance. In many cases, the nuclei tend to be oval to elongated and hyperchromatic. The amount of cytoplasm ranges from scant, with thin and tapering processes, to more eosinophilic broad processes. The tumour has a characteristic appearance of perivascular pseudorosette formation in which stout, non-tapering cell processes of astrocytes radiate towards a central, often hyalinised, blood vessel (Fig. 4.25).[72,73] Astroblastomas range from those with few mitoses and little proliferation to other tumours which have a high mitotic rate and cellular atypia. Immunocytochemistry reveals expression of GFAP, vimentin and S-100 in the tumour cells and electron microscopy reveals 10 nm intermediate filaments in the cell processes.[72,74] Although the pure form of astroblastoma is rare, areas that resemble astroblastoma may be seen in glioblastomas.

Concerning *differential diagnosis*, the most important consideration in astroblastomas is to distinguish them from ependymomas. The perivascular pseudorosettes in astroblastomas are rather different from those in

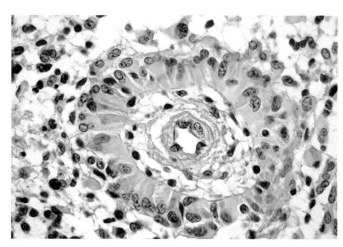

Fig. 4.25 **Astroblastoma.** Tumour cells surround and send out broad processes to a central vessel. The background tumour cells are characteristically loosely arranged. H & E.

ependymomas. In astroblastomas, the perivascular cell processes are thick and chunky, whereas in ependymomas, halos of very fine GFAP positive processes are arranged around blood vessels. Perhaps the most important technique for distinguishing astroblastomas from ependymomas is electron microscopy; ependymomas contain cilia which are absent in astroblastomas.

The *prognosis* of astroblastoma is best judged on its mitotic rate, the Ki-67/MIB-1 labelling index, the size and site of the tumour and its extent of surgical excision. Those tumours with a high proliferation rate behave clinically in a similar way to anaplastic astrocytoma.

Diffuse astrocytic tumours

Classification and grading

The diffuse, fibrillary astrocytomas are often separated from the 'other' astrocytomas for practical and, to some extent, biological reasons, since they are by far the most common type of astrocytoma. These tumours have been termed 'diffuse' because of their tendency to infiltrate the brain parenchyma in a diffuse manner, but this property is not unique to the diffuse, fibrillary astrocytomas. Similarly, while they have been termed 'fibrillary' to highlight their fibrillary histopathological nature, such fibrillar characteristics are not unique to these astrocytic tumours. Nonetheless, diffuse, fibrillary astrocytomas are recognised histologically by their irregular and atypical astrocytic glial nuclei scattered in a glial fibrillary background.

Distinction of diffuse astrocytomas from other astrocytic tumours such as pilocytic astrocytoma, PXA and subependymal giant cell astrocytoma is, however, not absolute. For instance, a seemingly distinct tumour such as the PXA can recur as a typical glioblastoma.

Astrocytic components also figure prominently in a number of 'mixed' tumours in which there is a mixture of neoplastic astrocytic cells and non-astrocytic tumour cells. Included under the rubric of 'mixed' tumours would be entities such as ganglioglioma, in which astrocytoma and neoplastic neurons co-mingle, and oligoastrocytoma, in which astrocytoma merges with oligodendroglioma. Again, however, these 'mixed' tumours may overlap with the group of diffuse astrocytomas, including at the molecular genetic level (see below).

Overview of grading schemes

Grading schemes for diffuse, fibrillary astrocytomas have proliferated almost as rapidly as the glioblastoma itself. From a historical point of view, there are two schools of astrocytoma grading, one begun by Bailey and Cushing in the late 1920s[75] and one by Kernohan in the late 1940s.[76] Most of the currently used systems are derived directly or indirectly from one of these two original systems. Some of the better known grading schemes are tabulated below. From the table, it is apparent that there are two major types of grading system: those that use numbers (left side of Table 4.4) and those that use names (right side of Table 4.4). The grading systems that use numbers trace their ancestry to the Kernohan scheme, while those that use names are largely derived from the Bailey and Cushing scheme.

The Kernohan types of system are based on the notion of dedifferentiation, implying that higher grades of tumours arise through a process of progressive dedifferentiation or anaplasia from lower grades: a grade 4 tumour is more 'anaplastic' or dedifferentiated than a grade 2. At the theoretical heart of such a scheme is the concept that glioblastoma (grade 4) arises from lower grade astrocytoma. In fact, this can occur in clinical practice; a patient who originally had a grade 2 tumour may present a few years later with a grade 4 lesion. Most of the grading schemes that use numbers (left side of table) are based on this idea. The table also illustrates that the original Kernohan scheme attempted to subclassify higher grade astrocytomas, reserving two grades for glioblastoma. Because the original Kernohan scheme has proved somewhat impractical, it has fallen out of favour with most neuropathologists.

The Bailey and Cushing classification scheme, on the other hand, was based on the concept that the neoplastic cells resemble their histogenetic counterparts. The existence, however, of a distinct 'astroblast' or 'glioblast' in the normal development of the human brain still remains an area of controversy. Nonetheless, the current division of diffuse, fibrillary astrocytomas into astrocytoma, anaplastic astrocytoma and glioblastoma theoritically reflects these original concepts. (The term 'astroblastoma' is now reserved for a specific type of astrocytic tumour, and has been replaced in this context by 'anaplastic astrocytoma' or 'malignant astrocytoma'.) The three tiered, Ringertz type systems are the most popular of these systems.[76–80] This modified Ringertz system[80] is also used by the WHO, and correlates with the WHO grades II–IV.[17] It is of interest that these grading systems do not necessarily imply progression of lower grade tumours to higher grade tumours; it remains possible that some higher grade tumours such as the glioblastoma arise 'de novo'. In fact, in clinical practice, most patients with glioblastoma present with a rapidly growing mass, without any history of a prior lower grade lesion.

One further confusing feature of some numerical grading systems for adult, supratentorial astrocytomas is that they run from grade II to grade IV, and do not really include a grade I. In the WHO system, this is because the grade I designation is reserved for benign tumours such as the pilocytic astrocytoma, which is completely different from the diffuse, fibrillary astrocytoma.[82] In the St Anne/Mayo scheme, the essential absence of a grade 1 reflects the inability to diagnose an astrocytoma without at least one of the four criteria (see discussion below). Because cytological atypia is, for all intents and purposes, necessary to diagnose an astrocytoma, the lowest possible St Anne/Mayo grade has one of the four histological features and is therefore grade 2.

WHO grading system

The WHO grading system is a readily applicable and simple system for the assessment of all brain tumours, including astrocytomas. For the diffuse, fibrillary astrocytic tumours, the WHO system recognises diffuse astrocytoma as grade II of IV, anaplastic astrocytoma as

Table 4.4 Grading schemes for diffuse fibrillary dystrocytomas

Kernohan 1949	St A/M current	WHO current	Ringertz current	UCSF current	Bailey and Cushing 1926, 1930
1	2	II	Astrocytoma	MoAA	Astrocytoma
2	3	III	Anaplastic astrocytoma	HAA	Astroblastoma
3	4	IV	GBM	GBM	Spongioblastoma multiforme
4					

GBM, glioblastoma multiforme; HAA, highly anaplastic astrocytoma; UCSF, University of California, San Francisco (compare with WHO 2000 classification in Table 4.1a); MoAA, moderately anaplastic astrocytoma; St A/M, St Anne/Mayo

grade III of IV, and glioblastoma as WHO grade IV of IV. (WHO grade I is reserved for pilocytic astrocytomas and other biologically benign tumours.) The 1993/2000 revised WHO classifications adopted some features of the St Anne/Mayo system, which has made the revised WHO approach more objective than the 1979 WHO system. Nonetheless, the 1993/2000 WHO grading schemes retain a healthy amount of subjectivity. For some neuropathologists, the latitude provided by the WHO definitions is a welcome opportunity to infuse some clinicopathological experience into evaluating these tumours.

The WHO defines grade II diffuse astrocytoma as 'an astrocytic neoplasm characterised by a high degree of cellular differentiation, slow growth and diffuse infiltration of neighbouring brain structures.[17]

Grade III anaplastic astrocytoma is defined by the WHO as 'a diffusely infiltrating astrocytoma with focal or dispersed anaplasia and a marked proliferative potential.[17] The definition is slightly openended; significantly, it does not *require* the presence of increased cellularity, nuclear atypia, pleomorphism and mitotic activity, but implies only that they may be present. The absence of necessary features therefore allows the diagnosis of anaplastic astrocytoma, WHO grade III, solely on the basis of the pathologist perceiving histological features of anaplasia. Thus, a moderately hypercellular tumour (i.e. an increase in nuclear : cytoplasmic ratio) with moderately anaplastic nuclei may be designated grade III in the absence of mitotic figures. Significantly, the WHO criteria prohibit the presence of vascular proliferation and necrosis in grade III tumours: 'vascular proliferation and necrosis are absent'.[17] The presence of either of these two histological features necessitates an upgrade to WHO grade IV. This is a significant departure from previous popular grading schemes which have allowed endothelial (microvascular) proliferation in grade III anaplastic astrocytomas. The insistence on a diagnosis of glioblastoma, WHO grade IV, in the presence of vascular proliferation alone is supported by recent clinicopathological studies demonstrating that glioblastomas diagnosed on the basis of vascular proliferation alone follow clinical courses similar to glioblastomas with necrosis.[83]

Grade IV glioblastoma (the WHO uses the term 'glioblastoma' rather than 'glioblastoma multiforme') is defined by the WHO as 'the most malignant astrocytic tumour, composed of poorly differentiated neoplastic astrocytes. Histopathological features include cellular pleomorphism, nuclear atypia, brisk mitotic activity, vascular thrombosis, microvascular proliferation and necrosis.' Essential for the histological diagnosis is the presence of microvascular proliferation and/or necrosis.[17,81] This defintion is the most exact of the three grades and allows the diagnosis of WHO IV on the basis of either vascular proliferation or necrosis. Nonetheless, the type of necrosis is not specified; either geographic, infarctive necrosis or necrosis with pseudopalisading is sufficient. Nor is a definition of vascular proliferation offered. Thus, again, there is some latitude in cases with plump endothelium that may fall short, in the eyes of some pathologists, of frank vascular proliferation.

St Anne/Mayo grading system

This recently popularised grading system is a simple, objective and reproducible scheme for grading adult, supratentorial, diffuse, fibrillary astrocytomas.[84] Originally described by Daumas-Duport in the early 1980s,[85] the scheme has been referred to as the Daumas-Duport system, but has more recently been termed the St Anne/Mayo system.[82,86] *It is important to note that the system was designed for use on adult, supratentorial, diffuse, fibrillary astrocytomas, and has not been evaluated in the assessment of other astrocytomas.* The system is based on assessing the presence or absence of only four histological features (note the acronym 'AMEN'):

1. atypia (cytological)
2. mitotic figures
3. endothelial proliferation
4. necrosis

If no features are present, the astrocytoma is a grade 1. (Note that the St Anne/Mayo system uses Arabic numerals, rather than the Roman numerals used by the WHO.) As stated above, because it is difficult to diagnose an astrocytoma without at least some cytological atypia, grade 1 tumours are essentially not found in the St Anne/Mayo scheme. If one feature is present, the tumour is designated grade 2. This feature is most commonly cytological atypia, for the above-stated reason. If two features are present, the tumour is designated grade 3. This second feature is usually mitotic activity. The presence of even a single mitotic figure is presumed to be of enough importance to change a tumour from a grade 2 to a grade 3, although the ability to find a single mitosis is obviously subject to sampling error.[87] If either three or four features are present, the tumour is a grade 4. The system is summarised in Table 4.5.

The grading system is simple, since it assesses the presence or absence of four histological features that are well known to all pathologists. The system is therefore also relatively objective. Because of these two features, simplicity and objectivity, the system should

Table 4.5 St Anne/Mayo grading system

Four features	If	Then ....
Atypia	1 feature present	grade 2
Mitotic figures	2 features present	grade 3
Endothelial proliferation	3, 4 features present	grade 4
Necrosis		

provide a means of standardising astrocytoma grading between different centres, including centres without neuropathologists.

There are, however, some potential problems with the St Anne/Mayo scheme. The system may assign lower grades than the WHO scheme in two important situations.

1. In a case with cytological atypia and necrosis, but without either mitotic figures or endothelial proliferation, the St Anne/Mayo would assign a grade 3. However, it has been shown in numerous studies that necrosis alone is sufficient to assign a tumour to the highest grade.[88,89] One study of the St Anne/Mayo system showed that those 'grade 3' tumours with atypia and necrosis did as poorly as grade 4 tumours.[90] Therefore, the St Anne/Mayo system tends to undergrade tumours with just atypia and necrosis.

2. Similarly, the St Anne/Mayo system may undergrade densely cellular tumours with atypical nuclei but without mitotic figures. These tumours are assigned a grade 2, but appear to be highly malignant histologically and would be assigned a grade III by the WHO. The subjective opinion of most neuropathologists is that these tumours would be more appropriately designated grade III.

It is important to realise that such discrepancies are not common, and there is in general good concordance between the two systems, especially given the recent adjustments to the WHO system.[82] The most discordant grading, in our experience, has been in the distinction of grade II/2 from grade III/3 tumours.[91] As mentioned above, the WHO will allow a grade III designation in hypercellular tumours without mitotic activity, while the St Anne/Mayo system requires mitotic activity. We have found that clinical course and proliferative activity, as measured by Ki-67/MIB-1 labelling indices, is more accurately reflected by the WHO grade of III in these cases.[91]

Terminology

Undoubtedly grading systems are useful for the communication of diagnostic and prognostic information between pathologists and clinicians, but there is potential for confusion in the terminology for astrocytic tumours due to the many different histological systems of nomenclature and grading. The terms 'low grade glioma' or 'low grade astrocytoma' are occasionally used but these terms do not distinguish diffuse astrocytomas from pilocytic astrocytomas which have a different prognosis and biological behaviour.[16] In order to avoid any possible confusion in the present account of astrocytic tumours, we will follow the terminology used in the WHO

1993/2000 classifications.[17,81] It is, however, recognised that the WHO classification (Table 4.1) is not perfect and that criteria adopted for adult tumours may not adequately fit childhood tumours.[92,93] The following terms will be used for diffuse astrocytic tumours:

Diffuse astrocytoma
    fibrillary, protoplasmic and gemistocytic subtypes
Anaplastic astrocytoma
Glioblastoma
    Variants:
       giant cell glioblastoma
       gliosarcoma
Gliomatosis cerebri

We leave the reader to adopt grading systems as required using Table 4.4 for conversions.

Diffuse astrocytoma

Diffuse astrocytomas are slowly growing, diffuse well differentiated tumours. They arise most commonly in the cerebral hemispheres of young adults, aged 20–40 years, but also occur in the pons, medulla and spinal cord, particularly in children and adolescents. Such tumours may present clinically with epilepsy, focal neurological signs and raised intracranial pressure. One of the major complications of cerebral diffuse astrocytomas is the high incidence of anaplastic change which may occur during the early stages of tumour growth or 5 or 10 years after presentation.[94–97]

Incidence

Diffuse astrocytomas constitute less than 10% of primary cerebral tumours,[94,98,99] but a higher proportion of primary brain stem and spinal cord tumours. There is a peak incidence of diffuse astrocytoma between 30 and 40 years of age, with an equal male and female sex ratio in adults but a slight male predominance under the age of 20 years (Fig. 4.26). Ten per cent of diffuse astrocytomas occur below the age of 20 and 60% between the ages of 20 and 45 years.[97]

Site

The majority of diffuse astrocytomas occur in the cerebral hemispheres with predilection for temporal lobes and frontal lobes (Fig. 4.27). Approximately 20% involve the central grey matter areas, such as the thalamus and basal ganglia. Most of the cerebellar, brain stem (Table 4.3) and spinal cord diffuse astrocytomas occur in children.[99]

Clinical features

The clinical signs and symptoms induced by diffuse astrocytomas depend largely upon the site within the CNS. They usually develop slowly but may present

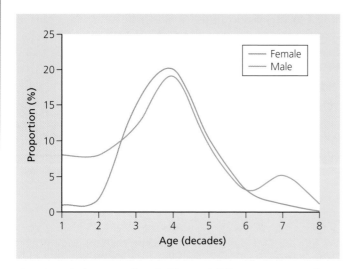

Fig. 4.26 **Relative age and sex incidence of diffuse astrocytomas.** (Data derived from Ref. 17).

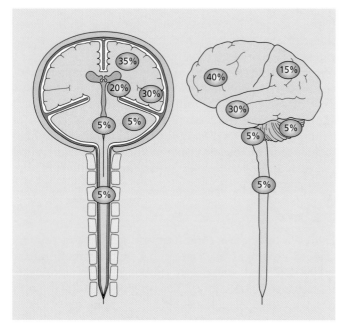

Fig. 4.27 **Preferential sites in the CNS for diffuse astrocytomas.**

suddenly with the onset of epilepsy. Frontal lobe tumours may induce changes in personality and diffuse astrocytomas arising more posteriorly in the cerebral hemispheres result in progressive hemiparesis due to invasion of tumour into the internal capsule. More centrally, diffuse astrocytomas involving the thalamus frequently present with raised intracranial pressure due to hydrocephalus from occlusion of the third ventricle. A similar effect may be induced by diffuse astrocytomas of the midbrain compressing the aqueduct of Sylvius or by tumour in the pons occluding the fourth ventricle. Within the brain stem, diffuse astrocytomas may induce cranial nerve palsies due to invasion of cranial nerve nuclei

around the aqueduct or in the floor of the fourth ventricle. Progressive bilateral motor signs may ensue due to invasion of tumour into the corticospinal tracts in the pons and medulla.[101] Similar bilateral corticospinal tract damage is induced by tumour in the spinal cord, although local invasion of the grey matter and damage to anterior horn cells may also be a feature resulting in muscle wasting in the arms thus mimicking such diseases as spinal muscular atrophy.

In some cases, diffuse astrocytomas develop in 'silent areas' of the brain and produce no focal neurological signs and patients may first present with signs and symptoms of raised intracranial pressure, such as headache, vomiting and drowsiness.[99] These may also be the symptoms of hydrocephalus resulting from occlusion of the ventricular system by an expanding tumour.

Diffuse astrocytomas invade surrounding tissue and, in some cases, seed through the subarachnoid space.[102–105] Such spread occurs particularly with tumours in the spinal cord and brain stem with seedlings distributed throughout the length of the spinal cord. Examination of the CSF in these cases shows an increase in protein content with an absence of inflammatory cells.[99] Although it is possible to detect astrocytoma cells in the CSF by cytospin cytology, the success rate is not high and should not be relied upon for definitively diagnosing spread of diffuse astrocytoma over the spinal cord. MRI may be required to detect such spread.

Radiology

A clear clinical history and a careful physical examination may give a firm indication of the presence of a tumour and its site. However, the definitive diagnosis is made by neurological imaging and histological examination of the biopsy. Prior to the introduction of CT scanning some 25 years ago, the expanding nature of a cerebral diffuse astrocytoma in older adults may have been detected by the displacement of a calcified pineal gland from the midline, or by distortion of the ventricular system as depicted on air encephalography or by displacement of cerebral vessels on angiography. Focal calcification may occur in diffuse astrocytomas and this may also be detected on skull X-ray.

Neuroimaging by CT scan and MRI is now the investigation of choice. These techniques produce not only information regarding the site and extent of the tumour but also, following contrast enhancement techniques, much information regarding the nature of the tumour may be obtained for diagnosis and management of the patient.[106–109] Positron emission tomography (PET) is used for functional studies such as glucose uptake and blood flow in tumours.

On CT scan, a diffuse cerebral astrocytoma appears as a black area of low density in which the shade of the blackness is intermediate between normal brain and the CSF in the ventricles. Such change in character of the tissue is probably due to the high water content of the tumour. The cerebral hemisphere involved may show expansion with shift of midline structures. Similar low density swelling is seen with diffuse astrocytomas in the midbrain, pons, medulla and spinal cord; these regions are best viewed on MRI, as CT scan is not the ideal technique to visualise structures in the posterior fossa. If focal calcification is present within the tumour, it appears as white spots on non-enhanced and enhanced CT scans. The injection of contrast medium tests the integrity of the 'blood–brain barrier', thus, as the blood vessels of diffuse astrocytomas tend to be well formed and have an intact 'blood–brain barrier' diffuse astrocytomas do not show contrast enhancement. If there are regions within an astrocytic tumour that are enhancing, it suggests that focal anaplastic change has occurred.

MRI may give a better image of the extent of diffuse astrocytoma. In T2-weighted images the tumour appears as a white area (Fig. 4.28), often expanding white matter and distorting the contours of the brain and the ventricles. MRI is particularly ideal for examining tumours in the midbrain, pons, medulla and spinal cord, as the extent and effects of the tumour can be viewed not only in horizontal section but also in the sagittal plane.

Pathology

Macroscopic features

Whatever its site in the brain or spinal cord, a diffuse astrocytoma at post-mortem appears as an expansion of the involved region and replacement of normal structures by pale, cream or grey, and sometimes gelatinous, tissue which may contain microcystic spaces or even a large cyst, particularly in cerebral diffuse astrocytomas (Figs 4.29 and 4.30). The cyst itself may contain straw coloured fluid which, in a formalin fixed brain, may be coagulated. Diffuse astrocytomas in the pons (Fig. 4.31) or spinal cord (Figs 4.32 and 4.33) often result in expansion of the affected area, engulfing or distorting surrounding structures (Fig. 4.33).

Post-mortem examination of a patient dying with an diffuse astrocytoma has a number of important purposes. It may be necessary to establish the cause of death either from raised intracranial pressure or due to inhalation pneumonia or cardiac arrest following involvement of the lower cranial nerves by tumour. Spinal cord tumours may result in bladder dysfunction and, eventually, chronic pyelonephritis and renal failure. In patients who have died in the postoperative period, the surgeon may be anxious to review the operation site and the results of the operation on the brain itself. The skin incision, the craniotomy flap or the burr hole should be examined carefully for signs of haemorrhage or infection but the

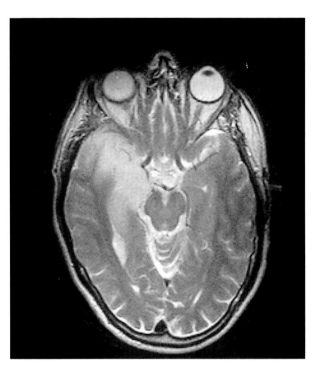

Fig. 4.28 **Diffuse astrocytoma**. MRI (T2-weighted image) showing diffuse expansion of the right temporal lobe by astrocytoma shown here as a white area.

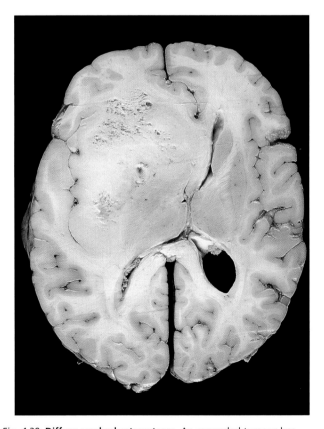

Fig. 4.29 **Diffuse cerebral astrocytoma**. An expanded tumour has distorted one hemisphere, resulting in midline shift and compression of the lateral ventricles. The tumour has ill-defined borders and shows microcystic change. Horizontal section of cerebral hemispheres.

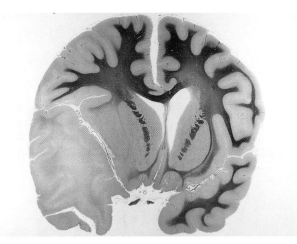

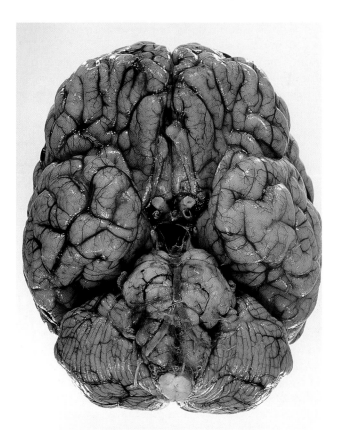

Fig. 4.30 **Diffuse astrocytoma.** A low power histological coronal section of both hemispheres. The myelin is stained blue. An astrocytoma has replaced the temporal lobe on the left and is diffusely invading the external capsule and the edge of the putamen. Some distortion of the brain is seen by shift of the midline towards the right. Klüver-Barrera stain.

Fig. 4.31 **Diffuse astrocytoma.** The pons is broad and has expanded anteriorly so that the basilar artery now occupies a groove in the front of the pons.

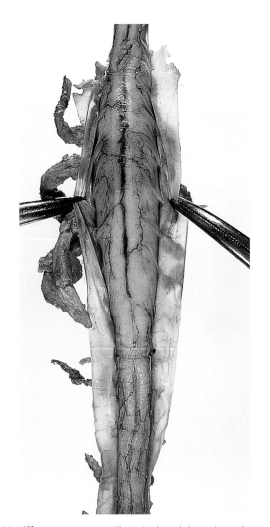

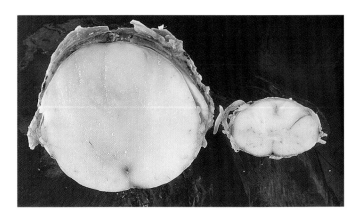

Fig. 4.33 **Diffuse astrocytoma.** Same tumour as Fig. 4.32 showing the relative enlargement induced by the expansion of the astrocytoma (left) compared with a section of normal cervical cord (right). 13-year-old patient.

brain itself should be fixed prior to detailed examination. Examination of the whole neuroaxis is advisable, particularly as diffuse astrocytomas may spread through the subarachnoid space particularly from spinal cord and posterior fossa tumours.

From the pathologists' point of view, one of the most important reasons for examining tumours at post-mortem is to maintain familiarity with the macroscopic

Fig. 4.32 **Diffuse astrocytoma.** The spinal cord shows irregular enlargement in the cervical region.

appearance of tumour tissue, the histological patterns of invasion of the tumour and the ways in which an astrocytic tumour may distort different regions of the CNS. These features are valuable for the interpretation of CT and MRI and for recognising different patterns of diffuse astrocytoma invasion that may be encountered in small surgical stereotactic biopsies, or at resection margins.

The brain at post-mortem may be increased in weight due to the bulk of the tumour and fluid within the tumour. Diffuse astrocytomas are rarely associated with extensive peritumoral oedema and the brain may only weigh 1300 or 1400 g rather than the gross increase in weight that is often seen with glioblastoma. The shape of the brain is best appreciated following 2 or 3 weeks fixation, suspended in buffered formalin. Expansion of the cerebral hemispheres results in flattening of the gyri, which is particularly well seen over the convexities of the hemispheres; the hemisphere involved by tumour may be irregularly swollen and quite noticeably softened. Examination of the base of the brain may reveal herniation of the uncus and parahippocampal gyrus through the tentorial opening. This is best observed following removal of the brain stem and cerebellum by a horizontal cut through the midbrain. One or two centimetres of herniated brain may be seen with a distinct groove marking the free edge of the tentorium cerebelli. The herniated portion of brain may be discoloured red or brown due to infarction; further infarction of the undersurface of the temporal lobe on the same side as the tumour may be present, due to compression of branches of the posterior cerebral artery that cross the groove and are thus compressed by the free edge of the tentorium cerebelli. The visual cortex may also be infarcted due to deprivation of its blood supply through compression of branches of the posterior cerebral artery. Although expansion of a supratentorial tumour rarely causes herniation of the cerebellar tonsils, this may occur if the patient has spent a period on the ventilator and hypoxic change has occurred in the cerebellum.

Diffuse astrocytomas of the midbrain, pons (Fig. 4.31) and medulla are characterised by expansion of these regions, visible from the external aspect of the brain stem. Soft gelatinous material may expand from the front of the pons and medulla and bury the basilar and vertebral arteries.

Coronal slices of the cerebral hemispheres reveal the extent of involvement by a cerebral diffuse astrocytoma and the degree of brain displacement (Fig. 4.30). A diffuse astrocytoma will either be softer or firmer than normal brain; thus, the limits of the tumour may be better defined by palpation than by visual inspection. Tumours frequently merge almost imperceptably with normal brain structures, causing only a slight blurring of the grey/white matter borders at the periphery of the

tumour but with complete replacement of structures in the centre. Increase in bulk of a diffuse astrocytoma in one hemisphere will result in distortion of the ventricular system, a shift of the midline towards the other side and herniation of the cingulate gyrus under the falx cerebri; this is in addition to the herniation of the parahippocampal gyrus through the tentorial opening.

Sectioning of the brain stem and cerebellum en bloc is probably the best way of examining most diffuse astrocytomas in this region. It allows the extent of tumour invasion from the brain stem into the middle cerebellar peduncles to be detected and the degree of compression of the fourth ventricle or invasion of the fourth ventricle to be appreciated.

Examination of the spinal cord should start with longitudinal incision of the dura and identification of the region of spinal cord expanded by diffuse astrocytoma. Seeding of tumour over the dorsal and ventral aspects of the cord can also be identified and is usually seen as gelatinous material, obscuring the nerve roots and blood vessels on the surface of the cord. Horizontal sections of the spinal cord in the region of the tumour show obliteration of the grey and white matter (Fig. 4.33). Below and above the region of the tumour, degeneration of the descending lateral corticospinal tracts or the ascending dorsal columns may be obvious macroscopically.

Intraoperative diagnosis

The major purposes of intraoperative histological study of tumour biopsies are *first* to establish that adequate tumour tissue has been obtained at biopsy for further study in paraffin sections or by research techniques and, *second*, to establish a diagnosis for the immediate management of the patient (see Chapter 3). It is well recognised that the accuracy of intraoperative rapid diagnosis is not as high as the more considered diagnosis from paraffin sections so care must be taken to only issue guidelines on the diagnosis from cryostat sections and smears and not a definitive opinion. It is also essential to ensure that enough material has been received to allow a firm diagnosis to be established at a later date. This may not be possible when the tumour is in a sensitive area such as the brain stem or spinal cord and the surgeon may need to reach a compromise between supplying enough tissue and the risk of inducing neurological deficit.

The two major techniques used for the rapid intraoperative diagnosis of diffuse astrocytomas are cryostat sections and smears.[110–112] Although each is valuable in its own right, they complement each other and are best used in combination; different views of the tumour can be obtained, thus increasing the accuracy of the diagnosis. Furthermore, material used for cryostat section can be stored deep frozen in a liquid nitrogen freezer for research purposes or, if necessary, can be placed in fixative for subsequent examination in paraffin sections. The techniques of cryostat sectioning and smear preparation are covered in Chapter 2.

Cryostat sections Portions of the biopsy for cryostat section should be carefully selected. It is usually most fruitful to examine discoloured, soft, gelatinous tissue or firm tissue within the biopsy; such tissue may be grey, white or cream coloured. In some cases, the astrocytoma may be so diffusely invading that the tissue is indistinguishable from normal brain. A selection of pieces can often be included in one cryostat block, but it is advisable to keep some material unfrozen as freezing may reduce the quality of the histology in subsequent paraffin sections. It is well worth perfecting the freezing technique and sectioning for brain tumour tissue as good quality sections are so much easier to interpret than those that are distorted by ice crystal formation or shattered during cutting.

The two important features to recognise in a cryostat section in the diagnosis of a diffuse astrocytoma are (a) the hyperchromatic, slightly enlarged nuclei of the tumour cells and (b) glial processes. The number of nuclei per unit area ('cellularity') may vary; it may be greater or less than normal brain tissue. Although the major staining technique for cryostat sections is H & E, haematoxylin–van Gieson can be valuable for identifying myelinated fibres (stained black) within tissue infiltrated by tumour. Reticulin stains may also be of value as most astrocytic tumours have little reticulin that is located only around the blood vessels.

Smears The smear technique is simple to perform and the presence of tumour tissue can be assessed at various stages of preparation.[110–112] For example, it is possible to select very small pieces of tissue (1 mm cubes or less) that are macroscopically abnormal, smear them and observe the pattern of smearing. Normal brain tissue is smoothly distributed on the slide, whereas, in general, pathological material produces some degree of clumping. This is not always the case with diffuse astrocytomas that may produce deceptively smooth smears, but a 'lumpy' smear is characteristically seen with glioblastoma. Following staining by toluidine blue or with H & E, the nature of the cell processes, the cell nuclei and the structure of blood vessels are well demonstrated (Fig. 4.34). The delicate astrocytic processes or the plump profiles of astrocytic cells and the variation in nuclear shape and size can be seen. A major feature of the tumour cell nuclei is their dense staining, a size that is often larger than normal and the irregularity of outline; nucleoli are usually small or absent. The lack of macrophages and the delicate nature of the astrocytic processes also helps to distinguish diffuse astrocytoma from reactive changes around an infarct or abscess. Blood vessels in diffuse astrocytomas are delicate with thin walled capillaries, and occasional arteries and veins. The capillary endothelial proliferation

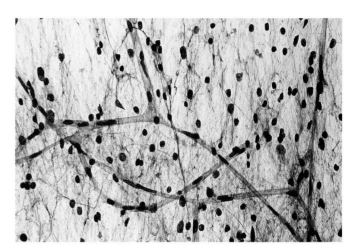

Fig. 4.34 **Diffuse astrocytoma**. Smear preparation reveals a population of cells with some variation in nuclear shape and size and with fine fibrillary processes. The blood vessels are thin walled and branched. Toluidine blue.

seen in glioblastoma is not a feature of diffuse astrocytomas. Even with tough astrocytoma tissue, which does not smear well, the edges of smeared fragments usually reveal the astrocytic nature of the tumour cells.

Histological features

The amount of tissue received from a biopsy varies, depending upon the type of operation. If the whole of the frontal or temporal lobe is removed, there is a good opportunity for examining the relationship between the tumour and surrounding tissue. However, as often happens, even when the operation entails removal of a large bulk of a diffuse astrocytoma, limited material is available for histological examination due to the suction techniques that may be used for removal of brain tumours at surgery. Adequate sampling of the tissue removed is desirable in order to detect anaplastic change within a diffuse astrocytoma.

There is an increasing trend for stereotactic biopsy techniques to be used for the diagnosis of brain tumours. In the hands of experienced operators, stereotactic biopsies can be extremely informative, as accurately targeted samples from different areas of the tumour will be available for histological evaluation and, although the samples are small, they should give a full picture of the histological appearances of the tumour. However, if samples are taken from inappropriate sites, interpretation, and thus diagnosis, may be difficult. A flow chart summarising the handling of a biopsy for the diagnosis of a CNS tumour is depicted in Chapter 2.

There is a moderate degree of variation in cell morphology in diffuse astrocytomas, and in the relationships between tumour cells and the surrounding CNS tissue. Many of the histological appearances can be evaluated in H & E stained sections but other techniques, including immunocytochemistry, are also very valuable in the assessment of diffuse astrocytomas. For the most part, the histological patterns and the cytology in diffuse astrocytomas mimic normal and reactive astrocytes. Care must be taken, therefore, to distinguish tumour cells from normal astrocytes and from reactive astrocytosis, particularly as astrocytomas diffusely infiltrate normal tissue and thus the tumour cells are intimately admixed with normal tissue elements. Necrosis and microvascular (capillary endothelial) proliferation are not features of diffuse astrocytomas and any areas of necrosis will raise the suspicion that the tumour has progressed to glioblastoma. Fig. 4.74 is a summary diagram showing the major histological and cytological features of astrocytic tumours in comparison to normal and reactive astrocytes.

Four key points to observe in the diagnosis of diffuse astrocytomas are:

1. Many of the diffuse astrocytoma tumour cells have hyperchromatic nuclei which are often larger than normal astrocyte nuclei, with a small or absent nucleolus and an irregular border quite unlike the smooth borders seen in normal or reactive astrocyte nuclei. Such hyperchromatic nuclei can be identified in H & E stained sections (Fig. 4.35).
2. The delicate tumour cell processes contain GFAP (Fig. 4.36).
3. Diffuse astrocytomas are composed of sheets of astrocytic cells, without the significant numbers of macrophages or microglia that would be a feature of reactive change.
4. Cells are often distributed in clumps rather than evenly dispersed as in normal tissue or in reactive astrocytosis.

Three major cytological patterns are observed in diffuse astrocytomas:

1. *Fibrillary astrocytomas* are composed of cells which resemble the fibrillary astrocytes of white matter and contain moderate amounts of GFAP in their processes.
2. *Protoplasmic astrocytomas* contain astrocytes which resemble the protoplasmic astrocytes that are normally present in the cerebral cortex; the cells contain few GFAP positive intermediate filaments in their processes.
3. *Gemistocytic* astrocytomas are composed of plump cells which bear some resemblance to reactive astrocytes. However, they usually have a more globular accumulation of paranuclear cytoplasm (Fig. 4.37) and fewer processes than reactive astrocytes (see Fig. 4.74). The term 'gemistocyte' has been widely used to describe cells as diverse as reactive astrocytes, or tumour cells within diffuse astrocytomas, anaplastic astrocytomas, and glioblastoma, so the term is not at all specific for tumour cells.

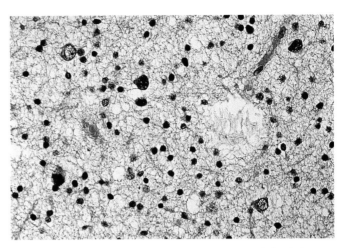

Fig. 4.35 Diffuse astrocytoma. Tumour cells, recognisable by their hyperchromatic nuclei, are diffusely invading brain, such that neurons, characterised by their pale nuclei, prominent nucleoli and basophilic cytoplasm are still seen within the tissue. The background fibrillary matrix is a mixture of tumour cells processes and myelinated axons. An area of microcystic change is also seen. H & E.

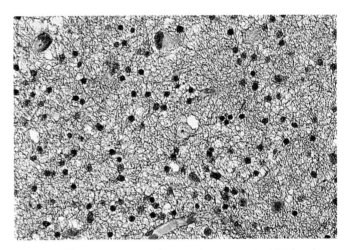

Fig. 4.36 Diffuse astrocytoma. The same tumour as Fig. 4.35 showing expression of GFAP in many of the processes and astrocytic tumour cells. Some tumour cells, characterised by their hyperchromatic nuclei, do not express GFAP (top). GFAP negative neurons are also seen (centre). Immunocytochemistry for GFAP.

Fibrillary astrocytoma is the commonest type of histological pattern seen in diffuse astrocytomas, although there may be some variation in histological appearance in these tumours, with the inclusion of other histological patterns, even within a small biopsy. The tumour cells have fine fibrillary processes, which may be closely packed together in sheaths; in other areas, the cells are more loosely packed with an extensive extracellular space between the fine fibrillary processes (Figs 4.34 and 4.35). Microcysts may occur in these tumours and are filled with fluid and varying amounts of mucinous protein. The nuclei show variation in shape and size compared with normal astrocytes and varying degrees of

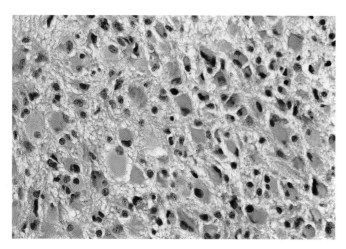

Fig. 4.37 Gemistocytic astrocytoma. The majority of the tumour cells are plump with copious paranuclear cytoplasm and variation in nuclear shape and size. There is a fine fibrillary background but the tumour cells do not have the broad processes typical of reactive astrocytes. H & E.

hyperchromasia (Fig. 4.34). Mitoses are absent or rare even in large areas of tumour biopsy. Immunocytochemistry reveals expression of GFAP and S-100 protein in the cell processes of fibrillary astrocytomas (Fig. 4.36). Ki-67/MIB-1 proliferation indices are generally less than 1–2% in fibrillary astrocytomas.[113–118]

Protoplasmic astrocytoma is uncommon as a pure histological pattern, although areas of protoplasmic astrocytoma may be seen scattered among other histological types. Composed of cells with moderately regular round nuclei with some hyperchromasia, cells in protoplasmic astrocytomas have fine processes with a low content of glial filaments. Nuclei are widely spaced and lakes of mucoid material and microcysts are a characteristic of this type of tumour. Immunocytochemistry reveals little GFAP in the processes and thus the connotation protoplasmic astrocytoma. It is important to recognise this histological pattern as part of the diagnostic spectrum of diffuse astrocytoma. The round nuclei of many of the tumour cells should not be confused with oligodendroglioma in which the cells are usually more closely packed and do not have the fine cytoplasmic processes of a protoplasmic astrocytoma. (MIB-1) proliferation indices are generally less than 1–2% in protoplasmic astrocytomas.[113–118]

Gemistocytic astrocytoma, in its pure form, is an uncommon subtype of diffuse astrocytoma. Plump gemistocytic astrocytic cells, with globular eosinophilic collections of paranuclear cytoplasm, may be present in a predominantly fibrillary or protoplasmic astrocytoma. In some tumours, however, the gemistocytes predominate and the tumour comes under the WHO classification of gemistocytic astrocytoma (Fig. 4.37). Tumour cells closely resemble reactive astrocytes but hyperchromasia and irregularity of the nuclei and the relatively few and rather short cell processes help to distinguish tumour cells from reactive gliosis (see Fig. 4.74) It must be recognised, however, that hyperchromatic nuclei and binucleate astrocytes do occur in longstanding reactive gliosis long after an episode of trauma or infarction.

Immunocytochemistry of gemistocytic astrocytomas shows strong expression of GFAP in the cell bodies and processes. Ki-67/MIB-1 indices are usually less than 5% but the plump gemistocytic astrocytes show a significantly lower rate of proliferation than fibrillary or protoplasmic astrocytic tumour components.[119] This suggests that gemistocytic tumour cells may not form part of the proliferating population.

Infiltration of normal brain tissue by diffuse astrocytoma

Although the histological pattern and the profusion of neoplastic cells in the central regions of diffuse astrocytomas may present little problem with diagnosis, stereotactic biopsies may contain tissue from the infiltrating edges of diffuse astrocytomas. Tumour cells may be interspersed with normal cell elements of cortex and white matter.[120] Infiltrating tumour cells are recognised mainly by their nuclei which are hyperchromatic, irregular in outline and often increased in size when compared with the nuclei of normal tissue cells. In addition to H & E staining, the haematoxylin van Gieson stain is a useful adjunct for identifying the normal elements of white matter – myelin sheaths (black) – into which the tumour cells are infiltrating. GFAP immunocytochemistry identifies the processes of fibrillary tumour astrocytes infiltrating the cortex but is less useful in the identification of fibrillary astrocytes in the white matter as there is GFAP in normal white matter astrocytes.

The patterns of brain infiltration by diffuse astrocytic tumours are similar to those of other diffuse gliomas and are highly characteristic. Although more commonly encountered in oligodendroglial tumours (see Chapter 5), they are also present in many astrocytomas and may thus be helpful in establishing a diagnosis of infiltrating astrocytoma when only the edge of the specimen is sampled. The patterns are known as 'secondary structures of Scherer' and include perineuronal satellitosis, perivascular growth, subpial infiltration and invasion along white matter tracts. Perineuronal satellitosis refers to the propensity of tumour cells to surround neurons as they infiltrate the cerebral cortex. This is often easily noted on low-power microscopic examination of samples that include cerebral cortex, sometimes quite strikingly in oligodendrogliomas. Notice must be taken of the site of the biopsy, as satellitosis of normal oligodendrocytes is commonly encountered in normal temporal lobe specimens. In astrocytomas, the cells are easily recognised by their irregular, hyperchromatic 'naked' nuclei. Perivascular growth is less common than perineuronal satellitosis, and should be distinguished from frank subarachnoid invasion in which cells can fill perivascular Virchow–

Robin spaces. Subpial infiltration is highly characteristic of diffuse gliomas and is essentially diagnostic when found; this is also more typical of oligodendrogliomas but can be found in diffuse astrocytomas as well. Invasion along white matter tracts is a common secondary structure, and is usually found in diffuse astrocytomas when adjacent white matter is sampled. When present, the tumour cells invading along white matter tracts often assume an elongated, 'piloid' appearance. If this is found as the only feature in a biopsy, the microscopic features may be identical to that of gliomatosis cerebri (see below).

Blood vessels within diffuse astrocytomas Particularly well demonstrated in reticulin stains, the blood vessels of diffuse astrocytomas are thin walled but not quite as delicate as those in normal brain. They do not show the glomeruloid microvascular proliferation of glioblastoma and they are not the multichannelled vessels seen in pilocytic astrocytomas. Occasionally lymphocytes are seen around blood vessels within diffuse astrocytomas but the macrophage and lymphocyte content within these tumours is usually very low.

Histology of post-mortem tissues The purposes of histological examination of a diffuse astrocytoma at post-mortem include confirmation of the diagnosis, characterisation of the normal structures involved by the tumour for clinicopathological correlation, and familiarisation with the variation in histological patterns that can occur within a diffuse astrocytoma and at its infiltrating edge. This is particularly important in order to maintain the skill for diagnosis on small stereotactic biopsy specimens. Blocks of tissue taken from cerebral hemispheres, brain stem and cerebellum and from spinal cord should not only include the relevant areas of tumour and invading edge, but they should also include anatomically recognisable structures so that histological sections can be correctly orientated in relation to the whole tumour and to the whole brain. H & E stained sections are valuable for the general histology of the tumour and surrounding brain and the Klüver-Barrera stain is ideal for demonstrating how the tumour has distorted normal brain tissue, particularly white matter (Fig. 4.30). Haematoxylin–van Gieson can be used for a similar purpose. Vascular structures within the tumour can be identified by reticulin staining. Immunocytochemistry for GFAP will establish the identity of astrocytic tumour cells and the presence of reactive astrocytosis within surrounding brain. Axons coursing through the tumour can be identified by neurofilament protein immunocytochemistry or by silver stains and the presence of axons and dendrites by synaptophysin immunocytochemistry.

Differential diagnosis

A more detailed section on differential diagnosis is given below related to the whole group of diffuse astrocytic tumours. It is sufficient here to say that the main differential diagnoses for low grade diffuse astrocytomas are reactive astrocytosis due to focal non-neoplastic brain damage and other diffuse gliomas. The major diffuse gliomas to be considered are low grade oligodendrogliomas and oligoastrocytomas and anaplastic astrocytomas. Differentiation from reactive astrocytosis is often difficult, especially in small stereotactic biopsies, but the relative absence of macrophages or other signs of inflammation and the presence of hyperchromatic astrocytic nuclei within the astrocytoma should allow the distinction to be made. The differential diagnosis with oligodendroglioma and oligoastrocytoma has become more problematic in recent years, as many pathologists have loosened their criteria for oligodendroglial tumours. In general, the more classical oligondendroglial appearances (see Chapter 5) appear more closely allied with the relevant clinical and genetic features of oligodendroglioma.[118] Finally, the absence of mitoses and anaplastic cells distinguishes grade II astrocytoma from anaplastic astrocytoma.

Therapy and prognosis

Diffuse astrocytomas rarely respond significantly to radiotherapy or chemotherapy but surgical removal of tumour bulk or drainage of cysts in diffuse astrocytomas may considerably improve the patient's symptoms, particularly if they are due to raised intracranial pressure.[32,122–126] Due to the diffuse infiltrating nature of a diffuse astrocytoma, it is rarely possible to completely excise the tumour and there are many areas, such as thalamus, internal capsule, brain stem and spinal cord where it is not possible to excise a tumour without damage to neural structures and unacceptable worsening of neurological deficits.

Many patients survive for a number of years with diffuse astrocytomas but the prognosis is uncertain, as anaplastic change occurs in the majority of cerebral diffuse astrocytomas after varying lengths of time, in some cases, as long as 5–10 years. Anaplastic change in diffuse astrocytomas is usually accompanied by a rapid deterioration in the patient's state and by the appearance of enhancing regions on CT scan or MRI. The prognosis of a diffuse astrocytoma[127] is related to the neurological state of the patient preoperatively (Karnofsky performance status) and the location of the tumour, as radical surgical removal is the most important factor in the management of this tumour, and radiotherapy.

Cerebral diffuse astrocytomas may eventually result in the patient's death, due either to raised intracranial pressure from the slowly growing diffuse tumour or following acceleration of growth due to anaplastic change. Diffusely invading astrocytomas of the brain stem usually result in a patient's death due to involvement of the nuclei of the lower cranial nerves such as the vagus, accessory and glossopharyngeal with disturbance of swallowing resulting in inhalation pneumonia.

Anaplastic astrocytoma

Anaplastic astrocytoma can be defined as a tumour which was initially a diffuse astrocytoma but has undergone anaplastic change. The anaplastic change may be focal and is characterised:

1. by rapid deterioration in the clinical state of a patient with a diffuse astrocytoma;
2. by focal enhancement on CT or MRI in an otherwise diffuse, non-enhancing astrocytoma;
3. on biopsy by the presence of anaplastic cells in an astrocytic tumour with high nuclear : cytoplasmic ratios, increased mitotic activity and raised Ki-67/MIB-1 proliferation indices. The prognosis of anaplastic astrocytoma is poor but sometimes better than that of glioblastoma; 50% of patients do not survive more than 1 year after diagnosis.

Incidence

The incidence and age of the onset of anaplastic astrocytoma largely mirrors that of diffuse astrocytoma, although patients are slightly older[17] (Fig. 4.38). Those tumours that first present as anaplastic astrocytomas are generally in a younger age group than those with glioblastomas but there is considerable overlap.

Site

As with diffuse astrocytomas, anaplastic astrocytomas arise mainly in the cerebral hemispheres (Fig. 4.39). Diffuse astrocytomas in the brain stem and spinal cord may cause death of the patient due to invasion perhaps before anaplastic change has occurred but anaplastic astrocytomas do occur at these sites; they are very rare in the cerebellum.

Clinical features

Clinical signs and symptoms depend upon the site of the tumour. In some cases, anaplastic astrocytoma is diagnosed de novo following the onset of signs of raised intracranial pressure, such as headache, drowsiness and vomiting but in many cases anaplastic change occurs after varying lengths of time (4–5 years) following the diagnosis of a diffuse astrocytoma.[99] In general, anaplastic change is suspected when there is an acceleration in clinical deterioration in a patient with a diffuse astrocytoma. Patients who have an anaplastic astrocytoma at first presentation may develop signs of raised intracranial pressure or progressive focal neurological signs.

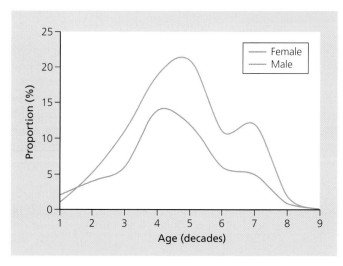

Fig. 4.38 **Relative age and sex incidence of anaplastic astrocytomas.** (Data derived from Ref 17).

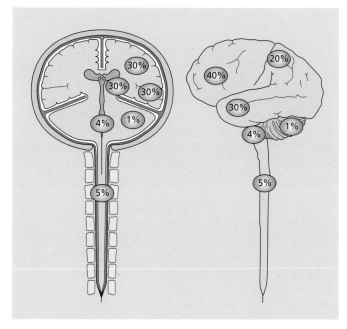

Fig. 4.39 **Preferential sites in the CNS for anaplastic astrocytomas.**

Radiology

With a clinical history of an expanding lesion in the cerebral hemispheres, brain stem or spinal cord, anaplastic astrocytoma is suspected when there is patchy diffuse enhancement on CT and MRI (Fig. 4.40), especially if this diffuse enhancement is focal within an otherwise non-enhancing low density lesion.[106,108] Thus, anaplastic astrocytoma can be distinguished from diffuse astrocytoma by its focal enhancement, although the converse is not true, as areas of anaplastic astrocytoma may be seen in some 40% of non-enhancing diffuse astrocytic tumours. Anaplastic astrocytoma can be separated from classical

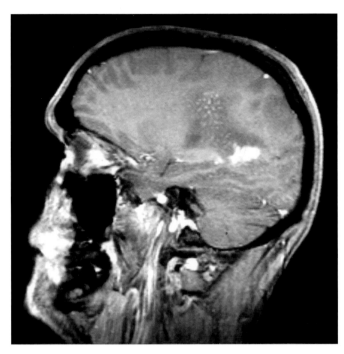

Fig. 4.40 **Anaplastic astrocytoma.** A contrast-enhanced MRI scan shows irregular enhancementof an ill-defined deep-seated anaplastic astrocytoma. The surrounding brain is oedematous, and enlarged Virchow–Robin spaces are present. (Courtesy of Dr D Collie, Edinburgh.)

glioblastoma by the absence of the ring enhancing pattern that is typical of glioblastoma.[106,108,109]

Pathology

The procedures for examining an anaplastic astrocytoma at autopsy are the same as for diffuse astrocytoma (see above).

Macroscopic features

Anaplastic astrocytomas are similar to diffuse astrocytoma in their macroscopic appearances, although the texture and colour of an anaplastic astrocytoma may be more variable. When examining a post-mortem brain, anaplastic astrocytomas are usually best detected by palpation, as the tumour is often soft and gelatinous but it may be firmer than normal brain. It is often only by histological evaluation of tissue sections that focal anaplastic change is detected by the presence of an increased nuclear : cytoplasmic ratio and mitoses. Anaplastic astrocytomas do not exhibit the areas of necrosis and haemorrhage so typical of glioblastoma.

Intraoperative diagnosis

If successful evaluation of an anaplastic astrocytoma is to be achieved at biopsy, it is advisable to have firm understanding between the pathologist and the surgeon. The target region for a stereotactic biopsy is preferably the area of enhancement on CT scans and this should be clearly indicated to the pathologist. If an open biopsy is performed, or there is partial removal of the tumour, as much tissue as possible should be sent to the pathology laboratory so that anaplastic areas can be identified through adequate sampling.

Diagnosis of anaplastic astrocytoma by a rapid intraoperative technique is usually easier in a well targeted stereotactic biopsy than in bulk tissue that has been removed at craniotomy. In cryostat sections, there is an increase in 'cellularity' (i.e. an increase in nuclear : cytoplasmic ratio) compared with a diffuse astrocytoma (Fig. 4.41). The nuclei are often rod shaped rather than the round hyperchromatic nuclei of a diffuse astrocytoma; finding mitoses within such tissue increases the confidence with which a diagnosis of anaplastic astrocytoma can be made. Blood vessels in cryostat sections and in smears are generally thin walled and do not show the glomeruloid microvascular proliferation of glioblastoma. Necrosis is not a feature of anaplastic astrocytoma. Cytology of the cells in smears[110–112] often reveals a relative lack of perinuclear cytoplasm and processes and emphasises the bipolar, rod shaped nature of many of the tumour cells. Care must be taken in the evaluation of cryostat sections and smears from anaplastic astrocytomas, particularly if no clear anaplastic features are seen; sampling error may mean that the anaplastic tissue has not been included in the cryostat section block or smear.

Histological features

In paraffin sections stained with H & E, typical areas of diffuse astrocytoma may be present in an anaplastic astrocytoma; in the regions of diffuse astrocytoma, the nuclei are well separated, round, and a proportion are enlarged to up to twice the normal size and hyperchromatic. The anaplastic areas are identified by the crowding together of tumour cell nuclei due to the relative lack of cytoplasm; many of the nuclei are rod shaped and hyperchromatic (Figs 4.41 and 4.42). Although mitoses may be uncommon, their presence is almost essential for establishing the diagnosis of anaplastic astrocytoma.

Blood vessels within anaplastic astrocytomas are, in general, thin walled although they may be larger than the fine vessels in diffuse astrocytomas but they do not have the features of glomeruloid microvascular proliferation seen in glioblastoma. By definition, the presence of necrosis would indicate a diagnosis of glioblastoma.[88,89] However, on rare occasions, small regions of infarct-like necrosis may be found in anaplastic astrocytomas in the absence of highly cellular tumour and in the absence of prior therapy. The significance of such necrosis is unclear.

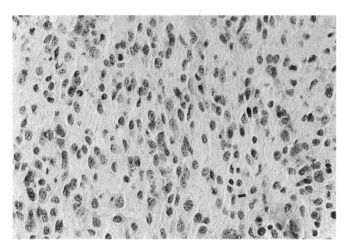

Fig. 4.41 Anaplastic astrocytoma. Focal pleomorphism with an increase in nuclear cytoplasmic ratio with crowding of cells and some rod shaped nuclear forms. Mitoses are present in this field and are the major indication of anaplastic change in a diffuse astrocytic tumour. H & E.

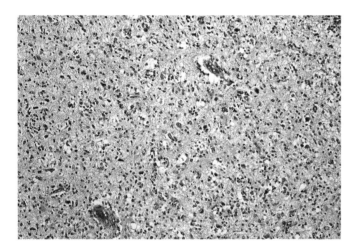

Fig. 4.42 Anaplastic astrocytoma. This cellular tumour exhibits diffuse anaplasia, with widespread nuclear pleomorphism and prominent blood vessels, but no evidence of necrosis. H & E.

Immunocytochemistry

Immunocytochemistry is valuable in anaplastic astrocytomas firstly for definitely identifying the cells as astrocytic by the presence of GFAP in the cytoplasm. Some cells may lack GFAP but usually do express vimentin and S-100 protein. Secondly, immunocytochemistry is useful for estimating proliferative activity with Ki-67/MIB-1 antibodies. Using a graticule, 1000 cells in the area of highest nuclear labelling can be counted and labelling indices above 3% raise the suspicion of anaplastic astrocytoma.[113–118,128] Most anaplastic astrocytomas have a labelling index of between 4 and 5% and overlap with diffuse astrocytoma on the one hand and glioblastoma on the other.

Some difficulty in diagnosis in anaplastic astrocytomas may be experienced when the tumour is composed mainly of plump gemistocytic cells. However, in most anaplastic astrocytomas of this type a proportion of rod shaped anaplastic nuclei are seen with small amounts of cytoplasm, mitoses and a Ki-67/MIB-1 labelling index within the range of 4–5% for anaplastic astrocytoma.

Therapy and prognosis

Surgical intervention for anaplastic astrocytoma is usually for diagnosis and palliative therapy for raised intracranial pressure. Despite surgical extirpation and radiotherapy, the prognosis of anaplastic astrocytoma is only slightly better than that of glioblastoma.[129] Mean survival times are typically of the order of 2 years from diagnosis.[17,129] Occasional anaplastic astrocytomas will respond to chemotherapy, but responses tend to be short-lived.

Glioblastoma

Previously termed *glioblastoma multiforme*, the name *glioblastoma* is now considered to be less cumbersome. Glioblastoma is a rapidly enlarging, anaplastic, astrocytic tumour with areas of necrosis and microvascular (capillary endothelial) proliferation. They arise mainly in patients over 50 years of age, produce rapidly progressing clinical signs and show ring enhancement on CT scan. Glioblastomas and have a poor prognosis, with a mean survival of less than 1 year,[130] although long term survival of up to 15 years has been reported.[131]

Incidence

With an annual incidence of two or three cases per 100 000 of the population per year[132] in Europe and North America, glioblastomas are the commonest primary intracranial tumours in adult neurosurgical practice. The widespread use of imaging techniques (CT and MRI) has increased the ease with which these tumours are identified and has increased the number of tumours biopsied for histological confirmation. Glioblastomas account for some 60% of all astrocytic tumours and 12–15% of all intracranial neoplastic lesions. Although they may occur at any age, glioblastomas are uncommon in children and have a peak incidence between 50 and 70 years[95] (Fig. 4.43). The annual peak incidence in southern Britain is 7.3:100 000 in the sixth decade, with a male predominance of approximately 3:2.[95]

Site

The cerebral hemispheres are the most common site for glioblastoma with some 70% arising in the frontal and temporal lobes and 20% in the parietal lobes[17,91,96] (Fig. 4.44). These tumours are uncommon in the occipital lobes and even less common in the brain stem, cerebellum and

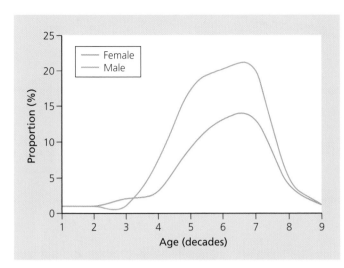

Fig. 4.43 **Relative age and sex incidence of glioblastomas**. (Data derived from Ref. 17).

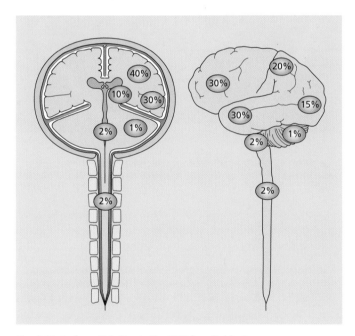

Fig. 4.44 **Preferential sites in the CNS for glioblastomas**.

spinal cord.[133] Occasionally, glioblastomas seed through the ventricular system and metastasise down the spinal cord; they rarely metastasise outside the CNS but there are a number of case reports of glioblastoma in cervical lymph nodes and other organs.[28]

Clinical features

The pattern of clinical presentation depends upon the site of the tumour and its rapidity of growth. Complications, such as haemorrhage and infarction in the tumour may result in sudden enlargement and raised intracranial pressure. Frontal lobe lesions are associated with intellectual deterioration, blunting of the personality and

loss of memory.[134] When sited more posteriorly in the hemispheres, glioblastomas may present with focal neurological signs of sensory impairment. The presenting sign may be seizures, although this is less common than with the well differentiated diffuse astrocytomas. If the tumour involves the internal capsule, hemiparesis may ensue; more focal paresis may be seen if just one region of the motor cortex itself is involved. As tumours enlarge within the cerebral hemisphere, CSF outflow through the foramina of Monro may be obstructed resulting in obstructive hydrocephalus, a rapid rise in intracranial pressure, and the onset of drowsiness, vomiting and, finally, coma. Temporal lobe glioblastomas may present with temporal lobe epilepsy or with raised intracranial pressure. Rarely, glioblastomas arise in the midbrain, pons or medulla; they may rapidly involve the corticospinal tracts, resulting in quadriparesis, or damage the lower cranial nerve nuclei causing cranial nerve palsies. Hydrocephalus due to obstruction of the fourth ventricle may ensue. Such complications are seen particularly in diffuse pontine astrocytomas in children. Glioblastomas in the spinal cord, either primary or metastatic,[105,133,135] interfere with corticospinal tract function and result in quadriparesis if they are in the cervical region or paraparesis if sited in the thoracic spinal cord or below. Glioblastomas in the cerebellum are rare and may present with ataxia or hydrocephalus due to compression of the fourth ventricle.[136,137]

Radiology

Glioblastomas enhance on CT scanning and MRI. Many present a typical scan appearance of ring enhancement due to a central area of necrosis surrounded by enhancing viable tumour; a low density area of oedema usually surrounds the tumour (Fig. 4.45). Distortion of the surrounding brain with shift of the midline and occlusion of the ventricles and hydrocephalus are well visualised on scans. Despite the typical appearance, glioblastoma may be confused on scans with other enhancing lesions within cerebral hemispheres, especially cerebral abscess, metastatic tumours, lymphoma, or even acute multiple sclerosis plaques (see section on differential diagnosis below). Although in some cases glioblastomas appear to be multifocal radiologically, there are, in almost every case, glioblastoma cells connecting the major tumour masses when the brain is examined by histology at post-mortem. The extent of peritumoral oedema and diffuse tumour extension around glioblastomas is well visualised by MRI (Fig. 4.46); much of the mass effect of a tumour may be due to oedema.

An estimate of the speed of enlargement of a glioblastoma is occasionally possible when a barely detectable lesion on a scan is seen to enlarge within 3–4 months to a ring enhancing 5 cm diameter lesion with central necrosis and peritumoral oedema.

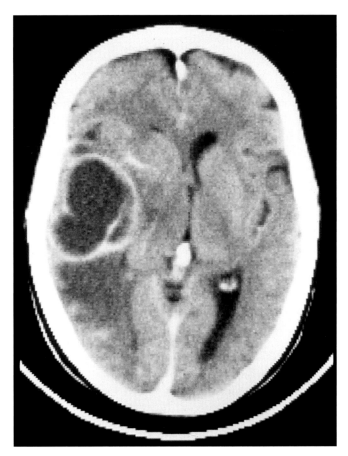

Fig. 4.45 **Glioblastoma**. CT scan showing a ring enhancing lesion in the right cerebral hemisphere resulting in distortion of the ventricular system and shift of the midline. Adjacent to the ring enhancing lesion is an area of decreased density, indicating oedema.

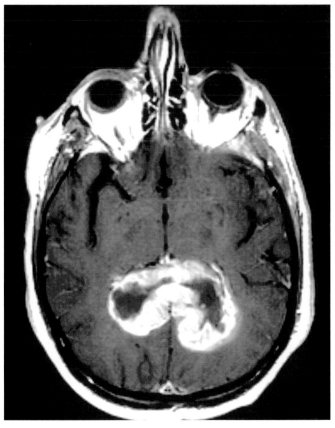

Fig. 4.46 **Glioblastoma**. This contrast-enhanced axial MRI scan shows a large bilateral butterfly glioblastoma, with marked peripheral enhancement and central necrosis. (Courtesy of Dr D Collie, Edinburgh.)

Pathology

Macroscopic features

The term 'multiforme' previously associated with glioblastoma applies as much to the heterogeneity of the macroscopic appearance of different regions of the tumour as to the histological diversity.

The location of a glioblastoma in an uncut post-mortem brain may be obvious from the assymetrical swelling of the cerebral hemispheres, with flattening of the cerebral gyri over the tumour. Palpation often reveals a soft patch of brain where tumour has approached the surface of the cortex and this area may be discoloured purple or dark grey (Fig. 4.47). Sometimes the gyri are irregularly broadened as the infiltrating edge of the tumour replaces cerebral cortex.

The shape and full extent of a glioblastoma is best examined in a brain that has been fixed for 4 weeks in formalin, as the slices retain their shape and the geography of the tumour. Small glioblastomas, up to 3 or 4 cm in diameter, may be circular in outline if they are centrally placed within the frontal (Fig. 4.48) and temporal lobes. As they increase in

size, the profile becomes irregular as the tumour progressively invades the hemisphere (Fig. 4.49). As tumour cells track along white matter pathways, a glioblastoma in one occipital or frontal lobe may pass across the corpus callosum anteriorly or posteriorly into the contralateral hemisphere (Fig. 4.50). Such a butterfly glioblastoma may be recognised on CT scans and MRI (Fig. 4.46), or it may appear as two separate tumours. Multifocal glioblastomas are sometimes observed, even in post-mortem brain slices, but usually there is intervening spread of tumour cells that can be detected microscopically.

A number of regions can be recognised in the cut surface of the glioblastoma which produce its multi-coloured appearance and correspond to the areas of enhancement or low density on CT scan. The central regions of a glioblastoma are frequently necrotic with a yellow granular appearance and focal haemorrhages; thrombosed vessels may be visible within the necrotic areas. In this way, glioblastoma can be distinguished from diffuse astrocytoma and anaplastic astrocytom in which areas of necrosis are not a feature. Small glioblastomas may appear very similar in appearance to isolated meta-

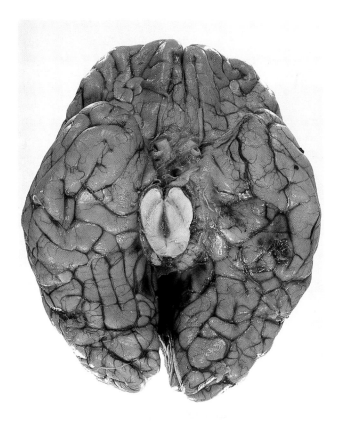

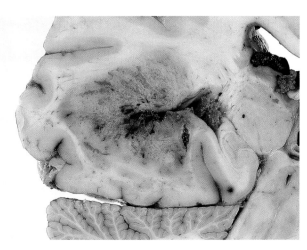

Fig. 4.49 **Glioblastoma**. The central area of the tumours is haemorrhagic and necrotic and the pink/grey tumour tissue is seen extending into the temporal lobe white matter.

Fig. 4.47 **Glioblastoma**. A patch of discolouration caused by a glioblastoma is seen laterally on the under surface of the temporal lobe. Enlargement of the left hemisphere is reflected in the compression of the brain stem and the presence of parahippocampal gyral herniation.

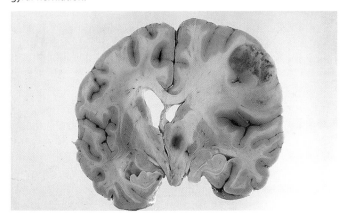

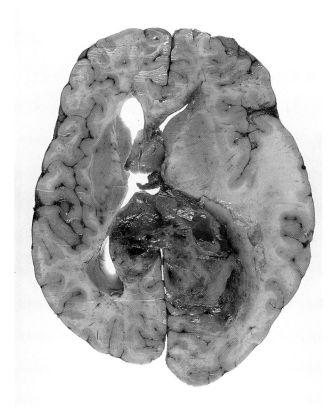

Fig. 4.48 **Glioblastoma**. A relatively small tumour 3–4 cm in diameter and circular in shape is seen peripherally in the posterior portion of the right frontal lobe. The tumour and its associated oedema has caused distortion of the brain and herniation of the right cingulate gyrus and the parahippocampal gyrus. Haemorrhage has occurred into the anterior portion of the thalamus.

Fig. 4.50 **Glioblastoma**. A butterfly pattern is shown extending from one occipital lobe to the other in this horizontal section of both cerebral hemispheres.

static carcinomas; in general, however, metastases are spherical with a circular outline, whereas glioblastomas over 2 cm or so in diameter are more irregular in shape. Viable tumour in glioblastoma is recognisable, usually as a grey, or sometimes purple, band of tissue at the peri- phery of the tumour. Glioblastomas may invade white matter tracts and spread for considerable distances along the fornices, corpus callosum and the optic radiation as well as diffusely through the hemispheric white matter. Even when the tumour appears to be sharply demarcated

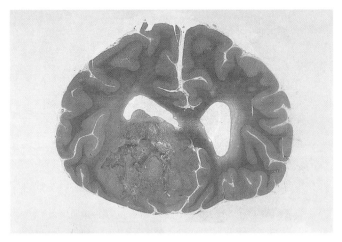

Fig. 4.51 Glioblastoma. Low power view of a histological section of both frontal lobes. The glioblastoma is expanding the inferior aspect of the frontal lobe on the left and is seen as a mixture of dark peripheral areas of friable tumour and a central, pale necrotic region. H & E.

from surrounding white matter and cortex macroscopically, invasion beyond the macroscopic limits of the tumour is usually seen in histological preparations.

The mass effect of a glioblastoma and its accompanying oedema and necrosis may distort the cerebral hemispheres in a number of ways (see Chapter 20). Those tumours involving the frontal lobes, extending back into the thalamus and basal ganglia may displace the hemisphere across the midline, compress the third ventricle and the foramina of Monro and result in dilatation of the occipital horns of the lateral ventricles (Fig. 4.51). If the tumour is in the upper part of the hemisphere, the cingulate gyrus is often herniated under the falx cerebri and may show focal infarction due to compression of the vessels on its surface. Downward displacement of the hemisphere is most prominent with temporal lobe glioblastomas and the uncus and parahippocampal gyrus become herniated through the tentorial opening, between the free edge of the tentorium cerebelli and the midbrain. Such herniation has a number of major effects. Initially, the oculomotor nerve becomes crushed by the herniated brain against the free edge of the tentorium cerebelli, resulting in paralysis of parasympathetic function in the eye and then a fixed and dilated pupil on the affected side. Subsequently, branches of the posterior cerebral artery crossing the inferior aspect of the temporal lobe may be occluded, due to compression between the herniated brain and the free edge of the tentorium cerebelli. Such compression results in ischaemia and infarction of the inferior aspect of the temporal lobe and of the occipital lobe, as far back as the visual cortex. Perhaps the most severe complication is compression of the midbrain, with the development of flame shaped haemorrhages, probably due to direct compression of venous drainage of the midbrain. Such haemorrhage is usually associated with unconsciousness and is seen in a proportion of patients dying with raised intracranial pressure, due to growth of a cerebral glioblastoma. One other effect of brain stem distortion due to herniation of the parahippocampal gyrus, is damage to the contralateral cerebral peduncle. This gives rise to the anomalous clinical signs in which hemiparesis may develop on the same side as the cerebral tumour. The pathological lesion is known as 'Kernohan's notch'. Distortion of other areas of the brain results in swelling of the affected region; in the posterior fossa this may result in compression of the fourth ventricle and supratentorial hydrocephalus. In the spinal cord, swelling due to glioblastoma may result in impairment of blood supply of surrounding regions of the cord with infarction.

The results of surgical resection or radiotherapy should be taken into account when assessing the effects of the tumour upon the brain at post-mortem. The resection cavity may remain as a cystic area with a gliotic discoloured wall or it may refill with tumour as the residual tumour regrows; such regrowth may be considerable and may reach the original bulk of the tumour within a few months. Spread of tumour through the CSF on the surface of the brain and spinal cord or through the ventricular system may be seen in such patients. The effect of radiotherapy is often to increase the amount of necrosis within the tumour. An increase in the amount of nuclear and cytoplasmic pleomorphism in tumour cells and the presence of endarteritis induced by the irradiation is seen by microscopy. There is no clear picture of the effects of systemic chemotherapy on the histology of glioblastomas but local infusion of chemotherapeutic agents into surgical cavities results in increased pleomorphism of the surviving tumour cells.[138]

Intraoperative diagnosis

The poor prognosis of glioblastoma, even after surgical removal and radiotherapy and chemotherapy, is a major factor influencing the management of these tumours. Some glioblastomas, particularly in the frontal and temporal regions may be excised by lobectomy for relief of symptoms and to reduce intracranial tumour bulk. In such operations, substantial amounts of tumour tissue may be available for rapid diagnosis, for research purposes and for paraffin embedding and electron microscopy. This, however, cannot be guaranteed because surgical techniques frequently dictate use of suction for removal of tumour tissue so that the amount taken as a biopsy may be very small.

With the introduction of stereotactic biopsy techniques, very specific areas of a glioblastoma can be sampled but the quality of the material depends largely on the experience of the surgeon and the accuracy with which the stereotactic biopsy is targeted. Ideally, a stereotactic biopsy should present the pathologist with diagnostic samples of tissue containing:

1. the enhancing rim of the tumour;
2. necrotic tissue from the centre of the tumour; and
3. oedematous brain tissue infiltrated by glioblastoma cells from outside the main enhancing ring of the tumour.

Such multisampling is ideal for comparing the pathology with the CT scan or MRI performed for the location of the biopsies. Planned biopsy sites are often marked on the appropriate scans by a cross. Perhaps more than in any other branch of pathology, it is essential for the pathologist to discuss the MRI or CT scans with the surgeon or radiologist. Lack of correlation of the pathology with the imaging can lead to very serious errors of diagnosis.

Much has been written in the past about the relative values of cytological smears and cryostat sections of cerebral tumours.[110,112] Given the importance of establishing a diagnosis intraoperatively for management of the patient, it is usually advisable to use both cryostat sections and smears for diagnosis.

Macroscopic inspection of stereotactic biopsy material is often useful in selecting material for smear diagnosis. The bright yellow colour of necrotic tissue is often apparent and viable tumour tissue may be more gelatinous and grey. Samples of tissue, up to 1 mm cube, can be placed on slides and smeared and the advantage of this technique is that the texture of the smear may indicate whether abnormal viable tumour tissue, necrotic tissue or non-tumorous brain tissue is present in the smear. Glioblastoma tumour tissue smears in a lumpy fashion as tumour cells tend to aggregate around the abnormal vessels within the tumour. Necrotic tissue is rather granular in its appearance, even in the unstained smear, and non-tumorous tissue, even if slightly gliotic, will be much smoother in its smear pattern than glioblastoma tumour tissue.

Smears Microscopic inspection at low power of toluidine blue or H & E stained smears of glioblastoma reveal a number of diagnostic features most important of which are:

1. the presence of abnormal blood vessels showing microvascular (capillary endothelial) proliferation (Fig. 4.52); such a feature is readily recognised as relatively large blood vessels that suddenly end as short, stubby, bulbous structures which, on higher power, are seen as glomeruloid structures formed from thin walled capillaries containing erythryocytes;
2. the presence of astrocytic cells with long, fine processes; such cells may exhibit considerable pleomorphism and range from bipolar spindle cells with rod shaped nuclei and long terminal cytoplasmic processes to multinucleate cells with copious cytoplasm and fine peripheral processes (Fig. 4.53).

Varying degrees of cytoplasmic and nuclear pleomorphism are seen in glioblastoma cells with nuclear hyper-

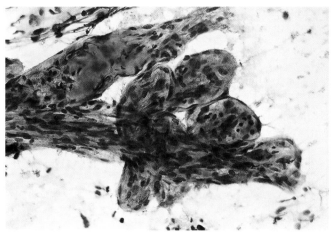

Fig. 4.52 **Glioblastoma**. A smear preparation showing enlarged blood vessels with club-like extensions of capillary epithelial proliferation. The erythrocytes in the vessels are blue–green in colour. Toluidine blue.

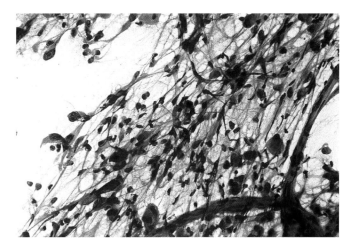

Fig. 4.53 **Glioblastoma**. A smear preparation showing astrocytic cells with long fine processes. The variation in nuclear shape and size with some large nuclei is an indication that this is tumour tissue. The cells have fewer processes than reactive astrocytes. Toluidine blue.

chromasia and moderately prominent nucleoli. Although mitoses may be seen in smears, they are not seen frequently enough to be reliable diagnostic markers. It is the background of the pleomorphic astrocytic tumour cell processes which is typical for glioblastoma.

Cryostat sections Tumour tissue that is properly frozen in liquid nitrogen is usually well preserved and can be subsequently fixed in formalin for paraffin sections. Therefore with a stereotactic biopsy in which no tumour is obvious macroscopically, all the cores from a stereotactic biopsy may be placed on the cryostat chuck for sectioning in the search for tumour tissue. If there is sufficient and obvious tumour tissue in the biopsy, however, it is advisable to keep some cores unfrozen for direct fixation in formalin. Freezing may interfere with subsequent interpretation of histological patterns of some tumours, particularly oligodendrogliomas. The main purposes of examining cryostat sections and smears are:

1. to establish the presence of tumour tissue in the biopsy for further definitive diagnosis in paraffin sections;
2. to give an opinion on the most probable tumour diagnosis to assist the surgeon in the immediate management of the patient; and
3. to detect the presence of another lesion (e.g. an abscess or a tumour such as meningioma) that is more amenable to surgical removal.

Meningiomas, if infarcted in the centre, may mimic the CT scan appearances and rapid clinical progression of the glioblastoma, but the two tumours are often more easily distinguished in a cryostat section than in a smear. Similarly, metastatic carcinoma is often more readily discerned in a cryostat section where the organoid patterns may be better preserved than in the smear. In some cases, the tissue may be too firm and tough to smear and cryostat sections are essential for intraoperative diagnosis. Hyperchromasia and pleomorphism of the nuclei are readily identified in cryostat sections, as are mitoses, although these may be relatively uncommon in glioblastoma. Pseudopalisading around areas of necrosis and larger areas of necrotic tissue can easily be identified, although microvascular proliferation is often easier to detect in smears than in cryostat sections.

Techniques other than H & E can be applied, often fairly rapidly, to cryostat sections. Particularly valuable are haematoxylin–van Gieson, which will identify bands of collagen and may help to exclude meningiomas and metastatic carcinomas, and reticulin stains which emphasise the lack of connective tissue in many areas of a glioblastoma and the positive feature of microvascular proliferation. Both these techniques can be performed within 10 min and may be extremely helpful in evaluating difficult biopsies. Immunocytochemistry for GFAP to confirm the astrocytic nature of the tumour can also be performed on the cryostat sections; this may take rather longer than the tinctorial stains but can be achieved within 30–45 min.

If tumour tissue is used for research purposes, and samples can be stored frozen in liquid nitrogen, the diagnostic cryostat sections are a valuable guide to the content of the tissue that will subsequently be used for research purposes.

Histological features

Large biopsy specimens taken from surgical lobectomies or from brain slices at post-mortem reveal the considerable diversity of histological appearance which justified the name glioblastoma 'multiforme'. It has now been recognised, largely from clinicopathological correlation studies, that certain criteria can be applied to a tumour to classify it as glioblastoma and to separate it from anaplastic astrocytoma.

Within an otherwise typical anaplastic astrocytoma, the following features necessitate a diagnosis of glioblastoma:

1. necrosis;
2. glomeruloid microvascular (capillary endothelial) proliferation.

Current surgical practice dictates that many biopsies are small and present only a glimpse of the whole structure of glioblastoma. Advantage can, therefore, be taken from the larger biopsies and autopsy specimens to gain experience of the overall histological organisation, (or disorganisation) of a glioblastoma. CT or MRI frequently demonstrates glioblastomas as ring enhancing lesions with a cystic or necrotic centre. When the whole tumour is viewed histologically, a central, often multifocal area of necrosis is surrounded by highly cellular tumour. Cytologically, the tumour cells are remarkably variable, and this variability is a hallmark of glioblastoma. Some tumours are strikingly pleomorphic, with large cells and small cells of different morphological appearance. Other tumours are more uniform, featuring large numbers of either giant or small cells (see sections on Giant cell glioblastoma and Small cell glioblastoma). The vast majority of glioblastomas, however, have a combination of malignant glial cell types, with notable pleomorphism, and with multinucleated giant cells mixed with small anaplastic cells (Figs 4.54 and 4.55). Mitotic figures are usually easily detected, including highly atypical forms, particularly in giant cell glioblastomas.

Tongues of necrosis extend into the viable rim of the tumour and are surrounded by regions of pseudopalisading in which the nuclei of tumour cells are aligned per-

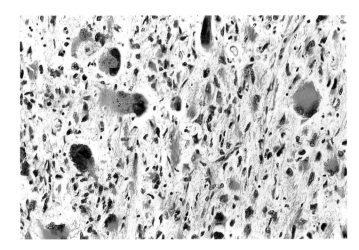

Fig. 4.54 **Glioblastoma**. The pleomorphic region in the centre of the glioblastoma showing multinucleated giant cells and rod shaped anaplastic glial cells. H & E.

pendicularly to the edge of the necrosis (Fig. 4.56). The pseudopalisading pattern of necrosis is quite typical for glioblastoma but is not unique – it can be seen in ana-plastic oligodendrogliomas and occasionally as small areas in atypical or malignant meningiomas. Within the larger, infarct-like regions of necrosis, it is often possible to recognise thrombosed arteries and veins, suggesting that the necrosis is a form of infarction. Although macro-phages may be present around the edges of necrotic areas, they are not as numerous as the macrophages that accumulate in areas of infarcted non-neoplastic brain or in acutely demyelinating multiple sclerosis plaques.[139,140] If it is only necrotic tissue that is present in a small biopsy, the relative absence of macrophages is often a good indication that the necrosis is from tumour tissue rather than from infarction. Nevertheless, such macrophage free necrosis is also seen in metastases, and occasionally in non-neoplastic lesions, so it cannot be used as a definite diagnostic criterion for glioblastoma (see section on Differential diagnosis below).

At the periphery of a glioblastoma, the tumour may appear to be relatively well circumscribed on macro-scopic and low power light microscopic inspection. At higher power, however, tumour cells are seen to infiltrate diffusely normal tissue often with alignment of tumour cells around neurons, around blood vessels and along the subpial surface of the cerebral cortex. The apparent sharp demarcation may be an indication of the rapid destruction of normal cell elements by the advancing edge of the glioblastoma. This relatively sharp border between tumour and normal brain is in contrast to diffuse astrocytomas in which tumour cells insinuate themselves for large distances between normal tissue elements. Characteristic of the advancing edge of the glioblastoma are the bipolar anaplastic glial cells with rod shaped hyperchromatic nuclei (Fig. 4.57). Such cells are seen well in H & E stained sections and in smear preparations. It is these cells that are the main proliferating element in a glioblastoma, whereas the more dramatic pleomorphic giant cells in the centre of the tumour often show less proliferative activity, and may exhibit abnormal mitoses. Cytologically, glioblastomas often contain cells of greatly varying appearances, ranging from giant cells to small, primitive cells. The varied cytological appearance is characteristic of glioblastoma, hence the old term 'multiforme'. Some tumours are dominated by either giant cells or small cells (see below).

Blood vessel alterations are characteristic of glio-blastoma. There are two major features of blood vessels in glioblastomas which distinguish them from blood vessels in normal brain in diffuse astrocytomas and anaplastic astrocytomas. One feature is large arteries or veins with intravascular thrombi, particularly in con-fluent, infarct-like regions of necrosis. The second feature is microvascular proliferation, defined as a proliferation of hyperplastic blood vessels in which the vessel wall is

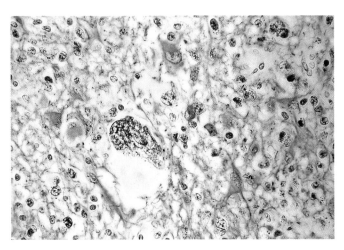

Fig. 4.55 **Glioblastoma**. Immunocytochemistry shows variation in expression of GFAP among glioblastoma cells. A large pleomorphic cell in the centre is devoid of GFAP expression, whereas smaller cells surrounding it are stained. Immunocytochemistry for GFAP.

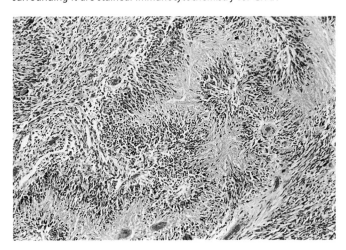

Fig. 4.56 **Glioblastoma**. Areas of necrosis are surrounded by pseudopalisades of tumour cells. This is typical of glioblastoma but not a constant feature in biopsies. H & E.

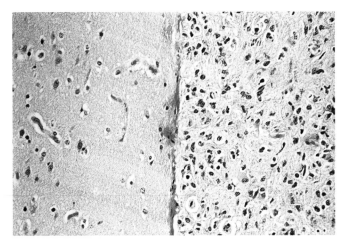

Fig. 4.57 **Glioblastoma**. On the right hand side is cerebral cortex infiltrated by rod shaped anaplastic glial tumour cells and to the left is normal cerebral cortex separated from the tumour by a sulcus in the centre. H & E.

two or more endothelial cells in thickness. Termed 'endothelial proliferation' in the past, it is now recognised that microvascular proliferation, as it progresses, involves smooth muscle and other vascular cells in addition to endothelial cells. Eventually, so-called 'glomeruloid' structures form, which are virtually pathognomonic of glioblastoma. These are multichannelled, nodular vascular structures that closely resemble, at least on low-power microscopic examination, renal glomeruli. As discussed below in the section on Biology, microvascular proliferation may be distributed throughout the viable areas of the tumour but is often most prominent adjacent to areas of necrosis. Appearing as glomeruloid tangles of capillaries with vessel walls more than one endothelial cell in thickness, some of which contain erythrocytes, microvascular proliferation is recognisable in H & E stained sections (Fig. 4.58) but is far better demonstrated in a reticulin stain (Fig. 4.59). In the majority of glioblastomas, the tumour cell areas are devoid of reticulin, which is only concentrated around vessels. Electron microscopy clearly shows single capillary buds in glioblastomas (Fig. 4.60) or the multiple capillary buds in larger areas of microvascular proliferation.[141,142] (Fig. 4.61)

Perivascular spaces, and in particular periarterial spaces, act as channels for the drainage of interstitial and oedema fluid from normal brain tissue[28] and from tumours in the brain.[140,141] Such spaces contain resident perivascular cells which act as histiocytes in the fluid drainage pathways and are upregulated around arteries within and adjacent to glioblastomas.[140] Glioblastomas, as well as other malignant gliomas, may also invade the subarachnoid space proper. This may be observed in biopsy or resection specimens that include superficial cerebral cortex and subarachnoid space. Involvement of the subarachnoid space presumably accounts for the ability of glioblastomas

to spread via the cerebrospinal fluid to produce 'drop metastases'. In such situations, it is not uncommon to find invasion of the adjacent brain or spinal cord parenchyma from such subarachnoid metastases.

Immunocytochemistry

The two most valuable immunocytochemical techniques for the diagnosis of glioblastoma are GFAP and Ki-67/MIB-1.

Expression of GFAP is variable within the tumour cells of glioblastoma. Many of the large pleomorphic cells show no expression of GFAP (Fig. 4.55) but this technique is valuable for identifying the astrocytic nature of other tumour cells and for distinguishing them from reactive

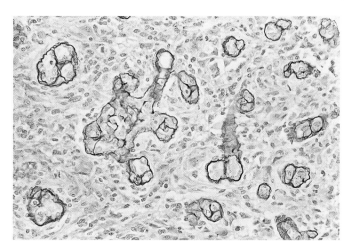

Fig. 4.59 **Glioblastoma**. Capillary endothelial proliferation well demonstrated by reticulin staining. Multiple capillary buds are bound together by connective tissue. Reticulin stain.

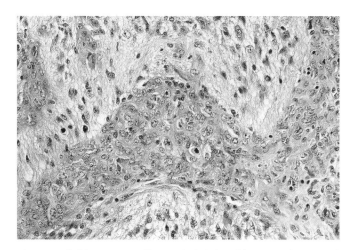

Fig. 4.58 **Glioblastoma**. Capillary endothelial proliferation. The mass of endothelial cells is more darkly stained than the surrounding glioblastoma cells. Some vessel lumina can be seen and they contain erythrocytes; mitoses are also present. H & E.

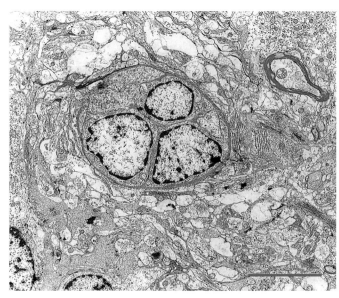

Fig. 4.60 **Glioblastoma**. A single capillary bud formed by endothelial cells but with no distinct lumen. Bar = 1 μm.

Immunocytochemistry for proliferation antigens such as Ki-67/MIB-1 (Fig. 4.62) can be very valuable for assessing proliferation in glioblastomas. The labelling index tends to be higher in glioblastomas than in diffuse astrocytomas and is often higher in glioblastomas than in anaplastic astrocytomas.[113,114,143] Levels between 5 and 10% labelled nuclei would be expected in glioblastoma, compared with 1–5% in diffuse astrocytomas. Anaplastic astrocytomas are intermediate with labelling indices of 4–5%.[24,128]

In studying the biology of glioblastoma, the distribution of macrophages, perivascular cells and lymphocytes within tumours can be characterised by use of the appropriate antibodies. Furthermore, growth factors such as VEGF and epidermal growth factor (EGF), and their receptors can be detected in a proportion of glioblastomas.[144–146] Blood vessel endothelium is well demonstrated by factor VIII related antigen or by lectin staining with *Ulex europeus*. These techniques will identify the endothelial linings to both normal and abnormal blood vessels within the tumours. Normal neural elements within the tumour can be identified using antibodies to neurofilament proteins and to synaptophysin.

Differential diagnosis

The more detailed aspects of differential diagnosis for glioblastoma are covered in the section devoted to diffuse astrocytic tumours as a group. However, it is appropriate to consider briefly here the relationship between imaging and the pathology differential diagnosis.

Although the diagnosis of glioblastoma often appears to be very clear from the CT and MRI, there are other lesions, some of which are not neoplastic, that may resemble glioblastoma on imaging. Chief among the non-neoplastic lesions are cerebral abscess, and less commonly infarction and multiple sclerosis, all of which can present as ring enhancing lesions on CT or MRI. Infarcted meningiomas, pilocytic astrocytomas and more malignant tumours such as metastases and malignant lymphoma may also resemble glioblastoma on imaging. Although very helpful to the pathologist in reaching the diagnosis, care must be taken not to put too much reliance on the imaging alone for the diagnosis of an intracranial lesion. The onus is therefore on the pathologist to ensure that enough tissue is received from the surgeon to establish the diagnosis of glioblastoma by the presence of an anaplastic astrocytic tumour with areas of necrosis and microvascular proliferation within the biopsy.

Therapy and prognosis

The outcome of glioblastoma depends largely upon the stage at which it is diagnosed, the site of the tumour and the age of the patient.[129,130] Most clinical surveys suggest that 50% of the patients will survive no longer than 1 year

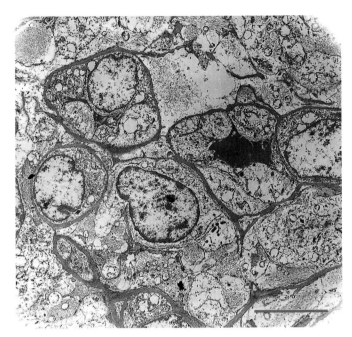

Fig. 4.61 **Glioblastoma**. Capillary endothelial proliferation characterised by multiple capillary buds bound together by connective tissue. Small lumina are seen in some of the buds. Bar = 1 μm.

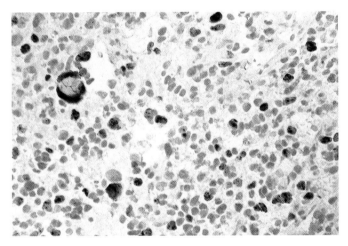

Fig. 4.62 **Glioblastoma**. A high proliferation index of darkly stained nuclei is shown in this immunocytochemical preparation. Ki-67/MIB-1.

astrocytes. Although many of the rod shaped anaplastic cells of the periphery of a glioblastoma do not express GFAP, there is usually a population of spindle shaped tumour cells and more globular tumour cells that do express GFAP. These cells may show positive staining in the perinuclear regions and in processes but, unlike reactive astrocytes, the processes are usually few in number and rather short. Rod shaped nuclei of the small infiltrating anaplastic glial cells in glioblastoma may be confused with microglia but the two cell types can be distinguished by the hyperchromasia of the tumour cell nuclei and by the expression of microglial markers, for example, PGM-1 (CD68) by the microglial cells.[139]

and almost all the patients with glioblastoma will not survive more than 2 years. Surgical excision and radiotherapy have some beneficial effect on the overall prognosis and they may increase the quality of life for the patient. Individuals under the age of 50 have a slightly longer survival time than those over 50 when treated by surgery and radiotherapy. Patients over the age of 65 years have a particularly poor prognosis. Glioblastomas deeply seated in the thalamus and basal ganglia, and thus inaccessible to surgical excision, have a poor prognosis, as do the rare glioblastomas in the posterior fossa. Glioblastomas in the frontal and temporal lobes, which are accessible to excision, may have a slightly longer survival time.

Symptomatic treatment by corticosteroids is often very effective initially in patients with glioblastoma. The mode of action of the steroids is unclear but they have an effect of reducing intracranial pressure and reducing the severity of symptoms due to these tumours in the early stages. After radiotherapy, many centres employ chemotherapy, but the results have not been marked.

Histological variants of glioblastoma

One of the major characteristics of glioblastoma is its wide variability in histological appearance. Thus it is very useful to have the basic criteria of an anaplastic glial tumour with microvascular proliferation and areas of necrosis for the diagnosis of this tumour. Nevertheless, there are particular histological variants of glioblastoma which are worthy of separate mention because of their very distinctive appearance and because of the discussion that has occurred regarding their biological behaviour. One of these tumours is *giant cell glioblastoma* which usually occurs in younger patients and, despite its bizarre appearance, may have a better prognosis than other types of glioblastoma. Another is *gliosarcoma* which, for many years, was viewed as a mixed astrocytic tumour and sarcoma, but has a similar prognosis and age range of presentation to glioblastoma. Gliosarcomas may be confused clinically with metastases or even with meningiomas.

Giant cell glioblastoma

Although this variant of glioblastoma is relatively rare, it may represent up to 5% of glioblastomas; it has a wider age range than other types of glioblastoma (Fig. 4.63) but is encountered more frequently in younger age groups (under 50 years).[17]

Clinically, patients present with a short history similar to that of other types of glioblastoma and usually without a protracted history suggestive of a pre-existing diffuse astrocytoma. Radiologically, giant cell glioblastomas enhance, and they may be localised to peripheral areas of the cerebral hemispheres. Giant cell glioblastomas appear

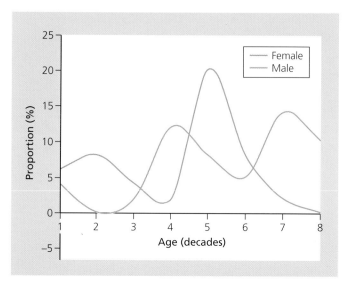

Fig. 4.63 **Relative age and sex incidence of giant cell glioblastomas.** (Data derived from Ref. 17).

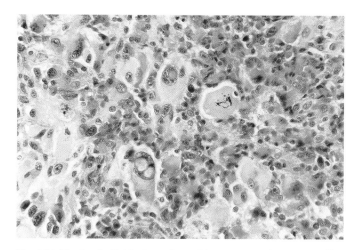

Fig. 4.64 **Giant cell glioblastoma.** Large bizarre astrocytic tumour cells are characteristic of this variant of glioblastoma. H & E.

to have a somewhat better prognosis than other glioblastomas,[147] especially in children[148] in whom they may be confused with PXA.[149]

The major pathological feature of these tumours is the presence of very large (often 500 µm in diameter) bizarre giant cells which express GFAP and S-100 protein[149] (Fig. 4.64). Pleomorphic, irregular nuclei are often multiple within tumour cells and many have large nucleoli. Admixed with the giant cells is a population of smaller tumour cells which show a higher proliferation rate (14–90%) than the giant cells.[150] There may be a prominent reticulin content throughout the tumour or in isolated regions. Atypical mitoses are frequently seen throughout the tumour and immunocytochemistry reveals variable expression of GFAP within tumour cell cytoplasm and p53 protein in giant cell nuclei.

Although giant cell glioblastomas often arise as primary glioblastomas, i.e. without a history of prior diffuse astrocytoma, they have genetic alterations more similar to secondary glioblastomas with frequent *TP53* mutations (see Biology and genetics section below).

Small cell glioblastoma

Unlike giant cell glioblastoma and gliosarcoma, small cell glioblastoma is not a variant of glioblastoma listed in the 2000 WHO classification. Nonetheless, the term is widely used by neuropathologists to describe a glioblastoma comprising predominantly small, anaplastic cells. The cells tend to be rather monomorphic, with small to medium-sized, hyperchromatic nuclei that are carrot-shaped, rounded or slightly elongated. The cells most closely resemble those found in primitive neuroectodermal tumours such as medulloblastomas or in anaplastic oligodendrogliomas. As with other glioblastomas, the tumours frequently display mitotic activity, microvascular prolieration and necrosis, including with pseudopalisading. GFAP immunohistochemistry will usually highlight only scattered positive cell processes, but stains for neuronal markers are negative.

Given the small, anaplastic cells, the major differential diagnostic considerations are a primitive neuroectodermal tumour and an anaplastic oligodendroglioma. Positivity for markers of neuronal and/or muscle differentiation would argue in favour of a primitive neuroectodermal tumour, as would young age of the patient. The presence of classical oligodendroglioma elsewhere in the specimen would, on the other hand, favour a diagnosis of anaplastic oligodendroglioma. In our experience, small cell glioblastomas lack the overall uniformity and organisation of anaplastic oligodendrogliomas, with more pleomorphic and slightly elongated nuclei that appear haphazardly arranged. Recent molecular genetic enquiries have promised to clarify this differential diagnosis as well, as approximately two-thirds of small cell glioblastomas exhibit amplification of EGFR.[151] This is important, as those anaplastic oligodendrogliomas with EGFR amplification are aggressive malignancies and are poorly responsive to chemotherapy.[152] Therefore, in a diagnostically challenging case, when the pathologist is unsure of whether to label the lesion a small cell glioblastoma or an anaplastic oligodendroglioma, a positive result for EGFR amplification would imply that the tumour would follow an aggressive course similar to a glioblastoma are, regardless of the pathological diagnosis.

Gliosarcoma

The essential pathological features of gliosarcomas, and other desmoplastic astrocytomas such as desmoplastic cerebral astrocytomas and gangliogliomas (see Chapter 8), are that spindle cell elements, rich in reticulin and poor in GFAP expression, surround islands of varying size composed of reticulin-free GFAP positive cells.[153–156] The vast majority of such tumours are gliosarcomas, although rare low grade fibrous astrocytomas or 'gliofibromas' have been reported.[154,155] These are discussed with the closely related entity, desmoplastic infantile, ganglioglioma,[156] in Chapter 8.

Gliosarcomas constitute some 2% of all glioblastomas.[153] The age range is similar to that of primary glioblastoma (Fig. 4.65); they are located almost exclusively in the cerebral hemispheres with a predilection for the temporal lobes (44%) but they occur in the parietal lobes (28%), frontal lobes (17%) and occipital lobes (11%).[153]

Clinically, there is usually a short history either with seizures or the onset of focal neurological signs. Gliosarcomas have a similar prognosis to glioblastoma.[153] Radiologically, those tumours that contain a large fibrous component may appear as a well circumscribed, enhancing lesions mimicking either a cerebral metastasis or a meningioma.

Gliosarcomas may be removed as circumscribed nodules which show prominent central necrosis and may be confused macroscopically with a metastasis or abscess. Difficulty may arise in establishing a rapid intraoperative diagnosis due to the prominence of the fibrous component. These tumours may be impossible to smear due to their firm consistency and are best examined by cryostat sectioning. Suspicion that the tumour is a gliosarcoma is raised by the presence of islands of glial cells with hyperchromatic pleomorphic nuclei surrounded by spindle cell elements. A reticulin stain on a cryostat section is extremely valuable in establishing the diagnosis as it identifies the fibrous

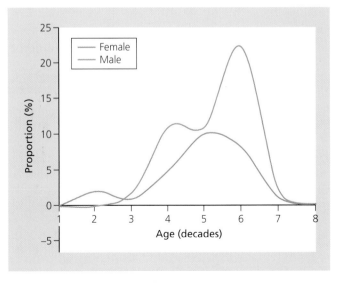

Fig. 4.65 **Relative age and sex incidence of gliosarcomas**. (Data derived from Ref. 17).

component and highlights the reticulin negative glial component. A firm diagnosis can be established on a cryostat section by immunocytochemistry for GFAP which will identify the glial component within the tumour.

Many glioblastomas contain small areas of fibrosis, particularly associated with blood vessels and many contain spindle shaped GFAP positive glial tumour cells. In order to conform to the descriptions of gliosarcoma, the tumour should be mainly composed of a biphasic pattern of spindle cells surrounded by reticulin staining and islands of poorly differentiated glial tumour cells which are free of reticulin (Figs 4.66 and 4.67). Often the tumour is a firm nodule with a central area of necrosis and glioblastoma cells infiltrating normal or oedematous brain at the edge of the fibrous nodule. Varying degrees of lymphocyte infiltration may be seen around vessels at the periphery of gliosarcomas.

The spindle cell element of gliosarcomas resembles a storiform pattern of malignant fibrous histiocytomas (Figs 4.66 and 4.67). Almost every cell is surrounded by reticulin and there is often some nuclear pleomorphism and mitoses in these areas. Immunocytochemistry reveals GFAP expression in a proportion of the spindle cells (Fig. 4.68)[157] mixed with GFAP negative cells.

In addition to the spindle cell elements, other tissues may be identified in gliosarcomas with the formation of cartilage, smooth muscle and striated muscle, bone and osteoid chondral tissue.[17] Epithelial elements have also been identified in gliosarcomas, some of which are squamoid.

Immunocytochemical identification of a proportion of the spindle cells in gliosarcoma as glial elements suggested that these tumours are from a common astrocytic origin.[157] Similar genetic changes have now been identified in both the glial and spindle cell ('sarcomatous') areas confirming the monoclonal origin of this astrocytic tumour. Identical mutations of the *TP53* tumour suppressor gene in the gliomatous and the sarcomatous components of gliosarcomas support a common origin from glial cells.[158] Similar genetic changes with gain of chromosome 7, loss of chromosome 10, deletions in chromosome 9p arm and alterations in chromosome 3 have been observed in classical glioblastomas and in gliosarcoma.[159]

The *prognosis* for gliosarcomas is similar to that of glioblastoma, despite the apparent demarcation of the tumour from surrounding brain at surgery. Gliosarcoma has a 35-week mean survival period compared with 41 weeks for glioblastoma.[152]

Other variants

Glioblastomas may have an extraordinarily large number of different histological appearances. Reports of rare variants abound in the literature, including heavily

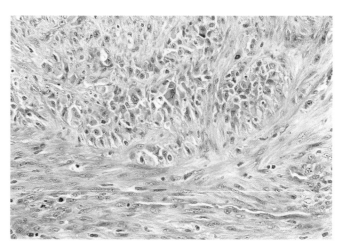

Fig. 4.66 Gliosarcoma. A spindle cell area (bottom) and more typical pleomorphic glial areas (top) are shown. H & E.

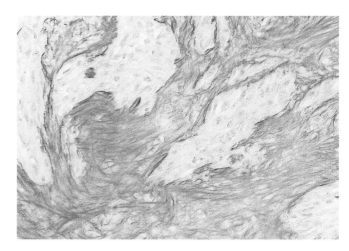

Fig. 4.67 Gliosarcoma. A similar field to Fig. 4.66 stained for connective tissue. Reticulin rich areas of spindle cells separate the reticulin free islands of more typical glial cells. Reticulin stain.

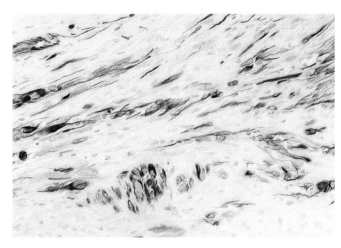

Fig. 4.68 Gliosarcoma. Rounded and stellate tumour cells express GFAP as do elongated spindle cells in the reticulin rich regions of this tumour. Immunocytochemistry for GFAP.

lipidised variants, granular cell tumours and 'sarcogliomas'. These are not common and are not recognised as clear variants by the 2000 WHO classification.

Heavily lipidised glioblastomas, as their name suggests, feature lipid droplets in many cells. These must be distinguished from pleomorphic xanthoastrocytomas by their lack of granular bodies, high mitotic index, rarity of cystic components and the generally infiltrative margins. Some lipidised glioblastomas exhibit a cohesive architecture with epithelioid nests and sheets of cells. These features may be accompanied by the expression of both cytokeratins and EMA (the 'lipid-rich epithelioid glioblastoma'), raising potential diagnostic confusion with metastatic carcinoma.[160] Careful study will usually reveal areas of more typical glioblastoma, with expression of GFAP in large tumour cells.

Granular cell glioblastomas contain large numbers of cells with granular cytoplasm that sometimes resemble foamy macrophages (Fig. 4.69). Alternatively, the granular cells can be quite large and have vaguely eosinophilic granules, more akin to the larger histiocytic cells seen in conditions such as Erdheim–Chester disease. This appearance can lead to diagnostic confusion. As the foamy granular cells in granular cell glioblastomas express GFAP (Fig. 4.70) and lack expression of microglial/macrophage markers such as CD68 (Fig. 4.71), they can usually be identified fairly readily as glial tumours.

'Sarcoglioma' is an ill-defined and rare entity related to glioblastoma.[161] This entity occurs in the unusual situation in which a mesenchymal tumour, typically in the meninges, is associated with an underlying glioma. The reported cases feature primary tumours such as haemangiopericytomas of the meninges and malignant astrocytic tumours. Originally, it was postulated that the glial tumour represented transformation of an exuberant astrocytic reaction to the overlying tumour. To our knowledge, however, none of these rare cases has been studied with molecular genetic techniques that could clarify their histogenesis. Possibilities include induction of an underlying glioma by the sarcomatous lesion, although this seems unlikely, or 'collision' tumours in an individual predisposed to intracranial tumour development for either hereditary or environmental reasons.

Gliomatosis cerebri

Many diffuse astrocytomas and anaplastic astrocytomas invade large areas of brain and are often widely distributed at clinical presentation. In gliomatosis cerebri, however, there is an even more diffuse spread of tumour cells, often involving both cerebral hemispheres or large areas of the brain stem or spinal cord. Although most cases of gliomatosis cerebri are described in adults,[162] the age range is from neonates to 83 years, with both sexes

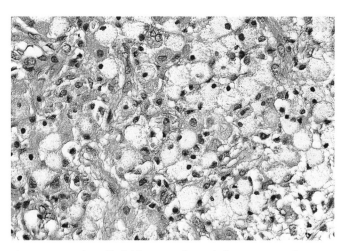

Fig. 4.69 **Granular cell glioblastoma**. The typical appearance of a granular cell glioblastoma showing multiple foamy cells resembling macrophages. H & E.

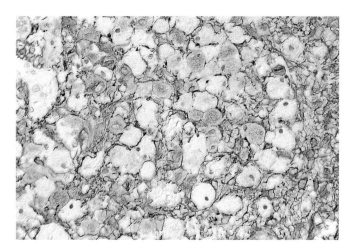

Fig. 4.70 **Granular cell glioblastoma**. Tumour cells, including some of the foamy cells, express GFAP. Immunocytochemistry for GFAP.

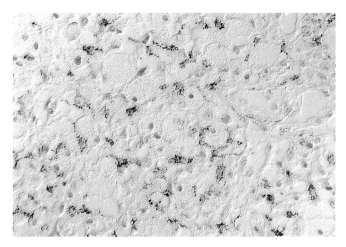

Fig. 4.71 **Granular cell glioblastoma**. Microglial cells are insinuated between the tumour cells but the large foamy cells do not stain for this macrophage marker. Immunocytochemistry for CD68.

affected equally (Fig. 4.72). The cerebral hemispheres are most commonly affected with a lower frequency of involvement of the brain stem, medulla and spinal cord.[163]

Clinically, patients present with features relating to the major area of tumour infiltration,[162] but most frequently with signs of corticospinal tract involvement, dementia, headache and seizures. Psychiatric problems may occur with lethargy, behavioural changes and psychosis. PET has been used to demonstrate decreased metabolism and disconnection of the cortex with gliomatosis cerebri.[164] Sensory deficits and pain are also described.

Radiological investigations revealed diffuse enlargement of affected areas of brain which appear as ill-defined areas of low density in CT scans and increased signal in T2-weighted MRI.[163,165] At post-mortem, areas of the CNS involved by gliomatosis cerebri show diffuse enlargement and blurring of grey matter–white matter borders. Occasionally, there is a distinct nodule of tumour.

Rapid intraoperative diagnosis and histological diagnosis on paraffin sections may present problems. The surgeon may have difficulty identifying a suitable target, although deep within an abnormal area in a T2-weighted MRI is often most fruitful.

Histologically, gliomatosis cerebri is characterised by the diffuse invasion of grey and white matter by spindle shaped cells with rod shaped nuclei orientated along white matter fibre tracts or along axons and terminal dendrites within the cerebral cortex (Fig. 4.73). Many of the rod shaped nuclei are hyperchromatic; mitoses may be seen but they are variable in number. Rarely, the cells of gliomatosis cerebri may have the appearance of oligodendroglioma.

Immunocytochemistry for GFAP shows variable and often poor staining of the tumour cells and the picture may be confused by the large number of reactive astrocytes present in the field. One of the major problems is confusion between tumour cells and microglia. Hyperchromasia of tumour cell nuclei is helpful in distinguishing between the two cell types but immunocytochemistry may be required to exclude a microglia reaction Ki-67/MIB-1 labelling may also be complicated by labelling of reactive cells as well as tumour cells. Published figures suggest that the Ki-67/MIB-1 labelling index is about 7%.[17]

The prognosis of gliomatosis cerebri is poor,[163] with a median survival of some 38 months which correlates with the Ki-67/MIB-1 labelling index of the tumour.[162]

The *differential diagnosis* of gliomatosis cerebri, at a clinical and radiological level, includes other diffuse or multifocal tumours of the brain, such as lymphoma,[166] as well as diffuse non-neoplastic conditions such as demyelinating diseases. Histologically, the primary difficulty can be the identification of the neoplastic cells, as they may be diffusely distributed among the normal grey and white matter structures of the brain. Their rod-shaped nuclei may also be confused with microglia.

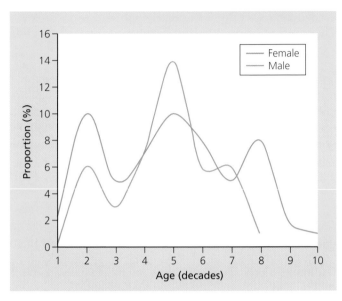

Fig. 4.72 **Relative age and sex incidence of gliomatosis cerebri**. (Data derived from Ref. 17).

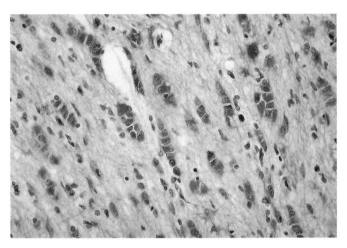

Fig. 4.73 **Gliomatosis cerebri**. Corpus callosum with diffusely infiltrating tumour cells, arranged in short chains, orientated along the white matter fibre tracts. Immunocytochemistry for GFAP.

Furthermore, it must be kept in mind that a diagnosis of gliomatosis cerebri is a clinicopathological one and dependent on radiological information. A biopsy of gliomatosis cerebri is indistinguishable from that of the margin of a diffusely infiltrative astrocytoma.

The histogenesis of gliomatosis cerebri is not clear. It is most likely, however, that gliomatosis does not represent a 'field effect' in which neoplastic transformation occurs throughout the brain. Gliomatosis most likely represents the most diffusely infiltrative type of diffuse astrocytoma, a clonal neoplastic lesion in which the tumour cells have a remarkable propensity for brain invasion without the ability to form a solid tumour in one location.

Differential diagnosis of diffuse astrocytic tumours

Because astrocytic tumours are so common and have a remarkably varied range of histological appearances, the differential diagnosis is wide. A summary diagram in Fig. 4.66 depicts the major features that distinguish astrocytic tumours from each other and from non-neoplastic astrocyte reactions within the brain.

Other differential diagnoses include a wide range of neoplastic lesions as well as several important non-neoplastic conditions. In many cases, the clinical and neuroradiological features narrow the differential diagnosis considerably, and the clinician may have a high index of suspicion that the biopsy will yield a diagnosis of astrocytic tumour; this is particularly true for typical, ring enhancing glioblastomas in older patients. However, a number of benign neoplasms and non-neoplastic processes may present with clinical and neuroradiological findings essentially indistinguishable from an astrocytic tumour, so that many other entities should be considered before proposing a histological diagnosis of astrocytic tumour. These entities are discussed below.

Differential diagnosis of non-neoplastic processes

It is of primary importance to exclude non-neoplastic processes that may mimic astrocytic tumours clinically and neuroradiologically, as the treatment of these diseases differs markedly from that of astrocytic tumours (Fig. 4.74). A high percentage of major misdiagnoses detected in neuropathology consultation practices are non-neoplastic cerebral conditions that have been diagnosed as neuroepithelial tumours.[167]

Reactive astrocytosis (gliosis)

Astrocytosis may accompany a variety of CNS conditions, from infarcts to infectious processes to neoplasms. Because reactive astrocytosis may be moderately hypercellular and may contain slightly irregular nuclei, it may resemble diffuse, fibrillary astrocytoma – or rarely anaplastic astrocytoma – on biopsy. There are some general morphological differences between acute and chronic reactive astrocytosis, and knowledge of these features helps in the distinction between astrocytic tumours and astrocytosis. In acute gliosis, astrocytes tend to have copious eosinophilic cytoplasm; in chronic gliosis, the astrocytic cytoplasm is not conspicuous and there is a background of densely packed, coarse fibrillary processes. Rosenthal fibres may be numerous in chronic gliosis, especially around syringomyelic cavities or around tumours such as craniopharyngiomas or haemangioblastomas. Although Rosenthal fibres may be confusing in the differential diagnosis of pilocytic astrocytoma, they

are not a problem in the diagnosis of adult, diffuse, fibrillary astrocytoma, since Rosenthal fibres are not characteristic of these tumours.

Several histological features help to distinguish diffuse astrocytomas from gliosis (Fig. 4.74). The most important feature is nuclear pleomorphism. Irregularly shaped nuclei, such as elongated nuclei or nuclei with grooves or multiple lobes, are highly suggestive of tumour cells. Hyperchromasia is also strongly suggestive of neoplasia, since reactive astrocytes tend to have more euchromatic nuclei with single prominent nucleoli. On the other hand, areas of longstanding reactive astrocytosis frequently show some degree of nuclear hyperchromasia similar to the 'ancient change' seen in longstanding Schwannomas (see Chapter 15) The distribution of cells also can be helpful. Irregularly distributed cells with an increase in nuclear : cytoplasmic ratio is more indicative of neoplasia than reactive gliosis, in which cells tend to be more regularly distributed. In addition, so-called 'secondary structures of Scherer'[168] – perineuronal satellitosis of tumour cells, subpial or subependymal spread of cells, and perivascular satellitosis – are also characterstic of neoplasia. Microcysts, although not present in all diffuse astrocytomas, are not seen in reactive gliosis.

In most diffuse astrocytomas, neoplastic cells tend not to have large amounts of eosinophilic cytoplasm (copious eosinophilic cytoplasm is typical of gemistocytic astrocytoma). As a result, the identification of scattered cells with extensive eosinophilic cytoplasm should quickly raise the possibility of a reactive gliosis. Reactive astrocytes tend to have many more processes than astrocytic tumour cells (Fig. 4.74). On the other hand, the absence of cytoplasm does not necessarily make an astrocyte neoplastic. Alzheimer Type 2 astrocytes, for instance, are found throughout the brain in metabolic imbalances such as hepatic encephalopathy. These polyploid non-neoplastic astrocytes have irregular nuclei and no visible cytoplasm, but have strikingly pale, vesicular rather than hyperchromatic nuclei. Fortunately, the types of metabolic processes that lead to the development of Alzheimer Type 2 astrocytes rarely lead to biopsy, so these cells are more often encountered in autopsy material than in surgical specimens.

A few further general caveats are important to keep in mind when deciding whether a biopsy represents a diffuse astrocytoma or a reactive process:

1. Macrophages are quite uncommon in astrocytic tumours, except in occasional anaplastic astrocytomas and in glioblastomas that have been treated or have extensive necrosis. Therefore, the identification of macrophages in a putatative 'diffuse astrocytoma' should raise the suspicion of a reactive process, such as an infarct or demyelinating disease such as multiple sclerosis.

2. Perineuronal satellitosis, while highly suggestive of infiltrating tumour (especially of oligodendroglioma), can be a normal feature of cerebral cortex, especially temporal lobe cortex; one must be sure that the perineuronal cells are atypical and present in greater numbers than usual.

3. Freezing may introduce a number of artefacts in brain tissue, such as nuclear atypia and cystic disruption of the tissue, that may simulate an astrocytic tumour. Therefore, the presence of some nuclear atypia in cryostat sections or in fixed, embedded sections of previously frozen tissue should be viewed with caution and should not be used as the sole criterion for diagnosing diffuse astrocytoma. For this reason, it may be advisable to retain some tissue unfrozen from all biopsy specimens so that this tissue can be quickly fixed for standard processing.

Acute demyelinating disease/multiple sclerosis

Multiple sclerosis is a demyelinating disease characterised clinically and radiologically by lesions that are separated in 'space and time'. Multiple sclerosis, however, can present clinically and radiologically as a single, enhancing, expansile lesion, thus raising the possibility of anaplastic astrocytoma.[169] This may lead to biopsy of an acutely demyelinated plaque. The initial key to the histological diagnosis of multiple sclerosis in this situation is the identification of foamy macrophages. Numerous macrophages are characteristic of acute multiple sclerosis plaques and, in the proper clinical situation, should strongly suggest the diagnosis of demyelinating disease. However, a sheet of macrophages, with their relatively small nuclei and foamy cytoplasm, may resemble an oligodendroglioma, with the 'fried egg' appearing cells, particularly on low power examination. However, cryostat sections of macrophages, with the attendant distortion of the freezing process, may create a resemblance to an astrocytic tumour as well. Oil red O staining for neutral lipid is very useful for identifying lipid filled macrophages in cryostat sections and distinguishing them from lipid poor tumour cells. Smear preparations are quite helpful for intraoperative diagnosis in this setting, allowing ready identification of macrophages with their characteristic nuclei and foamy, well defined cytoplasm without cell processes. Scattered lymphocytes support the diagnosis of multiple sclerosis, but can be seen in astrocytic tumours (particularly gemistocytic astrocytoma, pleomorphic xanthoastrocytomas and gangliogliomas) and in other demyelinating diseases such as progressive multifocal leucoencephalopathy (especially in AIDS patients – see below). Astrocytes are plentiful at the margins of multiple sclerosis plaques and appear reactive, with eosinophilic cytoplasm and often with distinct nucleoli. As discussed above, the identification of such reactive cells should divert one away from a diagnosis of glioma.

So-called Creutzfeldt cells may also be found at the periphery of acute multiple sclerosis plaques, and appear histologically ominous. These are probably astrocytic cells; they have large nuclei with a fragmented chromatin pattern that resembles an atypical dispersed mitotic figure. This resemblance is strengthened by the observation that such cells often label with the Ki-67/MIB-1 antibody, which recognises proliferating cells. The first, but unfortunately erroneous, reaction that they elicit is that such atypical mitotic figure-like cells must indicate anaplastic astrocytoma. Their distinctive appearance, however, should instead alert the pathologist to the correct diagnosis of probable demyelinating disease. The diagnosis of demyelinating disease can then be confirmed with a myelin stain (e.g. Luxol fast blue) to show loss of myelin and immunocytochemistry for neurofilament protein or a silver impregnation technique (e.g. Bodian) to show relative preservation of axons.

Progressive multifocal leucoencephalopathy

Progressive multifocal leucoencephalopathy (PML) is a destructive, demyelinating disease caused by the JC type of papovavirus. The disease is typically multifocal, and does not usually raise the differential diagnosis of astrocytic tumour. On occasion, however, lesions may be unifocal (often in the occipital lobe) and rapidly expanding, thus simulating a glioma. Since PML affects immunosuppressed patients, the emergence of AIDS has made PML more common, and a lesion that is sometimes biopsied. The virus predominantly affects oligodendroglia, and transforms their nuclei into enlarged, deeply basophilic, glassy appearing masses. These nuclei are pathognomonic of PML. By electron microscopy, immunocytochemistry and in situ hybridisation, such nuclei can be shown to contain the virus. The diagnostic nuclei typically surround an area of demyelination, which is characterised by loss of myelin, relative preservation of axons, and lipid laden macrophages. Inflammation tends to be scanty, although perivascular lymphocyte and plasma cell cuffing may be prominent in AIDS cases, and may obscure the diagnostic findings.[170]

In addition to the enlarged basophilic oligodendroglial nuclei, astrocytes may also be affected by the JC virus. In this situation, astrocytic nuclei become large and bizarre and, in every morphological respect, resemble neoplastic astrocytes. It is of interest that the JC virus is oncogenic in experimental animals; it has been used to induce experimental brain tumours, and is closely related to the tumorigenic SV40 virus. These nuclei, if encountered on a small biopsy and if numerous, have led to the erroneous diagnosis of diffuse astrocytoma. The key to correct diagnosis lies with the clinical history of immunosuppression, and in identifying the histological hallmarks of demyelination accompanied by the characteristic enlarged, deeply basophilic, glassy oligodendroglial or astrocytic nuclei.[171]

Cerebral infarction

Although the clinical and neuroradiological scenario usually allows the distinction of infarction from neoplasia, occasionally infarcts may be clinically or radiologically atypical, and raise the differential diagnosis of astrocytic tumour. The histological picture of cerebral infarct, as with infarcts in other areas of the body, varies with the age of the infarct. Most biopsied infarcts are acute or subacute. In these, the histological hallmarks are necrotic tissue characterised by eosinophilic 'red' hypoxic neurons with tissue pallor and fragmentation. Dark angular neurons are considered to be artefact and are commonly seen in biopsies of normal cerebral cortex; they therefore should not be considered as an indication of infarction. The type of inflammatory infiltrate correlates with the age of the infarct, with a few neutrophils in the early stages (24–48 h) and macrophages in the subacute (5 days) and later stages. When macrophages are numerous in an older infarct, the infarct will appear strikingly cellular, and may raise the differential diagnosis of glioma. Since macrophages have relatively small nuclei and foamy cytoplasm, a sea of macrophages may resemble an oligodendroglioma, with its 'fried egg' cells, on low power examination. The astrocytic response to infarction should conform to the reactive astrocytes described above under gliosis (Fig. 4.74), and should not be atypical. One further potential confusing feature of subacute infarction is endothelial proliferation. This may be rather intense at the periphery of an infarct as it begins to organise, and may suggest the endothelial proliferation of an oligodendroglioma or glioblastoma. These reactive vessels are not as thin walled and straight as those in oligodendroglioma. In addition, the vessels are often evenly spaced, and do not show piling up of endothelial cells into glomeruloid structures that is seen in the endothelial proliferation at the edge of a glioblastoma.

Toxoplasmosis

With the emergence of the AIDS epidemic, cerebral toxoplasmosis has become more frequent as a cause of intracranial mass lesions. Patients may, however, present *without* a clear history of AIDS or immunosuppression, and therefore toxoplasmosis should be entertained in the differential diagnosis of most necrotic mass lesions in the brain. Usually, these are multiple and are treated without biopsy, but toxoplasmosis may also present as a single, ring enhancing mass lesion that may clinically and radiologically simulate a glioblastoma. This situation may result in biopsy of a toxoplasma abscess. When diagnostic, the biopsy will show necrotic debris surrounded by gliotic brain with acute and chronic inflammation. Inspection of the surrounding brain parenchyma should demonstrate encysted forms of the organism, while free organisms can be identified in the parenchyma and in the central necrosis. Organisms can be identified on routine H & E stains, but may be more easily identified with Giemsa stains or immunohistochemical staining with anti-*Toxoplasma* antibodies.

On occasion, biopsies of toxoplasmosis may show only necrotic debris with small fragments of adjacent gliotic brain. If the gliosis appears cytologically atypical and organisms are not apparent, this may raise the differential diagnosis of glioblastoma. The pyknotic nuclear debris seen in glioblastomas may be difficult to distinguish from toxoplasma organisms. Immunocytochemistry for *Toxoplasma* may be helpful in making this distinction. The diagnosis of glioblastoma should therefore be made only if definite anaplastic glioblastoma cells are identified, and if immunocytochemistry for *Toxoplasma* is negative.

A final caveat is that encysted *Toxoplasma* organisms may rarely be found in essentially normal brain. We have on occasion seen isolated encysted organisms in normal brain at autopsy. More significantly, we have noted encysted *Toxoplasma* in the necrotic debris that accompanied a typical glioblastoma. For these reasons, we encourage the diagnosis of active toxoplasmosis to rest on the demonstration of more than a single encysted form and preferably on free organisms.

Intracerebral abscess

Intracerebral abscess is one of the most frequent radiological differential diagnoses for glioblastoma; the distinction is very important as abscesses are far more amenable to treatment than glioblastoma. In addition to *Toxoplasma*, a host of infectious organisms can cause intracerebral mass lesions. In developed countries, bacterial abscesses are the most common, while tuberculomas and cysticercal cysts are more common in other areas of the world.[172] These lesions can present as single, subacute, space occupying masses that are accompanied by substantial intracerebral oedema. When subacute, the organising, granulation and fibrous tissues at the margin of these abscesses can produce ring enhancement on neuroradiological studies. Patients can also present without systemic symptoms or signs (including fever) and without a definite infectious source. These confusing clinical and radiological features may necessitate a biopsy.

On histological examination, the purulent centre, replete with neutrophils, necrotic debris and perhaps microorganisms, is the initial key to diagnosis of a pyogenic abscess. Care must be taken to ensure appropriate bacterial culture of the pus or fragments of abscess wall; the responsibility usually lies with the pathologist making the cryostat section diagnosis. The wall of the intracerebral abscess should show three zones: the outer zone of gliotic brain, the middle zone of collagen rich granulation tissue, and the inner zone of purulent debris. The identification of collagen in a brain biopsy should alert the pathologist to the diagnosis, since very few processes in the brain lead to fibrosis (only brain abscess, trauma and neoplastic desmoplasia, e.g. gliosarcoma). 'Non-pyogenic' abscesses display many of these features, but often have additional histological characteristics. Tuberculomas, for instance, show the well known features of granulomatous inflammation, giant cells and caseous necrosis. Other organisms, such as *Cysticercus, Shistosoma, Nocardia* and amoeba are identified by their particular morphologies and staining properties. Special stains, cultures and serological studies should facilitate in identifying the organism responsible.

Radiation injury

Radiation injury to the nervous system (see Chapter 20) is characterised histologically by thickening and hyalinisation of small blood vessels, prominent endothelial cells, coagulative necrosis and reactive astrocytes that may have bizarre, enlarged nuclei. After large doses of radiation such as those used to treat astrocytic tumours (greater than 5000 or 6000 cGy), symptomatic radiation necrosis may follow. Histologically, this is characterised by extensive coagulative necrosis, calcification, haemorrhage and oedema, in addition to the above mentioned changes. Late delayed radiation necrosis typically occurs at least 6 months after treatment, and may clinically and radiologically resemble a recurrent glioblastoma. Although modern neuroimaging techniques such as PET scanning are proving to be useful in making the distinction between radiation necrosis and recurrent tumour, a biopsy is still necessary to make a definite diagnosis.

With a history of radiation (which should be available to the pathologist), the differential diagnosis is narrowed to three conditions: recurrent tumour, residual tumour and radiation necrosis. Recurrent tumour is defined as tumour that has arisen since therapy was last given. This diagnosis is the most straightforward histologically, featuring typical anaplastic astrocytoma or glioblastoma, often with aggregates of small, anaplastic cells and pseudopalisading around necrotic zones. Fortunately for the pathologist, the most important histological decision is often whether recurrent tumour is present. Residual tumour, on the other hand, is defined as tumour that was present at the time of radiation and is still present. It is thought that residual tumour cells are either not viable or not as robust as recurrent tumour. Residual tumour cells are enlarged, often with bizarre nuclei and eosinophilic cytoplasm, appearing cytologically similar to radiated tumour cells in other areas of the body. These are scattered throughout the biopsy, but are not densely aggregated. Often these cells accompany radiation necrosis, and it may be impossible to distinguish irradiated residual tumour cells from bizarre irradiated reactive astrocytes. These changes are discussed more extensively in Chapter 20.

Differential diagnosis of other neoplastic conditions

Metastatic carcinoma

Many metastatic carcinomas may be diagnosed with a fairly high degree of confidence in the presence of multiple lesions on neuroimaging and a history of a primary tumour. Solitary lesions in the absence of a primary lesion raise the differential diagnosis of a primary glioblastoma, particularly since these tumours are most common in the same age groups. Furthermore, some glioblastomas may present as apparently multiple masses on neuroradiological examination. While most carcinomas have distinctive epithelial features and are easily diagnosed histologically, poorly differentiated tumours may be difficult to distinguish on light microscopic examination from a glioblastoma. A well demarcated margin may support a diagnosis of carcinoma, but is not diagnostic as this may be seen, on rare occasions, in glioblastomas. The diagnosis is usually resolved by immunocytochemistry, with even in poorly differentiated carcinomas staining for cytokeratins and glioblastomas at least focally for GFAP. Sometimes, however, glioblastomas may stain for cytokeratins, particularly if an antikeratin antibody 'cocktail' is used. Using antibodies separately against high and low molecular weight keratins may solve any difficulties, since glioblastomas show cross reactivity for the antibodies against high molecular weight, but not low molecular weight, keratins. Typically, however, cytokeratin staining is only noted in tumours that stain for GFAP, which argues strongly for a glial tumour since GFAP staining in carcinomas is very rare. In remaining problematic cases, epithelial membrane antigen staining may be helpful in diagnosing carcinoma, or specific markers in tumours such as prostate or thyroid cancer. Finally, electron microscopy may be helpful in identifying specific intracellular organelles, but is rarely necessary (Chapter 12).

It is also important to mention that some glioblastomas may display epithelial features, and thereby mimic carcinoma. Such features include papillary and glandular structures and even squamoid foci. These features may be more common in gliosarcomas than in standard glioblastoma. In most cases, typical glioblastoma or gliosarcoma is present in other regions of the biopsy. In rare problematic cases, GFAP immunocytochemistry usually resolves the problem.

Primary CNS lymphoma

In large biopsy specimens, CNS lymphoma is easily distinguished from astrocytic tumours. However, in small biopsies that sample few cells, the distinction may be difficult. Often, a perivascular arrangment of cells suggests lymphoma, but infiltrating gliomas may display perivascular spread, one of the secondary structures of Scherer. Cytological evaluation is often diagnostic; for instance, on intraoperative touch or dab preparations, lymphoma cells have large, sometimes cleaved nuclei, often with prominent nucleoli or many clumped chromocentres, and a paucity of cytoplasm. The tumour cells are not cohesive. Immunocytochemistry is diagnostic, since lymphoma cells label for common leucocyte antigen and usually for B-cell markers, as opposed to GFAP in astrocytic tumours (Chapter 11).

Other astrocytic tumours

There may be considerable histological overlap between the diffuse, fibrillary astrocytomas and other astrocytic tumours such as pilocytic astrocytoma, PXA, subependymal giant cell astrocytoma, ganglioglioma and oligoastrocytoma. Since most of the above entities (with the exception of oligoastrocytoma and some PXAs) are slow growing and have a much better prognosis, the differential diagnosis with diffuse, fibrillary tumours is of great clinical importance. In many instances, a combined clinicopathological approach is most helpful in making these distinctions, since many tumours have characteristic clinical and neuroradiological features.

Pilocytic astrocytoma In many cases of pilocytic astrocytomas, the clinical history will be highly suggestive of pilocytic astrocytoma, for instance, tumours occurring in younger patients in the cerebellum, optic nerve or third ventricular region. Nonetheless, diffuse, fibrillary astrocytomas may involve these regions as well and may affect young patients. In most cases, pilocytic astrocytomas can be distinguished histologically from diffuse, fibrillary astrocytomas, when pilocytic astrocytomas have classical features such as a biphasic pattern with coarse fibrillary zones and spongy zones, Rosenthal fibres and granular bodies. Indeed, the presence of Rosenthal fibres or granular bodies should at least cast doubt upon a diagnosis of diffuse, fibrillary astrocytoma. Some pilocytic astrocytomas, however, do not have all of these features and such tumours may be difficult to distinguish from diffuse, fibrillary astrocytomas, especially if the pilocytic astrocytoma is in a cerebral hemisphere. In general, most pilocytic astrocytomas, even in the cerebral hemispheres, will contain coarse fibrillary regions with elongated, piloid tumour cells in the absence of mitotic activity. In most cases, at least some Rosenthal fibres or granular bodies will be present on careful inspection.

Pleomorphic xanthoastrocytoma In most cases, the differential diagnosis of PXA is quickly raised in an astrocytic tumour with more than moderate pleomorphism, particularly in tumours with bizarre, large cells. However, it is important to recall that some PXAs may have a prominent spindle cell component and that the possibility of PXA should probably at least be entertained in any superficially located tumour in a young patient that does not have classical diffuse, fibrillary features. In classical PXA, the diagnosis is relatively straightforward, with pleomorphic and lipid laden cells in the absence of histological features of anaplasia. Lipidised cells may be very rare or even absent in PXAs and therefore the lack of such cells does not argue strongly against a diagnosis of PXA. Furthermore, glioblastomas may be heavily lipidised, so that the presence of lipid does not necessarily imply that the tumour is a PXA. Gemistocytic astrocytomas have cells with copious cytoplasm, but the nuclei do not achieve the same degree of pleomorphism characteristic of PXA. Importantly, however, some PXAs demonstrate malignant features such as mitotic activity and necrosis. Furthermore, as PXAs may transform into typical glioblastomas, such lesions may be difficult to distinguish in particular from giant cell glioblastomas, especially since giant cell glioblastomas are often well demarcated, relatively superficial, occur in young patients, and may have conspicuous inflammation – features also typical for PXA. For this reason, in cases that display malignant histological features, the distinction from a diffuse, fibrillary astrocytoma may not be possible. In such cases, however, treatment often errs on the side of treating the tumour as if it were a diffuse, fibrillary astrocytoma. Inflammation may be prominent in these lesions, but does not help in the differential diagnosis with gemistocytic astrocytoma and giant cell glioblastoma, since these lesions may contain numerous perivascular inflammatory infiltrates.

Subependymal giant cell astrocytoma Because of the relative rarity of subependymal giant cell astrocytoma, its invariable location within or adjacent to the lateral ventricle and its close association with tuberous sclerosis, subependymal giant cell astrocytomas rarely presents a major diagnostic problem with diffuse, fibrillary astrocytoma. The relatively uniform appearance of the large, ganglioid tumour cells is histologically distinctive and diagnostic in the setting of tuberous sclerosis. Because of the variable expression of tuberous sclerosis, it is possible that subependymal giant cell astrocytomas may occur in the absence of known tuberous sclerosis and some authors have reported cases occurring in the absence of tuberous sclerosis. Subependymal giant cell astrocytomas may have prominent spindle cell regions, but these are usually plump spindle cells that merge with the typical ganglioid cells. The tumour cells in subependymal giant cell astrocytomas often label immunohistochemically with neuronal markers in addition to glial markers, providing a method of distinguishing diagnostically difficult cases.

Ganglioglioma These tumours often occur in patients in the first three decades of life, while diffuse, fibrillary astrocytomas typically affect patients in the fourth through seventh decades; nonetheless, cases of either tumour type may occur at any age. Clinically, patients with ganglioglioma may have a long history of seizures and, on neuroimaging, are often superficial and cystic, sometimes with thinning of the overlying calvarium. Macroscopically, a well demarcated tumour consisting of a mural nodule in a cyst argues for a ganglioglioma rather than a diffuse astrocytoma. On microscopic examination, a crisp border surrounded by reactive, sometimes hemosiderin laden brain confirms the macroscopic impression in many cases of ganglioglioma. Gangliogliomas often have a coarse fibrillary background, which is more coarse than that of typical diffuse astrocytomas and is more akin to that of pilocytic astrocytoma. Eosinophilic granular bodies may be plentiful, and Rosenthal fibres may be present, both features that are distinctly uncommon in diffuse astrocytomas. The presence of dense perivascular lymphocytic infiltrates and large, almost malformative blood vessels are also characteristic of ganglioglioma and less commonly noted in diffuse astrocytomas (Chapter 9).

The diagnosis of ganglioglioma, however, rests on the demonstration of neoplastic ganglion cells. In most cases, these are readily appreciated on microscopic examination, often as clusters of pleomorphic neuronal cells with Nissl substance. In some cases, it may be difficult to distinguish true neoplastic ganglion cells from neurons entrapped by a diffuse, infiltrating tumour. Because gangliogliomas are rarely infiltrative, finding regions with clear cortical infiltration makes a diagnosis of ganglioglioma unlikely and we have found this a reliable method for distinguishing these entities in the uncommon difficult case. Some authors have suggested that synaptophysin immunopositivity provides a specific method for detecting neoplastic ganglion cells, with neoplastic ganglion cells displaying punctate staining below the cell membrane and non-neoplastic cells remain unlabelled.[173] More recent studies have cast doubt on the utility of this approach, by demonstrating many types of normal neurons that have a similar immunohistochemical staining pattern for synaptophysin.[174,175] We have, in turn, not found synaptophysin staining useful in diagnosing ganglion cell tumours and express concern that the use of synaptophysin positivity as a sole criterion for diagnosing a ganglion cell tumour risks misdiagnosing some diffuse, fibrillary astrocytomas as ganglion cell lesions.

Oligodendrogliomas and oligoastrocytomas (mixed gliomas) The distinction of oligodendroglioma and oligoastrocytoma from pure diffuse astrocytoma is of prognostic significance, since the presence of oligodendroglial

features in a glioma appears to signify a better prognosis.[78,86,122,176,177] It is also now clear that oligodendrogliomas, particularly anaplastic oligodendrogliomas, are chemosensitive tumours.[178] Patients with well differentiated oligodendrogliomas,[179] oligoastrocytomas,[180] and anaplastic oligoastrocytomas,[181] may also respond dramatically to chemotherapy. Thus, the distinction of oligodendroglioma and oligoastrocytoma from pure diffuse astrocytoma is now of therapeutic significance, placing increased pressure on the pathologist to decide, 'Is there an oligodendroglial component?'

The histopathological diagnosis of oligodendroglioma remains controversial and subjective.[118,182] Given the lack of an objective marker for oligodendroglial differentiation, there are no universally accepted criteria for diagnosing the histologically atypical lesions. Thus, even among neuropathologists, different thresholds exist for the diagnosis of oligodendroglial components in a glioma. The generally accepted histological features of oligodendroglioma are moderate to marked increased nuclear:cytoplasmic ratio (hypercellularity), round nuclei with perinuclear halos, and a background that is rich in delicate, branching vessels and poor in fibrillar processes. Calcification, in the form of calcospherites, is also a characteristic of oligodendroglioma. However, none of these histological features is unique to oligodendroglioma, and some oligodendroglial tumours, especially anaplastic variants, can have very few of these characteristics. For instance, the classical 'fried egg' appearance of oligodendroglial cells with perinuclear halos is not always present, particularly in specimens which have been frozen. Thus, the uniform and round nature of the tumour cells is, in many cases, the key to raising the possibility of an oligodendroglial component. Often oligodendroglial tumour cells, with characteristic oligodendroglial nuclei, will have small eccentric rounded tufts of eosinophilic cytoplasm, forming so-called 'mini-' or 'microgemistocytes'; this feature should not distract the pathologist to a diagnosis of astrocytic tumour. Anaplastic tumours may assume a number of histological patterns not classically associated with oligodendrogliomas, such as a spindled appearance to many of the nuclei.

There is also argument over how much oligodendroglioma is necessary to diagnose oligoastrocytoma, over whether oligoastrocytoma can be diagnosed in cases where the components are intermixed rather than distinctly separated, and even over whether oligoastrocytoma even exists. There also remains a substantial 'grey zone' between anaplastic oligodendrogliomas and glioblastomas, with some authors diagnosing glioblastoma in an anaplastic oligodendroglioma with perinecrotic pseudopalisading, and others retaining the term anaplastic oligodendroglioma for such tumours. Significantly, classical anaplastic oligodendroglial tumours that also have perinecrotic pseudopalisading may respond to chemotherapy;[183] it would therefore seem prudent to include such tumours under the 'oligodendroglioma' rubric in order to alert the neuro-oncologist to the possible beneficial role for chemotherapy in such a patient.

The concept that molecular genetic alterations may provide such markers of oligodendroglioma is tantalising but still in the early stages of development. Approximately two-thirds of oligodendrogliomas and anaplastic oligodendrogliomas display co-ordinate allelic losses of chromosomes 1p and 19q.[183–185] Astrocytic tumours, on the other hand, while having loss of chromosome 19q in about 50% of cases,[186,187] do not commonly lose chromosome 1p.[188] Thus, the combined loss of chromosomes 1p and 19q may be a useful marker of oligodendroglial gliomas[118]. Significantly, combined allelic loss of chromosomes 1p

and 19q appears to mark chemosensitive anaplastic oligodendrogliomas,[183] suggesting again that this molecular genetic signature may be a practical tumour marker in neuro-oncology practice (Chapter 5).

Biology and genetics of diffuse astrocytic tumours

Diffuse astrocytoma

Tumorigenesis is a multistep process in which cells become immortalised, proliferate, invade and modulate their environment. Over the past few years, molecular biological studies have provided insights into the basic mechanisms underlying astrocytic tumour formation and progression[189]

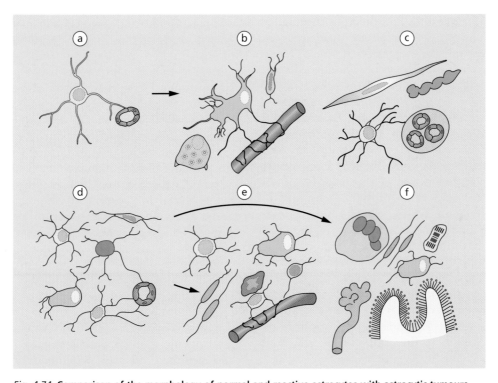

Fig. 4.74 **Comparison of the morphology of normal and reactive astrocytes with astrocytic tumours with a summary of the histological progression from diffuse astrocytoma to anaplastic astrocytoma or glioblastoma. (a)** Normal astrocyte and blood vessel. **(b)** Reactive astrocyte with extensive paranuclear cytoplasm and stout processes. A foamy macrophage and elongated microglial cell are also shown. **(c)** Pilocytic astrocytoma with a strap-like pilocytic cell and an irregular Rosenthal fibre. Some cells are stellate and their processes coat the glia limitans of the blood vessels. Multiple capillary channels are seen in this tumour. **(d)** Diffuse astrocytoma. The tumour cells may take many forms but are recognisable by their hyperchromatic nuclei. Some tumour cells have fine stellate processes and others are plump cells with fewer processes than reactive astrocytes. Normal astrocytes may be admixed with the tumour cells. Diffuse astrocytoma may evolve into either anaplastic astrocytoma or glioblastoma. **(e)** Anaplastic astrocytoma is similar in histology to diffuse astrocytoma except that the cells are more crowded together due to an increase in nuclear : cytoplasmic ratio. Mitoses are present and rod shaped anaplastic cells may be seen, together with the stellate and plump astrocytes with hyperchromatic nuclei seen in a diffuse astrocytoma. **(f)** Glioblastoma consists of a variety of cell types of which the rod shaped anaplastic cells are the most characteristic. Near the centre of the tumour the cells may be large and multinucleate and, in other areas, they may have a plump morphology. Mitoses are seen and there is microvascular (capillary endothelial) proliferation, pseudopalisading and areas of necrosis.

(Fig. 4.74). The cell of origin of diffuse astrocytomas remains undetermined, with some arguments implicating mature astrocytes and others suggesting residual precursor cells. Nonetheless, this enigmatic progenitor cell must somehow undergo oncogenic transformation to form a diffuse astrocytoma. Malignant progression almost inevitably follows; in the case of so-called secondary glioblastoma, progression typically occurs a few years after the formation of a diffuse astrocytoma; in the case of primary (or clinically de novo) glioblastomas, malignant transformation appears to occur soon after the initial transforming event.

One requirement for oncogenesis is the induction of deregulated growth. Candidates for inducing such growth are the platelet-derived growth factors (PDGF) and their receptors. PDGF ligand and receptor overexpression, predominantly of the A-chain of the ligand and the α-chain of the receptor, are early and frequent events in glioma formation, suggesting an autocrine stimulatory loop.[190] The mechanisms responsible for overexpression in most cases have not been elucidated, although rare anaplastic astrocytomas and glioblastomas display amplification of the gene encoding the PDGF alpha-receptor.[191] Activation of the PDGF system provides a growth stimulus to glial cells,[192] raising the possibility that cognate overexpression of PDGF A-chains and alpha-receptors may overcome growth control in astrocytoma precursor cells. Other growth factors may contribute as well, as high expression of a number of growth factors – such as epidermal growth factor (EGF), fibroblast growth factor (FGF), transforming growth factor-alpha (TGF-alpha) and insulin-like growth factors – has been noted in diffuse astrocytomas, although most of these growth factors are only highly overexpressed in anaplastic astrocytomas and glioblastomas.

Deregulated growth, however, leads to apoptosis if the cell has an intact mechanism for sensing cell cycle aberrations. Thus, a second central aspect of cell transformation is abrogation of the apoptotic or cell death response. One mechanism by which this may occur is inactivation of the *TP53* gene. The *TP53* gene on chromosome 17p encodes the p53 protein, which has an integral role in a number of cellular processes, including apoptosis, cell cycle arrest, response to DNA damage and angiogenesis. Inactivation of *TP53*, usually by mutation of one copy and chromosomal loss of the remaining allele, occurs in approximately one-third of human diffuse astrocytomas, anaplastic astrocytomas and glioblastomas.[9] These mutations are primarily missense mutations and target the evolutionarily conserved domains in exons 5, 7 and 8. Particular hotspots for mutations include codons 175, 248 and 273, in which C to T transitions are most likely the result of spontaneous deamination of 5-methylcytosine residues. These mutations affect p53 residues that are crucial for DNA binding, presumably

leading to loss of p53 mediated transcriptional activity.[193] Interestingly, cortical astrocytes from mice bearing only one *TP53* allele behave like normal astrocytes until they lose the wild type *TP53* allele, at which time they acquire in vitro characteristics of transformed cells.[194,195]

Amplification of the *MDM2* oncogene, an upstream inhibitor of p53 function, may be another means of abrogating p53 function in human gliomas, but amplification of this oncogene is restricted to a relatively small percentage of anaplastic astrocytomas and glioblastomas.[196,197] Curiously, some diffuse astrocytomas accumulate wild type p53 protein in their nuclei,[198] with attendant upregulation of p21 expression.[199] Interestingly, those gliomas that accumulate wild type p53 are more likely to express the bcl-2 antiapoptotic protein.[200] Overexpression of bcl-2 may have similar effects to p53 inactivation since both processes would impair the ability of cells to undergo apoptosis. Abrogation of the cell death response by any of these mechanisms presumably allows growth stimulated astrocytic clones to survive in the face of deregulated proliferation. Indeed, the correlation between PDGF alpha-receptor overexpression and chromosome 17p events[191] hints at that p53 inactivation may be selected for only if increased proliferation has been occasioned by PDGF activation. Indeed, cortical astrocytes from p53-deficient mice rapidly acquire the in vitro characteristics of transformed cells, particularly in the presence of certain growth factors.[194,195]

p53 inactivation may also be integral in establishing the potential for additional genomic instability, eventually allowing for the selection of more malignant clones.[201] Indeed, genomic instability, as evidenced by gene amplification and aneuploidy, appears directly related to loss of p53.[194] In this regard, the initial genetic alterations of diffuse astrocytomas, particularly those inactivating p53, can be thought of as the events that remove the 'gatekeeper', allowing further tumorigenic changes to occur.[202] Cells that had undergone the initial tumorigenic changes would display a slow net growth and yet have an high likelihood of undergoing progression to a more malignant lesion – features characteristic of diffuse astrocytomas.

The ability to invade diffusely is a cardinal feature of diffuse astrocytoma and is a phenotype acquired early, by the time the tumour is grade II. Much work has been done on the biology of invasion, but it has been hampered by lack of wholly representative models.[120] Human astrocytoma cells are able to attach to and migrate along a variety of extracellular matrix substances via interactions between cell surface and extracellular molecules. Among the cell surface adhesion molecules, CD44 and neural cell adhesion molecule are expressed in astrocytomas and influence migration and invasion in in vitro assays. Specific integrins, a family of dimeric cell surface molecules, are also expressed on astrocytomas and mediate interactions with extracellular molecules such as vitronectin. Disruption of specific integrin–matrix interactions impedes astrocytoma invasion in experimental systems. Growth factors, such as PDGF, EGF, FGF, TGF-alpha and hepatocyte growth factor, are also expressed in astrocytomas and have been shown to increase invasion in vitro. Expression of particular proteases, including metalloproteinases, urokinase-type plasminogen activator and cathepsins, also appears necessary for invasion, for digestion of extracellular matrix components. Thus, glioma cells express a complex set of molecules that are still only barely understood, enabling their insidious migration into the cerebral parenchyma.

Allelic loss of chromosome 22q is found in approximately 20–30% of diffuse astrocytomas,[203,204] implying that a diffuse astrocytoma tumour suppressor gene resides on this chromosome. Little is known about the precise location of this putative gene, and deletion mapping studies have produced conflicting results.[205,206] The neurofibromatosis 2 (*NF2*) gene, while a tempting candidate gene, has been excluded.[206,207]

Anaplastic astrocytoma

The transition to anaplastic astrocytoma is associated with inactivation of tumour suppressor genes on chromosomes 9p, 11p, 13q and 19q (Fig. 4.75), as allelic losses of these chromosomes are common in anaplastic astrocytoma and glioblastoma, but rare in diffuse astrocytoma. Two of these chromosomal loci contain known tumour suppressor genes: the *CDKN2A/p16* gene on chromosome 9p and the *RB* gene on chromosome 13q. These genes encode proteins that are components of a crucial cell cycle regulatory pathway involving p16, cyclin dependent kinase 4 (cdk4, encoded by the *CDK4* gene on chromosome 12q), cyclin D1 and pRb. At least half of all anaplastic astrocytomas and the vast majority of glioblastomas appear to have alterations affecting at least one component of the p16-cdk4/cyclin D1-pRb pathway.[208–215] The most common alteration appears to be inactivation of *CDKN2A/p16*, occurring in 33–68% of glioblastoma and in approximately 75–90% of glioblastoma cell lines.[208,210–212,216,217] Such inactivation is usually achieved by homozygous deletion of the gene, although point mutations and methylation of 5′ CpG islands are rare alternative mechanisms.[214,218,219] The next most common alterations of the p16-cdk4-cyclin D1-pRb pathway are pRb inactivation, occurring in about 20–30% of anaplastic astrocytomas and glioblastomas,[214,215,220] and *CDK4* gene amplification and overexpression, occurring in 10–15% of anaplastic astrocytomas and glioblastomas.[197,212,215, 221,222]

These molecules function in a regulatory pathway that controls the G1 to S phase transition of the cell cycle. The simplest schema suggests that p16 inhibits the

cdk4/cyclin D1 complex, preventing cdk4 from phosphorylating pRb, and thus ensuring that pRb maintains G1 arrest.[223–227] Disruption of this pathway, with subsequent deregulated progression into S phase, may occur if *CDKN2A/p16* or pRb are inactivated or if cdk4 or cyclin D1 are overexpressed, suggesting that perturbation of any individual component will have an oncogenic effect.[223–227] In anaplastic astrocytomas and glioblastomas, in fact, these genetic changes are often alternative events, rarely occurring together in the same tumours.[212,214,215] Significantly, however, those tumours with chromosome 9p21/*CDKN2A/p16* deletions have significantly higher proliferation indices than those tumours without deletions.[228] One possible explanation is that the homozygous deletions of chromosome 9p21 disrupt two additional cell cycle regulatory molecules: the alternative *CDKN2A/p16* transcript[229,230] known as p19ARF[231] and the nearby *CDKN2B* gene-encoded p15.[228]

Thus, a key event in the transition to anaplastic astrocytomas and glioblastomas is the elimination of a critical cell cycle regulatory pathway or pathways (Fig. 4.75). Disruption of this checkpoint has a number of clinicopathological correlates. From a neuropathological point of view, mitotic activity is characteristic of anaplastic astrocytomas and glioblastomas, but not diffuse astrocytomas (WHO grade II or St Anne/Mayo grade 2). From a clinical point of view, patients with anaplastic

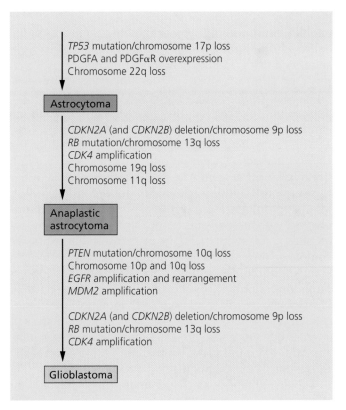

Fig. 4.75 **Molecular genetics of astrocytic tumours.**

astrocytomas and glioblastomas have a substantially poorer prognosis than those with diffuse astrocytomas. All of these observations argue that release of this critical cellular brake underlies the marked increase in proliferative activity that accompanies progression to anaplastic astrocytoma.

Some of the other genetic events do not yet fit so neatly into the arena of cell cycle regulation. The putative chromosome 19q tumour suppressor gene, for instance,[187,232-234] has not yet been identified and its function thus remains unknown. Nonetheless, its function must be integral to diffuse astrocytoma progression since allelic loss of chromosome 19q occurs in about 50% of anaplastic astrocytomas and glioblastoma.[187] Allelic loss of chromosome 11p also occur in about 25% of anaplastic astrocytomas and glioblastomas, suggesting the presence of a glioma tumour suppressor gene on this chromosome as well. Deletion mapping studies have suggested that the gene lies toward the telomere of the short arm, at 11p15.5,[235,236] but this gene has also not yet been identified.

Glioblastoma

Malignant progression to glioblastoma is associated with inactivation of tumour suppressor genes on chromosome 10 and amplification of the EGF receptor (*EGFR*) gene,[146,203,204] and less commonly, chromosomal losses of 4q, 9p, 11p and 13q, chromosomal gains of 1q, 6p and 20q, and amplification sites on 1q2, 4q, 7q, 12p, 13q, 18p and 22q.[237,238] Chromosome 10 loss occurs in 60–85% of glioblastomas, with most cases showing allelic loss of the entire chromosome. Deletion mapping studies have suggested that at least two tumour suppressor gene lie on the long arm,[239-242] with yet another, less commonly involved tumour suppressor genes on the short arm.[146,241,243] The recent cloning of the *PTEN/MMAC1* gene on chromosome 10q23 and the documentation of *PTEN/MMAC1* mutations in glioblastomas,[244,245] as well as the *DMBT1* gene on chromosome 10[246] will focus activity on these particular genes in glioblastomas, but other chromosome 10 glioma suppressor genes must also exist. The *PTEN/MMAC1* product is a protein tyrosine phosphatase, with tumour suppressor activity being dependent on phosphatase activity.[247] The protein also has extensive homology to tensin, a protein that interacts with actin filaments at focal adhesions. Thus, PTEN could suppress tumour cell growth by antagonising protein tyrosine kinases and regulate tumour cell mobility and intercellular interactions by affecting the cytoskeleton. Loss of at least one chromosome 10q tumour suppressor gene appears to upregulate angiogenesis via decreased expression of the antiangiogenic thrombospondin-1.[248]

The *EGFR* gene is amplified in approximately 40% of all glioblastomas, resulting in overexpression of EGFR, a transmembrane receptor tyrosine kinase.[146,249,250]

Approximately one-third of glioblastomas with *EGFR* gene amplification also have gene rearrangements, the most common mutation deleting exons 2 through 7. This deletion leads to a truncated, constitutively active mutant. EGFR overexpression is also commonly accompanied by expression of the EGFR ligands, EGF and TGF-alpha. Autocrine and paracrine EGFR activation and/or expression of constitutively active EGFR mutants facilitate cellular growth, with some studies showing that EGFR activation may lead to upregulation of VEGF[251] and others demonstrating that specific EGFR mutants increase cellular proliferation and decrease apoptosis.[252]

Molecular biological inquiries have begun to piece together relationships between some of the cardinal histological features of glioblastoma, such as necrosis, angiogenesis and cellular proliferation. The critical histological finding that allows the diagnosis of glioblastoma is necrosis; as an independent prognostic factor, the presence of necrosis clearly implies a bad prognosis.[85,86] The biological correlate of this observation is that by the time necrosis occurs in diffuse astrocytic tumours, the tumour cells have achieved a highly malignant state, since tumour necrosis itself does not result directly in aggressive behaviour. This malignant state may be effected by a vicious cycle involving necrosis induced hypoxia and various angiogenic and growth factors (Fig. 4.75).

Anaplastic astrocytomas contain rapidly dividing cells with high metabolic demands and small regions of necrosis may develop in areas where there is insufficient blood supply. Larger areas of necrosis may arise from vascular thrombosis secondary to coagulation abnormalities, which are common in patients with glioblastoma. These necrotic zones in turn lead to hypoxia in the surrounding tissues. Alternatively, high metabolic activity within a tumour may itself lead to hypoxia before necrosis has occurred.[253-255] Hypoxia itself has a number of sequelae. Hypoxia appears to upregulate the expression of angiogenic factors, particularly the potent VEGF,[255] which eventually leads to endothelial proliferation to counter the hypoxic insult.

Other growth factors that are highly expressed in malignant astrocytic tumours – such as FGFs, TGFs and PDGF-beta – are also angiogenic and may facilitate vascular proliferation via angiogenic growth factor receptors that are expressed by endothelial cells in gliomas. Hypoxic cell death may additionally lead to release of growth factors from the dying cells. Furthermore, hypoxia may act as a selective force to allow emergence of resistant, and thus highly malignant, clones of tumour cells. Interestingly, hypoxia will select for those apoptosis resistant tumour cells bearing inactivated p53.[253] Expression of some growth factors – such as VEGF, also known as vascular permeability factor – may also lead to the development of tumoural oedema, by altering vascular permeability.

Such vessels, at least in the early stages of reavascularisation, appear to arise from the co-opting of local vessels.[256] At some, probably later stage, however, the cells composing these hyperplastic vessels most likely arise from bone marrow-derived precursor cells that undergo vascular differentiation.[257]

Hypoxia may therefore facilitate angiogenesis, release of growth factors and emergence of highly malignant clones. Some of these biological events can be readily appreciated histologically in glioblastomas, in which regions of necrosis are often surrounded by proliferating cells, which in turn are surrounded by garlands of proliferating blood vessels. The sum of such effects is enhanced tumorigenic potential at the cellular level.[254] In this manner, there must emerge, at the microenvironmental level, increasingly malignant subclones. This hypothesis would provide a simple explanation for the marked heterogeneity noted histologically in glioblastomas and a possible explanation for the marked resistance to conventional cytotoxic therapies seen clinically in patients with glioblastomas.

Clinical–pathological–genetic subsets of glioblastoma

While the malignant progression of diffuse astrocytoma is associated with distinct sets of genetic changes, some genetic alterations occur in mutually exclusive manners. Such observations raise the possibility that genetic subsets of glioblastoma exist and that, perhaps, genetic analysis may provide clinically useful information. The most salient example of the ability to divide glioblastomas into genetic subsets is the *TP53* mutation–*EGFR* amplification dichotomy: *TP53* mutations and *EGFR* amplification almost never occur in the same tumour.[258,259] In unselected series of glioblastomas, approximately one-third have p53 inactivation, one-third have *EGFR* gene amplification, and one-third have neither of these changes. Moreover, many of the other genetic events ally themselves with either *TP53* mutations or *EGFR* amplification. For instance, PDGF alpha-receptor overexpression and *RB* gene alterations are associated with *TP53* mutations, while *CDKN2A/p16* deletions and *MDM2* amplification are associated with *EGFR* amplification.[191,260–262] Thus, there appear to be multiple distinct genetic pathways to glioblastoma.[263]

It has long been observed that some glioblastomas arise in the setting of a prior diffuse, fibrillary astrocytoma or anaplastic astrocytoma, while other glioblastomas occur de novo, i.e. without a clear clinical history or pathological evidence of a prior diffuse astrocytoma. Those glioblastomas occurring in the setting of a prior diffuse astrocytoma have been termed *secondary glioblastomas*; those without, *primary* or *de novo glioblastomas*. It is important to emphasise, however, that primary glioblastomas may in fact arise from a diffuse astrocytoma or anaplastic astrocytoma, but, if so, develop quickly so that they appear clinicopathologically as primary glioblastomas.

Secondary glioblastomas typically present in adult patients who are younger, often in their fourth or fifth decades. Primary glioblastomas, while occurring at all ages, account for nearly all patients in their sixth or seventh decades. At the same time, clinicopathologically defined secondary glioblastomas are substantially less common than primary tumours, accounting for only about 20% of all glioblastomas. Although the effect of age on glioblastoma prognosis is well known, with younger patients faring considerably better than older, secondary glioblastomas also appear to have a better prognosis. Once a glioblastoma develops, the presence of a diffuse astrocytoma suggests a more favourable course.[264] Thus, although the factors are somewhat interwoven, it is clear that young age and prior diffuse astrocytoma suggest a different type of glioblastoma from the typical de novo tumours that occur in older adults.

In a parallel manner, those glioblastomas with *TP53* mutations occur in adults of a significantly younger age than those glioblastomas with *EGFR* gene amplification.[9,258] Furthermore, secondary glioblastomas have a much higher incidence of *TP53* mutations than do primary glioblastomas. Thus, *TP53* mutations may provide a molecular marker for secondary glioblastoma,[17] occurring in almost three-quarters of such cases (Fig. 4.68).[265,266] To some extent, this seems intuitive since p53 inactivation is closely associated with formation of diffuse astrocytomas,[267] and not with malignant progression.[265,266] One particular type of usually secondary glioblastoma that is closely associated with *TP53* gene mutations is the brain stem glioblastoma typically seen in children.[268]

EGFR gene amplification, on the other hand, is quite rare in secondary glioblastomas, in glioblastomas occurring in young adults and in brain stem glioblastomas in children. Those glioblastomas with *EGFR* amplification typically occur in older patients who do not have a history of preceding diffuse astrocytoma and in small cell glioblastoma[151]. Thus, *EGFR* gene amplification associated glioblastomas may arise either de novo, or rapidly from a pre-existing tumour. In patients in their seventh decade, *EGFR* gene amplification may occur in over 50% of tumours.

The correlation of primary glioblastoma with *EGFR* gene amplification, however, is not as tight as that of *TP53* mutations and secondary glioblastoma. As many as one-quarter of clinicopathologically defined primary glioblastomas have *TP53* gene mutations (Fig. 4.76). One subset of tumours that emerges from this *TP53* mutation predominant primary glioblastoma group is the giant cell glioblastoma. As discussed above, giant cell

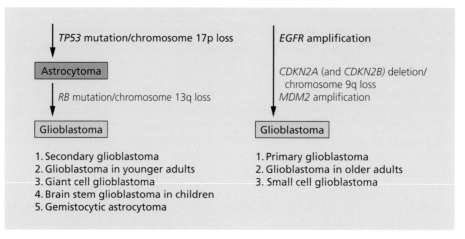

Fig. 4.76 **Molecular genetic subsets of glioblastoma.**

glioblastomas are a clinicopathogically distinct subtype of glioblastoma that arises as a well demarcated mass in younger adults and features large, bizarre astrocytic cells. These tumours almost invariably have *TP53* gene mutations.[269] The formation of such multinucleated, pleomorphic cells is most likely related to p53 inactivation itself, perhaps because of disruption of centrosome duplication or mitotic spindle control, which involves p53 function. Furthermore, the induction of brain tumours in p53 deficient mice using ethylnitrosurea yields tumours that are highly reminiscent of giant cell glioblastomas, but such tumours do not arise when these carcinogens are given to wild type mice.[270] Another subtype of malignant astrocytoma that may also have an unusually high incidence of *TP53* mutation are gemistocytic astrocytomas, although the mechanism whereby *TP53* mutation would lead to gemistocytic cells remains uncertain. Finally, it is important to recall that rare glioblastomas could arise from oligodendrogliomas and oligoastrocytomas, and these have their own unique genetic antecedents (see[263,271] and Chapter 5).

Unfortunately, the clinical relevance of these molecular genetic subsets has not yet been evaluated in a large, prospective study. To date, small, retrospective studies of genetic parameters and patient prognosis have revealed a few associations, but no clear correlations of genotype with tumour behaviour.[9,259,272,273] This contrasts with oligodendroglial tumours, for which molecular analysis is able to distinguish chemosensitive, good prognosis tumours from those which do not respond to chemotherapy and follow an aggressive course (see Chapter 5). Nonetheless, the ability of molecular investigations to assess biological events in human astrocytic tumours raises the possibility that new approaches to diagnosis and treatment will be based on an understanding of causative biological phenomena.

REFERENCES

Astrocytes and astrocytic tumours

1. Berry M, Butt AM. Structure and function of glia in the central nervous system. In: Graham DI, Lantos PL, eds. Greenfield's Neuropathology, 6th edn. London: Arnold, 1997; pp 63–83
2. Tsacopoulos M, Magistretti P. Metabolic coupling between glia and neurons. J Neurosci, 1996; 16:877–885
3. Kreuzberg GW, Blakemore WF, Graeber MB. Cellular pathology of the central nervous system. In: Graham DI, Lantos PL, eds. Greenfield's Neuropathology, 6th edn. London: Arnold, 1997; pp 85–156
4. Knudsen AG. All in the (cancer) family. Nat Genet, 1993; 5:103–104
5. Dirven CMF, Tuerlings J, Molenaar WM et al. Glioblastoma multiforme in four siblings: a cytogenetic and molecular genetic study. J Neurooncol, 1995; 24:251–258
6. van Meyel DJ, Ramsay DA, Chambers AF et al. Absence of hereditary mutations in exons 5 through 9 of the TP53 gene and exon 24 of the neurofibromin gene in families with glioma. Ann Neurol, 1994; 35:120–122
7. Lubbe J, von Ammon K, Watanabe K et al. Familial brain tumour syndrome associated with a p53 germline deletion of codon 236. Brain Pathol, 1995; 5:15–23
8. Malkin D, Li FP, Strong LC et al. Germ line TP53 mutations in a familial syndrome of breast cancer, sarcomas, and other neoplasms. Science, 1990; 250:1222–1228
9. Louis DN. The TP53 gene and protein in human brain tumors. J Neuropathol Exp Neurol, 1994; 53:11–21
10. Listernick R, Louis DN, Packer RJ et al. Optic pathway gliomas in children with neurofibromatosis 1: Consensus statement from the NF1 Optic Pathway Glioma Task Force. Ann Neurol, 1997; 41:143–149
11. von Deimling A, Louis DN, Menon AG et al. Deletions on the long arm of chromosome 17 in pilocytic astrocytoma. Acta Neuropathol, 1993; 86:81–85
12. Li Y, Bollag G, Clark R et al. Somatic mutations in the neurofibromatosis 1 gene in human tumors. Cell, 1992; 69:275–281
13. Hamilton SR, Liu B, Parsons RE et al. The molecular basis of Turcot's syndrome. New Eng J Med, 1995; 332:839–847
14. Taylor MD, Perry J, Zlatescu MC et al. hPMS2 exon 5 mutation and malignant glioma: case report and molecular genetic study. J Neurosurg, 1999; 90:946–950
15. Bahuau M, Vidaud D, Jenkins RB et al. Germ-line deletion involving the INK4 locus in familial proneness to melanoma and nervous system tumors. Cancer Res, 1998; 58:2298–2303

Pilocytic astrocytoma

16. Giannini C, Scheithauer BW. Classification and grading of low-grade astrocytic tumors in children. Brain Pathol, 1997; 7:785–798

17. Kleihues P, Cavenee WK. Pathology and Genetics of tumours of the nervous system. Lyon: IARC, 2000
18. Kayama T, Tominaga T, Yoshimoto T. Management of pilocytic astrocytoma Neurosurg Rev, 1996; 19:217–220
19. Fisher PG, Breiter SN, Carlson BS et al. A clinicopathological reappraisal of brain stem tumor classification. Identification of pilocytic astrocytoma and fibrillary astrocytoma as distinct entities. Cancer, 2000; 89:1569–1576
20. Alshail E, Rutka JT, Becker LE et al. Optic chiasmatic-hypothalamic glioma. Brain Pathol, 1997; 7:799–806
21. Reardon DA, Gajjar A, Sanford RA et al. Bithalamic involvement predicts poor outcome among children with thalamic tumors. Pediatr Neurosurg, 1998; 29:29–35
22. Dirven CM, Mooij JJ, Molenaar WM. Cerebellar pilocytic astrocytoma: a treatment protocol based upon analysis of 73 cases and a review of the literature. Childs Nerv Syst, 1997; 13:17–23
23. Ganju V, Jenkins RB, O'Fallon JR et al. Prognostic factors in gliomas. A multivariate analysis of clinical, pathologic, flow cytometric, cytogenetic and molecular genetic markers. Cancer, 1994; 74:920–927
24. Giannini C, Scheithauer BW, Burger PC et al. Cellular proliferation in pilocytic and diffuse astrocytomas. J Neuropathol Exp Neurol, 1999; 58:46–53
25. Ito S, Hoshino T, Shibuya M et al. Proliferative characteristics of juvenile pilocytic astrocytomas determined by bromodeoxyuridine labeling. Neurosurgery, 1992; 31:413–419
26. Huber G, Glas B, Hermes M. Computerised tomographic and magnetic resonance tomographic findings in pilocytic astrocytoma. Rofo Fortschr Geb Rontgenstr Neuen Bildgeb Verfahr, 1997; 166:125–132
27. Rollins NK, Nisen P, Shapiro KN. The use of early postoperative MR in detecting residual juvenile cerebellar pilocytic astrocytoma. Am J Neuroradiol, 1998; 19:151–156
28. Weller RO. Pathology of cerebrospinal fluid and interstitial fluid of the CNS: significance for Alzheimer disease, prion disorders and multiple sclerosis. J Neuropathol Exp Neurol, 1998; 57:885–894
29. Leung SY, Chan AS, Wong MP et al. Expression of vascular endothelial growth factor and its receptors in pilocytic astrocytoma. Am J Surg Pathol, 1997; 21:941–950
30. Pollack IF, Albright AL. Management of pediatric brain tumors. Neurosurg Q, 1996; 6:116–136
31. Campbell JW, Pollack IF. Cerebellar astrocytomas in children. J Neurooncol 1996; 28:223–231
32. Gajjar A, Sanford RA, Heideman R et al. Low-grade astrocytoma: a decade of experience at St. Jude Children's Research Hospital. J Clin Oncol, 1997; 15:2792–2799
33. Tomlinson FH, Scheithauer BW, Hayostek CJ et al. The significance of atypia and histologic malignancy in pilocytic astrocytoma of the cerebellum: a clinicopathologic and flow cytometric study. J Child Neurol, 1994; 9:301–310
34. Ishii N, Sawamura Y, Tada M et al. Absence of TP53 gene mutations in a tumor panel representative of pilocytic astrocytoma diversity using a TP53 functional assay. Int J Cancer, 1998; 76:797–800
35. Tacconi L, Farah JO, Rossi ML et al. Neurohypophyseal pilocytic astrocytoma invading the skull base. Br J Neurosurg, 1999; 13:614–617
36. Tihan T, Fisher PG, Kepner JL et al. Pediatric astrocytomas with monomorphous pilomyxoid features and a less favorable outcome. J Neuropathol Exp Neurol, 1999; 58:1061–1068
37. Platten M, Giordano MJ, Dirven CMF et al. Upregulation of specific *NF1* gene transcripts in sporadic pilocytic astrocytomas. Am J Pathol, 1996; 149:621–627
38. Tihan T, Davis R, Elowitz E et al. Practical value of Ki-67 and TP53 labeling indexes in stereotactic biopsies of diffuse and pilocytic astrocytomas. Arch Pathol Lab Med, 2000; 124:108–113

Subependymal giant cell astrocytoma

39. Al Saleem T, Wessner LL, Scheithauer BW et al. Malignant tumors of the kidney, brain, and soft tissues in children and young adults with the tuberous sclerosis complex. Cancer, 1998; 83:2208–2216
40. Short MP, Richardson EP, Haines JL et al. Clinical neuropathological, and genetic aspects of the tuberous sclerosis complex. Brain Pathol, 1995; 5:173–180
41. Gyure KA, Prayson RA. Subependymal giant cell astrocytoma: a clinicopathologic study with HMB45 and MIB-1 immunohistochemical analysis. Mod Pathol, 1997; 10(4):313–317
42. Yamanouchi H, Jay V, Rutka JT et al. Evidence of abnormal differentiation in giant cells of tuberous sclerosis. Pediatr Neurol, 1997; 17:49–53
43. Yamanouchi H, Ho M, Jay V et al. Giant cells in cortical tubers in tuberous sclerosis showing synaptophysin-immunoreactive halos. Brain Develop, 1997; 19:21–24
44. Green AJ, Smith M, Yates JRW. Loss of heterozygosity on chromosome 16p13.3 in hamartomas from tuberous sclerosis patients. Nat Genet, 1994; 6:193–196
45. Green AJ, Johnson PH, Yates JR. The tuberous sclerosis gene on chromosome 9q34 acts as a growth suppressor. Hum Mol Genet, 1994; 3:1833–1834
46. Turgut M, Akalan N, Ozgen T et al. Subependymal giant cell astrocytoma associated with tuberous sclerosis: diagnostic and surgical characteristics of five cases with unusual features. Clin Neurol Neurosurg, 1996; 98:217–221

Pleomorphic xanthoastrocytoma

47. Kepes JJ, Rubinstein LJ, Eng LF. Pleomorphic xanthoastrocytoma: a distinctive meningocerebral glioma of young subjects with a relatively favorable prognosis. Cancer, 1979; 44:1839–1852
48. Kepes JJ, Louis DN, Giannini C et al. Pleomorphic xanthoastrocytoma. In: Kleihues P, Cavenee WK, eds. World Health Organization classification of tumours of the central nervous system. Lyon: IARC 2000
49. Kepes JJ. Pleomorphic xanthoastrocytoma: the birth of a diagnosis and concept. Brain Pathol, 1993; 3:269–274
50. Giannini C, Scheithauer BW, Burger PC et al. Pleomorphic xanthoastrocytoma: what do we really know about it? Cancer, 1999; 85:2033–2045
51. Kubo O, Sasahara A, Tajika Y et al. Pleomorphic xanthoastrocytoma with neurofibromatosis type 1: case report. Noshuyo Byori, 1996; 13:79–83
52. Ozek MM, Sav A, Pamir MN et al. Pleomorphic xanthoastrocytoma associated with von Recklinghausen neurofibromatosis. Childs Nerv Syst, 1993; 9:39–42
53. Wasdahl DA, Scheithauer BW, Andrews BT et al. Cerebellar pleomorphic xanthoastrocytoma: case report. Neurosurgery, 1994; 35:947–950
54. Mallucci C, Lellouch Tubiana A, Salazar C et al. The management of desmoplastic neuroepithelial tumours in childhood. Childs Nerv Syst, 2000; 16:8–14
55. Kepes JJ, Kepes M, Slowik F. Fibrous xanthomas and xanthosarcomas of the meninges and the brain. Acta Neuropathol, 1973; 23:187–199
56. Chakrabarty A, Mitchell P, Bridges LR et al. Malignant transformation in pleomorphic xanthoastrocytoma – a report of two cases. Br J Neurosurg, 1999; 13:516–519
57. Kepes JJ, Rubinstein LJ, Ansbacher L et al. Histopathological features of recurrent pleomorphic xanthoastrocytoma: further corroboration of the glial nature of this neoplasm. Acta Neuropathol, 1989; 78:585–593
58. Macaulay RJ, Jay V, Hoffman HJ et al. Increased mitotic activity as a negative prognostic indicator in pleomorphic xanthoastrocytoma. J Neurosurg, 1993; 79:761–768
59. Pahapill PA, Ramsay DA, Del Maestro RF. Pleomorphic xanthoastrocytoma: case report and analysis of the literature concerning the efficacy of resection and the significance of necrosis. Neurosurgery, 1996; 38:822–828
60. Prayson RA, Morris HH, 3rd. Anaplastic pleomorphic xanthoastrocytoma. Arch Pathol Lab Med, 1998; 122:1082–1086
61. Kepes JJ, Rubinstein LJ. Malignant gliomas with heavily lipidized (foamy) tumour cells: a report of three cases with immunoperoxidase study. Cancer, 1981; 47:2451–2459
62. Kordek R, Biernat W, Sapieja W et al. Pleomorphic xanthoastrocytoma with a gangliomatous component: an immunohistochemical and ultrastructural study. Acta Neuropathol, 1995; 89:194–197
63. Lindboe CF, Cappelen J, Kepes JJ. Pleomorphic xanthoastrocytoma as a component of a cerebellar ganglioglioma: case report. Neurosurgery, 1992; 31:353–355
64. Paulus W, Lisle DK, Tonn JC et al. Molecular genetic alterations in pleomorphic xanthoastrocytoma. Acta Neuropathol, 1996; 91:293–297
65. Geddes JF, Swash M. Hugh Cairns, Dorothy Russell and the first pleomorphic xanthoastrocytoma? Br J Neurosurg, 1999; 13:174–177

66. Weldon Linne CM, Victor TA, Groothuis DR et al. Pleomorphic xanthoastrocytoma. Ultrastructural and immunohistochemical study of a case with a rapidly fatal outcome following surgery. Cancer, 1983; 52:2055–2063

Chordoid glioma

67. Brat DJ, Scheithauer BW, Staugaitis SM et al. Third ventricular chordoid glioma: a distinct clinicopathological entity. J Neuropathol Exp Neurol, 1998; 57:283–290
68. Pomper MG, Passe TJ, Burger PC, Scheithauer B, Brat DJ. Chordoid glioma: a neoplasm unique to the hypothalamus and anterior third ventricle. Am J Neuroradiol, 2001; 22:464–469
69. Vajtai I, Varga Z, Scheithauer BW et al. Chordoid glioma of the third ventricle: Confirmatory report of a new entity. Hum Pathol, 1999; 30:723–726
70. Cenacchi G, Roncaroli F, Cerasoli S et al. Chordoid glioma of the third ventricle: an ultrastructural study of three cases with a histogenetic hypothesis. Am J Surg Pathol, 2001; 25:401–405
71. Reifenberger G, Weber T, Weber RG et al. Chordoid glioma of the third ventricle: immunohistochemical and molecular genetic characterization of a novel tumor entity. Brain Pathol, 1999; 9:617–626

Astroblastoma

72. Husain AN, Leestma JE. Cerebral astroblastoma: Immunohistochemical and ultrastructural features. Case report. J Neurosurg, 1986; 64:657–661
73. Yunten N, Ersahin Y, Demirtas E et al. Cerebral astroblastoma resembling an extra-axial neoplasm. J Neuroradiol, 1996; 23:38–40
74. Kujas M, Faillot T, Lalam T et al. Astroblastomas revisited. Report of two cases with immunocytochemical and electron microscope study. Histogenetic considerations. Neuropathol Appl Neurobiol, 2000; 26:295–300

Diffuse astrocytoma/anaplastic astrocytoma

75. Bailey P, Cushing H. A classification of the tumors of the glioma group on a histogenetic basis with a correlated study of prognosis. Philadelphia: JB Lippincott, 1928
76. Kernohan JW, Mabon RF, Svien HJ et al. A simplified classification of gliomas. Proc Staff Meet Mayo Clin, 1949; 24:71–75
77. Burger PC, Scheithauer BW, Vogel FS. Surgical pathology of the nervous system and its coverings, 3rd edn. New York: Churchill Livingstone, 1991
78. Russell DS, Rubinstein LJ. Pathology of tumours of the nervous system, 5th edn. Baltimore: Williams & Wilkins, 1989
79. Burger PC, Scheithauer BW. Tumors of the central nervous system. Washington, DC: Armed Forces Institute of Pathology, 1994
80. Ringertz N. Grading of gliomas. Acta Pathol Microbiol Scand, 1950; 27:51–64
81. Kleihues P, Burger PC, Scheithauer BW. Histological typing of tumours of the central nervous system. Berlin: Springer-Verlag; 1993
82. Kleihues P, Burger PC, Scheithauer BW. The new WHO classification of brain tumours. Brain Pathol, 1993; 3:255–268
83. Barker FG, Davis RL, Chang SM et al. Necrosis as a prognostic factor in glioblastoma multiforme. Cancer, 1996; 77(6):1161–1166
84. Daumas-Duport C, Scheithauer B, O'Fallon J et al. Grading of astrocytomas. A simple and reproducible method. Cancer, 1988; 62:2152–2165
85. Daumas-Duport C, Monsaigeon V, Szilka G. Serial stereotactic biopsies: a double histologic code of gliomas according to malignancy and 3D configuration as an aide to therapeutic decision and assessment of results. Appl Neurophysiol, 1982; 45:431–437
86. Shaw EG, Scheithauer BW, O'Fallon JR et al. Oligodendrogliomas: the Mayo Clinic experience. J Neurosurg, 1992; 76:428–434
87. Glantz MJ, Burger PC, Herndon JE et al. Influence of the type of surgery on the histologic diagnosis in patients with anaplastic gliomas. Neurology, 1991; 41:1741–1744
88. Burger PC, Vogel FS, Green SB et al. Glioblastoma multiforme and anaplastic astrocytoma: pathologic criteria and prognostic implications. Cancer, 1985; 56:1106–1111
89. Burger PC, Green SB. Patient age, histologic features and length of survival in patients with glioblastoma multiforme. Cancer, 1987; 59:1617–1625

90. Kim TS, Halliday AL, Hedley-Whyte ET et al. Correlates of survival and the Daumas-Duport grading system for astrocytomas. J Neurosurg, 1991; 70:27–37
91. Hsu DW, Louis DN, Efird J et al. The use of MIB-1 (Ki-67) immunoreactivity in differentiating grade II and III gliomas. J Neuropathol Exp Neurol, 1997; 56:857–865
92. Gilles FH, Brown WD, Leviton A et al. Limitations of the World Health Organization classification of childhood supratentorial astrocytic tumors. Children Brain Tumor Consortium. Cancer, 2000; 88:1477–1483
93. Gilles FH, Leviton A, Tavare CJ et al. Definitive classes of childhood supratentorial neuroglial tumors. The Childhood Brain Tumor Consortium. Pediatr Dev Pathol, 2000; 3:126–139
94. Collins VP. Gliomas. Cancer Surv, 1998; 32:37–51
95. Shafqat S, Hedley Whyte ET, Henson JW. Age-dependent rate of anaplastic transformation in low-grade astrocytoma. Neurology, 1999; 52:867–869
96. Ohgaki H, Schauble B, zur Hausen A et al. Genetic alterations associated with the evolution and progression of astrocytic brain tumours. Virchows Arch, 1995; 427:113–118
97. Piepmeier J, Christopher S, Spencer D et al. Variations in the natural history and survival of patients with supratentorial low-grade astrocytomas. Neurosurgery, 1996; 38:872–878
98. Barker DJ, Weller RO, Garfield JS. Epidemiology of primary tumours of the brain and spinal cord: a regional survey in southern England. J Neurol Neurosurg Psychiatry, 1976; 39:290–206
99. Schiffer D. Brain tumors. Pathology and biological correlates. Berlin: Springer-Verlag, 1993
100. McKinney PA, Parslow RC, Lane SA et al. Epidemiology of childhood brain tumours in Yorkshire, UK, 1974–95: geographical distribution and changing patterns of occurrence. Br J Cancer, 1998; 78:974–979
101. Squires LA, Constantini S, Miller DC et al. Diffuse infiltrating astrocytoma of the cervicomedullary region: clinicopathologic entity. Pediatr Neurosurg, 1997; 27:153–159
102. Perez MJ, Lorenzo G, Munoz A et al. Low grade disseminated astrocytoma in childhood. Rev Neurol, 1997; 25:877–881
103. Perrin RG, Bernstein M. Iatrogenic seeding of anaplastic astrocytoma following stereotactic biopsy. J Neurooncol, 1998; 36:243–246
104. Singh M, Corboy JR, Stears JC et al. Diffuse leptomeningeal gliomatosis associated with multifocal CNS infarcts. Surg Neurol, 1998; 50:356–362
105. Materlik B, Steidle Katic U, Wauschkuhn B et al. Spinal metastases of malignant gliomas. Strahlenther Onkol, 1998; 174:478–481
106. Afra D, Osztie E. Histologically confirmed changes on CT of reoperated low-grade astrocytomas. Neuroradiology, 1997; 39:804–810
107. Tamura M, Shibasaki T, Zama A et al. Assessment of malignancy of glioma by positron emission tomography with ^{18}F-fluorodeoxyglucose and single photon emission computed tomography with thallium-201 chloride. Neuroradiology, 1998; 40:210–215
108. Girard N, Wang ZJ, Erbetta A et al. Prognositic value of proton MR spectroscopy of cerebral hemisphere tumors in children. Neuroradiology, 1998; 40:121–125
109. Schwarzmaier HJ, Yaroslavsky IV, Yaroslavsky AN. Treatment planning for MRI-guided laser-induced interstitial thermotherapy of brain tumors—the role of blood perfusion. J Magn Reson Imaging, 1998; 8:121–127
110. Shah AB, Muzumdar GA, Chitale AR et al. Squash preparation and frozen section in intraoperative diagnosis of central nervous system tumors. Acta Cytol, 1998; 42:1149–1154
111. Gonzalez Campora R, Haynes LW, Weller RO. Scanning electron microscopy of malignant gliomas. A comparative study of glioma cells in smear preparations and in tissue culture. Acta Neuropathol, 1978; 41:217–221
112. Slowinski J, Harabin Slowinska M, Mrowka R. Smear technique in the intraoperative brain tumor diagnosis: Its advantages and limitations. Neurol Res, 1999; 21:121–124
113. Raghavan R, Steart PV, Weller RO. Cell proliferation patterns in the diagnosis of astrocytomas, anaplastic astrocytomas and glioblastoma multiforme: a Ki-67 study. Neuropathol Appl Neurobiol, 1990; 16:123–133
114. Enestrom S, Vavruch L, Franlund B et al. Ki-67 antigen expression as a prognostic factor in primary and recurrent astrocytomas. Neurochirurgie, 1998; 44:25–30

115. Kordek R, Biernat W, Alwasiak J et al. Proliferating cell nuclear antigen (PCNA) and Ki-67 immunopositivity in human astrocytic tumours. Acta Neurochir, 1996; 138:509–512

116. Litofsky NS, Mix TC, Baker SP et al. Ki-67 (clone MIB-1) proliferation index in recurrent glial neoplasms: no prognostic significance. Surg Neurol, 1998; 50:579–585

117. Pierce E, Doshi R, Deane R. PCNA and Ki-67 labelling indices in pre-irradiated and post-irradiated astrocytomas: a comparative immunohistochemical analysis for evaluation of proliferative activity. Mol Pathol, 1998; 51:90–95

118. Prayson RA, Estes ML. MIB1 and TP53 immunoreactivity in protoplasmic astrocytomas. Pathol Int, 1996; 46:862–866

119. Kros JM, Schouten WC, Janssen PJ et al. Proliferation of gemistocytic cells and glial fibrillary acidic protein (GFAP)-positive oligodendroglial cells in gliomas: a MIB-1/GFAP double labeling study. Acta Neuropathol, 1996; 91:99–103

120. Pilkington GJ. Tumour cell migration in the central nervous system. Brain Pathol, 1994; 4:157–166

121. Sasaki H, Zlatescu MC, Betensky RA et al. Histopathological-molecular genetic correlations in referral pathologist-diagnosed low-grade 'oligodendroglioma.' J Neuropathol Exp Neurol, 2002; 61:58–63

122. Medbery CA, Straus KL, Steinberg SM et al. Low-grade astrocytomas: treatment results and prognostic variables. Int J Radiat Oncol Biol Phys, 1998; 15:837–841

123. Goh KY, Velasquez L, Epstein FJ. Pediatric intramedullary spinal cord tumors: is surgery alone enough? Pediatr Neurosurg, 1997; 27:34–39

124. Grabb PA, Lunsford LD, Albright AL et al. Stereotactic radiosurgery for glial neoplasms of childhood. Neurosurgery, 1996; 38:696–701

125. Inoue HK, Kohga H, Zama A et al. Pathobiology of cerebral gliomas in children and the role of radiosurgery. Stereotact Funct Neurosurg, 1996; 66(Suppl 1):278–287

126. van Veelen ML, Avezaat CJ, Kros JM et al. Supratentorial low grade astrocytoma: prognostic factors, dedifferentiation, and the issue of early versus late surgery. J Neurol Neurosurg Psychiatry, 1998; 64:581–587

127. Nakamura M, Konishi N, Tsunoda S et al. Analysis of prognostic and survival factors related to treatment of low-grade astrocytomas in adults. Oncology, 2000; 58:108–116

128. Montine TJ, Vandersteenhoven JJ, Aguzzi A et al. Prognostic significance of Ki-67 proliferation index in supratentorial fibrillary astrocytic neoplasms. Neurosurgery, 1994; 34:674–678

129. Dropcho EJ, Soong SJ. The prognostic impact of prior low grade histology in patients with anaplastic gliomas: a case-control study. Neurology, 1996; 47:684–690

Glioblastoma

130. Davis FG, Freels S, Grutsch J et al. Survival rates in patients with primary malignant brain tumors stratified by patient age and tumor histological type: an analysis based on surveillance, epidemiology, and end results (SEER) data, 1973–1991. J Neurosurg, 1998; 88:1–10

131. Scott JN, Rewcastle NB, Brasher PM et al. Long-term glioblastoma multiforme survivors: a population-based study. Can J Neurol Sci, 1998; 25:197–201

132. Fleury A, Menegoz F, Grosclaude P et al. Descriptive epidemiology of cerebral gliomas in France. Cancer, 1997; 79:1195–1202

133. Merchant TE, Nguyen D, Thompson SJ et al. High-grade pediatric spinal cord tumors. Pediatr Neurosurg, 1999; 30:1–5

134. Pollak L, Gur R, Walach N et al. Clinical determinants of long-term survival in patients with glioblastoma multiforme. Tumori, 1997; 83:613–617

135. Buhl R, Barth H, Hugo HH et al. Spinal drop metastases in recurrent glioblastoma multiforme. Acta Neurochir, 1998; 140:1001–1005

136. Katz DS, Poe LB, Winfield JA et al. A rare case of cerebellar glioblastoma multiforme in childhood: MR imaging. Clin Imaging, 1995; 19:162–164

137. Kuroiwa T, Numaguchi Y, Rothman MI et al. Posterior fossa glioblastoma multiforme: MR findings. Am J Neuroradiol, 1995; 16:583–589

138. Garfield J, Dayan AD, Weller RO. Postoperative intracavitary chemotherapy of malignant supratentorial astrocytomas using BCNU. Clin Oncol, 1975; 1:213–222

139. Tran CT, Wolz P, Egensperger R et al. Differential expression of MHC class II molecules by microglia and neoplastic astroglia: relevance for the escape of astrocytoma cells from immune surveillance. Neuropathol Appl Neurobiol, 1998; 24:293–301

140. Kida S, Ellison DW, Steart PV et al. Characterization of perivascular cells in astrocytic tumours and peritumoral oedematous brain. Neuropathol Appl Neurobiol, 1995; 21:121–129

141. Weller R, Foy M, Cox S. The development and ultrastructure of the microvasculature in malignant gliomas. Neuropathol Appl Neurobiol, 1977; 3:307–322

142. Weller RO, Griffin RL. Transmission and scanning electron microscopy of the microcirculation of gliomas. Adv Neurol, 1978; 20:569–575

143. Onda K, Davis RL, Shibuya M et al. Correlation between the bromodeoxyuridine labeling index and the (MIB-1) and Ki-67 proliferating cell indices in cerebral gliomas. Cancer, 1994; 74:1921–1926

144. Plate KH, Mennel HD. Vascular morphology and angiogenesis in glial tumors. Exp Toxicol Pathol, 1995; 47:89–94

145. Machein MR, Kullmer J, Fiebich BL et al. Vascular endothelial growth factor expression, vascular volume, and capillary permeability in human brain tumors. Neurosurgery, 1999; 44:732–741

146. von Deimling A, Louis DN, von Ammon K et al. Association of epidermal growth factor receptor gene amplification with loss of chromosome 10 in human glioblastoma multiforme. J Neurosurg, 1992; 77:295–301

Variants of glioblastoma

147. Meyer Puttlitz B, Hayashi Y, Waha A et al. Molecular genetic analysis of giant cell glioblastomas. Am J Pathol, 1997; 151:853–857

148. Klein R, Molenkamp G, Sorensen N et al. Favorable outcome of giant cell glioblastoma in a child. Report of an 11-year survival period. Childs Nerv Syst, 1998; 14:288–291

149. Katoh M, Aida T, Sugimoto S et al. Immunohistochemical analysis of giant cell glioblastoma. Pathol Int, 1995; 45:275–282

150. Huang MC, Kubo O, Tajika Y et al. A clinico-immunohistochemical study of giant cell glioblastoma. Noshuyo Byori, 1996; 13:11–16

151. Burger PC, Pearl DK, Aldape K et al. Small cell architecture – a histological equivalent of EGFR amplification in glioblastoma multiforme? J Neuropathol Exp Neurol, 2001; 60:1099–1104

152. Ino Y, Betensky RA, Zlatescu MC et al. Molecular subtypes of anaplastic oligodendroglioma: implications for patient management at diagnosis. Clin Cancer Res, 2001; 7:839–845

153. Galanis E, Buckner JC, Dinapoli RP et al. Clinical outcome of gliosarcoma compared with glioblastoma multiforme: North Central Cancer Treatment Group results. J Neurosurg, 1998; 89:425–430

154. Prayson RA. Gliofibroma: a distinct entity or a subtype of desmoplastic astrocytoma? Hum Pathol, 1996; 27:610–613

155. Sharma MC, Gaikwad S, Mehta VS et al. Gliofibroma: Mixed glial and mesenchymal tumour. Report of three cases. Clin Neurol Neurosurg, 1998; 100:153–159

156. Louis DN, von Deimling A, Dickersin G et al. Desmoplastic cerebral astrocytoma of infancy: a histopathological, immunohistochemical, ultrastructural and molecular genetic study. Hum Pathol, 1992; 23:1402–1409

157. Jones H, Steart PV, Weller RO. Spindle-cell glioblastoma or gliosarcoma? [see comments]. Neuropathol Appl Neurobiol, 1991; 17:177–187

158. Biernat W, Aguzzi A, Sure U et al. Identical mutations of the TP53 tumour suppressor gene in the gliomatous and the sarcomatous components of gliosarcomas suggest a common origin from glial cells. J Neuropathol Exp Neurol, 1995; 54:651–656

159. Boerman RH, Anderl K, Herath J et al. The glial and mesenchymal elements of gliosarcomas share similar genetic alterations. J Neuropathol Exp Neurol, 1996; 55:973–981

160. Rosenblum MK, Erlandson RA, Budzilovitch GN. The lipid-rich epitheliod glioblastoma. Am J Surg Pathol, 1991; 15:925–934

161. Lalithia VS, Rubinstein LJ. Reactive glioma in intracranial sarcoma: a form of mixed sarcoma and glioma ('sarcoglioma'): report of eight cases. Cancer, 1979; 43:246–257

Gliomatosis cerebri

162. Kim DG, Yang HJ, Park IA et al. Gliomatosis cerebri: Clinical features, treatment, and prognosis. Acta Neurochir, 1998; 140:755–762

163. Ponce P, Alvarez Santullano MV, Otermin E et al. Gliomatosis cerebri: Findings with computerised tomography and magnetic resonance imaging. Eur J Radiol, 1998; 28:226–229

164. Plowman PN, Saunders CAB, Maisey MN. Gliomatosis cerebri: Disconnection of the cortical grey matter, demonstrated on PET scan. Br J Neurosurg, 1998; 12:240–244

165. Keene DL, Jimenez C, Hsu E. MRI diagnosis of gliomatosis cerebri. Pediatr Neurol, 1999; 20:148–151

166. Furusawa T, Okamoto K, Ito J et al. Primary central nervous system lymphoma presenting as diffuse cerebral infiltration. Radiat Med Med Imaging Radiat Oncol, 1998; 16:137–140

Differential diagnosis of glioblastoma

167. Bruner JM, Inouye L, Fuller GN et al. Diagnostic discrepancies and their clinical impact in a neuropathology referral practice. Cancer, 1997; 79:796–803

168. Scherer HJ. Structural development in gliomas. Am J Cancer, 1938; 34:333–351

169. Kepes JJ. Large focal tumour-like demyelinating lesions of the brain: intermediate entity between multiple sclerosis and acute disseminated encephalomyelitis? A study of 31 patients. Ann Neurol, 1993; 33:18–27

170. Hair LS, Nuovo G, Powers JM et al. Progressive multifocal leukoencephalopathy in patients with human immunodeficiency virus. Hum Pathol, 1992; 23:663–667

171. Ueki K, Richardson EP, Henson JW et al. In situ PCR detection of JC virus in PML. Ann Neurol, 1994; 36:670–673

172. Recht L, Louis DN. Case records of the Massachusetts General Hospital "Cerebral schistosomiasis". New Eng J Med, 1996; 335:1906–1914

173. Miller DC, Koslow M, Budzilovich GN et al. Synaptophysin: a sensitive and specific marker for ganglion cells in central nervous system neoplasms. Am J Surg Pathol, 1990; 21:271–276

174. Quinn B. Synaptophysin staining in normal brain: importance for diagnosis of ganglioglioma. Am J Surg Pathol, 1998; 22:550

175. Zhang PJ, Rosenblum MK. Synatophysin expression in the human spinal cord Diagnostic implications of an immunohistochemical study. Am J Surg Pathol, 1996; 20:273–276

176. Wallner KE, Gonzales M, Sheline GE. Treatment of oligodendrogliomas with or without postoperative irradiation. J Neurosurg, 1988; 68:684–688

177. Smith MT, Ludwig CL, Godfrey, AD et al. Grading of oligodendrogliomas. Cancer, 1983; 52:2107–2114

178. Cairncross JG, Macdonald DR, Ramsay DA, Aggressive oligodendroglioma: a chemosensitive tumour. Neurosurgery, 1992; 31:78–82

179. Mason WP, Krol GS, DeAngelis LM. Low-grade oligodendroglioma responds to chemotherapy. Neurology, 1996; 46:203–207

180. Glass J, Hochberg FH, Gruber ML et al. The treatment of oligodendrogliomas and mixed oligodendroglioma-astrocytomas with PCV chemotherapy. J Neurosurg, 1992; 76:741–745

181. Kim L, Hochberg FH, Thornton AF et al. PCV (procarbazine, CCNU, vincristine) therapy of grade III and grade IV oligoastrocytoma. J Neurosurg, 1996; 85:602–607

182. Coons SW, Johnson PC, Scheithauer BW et al. Improving diagnostic accuracy and interobserver concordance in the classification and grading of primary gliomas. Cancer, 1997; 79:1381–1393

183. Cairncross JG, Ueki K, Zlatescu MC et al. Specific chromosomal losses predict chemotherapeutic response and survival in patients with anaplastic oligodendrogliomas. J Natl Cancer Inst, 1998; 90:1473–1479

184. Reifenberger J, Reifenberger G, Liu L et al. Molecular genetic analysis of oligodendroglial tumours shows preferential allelic deletions on 19q and 1p. Am J Pathol, 1994; 145:1175–1190

185. Kraus JA, Koopman J, Kaskel P et al. Shared allelic losses on chromosomes 1p and 19q suggest a common origin of oligodendroglioma and oligoastrocytoma. J Neuropathol Exp Neurol, 1995; 54:91–95

186. Rubio M-P, Correa KM, Ueki K et al. The putative glioma tumour suppressor gene on chromosome 19q maps between APOC2 and HRC. Cancer Res, 1994; 54:4760–4763

187. Rosenberg JE, Lisle DK, Burwick JA et al. Refined deletion mapping of the chromosome 19q glioma tumour suppressor gene to the D19S412-STD interval. Oncogene, 1996; 13:2483–2485

188. Maintz D, Fiedler K, Koopman J et al. Molecular genetic evidence for subtypes of oligoastrocytomas. J Neuropathol Exp Neurol, 1997; 56:1098–1104

Biology and molecular genetics

189. Louis DN, A molecular genetic model of astrocytoma histopathology. Brain Pathol, 1997; 7:755–764

190. Hermanson M, Funa K, Hartman M et al. Platelet-derived growth factor and its receptors in human glioma tissue: expression of messenger RNA and protein suggests the presence of autocrine and paracrine loops. Cancer Res, 1992; 52:3213–3219

191. Hermanson M, Funa K, Westermark B et al. Association of loss of heterozygosity on chromosome 17p with high platelet-derived growth factor α receptor expression in human malignant gliomas. Cancer Res, 1996; 56:164–171

192. Heldin C-H. Structural and functional studies on platelet-derived growth factor. EMBO J, 1992; 11:4251–4259

193. Cho Y, Gorina S, Jeffrey PD et al. Crystal structure of a TP53 tumour suppressor-DNA complex: understanding tumorigenic mutations. Science, 1994; 265:346–355

194. Yahanda AM, Bruner JM, Donehower LA et al. Astrocytes derived from TP53-deficient mice provide a multistep in vitro model for development of malignant gliomas. Mol Cell Biol, 1995; 15:4249–4259

195. Bogler O, Huang H-JS, Cavenee WK. Loss of wild-type TP53 bestows a growth advantage on primary cortical astrocytes and facilitates their in vitro transformation. Cancer Res, 1995; 55:2746–2751

196. Reifenberger G, Liu L, Ichimura K et al. Amplification and overexpression of the MDM2 gene in a subset of human malignant gliomas without TP53 mutations. Cancer Res, 1993; 53:2736–2739

197. Reifenberger G, Ichimura K, Reifenberger J et al. Refined mapping of 12q13-q15 amplicons in malignant gliomas suggests CDK4/SAS and MDM2 as independent amplification targets. Cancer Res, 1996; 56:5141–5145

198. Rubio M-P, von Deimling A, Yandell DW et al. Accumulation of wild-type TP53 protein in human astrocytomas. Cancer Res, 1993; 53:3465–3467

199. Ono Y, Tamiya T, Ichikawa T et al. Accumulation of wild-type TP53 in astrocytomas is associated with increase p21 expression. Acta Neuropathol, 1997; 94:21–27

200. Alderson LM, Castleberg RL, Harsh GR et al. Human gliomas with wild-type TP53 express bcl-2. Cancer Res, 1995; 55:999–1001

201. Sidransky D, Mikkelsen T, Schwechheimer K et al. Clonal expansion of TP53 mutant cells is associated with brain tumor progression. Nature, 1992; 355:846–847

202. Kinzler KW, Vogelstein B. Lessons from hereditary colorectal cancer. Cell, 1996; 87:159–170

203. James CD, Carlblom E, Dumanski JP et al. Clonal genomic alterations in glioma malignancy stages. Cancer Res, 1988; 48:5546–5551

204. Fults D, Pedone CA, Thomas GA et al. Allelotype of human malignant astrocytoma. Cancer Res, 1990; 50:5784–5789

205. Rey JA, Bello MJ, Jiménez-Lara AM et al. Loss of heterozygosity for distal markers on 22q in human gliomas. Int J Cancer, 1992; 51:703–706

206. Hoang-Xuan K, Merel P, Vega F et al. Analysis of the NF2 tumor-suppressor gene and of chromosome 22 deletions in gliomas. Int J Cancer, 1995; 60:478–481

207. Rubio M-P, Correa KM, Ramesh V et al. Analysis of the neurofibromatosis 2 (NF2) gene in human ependymomas and astrocytomas. Cancer Res, 1994; 54:45–47

208. Jen J, Harper W, Bigner SH et al. Deletion of p16 and p15 genes in brain tumors. Cancer Res, 1994; 54:6353–6358

209. Giani C, Finocchiaro G. Mutation rate of the CDKN2 gene in malignant gliomas. Cancer Res, 1994; 54:6338–6339

210. Dreyling MH, Bohlander SK, Adeyanju MO et al. Detection of CDKN2 deletions in tumor cell lines and primary glioma by interphase fluorescence in situ hybridization. Cancer Res, 1995; 55:984–988

211. Moulton T, Samara G, Chung W et al. MTS1/p16/CDKN2 lesions in primary glioblastoma multiforme. Am J Pathol, 1995; 146:613–619

212. Schmidt EE, Ichimura K, Reifenberger G et al. CDKN2 (p16/MTS1) gene deletion or CDK4 amplification occurs in the majority of glioblastomas. Cancer Res, 1994; 54:6321–6324

213. Walker DG, Duan W, Popovic EA et al. Homozygous deletions of the multiple tumor suppressor gene 1 in the progression of human astrocytomas. Cancer Res, 1995; 55:20–23

214. Ueki K, Ono Y, Henson JW et al. CDKN2/p16 or RB alterations occur in the majority of glioblastomas and are inversely correlated. Cancer Res, 1996; 56:150–153

215. He J, Olson JJ, James CD. Lack of p16^{INK4} or retinoblastoma protein (pRb), or amplification-associated overexpression of cdk4 is observed in distinct subsets of malignant glial tumors and cell lines. Cancer Res, 1995; 55:4833–4836

216. Kamb A, Gruis NA, Weaver-Feldhaus J et al. A cell cycle regulator potentially involved in genesis of many tumor types. Science, 1994; 264:436–440

217. Nobori T, Miura K, Wu DJ et al. Deletions of the cyclin-dependent kinase-4 inhibitor gene in multiple human cancers. Nature, 1994; 368:753–756

218. Ueki K, Rubio M-P, Ramesh V et al. MTS1/CDKN2 gene mutations are rare in primary human astrocytomas with allelic loss of chromosome 9p. Hum Mol Genet, 1994; 3:1841–1845

219. Merlo A, Herman JG, Mao L et al. 5′CpG island methylation is associated with transcriptional silencing of the tumor suppressor p16/CDKN2/MTS1. Nat Med, 1995; 1:686–692

220. Henson JW, Schnitker BL, Correa KM et al. The retinoblastoma gene is involved in malignant progression of astrocytomas Ann Neurol, 1994; 36:714–721

221. Ichimura K, Schmidt EE, Goike HM et al. Human glioblastomas with no alterations of the CDKN2 (p16^{INK4A}, MTS1) and CDK4 genes have frequent mutations of the retinoblastoma gene. Oncogene, 1996; 13:1065–1072

222. Reifenberger G, Reifenberger J, Ichimura K et al. Amplification of multiple genes from chromosomal region 12q13-14 in human malignant gliomas: preliminary mapping of the amplicons shows preferential involvement of CDK4, SAS, and MDM2. Cancer Res, 1994; 54:4299–4303

223. Serrano M, Hannon GJ, Beach D. A new regulatory motif in cell-cycle control causing specific inhibition of cyclin D/CDK4. Nature, 1993; 366:704–707

224. Medema RH, Herrera RE, Lam F et al. Growth suppression by p16^{ink4} requires functional retinoblastoma protein. Proc Natl Acad Sci U S A, 1995; 92:6289–6293

225. Koh J, Enders GH, Dynlacht BD et al. Tumour-derived p16 alleles encoding proteins defective in cell-cycle inhibition. Nature, 1995; 375:506–510

226. Lukas J, Parry D, Aagaard L et al. Retinoblastoma-protein-dependent cell-cycle inhibition by the tumour suppressor p16. Nature, 1995; 375:503–506

227. Lukas J, Aagaard L, Strauss M et al. Oncogenic aberrations of p16$^{INK4/CDKN2}$ and cyclin D1 cooperate to deregulate G1 control. Cancer Res, 1995; 55:4818–4823

228. Ono Y, Tamiya T, Ichikawa T et al. Malignant astrocytomas with homozygous CDKN2/p16 gene deletions have higher Ki-67 proliferation indices. J Neuropathol Exp Neurol, 1996; 55:1026–1031

229. Mao LAM, Bedi G, Shapiro GI et al. A novel p16^{INK4A} transcript. Cancer Res, 1995; 55:2995–2997

230. Stone S, Jiang P, Dayananth P et al. Complex structure and regulation of the *p16 (MTS1)* locus. Cancer Res, 1995; 55:2988–2994

231. Quelle DE, Zindy F, Ashmun RA et al. Alternative reading frames of the INK4a tumor suppressor gene encode two unrelated proteins capable of cell cycle arrest. Cell, 1995; 83:993–1000

232. Yong WH, Chou D, Ueki K et al. Chromosome 19q deletions in human gliomas overlap telomeric to D19S219 and may target a 425 kb region centromeric to D19S112. J Neuropathol Exp Neurol, 1995; 54:622–626

233. Yong WH, Ueki K, Chou D et al. Cloning of a highly conserved human protein serine threonine phosphatase gene from the glioma candidate region on chromosome 19q13.3. Genomics, 1995; 29:533–536

234. Ueki K, Ramaswamy S, Billings SJ et al. ANOVA, a putative astrocytic RNA-binding protein gene that maps to chromosome 19q13.3. Neurogenetics, 1997; 1:31–36

235. Sonoda Y, Iizuka M, Yasuda J et al. Loss of heterozygosity at 11p15 in malignant glioma. Cancer Res, 1995; 55:2166–2168

236. Fults D, Petronio J, Noblett BD et al. Chromosome 11p15 deletions in human malignant astrocytomas and primitive neuroectodermal tumors. Genomics, 1992; 14:799–801

237. Schrock E, Thiel G, Lozanova T et al. Comparative genomic hybridization of human malignant gliomas reveals multiple amplification sites and nonrandom chromosomal gains and losses. Am J Pathol, 1994; 144:1203–1218

238. Weber RG, Sabel M, Reifenberger J et al. Characterization of genomic alterations associated with glioma progression by comparative genomic hybridization. Oncogene, 1996; 13:983–994

239. Fults D, Pedone C. Deletion mapping of the long arm of chromosome 10 in glioblastoma multiforme. Genes Chromosomes Cancer, 1993; 7(3):173–177

240. Rasheed BKA, Fuller GN, Friedman AH, Bigner DD, Bigner SH. Loss of heterozygosity for 10q loci in human gliomas. Genes Chromosomes Cancer, 1992; 5:75–82

241. Karlbom AE, James CD, Boethius J et al. Loss of heterozygosity in malignant gliomas involves at least three distinct regions on chromosome 10. Hum Genet, 1993; 92:169–174

242. Rasheed BKA, McLendon RE, Friedman HS et al. Chromosome 10 deletion mapping in human gliomas: a common deletion region in 10q25. Oncogene, 1995; 10:2243–2246

243. Kimmelman AC, Ross DA, Liang BC. Loss of heterozygosity of chromosome 10p in human gliomas. Genomics, 1996; 34:250–254

244. Steck PA, Pershouse MA, Jasser SA et al. Identification of a candidate tumour suppressor gene, MMAC1, at chromosome 10q23.3 that is mutated in multiple advanced cancers. Nature Genet, 1997; 15:356–362

245. Li J, Yen C, Liaw D et al. PTEN, a putative protein tyrosine phosphatase gene mutated in human brain, breast and prostate cancer. Science, 1997; 275:1943–1947

246. Mollenhauer J, Wiemann S, Scheurlen W et al. DMBT1, a new member of the SRCR superfamily, on chromosome 10q25.3–26.1 is deleted in malignant brain tumours. Nat Genet, 1997; 17:32–39

247. Furnari FB, Lin H, Huang HS et al. Growth suppression of glioma cells by PTEN requires a functional phosphatase catalytic domain. Proc Natl Acad Sci U S A, 1997; 94:12479–12484

248. Hsu SC, Volpert OV, Steck PA et al. Inhibition of angiogenesis in human glioblastomas by chromosome 10 induction of thrombospondin-1. Cancer Res, 1996; 56:5684–5691

249. Ekstrand AJ, James CD, Cavenee WK et al. Genes for epidermal growth factor receptor, transforming growth factor α, and epidermal growth factor and their expression in human gliomas in vivo. Cancer Res, 1991; 51:2164–2172

250. Wong AJ, Bigner SH, Bigner DD et al. Increased expression of the epidermal growth factor receptor gene in malignant gliomas is invariably associated with gene amplification. Proc Natl Acad Sci U S A 1987; 84:6899–6903

251. Goldman CK, Kim J, Wong WL et al. Epidermal growth factor stimulates vascular endothelial growth factor production by human malignant glioma cells: a model of glioblastoma multiforme pathophysiology. Mol Biol Cell, 1993; 4:121–133

252. Nagane M, Coufal F, Lin H et al. A common mutant epidermal growth factor receptor confers enhanced tumorigenicity on human glioblastoma cells by increasing proliferation and reducing apoptosis. Cancer Res, 1996; 56:5079–5086

253. Graeber TG, Osmanian C, Jacks T et al. Hypoxia-mediated selection of cells with diminished apoptotic potential in solid tumors. Nature, 1996; 379:88–91

254. Kinzler KW, Vogelstein B. Life (and death) in a malignant tumor. Nature, 1996; 379:19–20

255. Plate KH, Breier G, Risau W. Molecular mechanisms of developmental and tumor angiogenesis. Brain Pathol, 1994; 4:207–218

256. Holash J, Maisonpierre PC, Compton D et al. Vessel cooption, regression, and growth in tumors mediated by angiopoietins and VEGF. Science, 1999; 284:1994–1998

257. Lyden D, Hattori K, Dias S, et al. Impaired recruitment of bone-marrow-derived endothelial and hematopoietic precursor cells blocks tumor angiogenesis and growth. Nature Med, 2001; 7:1194–1201

258. von Deimling A, von Ammon K, Schoenfeld D et al. Subsets of glioblastoma multiforme defined by molecular genetic analysis. Brain Pathol, 1993; 3:19–26

259. Rasheed BKA, McLendon RE, Herndon JE et al. Alterations of the TP53 gene in human gliomas. Cancer Res, 1994; 54:1324–1330

260. Fleming TP, Saxena A, Clark WC et al. Amplification and/or overexpression of platelet-derived growth factor receptors and

epidermal growth factor receptor in human glial tumors. Cancer Res, 1992; 52:4550–4553

261. Biernat W, Kleihues P, Yonekawa Y et al. Amplification and overexpression of MDM2 in primary (de novo) glioblastomas. J Neuropathol Exp Neurol, 1997; 56:180–185

262. Hayashi Y, Ueki K, Waha A et al. Association of EGFR gene amplification and CDKN2 (p16/MTS1) gene deletion in glioblastoma multiforme. Brain Pathol, 1997; 7:871–875

263. Louis DN, Gusella JF. A tiger behind many doors: multiple genetic pathways to malignant glioma. Trends Genet, 1995; 11:412–415

264. Winger MJ, Macdonald DR, Cairncross JG. Supratentorial anaplastic gliomas in adults: the prognostic importance of extent of resection and prior low-grade glioma. J Neurosurg, 1989; 71:487–493

265. Watanabe K, Tachibana O, Sato K et al. Overexpression of the EGF receptor and TP53 mutations are mutually exclusive in the evolution of primary and secondary glioblastomas. Brain Pathol, 1996; 6:217–223

266. Reifenberger J, Ring GU, Gies U et al. Analysis of p53 mutation and epidermal growth factor receptor amplification in recurrent gliomas with malignant progression. J Neuropathol Exp Neurol, 1996; 55:822–831

267. von Deimling A, Eibl RH, Ohgaki H et al. TP53 mutations are associated with 17p allelic loss in grade II and grade III astrocytoma. Cancer Res, 1992; 52:2987–2990

268. Louis DN, Rubio M-P, Correa K et al. Molecular genetics of pediatric brain stem gliomas. Application of PCR techniques to small and archival brain tumor specimens. J Neuropath Exp Neurol, 1993; 52:507–515

269. Meyer-Puttlitz B, Hayashi Y, Waha A et al. Molecular genetic analysis of giant cell glioblastomas. Am J Pathol, 1997; 151:853–857

270. Oda H, Zhang S, Tsurutani N et al. Loss of TP53 is an early event in induction of brain tumours in mice by transplacental carcinogen exposure. Cancer Res, 1997; 57:646–650

271. Louis DN, Cavenee WK. Molecular biology of central nervous system tumors. In: DeVita VT, Hellman S, Rosenberg SA, eds. Cancer: principles and practice of oncology, 5th edn. Philadephia: Lippincott-Raven, 1997; pp 2013–2022

272. Chung RY, Whaley J, Kley N et al. TP53 mutation and chromosome 17p deletion in human astrocytomas. Genes Chromosomes Cancer, 1991; 3:323–331

273. Leenstra S, Bijlsma EK, Troost D et al. Allele loss on chromosomes 10 and 17p and epidermal growth factor receptor gene amplification in human malignant astrocytoma related to prognosis. Br J Cancer, 1994; 70:684–689

5 Oligodendrogliomas and oligoastrocytomas

The common feature of oligodendrogliomas and oligoastrocytomas is the dominant presence of cells which cytologically resemble normal oligodendrocytes. Historically,[1] the suggestion that these tumours were differentiated along oligodendroglial lines came from three main observations:

1. The tumour cells have rounded nuclei arranged in a uniform, evenly spaced pattern, reminiscent of normal oligodendroglia.
2. The artefactual vacuolation of cytoplasm seen in formalin fixed histological preparations is identical to that seen with interfascicular oligodendrocytes.
3. Silver staining, optimised to detect normal oligodendroglial processes, also reveals similar cell processes in these neoplasms.

To some extent, this suggestion has been confirmed by in situ hybridisation approaches, which have demonstrated transcripts of myelin-associated genes in oligodendrogliomas[2]. Other investigations, however, particularly analysis with immunohistochemical techniques, have shown that the pattern of differentiation in this type of tumour is less certainly oligodendroglial. For instance, markers that identify normal oligodendroglial cells do not typically detect cells in so-called oligodendrogliomas.[3,4] In addition, these tumours frequently show evidence of astroglial differentiation, as evidenced by glial fibrillary acidic protein (GFAP) expression[5,6] and some tumours with an oligodendroglial appearance have been shown to be unequivocally neuronal or ependymal.[7,8] Because several other tumours mimic the appearance of oligodendroglioma, it is important that the diagnosis of oligodendroglioma be made after the exclusion of other possible tumours.

Excluding the lesions now recognised to be neuronal or ependymal, it has been proposed that oligodendroglial tumours represent a continuum of glial differentiation from GFAP negative cells through cells containing GFAP but still cytologically resembling oligodendroglia, through to cells recognisably astrocytic in cytology and nuclear characteristics.[5,6,9] Tumours which are composed purely of the rounded oligodendroglial-like cells are termed oligodendrogliomas, while tumours also containing differentiated astrocytic cells are termed oligoastrocytomas. In the World Health Organisation (WHO) classification, oligodendrogliomas are divided into two groups: WHO grade II oligodendrogliomas and WHO grade III anaplastic oligodendrogliomas. Oligoastrocytomas are similarly divided into WHO grade II oligoastrocytomas and WHO grade III anaplastic oligoastrocytomas.[10]

Despite the uncertainties which still exist as to the precise line of differentiation in this type of tumour, these lesions are most conveniently discussed as a distinct group. As discussed below, molecular genetic analyses have shown remarkable similarities among tumours in this large group, but have suggested that only some of the tumours designated histologically as oligoastrocytomas are closely allied with the pure oligodendrogliomas. In the following discussion, oligodendrogliomas will be presented and any differences related to oligoastrocytomas are highlighted separately.

Incidence

The cited frequency of oligodendroglial tumours varies in different series. An often quoted series of 208 patients with histologically confirmed oligodendrogliomas in Norway concluded that they represented just under 5% of all primary brain tumours. Other series have cited comparable incidences of 7.9% of all gliomas,[11] or higher, 18.8% of all gliomas.[12] More recent series, however, have stressed the difficulty of histologically identifying oligodendroglial tumours, and have suggested that these tumours are under-recognised and may comprise up to 25% of all gliomas.[13] The increased interest by neuro-oncologists in oligodendrogliomas, given their relative chemosensitivity, has placed an increased burden on neuropathologists to recognise oligodendroglial elements in diffuse cerebral gliomas. As a result, the frequency of diagnosis of oligodendroglioma and oligoastrocytoma has certainly increased in most clinical practices over the past 10 years. Until an objective marker exists for these tumours, the actual incidence of oligodendroglioma and oligoastrocytoma will remain speculative.

Most oligodendroglial or mixed gliomas arise between the ages of 35 and 55 with a peak at around 45 years and a male–female ratio of 1.5 to 2.1.[12,14] There is also an important smaller peak of incidence in infancy and childhood,[15,16] with 6% of diagnosed oligodendrogliomas occurring in children.[14] The majority of low grade tumours occur in patients under 40 years of age, whereas most high grade tumours occur in those over 40 years of age.[17]

Site

The majority of oligodendrogliomas arise in the periphery of the cerebral hemispheres in the frontal, parietal, temporal and occipital lobes in a ratio of about 3 : 2 : 2 : 1.[15,18,19] Rarely, multiple oligodendrogliomas have been reported[20,21] as has diffuse cerebral infiltration similar to gliomatosis cerebri.[22–24] Reports of intraventricular oligodendroglioma must now be reviewed since a large number of such tumours have been found, on review, to be central neurocytomas.[7,25–27]

Uncommonly, cerebellar oligodendrogliomas have been reported.[28–30] However as some patterns of pilocytic astrocytoma and clear cell ependymoma closely mimic the light microscopic appearance of oligodendroglioma, these must be excluded before a diagnosis of cerebellar oligodendroglioma is made.[8] Oligodendroglioma also occurs rarely in the brain stem[24,31] and spinal cord, where there is a slightly lower average age than with other gliomas.[22,32–35]

Extracerebral oligodendrogliomas have been described related to the meninges.[36,37] However the possibility of confusion with certain patterns of meningioma, particularly the clear cell variant, must always be considered.[38] They have also been recorded in heterotopic brain tissue[39] and optic nerve.[40]

Aetiology

As with most types of malignant glioma, the aetiology of oligodendrogliomas remains unclear. No causative environmental agents have been identified, although a case associated with previous irradiation has been reported.[41] Cases developing at the site of previous cerebral contusions have been reported, fulfilling the criteria for traumatic origin of a cerebral tumour,[42] but these associations remain anecdotal. Cases associated with multiple sclerosis have been rarely reported.[43]

Familial oligodendrogliomas have been documented,[44–46] and oligodendrogliomas have been reported in the setting of hereditary brain tumour syndromes. For instance, germline mutations of the *hPMS2* gene have been noted in one family with oligodendroglioma-like malignant gliomas and colonic tumours.[47]

Clinical features

Headache is the most common symptom, followed by seizures, visual loss, motor weakness and cognitive decline. Less common manifestations are ataxia, haemorrhage, stroke, and signs of leptomeningeal involvement from cerebrospinal fluid tumour spread. Seizures, including chronic intractable epilepsy, are a common clinical manifestation (87% of cases).[15,48,49] Symptoms are not generally related to tumour grade,[17] although lower grade tumours may come to diagnosis after a long history of seizures. Oligodendrogliomas may also present with large intratumoral haemorrhage and, among the malignant gliomas, such a presentation is perhaps most characteristic of oligodendrogliomas.[50–52] Finally, oligodendrogliomas may also present with death as the first indication of cerebral tumour and this has been cited to account for about 20% of such cases in one forensic series.[53]

Imaging features

On computerised tomography (CT), oligodendrogliomas are usually hypo- or isodense with respect to adjacent white matter. There is frequent calcification, usually most evident around the periphery and cortical aspect of the lesion (Fig. 5.1), but some oligodendrogliomas may resemble a so-called 'brain stone' with their diffuse,

dense mineralisation. Indeed, dense calcification in a parenchymal lesion should raise oligodendroglioma high in the differential diagnosis. Calvarial erosion may be seen overlying lesions, attributed to the peripheral location and slow growth rate of most oligodendrogliomas. Approximately half of all oligodendrogliomas show ill-defined faint enhancement (Fig. 5.2). Such enhancement is usually related to solid foci of high grade tumour, but rarely focal enhancement may be seen in low grade lesions. Peritumoral low attenuation is usually absent or mild and could represent either diffuse white matter spread of tumour or oedema. Involvement of cortex overlying a hemispheric tumour as ill-defined thickening is often suggestive that the underlying lesion is an oligodendroglioma.[18,54,55] Magnetic resonanance usually shows oligodendrogliomas as hypointense lesions on T1-weighted images and hyperintense lesions on T2-weighted scans.[18,54] In paediatric tumours calcification, contrast enhancement, and oedema are seen much less frequently than in adults, and reflect a generally higher proportion of low grade tumours.[56]

Pathology

Macroscopic features

Oligodendrogliomas are typically solid, soft, tan-to-pink-coloured tumours. Some lesions have a gelatinous texture

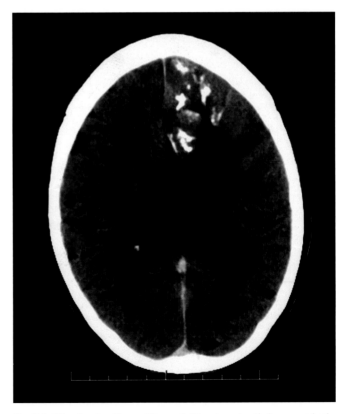

Fig. 5.1 **Oligodendroglioma.** CT scan (without contrast) shows marked calcification within an ill-defined frontal oligodendroglioma.

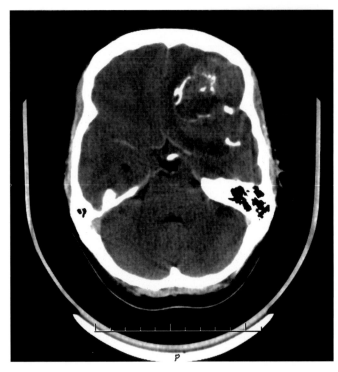

Fig. 5.2 Anaplastic oligodendroglioma. CT scan with contrast shows irregular enhancement and calcification in a frontal anaplastic oligodendroglioma, which exerts a substantial mass effect on the brain.

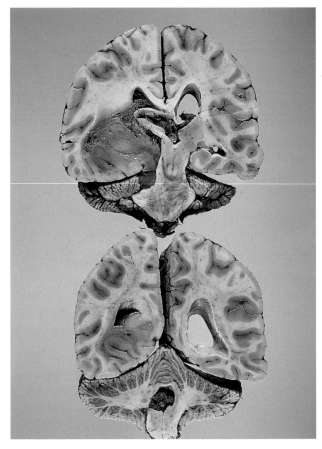

Fig. 5.3 Oligodendroglioma. A poorly defined tumour with a pale grey colour is seen replacing the temporal lobe.

which has been related to accumulation of extracellular mucopolysaccharide within the tumour.[57] Most tumours are macroscopically poorly circumscribed and blend imperceptibly into adjacent structures, without cyst formation, necrosis or haemorrhage (Fig. 5.3).[14] A common pattern of growth is diffuse infiltration of the cerebral cortex overlying a lesion originating in the hemispheric white matter, to produce a dome shaped lesion bulging out from between normal gyri. Thus, the appearance of a single expanded gyrus is highly characteristic of oligo-dendroglioma. This pattern of growth of oligodendroglial tumours may also result in extension into the lepto-meninges and even involvement of dura, leading to a mistaken impression of an infiltrative meningeal tumour. Calcification is encountered macroscopically in about 50% of all oligodendrogliomas and is usually detected as a gritty texture on cutting or while preparing brain smears.

Macroscopic cysts may occur in a small proportion of tumours.[18,58] Necrosis in oligodendrogliomas is mainly seen in high grade or anaplastic tumours, being seen in less than 10% of cases[54] (Fig. 5.4). Haemorrhage is not uncommon in oligodendrogliomas. In one study the highest haemorrhage rate for primary brain tumours was 29.2% for mixed oligoastrocytoma.[51] This has been related to the structure of small blood vessels in the tumour.[52] Uncommonly, oligodendrogliomas are multifocal[20,21] or occur as a diffuse cerebral infiltration similar to gliomatosis cerebri.[22–24]

Intraoperative diagnosis

Oligodendrogliomas usually smear well and produce a uniform, even smear (Fig. 5.5). Sometimes micro-calcifications are felt as a gritty sensation when making the smear. Cytologically, the best clue to the diagnosis of oligodendroglioma is the presence of rounded nuclei in cells having few processes (Fig. 5.6). The presence of a few classical astrocytic cells with angulated or lobated nuclei is to be expected in oligodendroglioma and does not exclude the diagnosis. Once the cytology features have suggested the diagnosis, a search will usually reveal characteristic fine capillaries (Fig. 5.5). Unlike some other types of glioma, cells of oligodendroglioma generally tend not to remain in close association with vessels but strip off in smear preparations.

Because freezing may markedly distort the nuclei in oligodendrogliomas (Table 5.1) and cause them to lose their classic, rounded appearance, it is best to preserve some portion of the biopsy as non-frozen tissue. None-theless, frozen sections may be useful in confirming the architectural patterns characteristic of oligodendrogliomas. In frozen sections, the cytoplasmic vacuolation that is often helpful in fixed material is not seen (Fig. 5.7). While

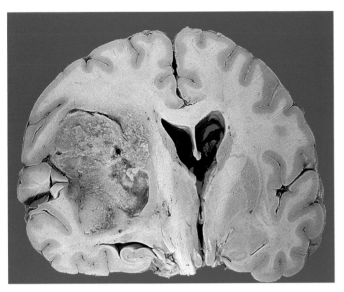

Fig. 5.4 **Anaplastic oligoastrocytoma**. This anaplastic oligoastrocytoma shows necrosis and has caused considerable mass effect.

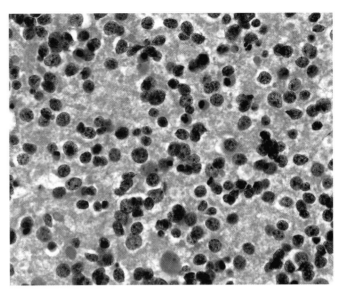

Fig. 5.6 **Oligodendroglioma**. Smear of oligodendroglioma viewed at high magnification. Tumours tend to produce an even spread of cells with rounded nuclei and little cytoplasmic detail. H & E.

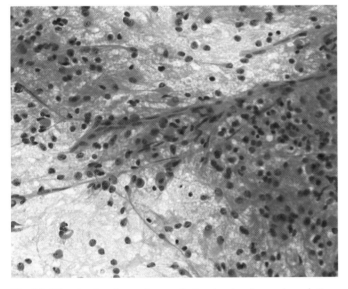

Fig. 5.5 **Oligodendroglioma**. Smear of oligodendroglioma viewed at low magnification. Small branching capillaries are prominent. H & E.

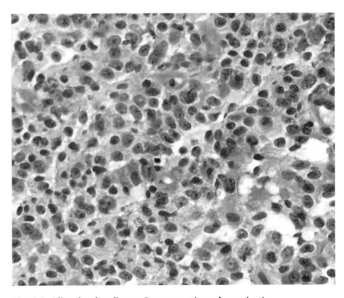

Fig. 5.7 **Oligodendroglioma**. Frozen section of anaplastic oligodendroglioma. Note absence of cytoplasmic vacuolation and that while nuclei generally have rounded contours, this is less well defined than when compared to fixed material. H & E.

the best clue to the diagnosis of oligodendroglioma is the presence of rounded neoplastic nuclei, as mentioned above, the nuclear shape may be distorted by freezing. For this reason, the frozen section diagnosis of oligodendroglioma is usually reliable only in lesions with high cellularity in which the dense, uniform cellularity, branching vasculature and calcifications are often found; in lesions of moderate cellularity, however, the presence of other cell types and reactive cells frequently obscures the diagnosis. If cortex is included with the specimen, neuronal satellitosis is often a feature which suggests the diagnosis.

Table 5.1 Difficulties in the intraoperative diagnosis of oligodendrogliomas

1. Frozen sections can artefactually cause oligodendroglioma nuclei to look more angular, irregular and heterochromatic, and thus more astrocytic
2. Perinuclear halos, the artefact of cytoplasmic vacuolation characteristic of oligodendrogliomas, are not seen in frozen sections or smears
3. Some ependymal and neuronal tumours closely mimic oligodendroglioma

As there is often difficulty in distinguishing low grade astrocytoma from oligodendroglioma on smear and frozen section a label of 'low grade glioma – possibly oligodendroglioma' is appropriate for intraoperative diagnosis, pending a firm diagnosis after inspection of fixed tissue. If there is nuclear pleomorphism, hyperchromatic nuclei, and mitoses in addition to features suggestive of oligodendroglioma, an intraoperative diagnosis of 'high grade glioma – possibly anaplastic oligodendroglioma' is appropriate.

In view of the overlap in appearance of lesions which mimic oligodendroglioma it is sensible to preserve material for electron microscopy. This is especially true when a lesion is from a site which would be unusual for an oligodendroglioma or for lesions close to the ventricular system where a diagnosis of neurocytoma or ependymoma are major possibilities.

Histological features

Oligodendroglioma Oligodendrogliomas are composed of glial cells with uniform rounded or slightly oval shaped nuclei, small amounts of cytoplasm and small numbers of cell processes. The key features of the glial cells that distinguish them from astrocytes are the relative paucity of cell processes and the rounded nature of the nuclei. Because there are varied architectural patterns for oligodendrogliomas, the recognition of classical oligodendroglial cytological features is integral to proper diagnosis.

Oligodendroglioma should be entertained as a possible diagnosis when a moderately cellular, diffusely infiltrative glioma has a somewhat uniform cytological appearance at low power. Most anaplastic astrocytomas and nearly all glioblastomas are characterised by a heterogeneous appearance at low power, but oligodendrogliomas are often remarkable for their cellular homogeneity, even in large resection specimens. Most lesions boast high cellularity, with closely apposed cells that form monotonous sheets with minimal intervening background fibrillarity (Fig. 5.8). Other lesions, however, are more infiltrative, particularly at the margins of the tumour; such cases may be of relatively low cell density with cells generally separated in an eosinophilic background of normal neuropil (Fig. 5.9).

As mentioned above, cytological features are essential to diagnosis. The cells of oligodendrogliomas are fairly monotonous and the nuclei have crisp membranes, a speckled chromatin pattern, and one or more small nucleoli. Nuclei may vary a little in size but the presence of hyperchromatic nuclei or pleomorphism should prompt consideration of anaplastic oligodendroglioma. The cytoplasm of cells in well fixed tissues is generally indistinct (Fig. 5.10). However, in tissues that have taken some time to fix, an important artefact develops – the so-

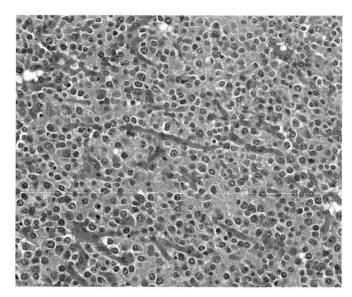

Fig. 5.8 **Oligodendroglioma**. Most tumours are composed of closely apposed cells that form monotonous sheets with minimal intervening background fibrillarity. H & E.

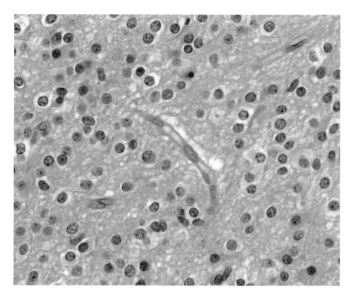

Fig. 5.9 **Oligodendroglioma**. Some tumours have a relatively low cell density, with cells generally separated in an eosinophilic background of normal neuropil. H & E.

called 'perinuclear halo', which is probably related to autolytic cytoplasmic vacuolation (Fig. 5.11). This distinctive pattern has been likened to 'frog spawn', 'fried eggs' or 'poached eggs'. Although artefactual and certainly not pathognomonic, the perinuclear halo is highly characteristic of oligodendroglioma. In some tumours, perinuclear halos may only be focally prominent, often in regions of cortical infiltration.

Astrocytic cells are virtually always present within oligodendrogliomas, particularly adjacent to large blood vessels. These are often clearly reactive in appearance, with oval, euchromatic nuclei, a large nucleolus, and

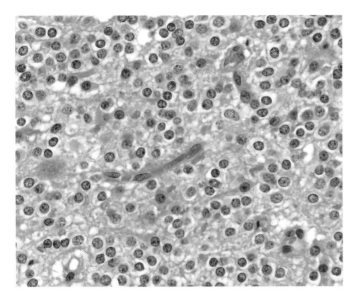

Fig. 5.10 **Oligodendroglioma**. In well fixed material cells are monotonous and nuclei have crisp membranes with a speckled chromatin pattern, and one or more small nucleoli. The cytoplasm is generally indistinct but when visible has a slightly granular eosinophilic texture. H & E.

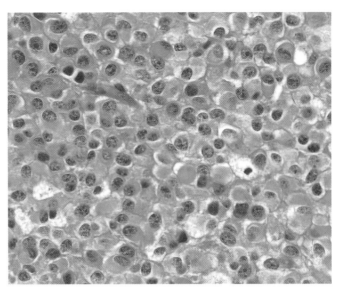

Fig. 5.12 **Oligodendroglioma**. This tumour contains many so-called minigemistocytes with a typically rounded cytoplasmic mass about the same size as the nucleus, composed of whorled, GFAP positive intermediate filaments – also shown stained with GFAP in Fig. 5.32 H & E.

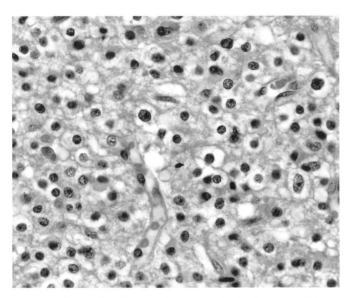

Fig. 5.11 **Oligodendroglioma**. In this tumour the 'perinuclear halo' artefact is pronounced. H & E.

branching GFAP positive cytoplasmic processes. A large proportion of astrocytic cells with atypical, neoplastic appearing nuclei, however, should prompt consideration of oligoastrocytoma (see below).

True astrocytic cells must be distinguished from 'minigemistocytes' or 'microgemistocytes' (Fig. 5.12). Minigemistocytes are cells with oligodendroglial tumour nuclei but with conspicuous eccentric eosinophilic cytoplasm; the cytoplasm is typically rounded and about the same size as the adjacent nuclei, and is composed of whorled, GFAP positive intermediate filaments. Such

cells are essentially diagnostic of oligodendrogliomas, and do not necessitate a change of diagnosis to oligo-astrocytoma. In our experience, however, the finding of extensive sheets of microgemistocytes usually heralds the presence of anaplastic change, and often is accompanied by frank gemistocytic astrocytoma, requiring a diagnosis of anaplastic oligoastrocytoma. GFAP positive oligo-dendroglial cells have also been described that are not microgemistocytic, but rather feature a delicate, even rim of GFAP positivity around a typical oligodendroglial tumour nucleus.[5]

Another characteristic feature of oligodendrogliomas at low power is the capillary vascular pattern. The vessels of oligodendrogliomas are typically numerous, with thin walled, straight and branching segments and small arcs, likened to 'chicken wire' (Fig. 5.8). This may cause the tumour cells to appear packaged into groups between the delicate arching capillaries and when prominent, can almost resemble the 'zellballen' pattern of paraganglioma (Fig. 5.13). This characteristic vascular pattern is often maintained in high grade oligodendrogliomas as well, and may be one key to diagnosis. Microscopic calcifi-cation is present in many, if not most cases of oligodendroglioma, even when not visible grossly or on neuroimaging. Calcification usually occurs as small calcospherites (Fig. 5.14), less commonly as larger masses of calcium and rarely as a component of metaplastic bone. Often, microscopic calcification can be detected along small tumoral vessels.

Oligodendrogliomas may either diffusely infiltrate white matter or may be relatively well circumscribed (Fig. 5.15). Some tumours stop abruptly at the junction of

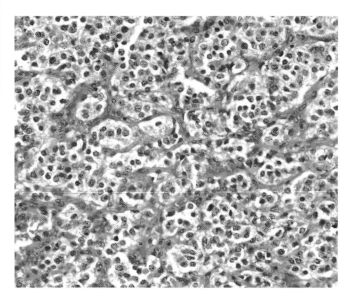

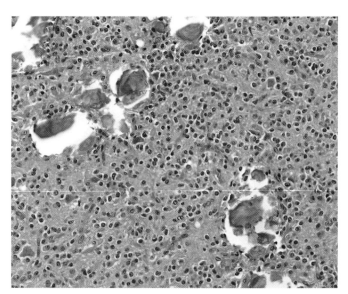

Fig. 5.13 **Oligodendroglioma**. In some tumours the vascular network delineates small tumour islands, reminiscent of the arrangement in a paraganglioma. H & E.

Fig. 5.14 **Oligodendroglioma**. Calcospherites are seen in a large proportion of oligodendrogliomas. In routine sections they often partly tear out of the section, as seen here. H & E.

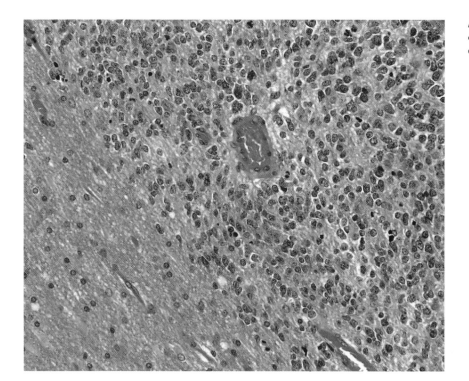

Fig. 5.15 **Oligodendroglioma.** In some oligodendrogliomas there is a sharp line of demarcation with adjacent white matter. H & E.

cortex and subcortical white matter, but most tumours infiltrate the cortex. Indeed, some tumours appear to involve the cortex preferentially. Cortical infiltration occurs in a characteristic pattern, with neoplastic glial cells aggregating around well preserved cortical neurons, termed 'neuronal satellitosis' (Fig. 5.16), or around cortical blood vessels. Another frequent pattern of growth is for neoplastic cells to proliferate and form masses in the subpial layer (Fig. 5.16), often extending horizontally in this layer beyond the macroscopically visible limits of the tumour. These secondary structures are highly characteristic of oligodendrogliomas and, while not specific, their presence should immediately prompt consideration of oligodendroglioma. As mentioned above, perinuclear halos may be particularly prominent in these cortically infiltrative portions of the tumour.

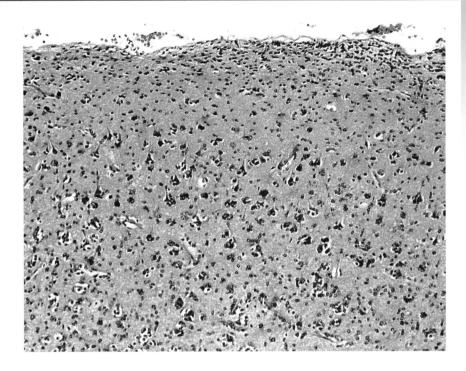

Fig. 5.16 **Oligodendroglioma.** This low magnification image emphasises satellitism of neurons in the cerebral cortex as well as subpial growth of tumour. H & E.

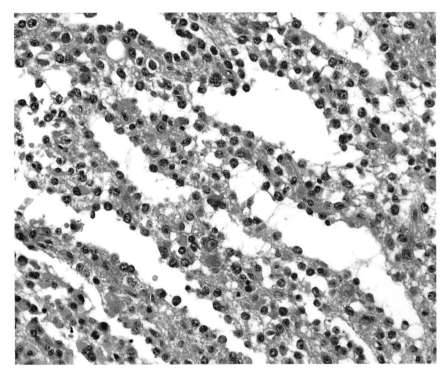

Fig. 5.17 **Oligodendroglioma.** Microcystic change is commonly seen in oligodendrogliomas and when involving the cortex can resemble structures seen in dysembryoplastic neuroepithelial tumour. H & E.

Other changes may be superimposed on this basic growth pattern. For instance, microcystic change is common (Fig. 5.17) in low grade oligodendrogliomas, with the spaces either empty or containing pale staining material. Some tumours accumulate mucopolysaccharide in between cells (mucinous change) which can be stained with periodic acid–Schiff (PAS). Signet ring cell oligodendroglioma has also been described, in which aggregates of signet ring cells, negative for GFAP are evident.[60,61] Other tumours may focally demonstrate a 'polar spongioblastoma' pattern, with neoplastic cells arranged in rhythmic palisades (Fig. 5.18).

Tumours containing crystals positive with PAS staining, possibly derived from the endosome–lysosome system, have been described.[62] An oligodendroglial tumour composed largely of eosinophilic granular cells has also been described,[63] and it is not uncommon for oligodendrogliomas to contain scattered cells containing fine eosinophilic refractile material that appears tinctorially similar to Rosenthal fibres.

Mitoses are not seen or are rare in low grade oligodendrogliomas, as is pleomorphism, microvascular proliferation and necrosis. The presence of these features should prompt consideration of anaplastic oligo-dendroglioma (see below).

Anaplastic oligodendroglioma The criteria for the diagnosis of anaplastic oligodendroglioma remain ill defined. In contrast to the diffuse astrocytic gliomas, one cannot draw strict divisions between low grade oligo-dendroglioma and anaplastic oligodendroglioma based solely on the presence or absence of individual histological features. In general, anaplastic oligodendroglioma is diagnosed when an oligodendroglial tumour shows at least some of the following features: high cell density, moderate pleomorphism with anaplastic nuclei, prominent mitotic activity, microvascular proliferation and necrosis (Figs 5.19–5.22). Histological features of anaplasia may be quite focal within oligodendrogliomas, in accordance with the neuroradiological observations that enhancement may also be focal within these tumours. For this reason, it is important to sample oligodendroglioma resection specimens extensively for histological examination.

High cell density may be diffuse or focal in oligo-dendrogliomas. When cell density is diffusely very high, with nuclei nearly abutting one another, other features of anaplasia are usually evident. Other cases, however, may show distinct nodules of marked hypercellularity, which may or may not contain other features of anaplasia.

The nuclei in anaplastic oligodendroglioma generally retain their rounded contours, but show moderate pleomorphism and hyperchromatism. The normally delicate chromatin pattern is replaced by a clumped coarse pattern, often with prominent nuceoli. In some high grade oligodendrogliomas, the nuclei become more elongate and appear almost spindled, sometimes with short bipolar cytoplasmic processes (Fig. 5.23). Such spindle cell oligodendrogliomas typically are uniformly hypercellular and have a conspicuous delicate branching or plumper branching vasculature, which lends a oligodendroglioma-like look to the low power appearance. The cells in these spindle cell oligodendrogliomas often face in the same direction, as opposed to spindle cell glioblastomas which feature such cells in a more haphazard arrangement. Pleomorphism may be even more marked in some high grade lesions, and multinucleated giant cells may be found, often with circumferentially arranged nuclei (Touton-like giant cells).

Mitotic activity is usually prominent in anaplastic oligodendrogliomas (Fig. 5.20), but exact mitotic counts necessary or sufficient for the diagnosis are not available. As discussed below, MIB-1 proliferation indices are elevated in most anaplastic oligodendrogliomas and correlate with malignancy grade and behaviour. Unfortunately, given the substantial variability in MIB-1 counts between laboratories, recommendations for cut-off values cannot be universal.

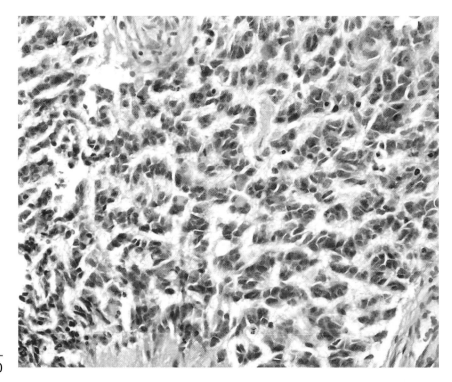

Fig. 5.18 Oligodendroglioma. In some tumours a palisaded pattern can be identified. H & E.

Fig. 5.19 **Anaplastic oligodendroglioma**. Anaplastic oligodendroglioma with high cellularity, nuclear pleomorphism and vascular proliferation. H & E.

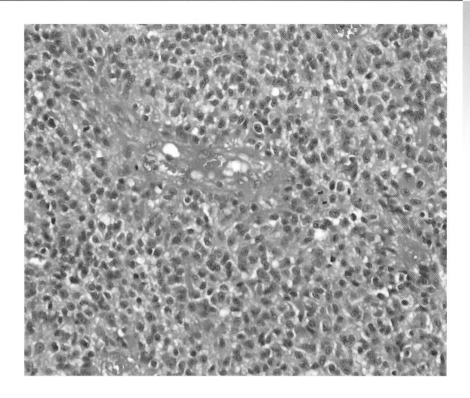

Fig. 5.20 **Anaplastic oligodendroglioma**. Nuclei generally have rounded contours, but show moderate pleomorphism and hyperchromatism. Chromatin has a clumped coarse pattern often with prominent nucleoli. Mitoses and apoptotic figures are prominent. H & E.

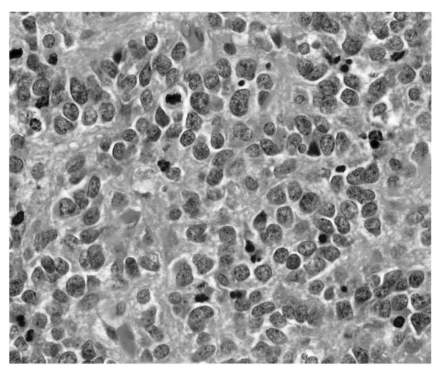

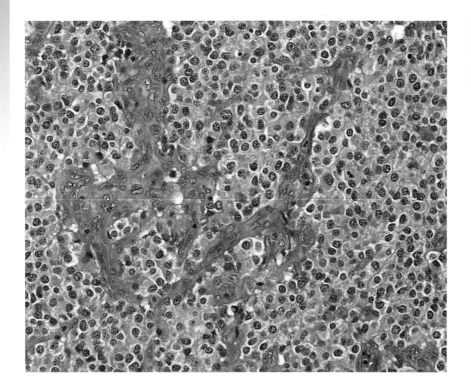

Fig. 5.21 **Anaplastic oligodendroglioma.** Microvascular proliferation is common in anaplastic oligodendrogliomas but may also be seen in some oligodendrogliomas that lack any other atypical histological features. H & E.

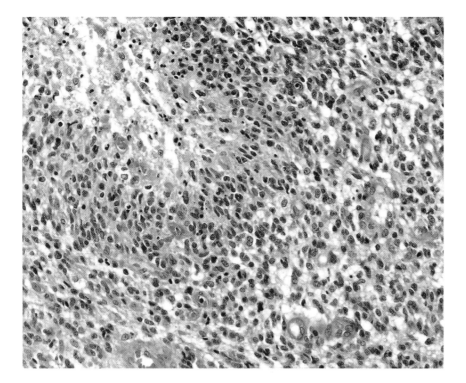

Fig. 5.22 **Anaplastic oligodendroglioma.** Focal necrosis with a palisaded pattern in an anaplastic oligodendroglioma. H & E.

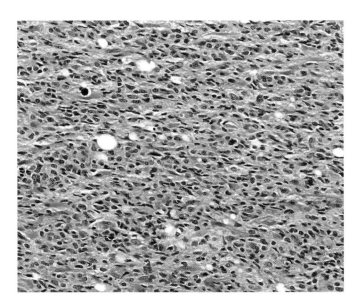

Fig. 5.23 **Anaplastic oligodendroglioma.** Spindle cell anaplastic oligodendrogliomas are hypercellular with the elongated neoplastic cells tending to face in the same direction, as opposed to spindle cell glioblastomas which feature cells in a haphazard arrangement. H& E.

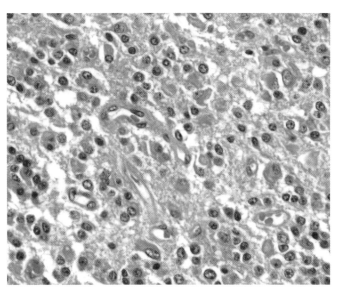

Fig. 5.24 **Astrocytes in oligodendroglioma.** In many oligodendrogliomas a small number of astrocytes are nearly always seen, as here, especially adjacent to vessels. Some workers require a defined proportion of tumour to be composed of astrocytes before calling it an oligoastrocytoma. H & E.

Microvascular proliferation is common in anaplastic oligodendrogliomas, but may be found in lower grade tumours as well (Fig. 5.19). The vascular proliferation ranges from increased cellularity of the branching capillaries to garlands of frank glomeruloid vessels that are similar to glioblastoma. Similarly, the necrosis found in anaplastic oligodendrogliomas may be similar to that found in glioblastoma, ranging from simple infarctive necrosis to complex, geographic necrosis with perinecrotic pseudopalisading of tumour cells (Fig. 5.22).

Oligoastrocytoma Oligoastrocytoma is characterised by a mixture of oligodendroglioma and astrocytoma. In neither element is there evidence of anaplastic change, such as nuclear pleomorphism, significant mitotic activity, microvascular proliferation or necrosis.

The diagnosis of oligoastrocytoma is fraught with difficulty and, as such, the frequency with which this diagnosis is made varies widely between institutions. One problem in making the distinction between an oligodendroglioma and an oligoastrocytoma is that virtually all oligodendrogliomas contain astroglial cells (see above), which is particularly evident when immuno-histochemistry is used to reveal astroglial lineage. Some of these cells are reactive astrocytes forming part of the tumour stroma, but others may be neoplastic. In general, reactive 'stromal' astrocytes occur in low density, tend to be adjacent to vessels, and are usually isolated or in small groups (Fig. 5.24). On the other hand, true neoplastic astroglial cells occur in one of two fairly distinct patterns: as sheets of cells or as cells intimately admixed with the oligodendroglial component (Figs 5.25 and 5.26).

These two patterns present different problems in the diagnosis of oligoastrocytoma. Those tumours that have distinct regions of classical oligodendroglioma and classical astrocytoma, often directly abutting one another, are most easily diagnosed as oligoastrocytoma. Unfortunately, such biphasic tumours constitute only a small minority of lesions for which the diagnosis of oligoastrocytoma is entertained. These biphasic tumours often contain cells transitional between oligodendroglial and astrocytic tumour cells in the specimen, sometimes at the junction of the two components (Fig. 5.26). As mentioned above, transitional cells can sometimes have the appearance of microgemistocytes, particularly in higher grade oligoastrocytomas.

The 'diffuse' or 'intermingled' form of oligoastrocytoma features oligodendroglial and astrocytic tumour cells intimately admixed. Given the necessity of cellular uniformity and round nuclei for the diagnosis of oligo-dendroglioma, such a mixed cell population obviously makes it more difficult to recognise an oligodendroglial component. On the contrary, some pathologists allow for a fair degree of pleomorphism in an otherwise typical oligodendroglioma and would consider the possibly astro-cytic nuclei as slightly pleomorphic oligodendroglioma nuclei; this approach would make it more difficult to recognise the astrocytic component. As a result, there are markedly different thresholds for the diagnosis of oligoastrocytoma, with some pathologists grouping most such tumours as oligodendrogliomas, others favouring a diagnosis of astrocytoma for such cases, and a third group often making the diagnosis of oligoastrocytoma. Until more objective markers are identified, the diagnosis of these admixed oligoastrocytomas will remain controversial.

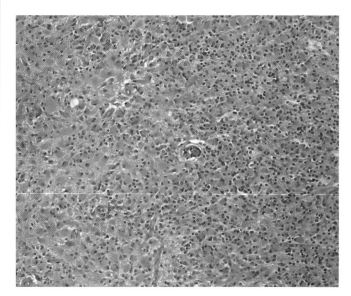

Fig. 5.25 **Oligoastrocytoma.** On the right, tumour is composed of a mixture of oligodendroglial-like and astroglial-like cells which gives way to a gemistocytic-pattern astrocytoma on the left. Other areas of tumour had a pure oligodendrogliomatous pattern. H & E.

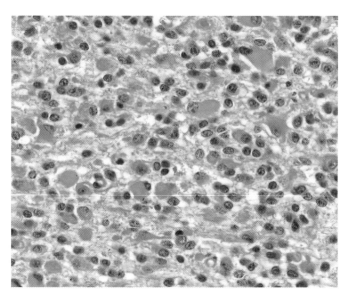

Fig. 5.26 **Oligoastrocytoma.** In some areas of oligoastrocytoma, cells with transitional appearances between oligodendrogliomatous and astrocytomatous cells are present. H & E.

Fortunately, molecular genetic approaches may be promising, with some oligoastrocytomas having genetic features characteristic of oligodendroglioma and others having genetic features typical of astrocytoma (see below).[64]

Another problem in making the diagnosis of oligoastrocytoma is defining a cut-off value for either an oligodendroglial or astrocytic component. It is obvious that any definition of a cut-off point based on number and disposition of astrocytic elements in an oligodendroglial tumour is arbitrary. The arbitrary nature of the decision is reinforced by data on the cell biology of oligodendroglial tumours which suggests a spectrum of differentiation between the oligodendroglial-like cell through transitional cells to astroglial cells.[5] Different authors cite ranges between 10 and 25% for the minimum proportion required to classify a tumour as oligoastrocytoma. This problem is made worse when considering potential sampling errors from stereotactic biopsy samples. We favour the approach of diagnosing oligoastrocytoma if both components are definitely present, regardless of the percentages of each component in the available, examined sections.

Anaplastic oligoastrocytoma In anaplastic oligoastrocytomas there is again a mixture of tumour with both oligodendroglial and astroglial characteristics. Anaplastic change (nuclear pleomorphism, mitoses, microvascular proliferation or necrosis) may be in the oligodendroglial component, the astroglial component or both (Figs 5.27 and 5.28). In most cases the anaplastic change is present in both components.

The problems of defining when a tumour is truly mixed holds true for anaplastic oligoastrocytoma as well as for

oligoastrocytoma (see discussion above). In contrast to low grade oligoastrocytoma, however, anaplastic oligoastrocytomas more often have distinct oligodendroglial and astrocytic components, with intimately admixed forms far less common. As mentioned above, one particular pattern is to find classical oligodendroglioma, sheets of microgemistocytes and then regions of gemistocytic astrocytoma, with anaplastic features in one or more of the regions. The difficult differential diagnosis with glioblastoma is discussed below.

Immunohistochemistry

Immunohistochemistry has a limited role in the diagnosis of oligodendroglioma. Unfortunately, no immunohistochemical markers have proven reliable for identifying oliogdendroglial differentiation in routine human oligodendroglioma specimens. For example, while some oligodendrogliomas express myelin related genes at the mRNA level,[2] immunoreactivity for myelin basic protein has been inconsistent.[3,65] Given the lack of diagnostic markers for oligodendroglioma, immunohistochemistry is primarily useful for excluding other entities, rather than for diagnosing oligodendroglioma.

GFAP is expressed in many oligodendrogliomas,[5] with four types of positive cells:

1. reactive astroglial cells, often adjacent to blood vessels (Fig. 5.29);
2. neoplastic cells with astrocytic morphology (Fig. 5.30);
3. neoplastic cells with oligodendroglial morphology (Fig. 5.31);
4. microgemistocytic neoplastic cells (Fig. 5.32).[3,66]

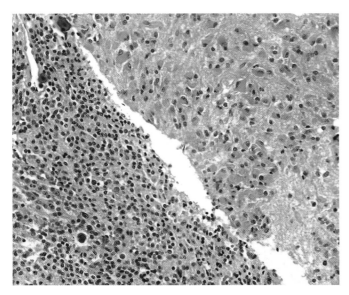

Fig. 5.27 **Anaplastic oligoastrocytoma.** In this sample two adjacent fragments from the same glioma show clear oligodendrogliomatous and astrocytomatous components. There was evidence of mitoses, pleomorphism and vascular proliferation in the astroglial component. H & E.

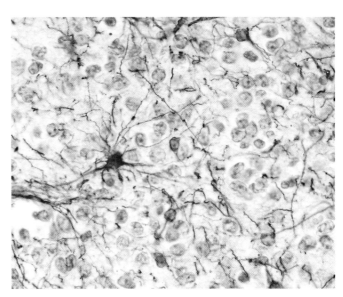

Fig. 5.29 **Oligodendroglioma.** Finely processed GFAP-stained reactive astroglial cells are commonly seen in oligodendrogliomas, whereas in most cases the majority of neoplastic cells are GFAP negative.

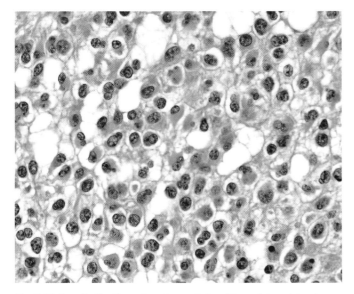

Fig. 5.28 **Anaplastic oligoastrocytoma.** Cells with a minigemistocyte morphology are often seen in anaplastic oligoastrocytomas at the interface between oligodendroglial and astroglial areas. H & E.

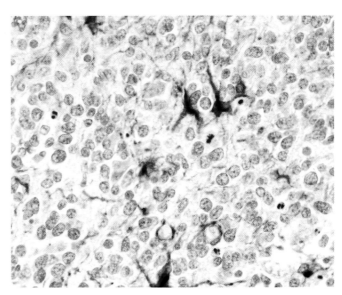

Fig. 5.30 **Anaplastic oligodendroglioma.** A small number of neoplastic cells with astrocytic morphology stain for GFAP and are seen in this anaplastic oligodendroglioma.

While GFAP immunohistochemistry may be useful in identifying microgemistocytes, its primary utility involves the identification of astrocytoma or astrocytic components, since astrocytic elements will usually show extensive GFAP immunolabelling of cells with broad and/or branching cell processes.

Over 90% of oligodendrogliomas show Leu7 positivity,[3,67] but other neuroepithelial tumours also show immunoreactivity with this antibody and therefore it is not of great diagnostic use.[3] Other markers expressed in oligodendrogliomas, but not specific to them, include alpha-B crystallin,[68] S-100 protein[69] and neurone specific enolase.[70] KP-1 immunoreactivity is seen in macrophages within oligodendrogliomas.[71]

Some tumours that appear to meet standard histological criteria for oligodendroglioma have been shown to express immunohistochemical markers of neuronal differentiation. In one series, 6% of tumours expressed synaptophysin and 31% showed expression of neurofilament proteins. The tumours showing neuronal

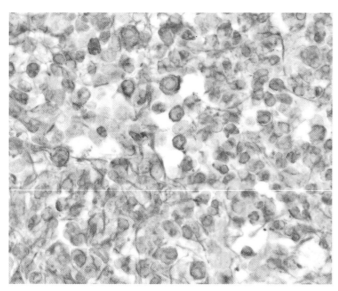

Fig. 5.31 **Oligodendroglioma.** While most cells in an oligodendroglioma are GFAP negative, some tumours as here show extensive GFAP immunoreactivity as ring-like profiles around the nucleus.

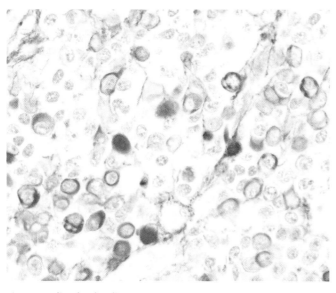

Fig. 5.32 **Oligodendroglioma.** Microgemistocytic neoplastic cells can be seen in some oligodendrogliomas. GFAP immunohistochemistry.

markers were not shown to differ in biological behaviour from those not expressing such markers.[72] However, similar findings have not been been reported in other series,[73] and it is important to recall that immunohistochemical positivity does not necessarily directly imply biological expression or differentiation.

Grading of oligodendroglial tumours

Several proposals have been made for the histological grading of oligodendroglial tumours, but most have focused on pure oligodendrogliomas rather than oligo-

astrocytomas. In general, most of the grading schemes divide oligodendroglial tumours into low grade and high grade lesions and emerge as essentially two-tier systems. Accordingly, the WHO only distinguishes two grades: WHO grade II, corresponding to oligodendroglioma and oligoastrocytoma; and WHO grade III, corresponding to anaplastic oligodendroglioma and anaplastic oligo-astrocytoma. The WHO system is somewhat subjective in its grading criteria, defining anaplastic oligodendroglioma as 'a well differentiated, diffusely infiltrating tumour composed of cells morphologically resembling oligodendroglia', and anaplastic oligodendroglioma as 'an oligodendroglioma with focal or diffuse histological features of malignancy, such as increased cellularity, cytological atypia, and high mitotic activity; microvascular proliferation and necrosis may be present'.[10] This allows considerable leeway in assigning the designation 'anaplastic' and remains a practical approach, but unfortunately does not address the issue of cases that fall intermediate between grade II and anaplastic grade III. In our experience, cases with worrying features that fall short of being frankly anaplastic are not uncommon, and attention to clinical and neuroradiological features (e.g. enhancement) may be needed to clarify if the tumour will follow an indolent or more aggressive course.

The Smith grading system separates oligodendroglial tumours into four groups, based on assessment of endothelial proliferation, necrosis, nuclear : cytoplasmic ratio, high cell density and pleomorphism – notably omitting mitotic activity as a major variable. In a large series of cases, 23% were grade A (low grade), 49% grade B, 22% grade C and 6% grade D (high grade). For this system, there is a good correlation with survival, with median survivals being: 94 months for grade A; 51 months for grade B; 45 months for grade C; and 17 months for grade D.[59] Two-thirds of patients with grade A tumours are under 40 years of age, while 83% of patients with grade D tumours are over 40 years of age.[17] If the features of cell density, pleomorphism and necrosis are evaluated by simple presence/absence scoring, with the reduction from four grades to three, this grading system has also proved useful.[74]

The Kernohan grading scheme and the St Anne/Mayo grading scheme (see Chapter 4) can also be applied to oligodendrogliomas and show correlation with survival. In a large series, patients with grade 1 or 2 tumours by either grading method had a median survival time of 9.8 years with 5- and 10-year survival rates of approximately 75% and 46%, respectively. Those patients with grade 3 or 4 tumours had a median survival time of 3.9 years, with 5- and 10-year survival rates of approximately 41% and 20%, respectively.[75]

A two grade scheme has also been proposed that incorporates neuroimaging features as well as histology.

Grade A tumours are characterised by absence of endothelial hyperplasia and/or contrast enhancement on imaging while grade B tumours are characterised by endothelial hyperplasia and/or contrast enhancement on imaging. Median survival for grade A lesions was 11 years while that for grade B lesions was 3.5 years. Five-year and 8-year survival rates were 89% and 60% for grade A and 33% and 15% for grade B. While the presence of microvascular proliferation was correlated with survival, in this series nuclear atypia, necrosis and mitoses were not predictive of survival.[76]

Proliferation indices

Ki-67/MIB-1 immunostaining has shown oligodendrogliomas to have low proliferation rates, generally about 1%, with more anaplastic forms having labelling indices in the range of 7–10%, or higher.[77] Some studies have suggested that the MIB-1 proliferation index adds prognostic information independent of patient's age, tumour site and grade,[78] but other work has denied that stratification of cases by cell proliferation index can predict survival independently when other factors are considered.[79,80]

Given the clear association between tumour grade and proliferation, MIB-1 immunohistochemistry remains a useful adjunct in the evaluation of oligodendroglial tumours, particularly those lesions for which grading appears intermediate.

Flow cytometry of oligodendrogliomas has shown that about 30% are diploid, 39% are tetraploid, and 31% are aneuploid with no correlation with survival.[81]

Electron microscopy

Ultrastructural examination has shown that the cells comprising oligodendrogliomas can be divided into four main types:[6,9,82–88]

1. Cells with large round or ovoid nuclei and scanty cytoplasm.
2. Cells with abundant cytoplasm, rich in organelles including crystalline bodies, microtubules, concentric membranous laminations or whorls and prominent elongated mitochondria. The cytoplasm of this type of cell is generally rich in ribosomes and glycogen granules with no discernible intermediate filaments; the concentric laminations, while characteristic of oligodendrogliomas, have been seen in other types of glioma.[82]
3. Minigemistocytes, in which intermediate filaments are arranged in parallel bundles.
4. Astrocytic cells exhibiting long fibrillary cellular processes.

In addition to these features an unusual pattern of a signet ring cell oligodendroglioma has been described in which, ultrastructurally, the cytoplasm was filled with dilated cisternae of rough endoplasmic reticulum containing granular material.[61] A granular cell variant of oligodendroglioma has also been described in which cells contain abundant electron dense material in lysosome-like bodies.[63]

As discussed in the section on differential diagnosis, ultrastructural examination is useful in the differential diagnosis between oligodendrogliomas, clear cell ependymomas and neurocytomas.[89,90]

Molecular biology

The cell of origin of oligodendrogliomas remains controversial. A common progenitor cell, the O2A progenitor, is believed to give rise to both galacto-cerebroside containing oligodendrocytes and GFAP containing type 2 astrocytes in development, at least within the rat optic nerve. It has therefore been tempting to suggest that oligodendrogliomas and oligoastrocytomas are derived from such O2A progenitor cells. As discussed above, oligodendroglial tumours may show divergent differentiation, and it is therefore likely that they arise from pleuripotential precursor cells.[91] Indeed, the generation of mouse models of oligodendroglioma and oligoastrocytoma that oncogenically target precursor cells adds strong support to this hypothesis.[92] Cells derived from these tumours may be forced in vitro to follow either astrocytic or oligodendroglial paths of differentiation.[93]

Oligodendrogliomas have characteristic genetic abnormalities along with genetic changes common to many types of malignant glioma. Allelic losses of chromosomal arms 1p and 19q are typical of oligodendrogliomas,[94–98] occurring in about 70% of oligodendrogliomas and anaplastic oligodendrogliomas.[80,96,97,99] The precise genes on 1p and 19q involved in oligodendroglioma pathogenesis remain unknown. These allelic losses are tightly linked with one another, so that allelic loss of chromosome 19q is found in nearly all tumours with loss of 1p. Nonetheless, while combined loss of 1p and 19q is quite characteristic of oligodendroglial tumours, it is important to note that allelic losses of 1p and 19q, and rarely both, can occur in astrocytic gliomas as well. In other words, combined allelic loss of 1p and 19q is not 'diagnostic' of oligodendroglioma in the absence of oligodendroglial histopathology. Combined loss of 1p and 19q is a statistically significant predictor of prolonged survival in patients with pure oligodendroglioma, independent of tumour grade.[100] Comparative genomic hybridisation has also shown frequent loss of chromosomes 4, 14, 15 and 18 in oligodendrogliomas.[97]

As oligodendrogliomas progress to anaplastic tumours, they undergo similar genetic alterations to astrocytic gliomas. For example, *TP53* gene mutations are rare in low grade oligodendrogliomas,[64] but are found in about 20% of anaplastic oligodendrogliomas.[80] Similarly, *CDKN2A/p16* deletions and loss of chromosome 10 occur in 15–25% of high grade oligodendrogliomas.[80]

For anaplastic oligodendrogliomas, molecular genetic analysis can be used to identify genetic subsets with markedly different clinical courses.[80,101] Those anaplastic oligodendrogliomas with allelic loss of chromosome 1p, or combined allelic losses of 1p and 19q, are nearly always responsive to PCV (procarbazine, CCNU and vincristine) chemotherapy, while those without these genetic changes respond far less commonly and usually less completely. In addition, those patients whose high grade oligodendrogliomas have allelic loss of chromosome 1p, or combined losses of 1p and 19q, have much longer survival times, with median overall survivals of 10 years compared to approximately 2 years for those patients whose tumours lack these changes.[80] Those tumours without 1p and 19q loss are more likely to have other progression-associated genetic changes, such as loss of chromosome 10, deletions of the *CDKN2A/p16* gene and *TP53* mutations. Immunohistochemical assessments of p53 and p16 expression have produced varied results in high grade oligodendrogliomas, and the immuno-histochemical associations with prognosis have not been as marked as the molecular genetic correlations.[80,102] Thus, molecular diagnostic testing for allelic losses of chromosome 1p, or 1p and 19q, offers potentially important clinical information and has already been incorporated into the clinical armamentarium for evaluting human glioma specimens.

The biological relationship between oligoastrocytoma and oligodendroglioma remains a subject of debate. Recent mouse models have raised the intriguing hypothesis that oligoastrocytomas and oligodendrogliomas may arise from similar oncogenic events occurring in different precursor cells.[91,92] Nevertheless, the genetic underpinnings of oligoastrocytoma are less well defined than those of pure oligodendroglioma, and interpretation of the available data must be moderated by knowledge that the criteria used to include tumours as oligo-astrocytomas may vary greatly between studies. For those oligoastrocytomas that are biphasic in appearance, microdissection of the oligodendroglial and astrocytic components have revealed identical genetic alterations, essentially confirming the monoclonal nature of these lesions.[103] The old notion that these may represent 'collision tumours' is no longer tenable. Many oligoastrocytomas have genetic features in common with oligodendrogliomas, namely allelic losses of 1p and 19q. There is also an inverse correlation in oligoastrocytomas between 1p and 19q allelic losses and *TP53* mutations.[64] This suggests that there are two molecular subtypes of oligoastrocytoma: one with 1p and 19q losses that is more closely aligned to oligodendrogliomas, and another with

TP53 mutations that is genetically more similar to fibrillary astrocytoma. It remains to be seen, however, whether these two genetic types of oligoastrocytoma are associated with different clinical behaviours.

Differential diagnosis

The diagnosis of an oligodendroglial neoplasm is often straightforward, but the increased clinical relevance of recognising oligodendroglial components in gliomas has resulted in a wider range of tumours being diagnosed under the rubric of oligodendroglial tumours. This widening spectrum of 'oligodendrogliomas' has, to some extent, blurred the margins between oligodendroglioma, oligoastrocytoma and even diffuse astrocytoma, and it remains to be seen how effective molecular genetic criteria will be in re-establishing these divisions (see above). There can also be problems in recognising the essential cytological features of oligodendrogliomas, especially when dealing with small biopsy samples that have been frozen for intraoperative consultation (see above), and it is therefore recommended that tissue be preserved unfrozen for paraffin sections. As with all histological diagnoses, attention to clinical and imaging features will often provide important clues to a correct diagnosis. The site of a lesion can give a good indication as to the differential diagnosis of a neoplasm with an oligodendroglial or 'clear cell' appearance, i.e. a ventricular tumour raises the differential diagnosis of central neurocytoma, whereas a superficial lesion brings up clear cell meningioma as a possibility (Table 5.2).

Astrocytomas

In the cerebral hemispheres, there can be confusion between fibrillary and protoplasmic astrocytomas (see Chapter 4) and oligodendroglioma, especially when dealing with stereotactic biopsy samples. The confusion with fibrillary astrocytoma occurs most often in the setting of a biopsy that has been entirely frozen, yielding nuclear pleomorphism in an oligodendroglioma. GFAP immunohistochemistry may be useful in distinguishing these entities if there is conspicuous staining of the extended cell processes of a fibrillary astrocytoma. However, caution must be taken not to mistake the normal

Table 5.2 Differential diagnosis of oligodendroglial neoplasms

Astrocytomas
Glioblastoma
Central neurocytoma
Dysembryoplastic neuroepithelial tumour
Clear cell ependymoma
Clear cell meningioma
Reactive conditions: inflammation, infarction
'Oligodendrogliosis'

fibrillarity of the background neuropil in infiltrating oligodendrogliomas with the tumour fibrillarity of an astrocytoma. The presence of rounded, cytologically characteristic nuclei should prompt one to consider a diagnosis of oligodendroglioma or oligoastrocytoma, particularly if there is a delicate branching vasculature and/or calcification.

Protoplasmic astrocytomas share with oligodendrogliomas a tendency for rounded nuclei, microcysts and sometimes a clear cell pattern. Careful inspection of cytology will reveal eccentricity of nuclei and a more delicate chromatin network in the astrocytoma. Nuclei sit at the intersections of a web of cell processes, often GFAP positive, in protoplasmic astrocytomas, not in the spaces as in the oligodendroglioma. Protoplasmic astrocytomas will not have the characteristic arborising fine vascular pattern seen in oligodendroglial tumours.

Many pilocytic cerebellar astrocytomas have oligodendroglial-like appearance (see Chapter 4) but realisation of the rarity of oligodendroglial tumours at this site should prompt careful consideration before making this diagnosis. Similarly, in the brain stem and spinal cord, detailed investigation including immunohistochemistry and electron microscopy is warranted in any tumour before it is considered as an oligodendroglioma.

Glioblastoma

The differential diagnosis between some anaplastic oligodendrogliomas or anaplastic oligoastrocytomas and glioblastoma is a thorny issue. The 2000 WHO consensus[10] supported the view that the diagnosis of glioblastoma should be reserved for astrocytic gliomas. The notion of an oligodendroglioma or anaplastic oligodendroglioma progressing to glioblastoma is not consistent with this approach, and it thus discourages the term 'glioblastoma' in the setting of a tumour with clear oligodendroglial features. It has become customary to search extensively in any diffuse glioma specimen for any areas in the lesion with rounded nuclei that could represent anaplastic oligodendroglioma, since the therapeutic and prognostic features of anaplastic oligodendroglioma differ markedly from those of glioblastoma. In this regard, it is not uncommon to be asked to review the slides from a patient who has done very well after therapy for a supposed glioblastoma and to realise, only in retrospect, that the lesion was an anaplastic oligodendroglial lesion.

The presence of necrosis, including necrosis with pseudopalisading and microvascular proliferation remains consistent with a diagnosis of anaplastic oligodendroglioma and does not necessitate a diagnosis of glioblastoma. Indeed, anaplastic oligodendrogliomas with pseudopalisading necrosis may respond well to PCV chemotherapy.[80] In general, such anaplastic oligodendrogliomas differ from glioblastomas in their homogeneous appearance on low power examination and their relatively uniform, predominantly rounded nuclei on high power examination; as their old name, 'glioblastoma multiforme' suggested, glioblastomas are archtecturally and cytologically heterogeneous lesions.

More problematic, however, is the designation of cases of typical glioblastoma in which careful examination reveals regions suggestive of high grade oligodendroglioma. Such lesions contain areas of small cells that raise the differential diagnosis of anaplastic oligodendroglioma or so-called 'small cell' glioblastoma. The correct diagnosis for such cases remains unclear, and molecular genetic analysis of these problematic lesions in the future may clarify their nosology. In the meanwhile, we do not advocate the use of the term 'anaplastic oligodendroglioma' for these questionable cases; rather we diagnose such cases as glioblastoma but add in the report that a minor oligodendroglial component may be present.

Reactive conditions

Aside from other diffuse gliomas, the most important differential diagnosis concerns reactive conditions, including demyelinating diseases, subacute cerebral infarcts and infectious conditions. The key to recognising such entities is the identification of inflammatory cells, notably macrophages. Most inflammatory conditions are easily distinguished from diffuse gliomas (see Differential diagnosis section in Chapter 4), but those with sheets of macrophages may histologically resemble densely cellular, homogeneous tumours. The rounded nuclei of macrophages and their vacuolated cytoplasm can create striking similarities to oligodendroglioma. Macrophages, however, are easily identified on smear preparations as non-cohesive cells with a small nucleus and bubbly or granular cytoplasm. On paraffin sections, attention should also be paid to these cytological features, since macrophages typically have well-defined cell borders, as opposed to oligodendroglioma cells. Immunohistochemistry for macrophage markers, such as KP-1/CD68, can confirm the presence of macrophages. Additional diagnostic stains, such as a myelin and axonal stain for demyelinating disease, identification of ischaemic neurons and infarcted tissue in cerebral infarcts, and special stains for organisms in infectious conditions, will confirm these differential diagnoses.

Central neurocytoma

Central neurocytomas (see Chapter 8) may be confused with oligodendrogliomas since the two lesions can appear virtually identical on light microscopic examination. The nuclei of neurocytomas, however, tend to have a more delicate chromatin pattern and the background stroma has a delicate, neuropil-like quality, often forming fibrillary, nuclear free zones. Neurocytomas are primarily tumours of the third and lateral ventricles, and neurocytoma must therefore be considered as a diagnosis for any oligodendroglioma-like tumour occurring in these locations; however, neurocytomatous tumours have been reported in other sites, including the hemispheres and spinal cord and must therefore at least be considered as a possibility in the differential diagnosis of oligodendroglioma in a wide variety of sites. The main guard against mistaking a neurocytoma for an oligodendroglioma is consideration of the site of the tumour and performing immunohistochemistry for neuronal markers such as synaptophysin. Caution must be taken, however, not to confuse synaptophysin staining of the normal intervening neuropil in an infiltrative oligodendroglioma with the true tumour cell positivity of a neurocytoma. Ultrastructural examination will also prove useful in the differential diagnosis of neurocytoma, but caution must again be exercised not to misinterpret the neuronal processes of normal neuropil as evidence of neuronal differentiation in a tumour.

Dysembryoplastic neuroepithelial tumour (DNT)

Oligodendrogliomas and DNTs share the presence of closely packed rounded tumour cells having perinuclear halos. While imaging features and anatomic site should raise the possibility that a lesion may be a DNT (Chapter 8) rather than an oligodendroglioma, low grade oligodendrogliomas may also present as masses in patients with a long history of seizures. Histologically, oligodendrogliomas may be multinodular and may be primarily intracortical, further emphasising the similarities with DNT. Nonetheless, oligodendrogliomas are diffusely infiltrative lesions and clear evidence of cortical invasion (perineuronal satellitosis and subpial growth) or diffuse white matter involvement argues for a diagnosis of oligodendroglioma. In this regard, the finding of 'floating neurons' in DNTs should not be mistaken for cortical infiltration by an oligodendroglioma. Finally, immunohistochemistry may be of some use in this differential diagnosis, with DNTs staining more convincingly for neuronal markers such as NeuN.[73]

The description of non-specific histological forms of DNT, with diagnosis based almost entirely on clinical and neuroimaging features,[104] potentially increases the diagnostic difficulty in such lesions, but we do not advocate the diagnosis of DNT in the absence of histological evidence of the specific glioneuronal element (Chapter 8).

Clear cell ependymoma

Clear cell ependymoma has been described in sites frequented by regular ependymomas (Chapter 6). The diagnostic possibility of ependymoma should be prompted by location of the lesion as well as histology. The most reliable way to ascertain this diagnosis is by ultrastructural examination. In cases where the only sample is in a wax block, re-embedding a portion taken from this block is very useful as the ultrastructural features of ependymal differentiation are well preserved even after re-embedding in resin.

Clear cell meningioma

Clear cell areas in a meningioma may resemble an oligodendroglioma and when in an unusual anatomic site, even the imaging may have suggested a glioma rather than a meningioma. The surgical findings and a histological search for typical areas of meningioma will usually resolve the problem. EMA immunoreactivity and meningothelial ultrastructural features are also useful aids in the diagnosis of clear cell meningioma (see Chapter 13).

Reactive oligodendroglial proliferation and 'angioglioma'

Oligodendroglial proliferation associated with prominent angiomatous vascularity has been reported several times.[102–108] An heroic review of over 1000 vascular malformations revealed eight cases containing an abnormal but non-neoplastic overgrowth of oligodendroglia 'oligodendrogliosis'. Two histological patterns were suggested; one appeared to be a malformative disposition of oligodendroglia as an integral part of the arteriovenous malformation. The other pattern possibly represented the effect of chronic ischaemia causing condensation of involved white matter.[107] Between 4 and 12% of low grade gliomas contain prominent angioma-like blood vessels and so-called 'angiogliomas' probably just represent unusually vascular gliomas. The behaviour of such lesions does not differ from those of similar gliomas without angioma-like vessels.[107]

Therapy and prognosis

Most patients who die of oligodendroglioma or mixed oligoastrocytoma do so because of local tumour recurrence without distant spread.[109] CSF seeding and leptomeningeal dissemination has been described in several series.[17,110,111] Intramedullary spread in the spinal cord via the CSF pathways is not uncommon.[109,112] Anaplastic oligodendroglioma has also been described as causing systemic metastases.[113,114]

Survival in patients with oligodendroglioma is potentially related to many factors including the patient age, sex, cognitive decline, seizures, intracranial hypertension and/or neurological deficits; tumour site, size, laterality, enhancement on neuroimaging; pathological grade and cytological features; molecular abnormalities such as allelic losses of chromosome 1p; and the extent of surgical resection, irradiation or chemotherapy.

The strongest prognostic factor in oligodendroglioma seems related to tumour grade. Using the St Anne/Mayo grading system, median survival and 5- and 10-year survival rates for low grade oligodendroglioma were 9.8 years, 73% and 49%; and for mixed oligoastrocytoma 7.1 years, 63% and 33%, respectively. Median survivals and 5- and 10-year survival rates for high grade tumours were 4.5 years, 45% and 15% for the oligodendrogliomas and for oligoastrocytomas, the overall median survival was 5.8 years and the 5-, 10- and 15-year survival rates were 55%, 29% and 17%, respectively.[112] When stratified according to Kernohan grade, patients with grades 1 and 2 tumours had a median survival of approximately 6.3 years, and 5- and 10-year survival rates of 58% and 32%, compared to 2.8 years 36% and 9%, respectively for patients with grades 3 and 4 tumours.[113] Other studies have reported similar findings.[17,59,75,109,117–119]

Patients who are diagnosed under the age of 40 years have a better prognosis than those in older age groups.[14,75,109,116,119] Patients who present with cognitive decline or hemiparesis have a worse prognosis.[14]

The role of radiation therapy for oligodendrogliomas has been uncertain with reports of increased survival as well as those showing no benefit. However, meta-analysis of the literature related to radiation therapy has demonstrated a survival advantage for surgery with radiation therapy compared to surgery only (5-year survival 56% vs 42%).[118] A study of patients treated for oligodendrogliomas in Norway from 1953 to 1977 has shown that survival was significantly prolonged if postoperative irradiation was performed (27% vs 36% at 5 years; 14% vs 17% at 8 years),[120] while no statistically significant benefit in survival was attributed to postoperative irradiation in other studies.[109,121]

Some anaplastic oligodendrogliomas are remarkably sensitive to PCV chemotherapy,[122] particularly a subgroup of rapidly enlarging, contrast enhancing, histologically anaplastic lesions that have been grouped as 'aggressive oligodendrogliomas'.[123,124] This group can be genetically separated into at least two therapeutic and prognostic subsets based on allelic loss of chromosome 1p and 19q (see above). Allelic loss of 1p is a statistically significant predictor of chemosensitivity, and combined loss involving chromosomes 1p and 19q is statistically significantly associated with both chemosensitivity and longer recurrence free survival after chemotherapy.[80,101] Since some anaplastic oligoastrocytomas[125,126] and low grade oligodendrogliomas[127] also respond to PCV chemotherapy, it will be of interest to determine whether such chromosomal changes correlate with clincial features in these tumours as well.[128] It is therefore encouraging that some data suggest that allelic loss of 1p

may correspond with low grade oligodendrogliomas having a better prognosis.[100] Indeed, a recent paper suggests that genotyping may not only improve classification of low grade oligodendrogliomas, but may provide an estimate of whether these tumours will respond to chemotherapy when they transform to more aggressive lesions.[129] Such advances lay the groundwork for genotyping to become an integral part of oligodendroglioma diagnosis.

REFERENCES

1. Bailey P, Bucy P. Oligodendrogliomas of the brain. J Pathol Bacteriol, 1929; 32:735–751
2. Golfinos JG, Norman SA, Coons SW et al. Expression of the genes encoding myelin basic protein and proteolipid protein in human malignant gliomas. Clin Cancer Res, 1997; 3:799–804
3. Nakagawa Y, Perentes E, Rubinstein LJ. Immunohistochemical characterization of oligodendrogliomas: An analysis of multiple markers. Acta Neuropathol, 1986; 72:15–22
4. Kashima T, Tiu SN, Merrill JE et al. Expression of oligodendrocyte-associated genes in cell lines derived from human gliomas and neuroblastomas. Cancer Res, 1993; 53:170–175
5. Herpes M, Budka H. Glial fibrillary acidic protein (GFAP) in oligodendroglial tumours: Gliofibrillary oligodendroglioma and transitional oligoastrocytoma as subtypes of oligodendroglioma. Acta Neuropathol, 1984; 64:265–272
6. Kamitani H, Masuzawa H, Sato J et al. Astrocytic characteristics of oligodendroglioma. Fine structural and immunohistochemical studies of two cases. J Neurol Sci, 1987; 78:349–355
7. Barbosa MD, Balsitis M, Jaspan T et al. Intraventricular neurocytoma: A clinical and pathological study of three cases and review of the literature. Neurosurgery, 1990; 26:1045–1054
8. Kawano N, Yada K, Yagishita S. Clear cell ependymoma. A histological variant with diagnostic implications. Virchows Arch (A) Pathol Anat Histopathol, 1989; 415:467–472
9. Kamitani H, Masuzawa H, Sato J et al. Mixed oligodendroglioma and astrocytoma: fine structural and immunohistochemical studies of four cases. J Neurol Sci, 1988; 83:219–225
10. Reifenberger G, Kros J, Burger P et al. Oligodendroglial tumours and mixed gliomas. In: Kleihues P, Cavenee WK, eds. Pathology and genetics of tumours of the nervous system. Lyon: IARC Press 2000; pp. 55–69
11. Helseth A, Mork SJ. Neoplasms of the central nervous system in Norway. III. Epidemiological characteristics of intracranial gliomas according to histology. APMIS, 1989; 97:547–555
12. Zulch K. Brain tumours. Their biology and pathology. 3rd edn. Berlin: Springer, 1986
13. Coons SW, Johnson PC, Scheithauer BW et al. Improving diagnostic accuracy and interobserver concordance in the classification and grading of primary gliomas. Cancer, 1997; 79:1381–1393
14. Mork SJ, Lindegaard KF, Halvorsen TB et al. Oligodendroglioma: incidence and biological behavior in a defined population. J Neurosurg, 1985; 63:881–889
15. Chin HW, Hazel JJ, Kim TH et al. Oligodendrogliomas. I. A clinical study of cerebral oligodendrogliomas. Cancer, 1980; 45:1458–1466
16. Favier J, Pizzolato GP, Berney J. Oligodendroglial tumors in childhood. Childs Nerv Syst, 1985; 1:33–38
17. Ludwig CL, Smith MT, Godfrey AD et al. A clinicopathological study of 323 patients with oligodendrogliomas. Ann Neurol, 1986; 19:15–21
18. Lee YY, Van TP. Intracranial oligodendrogliomas: imaging findings in 35 untreated cases. Am J Roentgenol, 1989; 152:361–369
19. Tice H, Barnes PD, Goumnerova L et al. Pediatric and adolescent oligodendrogliomas. AJNR Am J Neuroradiol, 1993; 14:1293–1300
20. Ogasawara H, Kiya K, Uozumi T et al. Multiple oligodendroglioma – case report. Neurol Med Chir, 1990; 30:127–131
21. Barnard RO, Geddes JF. The incidence of multifocal cerebral gliomas. A histologic study of large hemisphere sections. Cancer, 1987; 60:1519–1531

22. Fortuna A, Celli P, Palma L. Oligodendrogliomas of the spinal cord. Acta Neurochir, 1980; 52:3–4
23. Balko MG, Blisard KS, Samaha FJ. Oligodendroglial gliomatosis cerebri. Hum Pathol, 1992; 23:706–707
24. Pitt MA, Jones AW, Reeve RS et al. Oligodendroglioma of the fourth ventricle with intracranial and spinal oligodendrogliomatosis: a case report. Br J Neurosurg, 1992; 6:371–374
25. Nishio S, Tashima T, Takeshita I et al. Intraventricular neurocytoma: Clinicopathological features of six cases. J Neurosurg, 1988; 68:665–670
26. Kim DG, Chi JG, Park SH et al. Intraventricular neurocytoma: clinicopathological analysis of seven cases. J Neurosurg, 1992; 76:759–765
27. Yuen ST, Fung CF, Ng TH et al. Central neurocytoma: its differentiation from intraventricular oligodendroglioma. Childs Nerv Syst, 1992; 8:383–388
28. Gittens WO, Huestis WS, Sangalang VE. Oligodendroglioma of the cerebellum. Surg Neurol, 1980; 13:237–240
29. Packer RJ, Sutton LN, Rorke LB. Oligodendroglioma of the posterior fossa in childhood. Cancer, 1985; 56:195–199
30. Holladay FP, Fruin AH. Cerebellar oligodendroglioma in a child. Neurosurgery, 1980; 6:552–554
31. Koeppen AH, Cassidy RJ. Oligodendroglioma of the medulla oblongata in a neonate. Arch Neurol, 1981; 38:520–523
32. Pagni CA, Canavero S, Gaidolfi E. Intramedullary 'holocord' oligodendroglioma: case report. Acta Neurochir, 1991; 113:96–99
33. Merchant TE, Nguyen D, Thompson SJ et al. High-grade pediatric spinal cord tumors. Pediatr Neurosurg, 1999; 30:1–5
34. Nam DH, Cho BK, Kim YM et al. Intramedullary anaplastic oligodendroglioma in a child. Childs Nerv Syst, 1998; 14:127–130
35. Ushida T, Sonobe H, Mizobuchi H et al. Oligodendroglioma of the 'widespread' type in the spinal cord. Childs Nerv Syst, 1998; 14:751–755
36. Zentner J, Anagnostopoulos J, Gilsbach J. Solitary intracranial extracerebral glioma. Neurochirurgia, 1988; 31:101–103
37. Shuangshoti S, Kasantikul V, Suwanwela N et al. Solitary primary intracranial extracerebral glioma. Case report. J Neurosurg, 1984; 61:777–781
38. Mhiri C, Ben RT, Djindjian M et al. Pseudooligodendrogliomatous meningioma. Report of 2 cases and review of the literature. Neurochirurgie, 1991; 37:398–402
39. Bossen EH, Hudson WR. Oligodendroglioma arising in heterotopic brain tissue of the soft palate and nasopharynx. Am J Surg Pathol, 1987; 11:571–574
40. Lucarini C, Tomei G, Gaini SM et al. A case of optic nerve oligodendroglioma associated with an orbital non-Hodgkin's lymphoma in adult. Case report. J Neurosurg Sci, 1990; 34:319–321
41. Huang CI, Chiou WH, Ho DM. Oligodendroglioma occurring after radiation therapy for pituitary adenoma. J Neurol Neurosurg Psychiatry, 1987; 50:1619–1624
42. Perez DC, Cabello A, Lobato RD et al. Oligodendrogliomas arising in the scar of a brain contusion. Report of two surgically verified cases. Surg Neurol, 1985; 24:581–586
43. Gordana MT, Mauro A, Soffietti R et al. Association between multiple sclerosis and oligodendroglioma. Case report. Ital J Neurol Sci, 1981; 2:403–409
44. Bhatt AR, Mohanty S, Sharma V et al. Familial gliomas: a case report. Neurology, 1999; 47:136–138
45. Ferraresi S, Servello D, De LL et al. Familial frontal lobe oligodendroglioma. Case report. J Neurosurg Sci, 1989; 33:317–318
46. Kros JM, Lie ST, Stefanko SZ. Familial occurrence of polymorphous oligodendroglioma. Neurosurgery, 1994; 34:732–326
47. Taylor MD, Perry J, Zlatescu MC et al. The hPMS2 exon 5 mutation and malignant glioma. Case report. J Neurosurg, 1999; 90:946–950
48. Varma RR, Crumrine PK, Bergman I et al. Childhood oligodendrogliomas presenting with seizures and low-density lesions on computerised tomography. Neurology, 1983; 33:806–808
49. Morris HH, Estes ML, Gilmore R et al. Chronic intractable epilepsy as the only symptom of primary brain tumor. Epilepsia, 1993; 34:1038–1043
50. Harada K, Kiya K, Matsumura S et al. Spontaneous intracranial hemorrhage caused by oligodendroglioma. A case report and review of the literature. Neurol Med Chir, 1982; 22:81–84
51. Kondziolka D, Bernstein M, Resch L et al. Significance of hemorrhage into brain tumors: Clinicopathological study. J Neurosurg, 1987; 67:852–857
52. Liwnicz BH, Wu SZ, Tew JJ. The relationship between the capillary structure and hemorrhage in gliomas. J Neurosurg, 1987; 66:536–541
53. DiMaio SM, DiMaio V, Kirkpatrick JB. Sudden unexpected deaths due to primary intracranial neoplasms. Am J Forensic Med Path, 1980; 1:29–45
54. Margain D, Peretti VP, Perez CA et al. Oligodendrogliomas. J Neuroradiol, 1991; 18:153–160
55. Daumas-Duport C, Monsaigneon V, Blond S et al. Serial stereotactic biopsies and CT scan in gliomas: correlative study in 100 astrocytomas, oligo-astrocytomas and oligodendrocytomas. J Neurooncol, 1987; 4:317–328
56. Tice H. Barnes PD, Goumnerova L et al. Pediatric and adolescent oligodendrogliomas. Am J Neuroradiol, 1993; 14:1293–1300
57. Feigin I. The mucopolysaccharides of the ground substance of the human brain. J Neuropathol Exp Neurol, 1980; 39:1–12
58. Kikuchi K, Kamisato N, Kowada M et al. Large cystic oligodendroglioma in childhood. Report of operated cases. Childs Nerv Syst, 1985; 10:329–334
59. Smith MT, Ludwig CL, Godfrey AD et al. Grading of oligodendrogliomas. Cancer, 1983; 52:2107–2114
60. Kros JM, van den Brink WA, van Loon-van Luyt JJ et al. Signet-ring cell oligodendroglioma–report of two cases and discussion of the differential diagnosis. Acta Neuropathol, 1997; 93:638–643
61. Mikami Y, Shirabe T, Hata S et al. Oligodendroglioma with signet-ring cell morphology: a case report with an immunohistochemical and ultrastructural study. Pathol Int, 1998; 48:144–150
62. Luis SJ, Ramon S, Agueras S et al. Crystals in an oligodendroglioma: An optical, histochemical, and ultrastructural study. Ultrastruct Pathol, 1990; 14:151–159
63. Chorneyko K, Maguire J, Simon GT. Oligodendroglioma with granular cells: a case report. Ultrastruct Pathol, 1998; 22:79–82
64. Maintz D, Fiedler K, Koopmann J et al. Molecular genetic evidence for subtypes of oligoastrocytomas. J Neuropathol Exp Neurol, 1997; 56:1098–1104
65. Tanaka J, Hokama Y, Nakamura H. Myelin basic protein as a possible marker for oligodendroglioma. Acta Pathol, 1988; 38:1297–1303
66. Kros JM, Van Eden CG, Stefanko SZ et al. Prognostic implications of glial fibrillary acidic protein containing cell types in oligodendrogliomas. Cancer, 1990; 66:1204–1212
67. Motoi M, Yoshino T, Hayashi K et al. Immunohistochemical studies on human brain tumors using anti-Leu 7 monoclonal antibody in paraffin-embedded specimens. Acta Neuropathol, 1985; 66:75–77
68. Aoyama A, Steiger RH, Frohli E et al. Expression of alpha B-crystallin in human brain tumors. Int J Cancer, 1993; 55:760–764
69. Hayashi K, Hoshida Y, Horie Y et al. Immunohistochemical study on the distribution of alpha and beta subunits of S-100 protein in brain tumors. Acta Neuropathol, 1991; 81:657–663
70. Vinores SA, Bonnin JM, Rubinstein LJ et al. Immunohistochemical demonstration of neuron-specific enolase in neoplasms of the CNS and other tissues. Arch Pathol Lab Med, 1984; 108:536–540
71. Rossi ML, Buller J, Heath SA et al. Monocyte/macrophage infiltrate in 41 oligodendrogliomas. Paraffin-wax study. Path Res Pract, 1991; 187:2–3
72. Wharton SB, Chan KK, Hamilton FA et al. Expression of neuronal markers in oligodendrogliomas: an immunohistochemical study. Neuropathol Appl Neurobiol, 1998; 24:302–308
73. Wolf HK, Buslei R, Blumcke I et al. Neural antigens in oligodendrogliomas and dysembryoplastic neuroepithelial tumors. Acta Neuropathol, 1997; 94:436–443
74. Kros JM, Troost D, Van EC et al. Oligodendroglioma. A comparison of two grading systems. Cancer, 1988; 61:2251–2259
75. Shaw EG, Scheithauer BW, O'Fallon JR et al. Oligodendrogliomas: the Mayo Clinic experience. J Neurosurg, 1992; 76:428–434

76. Daumas-Duport C, Tucker ML, Kolles H et al. Oligodendrogliomas. Part II: A new grading system based on morphological and imaging criteria. J Neurooncol, 1997; 34:61–78

77. Boker DK, Stark HJ. The proliferation rate of intracranial tumors as defined by the monoclonal antibody KI 67. Application of the method to paraffin embedded specimens. Neurosurg Rev, 1988; 11:267–272

78. Kros JM, Hop WC, Godschalk JJ et al. Prognostic value of the proliferation-related antigen Ki-67 in oligodendrogliomas. Cancer, 1996; 78:1107–1113

79. Wharton SB, Hamilton FA, Chan WK et al. Proliferation and cell death in oligodendrogliomas. Neuropathol Appl Neurobiol, 1998; 24:21–28

80. Cairncross JG, Ueki K, Zlatescu MC et al. Specific genetic predictors of chemotherapeutic response and survival in patients with anaplastic oligodendrogliomas. J Natl Cancer Inst, 1998; 90:1473–1479

81. Kros JM, van EC, van Eden CJ et al. Prognostic relevance of DNA flow cytometry in oligodendroglioma. Cancer, 1992; 69:1791–1798

82. Kamitani H, Masuzawa H, Sato J et al. Ultrastructure of concentric laminations in primary human brain tumors. Acta Neuropathol, 1986; 71:1–2

83. Baloyannis S. The fine structure of the isomorphic oligodendroglioma. Anticancer Res, 1981; 1:243–248

84. Kros JM, de Jong AA, van de Kwast TH. Ultrastructural characterization of transitional cells in oligodendrogliomas. J Neuropathol Exp Neurol, 1992; 51:186–193

85. Sarkar C, Roy S, Tandon PN. Oligodendroglial tumors. An immunohistochemical and electron microscopic study. Cancer, 1988; 61:1862–1866

86. Liberski PP. The ultrastructure of oligodendroglioma: personal experience and the review of the literature. Folia Neuropathol, 1996; 34:206–211

87. Cervos-Navarro J, Ferszt R, Brackertz M. The ultrastructure of oligodendrogliomas. Neurosurg Rev, 1981; 4:17–31

88. Min KW, Scheithauer BW. Oligodendroglioma: the ultrastructural spectrum. Ultrastruct Pathol, 1994; 18:47–60

89. Cenacchi G, Giangaspero F, Cerasoli S et al. Ultrastructural characterization of oligodendroglial-like cells in central nervous system tumors. Ultrastruct Pathol, 1996; 20:537–547

90. Langford LA. Central nervous system neoplasms: indications for electron microscopy. Ultrastruct Pathol, 1996; 20:35–46

91. Louis DN, Holland ES, Cairncross JG. Glioma classification: a molecular reappraisal. Am J Pathol 2001; 159:779–786

92. Dai C, Celestino JC, Okada Y et al. PDGF autocrine stimulation dedifferentiates cultured astrocytes and induces oligodendrogliomas and astrocytomas from neural progenitors and astrocytes in vivo. Genes Dev 2001; 15:1913–1925

93. Dyer CA, Philibotte T. A clone of the MOCH-1 glial tumor in culture: multiple phenotypes expressed under different environmental conditions. J Neuropathol Exp Neurol, 1995; 54:852–863

94. von Deimling A, Louis DN, von Ammon K et al. Evidence for a tumor suppressor gene on chromosome 19q associated with human astrocytomas, oligodendrogliomas, and mixed gliomas. Cancer Res, 1992; 52:4277–4279

95. Kros JM, van Run PR, Alers JC et al. Genetic aberrations in oligodendroglial tumours: an analysis using comparative genomic hybridization (CGH). J Pathol, 1999; 188:282–288

96. Smith JS, Alderete B, Minn Y et al. Localization of common deletion regions on 1p and 19q in human gliomas and their association with histological subtype. Oncogene, 1999; 18:4144–4152

97. Bigner SH, Matthews MR, Rasheed BK et al. Molecular genetic aspects of oligodendrogliomas including analysis by comparative genomic hybridization. Am J Pathol, 1999; 155:375–386

98. Jeuken JW, Sprenger SH, Wesseling P et al. Identification of subgroups of high-grade oligodendroglial tumors by comparative genomic hybridization. J Neuropathol Exp Neurol, 1999; 58:606–612

99. Rosenberg JE, Lisle DK, Burwick JA et al. Refined deletion mapping of the chromosome 19q glioma tumor suppressor gene to the D19S412-STD interval. Oncogene, 1996; 13:2483–2485

100. Smith JS, Perry A, Borell TJ et al. Alterations of chromosome arms 1p and 19q as predictors of survival in oligodendrogliomas, astrocytomas, and mixed oligoastrocytomas. J Clin Oncol, 2000; 18:636–645

101. Ino Y, Betensky RA, Zlatescu MC et al. Molecular subtypes of anaplastic oligodendroglioma: implications for patient management at diagnosis. Clin Cancer Res 2001; 7:839–845

102. Miettinen H, Kononen J, Sallinen P et al. CDKN2/p16 predicts survival in oligodendrogliomas: comparison with astrocytomas. J Neurooncol, 1999; 41:205–211

103. Kraus JA, Koopmann J, Kaskel P et al. Shared allelic losses on chromosomes 1p and 19q suggest a common origin of oligodendroglioma and oligoastrocytoma. J Neuropathol Exp Neurol, 1995; 54:91–95

104. Daumas-Duport C, Varlet P, Bacha S et al. Dysembryoplastic neuroepithelial tumors: nonspecific histological forms – a study of 40 cases. J Neurooncol, 1999; 41:267–280

105. Chee CP, Johnston R, Doyle D et al. Oligodendroglioma and cerebral cavernous angioma. Case report. J Neurosurg, 1985; 62:145–147

106. Fischer EG, Sotrel A, Welch K. Cerebral hemangioma with glial neoplasia (angioglioma?). Report of two cases. J Neurosurg, 1982; 56:430–434

107. Lombardi D, Scheithauer BW, Piepgras D et al. 'Angioglioma' and the arteriovenous malformation-glioma association. J Neurosurg, 1991; 75:589–596

108. Tews DS, Bohl JE, Van Lindert E et al. Association of oligodendroglioma-like cell proliferation and angiomatous vasculature – coincidence or pathogenetically related lesions? Clin Neuropathol, 1998; 17:69–72

109. Nijjar TS, Simpson WJ, Gadalla T et al. Oligodendroglioma. The Princess Margaret Hospital experience (1958–1984). Cancer, 1993; 71:4002–4006

110. Natelson SE, Dyer ML, Harp DL. Delayed CSF seeding of benign oligodendroglioma. South Med J, 1992; 85:1011–1012

111. Civitello LA, Packer RJ, Rorke LB et al. Leptomeningeal dissemination of low-grade gliomas in childhood. Neurology, 1988; 38:562–566

112. Van VV, Calliauw L, Caemaert J. Intramedullary spread of a cerebral oligodendroglioma. Surg Neurol, 1988; 30:476–481

113. Dawson TP. Pancytopaenia from a disseminated anaplastic oligodendroglioma. Neuropathol Appl Neurobiol, 1997; 23:516–520

114. Macdonald DR, O'Brien RA, Gilbert JJ et al. Metastatic anaplastic oligodendroglioma. Neurology, 1989; 39:1593–1596

115. Shaw EG, Scheithauer BW, O'Fallon JR. Supratentorial gliomas: a comparative study by grade and histologic type. J Neurooncol, 1997; 31:273–278

116. Shaw EG, Scheithauer BW, O'Fallon JR et al. Mixed oligoastrocytomas: a survival and prognostic factor analysis. Neurosurgery, 1994; 34:577–582; discussion 582

117. Celli P, Nofrone I, Palma L et al. Cerebral oligodendroglioma: prognostic factors and life history. Neurosurgery, 1994; 35:1018–1034; discussion 1034–1035

118. Shimizu KT, Tran LM, Mark RJ et al. Management of oligodendrogliomas. Radiology, 1993; 186:569–572

119. Kros JM, Pieterman H, van Eden CG et al. Oligodendroglioma: the Rotterdam-Dijkzigt experience. Neurosurgery, 1994; 34:959–966; discussion 966

120. Lindegaard KF, Mork SJ, Eide GE et al. Statistical analysis of clinicopathological features, radiotherapy, and survival in 170 cases of oligodendroglicma. J Neurosurg, 1987; 67:224–230

121. Bullard DE, Rawlings CI, Phillips B et al. Oligodendroglioma. An analysis of the value of radiation therapy. Cancer, 1987; 60:2179–2188

122. Cairncross JG, Macdonald DR. Successful chemotherapy for recurrent malignant oligodendroglioma. Ann Neurol, 1988; 23:360–364

123. Cairncross JG, Macdonald DR, Ramsay DA. Aggressive oligodendroglioma: a chemosensitive tumor. Neurosurgery, 1992; 31:78–82

124. Macdonald DR, Gaspar LE, Cairncross JG. Successful chemotherapy for newly diagnosed aggressive oligodendroglioma. Ann Neurol, 1990; 27:573–574

125. Glass J, Hochberg FH, Gruber ML et al. The treatment of oligodendrogliomas and mixed oligodendroglioma-astrocytomas with PCV chemotherapy. J Neurosurg, 1992; 76:741–745

126. Kim L, Hochberg FH, Thornton AF et al. Procarbazine, lomustine, and vincristine (PCV) chemotherapy for grade III and grade IV oligoastrocytomas, J Neurosurg, 1996; 85:602–607

127. Mason WP, Krol GS, DeAngelis LM. Low-grade oligodendroglioma responds to chemotherapy. Neurology, 1996; 46:203–207

128. Mason W, Louis DN, Cairncross JG. Chemosensitive gliomas in adults: which ones and why? J Clin Oncol, 1997; 15:3423–3426

129. Sasaki H, Zlatescu MC, Betensky RA et al. Histopathological–molecular genetic correlations in referral pathologist-diagnosed low-grade 'oligodendroglioma'. J Neuropathol Exp Neurol, 2002; 61:58–63

6 Ependymal and choroid plexus tumours

Ependymal tumours

A modified version of the current World Health Organisation (WHO) classification of ependymal tumours[1] is shown in Table 6.1. In contrast to the WHO scheme, ectopic ependymomas have been separately itemised in view of their particular clinical and prognostic features. The WHO does not include ependymoblastomas with other ependymal tumours but classifies them as embryonal neoplasms, alongside other primitive neuroectodermal tumours. In the older literature the concept of ependymoblastoma has often been poorly defined, embracing a wide spectrum of anaplastic ependymal tumours without specific histological features.[2] However, there are good arguments for reserving the term ependymoblastoma to describe a specific type of primitive neuroepithelial neoplasm related to ependymomas[3,4] and a full account of this entity can be found in Chapter 7.

Ependymoma and anaplastic ependymoma

Incidence

The overall incidence of ependymomas in large series has been quoted as being 4.7% of all central nervous system (CNS) tumours[5] and 9.1% of all gliomas.[6] Amongst gliomas, ependymomas are relatively more common in the spinal cord, constituting between 32 and 43% of all intraspinal glial tumours.[7,8] The incidence also varies with patient age and most childhood studies give an overall incidence of around 10% of all CNS tumours[9,10] with a peak incidence in infants up to 5 years of age.[11] There is some evidence of a sex bias in ependymoma incidence statistics, most series giving a male preponderance.[2,5]

Site

Although often related topographically to the ventricular cavities, ependymomas may occur anywhere in the neuraxis. The proportion quoted as being intracranial varies from about 50 to 70% of all cases[7,11] and in most series the posterior fossa is the commonest site, accounting for up to about 70% of intracranial examples.[7,12] Of the posterior fossa tumours about half take origin from the floor of the fourth ventricle,[13] the remainder being sited in the roof and lateral recesses, or being too large for the point of origin to be certain.[12] Supratentorial tumours are most commonly related to the lateral ventricles, especially the trigone area, but rarely may occur in the third ventricle.[14] In addition, a small proportion of supratentorial ependymomas are entirely intracerebral, and show no obvious continuity with a ventricular cavity.[12] Spinal cord ependymomas may occur at cervical and upper thoracic levels but are more often located in the cauda equina

Table 6.1 Classification of ependymal tumours

1. *Ependymoma*
   Cellular
   Epithelial
   Papillary
   Clear cell
   Mixed
2. *Anaplastic ependymoma*
3. *Myxopapillary ependymoma*
4. *Subependymoma*
5. *Ectopic ependymoma*
   Parasacral
   Intra-abdominal

Note Ependymoblastomas are classified with other embryonal tumours, see Chapter 7

region, where they are frequently of myxopapillary type.[11,14] The site incidence of ependymomas varies with patient age (Fig. 6.1). In children, the tumours are mostly intracranial[7,11] with a particular predilection for the posterior fossa,[15] whilst in adults intracranial examples are more often supratentorial in location.[5,14] Adult ependymomas also account for the vast majority of spinal cord examples.[7,14] Thus, in one study the mean age of posterior fossa, supratentorial and spinal ependymomas was quoted as 7, 17 and 41 years respectively.[16]

Aetiology

Ependymomas are often regarded as taking origin from a single differentiated ependymal cell,[5] but there is ultrastructural evidence that they may derive either from less mature cells at differing stages of ependymal development[17] or from a common ependymoglial precursor cell related to the ependymal tanycyte of lower order species.[18] The influence of genetic factors on the aetiology of ependymomas is suggested by rare congenital examples[19] and familial occurrences of the tumour.[20] Adult ependymoma cells commonly show allelic losses of chromosome 22q, suggesting the presence of a tumour suppressor gene.[21,22] This has not yet been characterised but appears to be distinct from the gene for neurofibromatosis type 2.[22] In familial ependymoma pedigrees, non-neoplastic cells have shown a normal karyotype,[23] but de novo constitutional loss from chromosome 22 has been reported in one patient developing a sporadic ependymoma in childhood.[21] Rather confusingly, the cells of most childhood tumours have shown a different cytogenetic pattern from adult tumours, with allelic losses in a variety of differing chromosomes but only rare involvement of 22q.[24,25]

Clinical features

Intracranial ependymomas, especially those in the posterior fossa or near the foramen of Monro, commonly cause cerebrospinal fluid (CSF) obstruction and present with headache, vomiting and papilloedema due to acute

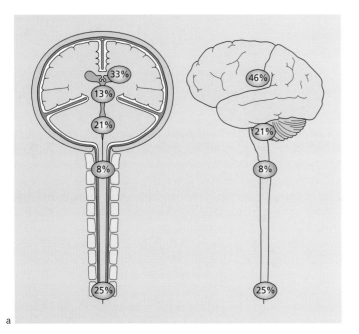
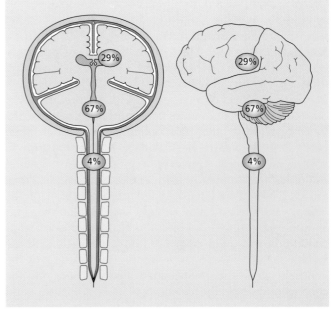

a   b

Fig. 6.1   **Distribution of ependymomas in relation to site and age. (a)** Adults. **(b)** Children.

hydrocephalus and raised intracranial pressure.[26] In posterior fossa tumours there may be an antecedent history of ataxia and visual disturbance, and if the tumour extends down through the foramen magnum, neck pain and stiffness may also be an early feature.[27] Epileptic seizures are more common with supratentorial lesions and occur in about one-third of cases.[28] Intraspinal ependymomas often present with a relatively long history spanning several years,[11] back pain being the most frequent clinical symptom.[29]

Radiology

Ependymomas may be imaged using either computerised tomography (CT) or magnetic resonance (MR) scans, but MRI is much better at delineating the extent of posterior fossa tumours[30,31] (Fig. 6.2) and is practically obligatory for spinal lesions. With intracranial tumours, CT scanning shows distinctive, multiple small foci of tumour calcification in up to half of cases[32] and cystic areas may also be found.[33] The tumour tissue is usually isodense or hyperdense on CT scanning, with moderate to intense, patchy enhancement after contrast medium is given.[34] Using MRI, ependymomas are typically isodense with brain in T1-weighted images, but hyperdense in T2-weighted sequences with variably intense gadolinium enhancement.

Pathology

Macroscopic features

Ependymomas are typically reddish-grey in colour and form nodular or lobulated masses. Excepting the most

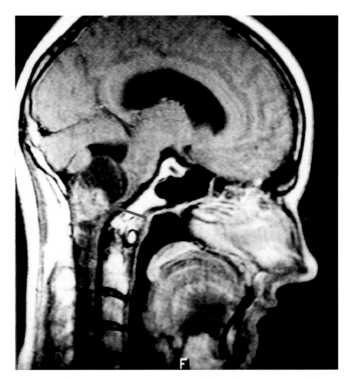

Fig. 6.2   **Ependymoma.** T1-weighted MRI scan of a fourth ventricle ependymoma with extension into the cisterna magna. The lower part of the lesion is enhancing after administration of contrast medium (arrow).

anaplastic lesions, they are usually well demarcated tumours, displacing adjacent brain tissue by expansion and giving a good surgical plane of cleavage. This is especially true of spinal examples, which may be so circumscribed as to permit a complete surgical enucleation.

On cut section, the tumour tissue is soft and homogeneous or granular in texture, and may have a gritty feel due to widespread microscopic calcification, especially in supratentorial examples. Areas of haemorrhage are only occasionally seen. Extensive cystic cavities can be present, especially in the larger cerebral lesions. Some of these may take the form of a large cyst with a mural nodule.[35] Supratentorial ependymomas usually arise close to the ventricular wall, and most examples extend at least partly into the ventricular cavity as a polypoid growth with a broad base. However, a proportion of cerebral examples are apparently entirely extraventricular. These are typically sited lateral to the trigone region of the lateral ventricle, and may be very large, extending as far as the pial surface.[2] Posterior fossa ependymomas commonly grow out from the fourth ventricle into the subarachnoid space.[36] Those arising in the floor of the ventricle show a marked tendency to protrude into the cisterna magna via the foramen of Luschka (Fig. 6.3), and may extend down through the foramen magnum, enveloping and compressing the medulla and upper cervical cord.[37] Less commonly, the tumours arise in a lateral recess of the ventricle and emerge as a polypoid growth in the cerebellopontine angle.[38]

Spinal cord ependymomas are usually discrete, elongate, sausage-like masses with a smooth surface. Intramedullary examples produce a fusiform expansion of the cord, and may extend over several segments (Fig. 6.4). The cauda equina tumours are especially well circumscribed, displacing or enveloping spinal roots and appearing quite separate from the cord. They are most often myxopapillary in type (see p. 158). Spinal cord ependymomas at any site, including the cauda equina, may be associated with an elongate, syrinx-like cavity in the spinal cord tissue above or below the level of the tumour.

Intraoperative diagnosis

Ependymomas are nearly always soft enough for rapid smear preparations to be made, and in most cases this is an ideal technique for intraoperative diagnosis. At low magnification, ependymoma smears usually show a striking papillary pattern, with cells clinging closely to the branching blood vessels. Since the vessels always smear out longitudinally, perivascular pseudorosettes are not visible in cross section but take the appearance of a longitudinal palisade of cell nuclei either side of the vessels (Fig. 6.5). This gives the papillary formations a denser, more organised appearance than those of astrocytoma smears. At higher magnification, the palisaded nuclei show a rather ill-defined orientation to the central vessels and are heaped up several layers in depth. The

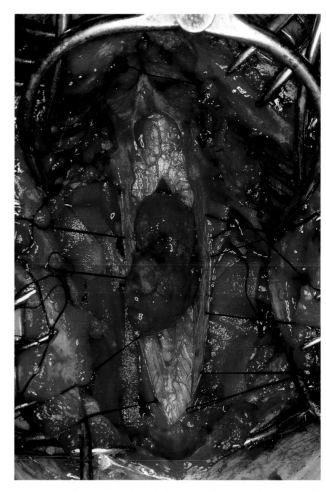

Fig. 6.4 **Ependymoma.** Intramedullary ependymoma of the cervical spinal cord. The lesion is being surgically removed via a median posterior excision and has a good plane of cleavage with the surrounding cord tissue.

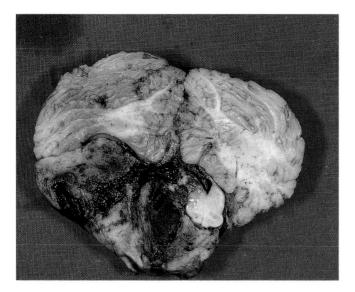

Fig. 6.3 **Ependymoma.** There is extensive growth out of the foramen of Luschka on one side, with compression and displacement of the adjacent cerebellum and medulla.

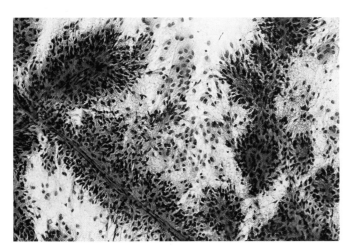

Fig. 6.5 **Ependymoma.** Smear preparation. The tumour cells cling to blood vessels in papillary palisades. Toluidine blue.

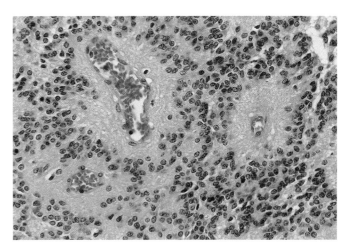

Fig. 6.6 **Ependymoma.** Tumour showing perivascular pseudorosettes. H & E.

cell nuclei are round in shape and usually larger than those seen in astrocytoma smears, and frequently have rather pale chromatin with one or more distinct nucleoli. There is an obvious fibrillary stroma, both adjacent to vessels and at the margins of the perivascular formations. Ependymoma cells usually exhibit a tendency to smear out individually, away from the papillary masses, and can show distinct perinuclear cytoplasm, sometimes with a tapering unipolar cell process. True ependymal rosettes or tubules are not usually visible in smear preparations.

When using frozen sections, intraoperative diagnosis depends largely on the demonstration of typical perivascular pseudorosettes, also seen in paraffin sections. Elsewhere, the rounded, ependymal nuclei are arranged in a characteristically monotonous pattern, but tubular rosettes may also be visible if these are a feature of the tumour concerned. Frozen sections can also be useful in assessing features of malignancy, including focal necrosis and vascular endothelial proliferation (see below).

Histological features

The histological appearance of ependymomas varies considerably, both within a single lesion and from one tumour to another. Typical ependymomas can have a predominantly cellular or epithelial growth pattern, or a mixture of the two, and some lesions may also show papillary or clear cell features. There are, however, a number of histological features fundamental to the diagnosis of ependymoma, regardless of the predominating architectural pattern. The cell nuclei are uniform and rounded in shape with well defined margins and a delicate, punctate chromatin pattern. There are often prominent nucleoli. Mitotic figures are usually infrequent in most low grade ependymomas, but may be occasionally encountered in the more cellular examples, especially those from a younger age group.[11] When present in any

number, mitoses should arouse suspicion of an increased malignant potential (see below). In histological sections the tumour cell cytoplasmic boundaries are usually poorly defined, and in most areas the nuclei appear embedded in a background of closely meshed, fibrillar stroma. This stains blue/purple with phosphotungstic acid haematoxylin (PTAH). Rosenthal bodies or fibres may be present in the stroma and have an intense dark blue or black colour with this stain. The cellularity varies widely, but tends to be highest in infantile posterior fossa tumours and supratentorial examples with other features of malignancy. Small blood vessels are usually quite abundant and thin walled, although a degree of vascular intimal proliferation may be found even in low grade examples.

The commonest and most important architectural feature of ependymomas is the *perivascular pseudorosette* (Fig. 6.6). Seen in cross section this consists of a broad circumferential zone around blood vessels which is devoid of cell nuclei and shows a distinct radial arrangement of tapering fibrillar cell processes, particularly apparent on PTAH staining (Fig. 6.7). These pseudorosettes are found in nearly all typical ependymomas and may be the only specialised architectural feature in some tumours. *True ependymal rosettes*, or tubules, are relatively uncommon by comparison, and are most often encountered in posterior fossa tumours in younger age groups, where it is claimed they are associated with a poorer prognosis.[11] They consist of a small central lumen surrounded by a ring of ependymal cells with an epithelial appearance and apical orientation (Fig. 6.8). These cells are of columnar or cuboidal type with central nuclei and well defined lateral and apical cell margins. Cilia may project from the apical cell surfaces into the lumen. *Ependymal canals or slit-like spaces* are closely related to the tubular rosettes. They are also relatively infrequent compared to perivascular pseudorosettes, and consist of narrow,

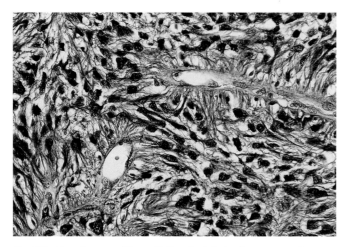

Fig. 6.7 **Ependymoma.** The radially orientated cell processes of perivascular pseudorosettes are strongly stained using PTAH.

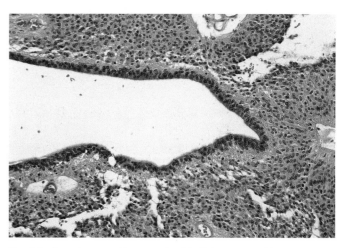

Fig. 6.9 **Ependymoma.** Tumour of epithelial pattern, with an ependymal lined canal. H & E.

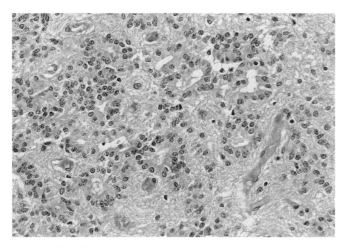

Fig. 6.8 **Ependymoma.** An example showing true ependymal rosettes (tubules). H & E.

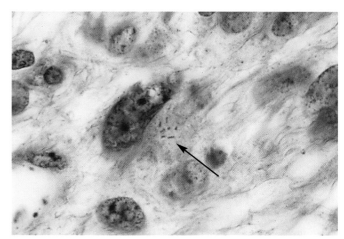

Fig. 6.10 **Ependymoma.** A cluster of blepharoplasts are visible adjacent to the nucleus of the large cell in the centre of the field (arrow). PTAH.

sometimes branching clefts lined by cells similar to those forming the tubules (Fig. 6.9). They are often a particular feature of intramedullary spinal ependymomas.[2] Cilia may again project from their luminal surfaces.

Reticulin is confined to blood vessel walls in typical ependymomas of all histological patterns, and no basement membrane is demonstrated in association with the basal layer of ependymal cells lining rosettes or canals. *Blepharoplasts* are small clusters of ciliary basal bodies, and are visible in some ependymomas as tiny punctate or ovoid intracytoplasmic bodies using a PTAH stain and a high magnification objective lens (Fig. 6.10). They are most often found in tumours showing tubular rosettes or ependymal canals and are typically sited next to the apical side of the nuclei of the cells lining those structures. They may also be found in other areas of tumour, again in a perinuclear location. Focal calcifications are not uncommonly present in ependymomas, especially those located supratentorially. Large cystic cavities, lined non-specifically by compressed tumour tissue may also be found, again more often in supratentorial lesions.

Histological variants of ependymoma

Cellular ependymomas These tumours show a prominent pattern of perivascular pseudorosettes separated by dispersed cell nuclei embedded in a fibrillar stroma (Fig. 6.11). Ependymal rosettes and canals are absent or extremely scarce. This is the most common pattern encountered in routine diagnostic practice and is frequently 'pure' rather than mixed with another histological pattern.

Epithelial ependymomas A predominance of tubular ependymal rosettes and ependymal lined canals is shown (Figs 6.8 and 6.9). They are more frequently found in childhood, especially in the posterior fossa, and often have an increased mitotic rate.[11] In practice, many examples show a mixed pattern, with some areas of dispersed cell nuclei and perivascular pseudorosettes.

Fig. 6.11 **Cellular ependymoma.** There are numerous perivascular pseudorosettes, but the tumour lacks ependymal lined tubules or canals. H & E.

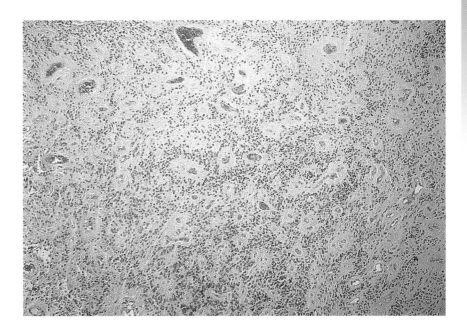

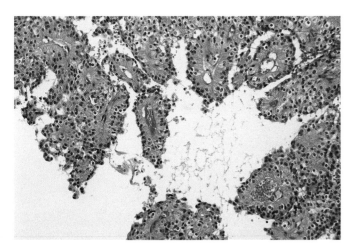

Fig. 6.12 **Papillary ependymoma** . Branching fibrovascular cores are surrounded by an epithelial-like layer of ependymal cells. H & E.

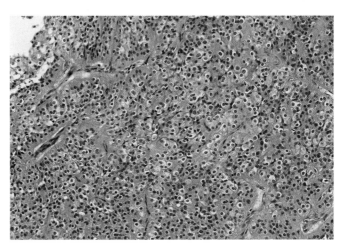

Fig. 6.13 **Clear cell ependymoma.** The sheets of clear cells with small central nuclei are reminiscent of an oligodendroglioma. H & E.

Papillary ependymomas.[2,39] These are a rare but distinctive histological variant, with branching fibrovascular cores covered by an epithelial-like layer of ependymal cells (Fig. 6.12). The basal aspects of the cells are not associated with a basement membrane, and radiating fibrillar processes are still present between the cell bodies and the underlying connective tissue. Despite this, care must be taken to distinguish these lesions from choroid plexus tumours. Ependymomas of this pattern are most frequently encountered in a fourth ventricle lateral recess or cerebellopontine angle, although they have been described elsewhere.[40] There is no association with increased grade of malignancy.[2]

Clear cell ependymomas This is another uncommon histological variant showing sheets of tumour cells with small central nuclei, optically clear cytoplasm and well defined cytoplasmic margins (Fig. 6.13). There are no pseudorosettes or other ependymal architectural features. The appearances are similar to oligodendroglioma, but electron microscopic studies have confirmed that the cells are ependymal in nature, with microvilli and cilia.[41,42] This histological pattern is usually encountered as a focal change in an otherwise typical ependymoma, but some lesions may be entirely clear cell in pattern, especially those arising in the region of the foramen of Monro.[2,5] When dealing with tumours at this site, it should be noted that central neurocytomas (see Chapter 8) may show both clear cell change and ependymal type perivascular pseudorosettes, and are easily confused with ependymomas on purely histological grounds. There is no known prognostic significance attached to clear cell change in ependymomas.

Mixed ependymomas This term may be used for tumours showing a mixture of histological patterns, usually combining cellular and epithelial features, although the cellular pattern may also be found in conjunction with papillary or clear cell change.

Cartilaginous ependymomas Very rarely, ependymomas may contain cartilage and sometimes bone.[43] These are usually posterior fossa tumours in children and enclose multiple separate nodules of mature or immature hyaline cartilage surrounded by a rim of collagenous stroma. The cartilage may surround bony trabeculae,[43] or have a uniform immature appearance similar to chondroma.[44] The intervening tumour is often notable for showing a mixture of ependymomatous and more astrocytic areas. No teratoid elements are present and the cartilage is thought to arise from entrapped mesenchymal elements in the tumour.[43]

Melanotic ependymomas These very uncommon tumours appear brown or black in colour macroscopically and are histologically typical except for the presence of melanin pigment.[45,46] The pigment has normal staining characteristics and is located within tumour cell cytoplasm. Ultrastructurally, primary melanosomes have been demonstrated within rosette forming cells, confirming that the melanin is produced by the neoplastic ependymal cells themselves.[45]

Grading of malignancy and anaplastic ependymoma

As with other primary glial tumours, ependymomas show a clinical and histological spectrum of malignancy, and there have been numerous attempts at defining a satisfactory grading system over the years.[5,6] The term anaplastic ependymoma is now often used to embrace all definitely malignant ependymal tumours,[2] although there are arguments for regarding ependymoblastomas as a distinct entity[47] and these tumours are described separately in Chapter 7. Depending on individual interpretation of the grading system used, the proportion of ependymomas described as anaplastic or grade III/IV lesions has varied from 7[7] to 21%.[48] In one series, 79% of ependymomas were regarded as being grade I/II, whilst another large study concluded that all typical ependymomas should be classed grade II or III, none showing a sufficiently benign clinical course to warrant grade I.[49] When considering the grading of malignancy in ependymomas, it should certainly be remembered that even lesions appearing histologically benign have the capacity to recur locally and seed the CSF pathways.[50]

Histologically, evidence of malignancy varies from a simple increase in cellularity and mitotic rate, through to complete loss of ependymal differentiation and an appearance that is indistinguishable from glioblastoma (Fig. 6.14). The more anaplastic ependymomas may thus show cellular pleomorphism with giant and multi-nucleated cells, vascular endothelial proliferation, focal tumour necrosis, and a tendency towards both macroscopic and histological infiltration of adjacent brain (Table 6.2). A high mitotic rate, large areas of necrosis and complete loss of differentiation appear to be particularly important histological features and have been statistically linked to poor prognosis in posterior fossa lesions.[51] Anaplastic change is more common in children, and in most studies has been described in around 25% of all juvenile ependymomas,[9,14] although some childhood studies have quoted a figure as high as 69%.[52] Anaplasia in childhood ependymomas is most commonly encountered in posterior fossa lesions[9] or large intracerebral, paraventricular tumours.[2] In any age group, histological and clinical evidence of malignancy is much less commonly encountered in ependymomas located in the spinal cord compared to intracranial sites.[53]

Immunocytochemistry

Between 70% and 80% of ependymomas show positive staining with antibodies to glial fibrillary acidic protein (GFAP).[54,55] The pattern of staining is variable, but typically includes scattered cell perikarya, individual cell processes, and the radiating fibrillary areas in perivascular

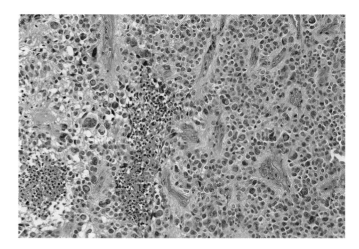

Fig. 6.14 **Anaplastic ependymoma.** The tumour shows cytological pleomorphism, focal necrosis and vascular endothelial proliferation. Poorly formed perivascular pseudorosettes are still apparent. H & E.

Table 6.2 Features associated with increased likelihood of malignancy in ependymomas

1. Posterior fossa or large intracerebral tumours in childhood
2. Epithelial pattern with tubular rosettes
3. Significant mitotic rate
4. Cytological pleomorphism
5. Vascular endothelial proliferation
6. Tumour necrosis
7. Diffuse infiltration of adjacent brain tissue

pseudorosettes[56] (Fig. 6.15). The cell bodies lining tubular rosettes and canals are usually unstained.[57] Antibodies to vimentin almost invariably stain ependymomas, with a pattern similar to that of GFAP.[58] A smaller proportion of tumours also show S-100 protein immunoreactivity,[59] although this may be less marked in the perivascular rosettes.[57] Depending on the source and type of antibody used, epithelial membrane antigen (EMA) immunoreactivity is found in a proportion of ependymomas, and as with normal ependyma, the staining is confined to the luminal surfaces of cells forming rosettes and canals[56,60] (Fig. 6.16). There is no apparent correlation of immunoreactivity for GFAP with the grade of malignancy[55] and anaplastic ependymomas may show either enhanced GFAP expression[61] or complete loss of staining.[62] Low grade ependymomas are negatively stained with cytokeratin antibodies,[63] making an important distinction from choroid plexus tumours, especially in the case of papillary ependymomas.[64] Occasional cells expressing cytokeratin immunoreactivity have been described in

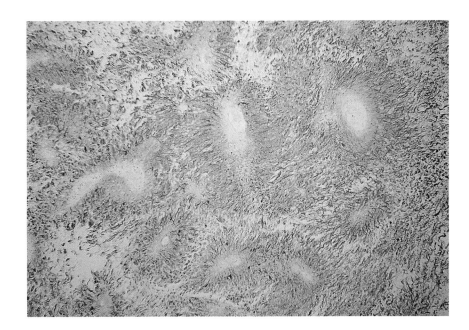

Fig. 6.15 Ependymoma. There is strong staining of the radiating fibrillary processes of perivascular pseudorosettes using immunocytochemistry for GFAP.

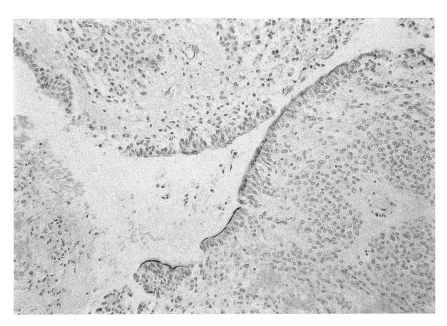

Fig. 6.16 Ependymoma. Immunocytochemical staining for EMA is confined to the apical surfaces of cells lining an ependymal canal.

some anaplastic ependymomas, probably due to aberrant epithelial differentiation.[62] However, such cytokeratin expression is very sparse by comparison with choroid plexus tumours and metastatic papillary adenocarcinomas, and thus unlikely to cause diagnostic confusion.[64]

Electron microscopy (Table 6.3)

Ultrastructurally the perikarya of ependymoma cells are arranged in closely knit, mosaic like clusters. These are separated by prominent areas of interlacing cell processes containing variable amounts of 20 nm microtubules and glial filaments.[65,66] Typical cells have rounded or polygonal nuclei showing dispersed, finely granular chromatin and well defined nucleoli. There is abundant electron lucent cytoplasm containing rather scanty organelles, including glycogen granules.[65] The most characteristic ultrastructural feature of ependymomas is the *intercellular microrosette*, formed from the apical surfaces of two or more cells which enclose a variable sized lumen (Fig. 6.17). Microvillous processes project from the cell surfaces into the lumen, usually as a complex interdigitating meshwork which partly or entirely occludes the luminal space. The cells forming microrosettes are joined near their luminal surfaces by junctional complexes similar to those seen in normal ependymal epithelium.[67] Zonulae adherentes are the most prominent component of these complexes, often with a single zonula ocludentes between the apical cell surface and the adherentes junctions. Desmosomes may also be found, either associated with these junctional complexes or occurring independently.[68] Cilia are sometimes associated with the microrosettes, but whilst they can be abundant in some cases,[69] they are frequently very sparse or not identified at all.[17,70] When present, the cilia either project into the rosette lumen or appear entirely buried within the adjacent cytoplasm.[69] Cilia in ependymomas typically have a normal glial type configuration of nine peripheral and two central tubules, but aberrant configurations of the axial skeleton may also be encountered.[71]

Table 6.3   Ultrastructural features associated with ependymomas

1. Separate, mosaic-like clusters of cells
2. Electron lucent cytoplasm containing glycogen
3. Prominent meshwork of interlacing cell processes containing glial filaments
4. Apical–basal polarisation of cell structure
5. Apical microvilli ⎫
6. Junctional complexes ⎬ Isolated or as part of an ependymal microrosette
7. Cilia/basal bodies ⎭
8. Basement membrane confined to blood vessels
9. Capillary endothelial cell fenestration

Microrosettes and associated ependymal specialisations are the most striking and frequently described ultrastructural features of ependymomas, but many tumour samples are dominated by large areas composed entirely of the interlacing cell processes.[66] Some of these processes are thought to arise from the opposite pole of the cells with apical surfaces contributing to microrosettes,[70] but many contain abundant glial filaments and are probably derived from the astrocytic type cells frequently encountered in ependymomas[17] (Fig. 6.17). These cells give rise to multipolar glial processes and contain abundant perikaryal cytoplasmic glial filaments, without any evidence of ependymal specialisation.

In poorly differentiated ependymal tumours, well formed microrosettes and cilia are even less likely to be encountered, but careful ultrastructural study may still reveal ependymal clues, including isolated clusters of microvilli or small intercellular spaces associated with isolated intercellular junctions. Intracytoplasmic glycogen and ciliary basal bodies are not specific features but may also be helpful in these circumstances.[65]

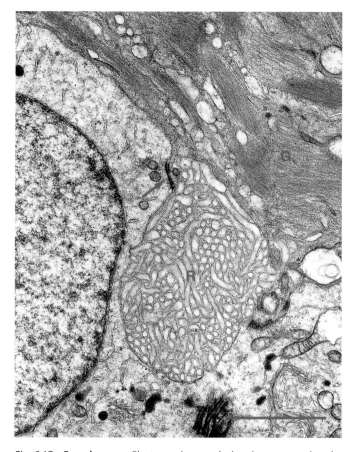

Fig. 6.17   **Ependymoma.** Electron micrograph showing an ependymal microrosette (R). The surrounding cells are joined by apical junctional complexes (arrow). An adjacent area shows interlacing processes filled with glial filaments (G). Bar = 2 µm.

Proliferation indices

Flow cytometry of ependymomas has shown some evidence of correlation with histological grade. Tumours graded I or II exhibit only minor changes in cytometry, but grade III lesions may demonstrate aneuploid or polyploid features.[72] However, this correlation is less obvious in spinal lesions, and some histologically low grade spinal cord ependymomas have had clearly polyploid DNA histograms.[72] Bromodeoxyuridine labelling may also prove useful in predicting the clinical behaviour of ependymomas. In one study, just over half the intracranial tumours and all the spinal ones had a labelling index of less than 1, which correlated with low grade histology and a good clinical outcome.[73] By contrast, three intracranial tumours which recurred all showed labelling indices of greater than 3, although only one of these showed histological evidence of malignancy at the time of initial surgery. A similar correlation can be shown between tumour grade and Ki-67/MIB-1 labelling, although in this instance a significant difference has been found between the labelling index of spinal tumours and non-anaplastic intracranial ones.[74]

Tissue culture

Most in vitro studies of ependymoma have shown a predominantly epithelial growth pattern in culture, with separate groups of uniform, polygonal cells arranged in sheets similar to those seen in cultures of normal ependymal cells.[75,76] In some studies, however, the cells have shown abundant fibrillar cytoplasmic processes,[77] and a population of piloid astrocyte-like cells has been reported in cultures of spinal cord ependymomas.[78] Transitions between the astrocytic and epithelial cell types have also been observed,[79] and one study has described a reversible astrocytic transformation of the epithelial cell sheets following treatment of the culture with dibutyryl cyclic adenosine monophosphate (AMP) and cytochalasin B.[75] Such observations suggest that the astrocytic elements seen in culture and on electron microscopy of biopsy tissue are an integral part of a single neoplastic cell line, rather than the result of mixed cell origin. The ependymal nature of the epithelial cell sheets has been borne out by longer term culture studies, which have shown development of rosettes and specific ependymal differentiation along the margins of the explants.[80]

Differential diagnosis

The most important tumour types involved in the differential diagnosis of ependymoma are listed in Table 6.4.

Astrocytoma

Distinction from a fibrillary astrocytoma may occasionally cause problems where an ependymoma shows a cellular

Table 6.4 Differential diagnosis of ependymoma

1. Astrocytoma
2. Choroid plexus papilloma
3. Metastatic adenocarcinoma
4. Medulloblastoma
5. Medulloepithelioma
6. Astroblastoma
7. Pineocytoma
8. Oligodendroglioma
9. Central neurocytoma

pattern without well formed perivascular pseudorosettes. This can be made more difficult if the amount of available tissue is very limited, as for example with a diagnostic sampling of an intrinsic spinal cord tumour. The radiological circumscription of ependymomas and their tendency to show a surgical plane of cleavage are often useful distinguishing features in these circumstances. Histologically, the cell nuclei in ependymomas tend to be rounder and more uniform than those in astrocytomas, with a finer chromatin pattern and more frequent, prominent nucleoli. Perivascular orientation may be prominent in some astrocytomas, but the appearances differ from those of ependymal pseudorosettes in showing broader foot processes abutting the vessel wall, with less marked radial orientation of the processes and a narrower, less well defined anucleate zone around the vessel. A careful search for ependymal tubular rosettes should always be made, because although they can be absent or very infrequent in many ependymomas, they act as a clear distinguishing feature from astrocytomas if any are found. As a last resort, electron microscopy may be useful in the distinction from astrocytomas, since microrosettes or isolated tufts of microvilli associated with cell junctions may be found in ependymomas that lack any distinctive ependymal architecture in paraffin sections.

Choroid plexus papillomas

These form an important differential diagnosis of ependymoma, especially when the latter has a more pronounced papillary pattern.[2] Like ependymomas, choroid plexus tumours are particularly common in children, typically occur in ventricle related sites, and are usually well circumscribed both grossly and histologically. Using routine stains, choroid plexus tumours usually show a greater degree of epithelial organisation around the vascular papillae than ependymomas, and there are often some areas with only a single layer of cells. There is usually a greater degree of apical–basal orientation and the cells have relatively well defined cytoplasmic margins. Also in contrast to ependymomas, there is a continuous basement membrane below the epithelial layer (a reticulin stain is useful here), often with appreciable amounts of perivascular collagenous tissue. There is no fibrillary stroma like that seen in ependymal perivascular pseudorosettes, and neither tubular rosettes or epithelial lined slits are found. Using immunocytochemical stains, antibodies for S-100 protein and EMA may show positive staining elements in both tumour types and are usually not helpful. GFAP immunostaining may show occasional positive cell bodies in choroid plexus tumours but will emphasise the absence of glial cell processes and perivascular fibrillary areas. Cytokeratins are usually widely expressed in choroid plexus tumours, but this is very rare even in malignant ependymomas and has not been seen in those with a papillary pattern.[64] Finally, immunocytochemical expression of transthyretin or carbonic anhydrase C is perhaps the most specific way of demonstrating that a tumour is of choroid plexus rather than ependymal origin, although it may be difficult to demonstrate in the most anaplastic tumours.

Metastatic adenocarcinoma

In adults, a para- or intraventricular carcinoma metastasis may easily be confused with papillary forms of ependymoma. As with choroid plexus tumours, metastases will differ histologically in showing a subepithelial, reticulin positive basement membrane and a complete lack of fibrillary stroma. Tubular acini in metastatic adenocarcinomas differ from ependymal tubular rosettes in the absence of cilia or blepharoplasts, and are often the site of mucin production. Metastatic lesions usually have a greater degree of macroscopic brain infiltration at their margins, although this can also be seen in high grade ependymomas. In contrast to ependymomas, most adenocarcinomas show substantial cytokeratin staining using immunocytochemistry, but GFAP expression is confined to entrapped reactive glial elements, mostly near the margins of the lesion. The use of antibodies to EMA under these circumstances is probably best avoided, as positive staining is not uncommon in ependymomas of more epithelial histological pattern.

Medulloblastoma

Medulloblastoma needs to be considered in the differential diagnosis of anaplastic ependymoma of the fourth ventricle, especially in children (see also ependymoblastoma in Chapter 7). In contrast to ependymomas, there are no perivascular pseudorosettes in medulloblastomas and there is usually a much less conspicuous fibrillary stroma. The rosettes in medulloblastomas have a solid fibrillary core without a central lumen, and tubules are not found unless there is retinoblastic differentiation. Desmoplastic medulloblastomas often appear macroscopically circumscribed like ependymomas, but may be easily distinguished histologically by their abundant reticulin content. Microscopic infiltration of cerebellum

by medulloblastomas is usually much more diffuse than that seen in all but the highest grade ependymomas. Immunocytochemically, medulloblastomas do not show the EMA expression often seen in ependymomas, and they frequently express immunopositivity for neuron specific enolase and other neuronal antigens such as PGP9.5 Antibodies to GFAP can show quite widespread positive staining in medulloblastomas with astrocytic differentiation, and should be interpreted with care.

Medulloepithelioma

Although very rare, these tumours are grossly well circumscribed like ependymomas and may be confused histologically with papillary ependymoma due to their tubular pattern and epithelial organisation. Unlike ependymomas, however, the perivascular epithelial layer in medulloepitheliomas has a distinctive pseudostratified organisation, with an underlying reticulin positive basement membrane. The apical surfaces of the cells have distinct, well defined cell membranes but there are no cilia or blepharoplasts. It should be noted that many medulloepitheliomas show varied combinations of glial and neuroblastic differentiating activity, occasionally including the formation of ependymal rosettes.[81] Areas of typical medulloepithelioma are usually still present, however, and the ependymal rosettes described have been more like those of ependymoblastoma, with multiple cell layers and mitotic figures.

Astroblastoma

Like ependymomas, astroblastomas are commonest in younger age groups. They can be paraventricular or even intraventricular, and are usually well circumscribed macroscopically. Histologically, they also form perivascular rosettes, but these differ from ependymal ones in showing broader radial processes which have a terminally expanded footplate rather than a tapering outline, and are not stained with PTAH. Astroblastoma cell nuclei are usually more irregular than in ependymoma, with a coarser chromatin pattern. Also in contrast to ependymoma, the areas between the perivascular rosettes is distinctly rarefied, with only scanty spindle or stellate cells rather than solid fibrillary stroma. Astroblastomas do not show true tubular rosettes or epithelial lined slits, but like ependymomas they may express widespread immunoreactivity for GFAP.

Pineocytoma

This needs to be considered as a differential diagnosis of ependymoma in a posterior third ventricle site. Like ependymomas, pineocytomas are well circumscribed, often calcified and may project into the ventricular cavity.

Histologically, they can also show a perivascular papillary pattern, but the scanty radial processes are club ended and react positively with silver impregnations rather than glial stains. Difficulty may arise if a pineocytoma shows a predominant pattern of large pineocytomatous rosettes, which at first glance may be confused with ependymal pseudorosettes. However, the solid pineocytomatous rosettes can be distinguished by their lack of constant relationship to a central blood vessel and the absence of radial orientation of the fibrillar stroma. Moreover, the centres of the rosettes do not stain with PTAH or antibodies to GFAP, although there may be extensive immunoreactivity for glial GFAP elsewhere in pineocytomas.

Oligodendroglioma

The difficulty here lies in the distinction from ependymomas with extensive clear cell change. In terms of site, oligodendrogliomas are more often superficial tumours whereas clear cell ependymomas are typically deep seated lesions, occurring especially in the foramen of Monroe region (see also central neurocytoma, below). On histological grounds alone it can be very difficult to distinguish the clear cell variant of ependymoma from oligodendroglioma, but many cases show more typical ependymomatous areas, and it may be worth examining more tissue blocks or deeper levels to look for these. Failing this, electron microscopy is likely to be useful, since the clear cells in ependymomas show typical ultrastructural ependymal features, including cilia, microvilli and junctional complexes.

Central neurocytoma

These tumours occur in the third ventricle and septal area, predominantly in younger age groups, and may exhibit clear cell change or ependymal type perivascular pseudorosettes (see Chapter 8). Distinction from typical or clear cell ependymomas at this site is often not possible using routine stains, and relies on the results of immunocytochemistry and electron microscopy. Central neurocytomas differ from ependymomas in their consistent immunocytochemical expression of synaptophysin and neuron specific enolase, and a majority are unstained with antibodies to GFAP. Ultrastructurally, central neurocytomas can be distinguished from ependymomas by evidence of neuroblastic differentiation, including synapses, neurosecretory dense core vesicles and neuritic processes containing microtubules.

Therapy

Surgical resection is the mainstay of treatment for ependymomas and needs to be as radical as possible, since the completeness of primary excision strongly influences prognosis.[82,83] Unfortunately, whilst a total macroscopic removal is often possible with spinal tumours[84] the site of many intracranial ependymomas precludes total excision, especially with lesions arising in the floor of the fourth ventricle.[27] Even where radical excision has proved possible, postoperative radiotherapy has played an important part in the management of older children and adults, and has dramatically improved long term survival.[50] Local fields have usually been considered adequate for low grade supratentorial tumours and most spinal ones,[85] but because of the risks of CSF dissemination, prophylactic craniospinal axis treatment has traditionally been recommended for posterior fossa ependymomas and supratentorial lesions which are of high grade.[52,91] The role of chemotherapy remains controversial, although ependymomas appear to be relatively refractory to this form of treatment. The long term survival of children with posterior fossa tumours has not been improved by the addition of chemotherapy to postoperative craniospinal irradiation[85] and there have been disappointing results using high dose chemotherapy in children with relapsed disease.[86] However, some success has been reported in very young infants receiving primary postoperative chemotherapy without radiotherapy.[87]

Prognosis

Ependymomas of all grades show a marked tendency to recur locally, particularly if incompletely excised,[50,88] and this is the commonest cause of an initial deterioration after primary treatment.[27] Of equal importance is the undoubted ability of ependymomas to spread throughout the subarachnoid space. The incidence of CSF seeding has been variously quoted as occurring in anything between about 5% of cases[89] to 75% of cases,[90] although most large reviews suggest that clinical evidence of seeding is probably found in approximately 12% of all ependymomas.[50,91] There is a significant rate of seeding in histologically low grade ependymomas[52] but dissemination in the CSF pathways is most likely to occur with anaplastic tumours[92] and those sited in the posterior fossa.[52] CSF seeding usually follows local recurrence at the primary excision site, suggesting that it may be initiated by surgical intervention.[93] Much less frequently, ependymomas may metastasise outside the CNS,[94] with cervical lymph nodes and lungs as the commonest sites for secondary deposits.[36,95] The primary lesions in such cases have usually been intracranial and high grade,[96,97] although systemic metastases have been reported in association with primary spinal cord sites[98] and initially low grade tumours.[99] As with CSF seeding, most cases of systemic spread have followed primary surgical intervention and local recurrence of tumour.[95,97]

Using a combination of surgery and radiotherapy, the overall 5-year survival rate for ependymomas is usually quoted at about 50–60%.[48,100] Longer term survival figures are less optimistic, and rarely exceed 40%.[100,101] Survival varies with both patient age and tumour site, and most studies agree that posterior fossa lesions have a worse prognosis than supratentorial ones,[16] especially in children and infants.[11,89] An exception to this trend are the large extraventricular cerebral ependymomas, which are more often anaplastic and again carry a very poor prognosis.[2] Spinal ependymomas usually have a more favourable outlook than cranial ones,[11] with figures of up to 83% for 5-year survival[102] and many cases surviving over 10 years.[103] The grade of malignancy is another important factor affecting prognosis in ependymomas.[104,105] For more malignant ependymomas, the 5-year survival rate is often quoted as less than 30%, in contrast to figures of up to 70% for lesions of low histological grade.[48] In practical terms, therefore, the prognosis for patients with ependymomas will be determined by the combined effect of several interlinked variables, most notably histological grade, age, site and the completeness of the primary surgical excision.[82]

Myxopapillary ependymoma

This variant of ependymoma occurs predominantly in the region of the filum terminale and has a highly distinctive histological appearance. It is listed as an independent subgroup of ependymal tumours in the WHO classification.[1] The recognition of these tumours as a distinct entity is of considerable clinical importance, since they are more amenable to radical surgical resection than most other forms of ependymoma and their particular biological behaviour has specific implications for both therapy and prognosis. They should not be confused with papillary forms of typical ependymoma which lack the striking myxoid change and do not have the same favourable prognosis.

Incidence and site

In most series, myxopapillary ependymomas account for approximately 5% of all ependymal tumours,[106] but in the spinal canal this proportion rises to around 17%.[7] In the cauda equina region alone they account for up to 50% of ependymomas[107] and the vast majority are found at this location, usually attached to the filum terminale.[11,108] The remaining neuraxial examples have been described with almost anecdotal frequency at a number of more cephalic sites, including the lateral ventricles and thoracolumbar spinal roots.[109,110] Outside the CNS the myxopapillary variant is by far the commonest type of ependymoma found in pre- or postsacral ectopic sites (see p. 166). It

should be emphasised that not all ependymomas occurring in the cauda equina are of the myxopapillary variety, both typical and non-myxoid papillary ependymomas being well described at this site.[7] The age at presentation for myxopapillary lesions ranges from 6 to 82 years,[111] but there is a tendency for the tumour to present relatively more often in young adults, with a mean age in the mid fourth decade of life.[108,111] As with typical ependymomas, there is evidence for a slight sex bias towards males.[111]

Aetiology

Cauda equina myxopapillary ependymomas are assumed to arise from the ependymal cell nests normally present in the filum terminale.[112] The reason for the striking myxopapillary appearance in these tumours, however, is not entirely certain. Their light microscopic features suggest a progressive distortion of normal ependymoma architecture by an accumulation of myxoid material in perivascular spaces.[2] Both direct secretion by the tumour cells[113] and vascular extravasation via endothelial fenestrations[114] have been postulated as a mechanism for this myxoid deposition, but there is ultrastructural evidence that the material may actually result from excess basement membrane production around the tumour cells.[115] Collagenous elements abut directly onto ependymal cells in the normal filum terminale[113] and it has been suggested that this abnormal juxtaposition of collagen may induce basement membrane production.[115] In support of this hypothesis tissue culture studies of rat spinal cord have demonstrated basement membrane production where neuroglial elements interface with substrate collagen[116] and organ culture of myxopapillary ependymomas has shown an increase in basement membrane material closely related to the collagen of the extracellular space.[117]

Clinical features

As with other types of ependymoma in the cauda equina region, myxopapillary ependymomas of the filum terminale most commonly present with pain in the lower back or coccygeal region, which is sometimes accompanied by sciatic radiation or other evidence of lumbosacral radiculopathy. There may be associated lower limb sensory disturbance with a low lumbar sensory level in some cases, and urinary sphincter disturbances can also occur.[107,108] There is typically a long antecedent history, which may span several years[11] but a small proportion of cases present acutely due to massive haemorrhage into the tumour or subarachnoid space.[107]

Radiology

Radiological diagnosis traditionally used myelography to demonstrate a complete block to the passage of contrast medium in the lumbar region.[107,111] More recently, however, myelography has been superseded by MRI scanning, which is now undoubtedly the best technique for imaging cauda equina myxopapillary ependymomas.[108] In contrast to non-myxopapillary ependymomas, a significant proportion of cases are hyperintense in T1-weighted images.[118]

Pathology

Macroscopic features

Cauda equina region myxopapillary ependymomas are usually elongate, sausage shaped tumours with a smooth, lobulated surface. They can be very large by the time of clinical presentation, and lesions over 10 cm in length are not unusual.[108] The larger examples may be associated with deformity or erosion of the sacrum. The majority of myxopapillary ependymomas at this site are well defined lesions, appearing almost encapsulated macroscopically, and displacing or compressing the adjacent cauda equina nerve roots. Some examples, however, may infiltrate and envelope the nerve roots, and massive extension into the adjacent extravertebral tissues has also been documented. The cut section often reveals areas of old or recent haemorrhage, but there is less tendency to gritty calcification than with typical ependymomas.

Intraoperative diagnosis

Most myxopapillary ependymomas are soft enough to make smear preparations and have a highly distinctive cytological appearance. At low power, smears show organised papillary structures, with palisades of tumour cells arranged around branching vessels, similar to those seen in typical ependymomas. In myxopapillary lesions, however, the perivascular gliofibrillary stroma is largely replaced by abundant mucinous matrix, which is strongly metachromatic on toluidine blue staining (Fig. 6.18). Some of the papillary structures may lack a central blood vessel, and when smeared in cross section give the appearance of a solid, metachromatic, mucinous core surrounded by one or more layers of ependymal cells. The tumour cells have large, rounded and vesicular nuclei similar to those seen in typical ependymoma, and again often contain prominent nucleoli.

Histological features

The most characteristic areas of myxopapillary ependymoma are made up of numerous small papillary structures, each surrounded by well defined cuboidal or columnar cells, usually in a single layer. These cells have rounded, ependymal type nuclei with distinct margins and a delicate chromatin meshwork, but they lack obvious cytoplasmic processes. The cores of the papillae consist either of a central blood vessel surrounded by mucinous

matrix, or are entirely filled by the matrix (Fig. 6.19). The matrix is metachromatic when stained with toluidine blue and strongly positive with connective tissue mucin stains such as Alcian blue (Fig. 6.20). Where central blood vessels are present there is often extensive thickening and hyalinisation of the vessel wall, which may be associated with iron pigment and evidence of previous haemorrhage. Other areas of the tumour show a looser structure, with tumour cell nuclei embedded in a meshwork of fine cytoplasmic processes which stain with PTAH. These processes enclose numerous microcystic spaces and are arranged in a radial fashion around the outer basement membrane of blood vessels. In such areas, the perivascular spaces are often enlarged, and appear empty or contain only very scanty mucinous matrix (Fig. 6.21). Occasionally, there may also be more compact gliofibrillar areas resembling those of typical ependymomas, with peri-

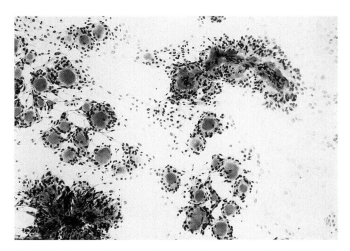

Fig. 6.18 **Myxopapillary ependymoma.** Smear preparation. Well organised cuffs of tumour cells are arranged around metachromatic, mucinous central cores. Toluidine blue.

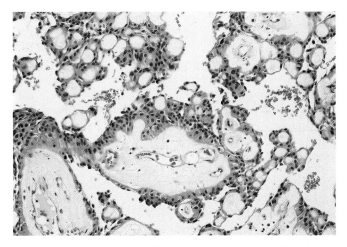

Fig. 6.19 **Myxopapillary ependymoma.** The tumour has a distinctive papillary architecture. Some of the mucinous cores also contain blood vessels. H & E.

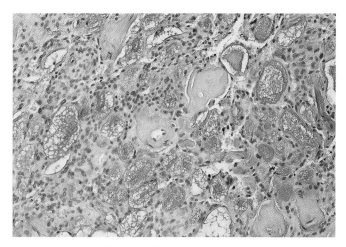

Fig. 6.20 **Myxopapillary ependymoma.** The central cores of the papillary formations stain strongly with stains for connective tissue mucin. PAS–Alcian blue.

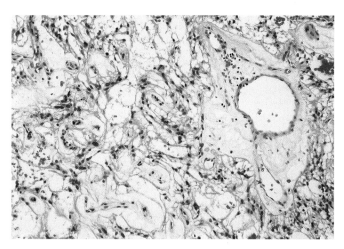

Fig. 6.21 **Myxopapillary ependymoma.** A looser area of tumour with a meshwork of fine cytoplasmic processes enclosing microcystic spaces. Perivascular spaces are enlarged and contain mucinous material. H & E.

vascular pseudorosettes or even true ependymal rosettes.[119] Most myxopapillary ependymomas have sharply defined histological margins, although some may enclose nerve roots, and a proportion are surrounded by a condensed connective tissue capsule.[111] Mitotic figures are not usually seen and myxopapillary ependymomas of the cauda equina are generally regarded as tumours of very low grade, corresponding to grade I in the WHO classification.[2]

Immunocytochemistry

In the more fibrillary areas, myxopapillary ependymomas show strong immunopositivity with antibodies to vimentin and GFAP.[64] In the papillary areas, however, the cells surrounding myxoid cores may be unstained or only patchily stained with antibodies to GFAP.[61] Scanty positive staining of tumour cells with an antibody to S-100 protein has been reported,[61] but despite the epithelial

appearance of the papillary structures, there is no reaction with antibodies to cytokeratin.[64,120] This is an important distinction from other papillary and myxoid tumours such as metastatic adenocarcinomas, choroid plexus tumours and chordomas.

Electron microscopy

Ultrastructurally, many areas of myxopapillary ependymoma consist of stellate cells forming a loose meshwork of tenuous cell processes which contain abundant, glial type intermediate filaments. The cells and their processes are widely separated by expanded extracellular space, in contrast to typical ependymomas where the glial cell processes are normally closely packed together.[66] The largest areas of expanded extracellular space, including those around blood vessels, are bounded by an epithelial palisade of tumour cell bodies joined by junctional complexes near their apical surfaces (Fig. 6.22). As in typical ependymomas, these complexes include zonulae occludens and desmosomes in addition to zonulae adherentes. Septate junctions, normally only present in invertebrate species, have also been described in myxopapillary ependymomas and may represent a specific ultrastructural feature of this tumour.[121] The apical surfaces of the tumour cell palisades show ependymal specialisation with abundant microvilli and cilia, sometimes with abnormal configurations of axial tubules.[119] Occasionally, 'polar inversion' may be found, in which the microvillus-bearing apical surface of one cell abuts directly against the flattened basal surface of an adjacent cell[122] (Fig. 6.22). All the expanded extracellular spaces are lined by thickened, three-layered basement membrane which is a consistent ultrastructural feature of myxopapillary ependymomas.[66,115] The loose inner zone and compact middle layer of the membrane are narrow and well defined, but the outer zone is irregular and merges with the amorphous material and collagen in the extracellular space (Fig. 6.22).

Tissue culture

There have been few in vitro studies of myxopapillary ependymoma, but a report of one case has described an epithelial growth pattern similar to that seen with typical ependymomas.[117] An earlier study emphasised the glial morphology of the explants, with multipolar cells bearing delicate cytoplasmic processes.[122] In organ culture, differences from typical ependymoma have been more apparent, with the development of connective tissue cores covered by an epithelial layer of cells showing abundant reduplication of basement membrane material.[117]

Differential diagnosis

The most important tumour types involved in the differential diagnosis of myxopapillary ependymoma are listed in Table 6.5.

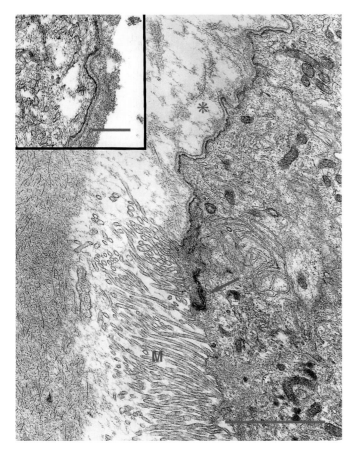

Fig. 6.22 **Myxopapillary ependymoma.** The apical surface of one palisaded tumour cell bears a profusion of microvilli (M). It is joined by an apical junctional complex (arrow) directly to the basal aspect of an adjacent cell (asterisk), demonstrating polar inversion. Electron micrograph. Bar = 2.0 μm. Inset: The tumour cell basement membranes have a characteristic three-layered structure, with a compact middle layer and a broad, irregular outer zone. Bar = 0.5 μm.

Table 6.5 Differential diagnosis of myxopapillary ependymoma

1. Cauda equina paraganglioma
2. Metastatic adenocarcinoma
3. Chordoma
4. Chondroma/chondrosarcoma

Paraganglioma

Cauda equina paragangliomas are usually well circumscribed, lobulated tumours within the sacral canal which can be difficult to distinguish from myxopapillary ependymomas on clinical, radiological or surgical grounds. Histologically, however, they lack the well organised papillary architecture and mucinous matrix of myxopapillary ependymomas and are usually easily identified by their typical pattern of cell nests enclosed by reticulin. Immunocytochemically, paragangliomas differ from ependymomas in their expression of neuronal antigens such as neuron specific enolase, neurofilament

protein and synaptophysin. Many also express cytokeratins. The results of immunocytochemical staining for GFAP should, however, be interpreted with care, since there may be positive staining sustentacular cells or filum terminale astrocytes within paragangliomas.

Choroid plexus tumours

Although choroid plexus tumours are unknown as primary lesions in the cauda equina region, they may occur anywhere in the neuraxis as CSF seedlings. They have a similar papillary architecture to that of myxopapillary ependymomas, and have many features in common at an ultrastructural level. The major histological differences are the absence of any mucinous or myxoid changes in the stroma of the papillary cores and the lack of a gliofibrillar component, best assessed by immunostaining for GFAP. Also unlike myxopapillary ependymomas, choroid plexus tumours exhibit consistent immunoreactivity with antibodies to cytokeratins, carbonic anhydrase and transthyretin.

Metastatic adenocarcinoma

Some metastases may show both mucinous lakes and a papillary architecture, but the gliofibrillary areas found in myxopapillary ependymomas are absent, and immunoreactivity to GFAP is limited to entrapped reactive glial elements. In addition, cilia are not usually found on the apical cell surfaces of metastases, either histologically or ultrastructurally. However, the most reliable method of distinguishing metastatic adeno-carcinomas from myxopapillary ependymomas is again the demonstration of immunoreactivity for cytokeratin.

Chordoma

Like myxopapillary ependymomas, these tumours are relatively common in the cauda equina region and show a prominent myxoid matrix which stains positively for connective tissue mucins. However, the matrix is usually more abundant in chordomas and the cells are arranged in dispersed cords or strands rather than papillary formations. Moreover, the tumour cells are typically more pleomorphic than those of myxopapillary ependymomas and show a distinctive 'physaliphorous' pattern of cytoplasmic vacuolation (see Chapter 18). Immunocytochemically, chordomas lack intrinsic gliofibrillary elements and stain positively with immunocytochemistry for cytokeratins. Ultrastructurally, chordoma cells may be distinguished by the absence of apical cell specialisations, including cilia and microvilli.

Cartilaginous tumours

The matrix in cartilaginous tumours shows a similar toluidine blue metachromasia and alcianophilia to that in myxopapillary ependymomas, but most chondromas and low grade chondrosarcomas can be easily distinguished by the presence of typical cartilaginous architecture, with dispersed tumour cells in lacunar spaces. Myxoid variants of chondrosarcoma differ in showing cords and strands of cells within the matrix, but still lack a papillary structure. Most cartilaginous tumours are not immunoreactive for cytokeratins, but they can be distinguished from ependymomas by the lack of GFAP immunostaining, and if necessary by the absence of cilia, microvilli or other ependymal features at ultrastructural level.

Therapy and prognosis

Although generally regarded as being of lower grade malignancy than their more typical counterparts, myxopapillary ependymomas still show the same tendency to recur locally and seed in the CSF pathways, and may even metastasise to systemic sites.[106,107] By comparison with typical ependymomas, however, both local recurrences and distant metastases tend to occur at longer intervals after primary therapy, and remissions of over 10 years are not unusual before the first manifestations of recurrent disease.[107]

The majority of cauda equina myxopapillary ependymomas are well circumscribed and surgically accessible, and total primary excision is the treatment of choice.[108,111] The relatively favourable prognosis associated with these tumours is at least partly related to the completeness of primary surgical excision, and in some series a 100% cure rate has been claimed where total removal has been possible.[108] In cases where there is widespread infiltration of the cauda equina, resection may be limited by the need to avoid mutilating the nerve roots[123] and should then be combined with local postoperative radiotherapy.[107,123] Disease free survival periods of up to 20 years have been reported in these circumstances.[123] However, in some long term follow-up studies the prognosis has been slightly less favourable because of late tumour recurrences,[107] even after apparently complete primary excision of encapsulated tumours.[111] In the largest published series of 70 cauda equina region myxopapillary ependymomas, the mean survival was 19 years after complete excision of the tumour and 14 years after partial excision, with an overall mortality of 6.5% as a result of multiple recurrences.[111]

Subependymoma

This rare, slow growing tumour is separately identified as a variant of ependymoma in the WHO classification.[1] Although the term subependymoma is now universally accepted, it should be noted that the older literature contains a number of synonyms, including subependymal glomerulate astrocytoma,[124] subependymal astrocytoma[125] and subependymal mixed glioma.[126]

Incidence

Approximately 50% of subependymomas are an incidental post-mortem finding[127] and such clinically silent tumours have been reported in 0.4% of 1000 consecutive autopsies.[128] The age at death of these asymptomatic patients ranges from the fifth to the eighth decade, with a mean of 60 years.[127] The remaining patients present symptomatically during life, and account for approximately 0.7% of all intracranial neoplasms.[128] Unlike other ependymal tumours, symptomatic subependymomas are rare in childhood[129] and occur mostly after the age of 40 years, although their mean age of presentation is lower than the mean age at death in the clinically silent cases.[127,130] In both groups, there is a significant male predominance.[127,130]

Site

Subependymomas presenting as an incidental autopsy finding almost always arise in the fourth ventricle, although rare lateral ventricle examples have been described.[127] Of the symptomatic lesions, the commonest site is again the fourth ventricle, which accounts for about 70% of cases.[127] They may be attached either to the floor or the roof of the ventricular cavity.[127,130] Supratentorial subependymomas accounted for 27% of symptomatic cases in the largest published review.[127] These tumours usually arise in the walls of the lateral ventricles,[127] but about one-fifth take origin in the base of the septum pellucidum.[125,127] The septal tumours may grow outwards into the third and lateral ventricular cavities, and they frequently obstruct the foramina of Monro.[131] The spinal cord is an uncommon site for subependymomas, accounting for only 2% of all symptomatic cases.[127,132] Most are intramedullary lesions and occur in the cervical region[133,134] although both thoracolumbar[132] and extramedullary examples[135] have been described.

Aetiology

Ultrastructural studies have demonstrated unequivocal ependymal features in some of the cells in subependymomas,[136] and they are now usually regarded as a variant of typical ependymomas.[136,137] The very slow growth rate of subependymomas, however, has led to considerable speculation over their mode of development. Some authors have suggested they may derive from a reactive process in the subependymal tissues, a view supported by their frequent multiplicity and the examples which have arisen in close proximity to other tumours.[138,139] There have also been proposals that subependymomas are maldevelopmental or hamartomatous in origin, with familial examples,[140] simultaneous presentation in identical twins[141] and adjacent meningoglial heterotopia[142] all being quoted in support of this hypothesis. The cell of origin of subependymomas is also rather uncertain, although it seems most likely that they arise either from mature subependymal elements or persisting ependymoglial precurser cells in the subependymal layer.[143]

Clinical features

A symptomatic presentation occurs in practically all subependymomas of the spinal cord and foramen of Monro region, in about two-thirds of all supratentorial examples, and in about one-third of those arising in the fourth ventricle.[127] The duration of symptoms prior to presentation may be quite prolonged and is usually between 1 and 10 years.[127] The commonest cause of presentation is raised intracranial pressure due to obstructive hydrocephalus, which occurs in a majority of the symptomatic fourth ventricular cases and in about one-quarter of supratentorial tumours,[127] especially those in the region of the foramen of Monro.[144] Fourth ventricle subependymomas frequently have an antecedent history of poor balance, with gait or truncal ataxia, and may also present with visual disturbance or lower cranial nerve palsies.[127,130] In the spinal cord, subependymomas typically produce lower limb spasticity with an appropriate sensory level, and there may be sphincter dysfunction if the lesion is more caudally sited.[132]

Radiology

Radiologically, subependymomas typically appear as solid, isodense intraventricular lesions using CT.[130] Contrast enhancement is very inconstant, and may be entirely absent, irregular or diffuse.[130,145] Calcification is demonstrated radiologically in about half of the cases.[130] MR imaging is of particular value for subependymomas in the posterior fossa and spinal cord.[147] They are usually iso- or hypointense in T1-weighted images but hyperintense with T2-weighting with sparse or absent contrast enhancement.[27,146] Compared to typical ependymomas, subependymomas are more often entirely intraventricular and less frequently cystic or calcified,[145] but both the CT and MRI appearances are generally felt too similar to permit reliable radiological distinction between the two types of tumour.[147]

Pathology

Macroscopic features

Subependymomas found incidentally at autopsy are typically small, hard, whitish nodules, which are sharply circumscribed and project into the ventricular cavity. They are usually less than 1 cm in size[127] and may be multiple.[126] Those tumours presenting symptomatically are mostly larger, lobulated lesions, which fill the ventricular cavity and may be over 5 cm across[126] (Fig. 6.23). They more often show cysts, tumour haemorrhages and areas of calcification on cut section. The fourth ventricular symptomatic lesions frequently protrude out of the foramen of Magendie in a fashion similar to some typical ependymomas and may extend to fill the cerebellopontine angles and envelope the medulla.[130] Such large fourth ventricular lesions remain mostly well circumscribed, but some may lack a good plane of cleavage with the adjacent floor or walls of the ventricular cavity.

Intraoperative diagnosis

Subependymomas are usually too tough to make satisfactory smear preparations, and attempts at smearing the tumour tissue generally produce large masses of cell nuclei and dense fibrillary stroma which are too thick to be of any real diagnostic value. Frozen sections, by contrast, will generally reveal the typical histological architecture of the tumour and permit an intraoperative diagnosis to be made.

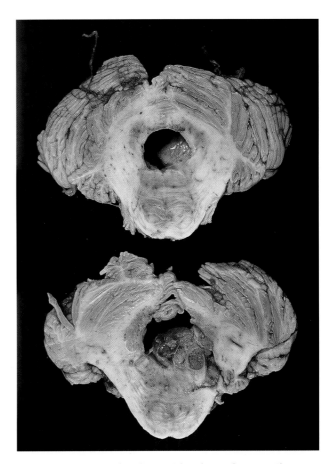

Fig. 6.23 **Symptomatic fourth ventricle subependymoma.** The tumour is densely adherent to the floor of the ventricle and projects upwards as a lobulated, well circumscribed mass.

Histological features

The tissue is quite sparsely cellular with tumour cell nuclei gathered into small clusters or nests, each widely separated by an abundant gliofibrillary stroma (Fig. 6.24). The nuclei are mostly ependymal in appearance, with well defined rounded or ovoid outlines and finely stippled chromatin. Paranuclear blepharoplasts are often demonstrable with PTAH staining. The clusters of nuclei are randomly arranged and there are no ependymal-type rosettes or canals in typical subependymomas. Distinct perivascular pseudorosettes are again not a typical feature of these tumours, although poorly formed examples may be found in some cases. The extensive gliofibrillary

stroma is positive staining with PTAH (Fig. 6.25) and may contain Rosenthal fibres. The fibrillary processes of the stroma are usually closely packed to form a dense meshwork, but some areas may show a looser texture with microcystic spaces. Degenerative changes are common, especially in the larger tumours, where there may be extensive areas of collagenous scarring, calcification and evidence of old and recent haemorrhage (Fig. 6.26). Although some cases may show pronounced nuclear pleomorphism,[128,148] mitotic figures are not present in typical subependymomas, which are regarded as very slow growing tumours, corresponding to grade I in the WHO grading system.[2] There is usually a

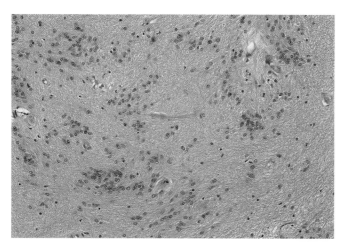

Fig. 6.24 **Subependymoma.** The tumour cell nuclei are gathered into loose clusters separated by abundant, dense, gliofibrillary stroma. H & E.

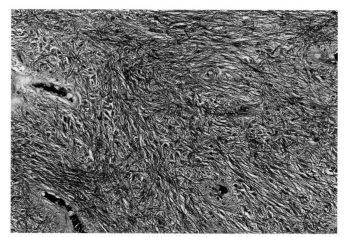

Fig. 6.25 **Subependymoma.** The gliofibrillary stroma is strongly stained with PTAH.

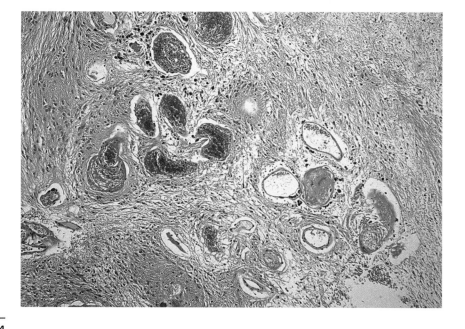

Fig. 6.26 **Subependymoma.** There is thrombosis and hyalinisation of blood vessels, with deposition of haemosiderin pigment. H & E.

circumscribed interface with adjacent nervous tissue, but some of the larger symptomatic tumours may show infiltrative behaviour, with lobules or finger-like extensions protruding deeply into the surrounding brain.[130] Of still more sinister prognostic significance are mixed tumours, which show an abrupt transition with areas of typical ependymoma, including ependymal tubules and well formed perivascular pseudorosettes (Fig. 6.27). Mixed tumours are said to account for up to 15% of symptomatic subependymomas.[127] They generally occur in younger patients and are associated with a more rapid and infiltrative growth pattern.[127,137]

Immunocytochemistry

Both the perinuclear cytoplasm and the gliofibrillary stroma of subependymomas show consistent, strong immunopositivity with antibodies to GFAP.[58,149] There is also a very similar pattern of immunocytochemical staining using antibodies to vimentin.[58]

Electron microscopy

Ultrastructurally, most areas of subependymoma consist of sheets of interweaving cell processes, almost entirely filled with glial type intermediate filaments (Fig. 6.28). Unlike astrocytomas, the cell processes are very closely packed together with little or no visible extracellular space, and are joined by zonula adherentes junctions.[143] They do not form astrocytoma-like foot processes around vascular basement membranes. Some of the tumour cell perikarya are similar to fibrous astrocytes, containing abundant cytoplasmic glial filaments, and these cells give rise to the fibrillary cell processes. Other cells show rudimentary ependymal differentiation, with short surface microvilli and occasional cilia[150] (Fig. 6.28). Although the microvilli are occasionally associated with zonula adherentes junctions, well formed ependymal-type microrosettes with junctional complexes are not usually seen except in mixed tumours with typical ependymomatous areas.[136]

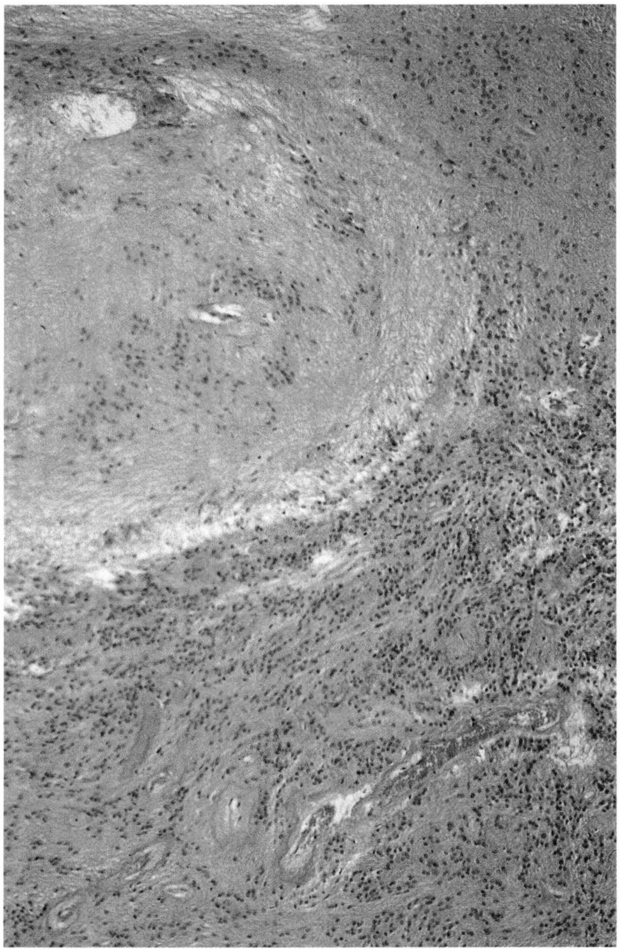

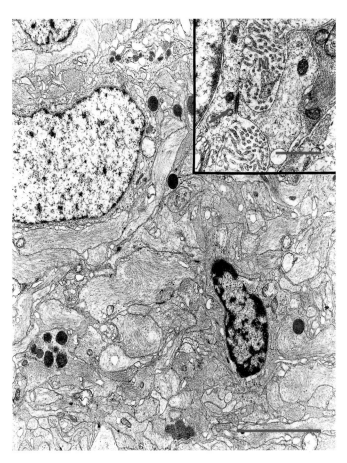

Fig. 6.27 **Mixed ependymoma and subependymoma.** Typical subependymoma (top) blends abruptly into more cellular, ependymoma-like tumour forming perivascular pseudorosettes. H & E.

Fig. 6.28 **Subependymoma.** Ultrastructurally, the tumour consists largely of closely packed cell processes filled with glial filaments. Electron micrograph. Bar = 4 μm. Inset: Some cells may show rudimentary ependymal differentiation, with surface microvilli (M) and associated junctional complexes (arrow) Bar = 1 μm.

Differential diagnosis

Fibrillary astrocytoma

This is the only tumour likely to be confused with subependymoma, but the distinction can be difficult in some cases, especially with intramedullary spinal cord lesions.[133] The presence of a surgical plane of cleavage may help identify subependymomas in this context, but histological distinction from astrocytoma relies largely on demonstrating the typical pattern of 'nested' nuclei and the presence of blepharoplasts. Where doubt remains, electron microscopy will nearly always reveal evidence of rudimentary ependymal differentiation in subependymomas. The close juxtaposition of fibrillary cell processes and absence of perivascular foot processes also aids ultrastructural distinction from fibrillary astrocytomas.

Therapy

Pure subependymomas with no ependymomatous component differ from other ependymal tumours in lacking any capacity for CSF dissemination or systemic metastasis.[2] Even where tumour excision is incomplete, there is little evidence of significant tumour regrowth after prolonged follow up[130] and the success of treatment depends largely on the accessibility of the tumour and the ability to perform an adequate but atraumatic surgical resection.

Total resection is usually possible in supratentorial cases, whether of septal or ventricular wall origin[27,151] and radiotherapy need not be considered.[152] For spinal cord subependymomas, atraumatic surgical removal is technically more difficult, but total or near total removal is often possible,[134,153] especially with the aid of a surgical laser and intraoperative electrophysiological monitoring of spinal cord function.[133] Fourth ventricle lesions pose more of a surgical problem, mainly because of the danger of damaging the vegetative control centres in the floor of the ventricle. Some of these lesions can be easily peeled away from their attachments, but in about half of cases total surgical excision is precluded by nodular infiltration or simply very tenacious attachment to the floor of the ventricle.[27,152] Surgery may have to be curtailed in such circumstances, especially where intraoperative disturbance of respiratory or cardiovascular autoregulation is encountered, and a ventriculoatrial shunt used to treat the obstructive hydrocephalus.[130] When incompletely excised tumours show a histological transition with ependymoma, postoperative radiotherapy is probably advisable.[152]

Prognosis

Prognosis in typical subependymomas is determined largely by surgical factors and is most favourable in the supratentorial lesions, where atraumatic, radical resection is usually possible.[152,154] For fourth ventricular lesions,

published perioperative mortality figures have varied between 30 and 50% of cases,[127,130] although many of these refer to the period before microsurgical technique was established.[154] The prognosis is worst in the largest tumours, especially those which are more rapidly growing and show a mixed histological pattern with ependymomatous areas.[127,152] For those surviving the perioperative period, the long term prognosis is usually very favourable in cases of pure subependymoma. Recurrences are rare and CSF seeding has not been recorded, even if there is radiologically demonstrable residual tumour.[130,154]

Ectopic ependymomas

Ependymomas occurring at primary sites outside the CNS are an uncommon but well documented phenomenon. They can be divided into two groups: those arising in the extraspinal sacral tissues and those originating in the pelvic abdominal cavity.

Parasacral ependymoma

Incidence and site

No incidence figures are available for primary ependymomas of the parasacral region, the largest published series having collected only seven cases.[155] They are, however, more common than ectopic astrocytic tumours at this site. The majority arise either subcutaneously over the posterior aspect of the sacrum or in the soft tissues anterior to it,[156] but examples within the sacral bones have also been described.[157]

Aetiology

Heterotopic ependymal cell nests are probably responsible for those tumours arising anteriorly,[156] whilst the posterior ones are thought to take origin from an embryological ependymal remnant known as the coccygeal medullary vestige.[122,158] This is a remnant of the caudal end of the developing neural tube, and is present in up to 50% of healthy infants,[159] especially where a skin dimple is present.[158,160] The vestige appears histologically as a small cluster of ependymal cells, often showing perivascular myxopapillary change, and is normally biologically indolent.[160]

Clinical features

The age of presentation ranges from infancy to the fifth decade of life with a peak incidence in the third decade.[155,156] Posterior lesions are usually visible and palpable as a subcutaneous mass, often clinically mistaken for a pilonidal sinus.[155,161] Anterior lesions produce the signs and symptoms of a lower abdominal tumour, sometimes with sphincter or sacral root disturbance.[156,162] Many of these tumours are only correctly diagnosed after surgery, but the mass can be well delineated preoperatively by MR or CT scans, and bony erosion of the sacrum may be seen radiologically with the larger lesions. MRI may also be useful in excluding a transdural connection.[156]

Pathology

The tumours are usually well circumscribed, lobulated masses lying within subcutaneous or retroperitoneal soft tissues, although there may be bony attachment or involvement in some cases.[154] Histologically, the majority are typical myxopapillary ependymomas, but occasional examples are non-myxoid papillary ependymomas or anaplastic ependymal tumours, including ependymoblastomas.[163,164] The myxopapillary lesions have histological, immunocytochemical and ultrastructural features indistinguishable from their intradural, cauda equina region counterparts.[122,155]

Differential diagnosis

As with the cauda equina lesions, parasacral myxopapillary ependymomas must be distinguished from other mucinous or myxoid lesions, such as chordomas, chondroid tumours and mucinous metastatic adenocarcinomas. However, the possibility of teratoma should also be considered at a parasacral site, especially if there is any radiological evidence of spina bifida. Where a well differentiated, papillary teratoid neoplasm is suspected, the most useful distinguishing features of ectopic ependymoma are likely to be the absence of recognisable tumour elements derived from germ cell lines other than the neuroectoderm, and the negative immunostaining of the epithelial elements with antibodies to cytokeratin. Negative immunocytochemical staining for teratoma related antigens may also be helpful, including carcinoembryonic antigen, alphafetoprotein and human chorionic gonadotropin.

Therapy and prognosis

Despite their innocent histological appearance, myxopapillary parasacral ependymomas are locally aggressive tumours with a marked tendency to local recurrence.[165,166] This may occur at very long intervals after primary excision, in some cases with a latency of up to 20 years.[155] There is also a significant risk of distant metastasis, with secondary deposits most commonly reported in lymph nodes and lungs.[167,168] The treatment of choice is primary surgical removal, which should be as early and complete as possible to try and prevent local recurrences.[158,169] Although the lesions often appear to shell out easily,[161] surgery should be radical, with wide excision margins.[165] Where the tumour is infiltrating too widely to permit complete surgical excision, local radiotherapy has been recommended postoperatively.[155] The prognosis will clearly depend on the histological type of the tumour, with anaplastic ependymomas carrying a worse prognosis than low grade ones. Even with myxopapillary tumours, however, metastases may occur in up to 20% of cases,[161] and although anecdotal survival of up to 25 years has been reported, the mean postoperative survival of cases in the literature has been estimated at about 10 years.[156]

Intra-abdominal ependymoma

Ectopic ependymomas within the abdominal cavity occasionally arise in the omentum,[170] but are more usually found in association with the female reproductive tract. Sites here include ovary, broad ligament, mesovarium and intersacral ligament.[171–173] The aetiology of these tumours is obscure, since ependymal cell nests are embryologically unlikely in this location, but an origin from a single germ cell line ovarian teratoma has been postulated for some cases.[174] Intra-abdominal ependymomas invariably occur in females, and the clinical presentation is typically in middle life.[171,175] Unlike the parasacral lesions, the histology is most often that of a typical ependymoma, with ependymal rosettes and perivascular pseudorosettes.[173,174] Papillary and anaplastic variants have also been described.[172,174] The important differential diagnosis of these lesions is serous carcinoma of the ovary, and the their ependymal nature needs to be confirmed by immunocytochemical staining for GFAP.[173,174] This may even be possible on cytological aspirates from the tumour.[170] Care should be taken in interpreting the results of immunoreactivity to cytokeratin, since some cases of ectopic ependymoma may show a positive reaction.[171]

Although intra-abdominal ependymomas frequently have a well differentiated histological appearance, they have the capacity to recur locally and metastasise.[172,173] Survival of up to 5 years has been reported, however, and there is some evidence that the prognosis may be linked to the extent of local tumour spread at the time of surgery.[173]

Choroid plexus tumours

Choroid plexus epithelium is a highly specialised tissue of secretory and absorptive function, and the tumours derived from it have many similarities with systemic papillomas and carcinomas. However, choroid plexus epithelium is of neuroepithelial derivation, sharing a common embryologic origin with ependymal cells, and there are good arguments for grouping choroid plexus tumours alongside ependymal neoplasms. In the current WHO classification they are listed under tumours of neuroepithelial tissue, with subdivision into carcinomas and benign papillomas. In contrast to gliomas, there is little evidence for a gradation of malignancy in choroid plexus tumours, and most choroid plexus carcinomas appear to represent primary malignancies, unrelated to a pre-existing benign papilloma. Although villous hypertrophy of the choroid plexus is not generally regarded as a neoplastic process, and therefore does not appear in tumour classifications, it has been included here because of its close relationship with true papillomas of the choroid plexus.

Choroid plexus papilloma

Incidence

Taken as a single group, choroid plexus tumours account for between 0.4 and 0.6% of all intracranial tumours,[176,177] but the incidence is up to 4% in children, and for the first year of life it is usually quoted as being between 9 and 12%.[178,179] This striking predilection for infants means that up to 50% of all choroid plexus tumours present at birth or during the first year of life.[180] In infancy, the sexes are equally represented, but there is a slight bias towards males when all age groups are considered together.[181]

Site

The majority of choroid plexus papillomas arise in the lateral and fourth ventricles, which together account for over three-quarters of cases[182,183] (Fig. 6.29). Those in the lateral ventricles are more often childhood tumours and are usually sited in the region of the trigone.[183,184] They sometimes extend through the foramen of Monro and may grow into the third ventricle or lateral ventricle on the opposite side.[184] In adults, the tumours most often

occur in the fourth ventricle[184] and may extend through the foramen of Luschka into the cerebellopontine angle.[183,184] Rarely the tumours may arise primarily in the cerebellopontine angle[185] and sometimes extend down into the cervical spinal canal.[186]

Aetiology

In adults, choroid plexus papillomas are presumed to take origin from differentiated choroid plexus epithelium, but it has been suggested that some infantile choroid plexus tumours may originate directly from more primitive ventricular lining elements which have retained bipotential differentiating capacity.[187] Certainly congenital cases of choroid plexus papilloma are not uncommon[188,189] and the greater tendency of congenital and infantile cases to be ciliated may be an indication that such tumours develop during the phase when the differentiating fetal choroid plexus is transiently ciliated.[187] Choroid plexus papillomas occur consistently in transgenic mice carrying the genes for Simian virus 40,[190] suggesting that the virus may play a role in tumorigenesis. This is supported by the isolation of SV40 DNA sequences from 50% of human papillomas[191] and by studies showing that the viral DNA sequences can be retrieved and used to infect cultured monkey kidney cells.[192]

Clinical features

In infants and young children, choroid plexus papillomas of the lateral ventricle typically present with progressive hydrocephalus.[181,183] The history is often quite short,[181] and there may also be progressive head enlargement.[193]

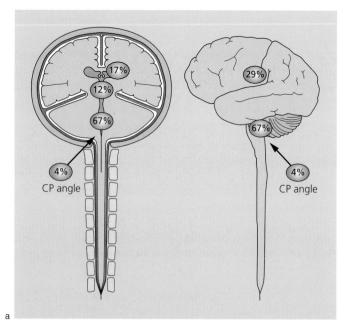

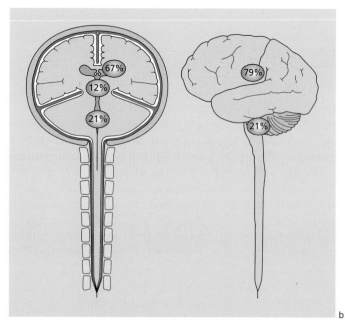

a   b

Fig. 6.29 **Distribution of choroid plexus papillomas in relation to site and age. (a)** Adults. **(b)** Children.

In adults with lateral ventricular tumours, there is usually a longer history which may include headache, paresis, cranial nerve palsies and progressive visual loss.[181,184] With fourth ventricular and cerebellopontine angle tumours, signs and symptoms of hydrocephalus are the most common presentation in all age groups, and may be accompanied by focal features such as ataxia, lower cranial nerve palsies and visual disturbances.[183,184] The hydrocephalus associated with choroid plexus papillomas is usually obstructive in the case of posterior fossa tumours, but up to 30% of lateral ventricle lesions show radiological evidence of a communicating hydrocephalus.[181] This may resolve entirely after complete excision of the tumour,[194] and there is now good evidence that overproduction of CSF by choroid plexus papillomas contributes significantly to tumour associated hydrocephalus, even when there is an element of mechanical obstruction.[181] Preoperative ventricular drainage has yielded much greater volumes of CSF than in cases of simple obstructive hydrocephalus with normal choroid plexus,[195] and ventricular perfusion studies have demonstrated up to 10-fold increases in preoperative CSF production, falling to normal following complete excision of the tumour.[196,197]

Radiology

CT typically reveals a hyperdense intraventricular tumour mass, often with speckled calcification. There is uniform, bright enhancement following administration of intravenous contrast media.[184,198] Using MRI, choroid plexus papillomas usually appear hypodense or isodense relative to brain using T1-weighted images (Fig. 6.30) and hyperdense with T2-weighting.[184,198] In addition to CT or MRI scans, preoperative angiography is often performed to determine the anatomy of the main feeding vessels.[184,199] These are usually choroidal or perforating branches in the case of lateral ventricle papillomas, and branches of the superior or posterior inferior cerebellar arteries for tumours sited in the fourth ventricle.[184,199]

Pathology

Macroscopic features

Choroid plexus papillomas are pinkish-grey masses with a friable, tufted surface resembling that of a cauliflower. On cut section they have a firm, granular texture which is frequently gritty due to extensive calcification. Some examples may show areas of old or recent haemorrhage within the tumour tissue. The tumour mass is usually entirely extraparenchymal and well demarcated from the surrounding brain tissue. Lateral ventricle papillomas often have a pedicle attachment to the choroid plexus in the trigone region. Fourth ventricular lesions may extend out of the lateral recesses and, like those arising in the

cerebellopontine angle, cause compression and distortion of the brain stem. Regardless of site, the tumours are nearly always associated with marked ventricular enlargement. This is usually generalised but may be asymmetric in some cases of lateral ventricle origin.

Intraoperative diagnosis

Choroid plexus papillomas usually make distinctive smear preparations, without the need to resort to frozen sections. The smear appearance closely resembles that of normal choroid plexus, with delicate, well defined papillary structures covered by a regular layer of cuboidal epithelium (Fig. 6.31). Mitotic figures and significant pleomorphism are not usually seen and should arouse suspicion that the lesion is a primary choroid plexus carcinoma or a metastasis. Papilloma tissue tends to be more prominently vascularised than normal choroid plexus, and in places the epithelium may be several cells thick instead of forming a single layer. Nevertheless, care must be taken not to misinterpret normal choroid plexus tissue incorporated into deep burr hole biopsies which inadvertently penetrate a ventricular cavity. The epithelial organisation, well organised papillary architecture and

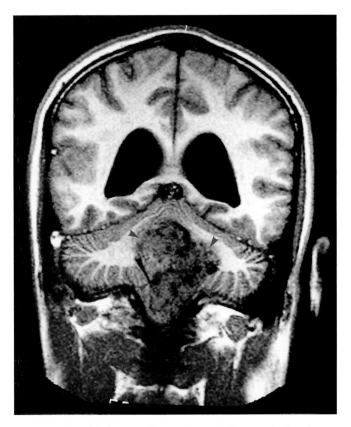

Fig. 6.30 **Choroid plexus papilloma.** Coronal MRI scan of a fourth ventricular tumour. The tumour fills the expanded ventricular cavity (arrowheads) and has a mottled, isodense appearance on this non-enhanced, T1-weighted image.

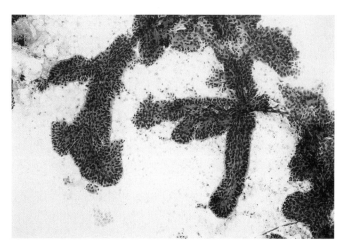

Fig. 6.31 **Choroid plexus papilloma.** Smear preparation. There is a well organised papillary architecture. The appearances are similar to those of normal choroid plexus, although the epithelial layer is often more than one cell in thickness. Toluidine blue.

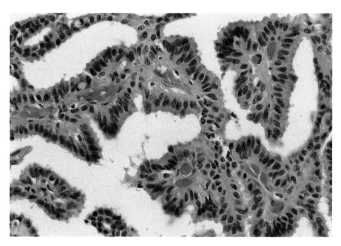

Fig. 6.32 **Choroid plexus papilloma.** The histological appearance is again similar to that of normal choroid plexus, with regular cuboidal epithelium around well vascularised papillary cores. H & E.

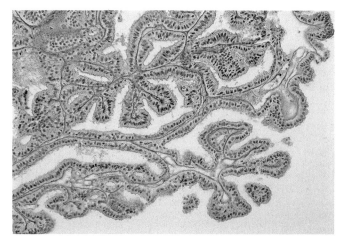

Fig. 6.33 **Choroid plexus papilloma.** The epithelial layer rests on a continuous basement membrane. Reticulin stain.

absence of gliofibrillary material usually make smears of choroid plexus papillomas easy to distinguish from those of ependymoma.

Histological features

Histological sections show sheets of papillary formations, each with a basic architecture similar to that of normal choroid plexus (Fig. 6.32). There is an epithelial layer of cuboidal or columnar cells with regular, rounded, centrally placed nuclei. In places the epithelium may be heaped up and more than one cell thick. The cells rest on a continuous basement membrane (Fig. 6.33). The papillary cores contain scanty collagenous tissue and a rich supply of thin walled blood vessels, and there are no gliofibrillary elements present. The papillary formations are closely packed together and are frequently cross cut or obliquely orientated. The apical surface of the epithelium may show cilia and blepharoplasts in some congenital and infantile examples, but cilia are not usually visible on light microscopy in adult tumours. In most cases, the tumour is histologically well circumscribed and does not breach the ventricular wall, although focal extension into adjacent brain tissue may occasionally be seen in some otherwise entirely benign papillomas. Mitotic figures are not usually found in benign choroid plexus papillomas, and suggest that malignant change may be taking place (Table 6.6). Tumours showing an appreciable mitotic rate may certainly be expected to recur, especially if the tumour is incompletely excised.[187] Typical benign papillomas, however, are regarded as grade I tumours in the WHO classification[182] and lack necrosis, a significant mitotic rate or overtly invasive features. Calcospherites are often abundant in the connective tissue stroma and there may be more extensive, confluent calcification in some cases. Examples with focal ossification have been reported,[200] especially in recurrent tumours following haemorrhage and fibrosis (Fig. 6.34). Rarely, the tumour cells may undergo striking oncocytic change,[201,202] which has also been found in non-neoplastic choroid plexus tissue.[203] Pigmented choroid plexus papillomas have also been reported, in which the tumour cells contain both Fontana stained, bleach sensitive melanin and periodic acid–Schiff (PAS) positive, autofluorescent lipofuscin pigment.[204,205] The melanin in these tumours is thought to derive from melanisation of

Table 6.6 Features suggesting malignancy in choroid plexus tumours

1. Loss of papillary architecture
2. Multilayered epithelium
3. Cytological pleomorphism
4. Mitoses
5. Tumour necrosis
6. Infiltration of adjacent brain

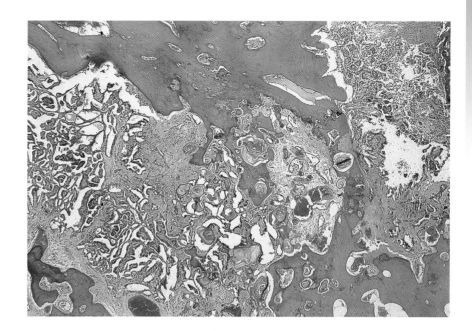

Fig. 6.34 **Choroid plexus papilloma.** Focal ossification is present in the stroma. H & E.

lipofuscin.[205] If there is evidence of mucous secretion, care must be taken not to misdiagnose metastatic adeno-carcinoma, but mucous secreting choroid plexus papillomas may certainly occur, with benign histology and evidence of transition from adjacent normal choroid plexus.[206] They usually contain tall, colomnar, mucous secreting goblet cells staining positively with PAS, and may show acinar structures[207,208] or a more typical papillary architecture.[206]

Immunocytochemistry

The vast majority of choroid plexus papillomas show uniform, strong immunoreactivity with antibodies to both cytokeratin[209,210] and vimentin[210] (Fig. 6.35 and Table 6.7). Most of the tumour cells can be shown to coexpress both antigens simultaneously.[211] A small but significant proportion of tumours also contain scattered cells in the epithelial layer which express immunoreactivity for GFAP.[210,212] Such cells occur in up to a half of all cases, and double labelling studies have shown coexpression of GFAP and cytokeratin in the same cells.[213,214] This phenomenon has been interpreted as evidence of ependymal differentiation in neoplastic choroid plexus cells.[215,216] Nearly all choroid plexus papillomas show consistent, diffuse positive immunostaining with anti-bodies to S-100 protein,[216,217] a feature which is not usually associated with carcinomas of the choroid plexus.[218] Normal choroid plexus is a unique site of transthyretin (prealbumin) synthesis in the CNS,[219] and choroid plexus papillomas also show consistent, intense immunoreactivity with antibodies to transthyretin.[212,220] There is a similar consistent immunoreactivity with antibodies to carbonic anhydrase C in both normal choroid plexus and choroid

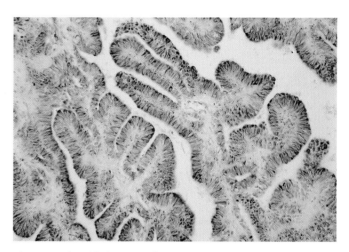

Fig. 6.35 **Choroid plexus papilloma.** The tumour cells are strongly stained using immunocytochemistry for cytokeratin.

Table 6.7 Immunocytochemistry of choroid plexus tumours

Antigen	Papilloma	Carcinoma
Cytokeratin	+	+
Epithelial membrane antigen	–	+ Variable
Carcinoembryonic antigen	–	+ Variable
Glial fibrillary acidic protein	Occasional cells	Occasional cells
S-100 protein	+	– Often
Carbonic anhydrase C	+	+
Transthyretin	+	+ Variable

plexus papillomas, but this has also been reported in other types of tumour, including some ependymomas and carcinomas.[221] Immunoreactivity for EMA has not been found in benign papillomas.[210]

Electron microscopy

Ultrastructurally, the epithelial cells in choroid plexus papillomas show well preserved apical–basal polarity, the apical surfaces bearing a profusion of microvilli (Fig. 6.36). Apical cilia are uncommon except in some congenital and infantile examples[222] and usually show a normal 9 + 2 arrangement of axial tubules.[223] The closely apposed lateral cell surfaces show complex interdigitations but are joined by junctional complexes only near the apical surface. The complexes consist of zonulae adherentes, desmosomes and tight junctions.[224] The basal surfaces of the cells are smooth and separated from perivascular collagen by a continuous basal lamina. The closely juxtaposed capillary vessels show membrane bridged endothelial cell fenestrations. As in normal choroid plexus tissue, the cytoplasmic matrix of adjacent tumour cells may show marked variation in electron density (Fig. 6.36), possibly reflecting differing states of cell hydration.[223,225] In infantile tumours there are often large pools of intracytoplasmic glycogen granules[222] and in adults the tumour cells frequently contain membrane bound, amorphous or lamellar intracytoplasmic inclusions, sometimes associated with filamentous material[225] (Fig. 6.36). These inclusions are also present in increasing size and complexity with ageing of the normal choroid plexus[223] and are probably autophagic in nature.

Tissue culture

Tissue culture of choroid plexus papillomas has consistently produced epithelial sheets of adherent, polygonal cells similar to those seen in cultures of other benign epithelial neoplasms.[226,227] In addition, there is evidence that prolonged culture can produce increasing differentiation in the tumour explants, with development of papillary structures resembling normal choroid plexus.[228] Microvilli, cytoplasmic interdigitation and occasional cilia have also been reported in one case.[229] In keeping with the secretory and absorptive function of normal choroid plexus, cultured papilloma cells may demonstrate intense pinocytic activity,[228] and the tumour cells also show evidence of phagocytic activity when cultures are treated with latex particles.[229]

Differential diagnosis

The regular, epithelial features of benign choroid plexus papillomas and their close histological resemblance to normal choroid plexus tissue normally make them easily distinguishable tumours, especially in view of their circumscribed, intraventricular location. However, other types of well differentiated, intraventricular papillary tumour need to be kept in mind, especially papillary ependymomas and metastatic adenocarcinomas.

Papillary ependymoma

These tumours may have a similar highly organised papillary architecture, but the cells show a less regular epithelial arrangement around the papillae than in choroid plexus papillomas. The individual cytoplasmic margins are relatively poorly defined in papillary ependymomas, and the continuous subepithelial basement membrane of choroid plexus tumours is absent. Cilia and blepharoplasts may be present in both tumour types, especially in children, but unlike choroid plexus tumours there is a prominent fibrillary stroma in the papillary cores of ependymomas, and little or no collagenous elements are present. The gliofibrillary material may be demonstrated using PTAH or immunocytochemistry for GFAP, although it should be remembered that a proportion of choroid plexus papillomas show scattered epithelial cell immunoreactivity for GFAP. Perhaps more usefully, immunocytochemical stains for cytokeratin, carbonic anhydrase C and transthyretin are practically always entirely negative in ependymomas but consistently positive in the epithelial cells of choroid plexus papillomas.

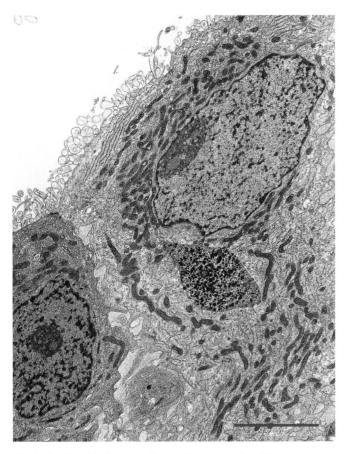

Fig. 6.36 **Choroid plexus papilloma.** Numerous microvillous processes cover the apical tumour cell surfaces. The two adjacent cells in this field show a marked difference in cytoplasmic density. A membrane bound autophagic body is present in the paler cell (asterisk). Electron micrograph. Bar = 4 μm.

Metastatic adenocarcinoma

In older age groups, the choroid plexus is a recognised site of systemic metastases, and using routine stains a well differentiated papillary adenocarcinoma may be difficult to distinguish from choroid plexus papillomas. The presence of goblet cells, mucin production and even acinar formations does not preclude the diagnosis of a primary choroid plexus tumour. Cilia and blepharoplasts may be helpful distinguishing features in some choroid plexus papillomas, but they are usually only seen in infantile examples, where carcinoma metastases are most unlikely. Moreover, both metastatic adenocarcinomas and primary choroid plexus tumours usually show widespread immunoreactivity with antibodies to both cytokeratins and transthyretin. The most reliable method of excluding a metastasis in difficult cases is the use of immunocytochemical staining for carbonic anhydrase C, which is always expressed by choroid plexus papillomas but not found in systemic adenocarcinomas.

Endolymphatic sac tumours

These recently defined tumours are low grade papillary adenocarcinomas arising from the endolymphatic sac epithelium in the bony labrinth of the middle ear.[230] Examples with intracranial spread have previously been mistaken for choroid plexus papillomas arising in the cerebellopontine angle, largely because of the histological similarities. However, even malignant choroid plexus tumours are most unlikely to invade the base of the skull and endolymphatic sac tumours may be distinguished immunocytochemically by the absence of transthyretin expression.

Therapy

Treatment of choroid plexus papillomas is aimed at radical primary surgical excision, which gives the greatest chance of long term cure, regardless of the age at presentation.[189,193] The excision needs to be as complete and meticulous as possible in order to reduce the risk of recurrence or CSF seeding.[231] Complete gross removal has been claimed for up to 90% of lateral ventricle papillomas, but the proportion is much lower for fourth ventricle tumours because of tenacious floor attachments or extension into the cerebellopontine angles.[184] Choroid plexus papillomas are not generally regarded as particularly radiosensitive tumours, and the role of radiotherapy in their treatment remains controversial.[232] There is probably little place for radiation treatment if a complete surgical removal has been achieved,[193] but there is some evidence that postoperative radiotherapy may be effective in reducing tumour size where only partial excision has been possible.[233] Some authorities have also advocated

craniospinal axis irradiation in cases showing radiological evidence of CSF seeding.[184]

The commonest complication associated with the treatment of choroid plexus papillomas is persistent postoperative hydrocephalus.[181] This occurs in a significant proportion of cases, even when there has been complete gross excision of the tumour.[234] The hydrocephalus is typically of communicating type and is due to fibrosis in the basal cistern leptomeninges secondary to chronic leakage of blood from the tumour into the CSF pathways.[181] Local recurrence of benign choroid plexus papillomas is uncommon after complete resection,[233] but where surgical removal has only been partial a significant number of cases require repeated surgical intervention at the primary site, even where postoperative radiotherapy is given.[181] For benign choroid plexus papillomas, seeding in the CSF pathways is again a rather uncommon complication, even in recurrent and partially excised cases,[193] and is said to occur in only about 7% of cases overall.[181] When seeding does occur, it tends to favour older age groups and may be delayed for several years after primary excision.[181,235]

Prognosis

Complete surgical removal of choroid plexus papillomas can be followed by long symptom free periods, in some cases amounting to a permanent cure.[181,236] The longer term prognosis is partly dependent on patient age, and thus indirectly linked to tumour site. For radically resected tumours in adults, most often fourth ventricular in location, symptom free follow up of up to 27 years has been reported with mean survival times of 9–13 years.[183,237] In children, the overall prognosis is less favourable, despite the greater chance of radical removal in lateral ventricle lesions.[183,184] Postoperative survival in infants is more likely to be associated with mental handicap or retardation, especially in those initially presenting with severe hydrocephalus.[181] Subtotal resection is associated with a poorer outcome in all age groups regardless of age,[181,232] although long term symptom free survival has been reported in occasional cases.[232]

Choroid plexus carcinoma

These rare tumours are sometimes referred to as 'malignant choroid plexus papillomas'. They are unequivocally malignant tumours in both clinical and pathological terms and may be regarded as being directly analogous with carcinomas arising in epithelial tissues elsewhere in the body.

Incidence

Choroid plexus carcinomas are extremely rare neoplasms and there is little reliable incidence data. Most reviews have found less than 50 cases documented in the literature where the diagnosis can be substantiated.[238,239] The tumours are more common in children than adults but still account for less than 20% of all choroid plexus neoplasms in children under 15 years[240] and only about 0.5% of all intracranial neoplasms in children less than 12 years.[241] The main peak of age incidence is about 2 years, but exceptional cases have been described in patients up to 60 years of age.[181]

Site

The overwhelming majority of childhood choroid plexus carcinomas arise in one or other lateral ventricle.[184,240] In adults, the tumours may also occur in the fourth ventricle, but the lateral ventricles are again a more common site.[238] Third ventricle lesions have been described but are anecdotal in frequency.[242] Lateral ventricle lesions may invade midline structures to involve the contralateral ventricular cavity,[243] whilst tumours arising in the fourth ventricle frequently extend out into the cerebellopontine angles.[239]

Aetiology

Most choroid plexus carcinomas present as de novo malignant tumours and documented transition between benign and malignant histology is very rare.[244,245] Occasionally, however, cases have been described where histologically malignant CSF seedings or local recurrences have followed primary excision of lesions with largely benign histological features.[187,245] This is said to be more likely if the primary papilloma exhibits a significant mitotic rate at the time of initial surgery.[187] Cytogenetic information is very sparse, but there is some evidence that choroid plexus carcinoma cells are most likely to be hyperhaploid, in contrast to the hyperdiploidy that characterises benign papillomas.[246]

Clinical features

The clinical history is usually shorter than for benign papillomas[184] and is under 6 months in about half of cases.[181] There is usually a rapid downhill course, with headache and vomiting as the most common symptoms.[181] Paresis or cranial nerve palsies occur in just over one-third of cases and hydrocephalus can be detected radiologically in about two-thirds of cases.[181,240] The hydrocephalus is more often obstructive in type, and evidence of CSF oversecretion is less frequently observed than in benign papillomas.[181] The appearances of choroid plexus carcinomas on CT and MRI scans are similar to those of benign papillomas, but with both types of scan there is said to be an increased heterogeneity of signal compared to the benign lesions.[184]

Pathology

Macroscopic features

Choroid plexus carcinomas are friable reddish-grey tumours which expand and distort the ventricular cavity and are often very large by the time of presentation. Massive spread of tumour nodules throughout the ventricular system and subarachnoid space is not an uncommon finding in autopsy studies[243] (Fig. 6.37). The tumours are usually at least partly circumscribed, but frequently show areas where they merge indistinctly with adjacent brain tissue, which is deeply infiltrated in some cases. The tumours have a varied consistency on cut section and often show large areas of central necrosis or haemorrhage.

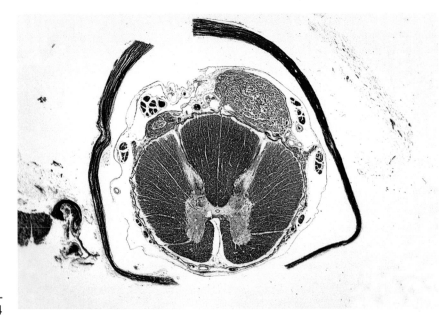

Fig. 6.37 **Choroid plexus carcinoma.** Autopsy spinal cord section from a patient dying with massive spread of tumour in the CSF pathways. Luxol fast blue-cresyl violet.

Intraoperative diagnosis

Smear preparations often show at least some tissue with a similar papillary and epithelial arrangement to that of benign papillomas, but with varying cytological evidence of malignancy. Even in clearly papillary lesions, the presence of frequent mitotic figures should alert suspicion that the lesion may turn out to be a choroid plexus carcinoma rather than a benign papilloma. More clearly malignant tumours show loss of papillary architecture, with marked pleomorphism, vascular proliferation and focal necrosis. In adults, the possibility of an adenocarcinoma metastasis in the choroid plexus needs to be kept in mind when such features are seen on the smears. The papillary architecture of poorly differentiated choroid plexus carcinomas is often more apparent in frozen sections than in smears and exuberant, glomeruloid vascular proliferation is frequently a particularly striking feature. Nevertheless, it may still not be possible to distinguish a choroid plexus carcinoma from a metastasis, which must remain the more likely diagnosis in older patients.

Histological features

The basic papillary architecture of benign papillomas is usually still apparent in some areas of choroid plexus carcinomas, although the growth pattern is generally more disorganised (Table 6.6, p. 170). The epithelial cells are less uniformly arranged around fibrovascular cores and mostly heaped up into several irregular layers (Fig. 6.38). A continuous subepithelial basement membrane is still apparent with reticulin staining, but apical cilia and blepharoplasts are not usually present, even in the infantile tumours. In addition, there are frequently areas of tumour which lack an obvious papillary organisation and consist of solid sheets of poorly differentiated epithelial cells. There is nearly always extensive histological invasion of adjacent brain tissue, and the tumour cells may infiltrate either diffusely or in solid epithelial clumps. There is usually abundant cytological evidence of malignancy, including cellular pleomorphism, nuclear hyperchromatism and atypia, multinucleation and tumour giant cells (Fig. 6.39). Mitotic figures are numerous and focal tumour necrosis may be present. Studies using immunocytochemistry with Ki-67/MIB-1 have shown as many as 60% of cells to be in a proliferative phase of the cell cycle in some choroid plexus carcinomas.[247] Immunocytochemistry has also shown an average growth fraction of 14%, by comparison with only 3.7% in benign papillomas.[248] Care should be taken with otherwise well differentiated, papillary, choroid plexus tumours which show only focal brain infiltration or occasional mitoses, since either feature may occur in benign papillomas without any subsequent evidence of malignant behaviour.[187] Mucous secretion has been

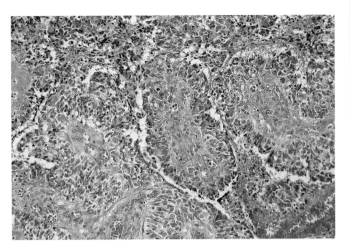

Fig. 6.38 **Choroid plexus carcinoma.** The epithelial layer is irregular and several cells thick. Both solid and papillary areas of tumour are present and there is prominent vascular endothelial proliferation. H & E.

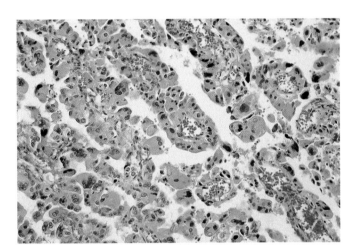

Fig. 6.39 **Choroid plexus carcinoma.** A papillary architecture is still apparent, but the tumour cells show marked cytological atypia. H & E.

described in some putative choroid plexus carcinomas, with a papillary or acinar growth pattern and goblet cells containing PAS staining material.[249] However, there is a danger of misdiagnosing metastatic adenocarcinoma in such circumstances, and great care is needed, especially in older patients (see Differential diagnosis, below). Like the benign papillomas, choroid plexus carcinomas may rarely show accumulation of pigment,[250,251] which is a mixture of Fontana stained, bleach sensitive melanin and lipofuscin. The melanin pigment is present within tumour cell cytoplasm, and is again thought to result from melanisation of lipofuscin.[250]

Immunocytochemistry

In common with their benign counterparts, choroid plexus carcinomas show consistent immunoreactivity with antibodies to cytokeratin,[213] and vimentin[210] (Table 6.7, p. 171). Focal immunostaining of the epithelial cells for GFAP is again present in some cases.[213] Most cases also show at least some staining with antibodies to transthyretin, although in poorly differentiated tumours this may be restricted to a small number of isolated cells[252] (Fig. 6.40). Immunocytochemical expression of EMA has been found in a proportion of choroid plexus carcinomas[210,212] (Fig. 6.41), whereas benign papillomas tested at the same time have not shown positive immunostaining for this antigen.[210] Also in contrast to the benign tumours, choroid plexus carcinomas often express immunoreactivity for carcinoembryonic antigen[212,218] and are more likely to lack expression of S-100 protein.[218] These last two features may relate to the degree of dedifferentiation in the malignant tumours.[218]

Electron microscopy

Ultrastructurally, areas of choroid plexus carcinoma can normally be found which retain many features of benign papillomas, including luminal orientation of cells, apical microvilli, junctional complexes, and a continuous basement membrane separating the basal cell surfaces from connective tissue elements.[253,254] Infantile cases may show pools of cytoplasmic glycogen,[253] but even in infants cilia are very rarely found compared to the benign tumours.[255] Depending on how the tumour is sampled, there are usually also extensive areas consisting of immature, poorly differentiated cells, lacking particular orientation or surface specialisation.[254]

Differential diagnosis

Metastatic adenocarcinoma

Choroid plexus carcinomas may be difficult to distinguish histologically from papillary adenocarcinoma, and metastasis to the choroid plexus from an undisclosed systemic primary tumour must be considered a more likely diagnosis in adult patients, especially if the lesion is obviously malignant or shows evidence of mucous production. Multifocal areas of tumour interspersed by normal looking choroid plexus are more likely to be the result of metastatic disease, whereas a genuine transition of tumour with non-neoplastic choroid plexus epithelium

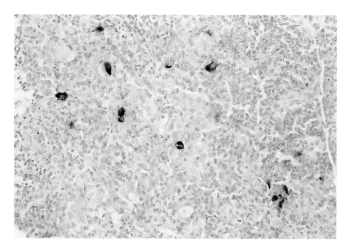

Fig. 6.40 Choroid plexus carcinoma. Most cases show some immunocytochemical expression of transthyretin, although in poorly differentiated tumours like this one the proportion of positively stained cells may be small.

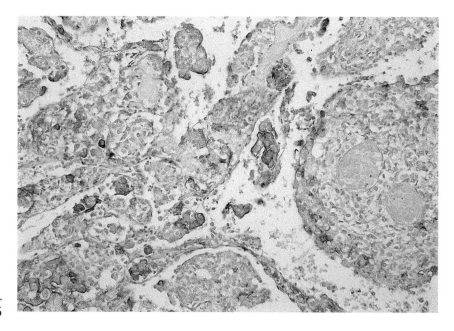

Fig. 6.41 Choroid plexus carcinoma. A proportion of the tumour cells are positively stained using immunocytochemistry for EMA.

is more suggestive of a primary lesion. Immunocyto-chemistry for epithelial antigens is clearly unhelpful in this context, but if immunoreactivity for carbonic anhydrase C, transthyretin or GFAP can be demonstrated, these will all help to identify positively a primary choroid plexus tumour.

Teratoma

Papillary forms of teratoma constitute an important differential diagnosis of choroid plexus carcinoma, especially in young male patients. Teratomas may metastasise to the choroid plexus from undisclosed primary sites, and readily identifiable teratoid elements may be lacking in such metastases, particularly in less well differentiated examples. Immunocytochemical stains for epithelial antigens, including carcinoembryonic antigen, may be positive in either entity and are likely to be unhelpful. Expression of carbonic anhydrase C and transthyretin is useful when present, but can be lacking in some poorly differentiated choroid plexus carcinomas. Positive immunocytochemical staining for alpha-fetoprotein and human chorionic gonadotropin may help identify some forms of germ cell neoplasm, but such antigens are inconstantly expressed in poorly differentiated lesions and a negative result must again be interpreted with caution.

Medulloepithelioma

In infants these tumours may be easily confused with choroid plexus carcinomas, and often show a similar gross circumscription and intraventricular location. The papillary, epithelial organisation of medulloepitheliomas is not unlike that of choroid plexus carcinomas, with a similarly well defined apical surface membrane, fibrovascular core and subepithelial basal lamina. The epithelial layer, however, has a characteristic pseudo-stratified organisation in medulloepithelioma, in contrast to the irregular, multilayered appearance seen in most choroid plexus carcinomas. A careful search should be made for histological evidence of glial or neuronal differentiation, which is present in about half of medullo-epithelioma cases. Immunocytochemical demonstration of transthyretin or carbonic anhydrase C may also help to distinguish choroid plexus carcinoma in these circumstances. Ultrastructurally, medulloepitheliomas show apical junctional complexes but lack the microvilli which can often be demonstrated in choroid plexus carcinomas.

Therapy

Radical surgical excision remains the primary treatment of choice for choroid plexus carcinomas,[184] but resection is frequently limited by local tumour infiltration and complete gross removal of tumour is generally only achieved in a minority of cases.[181,184] Both combination chemotherapy and radiotherapy are useful as adjunct therapies, although craniospinal irradiation seems to be more effective when leptomeningeal seeding is present.[256] Because of the deleterious effects of early irradiation, very young infants are usually treated with prolonged postoperative chemotherapy and delayed radiotherapy[257] or chemotherapy alone.[258]

Prognosis

In contrast to benign papillomas, choroid plexus carcinomas show a significant tendency to disseminate via the CSF pathways.[193] This is said to occur in up to two-thirds of cases,[243] regardless of the effectiveness of treatment of the primary tumour.[259] Malignant cells may be found in the CSF prior to surgical treatment[181] and many cases show massive, confluent dissemination throughout the ventricular system and subarachnoid space by the time of autopsy[243,259] (Fig. 6.37). Local extension of tumour out through the dura may also occur[260] and systemic metastases are not uncommon in longer survivors.[261,262]

Choroid plexus carcinomas are traditionally associated with a universally dismal prognosis, a majority of patients surviving less than 6 months from presentation in older series.[181,184] More recent use of postoperative chemotherapy in infants and children has resulted in longer disease free intervals,[257,258] but cure is still exceptional.[263] Death is usually related to complications of massive local recurrence or widespread CSF dissemination.[181] Patients in whom only partial excision of the tumour has been possible have the worst outcome, often dying within a few months of surgery, and the best chance of long term survival is where early and total excision of the tumour has been achieved.[193,258]

Villous hypertrophy of the choroid plexus

This extremely rare condition was first described in 1924[264] and is characterised by diffuse enlargement of the choroid plexuses. Only a handful of cases have been reported in the literature,[181] and most have presented at birth or shortly after, suggesting that a congenital process is involved.[265] The clinical presentation is that of hydrocephalus, which is of a communicating type in most cases and almost certainly the result of CSF oversecretion by the abnormal bulk of choroid plexus tissue. This has been supported by sequential falling of CSF outflow measurements following unilateral and subsequent bilateral excision of the abnormal tissue.[194] In most cases, the enlargement is confined to the choroid plexuses in the lateral ventricles,[181,194] but unlike bilateral choroid plexus papillomas, the process involves the entire length of the choroidal fissures, without circumscribed origin from a pedicle.[265] In occasional cases the fourth ventricle choroid plexus may also be involved.[266]

The gross appearance is that of enlarged but otherwise entirely typical choroid plexus tissue running the length of the dilated ventricles. The total mass of abnormal tissue may be up to 7.5 g, or 10 times the normal weight of the choroid plexuses for the age.[181] Histologically, the appearances are indistinguishable from normal choroid plexus, again suggesting that the lesion is a congenital hypertrophy and not a true neoplastic proliferation. Satisfactory treatment of the condition nonetheless requires complete excision of the enlarged choroid plexuses, which entails a significant operative risk in view of their extreme vascularity.[181] However, if a successful and complete excision is achieved, a permanent cure may be possible, with resolution of the hydrocephalus and no necessity for CSF shunting.[194,265]

REFERENCES

Ependymoma and anaplastic ependymoma

1. Kleihaus P, Burger PC, Scheithauer BW et al. Histological typing of tumours of the central nervous system, 2nd edn. Berlin: Springer, 1993
2. Zulch KJ Brain tumours. Their biology and pathology, 3rd edn. Berlin: Springer, 1986: pp 258–276
3. Mork SJ, Rubinstein LJ. Ependymoblastoma. A reappraisal of a rare embryonal tumour. Cancer, 1985; 55:1536–1542
4. Cruz-Sanchez FF, Haustein J, Rossi ML et al. Ependymoblastoma: A histological, immunohistological and ultrastructural study of five cases. Histopathology, 1988; 12:17–27
5. Arendt A. Ependymomas. In: Vinken PT, Bruyn GW, eds. Handbook of clinical neurology, vol. 18. Tumours of the brain and skull, part III. Amsterdam: North Holland, 1975: pp 105–150
6. Svein HJ, Mabon RF, Kernohan JW et al. Ependymoma of the brain: pathologic aspects. Neurology, 1953; 3:1–15
7. Mork SJ, Loken AC. Ependymoma. A follow-up study of 101 cases. Cancer, 1977; 40:907–915
8. Fried H, Skrzypczak J, Hohrein D. Spinal gliomas including ependymomas. Zentralbl Neurochir, 1988; 49:273–275
9. Kun LE, Kovnar EH, Sanford RA. Ependymomas in children. Pediatr Neurosci, 1988; 14:57–63
10. Madon E, Besenzon L, Brach-del-Prever A et al. Results of a multicenter retrospective study on pediatric brain tumours in Italy. Tumori, 1986; 72:285–292
11. Ilgren EB, Stiller CA, Hughes JT et al. Ependymomas: A clinical and pathologic study. Part I. Biologic features. Clin Neuropathol, 1984; 3:113–121
12. Namer IJ, Pamir MN, Benli K et al. Intracranial ependymomas. Study of 81 cases and comparison with the literature. Neurochirurgie, 1984; 30:153–158
13. Shuman RM, Alvord ECJ, Leech R. The biology of childhood ependymomas. Arch Neurol, 1975; 32:731–739
14. Barone BM, Elvidge AR. Ependymomas: A clinical survey. J Neurosurg, 1970; 33:428–438
15. Packer RJ, Schut L, Sutton LN et al. Brain tumours of the posterior cranial fossa in infants and children. In : Youmans JR, ed. Neurological surgery, 3rd edn. Philadelphia: WB Saunders, 1990: pp 3017–3039
16. Rawlings CE, Giangaspero F, Burger PC et al. Ependymomas: A clinicopathologic study. Surg Neurol, 1988; 29:271–281
17. Liu HM, McLone DG, Clark S. 1988; Ependymomas of childhood. Childs Brain, 1977; 3:281–296
18. Friede RL, Pollak A. The cytogenetic basic for classifying ependymomas. J Neuropathol Exp Neurol, 1978; 37:103–118
19. Heye N, Iglesias J, Huber S et al. Congenital ependymoma. Case

20. Savard ML, Gilchrist DM. Ependymomas in two sisters and a maternal male cousin with mosaicism with monosomy 22 in tumour. Pediatr Neurosci, 1989; 15:80–84
21. Park JP, Chaffee S, Noll WW et al. Constitutional de novo t(1;22)(p22;q11.2) and ependymoma. Cancer Genet Cytogenet, 1996; 86:150–152
22. Rubio MP, Correa KM, Ramesh V et al. Analysis of the neurofibromatosis 2 gene in human ependymomas and astrocytomas. Cancer Res, 1994; 54:45–47
23. Nijssen PC, Deprez RH, Tijssen CC et al. Familial anaplastic ependymoma: evidence of loss of chromosome 22 in tumour cells. J Neurol Neurosurg Psychiatry, 1994; 57:1245–1248
24. von Haken MS, White EC, Daneshvar-Shyesther L et al. Molecular genetic analysis of chromosome arm 17p and chromosome arm 22q sequences in sporadic pediatric ependymomas. Genes Chromosomes Cancer, 1996; 17:37–44
25. Neumann E, Kalousek DK, Norman MG et al. Cytogenetic analysis of 109 pediatric central nervous system tumours. Cancer Genet Cytogenet, 1993; 71:40–49
26. Dohrmann GJ, Farwell JR, Flannery JT. Ependymomas and ependymoblastomas in children. J Neurosurg, 1976; 45:273–283
27. Harsh GR, Wilson CB. Neuroepithelial tumours of the adult brain. In: Youmans JR, ed. Neurological surgery, 3rd edn. Philadelphia: WB Saunders, 1990: pp 3040-3136
28. Haller P, Patzold U. Diagnostic value of epileptic siezures for location and morphology of brain tumours: Contribution to preferred localisation of cerebral neoplasms. J Neurol, 1973; 203:311–336
29. Carragher AM, Heatley MK, Mirakhur M et al. A clinicopathological review of spinal ependymomas in Northern Ireland. Ulster Med J, 1990; 59:51–54
30. Griffin BR, Shuman WP Wisbeck W et al. Improved localization of infratentorial ependymoma by magnetic resonance imaging: Implications for radiation treatment planning. J Neurooncol, 1988; 6:147–155
31. Just M, Schwarz M, Higer HP et al. MR tomography in tumors of the posterior cranial fossa in childhood. Rofo Fortschr Geb Rontgenstr Neuen Bildgeb Verfahr, 1988; 148:195–199
32. Zee CS, Segall HD, Ahmadi J et al. Computed tomography of posterior fossa ependymomas in childhood. Surg Neuro, 1983; 20:221–226
33. Van-Tassel P, Lee YY, Bruner JM. Supratentorial ependymomas: Computed tomographic and pathologic correlations. J Comput Tomogr, 1986; 10:157–165
34. Armington WG, Osborn AG, Cubberley DA et al. Supratentorial ependymoma: CT appearance. Radiology, 1985; 157:367–372
35. Tomita T, McLone DG, Naidich TP. Mural tumors with cysts in the cerebral hemispheres of children. Neurosurgery, 1986; 19:998–1005
36. Liote H, Spaulding C, Vedrenne C et al. Thoracic metastases of ependymoma. Apropos of a case and review of the literature. Rev Pneumol Clin, 1988; 44:94–100
37. Courville CB, Broussahan SL. Plastic ependymomas of the lateral recess. Report of eight verified cases. J Neurosurg, 1961; 18:792–799
38. Kricheff II, Becker M, Schneck SA et al. Intracranial ependymomas: Factors influencing prognosis. J Neurosurg, 1964; 21:7–14
39. Zülch KJ, Kleinsasser O. Ortsgebundese Abireschungen in der Histologie und inc biologischen Verhalten der Ependymome. Zentralbl Allg Pathol, 1957; 97:59–66
40. Scharrer VE, Heiming E. Trabeculär-papilläres Ependymom über der Sakrokokzygeal region. Zentralbl Neurochir, 1974; 35:131–161
41. Kawano N, Yada K, Yagishita S. Clear cell ependymoma. A histological variant with diagnostic implications. Virchows Arch (A), 1989; 415:467–472
42. Kawano N, Yada K, Aihara M et al. Oligodendroglioma-like cells (clear cells) in ependymoma. Acta Neuropathol, (Berl), 1983; 62:141–144
43. Mathews T, Mooss Y. Gliomas containing bone and cartilage. J Neuropathol Exp Neurol, 1974; 33:456–471
44. Siqueira EB, Bucy PC. Chondroma arising within a mixed glioma. J Neuropathol Exp Neurol, 1966; 25:667–673
45. Rosenblum MK, Erlandson RA, Aleksic SN et al. Melanotic ependymoma and subependymoma. Am J Surg Pathol, 1990; 14:729–736
46. McCluskey JJ, Parker JC Jr, Brooks WH et al. Melanin as a component

report and immunohistochemical studies. Zentralbl Allg Pathol, 1989; 135:43–49

of cerebral gliomas. The melanotic cerebral ependymoma. Cancer, 1976; 37:2373–2379

47. Rubinstein LJ. The definition of the ependymoblastoma. Arch Pathol, 1970; 90:35–45

48. Shaw EG, Evans RG, Scheithauer BW et al. Postoperative radiotherapy of intracranial ependymoma in pediatric and adult patients. Int J Radiat Oncol Biol Phys, 1987; 13:1457–1462

49. Ernestus RI, Wilcke O, Schroder R. Intracranial ependymomas: Prognostic aspects. Neurosurg Rev, 1989; 12:157–163

50. Salazar OM. A better understanding of CNS seeding and a brighter outlook for postoperatively irradiated patients with ependymomas. Int J Radiat Oncol Biol Phys, 1983; 9:1231–1234

51. Figarella-Branger D, Gambarelli D, Dollo C et al. Infrantentorial ependymomas of childhood. Correlation between histological features, immunohistological phenotype, silver nucleolar organiser region staining values and post-operative survival in 16 cases. Acta Neuropathol (Berl) 1991; 82:208–216

52. Pierre-Kahn A, Hirsch JF, Roux FX et al. Intracranial ependymomas in childhood. Survival and functional results of 47 cases. Childs Brain, 1983; 10:145–156

53. Mork SJ, Risberg G, Krogness K. Anaplastic ependymomas. Neuropathol Appl Neurobiol, 1980; 6:307–311

54. Gottschalk J, Szymas J. Significance of immunohistochemistry for neurooncology. VI. Occurrence, localization and distribution of glial fibrillary acid protein (GFAP) in 820 tumours. Zentralbl Allg Pathol, 1987; 133:319–330

55. Pasquier B, Lachard A, Pasquier D et al. Glial fibrillary acidic protein and central nervous tumors. Immunohistochemical study of a series of 207 cases. 1: Astrocytomas. Glioblastomas. Ependymomas, Papillomas of the choroid plexus. Ann Pathol, 1983; 3:127–135

56. Cruz-Sanchez FF, Rossi ML, Esiri MM et al. Epithelial membrane antigen expression in ependymomas. Neuropathol Appl Neurobiol, 1988; 14:197–205

57. Kimura T, Budka H, Soler-Federsppiel S. An immunocytochemical comparison of the glia-associated proteins glial fibrillary acidic protein (GFAP) and S-100 protein (S100P) in human brain tumours. Clin Neuropathol, 1986; 5:21–27

58. Izukawa D, Lach B. Immunocytochemical analysis of intermediate filaments in human ependymal tumors. Can J Neurol Sci, 1988; 15:114–118

59. Nakamura Y, Becker LE, Marks A. Distribution of immunoreactive S-100 protein in pediatric brain tumors. J Neuropathol Exp Neurol, 1983; 42:136–145

60. Uematsu Y, Rojas-Corona RR, Llena JF et al. Distribution of epithelial membrane antigen in normal and neoplastic human ependyma. Acta Neuropathol (Berl), 1989; 78:325–328

61. Cruz-Sanchez FF, Rossi ML, Hughes JT et al. An immunohistological study of 66 ependymomas. Histopathology, 1988; 13:443–454

62. Kaneko Y, Takeshita I, Matsushima T et al. Immunohistochemical study of ependymal neoplasms: Histological subtypes and glial and epithelial characteristics. Virchows Archiv (A), 1990; 417:97–103

63. Miettinen M, Clark R, Virtanen I. Intermediate filament proteins in choroid plexus and ependyma and their tumors. Am J Pathol, 1986; 123:231–240

64. Ang LC, Taylor AR, Bergin D et al. An immunohistochemical study of papillary tumors in the central nervous system. Cancer, 1990; 65:2712–2719

65. Haustein J, Cruz-Sanchez F, Cervos-Navarro J. On the ultrastructure of ependymomas: A semiquantitative analysis of diagnostic criteria in 21 cases with special reference to glycogen as a marker. Neurosurg Rev, 1988; 11:67–76

66. Moss TH. Tumours of the nervous system. An ultrastructural atlas. Berlin: Springer, pp 17–23

67. Tani E, Higashi N. Intercellular junctions in human ependymomas. Acta Neuropathol (Berl), 1972; 22:295–304

68. Goebel HH, Cravioto H. Ultrastructure of human and experimental ependymomas. J Neuropathol Exp Neurol, 1972; 31:55–71

69. Ho KL. Abnormal cilia in a fourth ventricular ependymoma. Acta Neuropathol (Berl), 1986; 70:30–37

70. Friede RL, Pollak A. The cytogenetic basis for classifying ependymomas. J Neuropathol Exp Neurol, 1978; 37:103–118

71. Kubota T, Ishise J, Yamashima T et al. Abnormal cilia in a malignant ependymoma. Acta Neuropathol (Berl) 1986; 71:100–105

72. Spaar FW, Blech M, Ahyai A. DNA flow fluorescence-cytometry of ependymomas. Report on ten surgically removed tumours. Acta Neuropathol (Berl), 1986; 69:153–160

73. Nagashima T, Hoshino T, Cho KG et al. The proliferative potential of human ependymomas measured by in situ bromodeoxyuridine labeling. Cancer, 1988; 61:2433–2438

74. Schroder R, Ploner C, Ernestus RI. The growth potential of ependymomas with varying grades of malignancy measured by the Ki-67 labelling index and mitotic index Neurosurg Rev, 1993; 16:145–150

75. Nakagawa Y, Hirakawa K, Ueda K et al. Establishment of a human ependymoma cell line. No To Shinkei, 1983; 35:283–288

76. Batzdorf U, Pokress SM. Architectural features of ependymomas in tissue culture. J Neuropathol Exp Neurol, 1968; 27:333–347

77. Liss L. The use of tissue cultures in the study of brain tumours. Prog Exp Tumour Res, 1972; 17:93–110

78. Casentini L, Gullotta F, Momper U. Clinical and morphological investigations on ependymomas and their tissue culture. Neurochirugia (Stuttg), 1981; 24:51–56

79. Lumsden CE. The study by tissue culture of tumours of the nervous system. In: Russell DS, Rubinstein LJ, eds. Pathology of tumours of the nervous system, 3rd edn. London: Edward Arnold, 1971; pp 373–375

80. Vraa-Jenson J, Herman MM, Rubinstein LJ et al. In vitro characteristics of a fourth ventricle ependymoma maintained in organ culture systems. Neuropathol Appl Neurobiol, 1976; 2:349–364

81. Deck JHN. Cerebral medulloepithelioma with maturation into ependymal cells and ganglion cells. J Neuropathol Exp Neurol, 1969; 28:442–454

82. Papadopoulos DP, Giri S, Evans RG. Prognostic factors and management of intracranial ependymomas. Anticancer Res, 1990; 10:689–692

83. Fornari M, Pluchino F, Solero CL et al. Microsurgical treatment of intramedullary spinal cord tumours. Acta Neurochir Suppl (Wien), 1988; 43:3–8

84. Peschel RE, Kapp DS, Cardinale F et al. Ependymomas of the spinal cord. Int J Radiat Oncol Biol Phys, 1983; 9:1093–1096

85. Evans AE, Anderson JR, Lefkowitz-Boudreaux IB et al. Adjuvant chemotherapy of childhood posterior foss ependymoma: cranio-spinal irradiation with or without adjuvant CCCNU vincristine, and prednisilone: a Children's Cancer Group study. Med Pediatr Oncol, 1996; 27:8–14

86. Grill J Kulifa C, Doz F et al. A high-dose busulphan-thiotepa combination followed by autologous bone marrow transplantation in childhood recurrent ependymoma. A phase II study. Pediatr Neurosurg, 1996; 25:7–12

87. White L, Johnson H, Jones R et al. Postoperative chemotherapy without radiation in young children with malignant non-astrocytic brain tumours. A report from the Australia and New Zealand Childhood Cancer Study Group (ANZCCSG). Cancer Chemotherapy Pharmacol, 1993; 32:403–406

88. Tomita T, McLone DG, Das L et al. Benign ependymomas of the posterior fossa in childhood. Paediatr Neurosci, 1988; 14:277–285

89. Nazar GB, Hoffman HJ, Becker LE et al. Infratentorial ependymomas in childhood: Prognostic factors and treatment. J Neurosurg, 1990; 72:408–417

90. Ernestus RI, Wilcke O. Spinal metastases of intracranial ependymomas. Four case reports and review of the literature. Neurosurg Rev, 1990; 13:147–154

91. Bloom HJ. Intracranial tumours: Response and resistance to therapeutic endeavours. Int J Radiat Oncol Biol Phys, 1982; 8:1083–1113

92. Renaudin JW, DiTullio MV, Brown WJ. Seeding of intracranial ependymomas in children. Childs Brain, 1979; 5:408–412

93. Packer RJ, Siegel KR, Slaton LV et al. Leptomeningeal dissemination of primary central nervous system tumours of childhood. Ann Neurol, 1985; 18:217–221

94. Wakabayashi T, Yoshida J, Kuchiwaki H et al. Extraneural metastases of malignant ependymoma inducing atelectasis and superior vena cava syndrome. A case report and review of the literature. No Shinkei Geka, 1986; 14:59–65

95. Schreiber D, Schneider J, Heller T et al. Intracranial ependymoma with extraneural metastases. Zentralbl Allg Pathol, 1989; 135:57–64

96. Ferracini R, Manetto V, Poletti V et al. A cerebral ependymoma with extracranial metastases. Tumori, 1984; 70:389–392
97. Itoh J, Usui K, Itoh M et al. Extracranial metastases of malignant ependymoma. Case report. Neurol Med Chir (Tokyo), 1990; 30:339–345
98. Rubinstein LJ, Logan WJ. Extraneural metastases in ependymoma of the cauda equina. J Neurol Neurosurg Psychiatry, 1970; 33:763–770
99. Dunst J, Klinger M, Thierauf P. Ependymoma with cervical lymph node metastases. Klin Padiatr, 1987; 199:19–21
100. Di-Marco A, Campostrini F, Pradella R et al. Postoperative irradiation of brain ependymomas. Analysis of 33 cases. Acta Oncol, 1988; 27:261–267
101. Read G. The treatment of ependymoma of the brain or spinal canal by radiotherapy. A report of 79 cases. Clin Radiol, 1984; 35:163–166
102. Garret PG, Simpson WJ. Ependymomas: Results of radiation treatment. Int J Radiat Oncol Biol Phys, 1983; 9:1121–1124
103. Di-Marco A, Griso C, Pradella R et al. Postoperative management of primary spinal cord ependymomas. Acta Oncol, 1988; 27:371–375
104. Afra D, Muller W, Slowik F et al. Supratentorial lobar ependymomas: Reports on the grading and survival periods in 80 cases, including 46 recurrences. Acta Neurochir (Wien), 1983; 69:243–251
105. Chin HW, Hasel JJ, Kim TH et al. Intracranial ependymomas and ependymoblastomas. Strahlentherapie, 1984; 160:191–194

Myxopapillary ependymoma

106. Davis C, Barnard RO. Malignant behavior of myxopapillary ependymoma. Report of three cases. J Neurosurg, 1985; 62:925–929
107. Chan HSL, Becker LE, Hoffman HJ et al. Myxopapillary ependymoma of the filum terminale and cauda equina in childhood: Report of seven cases and review of the literature. Neurosurgery, 1984; 14:204–210
108. Rivierez M, Oueslati S, Philippon J et al. Ependymoma of the intradural filum terminale in adults. 20 cases. Neurochirurgie, 1990; 36:96–107
109. Sharma A. Myxopapillary ependymomas arising from nerve roots of the spinal cord. J Neurol Neurosurg Psychiatry, 1991; 54:563–564
110. Warnick RE, Raisanen J, Adornato BT et al. Intracranial myxopapillary ependymoma: case report. J Neurooncol, 1993; 15:251–256
111. Sonneland PR, Scheithauer BW, Onofrio BM. Myxopapillary ependymoma A clinicopathologic and immunocytochemical study of 77 cases. Cancer, 1985; 56:883–893
112. Tarlov IM. Structure of the filum terminale. Arch Neurol Psychiatry, 1938; 40:1–17
113. Miller C. The ultrastructure of the conus medullaris and filum terminale. J Comp Neurol, 1968; 132:547–566
114. Chow CW, Brittingham J. Perivascular pseudorosettes in childhood brain tumour: An ultrastructural and immunohistochemical study. Pathology, 1987; 19:12–16
115. Rawlinson DG, Herman MM, Rubinstein LJ. The fine structure of a myxopapillary ependymoma of the filum terminale. Acta Neuropathol (Berl), 1973; 25:1–13
116. Wolff JR, Hosli E, Hosli L. Basement membrane material and glial cells in spinal cord cultures of newborn rat. Brain Res, 1971; 32:198–202
117. Rawlinson DG, Rubinstein LJ, Herman MM. In vitro characteristics of a myxopapillary ependymoma of the filum terminale maintained in tissue and organ culture systems. Light and electron microscopic observations. Acta Neuropathol (Berl), 1974; 27:185–200
118. Kahan H, Sklar EM, Post MJ et al. MR characteristics of histopathological subtypes of spinal ependymoma. Am J Neuroradiol, 1996; 17:143–150
119. Specht CS, Smith TW, DeGirolami U et al. Myxopapillary ependymoma of the filum terminale. A light and electron microscopic study. Cancer, 1986; 58:310–317
120. Gottschalk J, Dopel SH, Schulz J et al. Significance of immunohistochemistry in neurooncology. V. Keratin as a marker for epithelial differentiation of primary and secondary intracranial and intraspinal tumours. Zentralbl Allg Pathol, 1987; 133:133–145
121. Ho KL. Intercellular septate-like junction of neoplastic cells in myxopapillary ependymoma of the filum terminale. Acta Neuropathol (Berl), 1990; 79:432–437
122. Wolff M, Santiago H, Dury MM. Delayed distant metastases from a subcutaneous sacrococcygeal ependymoma. Case report, with tissue culture, ultrastructural observations and review of the literature. Cancer, 1972; 30:1046–1067

123. Scott M. Infiltrating ependymomas of the cauda equina. Treatment by conservative surgery plus radiotherapy. J Neurosurg, 1974; 41:446–448

Subependymoma

124. Boykin FC, Cowen D, Ianucu CAJ. Subependymal glomerulate astrocytomas. J Neuropath Exp Neurol, 1954; 13:30–49
125. French JD, Bucy PC. Tumours of septum pellucidum. J Neurosurg, 1948; 5:433–449
126. Chason JL. Subependymal mixed gliomas. J Neuropathol Exp Neurol, 1956; 15:461–470
127. Scheithauer BW. Symptomatic subependymoma. Report of 21 cases with review of the literature. J Neurosurg, 1978; 49:689–696
128. Matsumura A, Ahyai A, Hori A et al. Intracerebral subependymomas. Clinical and neuropathological analyses with special reference to the possible existence of a less benign variant. Acta Neurochir (Wien), 1989; 96:15–25
129. Rea GL, Akerson RD, Rockswold GL et al. Subependymoma in a 2 1/2 year old boy. Case report. J Neurosurg, 1983; 59:1088–1091
130. Jooma R, Torrens MJ, Bradshaw J et al. Subependymomas of the fourth ventricle. Surgical treatment in 12 cases. J Neurosurg, 1985; 62:508–512
131. Nishio S, Fujiwara S, Tashima T et al. Tumors of the lateral ventricular wall, especially the septum pellucidum: Clinical presentation and variations in pathological features. Neurosurgery, 1990; 27:224–230
132. Guha A, Resch L, Tator CH. Subependymoma of the thoracolumbar cord. Case report. J Neurosurg, 1989; 71:781–787
133. Salcman M, Mayer R. Intramedullary subependymoma of the cervical spinal cord: Case report. Neurosurgery, 1984; 14:608–611
134. Vaquero J, Martinez R, Vegazo I et al. Subependymoma of the cervical spinal cord. Neurosurgery, 1989; 24:625–627
135. Matsumura A, Hori A, Spoerri O. Spinal subependymoma presenting as an extramedullary tumor: Case report. Neurosurgery, 1988; 23:115–117
136. Fu YS, Chen ATL, Kay S et al. Is subependymoma (subependymal glomerulate astrocytoma) an astrocytoma or an ependymoma? A comparative ultrastructural and tissue culture study. Cancer, 1974; 34:1992–2008
137. Russell DS, Rubinstein LJ. Pathology of tumours of the nervous system, 5th Edn. London: Edward Arnold, 1989: pp 192–219
138. Fenstermaker RA, Ganz E, Roessmann U. Giant invasive intracerebral dermoid tumour with subependymoma-like reaction: Case report. Neurosurgery, 1989; 25:646–648
139. Tolnay M, Kaim A, Probst A et al. Subependymoma of the third ventricle after partial resection of a craniopharyngioma and repeated postoperative irradiation. Clin Neuropathol, 1996; 15:63–66
140. Honan WP, Anderson M, Carey MP et al. Familial subependymomas. Br J Neurosurg, 1987; 1:317–321
141. Clarenbach P, Kleihues P, Metzel E et al. Simultaneous clinical manifestation of subependymoma of the fourth ventricle in identical twins. J Neurosurg, 1979; 50:655–659
142. Ho KL. Concurrence of subependymoma and heterotopic leptomeningeal neuroglial tissue. Arch Pathol Lab Med, 1983; 107:136–140
143. Moss TH. Observations on the nature of subependymoma: An electron microscopic study. Neuropathol Appl Neurobiol, 1984; 10:63–75
144. Hehman K, Norrell H, Howieson J. Subependymomas of the septum pellucidum. Report of two cases. J Neurosurg, 1968; 29:640–644
145. Stevens JM, Kendall BE, Love S. Radiological features of subependymoma with emphasis on computed tomography. Neuroradiology, 1984; 26:223–228
146. Maiuri F, Gangemi M, Iaconetta G et al. Symptomatic subependymomas of the lateral ventricles. Report of eight cases. Clin Neurol Neurosurg, 1997; 99:17–22
147. Spoto GP, Press GA, Hesselink JR et al. Intracranial ependymoma and subependymoma: MR manifestations. Am J Roentgenol, 1990; 154:837–845
148. Matsumura A, Ahyai A, Hori A. Symptomatic subependymoma with nuclear polymorphism. Neurosurg Rev, 1987; 10:291–293
149. Yamasaki T, Kikuchi H, Yamashita J et al. Subependymoma of the septum pellucidum radiologically indistinguishable from cavernous angioma. Case report. Neurol Med Chir; (Tokyo), 1989; 29:1020–1025
150. Azzarelli B, Rekate HL, Roessmann U. Subependymoma. A case report with ultrastructural study. Acta Neuropathol (Berl), 1977; 40:279–282

151. Yamasaki T, Kikuchi H, Higashi T et al. Two surgically cured cases of subependymoma with emphasis on magnetic resonance imaging. Surg Neurol, 1990; 33:329–335
152. Vaquero J, Herrero J, Cabezudo JM et al. Symptomatic subependymomas of the lateral ventricles. Acta Neurochirurg (Wein), 1980; 53:99–105
153. Jallo GI, Zagzag D, Epstein F. Intramedullary subependymoma of the spinal cord. Neurosurgery, 1996; 38:251–257
154. Ernestus RI, Schroder R. Clinical aspects of intracranial subependymoma. 18 personal cases and review of the literature. Neurochirurgia, 1993; 36:194–202

Ectopic ependymoma

155. Anderson MS. Myxopapillary ependymomas presenting in the soft tissue over the sacrococcygeal region. Cancer, 1966; 19:585–590
156. Morantz RA, Kepes JJ, Batnttzky S et al. Extraspinal ependymomas. Report of three cases. J Neurosurg, 1979; 51:383–391
157. Miralbell R, Louis DN, O'Keefe D et al. Metastatic ependymoma of the sacrum. Cancer, 1990; 65:2353–2355
158. Ciraldo AV, Platt MS, Agamanolis DP et al. Sacrococcygeal myxopapillary ependymomas and ependymal rests in infants and children. J Pediatr Surg, 1986; 21:49–52
159. Bale PM. Ependymal rests and subcutaneous sacrococcygeal ependymoma. Pathology, 1980; 12:237–243
160. Pulitzer DR, Martin PC, Collins PC et al. Subcutaneous sacrococcygeal ('myxopapillary') ependymal rests. Am J Surg Pathol, 1988; 12:672–677
161. Helwig EB, Stern JB. Subcutaneous sacrococcygeal myxopapillary ependymoma. A clinicopathologic study of 32 cases. Am J Clin Pathol, 1984; 81:156–161
162. Gerston KF, Suprun H, Cohen H et al. Presacral myxopapillary ependymoma presenting as an abdominal mass in a child. J Pediatr Surg, 1985; 20:276–278
163. Murphy MN, Dhalla SS, Diocee M et al. Congenital ependymoblastoma presenting as a sacrococcygeal mass in a newborn: An immunohistochemical, light and electron microscopic study. Clin Neuropathol, 1987; 6:169–173
164. Sanjuan-Rodriguez S, Gastejon-Casado J, Pimentel-Leo JJ et al. Extraspinal presacral ependymoblastoma. Ann Esp Pediatr, 1986; 24:333–335
165. Maiorana A, Fante R, Fano RA. Myxopapillary ependymoma of the sacrococcygeal region. Report of a case. Pathologica, 1989; 81:471–476
166. Prins BA, Landsman JN. Sacrococcygeal myxopapillary ependymoma. Neth J Surg, 1989; 41:47–48
167. Chou S, Soucy P, Carpenter B. Extraspinal ependymoma. J Pediatr Surg, 1987; 22:802–803
168. Kramer GW, Rutten E, Sloof J. Subcutaneous sacrococcygeal ependymoma with inguinal lymph node metastasis. Case report. J Neurosurg, 1988; 68:474–477
169. Timmerman W, Bubrick MP. Presacral and postsacral extraspinal ependymoma. Report of a case and review of the literature. Dis Colon Rectum, 1984; 27:114–119
170. Dekmezian RH, Sneige N, Ordonez NG. Ovarian and omental ependymomas in peritoneal washings: Cytologic and immunocytochemical features. Diagn Cytopathol, 1986; 2:62–68
171. Duggan MA, Hugh J, Nation JG et al. Ependymoma of the uterosacral ligament. Cancer, 1989; 64:2565–2571
172. Bell DA, Woodruff JM, Scully RE. Ependymoma of the broad ligament. A report of two cases. Am J Surg Pathol, 1984; 8:203–209
173. Kleinman GM, Young RH, Scully RE. Ependymoma of the ovary: Report of three cases. Hum Pathol, 1984; 15:632–638
174. Carlsson B, Havel G, Kindblom LG et al. Ependymoma of the ovary. A clinico-pathologic, ultrastructural and immunohistochemical investigation. A case report APMIS, 1989; 97:1007–1012
175. Grody WW, Nieberg RK, Bhuta S. Ependymoma-like tumour of the mesovarium. Arch Pathol Lab Med, 1985; 109:291–293

Choroid plexus tumours

176. Cushing H. Intracranial tumours. Illinois: Charles C. Thomas, 1932
177. Stanley P. Papillomas of the choroid plexus. Br J Radiol, 1968; 41:848–857
178. Jooma R, Hayward RD, Grant DN. Intracranial neoplasms during the first year of life: Analysis of one hundred consecutive cases. Neurosurgery, 1984; 14:31–41
179. Lellouch-Tubiana A, Pfister A, Da Lage C. Histologic classification and prevalence of tumors of the central nervous system in infants. Study of 100 excision samples. Ann Pathol, 1989; 9:195–198
180. Raimondi AJ, Tomita T. Brain tumours during the first year of life. Childs Brain, 1983; 10:193–207
181. Laurence KM. The biology of choroid plexus papilloma and carcinoma of the lateral ventricle. In : Virken PJ, Bruyn GW, eds. Handbook of clinical neurology, vol 17. Tumours of the brain and skull, Part II. Amsterdam: North Holland, 1974: pp 555–595
182. Zülch KJ. Brain tumours. Their biology and pathology. Heidelberg: Springer, pp 276–283
183. Bohm E, Strang R. Choroid plexus papillomas. J Neurosurg, 1961; 18:493–500
184. Harsh GR, Wilson CB. Neuroepithelial tumours of the adult brain. In: Youmans, JR, ed. Neurological Surgery, 3rd edn. Philadelphia: WB Saunders, 1990; pp 3040–3136
185. Kalangu K, Reznik M, Bonnal J. Choroid plexus papilloma of the cerebellopontine angle. Presentation of a case and review of the literature. Neurochirurgie, 1986; 32:242–247
186. Chan RC, Thompson GB, Durity FA. Primary choroid plexus papilloma of the cerebellopontine angle. Neurosurgery, 1983; 12:334–336
187. Russell DS, Rubinstein LJ. Pathology of tumours of the nervous system, 5th edn. London: Edward Arnold, 1989: pp 394–404
188. Buetow PC, Smirniotopoulos JG, Done S. Congenital brain tumours: A review of 45 cases. Am J Roentgenol, 1990; 155:587–593
189. Tomita T, Naidich TP. Successful resection of choroid plexus papillomas diagnosed at birth: Report of two cases. Neurosurgery, 1987; 20:774–779
190. Palmiter RD, Chen HY, Messing A et al. SV40 enhancer and large-T antigen are instrumental in development of choroid plexus tumours in transgenic mice. Nature, 1985; 316:457–460
191. Bergsagel D, Finegold MJ, Butel JS. DNA sequences similar to those of simian virus 40 in ependymomas and choroid plexus tumours of childhood. New Eng J Med, 1992; 326:988–993
192. Lednicky JA, Garcea RL, Bergsagel DJ et al. Natural simiam virus 40 strains are present in human choroid plexus and ependymoma tumours. Virology, 1995; 212:710–717
193. Bruce DA, Schut L, Sutton LN. Supratentorial brain tumours in children. In: Yeomans JR, ed. Neurological surgery, 3rd edn. Philadelphia: WB Saunders, 1990: pp 3000–3016
194. Budeman SK, Sullivan HG, Rosner MJ et al. Surgical removal of bilateral papillomas of the choroid plexus of the lateral ventricles with resolution of hydrocephalus. J Neurosurg, 1979; 50:677–681
195. Ray BS, Peck FC. Papilloma of the choroid plexus of the lateral ventricles causing hydrocephalus in an infant. J Neurosurg, 1956; 13:405–410
196. Eisenberg HM, McComb JG, Lorenzo AV. Cerebrospinal fluid overproduction and hydrocephalus associated with choroid plexus papilloma. J Neurosurg, 1974; 40:381–385
197. Milhorat TH, Hammock MK, Davis DA et al. Choroid plexus papillomas: Proof of cerebrospinal fluid overproduction. Childs Brain, 1976; 2:273–289
198. Coates TL, Hinshaw DB Jr, Peckman N et al. Pediatric choroid plexus neoplasms: MR, CT, and pathologic correlation. Radiology, 1989; 173:81–88
199. Raimondi AJ, Gutierrez FA. Diagnosis and surgical treatment of choroid plexus papilloma. Childs Brain, 1975; 1:81–115
200. Kawamata T, Kubo O, Kawamura H et al. Ossified choroid plexus papilloma: Case report. No Shinkei Geka, 1988; 16:989–994
201. Bonnin JM, Colon LE, Morowetz RB. Focal glial differentiation and oncocytic transformation in choroid plexus papilloma. Acta Neuropathol (Berl) 1987; 72:277–280
202. Stefano SZ, Vuzevski UD. Oncocytic variant of choroid plexus papilloma. Acta Neuropathol (Berl), 1985; 66:160–162
203. Kepes JJ. Oncocytic transformation of choroid plexus epithelium. Acta Neuropathol (Berl), 1983; 62:145–148
204. Reimund El, Sitton JE, Harkin JC. Pigmented choroid plexus papilloma. Arch Pathol Lab Med, 1990; 114:902–905
205. Yamazaki S, Ito U, Tomita H et al. Melanosis of choroid plexus papilloma of the lateral ventricle: A case report. No Shinkei Geka, 1987; 15:1033–1037
206. Hoenig EM, Ghatak NR, Hirano A et al. Multiloculated cystic tumour of the choroid plexus of the fourth ventricle. J Neurosurg, 1967; 27:574–579

207. Andreini L, Doglioni C, Giangaspero F. Tubular adenoma of choroid plexus. A case report. Clin Neuropathol, 1991; 10:137–140

208. Davis RL, Fox GE. Acinar choroid plexus adenoma. Report of a case. J Neurosurg, 1970; 33:587–590

209. Ang LC, Taylor AR, Bergin D et al. An immunohistochemical study of papillary tumors in the central nervous system. Cancer, 1990; 65:2712–2719

210. Cruz-Sanchez FF, Rossi ML, Hughes JT et al. Choroid plexus papillomas: An immunohistological study of 16 cases. Histopathology, 1989; 15:61–69

211. Doglion C, Dell'Orto P, Coggi G et al. Choroid plexus tumours. An immunocytochemical study with particular reference to the coexpression of intermediate filament proteins. Am J Pathol, 1987; 127:519–529

212. Matsushima T, Inoue T, Takeshita I et al. Choroid plexus papillomas: An immunohistochemical study with particular reference to the coexpression of prealbumin. Neurosurgery, 1988; 23:384–389

213. Mannoji H, Becker LE. Ependymal and choroid plexus tumours. Cytokeratin and GFAP expression. Cancer, 1988; 61:1377–1385

214. Kouno M, Kumanishi T, Washiyama K et al. An immunohistochemical study of cytokeratin and glial fibrillary acidic protein in choroid plexus papilloma. Acta Neuropathol (Berl), 1988; 75:317–320

215. Rubinstein LJ, Brucher JM. Focal ependymal differentiation in choroid ploexus papillomas. An immunoperoxidase study. Acta Neuropathol (Berl), 1981; 53:29–33

216. Taratuto AL, Molina H, Monges J. Choroid plexus tumours in infancy and childhood. Focal ependymal differentiation. An immunoperoxidase study. Acta Neuropathol (Berl), 1983; 59:304–308

217. Kinura T, Budka H, Soler-Federsppiel S. An immunocytochemical comparison of the glia-associated proteins glial fibrillary acidic protein (GFAP) and S-100 protein (S100P) in human brain tumours. Clin Neuropathol, 1986; 5:21–27

218. Coffin CM, Wick MR, Braut JT et al. Choroid plexus neoplasms. Clinicopathologic and immunohistochemical studies. Am J Surg Pathol, 1986; 10:394–404

219. Herbert J, Cavallaro T, Dwork AJ. A marker for primary choroid plexus neoplasms. Am J Pathol, 1990; 136:1317–1325

220. Kunishio K, Shiraishi T, Mishima N et al. Immunohistochemical study on distribution of transthyretin in normal human brain tissue and tumors. No To Shinkei, 1989; 41:245–249

221. Nakagawa Y, Perentes E, Rubinstein LJ. Non-specificity of anti-carbonic anhydrase C antibody as a marker in human neurooncology. J Neuropathol Exp Neurol, 1987; 46:451–460

222. Carter P, Beggs J, Waggener JD. Ultrastructure of three choroid plexus papillomas. Cancer, 1972; 30:1130–1136

223. Dohrmann GJ, Bucy PC. Human choroid plexus: A light and electron microscopic study. J Neurosurg, 1970; 33:506–516

224. Wakai S, Matsutani M, Mizutani H et al. Tight junctions in choroid plexus papillomas. Acta Neuropathol (Berl), 1979; 45:159–160

225. Moss TH. Tumours of the nervous system. An ultrastructural atlas. London: Springer, 1986: pp 43–49

226. Kersting G. Tissue culture of human gliomas. Prog Neurol Surg, 1968; 2:165–202

227. Unterharnscheidt FJ. Routine tissue culture of CNS tumours and animal implantation. Prog Exp Tumour Res, 1972; 17:111–150

228. Liss L. The use of tissue cultures in the study of brain tumours. Prog Exp Tumor Res, 1972; 17:93–110

229. Nakashima N, Goto K, Tsukidate K et al. Choroid plexus papilloma. Light and electron microscopic study. Virchows Arch (A), 1983; 400:201–211

230. Schick B, Kahle G, Krosbein H et al. Papillary tumour of the endolymphatic sac. HNO, 1996; 44:329–332

231. Spallone A, Pastore FS, Giuffre R et al. Choroid plexus papillomas in infancy and childhood. Childs Nerv Syst, 1990; 6:71–74

232. McGirr SJ, Ebersold MJ, Scheithauer BW et al. Choroid plexus papillomas: Long-term follow-up results in a surgically treated series. J Neurosurg, 1988; 69:843–849

233. Naguib MG, Chou SN, Mastri A. Radiation therapy of a choroid plexus papilloma of the cerebellopontine angle with bone involvement. Case report. J Neurosurg, 1981; 54:245–247

234. Husag L, Costabile G, Probst C. Persistent hydrocephalus following removal of choroid plexus papilloma of the lateral ventricle. Neurochirurgia (Stuttg), 1984; 27:82–85

235. Leys D, Pasquier F, Lejeune JP et al. Benign choroid plexus papilloma. 2 local recurrences and intraventricular seeding. Neurochirurgie, 1986; 32:258–261

236. Tacconi L, Delfini R, Cantore G. Choroid plexus papillomas: consideration of a surgical series of 33 cases. Acta Neurochirurg, 1996; 138:802–810

237. Guidetti B, Spallone A. The surgical treatment of choroid plexus papillomas: The results of 27 years experience. Neurosurg Rev, 1981; 4:129–137

238. Dohrmann GJ, Collias JC. Choroid plexus carcinoma: Case report. J Neurosurg, 1975; 43:225–232

239. Shankar SK, Banerjee AK, Verma K et al. Choroid plexus carcinoma. A case report. Neurol (India), 1976; 24:194–196

240. Laurence KM. The biology of choroid plexus papilloma in infancy and childhood. Acta Neurochirurg (Wein), 1979; 50:79–90

241. Felix I, Phudhichareonrat S, Halliday WC et al. Choroid plexus tumors in children: Immunohistochemical and scanning-electron-microscopic features. Pediatr Neurosci, 1987; 13:263–269

242. Sato K, Hayashi M, Kubota T et al. A case of large malignant choroid plexus papilloma in the third ventricle. Immunohistochemial and ultrastructural studies. No To Shinkei, 1989; 41:973–978

243. Lewis P. Carcinoma of the choroid plexus. Brain, 1967; 90:177–186

244. Casentini L, Rigobello L, Gerosa M et al. Choroid plexus carcinoma. Case report. Zentralbl Neurochir, 1979; 40:239–244

245. Masuzawa T, Shimabukuro H, Yoshimizu N et al. Ultrastructure of disseminated choroid plexus papilloma. Acta Neuropathol (Berl), 1981; 54:321–324

246. Li YS, Fan YS, Armstrong RF. Endoreduplication and telomeric association in a choroid plexus carcinoma. Cancer Genet Cytogenet, 1996; 87:7–10

247. Giangaspero F, Doglioni C, Rivano MT et al. Growth fraction in human brain tumors defined by the monoclonal antibody Ki-67. Acta Neuropathol (Berl), 1987; 74:179–182

248. Vajtai I, Varga Z, Aguzzi A. MIB-1 immunoreactivity reveals different labelling in low-grade and malignant epithelial neoplasms of the choroid plexus. Histopathology, 1996; 29:147–151

249. Tham KT, Wen HL, Teoh TB. A case of papillary adenocarcinoma of the choroid plexus. J Pathol, 1969; 99:321–324

250. Boesel CP, Suman JP. A pigmented choroid plexus carcinoma: Histochemical and ultrastructural studies. J Neuropathol Exp Neurol, 1979; 38:177–186

251. Lana-Peixotoma MA, Lagos J, Silbert SW. Primary pigmented carcinoma of the choroid plexus. A light and electron microscopic study. J Neurosurg, 1977; 47:442–450

252. Newbould MJ, Kelsey AM, Arango JC et al. The choroid plexus carcinomas of childhood: Histopathology, immunocytochemistry and clinicopathological correlation. Histopathology, 1995; 26:137–143

253. Anguilar D, Martin JM, Aneiros J et al. The fine structure of choroid plexus carcinoma. Histopathology, 1983; 7:939–946

254. Moss TH. Electron microscopic observations on malignant choroid plexus papilloma. Neuropathol Appl Neurobiol, 1983; 9:225–235

255. McComb RD, Burger PC. Choroid plexus carcinoma. Report of a case with immunohistochemical and ultrastructural observations. Cancer, 1983; 51:470–475

256. Geerts Y, Gabreels F, Lippens R et al. Choroid plexus carcinoma: a report of two cases and review of the literature. Neuropediatrics, 1996; 27:143–148

257. Duffner PK, Kun LE, Burger PC et al. Postoperative chemotherapy and delayed radiation in infants and very young children with choroid plexus carcinomas. The Pediatric Oncology Group. Pediat Neurosug, 1995; 22:189–196

258. Pierga JY, Kalifa C, Terrier-Lacombe MJ et al. Carcinoma of the choroid plexus: a pediatric experience. Med Pediat Oncol, 1993; 21:480–487

259. Griffin BR, Steward GR, Berger MS et al. Choroid plexus carcinoma of the fourth ventricle. Report of a case in an infant. Pediatr Neurosci, 1988; 14:134–139

260. Teng P, Papatheodorou C. Tumours of the cerebral ventricles in children. J Nerv Ment Dis, 1966; 142:87–93

261. Hayakawa I, Fujiwara K, Tsuchida T et al. Choroid plexus carcinoma with metastasis to bone. No Shinkei Geka, 1979; 7:815–818

262. Valladares JB, Perry RH, Kalbag RM. Malignant choroid plexus

papilloma with extraneural metastases. Case report. J Neurosurg, 1980; 52:251–255

263. Arico M, Raiteri E, Bossi G et al. Choroid plexus carcinoma: Report of one case with favourable response to treatment. Med Pediatr Oncol, 1994; 22:274–278

264. Davis LE. A physiopathologic study of the choroid plexus with a report of a case of villous hypertrophy. J Med Res, 1924; 44:521–534

265. Welch K, Strand R, Bresnan M et al. Congenital hydrocephalus due to villous hypertrophy of the telencephalic choroid plexuses. J Neurosurg, 1983; 59:172–175

266. Baar HS, Gacindo J. Bilateral papilloma of the choroid plexus. Maine Med Assoc, 1964; 6:95–99

7 Embryonal tumours

Tumours grouped under this heading (Table 7.1) are composed wholly, or in part, of undifferentiated cells with round or carrot shaped hyperchromatic nuclei, sparse fibrillary cytoplasm and a high mitotic rate. They mostly occur in children but a significant proportion of medulloblastomas also occur in adults. Considerable advances have been made in the treatment of embryonal tumours of the nervous system in recent years and the prognosis has improved.[1,2] Embryonal tumours have a propensity to spread widely through central nervous system tissue and through the cerebrospinal fluid (CSF) pathways.

The term *primitive neuroectodermal tumour (PNET)* has been used for many years to include a subgroup of embryonal tumours that is widely distributed throughout the CNS from retina and nose to cauda equina.[3] PNETs of the CNS are characterised by histologically undifferentiated cells which also show features of cytological differentiation, particularly towards neurons. A boost to the concept of PNET came with the introduction of immunocytochemistry which demonstrated divergent maturation within such tumours in the CNS, particularly with the expression of glial proteins (GFAP) and neuronal proteins (synaptophysin and neurofilament protein).[3] At its widest extent, the term 'primitive neuroectodermal tumour' included aesthesioneuroblastoma (see Chapter 18), retinoblastoma and pineoblastoma (see Chapter 9), in addition to the group of tumours currently included under the term PNET (Table 7.2). Molecular genetic studies,[4] however, have emphasised the differences between some of the better recognised PNET entities. For instance, certain hereditary tumour syndromes, which are attributable to defects in different tumour suppressor genes, predispose to distinct PNET phenotypes. Patients with constitutional retinoblastoma (*RB*) gene mutations have a predilection for retinoblastomas and pineoblastomas (Chapter 9) while patients with constitutional *PTCH* or *APC* gene mutations have a predilection for medulloblastoma (see Ch. 19). In addition, the sporadically occurring PNET tumour phenotypes often demonstrate different somatic genetic changes. Thus medulloblastoma often has defects of the short arm of chromosome 17 but atypical teratoid-rhabdoid tumours characteristically show loss of the long arm of chromosome 22.

Although the World Health Organisation (WHO) 2000 classification[5] includes the tumours shown in Table 7.1 within the group of embryonal tumours, only ependymoblastoma, medulloblastoma and supratentorial PNETs are included under the heading of primitive neuroectodermal tumour (Table 7.2). They show a range of cytological features of maturation and variable expression of proteins that are typical of mature neuroectodermal cells (Table 7.3). Medulloepithelioma and atypical teratoid-rhabdoid tumour have distinctly different histology from PNETs and also appear to have distinct genetic changes. Other tumours that have been included

under the term PNET in the past have been reallocated to different sections of the WHO classification. Pineoblastoma is now included with the pineal tumours (see Chapter 9), olfactory neuroblastoma (aesthesioneuroblastoma) has been grouped with neuroblastic tumours and, although mentioned in this chapter, polar spongioblastoma has been deleted from the WHO 2000 classification, as it is thought to be a cytological variation rather than a distinct entity.

Table 7.1 WHO 2000 – classification

Embryonal tumours
Medulloepithelioma
Ependymoblastoma
Medulloblastoma
  Desmoplastic medulloblastoma
  Large cell medulloblastoma
  Medullomyoblastoma
  Melanotic medulloblastoma
Supratentorial primitive
  neuroectodermal tumour (PNET)
  Neuroblastoma
  Ganglioneuroblastoma
(*Polar spongioblastoma*)
Atypical teratoid-rhabdoid tumour

Table 7.2 Primitive neuroectodermal tumours (PNET)

Ependymoblastoma
Medulloblastoma
  Desmoplastic medulloblastoma
  Large cell medulloblastoma
  Medullomyoblastoma
  Melanotic medulloblastoma
Supratentorial PNET
  Neuroblastoma
  Ganglioneuroblastoma

Table 7.3 Primitive neuroectodermal tumours

Cytological differentiation
  Undifferentiated
  Differentiated
    Neurons
      Ganglion cells
      Neuroblasts
    Astrocytes
    Ependyma
    Striated muscle

Immunocytochemistry
  Glial fibrillary acidic protein (GFAP)
  Synaptophysin
  Neurofilament protein
  Nestin
  Myoglobin or other muscle antigens

Medulloepithelioma

This is a highly malignant, primitive tumour, separated from PNETs by its distinctive architecture and extremely poor prognosis. The tumours are typified by a pseudo-stratified epithelium which appears to recapitulate the primitive medullary epithelium of the embryonic neural tube. Their other prominent characteristic is a capacity for differentiation into a wide variety of neuroepithelial and systemic cell lines.[6]

Incidence and site

Medulloepitheliomas are extremely rare tumours and their precise incidence is not known. The largest reported series has described eight patients[6] and most other documented examples have been single case reports. They are predominantly tumours of early childhood, but congenital cases have been reported[7] and exceptionally the presentation may be delayed until the second decade of life.[8] Up to half of all cases arise in association with one or other lateral ventricle but deep cerebral tumours not involving the ventricular lining are well described.[6] Isolated examples arising in the posterior fossa,[9] the pons[6] and the cauda equina[10] have also been reported.

Clinical features

These tumours are usually large at presentation and patients typically present with signs and symptoms of raised intracranial pressure, particularly vomiting and failure to thrive in infants.[6] Radiologically, the lesions usually appear as well defined masses with rather variable signal intensity. They may be either iso- or hypodense on both computerised tomography (CT) and magnetic resonance (MR) scans and the signal intensity may be uniform or non-homogeneous. Enhancement after administration of contrast media may be absent at first but develops during the later stages of tumour growth.[6]

Pathology

Macroscopic features

In post-mortem cases, medulloepitheliomas are usually seen as very large, well circumscribed masses with evidence of extensive haemorrhage and necrosis on cut section. Cystic spaces may also be present, and by the time of death widespread dissemination in the CSF pathway is often apparent.[6]

Histological features

The neuroepithelial component of medulloepitheliomas has a very distinctive histological appearance, charac-terised by well defined ribbons of pseudostratified epithelium folded into closely packed plates, papillary

structures and tubules (Fig. 7.1). The cytoarchitecture is said to resemble closely that of developing embryonic neural tube.[10] The cells vary from columnar to low cuboidal in shape and have indistinct cytoplasmic borders (Fig. 7.2). They have fairly uniform, ovoid nuclei with coarse chromatin and multiple nucleoli which are orientated perpendicularly across the epithelial ribbons (Fig. 7.3). Mitoses are always abundant and tend to be located in the cells nearer the inner epithelial surface, as in the primitive neural tube. The inner aspect of the epithelium is very crisply defined in routine stains but lacks cilia or a reticulin layer. The outer aspect, however, rests on a clearly visible reticulin stained membrane (Fig. 7.4).

The proportion of the specific neuroepithelial component varies widely from tumour to tumour, but in most cases there are also quite distinct areas composed of sheets of

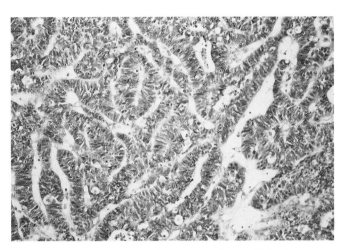

Fig. 7.1 **Medulloepithelioma.** These tumours have a distinctive architecture, with well defined ribbons of pseudostratified epithelium folded into plates, papillary structures and tubules. H & E.

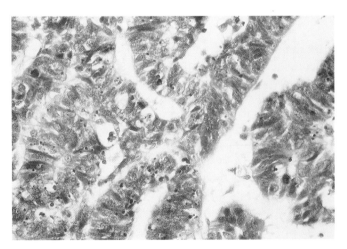

Fig. 7.2 **Medulloepithelioma.** Characteristic folded ribbons of pseudostratified epithelium are shown, sometimes enclosing tubular spaces. The cells are closely packed with indistinct cytoplasmic borders. H & E.

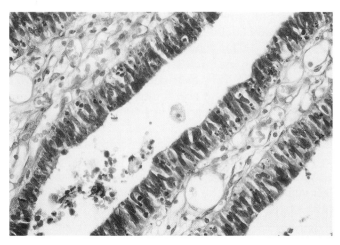

Fig. 7.3 **Medulloepithelioma.** The pseudostratified neuroepithelium is forming papillary structures with fibrovascular cores. The tumour cell nuclei are quite uniform with an elongate or ovoid shape and are orientated perpendicularly across the epithelial layer. H & E.

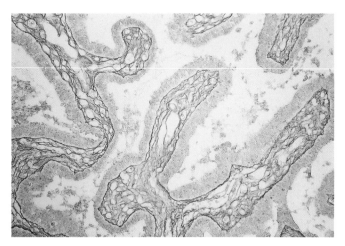

Fig. 7.4 **Medulloepithelioma.** The apical surface of the neuroepithelium lacks a basal lamina, but the basal surface rests on a continuous lamina which is reticulin positive. Reticulin preparation.

primitive cells showing evidence of a wide range of differentiation and maturation. Ependymoblastic rosettes, mature ependymal tubules, oligodendroglial-like cells and mature ganglion cells may all be encountered in these areas of tumour.[11–13] The degree of maturation in these differentiating areas can be quite striking, and in some cases an entire spectrum of both glial and neuronal differentiation from the most primitive to the most mature forms may be found within a single tumour.[7,8] In addition, some examples with differentiation into mature bone, cartilage and skeletal muscle have also been described.[11,13]

Immunocytochemistry

The cells in the neuroepithelial component of medullo-epitheliomas express vimentin and also show nestin immunoreactivity, which is largely confined to the basal aspect of the epithelial ribbons.[14] Focal expression of cyto-keratin, neurofilament protein and epithelial membrane antigen (EMA) may also be found in some cases, but the neuroepithelium cells do not stain with antibodies to glial fibrillary acidic protein (GFAP), S-100 protein or neuron specific enolase.[13,15,16] In the non-neuroepithelial areas of tumour, the results of immunocytochemistry will reflect the extent and variety of differentiation that is taking place. Depending on the degree of maturation in glial and neuronal elements, there may be varying degrees of staining with antibodies to GFAP, synaptophysin and neuron specific enolase in these areas, closely correlated with ganglionic and gliofibrillary features visible in tinctorial stains.

Electron microscopy

Ultrastructural studies show the neuroepithelial cells to be joined by lateral zonulae adherentes and confirm the absence of apical cilia and microvilli.[16,17] As suggested by light microscopy, the apical surface of the neuroepithelium also lacks basal lamina, but there is a distinct and continuous lamina covering the basal surfaces of the cells.

Differential diagnosis

Differentiating PNETs

The non-neuroepithelial areas of medulloepithelioma may be confused histologically with a number of differentiating embryonal tumours, and the key to this differential diagnosis lies in identification of the distinctive neuroepithelium found only in medulloepitheliomas. Selected primitive areas showing glial or neuronal differentiation may be impossible to distinguish from *neuroblastomas, medulloblastomas* or *ependymoblastomas*, but even here the divergence of differentiation will usually argue against such diagnoses. In a similar way, the presence of mature neuroglial elements is unlikely to be persuasive of astrocytoma, ependymoma or oligo-dendroglioma because of the intermingling of more primitive tissue and the divergent variety of elements present. In the end, however, a search around the biopsy will nearly always reveal areas of distinctive ribbon-like neuroepithelium to guide the pathologist away from an erroneous impression of a differentiating PNET or more mature neuroglial tumour.

Choroid plexus carcinomas

These tumours are also common in the lateral ventricles and may show a quite distinct papillary architecture with a superficial resemblance to the neuroepithelium of medulloepithelioma. Although the epithelium may be several cells in thickness, however, it usually lacks the uniform pseudostratified appearance of that in medulloepithelioma. Using immunocytochemistry, expression of cytokeratin is a much more constant and widespread feature in choroid plexus tumours, and even the most malignant examples can usually be specifically identified by cells expressing transthyretin.

Immature teratomas

These should also be included in the differential diagnosis as they may include primitive medullary epithelium. They can usually be distinguished from the neuroepithelial component of medulloepithelioma by the presence of tissue from other germ cell layers and by the variable expression of alpha-fetoprotein, carcinoembryonic antigen and placental alkaline phosphatase, depending on which other teratoid components are present.

Therapy and prognosis

Medulloepitheliomas are highly malignant, rapidly growing tumours with a very poor prognosis, the majority of patients dying within about 6 months of presentation. The best chance of longer term survival appears to correlate with total macroscopic surgical excision[6] but the role of adjuvant therapy is unknown. Seeding of tumour in the CSF pathways is a major complication[6,17] and in a majority of cases, prophylactic craniospinal axis irradiation is not possible because the presentation is in early infancy. Metastasis of tumour outside the nervous system has been documented in one case, with spread to regional lymph nodes.[18]

Ependymoblastoma

The term ependymoblastoma is used here to denote a rare group of highly malignant ependymal tumours which have a monotonous, primitive histological appearance, without the spectrum of anaplasia seen in ependymomas dedifferentiating towards glioblastoma.[19,20] Some authors have argued that ependymoblastomas are essentially ependymal in nature, albeit in a primitive fashion, and think that they should continue to be classified alongside other malignant ependymal tumours.[21] Other authorities take the view that ependymoblastomas are essentially PNETs showing evidence of ependymal differentiation, and have classified them with other PNETs such as medulloblastomas and neuroblastomas.[22,23] The latter arrangement conforms to the current WHO classification and is the one adopted here.

Incidence and site

Tumours with the true histological features of ependymoblastoma are extremely rare, and there have been too few reports in the literature to make any meaningful assessment of their statistical incidence. In contrast to typical ependymomas, ependymoblastomas are predominantly supratentorial, and many appear entirely intraparenchymal without any obvious relationship to a ventricular lining.[24] A smaller number arise in the posterior fossa[24] and occasional ectopic examples have been described in the sacral region, either anteriorly or subcutaneously.[25,26]

Aetiology

Ultrastructural studies have confirmed the basic ependymal lineage of ependymoblastomas,[27] but have also demonstrated the presence of very primitive ependymal-type cells comparable to those found in the developing neural tube of 3 week embryos.[20] It thus seems possible that ependymoblastomas derive from neoplastic change in a primitive medulloepithelial cell still at a very early stage of development, and are not simply the result of dedifferentiation in a more mature ependymal cell line.[19,20] The incidence of congenital ependymoblastoma is in keeping with this hypothesis.[25]

Clinical features

The majority of cases occur in infants under 5 years of age,[27] although occasional examples have been described in patients up to their mid-30s.[24] The median age of presentation is lower than for typical ependymomas and congenital examples are by no means uncommon.[24,28] There is usually a short clinical history relating to a rapidly expanding supratentorial mass lesion, with raised intracranial pressure, vomiting and papilloedema.[24] Neonates and younger infants may also show an abnormally large head.[24]

Radiology

The appearances on CT often differ from those of typical ependymomas in showing a higher attenuation prior to giving contrast medium and more intense contrast enhancement.[29] Calcification is less frequently seen radiologically and scans usually show rather indistinct tumour margins, with intense surrounding oedema. Using MRI, ependymoblastomas are hypodense in T1-weighted images, irregularly hyperdense with T2-weighting and show variable, patchy enhancement after administration of gadolinium.[30]

Pathology

Macroscopic features

Ependymoblastomas are often very large by the time of presentation, in some cases over 10 cm in diameter, especially in younger patients.[24] They usually appear grossly well circumscribed and on cut section may show cystic change, focal areas of necrosis and small foci of haemorrhage.

Histological features

There is typically a monotonous histological pattern with sheets of densely packed, small cells intersected by a mesh of thin walled blood vessels (Fig. 7.5). The tumour cells have a primitive, poorly differentiated appearance and are oval or spindle shaped. Nuclei are relatively large, rounded or ovoid in profile and show a coarse chromatin pattern. The tumour cell cytoplasm is scanty and indistinct, but may form delicate polar processes. There are abundant mitotic figures and focal necrosis is usually present (Fig. 7.5). The tumour lacks the disordered appearance of anaplasia seen in other malignant ependymomas, and features such as endothelial vascular proliferation, multinucleated cells, and bizarre cytological atypia are not usually found. The histological structure which distinguishes ependymoblastoma from other primitive neuroectodermal tumours is the ependymoblastic tubule, or rosette (Figs 7.6 and 7.7). Unlike typical ependymal rosettes, these are formed by multiple layers of tumour cells, the inner ones often in mitosis. They are

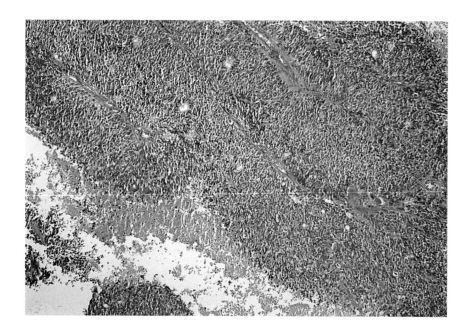

Fig. 7.5 Ependymoblastoma. The tumour is largely composed of monotonous sheets of closely packed, small cells. Necrosis is present in the bottom left of this field. H & E.

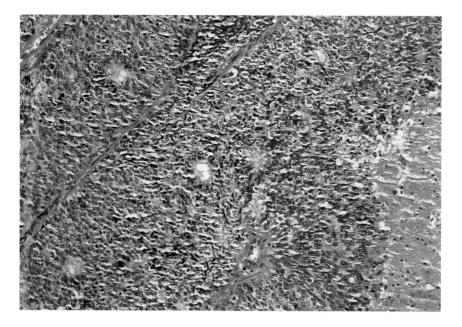

Fig. 7.6 Ependymoblastoma. Sheets of small, primitive looking cells are interrupted by several ependymoblastic rosettes. H & E.

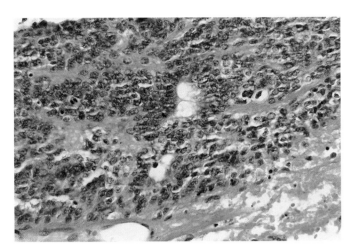

Fig. 7.7 **Ependymoblastoma.** Ependymoblastic rosettes are multilayered with well defined central lumina. Mitoses are often present in the cells forming these rosettes. H & E.

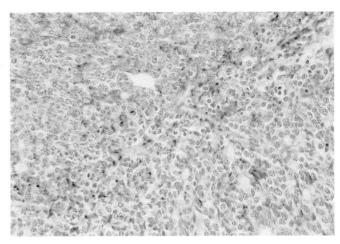

Fig. 7.8 **Ependymoblastoma.** Scattered tumour cells usually show expression of GFAP, but this is much less marked than in ependymomas.

arranged around a small central lumen and may also line longer, irregular shaped spaces. There is an internal limiting membrane, frequently bearing cilia, and juxtaluminal blepharoplasts may be seen with phosphotungstic acid haematoxylin staining. Ependymoblastic tubules are usually very numerous and easily found in all areas of the tumour. Typical, single layered ependymal rosettes may also be present, but the perivascular pseudorosettes which are the hallmark of most typical ependymomas are not a feature of ependymoblastomas. The margins of the tumour nearly always show widespread histological infiltration of adjacent brain tissue, despite the macroscopic impression of circumscription.

Immunocytochemistry

Many ependymoblastomas show at least some positive staining of tumour cells using antibodies to vimentin and S-100 protein, and this may include cells forming the ependymoblastic rosettes.[27,31] Some cases, however, entirely lack expression of S-100 protein.[32] Scanty immunoreactivity is usually found with antibodies to GFAP (Fig. 7.8), but this is much less marked than in typical ependymomas and largely confined to scattered, fine cell processes, mostly towards the tumour margins.[27] There is no immunoreactivity to EMA even around the luminal surfaces of ependymoblastic rosettes.[33] In contrast to many other primitive neuroectodermal tumours, including neuroblastomas and some medulloblastomas, no immunocytological evidence of neuronal differentiation has been found using antibodies to neurofilament protein and neuron specific enolase.[27]

Electron microscopy

Ultrastructural studies have demonstrated rather sparse intercellular microrosettes similar to those found in typical ependymomas, with tumour cells showing apical microvilli projecting into an intercellular lumen.[20,27] Cilia are associated with these structures, although they are frequently abortive or incomplete.[27] The junctional complexes linking the rosette forming cells are less structured than those seen in the microrosettes of typical ependymomas, and desmosomes have not been described.[20,27] Apart from those forming microrosettes, the tumour cells appear very poorly differentiated with large nuclei and little perinuclear cytoplasm.[27] Cytoplasmic organelles are scanty with a predominance of polysomes and free ribosomes. The ultrastructural appearance of these cells has been compared to that of developing ependymal precursor cells in early embryonic neural tubes.[20] In contrast to typical ependymomas, astrocyte-like cells and processes are not a conspicuous ultrastructural feature of ependymoblastomas.[27]

Differential diagnosis

Medulloblastoma

The distinction from ependymoblastoma relies essentially on the assessment of differentiating capacity in primitive neuroectodermal tumours. Medulloblastomas may show quite pronounced glial differentiation, but this is usually of spindle cell astrocytic pattern and specific features of ependymal differentiation are not usually found. The Homer–Wright rosettes present in many medulloblastomas differ from ependymoblastic rosettes in having a solid fibrillary core, without a luminal space, cilia or blepharoplasts (Fig. 7.9). They also lack the stratified arrangement seen in ependymoblastic rosettes. Unlike ependymoblastomas, many medulloblastomas show immunocytochemical evidence of neuroblastic differentiation, reacting with antibodies to neuronal antigens such as neuron

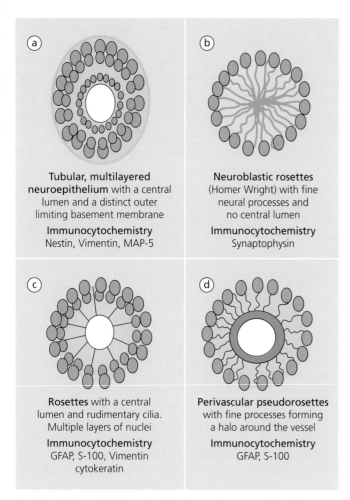

Tubular, multilayered neuroepithelium with a central lumen and a distinct outer limiting basement membrane
Immunocytochemistry
Nestin, Vimentin, MAP-5

Neuroblastic rosettes (Homer Wright) with fine neural processes and no central lumen
Immunocytochemistry
Synaptophysin

Rosettes with a central lumen and rudimentary cilia. Multiple layers of nuclei
Immunocytochemistry
GFAP, S-100, Vimentin cytokeratin

Perivascular pseudorosettes with fine processes forming a halo around the vessel
Immunocytochemistry
GFAP, S-100

Fig. 7.9 **Differential diagnosis of embryonal tumours.** The different types of tubule, rosette and pseudorosette are depicted in diagrammatic form. **(a)** Medulloepithelioma. **(b)** Medulloblastoma. **(c)** Ependymoblastoma. **(d)** Anaplastic ependymoma. (See also Chapter 2, Fig. 2.2)

specific enolase, synaptophysin and sometimes neurofilament protein. Antibodies to GFAP are unlikely to be helpful in distinguishing between the two tumour types, and immunopositivity in either case may in part relate to entrapped reactive astrocytic elements. Ultrastructural distinction from medulloblastoma relies on the demonstration of ependymal microrosettes, with their associated cilia, microvilli and junctional complexes.

Cerebral neuroblastoma

The differential diagnosis with ependymoblastoma is again a matter of assessing differentiation in primitive neuroectodermal tumours, although in this instance the presence or absence of neuroblastic features is of particular importance. The Homer Wright rosettes of neuroblastomas, like those of medulloblastomas, are solid structures which are readily distinguishable from ependymoblastic rosettes (Fig. 7.9). Ependymoblastomas

lack the argyrophilic neuritic processes often seen in neuroblastomas, and mature ganglion cells are never seen. Immunocytochemically, there is no expression of neuronal antigens such as neuron specific enolase and neurofilament protein. Ultrastructurally, ependymoblastomas again may be distinguished by the absence of neuroblastic features, particularly dense core vesicles, fine neuritic cell processes and synaptic structures.

Medulloepithelioma

Like ependymoblastomas, these are rapidly growing cerebral hemisphere tumours of infancy, which may be congenital and often relate to a lateral ventricle cavity. Histological confusion with ependymoblastomas may arise because of the epithelial organisation of tumour cell nuclei, with stratified cell layers and tubular formations (Fig. 7.9). However, the architecture of medulloepitheliomas is usually much more papillary than in ependymoblastomas, with a basement membrane under the epithelial layer and a variable connective tissue in the papillary cores. In undifferentiated medulloepithelioma, true rosettes with a central lumen are not present, and the apical surfaces of the cell layers lack cilia or blepharoplasts. It must be remembered, however, that many medulloepitheliomas show varied combinations of neuronal and glial differentiation, and ependymoblastic rosettes have occasionally been described under these circumstances.[34] This is usually a focal phenomenon, however, with juxtaposed areas of typical, undifferentiated medulloepithelioma.

Therapy and prognosis

Ependymoblastomas behave as highly malignant, primitive tumours and require radical surgery combined with radiotherapy or chemotherapy.[19] There is a marked tendency to local recurrence and primary surgical resection should be as complete as technically possible.[24] Postoperative craniospinal irradiation is usually recommended, except in very young infants, because of the high rate of dissemination in CSF pathways.[24,35] As with high grade typical ependymomas, the addition of postradiation chemotherapy has not been found to confer significant benefit.[36] Systemic metastases have been described in cases of ependymoblastoma, but only on an anecdotal basis.[37]

Histologically confirmed ependymoblastomas carry a worse prognosis than all but the most anaplastic of ependymomas.[38] Even with appropriate and aggressive therapy, death within 1 year is not unusual and the largest published series of 28 cases quoted an average survival of just 8 months.[39] Survival was not statistically influenced by the mode of treatment, although it tended to be longer in the cases receiving a combination of surgery, chemotherapy and radiotherapy.

Medulloblastoma

Medulloblastoma is the primitive neuroectodermal tumour of the cerebellum and is the most common intracranial PNET. It is a malignant, invasive, embryonal tumour arising mainly in children and showing a propensity to metastasise through the CSF pathways, and occasionally to distant organs such as lung and bone marrow. It should be noted that no such cell as a 'medulloblast' exists in modern embryonic terminology. Early descriptions of the tumour by Bailey and Cushing in the 1920s suggested that these tumours were derived from the external germinal layer of the cerebellum and, indeed, the infiltrating pattern of medulloblastoma certainly gives this impression. So far, however, there is only molecular evidence that the desmoplastic variant is so derived.

Incidence and site

Occurring with an approximate annual incidence of 0.5 per 100 000 children,[40] medulloblastomas account for some 20% of all brain tumours in children.[41] They have a peak incidence at 7 years of age (Fig. 7.10), with a slight male: female predominance (6.5:3.5). The majority of tumours (70%) occur under the age of 16 years and in adults, most tumours (80%) present between 21 and 40 years of age.[42] Although isolated examples in older age groups do occur, medulloblastomas are rarely seen over the age of 50.

The site of predilection for medulloblastoma in children is the cerebellar vermis, but as the tumour enlarges it projects laterally into the cerebellar hemispheres and anteriorly into the fourth ventricle. In adults, a proportion of the tumours arise in the more lateral portions of the cerebellum.[43]

Clinical features

Due to its site of origin and pattern of growth, medulloblastoma presents either with cerebellar ataxia or with raised intracranial pressure due to hydrocephalus resulting from occlusion of the fourth ventricle by the tumour. The latter is most common in infants and not infrequently constitutes a medical emergency. Treatment of the hydrocephalus may be a priority before surgical intervention or chemotherapy for the primary tumour is instituted. In the later stages of disease, clinical manifestations may be due to spread of the tumour through the CSF in the subarachnoid space, over the surface of the brain stem, the cerebellum, cerebral hemispheres and spinal cord.

Radiology

On CT scans (Fig. 7.11) medulloblastomas appear as solid or slightly mottled, brightly enhancing tumours in the

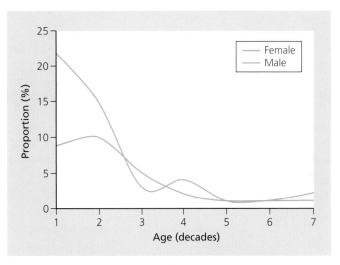

Fig. 7.10 **Medulloblastoma.** Relative age and sex distribution.

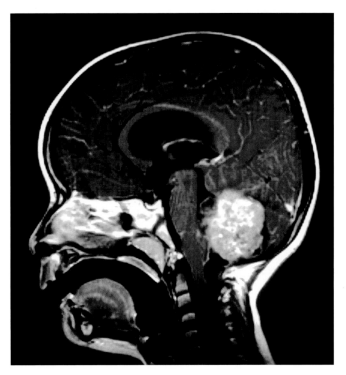

Fig. 7.11 **Medulloblastoma.** MRI scan of the cerebellum in a 5-year-old child. An enhancing midline tumour is present in the cerebellum with the typical enhancement pattern of medulloblastoma.

midline of the cerebellum. Extension into the fourth ventricle may occur and enhancing nodules of tumour may be seen on the surface of the brain or by MR imaging of the spinal cord either at presentation or in the later stages of the disease. In adults, medulloblastomas are seen as enhancing tumours often located more laterally in the cerebellar hemispheres. An assessment of spread at presentation is an important criterion for planning therapy and estimating the prognosis of the tumour. A thin layer of enhancement of the meninges due to the spread of tumour in this way may give the radiological appearances of meningitis. The differential diagnosis on radiology includes other enhancing tumours in the cerebellum and fourth ventricle, including ependymoma and pilocytic astrocytoma. Calcification may occur in all these tumours but the large, cystic component frequently seen in association with pilocytic astroctyoma is rarely present in association with medulloblastoma. In adults, the possibility of a metastasis as an enhancing lesion in the lateral aspects of the cerebellum must also be considered.

Pathology

Macroscopic features

Medulloblastomas vary in consistency. Some are soft, grey and gelatinous whereas the more desmoplastic tumours may be very firm. Although these firm tumours may appear to be relatively well circumscribed, invasion of the subarachnoid space around the cerebellar folia and of the cerebellar tissue itself, means that medulloblastomas are very rarely totally excised at surgery. Extension of the cerebellar medulloblastoma into the fourth ventricle is usually in continuity with the main tumour. At post-mortem, there may be varying degrees of tumour spread into the subarachnoid space. In the most severe cases, the brain may be encased by a layer of opalescent gelatinous tumour giving a 'sugar icing' effect over the cerebral hemispheres due to invasion of the subarachnoid space. Tumour may also extend down on to the surface of the spinal cord, giving a similar macroscopic appearance.

Intraoperative diagnosis

The site of the tumour gives a major clue to its nature, but during intraoperative diagnosis care must be taken to distinguish medulloblastoma from ependymoma, pilocytic astrocytoma and lymphoma. Medulloblastoma biopsy tissue is usually soft and grey, although the desmoplastic variants have a firmer consistency. In cryostat sections the tumour typically appears as sheets of cells with hyperchromatic nuclei and very little cytoplasm, giving a dark blue appearance to the section (Fig. 7.12). Individual nuclei vary moderately in shape and size and frequently the chromatin is diffuse and nucleoli may be very small. Mitoses and apoptotic cells are commonly seen in cryostat sections of medulloblastoma and there may be areas of necrosis and foci of calcification. Although occasional neuroblastic (Homer Wright) rosettes (Fig. 7.9) may be present, the perivascular pseudorosettes typical of ependymoma are not seen. The high nuclear:cytoplasmic ratio and mitoses in medulloblastoma help to distinguish it from pilocytic astrocytoma. Intraoperative smear preparations (Fig. 7.13) are also a useful diagnostic

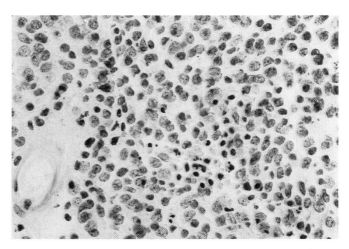

Fig. 7.12 **Medulloblastoma.** A cryostat section showing sheets of hyperchromatic nuclei with little cytoplasm. Mitoses may also be seen and areas of necrosis may be present. H & E.

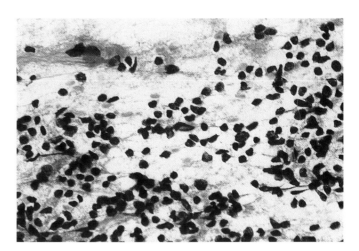

Fig. 7.13 **Medulloblastoma.** A smear shows dispersed cells with densely staining nuclei and few cell processes. Toluidine blue.

technique, showing a monolayer of discohesive, cytologically malignant cells with pleomorphic nuclei and a prominent degree of nuclear moulding where the cells abut each other.

In addition to the intraoperative diagnosis, cytospin preparations of lumbar CSF or ventricular CSF taken at the beginning of surgery are a useful method of staging tumour spread. Clumps of tumour cells are recognisable by the hyperchromatic nature of their nuclei, their very small nucleoli and the minimal amount of cytoplasm. Confirmation by immunocytochemistry may be possible using antibodies against GFAP or synaptophysin (Fig. 7.14).

Histological features

Medulloblastomas are composed of sheets of cells with a high nuclear:cytoplasmic ratio, hyperchromatic, and

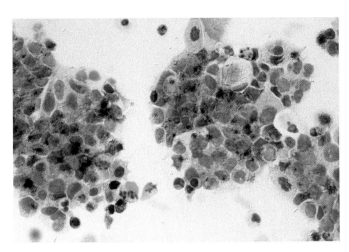

Fig. 7.14 **Medulloblastoma cells in CSF.** Compacted groups of cells expressing synaptophysin taken from the lumbar CSF of a patient with widespread medulloblastoma.

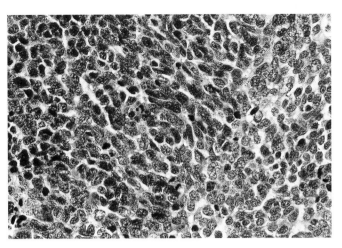

Fig. 7.15 **Medulloblastoma.** This tumour comprises sheets of cells with hyperchromatic nuclei and little cytoplasm. Mitoses and apoptosis are seen. H & E.

slightly angulated or oval nuclei showing a diffusely smudged chromatin pattern and a few small nucleoli (Fig. 7.15). The cytoplasm is sparse, eosinophilic and fibrillary. In some tumours, the nuclei are slightly less uniform in their staining and show some peripheral accumulation of chromatin. Various secondary structures may be seen in medulloblastomas. Neuroblastic rosettes (Homer Wright rosettes) are formed by an outer circle of tumour cell nuclei encircling a solid central filamentous area lacking a lumen (Figs 7.9 and 7.16). Tumour cell nuclei may also be arranged in rows with intervening bands of fibrillary cytoplasm creating a 'rhythmic pattern' (Fig. 7.17). In some tumours, pale staining islands of cells are seen in which the fibrillary cytoplasm is more abundant and the nuclei appear to be larger and rounder (Fig. 7.18). Immunocytochemistry has shown that cells in these islands usually express synaptophysin and have a lower proliferation index than the more classical areas of medulloblastoma.[44] High power microscopy of the cells in these 'pale islands' may also reveal cells with the cytological features of neurons with large, pale nuclei and prominent nucleoli (Fig. 7.19). The large numbers of mitoses typically found in the less mature areas of medulloblastomas are also appreciated at high magnification, as are the many cells that are undergoing apoptosis. From the main mass of tumour, medulloblastoma cells may spread through the subarachnoid space over the surface of the molecular layer of the cerebellum and then appear to reinvade the cerebellum either as single cells streaming along Bergmann glia or as nodules of tumour indenting the molecular layer (Fig. 7.20).

Reticulin stains reveal variable amounts of connective tissue within medulloblastomas. In many of the soft tumours in children, the main body of the tumour is devoid of reticulin but at sites where the tumour invades the subarachnoid space, it often induces the proliferation

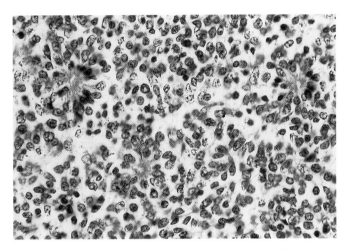

Fig. 7.16 **Medulloblastoma.** This tumour contains Homer Wright rosettes. The nuclei are arranged in circles and fibrillary processes project to the centre of the rosette. There is no lumen. H & E.

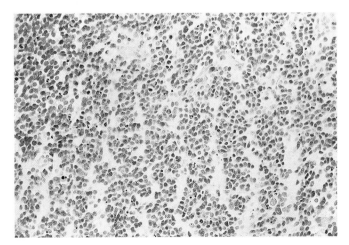

Fig. 7.17 **Medulloblastoma.** Nuclei are arranged in compact bands separated by cytoplasmic processes – the rhythmic pattern. H & E.

of connective tissue (Fig. 7.21). More abundant connective tissue is seen in reticulin stains of desmoplastic medullo-blastoma (see below) in which nests of tumour cells are surrounded by strands of connective tissue, accounting for the firm consistency of these tumours.

Immunocytochemistry

There can be few CNS tumours in which the results of immunocytochemical staining have engendered more discussion and speculation than medulloblastomas. A wide spectrum of immunocytochemical staining is seen in these tumours. Some tumours do not express any of the usual markers for normal neuroectodermal cells, whereas others show expression of multiple CNS proteins. The most valuable antibodies for confirming the diagnosis of medulloblastoma are directed against *synaptophysin* (a neuronal marker) and *GFAP* as a marker of astrocytes. Although some tumours are completely

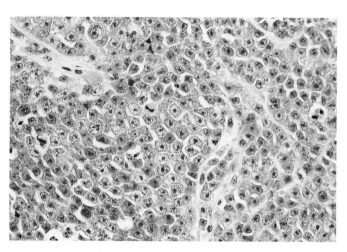

Fig. 7.19 **Medulloblastoma.** This cytological pattern in a medulloblastoma suggests neuronal differentiation. Although there is little cytoplasm, the cells have large nuclei with prominent nucleoli; mitoses are uncommon and Ki-67/MIB-1 labelling in this area was lower than in the more immature regions. H & E.

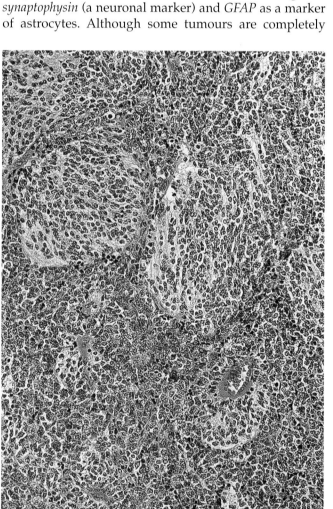

Fig. 7.18 **Medulloblastoma.** Among the diffuse sheets of cells with hyperchromatic nuclei and little cytoplasm are islands of tumour cells with more abundant cytoplasm. These pale areas usually show synaptophysin expression. H & E.

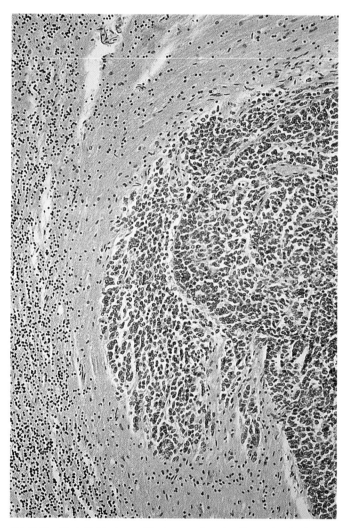

Fig. 7.20 **Medulloblastoma.** The tumour invades the molecular layer of the cerebellum from the subarachnoid space. H & E.

negative when stained with these antibodies, many medulloblastomas show either patchy or generalised staining with either one or both. Expression of synaptophysin in medulloblastomas may take several forms. In some tumours, there is diffuse staining of fine fibrillary cell processes. Staining may be patchy (Fig. 7.22) or confined to the circumscribed pale areas shown in Fig. 7.18. If there is cytological differentiation of ganglionic cells, they may express synaptophysin either in the cytoplasm (Fig. 7.23) or on the surface membrane. Such ganglion cells may also express the neuronal intermediate filament protein – *neurofilament protein* – and axonal structures may be present within medulloblastomas. Rosettes and cytoplasmic bands in rhythmic

areas of medulloblastoma may or may not express synaptophysin.

GFAP expression is also seen in two major patterns. In one pattern, spindle shaped or stellate GFAP positive cells are scattered through the tumour (Fig. 7.24), and could either represent stained medulloblastoma tumour cells or entrapped reactive astrocytes. Tumour cells can be identified by their hyperchromatic nuclei, perinuclear GFAP staining and their relatively few processes (Fig. 7.25). Often it is only islands of tumour cells that express GFAP within a medulloblastoma. Tumour cells may extend from the cerebellum into the subarachnoid space, in which case the cerebellar folium can often be identified by the presence of GFAP positive reactive astrocytes

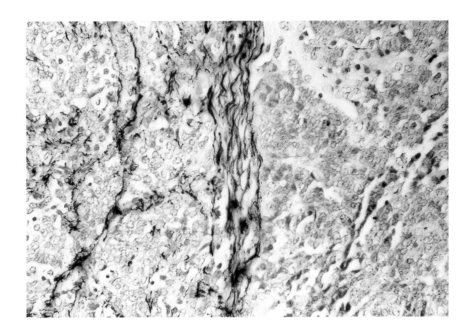

Fig. 7.21 **Medulloblastoma.** This field shows extension of medulloblastoma into the subarachnoid space. There is little reticulin associated with the tumour within the cerebellum (right) but in the subarachnoid space reticulin courses through the tumour (left). Reticulin stain.

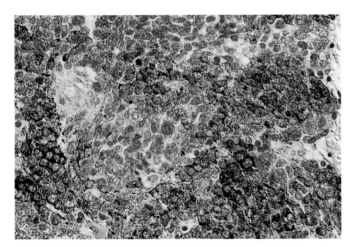

Fig. 7.22 **Medulloblastoma.** Patchy synaptophysin expression is seen with diffuse or granular staining of perinuclear cytoplasm. Immunocytochemistry for synaptophysin.

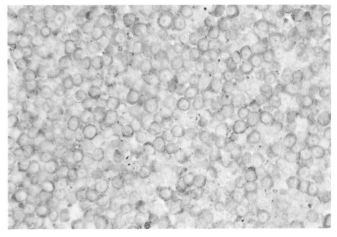

Fig. 7.23 **Medulloblastoma.** Same field as Fig. 7.19 showing synaptophysin expression in the cytoplasm of cells showing neuronal morphology. Immunocytochemistry for synaptophysin.

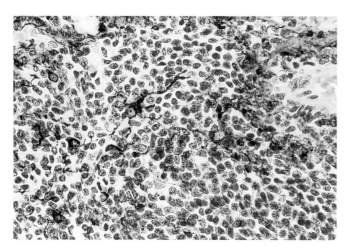

Fig. 7.24 **Medulloblastoma.** Expression of GFAP in tumour cells is shown with a thin rim of staining around the nucleus and the presence of stellate astrocytic cells within the tumour which could be entrapped reactive astrocytes. Immunocytochemistry for GFAP.

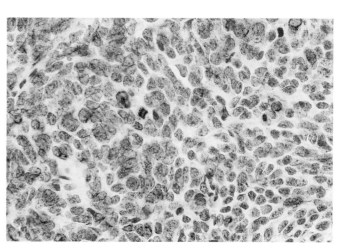

Fig. 7.25 **Medulloblastoma.** The tumour cells exhibit perinuclear expression of GFAP. Such staining can be patchy with individual tumours. Immunocytochemistry for GFAP.

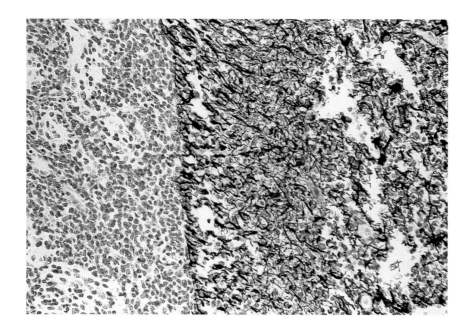

Fig. 7.26 **Medulloblastoma.** Diffuse invasion of cerebellar cortex and extension into the subarachnoid space. GFAP expression is seen within the astrocytes of the cerebellum but not by tumour cells in the subarachnoid space (left). Immunocytochemistry for GFAP.

within the brain tissue and an absence of GFAP expression by tumour cells in the subarachnoid space (Fig. 7.26). *Nestin* is expressed in neuroepithelial progenitor cells in the developing CNS, but is also expressed widely by many embryonic cells outside the CNS. It is an intermediate filament protein with a molecular weight of 210–240 kDa and is almost completely downregulated towards the end of gestation.[15] Among brain tumours, nestin expression has been described in medulloblastomas, astrocytomas, glioblastomas, ependymomas, gangliogliomas and meningiomas. Expression of the transmembrane *glucose transporter-1 protein* (GLUT-1) strongly suggests a stem cell origin for medulloblastomas.[45] Although none of the immunocytochemical techniques is

specific for medulloblastoma, a combination of histology, cytology and immunocytochemistry is valuable in making the diagnosis.

Electron microscopy

On ultrastructural examination, medulloblastoma cells frequently show a characteristic but non-specific nuclear morphology, with finely dispersed chromatin and very pronounced nuclear lobulation.[46] An interlacing meshwork of fine, electron lucent cell processes containing axial microtubules is often present between the cell nuclei, especially in areas showing solid rosettes. Bundles of intermediate glial filaments or collections of synaptic vesicles may be seen in some cases, as ultrastructural evidence of glial and neuroblastic differentiation.[46] However, such specific features may not be present in histologically and immunocytochemically undifferentiated areas of tumour and electron microscopy is therefore rarely of practical value in the diagnosis of medulloblastoma.

Proliferation indices

Mitoses are common in medulloblastomas, particularly in undifferentiated tumours where there may be two or more mitoses per high power field. Proliferation is less in areas showing cytological differentiation into neurons and in the 'pale islands' seen in a proportion of medulloblastomas (Fig. 7.18). Ki-67/MIB-1 immunocytochemistry is one reliable way of establishing a proliferation index in medulloblastomas (Fig. 7.27). The index is often greater than 20% and may be 50% in some foci.[47] There is also considerable apoptosis in medulloblastomas[48] and apoptotic tumour cells with condensed, fragmented nuclei are usually easier to find than mitotic figures.

Metastatic spread

Metastasis of neuroectodermal tumours from the CNS to other organs is very uncommon, but there are well documented cases of medulloblastoma metastasising to bone and lung.[49] Such spread usually follows surgical intervention or the insertion of a shunt into a ventricle.[50] Biopsies from metastases may be very small and fragmented particularly if taken as needle biopsies from bone, but groups of medulloblastoma cells may be detected by their hyperchromatic nuclei (Fig. 7.28). Identification of the tumour cells in both bone and lung may be facilitated by immunocytochemistry using anti-GFAP antibodies (Figs 7.29 and 7.30). Antisynaptophysin antibodies

are less valuable because peripheral neuroectodermal tumours such as paragangliomas are also positive. The range of differential diagnosis is usually not very wide but positive identification of metastatic medulloblastoma in lung and bone requires comparison of the immunocytochemical profile of the original tumour with the metastasis. Within the CNS, medulloblastoma spreads extensively through the subarachnoid space and groups of cells may be identified in lumbar CSF.[51] A cytological diagnosis is confirmed if the cells are expressing synaptophysin (Fig. 7.14) or GFAP.

Molecular biology

Sporadic medulloblastomas have been the subject of a number of studies investigating oncogenes, tumour

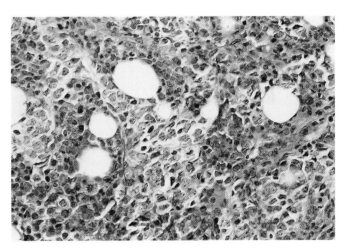

Fig. 7.28 **Metastatic medulloblastoma.** Metastases from medulloblastoma in bone marrow. Islands of hyperchromatic cells with little cytoplasm are seen mixed with marrow components that have more eosinophilic cytoplasm. H & E.

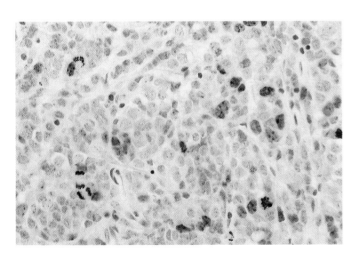

Fig. 7.27 **Medulloblastoma.** Cell proliferation as labelled by Ki-67/MIB-1. Labelling indices vary from 10 to 30% and are usually lower in areas of neuronal differentiation. Immunocytochemistry for MIB-1 proliferation antigen.

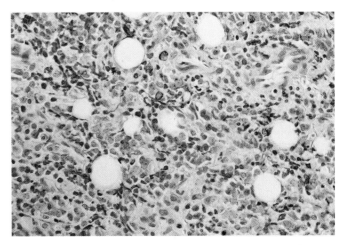

Fig. 7.29 **Metastatic medulloblastoma.** Same case as Fig. 7.28 showing GFAP expression in the metastatic tumour cells in bone marrow. Immunocytochemistry for GFAP.

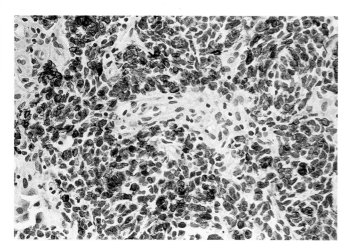

Fig. 7.30 **Metastatic medulloblastoma.** Strong expression of GFAP is shown within the tumour cells in the lung.

suppressor genes and regions of chromosomal loss. The most consistent finding has been isochromosome 17q on cytogenetic studies and the correlative allelic loss of chromosome 17p on molecular genetic analysis. The tumour suppressor gene on chromosome 17p that is inactivated by these genetic events has not been identified, but appears to map distal to the *TP53* tumour suppressor gene, which is only rarely altered in medulloblastomas. In addition to chromosome 17p loss, moderately common allelic losses have also been found on chromosomes 6q, 9q (see below), 11p and 16q. Among oncogenes, only amplification of the *C-MYC* oncogene has been noted with any regularity, but this is more common in medulloblastoma cell lines than in primary tumours.

The discovery of the genes underlying two tumour suppressor syndromes have shed light on the pathways involved in medulloblastoma tumorigenesis. Gorlin syndrome, a condition characterised by multiple basal cell carcinomas (also termed basal cell nevoid syndrome), bone cysts, ovarian fibromas, dysmorphic features and medulloblastomas was linked to a gene on the long arm of chromosome 9 (see Chapter 19). The responsible gene has been termed *PTCH*, a homologue of the *Drosophila* patched gene. Medulloblastomas often show allelic loss of chromosome 9q, with some papers suggesting that chromosome 9q loss occurs preferentially in desmoplastic variants of medulloblastoma and that patients with Gorlin syndrome preferentially develop desmoplastic medulloblastomas.[52] *PTCH* mutations have been documented in sporadic medulloblastomas.[53–55] The protein encoded by *PTCH* functions in the pathway initiated by the Sonic hedgehog protein (SHH). Other molecules in the *PTCH* pathway include smoothened (SMOH), and rare *SMOH* mutations have been documented in sporadic medulloblastomas.[56] The other condition linked to

medulloblastoma is Turcot syndrome, which is characterised by colonic and brain tumours (Chapter 19); patients with the adenomatous polyposis phenotype often develop medulloblastomas and these patients have mutations of the *APC* gene on chromosome 5q. Curiously, *APC* gene mutations and loss of chromosome 5q are rare in sporadic medulloblastomas. The APC protein operates in a molecular pathway that includes the beta-catenin protein, and rare mutations of beta-catenin gene have now been noted in sporadic medulloblastomas.[57] As other components of these two pathways are elucidated, it is likely that these components will be implicated in the genesis of medulloblastomas as well.

The question of whether molecular analyses can provide ancillary information for the management of medulloblastoma patients remains open. Some papers have suggested that patients whose tumours have loss of chromosome 17p may follow a more aggressive clinical course, but this has not been a universal finding and therefore assessment of chromosome 17p status has not achieved a place in the routine clinical management of medulloblastoma patients. Others have provided intriguing evidence that the level of expression of the trkC receptor may relate to prognosis, with those tumours showing high trkC expression following a more favourable course,[58] but this correlation awaits further confirmation.

A recent study based on DNA microarray gene expression data in medulloblastomas found that the clinical outcome appeared highly predictable on the basis of gene expression profiles at diagnosis.[58] The relevant genes included groups of genes influencing cerebellar differentiation (including TRKC and sodium channel genes) and extracellular matrix proteins (including elastin and collagen type V genes) in good prognosis cases, and cell proliferation and metabolism (including *MYBL*2 and *LDH*) in poor prognosis cases. These intriguing correlations await further confirmation.

Differential diagnosis

Medulloblastomas occur both in children and in adults; the age of the patient therefore should be carefully considered in the differential diagnosis of medulloblastoma (Table 7.4).

Table 7.4 Differential diagnosis of medulloblastoma

Children	Adults
Pilocytic astrocytoma	Haemangioblastoma
Ependymoma	Metastatic carcinoma
Haemangioblastoma	Vestibular Schwannoma
	Meningioma
	Lymphoma
	Pilocytic astrocytoma

Pilocytic astrocytoma

Pilocytic astrocytoma of the cerebellum is most commonly seen in children and young adults and presents either with cerebellar signs, such as ataxia, or with raised intracranial pressure due to compression of the fourth ventricle and obstruction of CSF resulting in hydrocephalus. Like medulloblastomas, pilocytic astrocytomas enhance in CT and MRI scans and calcification may occur in both types of tumour.

Histologically, however, pilocytic astrocytomas are quite distinct from medulloblastomas. The architectural pattern, lack of mitoses, abundant cytoplasm and the presence of Rosenthal fibres will all help to positively identify a pilocytic astrocytoma. Using immunocytochemistry, the filiform processes of cells in pilocytic astrocytoma are strongly GFAP positive, whereas GFAP staining may only be patchy in medulloblastoma and usually confined to perinuclear regions. Care must be taken not to confuse the reactive astrocytes in medulloblastoma with tumour cells. Ki-67/MIB-1 labelling for proliferation antigens is high (often over 20%) in medulloblastoma but low (under 2%) in pilocytic astrocytoma.

Ependymoma

Although ependymomas in the posterior fossa usually arise within the fourth ventricle, resulting in occlusion of the ventricular system and hydrocephalus, these tumours may also extend dorsally into the cerebellum. Because they enhance on CT and MRI, occur in children at a similar age and in a similar site to medulloblastoma, there may be problems with the diagnosis preoperatively. Care must be taken in the histological assessment of ependymoma and medulloblastoma, particularly as the treatment of these two tumour types is different. Well differentiated ependymomas may be easily distinguished from medulloblastoma, as the cells have abundant cytoplasm, nuclei of uniform size, few mitoses and well formed perivascular pseudorosettes or even true tubular rosettes. The picture may not be as clear with poorly differentiated (anaplastic) ependymomas in which there may be a high proliferation rate and a high nuclear : cytoplasmic ratio which can cause confusion with medulloblastoma. However the most useful distinguishing feature between ependymoma and medulloblastoma is the presence of perivascular pseudorosettes in ependymomas. These appear as anucleate fibrillar zones around vessels and express GFAP on immunocytochemistry. They are distinct from the neuroblastic (Homer Wright) rosettes in medulloblastoma (Fig. 7.9). Using electron microscopy, ependymomas may show the presence of cilia which is another distinguishing feature from medulloblastoma.

Haemangioblastoma

Haemangioblastomas are uncommon in children but in patients with von Hippel–Lindau syndrome they may arise at an early age (see Chapters 14 and 19). There is often no particular problem with the clinical differential diagnosis between haemangioblastoma and medulloblastoma, particularly if the haemangioblastoma has an associated cyst visible as an enhancing nodule on CT and MRI. However, in the absence of a cyst and a single enhancing nodule, cerebellar haemangioblastoma enters the differential diagnosis of medulloblastoma. Histologically, the cytology of the two tumours is distinct. Largely featureless sheets of hyperchromatic nuclei with sparse fibrillary cytoplasm and frequent mitoses in medulloblastoma can be distinguished from the histology of haemangioblastoma with its packets of cells surrounded by reticulin and well demarcated margins. Some confusion may occur, however, if medulloblastoma cells invade the subarachnoid space, where the tumour cells may be confused with rather more pleomorphic examples of haemangioblastoma. In frozen sections, haemangioblastomas contain lipid droplets in the cells when stained with Oil red O or Sudan dyes and this is not a feature of medulloblastoma. Immunocytochemistry may be helpful as haemangioblastoma cells do not express synaptophysin, usually present in medulloblastoma. Finally, the proliferation rate, either measured by mitoses or through MIB-1 labelling, is high (greater than 10%) in medulloblastoma but usually less than 1% in haemangioblastoma.

Metastatic carcinoma

Metastatic carcinoma and medulloblastoma both occur in the cerebellum in adults, and both appear on imaging as enhancing tumours often with areas of necrosis. Histologically, anaplastic carcinomas and small cell carcinomas of the lung may be easily confused with medulloblastoma. In rapid intraoperative diagnosis preparations, the epithelial cohesion and distinct cell borders of metastatic carcinoma cells may be distinguished from the diffuse fibrillary stroma in medulloblastoma but, ultimately, the differential diagnosis may depend upon immunocytochemistry. In contrast to most medulloblastomas, metastatic carcinomas usually express cytokeratin but not GFAP. Synaptophysin is less helpful, since small cell carcinomas of the lung may be synaptophysin positive, like medulloblastomas. Mitotic indices and Ki-67/MIB-1 labelling may be very similar in both metastatic carcinomas and medulloblastoma.

Vestibular Schwannoma

These typically present with deafness and tinnitus, and if large, with distortion of the fourth ventricle and supratentorial hydrocephalus. In some cases, medulloblastomas may mimic this presentation, particularly as an exophytic growth in the cerebellopontine angle. On biopsy, vestibular Schwannomas have a firm consistency, and are composed of spindle shaped cells surrounded individually by dense reticulin. The abundant fibrillary cytoplasm is S-100 positive, and GFAP negative on immunocytochemistry. The low proliferation rate in Schwannomas (less than 1%) will help to distinguish these tumours from medulloblastomas with their high proliferation rate and sheets of hyperchromatic cells, variably expressing synaptophysin and GFAP.

Meningioma

Meningiomas may also present in the cerebellopontine angle and because they enhance on CT and MR scans, they may occasionally be confused preoperatively with medulloblastoma. The histology in cryostat and paraffin sections in most cases of meningioma is distinct from medulloblastoma. However, in the more anaplastic meningiomas, the tumour may be composed of cells with hyperchromatic pleomorphic nuclei and a MIB-1 labelling index of over 5%. It is in these tumours that immunocytochemistry is valuable for the differential diagnosis. Meningiomas cells would typically express EMA but not synaptophysin or GFAP. Medulloblastomas are usually negative for EMA and many will express synaptophysin and GFAP. Furthermore, the majority of meningiomas are sharply demarcated from adjacent brain tissue, whereas medulloblastomas diffusely infiltrate surrounding cerebellum.

Malignant lymphoma

This is uncommon in the cerebellum, but it should be considered in the differential diagnosis of medulloblastoma, particularly in adults. Lymphomas typically appear in CT and MRI scans as well circumscribed enhancing nodules. Histologically, differentiation between medulloblastoma and lymphoma may pose a problem, particularly during rapid intraoperative diagnosis. The uniform nuclear morphology can produce a similar cytological appearance in both lymphoma and medulloblastoma and both tumours are typically composed of sheets of tumour cells with few organoid features. Touch preparations may be helpful in distinguishing between medulloblastoma and lymphoma during rapid intraoperative diagnosis, as the typical nuclear morphology in lymphomas may be well demonstrated. However, the certainty of differential diagnosis may require reticulin stains and immunocytochemistry on paraffin sections. Although reticulin bands may be present in desmoplastic medulloblastomas and those tumours that have invaded the subarachnoid space, reticulin in lymphomas is usually confined to blood vessels. In addition, the complex reduplication of reticulin in perivascular spaces is typical of lymphoma and not

usually seen in medulloblastoma. Immunocytochemistry for leucocyte common antigen and other lymphocyte subset markers and immunoglobulins should finally distinguish lymphoma from medulloblastoma.

Therapy and prognosis

Medulloblastomas show a high propensity to spread through the CSF and occasionally to metastasise to the lungs and bone. Treatment therefore is directed at the primary site in the cerebellum and the neuraxis according to the pattern of spread as assessed by MRI and CSF cytology.[51] Recent clinical trials have supported the use of radiation and chemotherapy as adjuvant treatment for medulloblastoma.[1,59] Such strategies result in an overall 5-year survival rate of 40–60% and a 5-year progression free survival rate of 12–29% but with neuropsychological deficits.[59] Occasional late recurrence of medulloblastoma after periods up to 19 years have been reported but this is very rare.[60]

Histological variants of medulloblastoma

In addition to classical medulloblastoma, there are a number of variants of medulloblastoma. One of these contains abundant connective tissue (desmoplastic medulloblastoma), whilst others incorporate cells with the morphology of striated muscle or pigment epithelium. These histological variants have such distinctive histological features that they are separately identified in the WHO classification (Table 7.1).

1. Desmoplastic medulloblastoma

This tumour shows a biphasic histological pattern. In the desmoplastic areas there are densely packed tumour cells with a high nuclear : cytoplasmic ratio and high proliferative activity which are embedded in a dense, intercellular reticulin network. Scattered through the tumour, however, are reticulin free islands in which the cells have more fibrillary cytoplasm, express synaptophysin and/or GFAP and show less proliferative activity (Figs 7.18 and 7.19). These areas resemble supratentorial PNETs (see below) rather than classical medulloblastoma. Desmoplastic medulloblastoma cells express the low affinity neurotrophin receptor, p75NTR.[61] Since this receptor is expressed by cells of the external granule cell layer of the fetal cerebellum, it has been suggested that desmoplastic medulloblastomas may arise from this cell layer.[61]

It is uncertain whether desmoplastic medulloblastomas have a more favourable prognosis than the classical medulloblastomas that lack the fibrous element.[42] However, there is some indication that desmoplastic tumours with extensive nodularity occurring in young children have a more favourable outcome than their more classical counterparts.[62] It is therefore important to recognise this histological variant.

2. Medullomyoblastoma

This tumour is a variant of medulloblastoma characterised by the presence of striated muscle cells. Although it was recognised in the 1930s, only some 40 cases have been described in the literature. Predominantly occurring in males, the majority of medullomyoblastomas occur in children between 2 and 10 years of age[63] although they may also occur in adults.[63] The cerebellar vermis is the commonest site, from which the tumour invades the fourth ventricle. Medullomyoblastomas sited more laterally in the cerebellar hemispheres are even less common. Because of their position, these tumours present with either a midline cerebellar syndrome or with signs of raised intracranial pressure, due to hydrocephalus from occlusion of the fourth ventricle. Medullomyoblastomas enhance on CT and MRI scans and cannot, therefore, be distinguished radiologically from classical medulloblastomas.[63–65] The growth potential and prognosis of medullomyoblastoma are similar to those of medulloblastoma.

Pathology

Macroscopically, medullomyoblastomas have a similar appearance to classical medulloblastomas, with a soft gelatinous consistency, a grey colour and granular areas of necrosis. *Intraoperative diagnosis* may be made on either smear or cryostat section preparations, through the recognition of medulloblastoma cells and the presence of strap-like striated muscle cells. *Histologically*, the muscle cells have a range of morphology (Figs 7.31 and 7.32). Some appear to be spherical eosinophilic cells with central nuclei (Fig. 7.32), whereas others are strap-like striated muscle fibres with cross striations (Figs 7.31 and 7.33). Such muscle cells may form groups or may be distributed evenly through the more primitive histological elements of the medulloblastoma. Using *immunocytochemical staining*, the striated muscle cells of medullomyoblastoma can be firmly identified through their expression of myoglobin (Fig. 7.33), desmin[65] and fast myosin.[66] The presence of synaptophysin and GFAP expression in the more primitive cells in these tumours confirms the presence of a medulloblastoma element. Although the muscle elements of the tumour show little proliferative activity, mitoses are frequent in the medulloblastoma areas and the Ki-67/MIB-1 labelling index is high. *Ultra-stuctural examination* reveals typical sarcomere structures in the striated muscle cells of these tumours (Fig. 7.34).[65] *Genetic studies* do not always show the same allelic loss on chromosomes 17p, 1q, and 9q that is seen in classical medulloblastomas.[67]

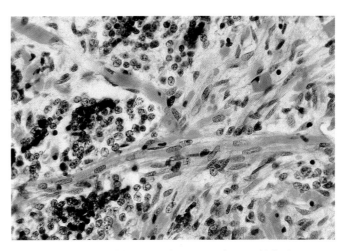

Fig. 7.31 **Medullomyoblastoma.** The tumour shows a biphasic pattern of tumour cells with small round nuclei and sparse fibrillary cytoplasm and larger cells with strap-like morphology and eosinophilic cytoplasm resembling striated muscle cells. H & E.

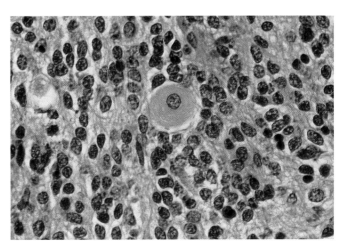

Fig. 7.32 **Medullomyoblastoma.** Small tumour cells are shown with round nuclei and some fibrillary cytoplasm surrounding a cell with extensive eosinophilic cytoplasm resembling a myoblast. H & E.

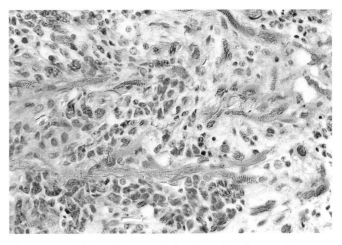

Fig. 7.33 **Medullomyoblastoma.** Striated muscle cells expressing myoglobin are admixed with more classical medulloblastoma cells.

Differential diagnosis

The presence of striated muscle cells in these tumours raises the possibility of teratoma and of primary rhabdomyosarcoma, but the absence of other mature tissue elements and the presence of the primitive neuroectodermal element in medullomyoblastomas can be used to exclude teratoma.

3. Melanotic medulloblastoma

This is a very rare tumour with histological features of classical medulloblastoma but with the presence of melanotic cells. The site and age distribution is similar to that of medulloblastoma.[68]

Histologically, melanotic cells appear as tubular epithelial structures or clusters in a tumour that otherwise resembles a classical medulloblastoma. (Fig. 7.35).[66,68–70] Ultrastructurally, tumour cells contain distinct melanosomes and immunocytochemically, melanotic cells may express S-100 protein.[66–68] It is possible that some of the melanotic cells arise from neural crest, whereas others may originate from the pigment layer of the retina and thus also from the neural tube. Melanotic cells may also be present in medullomyoblastoma.[66] The non-pigmented cells in these tumours show the typical immunocytochemical pattern of classical medulloblastoma and the tumour behaves in a similar way to medulloblastoma. Metastatic spread may be identified by pigmented tumour coating the surface of the brain. The prognosis is poor, with survival of 2–30 months.

4. Large cell medulloblastoma

This variant is seen in approximately 4% of medulloblastomas. The tumour cells have large nuclei with prominent nucleoli and more abundant cytoplasm than other medulloblastoma cells. However, there is also a high mitotic rate and areas of necrosis within this tumour.[5] These tumours are sometimes associated with *C-MYC* amplification, and may have a worse prognosis than standard medulloblastomas.

Supratentorial primitive neuroectodermal tumours (PNETs)

This designation arose out of the unifying concept of PNETs as poorly differentiated or undifferentiated neuroepithelial tumours which have the capacity for differentiation along multiple different cell lines.[71,72] Such tumours are relatively uncommon in the supratentorial compartment, and as discussed at the beginning of this chapter some of them can be separately classified according to specialised tissue of origin, as for example with retinoblastomas and pineoblastomas. The remaining examples are cerebral hemispheric tumours of no specific

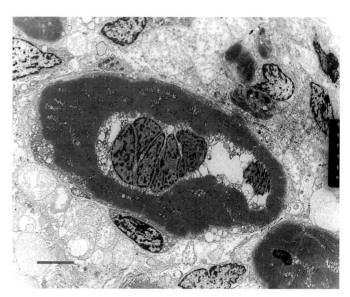

Fig. 7.34 **Medullomyoblastoma.** The ultrastructural appearances of a myoblast with central and peripheral nuclei and the presence of sarcomeric material in the cytoplasm are shown. Electron micrograph. Bar = 20 μm.

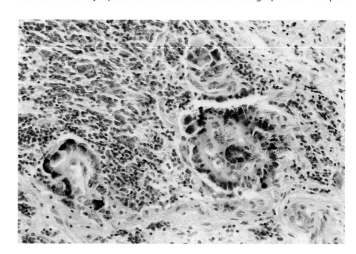

Fig. 7.35 **Melanotic medulloblastoma.** Melanotic tumour cells are admixed with medulloblastoma cells. The pigmented cells form epithelia often arranged in tubular structures. H & E.

site, which may be conveniently referred to simply as supratentorial PNETs, although in the past they have been called cerebral neuroblastomas[73] or even cerebral medulloblastomas.[74] Like all PNETs they are capable of multivaried differentiating activity, but in practice the majority of these lesions show a spectrum of differentiation along neuronal lineage.[75,76] Depending on the degree of neuroblastic and ganglionic maturation the WHO classification now recognises the terms cerebral neuroblastoma and cerebral ganglioneuroblastoma within the overall grouping of supratentorial PNETs.

Incidence and site

Supratentorial PNETs are rare tumours which probably account for less than 5% of all central nervous system embryonal tumours.[75,76] Some 80% of all cases present in the first decade of life, with 25% manifesting before 2 years of age.[75] There is no consistent sex predilection in reported series. By definition these tumours arise within the cerebral hemispheres or in the suprasellar region, and pineal examples are specifically excluded (see Ch. 9). It should be noted, however, that pathologically indistinguishable tumours can arise in a variety of other parts of the CNS, in addition to medulloblastomas of the cerebellum. Such unusually sited PNETs lie awkwardly in the current WHO classification, but have been described in such diverse locations as the pons[77] and the cauda equina.[78]

Clinical features

The presenting signs and symptoms are those of a large, rapidly expanding hemispheric mass lesion, with clinical evidence of raised intracranial pressure usually predominating.[79] In addition there may be seizures, focal neurological deficits appropriate to the location of the tumour and in infants, an enlarging head circumference. Suprasellar examples may cause visual and pituitary failure.[75,76] Radiologically, these tumours usually appear isodense to grey matter in CT and MRI images, enhance after administration of contrast media and may show cystic areas and focal mineralisation.[79] Central areas of non-enhancing necrosis may also be seen (Fig. 7.36).

Pathology

Macroscopic features

PNETs in the cerebrum may be very large at presentation and occupy much of one or both hemispheres (Figs 7.37 and 7.38). Macroscopically, they are soft grey tumours, although some may have a desmoplastic component and

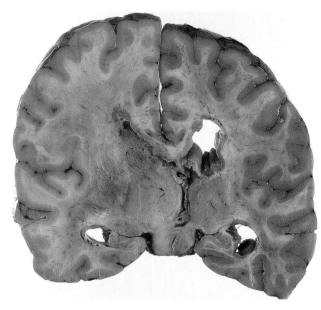

Fig. 7.37 **Supratentorial PNET.** Coronal section of the brain at post-mortem showing enlargement of the left hemisphere due to the presence of cerebral neuroblastoma.

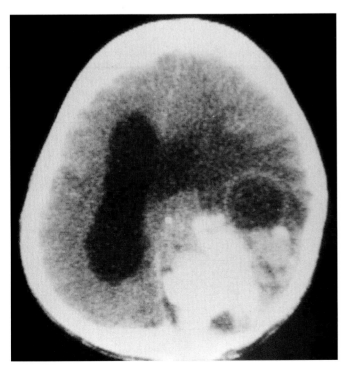

Fig. 7.36 **Supratentorial PNET.** An enhancing lesion is shown with a cystic area and darker areas of probable necrosis in this CT scan.

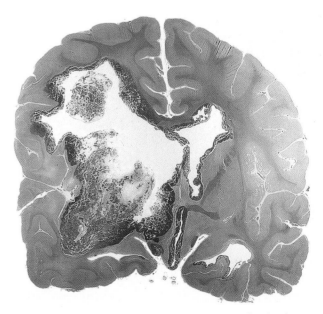

Fig. 7.38 **Supratentorial PNET.** Same case as Fig. 7.37 showing how the central region of the tumour is very fragile and has disappeared from the preparation. A basophilic rim of tumour surrounds the artefactual cavity. The tumour appears to be well circumscribed but it does, in fact, invade surrounding brain. H & E.

thus areas of firmer consistency. Central areas of the tumours are often granular and necrotic or cystic.

Intraoperative diagnosis

Like medulloblastomas, supratentorial PNETs are usually soft enough tumours to make good smear preparations. The cells easily smear into a monolayer and have pleomorphic nuclei which characteristically mould and indent each other. Mitoses are frequent. Depending on the degree of neuronal differentiation there may be a variable amount of finely filamentous tumour stroma, and in more mature ganglioneuroblastomas obvious large neuronal cells with ganglionic features are usually identifiable

Histological features

Poorly differentiated PNETs in the cerebrum have similar histological features to posterior fossa medulloblastomas. The tumour cells are usually arranged in featureless sheets when viewed at lower magnifications (Fig. 7.39). On closer examination, they have small, rounded, hyperchromatic nuclei and little discernible perinuclear cytoplasm (Fig. 7.40). Mitoses are variable in frequency but apoptotic nuclei are typically a prominent feature. Desmoplasia may be encountered in some examples with similar features to those seen in partly or wholly desmoplastic medulloblastomas (see above). Areas of haemorrhage, focal necrosis, calcification and melanin pigment may also be present in some cases. In very poorly differentiated examples, the tumour cell nuclei are

closely packed together with little background stroma, but areas of neuronal maturation are found in a significant proportion of supratentorial PNETs. With routine stains this is most commonly manifest as focal areas of decreased numbers of nuclei and more abundant filamentous stroma, sometimes referred to as 'pale islands' (Fig. 7.41). The tumour cell nuclei in these areas tend to be larger and may take on a neuronal appearance with pale chromatin and a distinct nucleolus (Fig. 7.42). The proportion of primitive and more differentiated areas varies considerably from case to case and, rather uncommonly, there are areas of very pronounced maturation containing large, sometimes atypical ganglion cells (Figs 7.43 and 7.44). As mentioned above, these tumours represent an extreme end of a spectrum of neuronal differentiation and are normally referred to as cerebral ganglioneuroblastomas.

Immunocytochemistry

The capacity of supratentorial PNETs to undergo neuronal differentiation is most clearly demonstrated by immunocytochemical staining. Even those tumours appearing entirely primitive in routine stains usually show widespread expression of neuronal epitopes such as synaptophysin and neuron specific enolase.[80] Immunostaining for such epitopes becomes more marked in the 'pale islands' of those tumours, confirming maturation along neuronal lines in these islands. Further evidence of neuronal differentiation may be evident using antibodies to neurofilament protein, microtubule associated protein 2 (MAP-2) and beta-tubulin.[81] Somewhat less often, focal

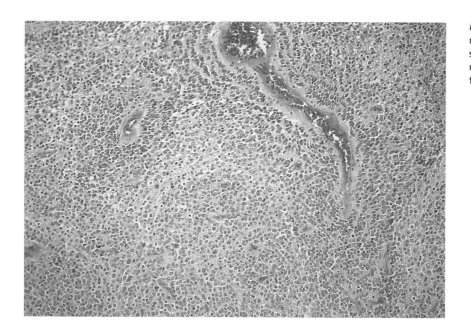

Fig. 7.39 **Supratentorial PNET.** At lower magnifications, poorly differentiated examples show closely packed tumour cells arranged in monotonous sheets, without specific architectural feaures. H & E.

immunostaining of tumour cells for GFAP may be found in apparently primitive areas of tumour, indicating divergent glial differentiation, and exceptionally immuno-staining for muscle antigens has also been described.[82] Expression of the transmembrane GLUT-1 strongly suggests a stem cell origin for supratentorial PNET.[45] Immunostaining with cell proliferation markers such as Ki-67/MIB-1 invariably shows a very high labelling index in the more primitive areas of tumour, even in examples where mitotic figures are hard to find.

Electron microscopy

Ultrastructural examination often, but not invariably, demonstrates dense core vesicles in supratentorial PNETs.[83,84] These become more abundant and easy to find

in tumours demonstrating a greater degree of neuronal differentiation and are accompanied by other ultrastructural evidence of neuroblastic lineage, including fine, electron lucent cell processes containing axial microtubules.[46] Synaptic vesicles or fully formed synapses have been reported in exceptional cases[85] and bundles of intermediate filaments in tumour cells probably represent glial differentiation.[46]

Molecular genetics

Isochromosome 17q and allelic loss of 17p, which is found in a high proportion of cerebellar medulloblastomas, is only rarely found in supratentorial PNETs[86] and although a variety of genetic abnormalities have been reported in these tumours, no consistent pattern has yet emerged.[87]

Differential diagnosis

Small cell glioblastoma

These tumours are relatively rare in infancy but present as large, rapidly growing hemispheric masses. Histologically, sheets of small primitive cells may be easily be confused with a poorly differentiated PNET. However, even small cell glioblastomas usually show distinguishing features such as glomeruloid microvascular proliferation and pseudo-palisades around foci of necrosis which are exceedingly rare in PNETs. The surest distinction is made using immuno-cytochemistry, since the consistent expression of neuronal antigens is not seen in glioblastomas.

Cerebral lymphoma

These may also be confused histologically with PNETs on account of their small, round cell cytology, although there

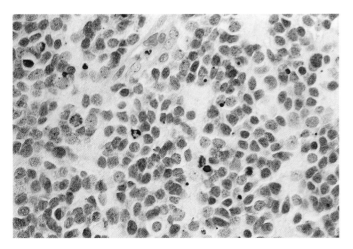

Fig. 7.40 **Supratentorial PNET.** As in medulloblastomas, supratentorial PNETs are composed of cells with hyperchromatic nuclei and poorly defined perinuclear cytoplasm. H & E.

Fig. 7.41 **Supratentorial PNET.** There are rounded areas with reduced numbers of nuclei and more abundant filamentous stroma, or so-called 'pale islands', which can give a nodular appearance at lower magnifications. These islands of maturation show enhanced immunocytochemical expression of neuronal antigens. H & E.

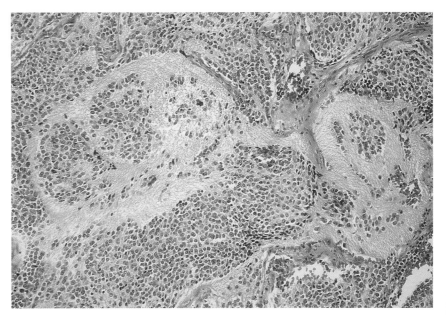

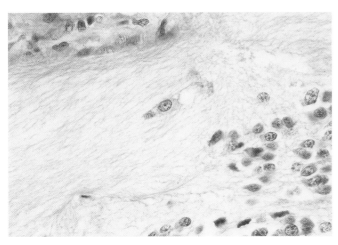

Fig. 7.42 **Supratentorial PNET.** The tumour cells in maturing 'pale islands' usually have larger nuclei with paler chromatin than those in the more primitive areas of tumour. Some may have a distinct nucleolus and discernible perinuclear cytoplasm, like the cell in the centre. H & E.

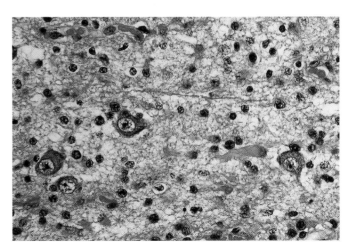

Fig. 7.44 **Supratentorial PNET.** This tumour is composed of mainly cells with small nuclei and many fibrillary processes but shows focal areas of ganglionic differentiation with groups of typical neurons. Unless these neuronal cells show cytological atypia (see Fig. 7.43), care must be taken not to mistake them for entrapped normal neurons. H & E.

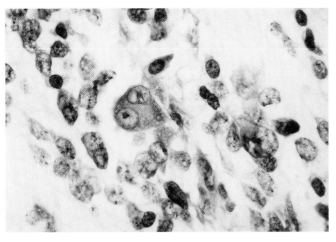

Fig. 7.43 **Supratentorial PNET.** In tumours showing more advanced neuronal differentiation, large ganglion cells can be found in the maturing 'pale islands'. Some have atypical cytological features, like this binucleate example. Cresyl violet stain.

is usually a much older age range of presentation. In intra-operative smear preparations, the best distinguishing cytological features are the lack of nuclear moulding which typifies PNETs, together with the presence of distinct rims of perinuclear cytoplasm. Histologically, lymphomas usually show a prominent population of small reactive lymphocytes and have a very diffuse pattern of marginal infiltration, with perivascular cuffing. Immunocytochemistry shows expression of lymphoid rather than neuronal antigens.

Ependymoblastoma

Both types of tumour tend to occur at deep cerebral sites and both show a tendency to seed in the CSF. Histologically,

ependymoblastomatous rosettes are one of the main distinguishing features as they are not present in supratentorial PNETs. Immunocytochemistry will again confirm the distinction, since neuronal antigens are not expressed by ependymoblastomas.

Ganglioglioma

These tumours will normally have a slower symptomatic onset in an older age group than supratentorial PNETs, but there is scope for confusing them both histologically and immunocytochemically with PNETs showing ganglionic and divergent glial differentiation. The important issue here is tissue sampling, and a careful search in biopsies from even the most differentiated PNET will reveal areas of primitive neuroblastic or undifferentiated tumour.

Neurocytoma

Again, these are usually tumours of an older age group and of less rapid growth than supratentorial PNETs, but some examples may contain ganglionic cells and need to be distinguished from PNETs showing neuronal maturation. As with ganglioglioma, the key lies in a careful search for areas of more primitive, undifferentiated tumour. In both cases cell elements will express neuronal antigens, but neurocytomas lack the primitive cytological appearance of the undifferentiated cells in PNETs.

Therapy and prognosis

Treatment of supratentorial PNETs follows similar lines to other types of PNET, including medulloblastoma. In infants and very young children, surgical debulking is combined with chemotherapy, sometimes with 'second look' surgery for residual or locally recurrent tumour once chemotherapy is complete.[75] Like other PNETs, supratentorial ones show a pronounced tendency to seed in the CSF pathways[88] and prophylactic craniospinal irradiation may be considered in older children. No correlation has been shown between the clinical behaviour of these tumours and the degree of differentiation demonstrated microscopically. Children with supratentorial PNETs have a considerably worse prognosis than medulloblastoma patients, with an overall 5-year survival rate of only 34%, less than half that for the infratentorial tumours.[89,90] Children presenting at less than 2 years of age are said to have a still worse prognosis.[75,91]

Polar spongioblastoma

Controversy exists as to whether this entity exists as a neoplasm in its own right, or whether it merely represents a histological pattern in regions of neoplasms which would otherwise be classified as another form of neuroepithelial tumour (usually astrocytoma or glioblastoma). The case reports which suggest that this is a distinct entity appear in the earlier literature, where polar spongioblastoma was described as a very rare neoplasm occurring mainly in children, with a peculiar histological appearance characterised by rows of unipolar or bipolar astrocytic spindle cells arranged in distinct palisades. Because it was felt to be only a histological variant of other tumours, polar spongioblastoma has been omitted from the WHO 2000 classification of Tumours of the Nervous System.[5]

Incidence, site and radiology

Some 14 cases of this tumour have been previously reported, 12 of which occurred in children.[92] The tumour predominantly affected the posterior fossa, especially the cerebellum, fourth ventricle or midbrain. Some tumours enhanced and others showed calcification on neuroradiology. Seeding into the spinal meninges has been described.[92]

Aetiology

There has been much speculation with regard to the histogenesis of these tumours but the generally accepted current opinion is that they represent an occasional growth pattern, usually affecting an otherwise ordinary astrocytic tumour.[93] Cerebellar examples are most likely to represent progressive differentiation in a primitive neuroectodermal tumour.[19] There is wide agreement that the polar spongioblastoma does not exist as a distinct entity.

Pathology

Histological features

The characteristic pattern of polar spongioblastomas consists of groups or rows of nuclei from which radiate fine, eosinophilic processes which give the tumour an alternating blue and pink appearance in H & E stained sections at low power. There is no direct relationship of the processes to blood vessels but care must be taken not to confuse this pattern with the pseudorosettes of ependymoma. Regions of tumours which correspond to the description of polar spongioblastoma can be identified in a range of glial tumours (particularly astrocytomas and glioblastomas), but may also occur in medulloblastomas and cerebral PNET. In some regions of the tumour, the polar spongioblastoma pattern can predominate, but a careful search of the tissue will usually allow identification of the primary tumour structure corresponding to the lesion from which the polar spongioblastoma pattern has been derived.

Immunocytochemistry

GFAP expression is seen in some cases, but there is expression of synaptophysin in others, probably reflecting the heterogenous tumours included in this histological variant.

Electron microscopy

Ultrastructural studies have revealed features of neuronal differentiation, including neurosecretory granules and synapse-like junctions,[93] and astrocytic features in some tumours.

Prognosis

The clinical behaviour of this entity will depend on the nature of the underlying neoplasm: in a previous series, this was reported to depend upon the proliferation index, the completeness of the excision at surgery, and the degree of spread throughout the neuraxis.[92]

Atypical teratoid-rhabdoid tumours

This rare tumour is composed of rhabdoid cells with or without elements of classical primitive neuroectodermal, epithelial or mesenchymal tumour. Most commonly arising in the kidney, it also occurs in the liver, thymus and the CNS.[94]

Incidence and site

These tumours occur mainly under the age of 18 years and usually within the first 2 years (median age 17 months in one large series).[95] Adult cases have also been reported, but are exceptional. A simultaneous presentation has been reported in two sisters of different ages, representing the first familial cases of this tumour in the CNS.[96] One case of atypical teratoid-rhabdoid tumour has been reported in a child with Canavan's disease, presumably by coincidence.[97] In children, atypical teratoid-rhabdoid tumours may be located in many different sites in the neuraxis but mainly in the cerebellum and cerebellopontine angle. The supratentorial compartment is less frequently the primary site for this neoplasm, but cases arising in the cerebral hemisphere have been reported, including occasional cases arising in the pineal region.[95,98] The tumour may also present as a spinal cord neoplasm.[99] Occasional patients present with multiple CNS metastases, involving both the infra- and supratentorial compartments, reflecting the aggressive nature of this neoplasm.[95]

Clinical features

The clinical signs and symptoms are very variable, depending on the site of the tumour and the age of the patient. In infants, the presenting features are often very non-specific, with vomiting and failure to thrive, in common with other posterior fossa neoplasms at this age.[95] Patients with disseminated disease at presentation will often have signs and symptoms relating to spinal 'drop' deposits as well as intracranial metastases. *Radiologically*, these tumours are hyperintense in CT scans, usually hypodense in MRI sequences and enhance after administration of contrast media[95] (Fig. 7.45). The size and location of these neoplasms is extremely variable (see above).

Pathology

Macroscopic features

Atypical teratoid-rhabdoid tumours have a similar gross appearance to that of primitive neuroectodermal tumours, with ill-defined margins and a soft fleshy consistency. Multiple foci of haemorrhage may be present, and necrosis is not uncommon. Calcification is a very uncommon feature. In autopsy cases of patients with disseminated disease, multiple, often superficial, tumour deposits may be present over the surfaces of the cerebrum, cerebellum and spinal cord.

Histological features

Histologically, the defining feature is groups of rhabdoid cells and epithelioid cells, with or without areas of typical smaller primitive neuroectodermal tumour cells.[95,99,100] The rhabdoid cell has a round or oval nucleus with an eccentric nucleolus and eccentric ball-like cytoplasm that is finely granular or homogeneous (Fig. 7.46). There is often a typical flask-like shape with a terminal filament (Fig. 7.47). The epithelioid elements may occur in the form of poorly formed glands, or may be set within a

myxoid stroma. The primitive neuroectodermal elements are extremely variable in their relative number and appearance, but most have been described as resembling a medulloblastoma. Other cell and tissue elements may occur in rhabdoid tumours, including mesenchymal areas, which may suggest a teratoid neoplasm. Haemorrhage is a common feature, but vascular endothelial proliferation is not characteristic of this tumour. Necrosis is often present, occasionally multifocal, but usually without surrounding nuclear pseudopalisading. Atypical teratoid-rhabdoid tumours are rapidly growing neoplasms, and both mitotic figures and apoptotic bodies are readily identifiable in all the cellular populations within the neoplasm.

Atypical teratoid-rhabdoid tumours have a propensity to invade and disseminate via the CSF pathway, and cytology has been used as both a diagnostic tool and to monitor tumour behaviour and recurrence. Typical cytological features of rhabdoid cells include the large size of the cells in the CSF, with eccentric nuclei and prominent nucleoli.[102]

Immunocytochemistry

Rhabdoid cells are polyphenotypic, expressing EMA, vimentin, smooth muscle actin, GFAP, neurofilament

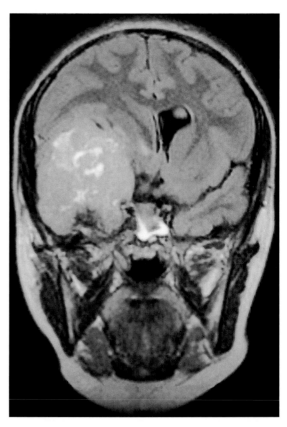

Fig. 7.45 **Atypical teratoid-rhabdoid tumour.** Contrast enhanced MRI scan of a large supratentorial atypical teratoid-rhabdoid tumour. There is variable enhancement within the tumour mass, which invades and displaces the adjacent temporal lobe.

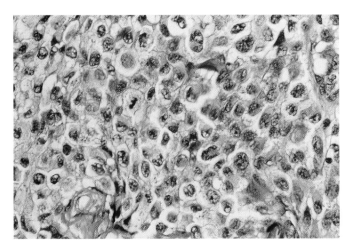

Fig. 7.46 Atypical teratoid-rhabdoid tumour. Sheets of cells are shown with abundant cytoplasm. Nuclei are often eccentrically placed and mitoses are frequent. H & E.

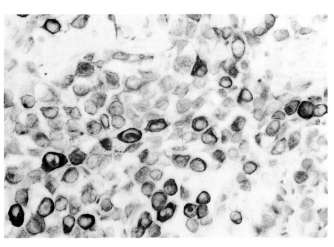

Fig. 7.47 Atypical teratoid-rhabdoid tumour. This tumour shows expression of cytokeratins and shows the typical morphology of the cells, often with small pointed terminal processes. Immunocytochemistry for low molecular weight cytokeratins (CAM 5.2).

Fig. 7.48 Atypical teratoid-rhabdoid tumour. Immunocytochemistry for smooth muscle actin. The walls of blood vessels and a large number of the tumour cells are stained, including the rhabdoid cells.

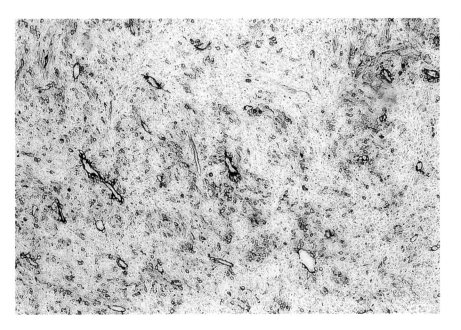

protein and cytokeratins[95,99,100] (Figs 7.47 and 7.48). They do not express desmin, but whorled bundles of intermediate filaments may be seen by electron microscopy. The other cellular components of the tumour exhibit immunocytochemical features appropriate to their cell type, for example, the primitive neuroectodermal component will stain strongly with antibodies to synaptophysin and neuron specific enolase. Proliferative activity is high, as is the labelling index with Ki-67/MIB-1, which had a mean of 63.9% in a recent study.[100]

Molecular biology

The precise origin of these tumours is still debated, but genetic studies suggest that they differ from typical PNET. Expression of the transmembrane GLUT-1 protein in atypical teratoid-rhabdoid tumours strongly suggests a stem cell origin.[45] Atypical teratoid-rhabdoid tumour shows monosomy for chromosome 22 and a tumour suppressor gene on 22q11.2 has been implicated in these tumours[95,102] as opposed to isochromosome 17q in PNETs. These tumours often have loss of chromosome 22q, and one case has been reported in a child with a ring chromosome 22.[103] However, while loss of chromosome 22q can be considered as supporting a diagnosis of atypical teratoid-rhabdoid tumours, it is neither specific nor completely sensitive since chromosome 22q loss can occur in other types of brain tumours and not all atypical teratoid-rhabdoid tumours have detectable chromosome 22q loss. The frequent loss of chromosome 22 in renal and systemic extrarenal rhabdoid tumours suggests the presence of a chromosome 22 tumour suppressor gene responsible for such lesions. The identification of the *INI1* gene confirmed this hypothesis, since mutations of this chromosome 22q gene are common in extracranial rhabdoid tumours.[104] This gene has also been implicated in intracranial atypical teratoid-rhabdoid tumours, both by somatic and by germline mutations.[105] The elucidation of the function of the protein encoded by the *INI1* gene may shed light of the pathogenesis of atypical teratoid-rhabdoid tumours. Furthermore, the demonstration of *INI1* gene mutations will serve as an important diagnostic criterion for such tumours in the future (see below).

Differential diagnosis

Atypical teratoid-rhabdoid tumours need to be distinguished form other malignant neoplasms in order that appropriate treatment and counselling are made available to the patient and their relatives. The most important differential diagnoses are:

Medulloblastoma/PNET

Since most cases of atypical teratoid-rhabdoid tumours present in the posterior fossa in infants, a clear distinction from medulloblastoma should be made. This is best achieved by the identification of the polyphenotypic rhabdoid cells on immunocytochemistry, particularly with antibodies to cytokeratins and smooth muscle actin, which usually give negative results in medulloblastomas. A PNET component can occur in atypical teratoid-rhabdoid tumours, but it is not usually the predominant histological feature. Supratentorial PNET can also be distinguished from atypical teratoid-rhabdoid tumours on the basis of immunocytochemisty, but molecular genetic studies for changes in chromosome 22q and the *INI1* gene (see above) may be used to help this distinction in cases of diagnostic uncertainty.

Choroid plexus carcinoma

Choroid plexus carcinomas may arise in the posterior fossa in infants, and can be distinguished from atypical teratoid-rhabdoid tumours on the basis of immunocyto-chemistry, since their polyphenotypic pattern of antigen expression is absent in choroid plexus carcinomas. Likewise, atypical teratoid-rhabdoid tumours usually do not express transthyretin, which is found in most choroid plexus carcinomas.

Malignant teratoma

The presence of admixed cell types (e.g. rhabdoid cells, epithelioid cells and PNET cells) in atypical teratoid-rhabdoid tumours may raise the suspicion of a malignant teratoma. This suspicion may be inadvertently reinforced by the polyphenotypic pattern of antigen expression. However, atypical teratoid-rhabdoid tumours do not express placental alkaline phosphatase, alpha-fetoprotein or any other germ cell tumour marker, and molecular genetic studies for changes in chromosome 22q and the *INI1* gene (see above) can be used to assist the diagnosis in difficult cases.

Glioblastoma

Clinically, atypical teratoid-rhabdoid tumours may be mistaken for glioblastomas, particularly when the lesion is large and in the supratentorial compartment. Histologically, the variety of cell types and the presence of large rhabdoid cells, along with the widespread haemorrhage, necrosis and mitotic activity in atypical teratoid-rhabdoid tumours can suggest that the tumour may be a glioblastoma. However, palisaded necrosis and vascular endothelial proliferation are not as common as in glioblastomas, and immunocytochemistry will aid diagnosis when the polyphenotypic pattern of antigen expression is demonstrated.

Therapy and prognosis

Atypical teratoid-rhabdoid tumours are clinically aggresive, very rapidly growing lesions which respond poorly to chemotherapy. The vast majority of infants and children with this tumour die within 1 year of presentation and the median postoperative survival in one large series was only 11 months.[95] Local recurrence and tumour dissemination via the CSF pathway, or both, were common terminal events. One recent small-scale study has reported a beneficial response to intensified therapy (high dose chemotherapy and autologous bone marrow transplant), with survivals of 19 and 46 months recorded.[106]

REFERENCES

1. Reddy AT, Packer RJ. Medulloblastoma. Curr Opin Neurol, 1999; 12:681–685
2. Grotzer MA, Janss AJ, Fung K et al. TrkC expression predicts good clinical outcome in primitive neuroectodermal brain tumors. J Clin Oncol, 2000; 18:1027–1035
3. Rorke LB, Trojanowski JQ, Lee VY et al. Primitive neuroectodermal tumors of the central nervous system. Brain Pathol, 1997; 7:765–784
4. Scheurlen WG, Schwabe GC, Joos S et al. Molecular analysis of childhood primitive neuroectodermal tumors defines markers associated with poor outcome. J Clin Oncol, 1998; 16:2478–2485
5. Kleihues P, Cavenee WK. Pathology and genetics of tumours of the nervous system. Lyon: IARC, 2000

Medulloepithelioma

6. Molloy PT, Yachnis AT, Rorke LB et al. Central nervous system medulloepithelioma: A series of eight cases including two arising in the pons. J Neurosurg, 1996; 84:430–436
7. Sato T, Shimoda A, Takahashi T et al. Congenital cerebellar neuroepithelial tumour with multiple divergent differentiations. Acta Neuropathol, 1980; 50:143–146

8. Scheithauer, BW, Rubinstein LJ. Cerebral medulloepithelioma. Report of a case with multiple divergent neuroepithelial differentiation. Childs Brain, 1979; 5:62–71

9. Best PV. Posterior fossa medulloepithelioma. J Neurol Sci, 1974; 22:511–518

10. Karch SB, Urich H. Medulloepithelioma: definition of an entity. J Neuropathol Exp Neurol, 1972; 31:27–53

11. Auer RN, Becker LE. Cerebral medulloepithelioma with bone, cartilage, and striated muscle. Light microscopic and immunohistochemical study. J Neuropathol Exp Neurol, 1983; 42:256–267

12. Deck JH. Cerebral medulloepithelioma with maturation into ependymal cells and ganglion cells. J Neuropathol Exp Neurol, 1969; 28:442–454

13. Caccamo DV, Herman MM, Rubinstein LJ. An immunohistochemical study of the primitive and maturing elements of human cerebral medulloepitheliomas. Acta Neuropathol, 1989; 79:248–254

14. Tohyama T, Lee VM, Rorke LB et al. Nestin expression in embryonic human neuroepithelium and in human neuroepithelial tumour cells. Lab Invest 1992; 66:303–313

15. Khoddami M, Becker LE. Immunohistochemistry of medulloepithelioma and neural tube. Pediatr Pathol Lab Med, 1997; 17:913–925

16. Troost D, Jansen GH, Dingemans KP. Cerebral medulloepithelioma – Electron microscopy and immunohistochemistry. Acta Neuropathol, 1990; 80:103–107

17. Pollak A, Friede RL. Fine structure of medulloepithelioma. J Neuropathol Exp Neurol, 1977; 36:712–725

18. Van Epps RR, Samuelson DR, McCormick DF et al. Cerebral medulloepithelioma. Case report. J Neurosurg, 1967; 27:568–573

Ependymoblastoma

19. Rubinstein LJ. The definition of the ependymoblastoma. Arch Pathol, 1970; 90:35–45

20. Langford LA. The ultrastructure of the ependymoblastoma. Acta Neuropathol, 1986; 71:136–141

21. Rubinstein LJ. Embryonal central neuroepithelial tumors and their differentiating potential. A cytogenetic view of a complex neuro-oncological problem. J Neurosurg, 1985; 62:795–805

22. Becker LE, Hinton D. Primitive neuroectodermal tumors of the central nervous system. Hum Pathol, 1983; 14:538–550

23. Sarkar C, Roy S, Tandon PN. Primitive neuroectodermal tumours of the central nervous system. An electron microscopic and immunohistochemical study. Indian J Med Res, 1989; 90:91–102

24. Mork SJ, Rubinstein LJ. Ependymoblastoma. A reappraisal of a rare embryonal tumour. Cancer, 1985; 55:1536–1542

25. Murphy MN, Dhalla SS, Diocee M et al. Congenital ependymoblastoma presenting as a sacrococcygeal mass in a newborn: An immunohistochemical, light and electron microscopic study. Clin Neuropathol, 1987; 6:169–173

26. Sanjuan-Rodriguez S, Gastejon-Casado J, Pimentel-Leo JJ et al. Extra-spinal presacral ependymoblastoma. Ann Esp Pediatr, 1986; 24:333–335

27. Cruz-Sanchez FF, Haustein J, Rossi ML et al. Ependymoblastoma: A histological, immunohistological and ultrastructural study of five cases. Histopathology, 1988; 12:17–27

28. Lipson A, Bale P. Ependymoblastoma associated with prenatal exposure to diphenylhydantoin and methylphenobarbitone. Cancer, 1985; 55:1859–1862

29. Armington WG, Osborn AG, Cubberley DA et al. Supratentorial ependymoma: CT appearance. Radiology, 1985; 157:367–372

30. Dorsay TA, Rovira MJ, Ho VB et al. Ependymoblastoma: MR presentation. Pediatr Radiol, 1995; 25:433–435

31. Cruz-Sanchez FF, Rossi ML, Hughes JT et al. An immunohistological study of 66 ependymomas. Histopathology, 1988; 13:443–454

32. Wada C, Kurata A, Hirose R et al. Primary leptomeningeal ependymoblastoma. Case report. J Neurosurg, 1986; 64:968–973

33. Uematsu Y, Rojas-Corona RR, Llena JF et al. Distribution of epithelial membrane antigen in normal and neoplastic human ependyma. Acta Neuropathol, 1989; 78:325–328

34. Deck JHN. Cerebral medulloepithelioma with maturation into ependymal cells and ganglion cells. J Neuropathol Exp Neurol, 1969; 28:442–454

35. Shyn PB, Campbell GA, Guinto FC Jr et al. Primary intracranial ependymoblastoma presenting as spinal cord compression due to metastasis. Childs Nerv Syst, 1986; 2:323–325

36. Ayan I, Darendelier E, Kebudi R et al. Evaluation of response to postradiation eight in one chemotherapy in childhood brain tumours. J Neurooncol, 1995; 26:65–72

37. Campbell AN, Chan HS, Becker LE et al. Extracranial metastases in childhood primary intracranial tumors. A report of 21 cases and review of the literature. Cancer, 1984; 53:974–981

38. Chin HW, Hasel JJ, Kim TH et al. Intracranial ependymomas and ependymoblastomas. Strahlentherapie, 1984; 160:191–194

39. Cervoni L, Celli P, Trillo G et al. Ependymoblastoma: a clinical review. Neurosurg Rev, 1995; 18:189–192

Medulloblastoma

40. Farwell JR, Dohrmann GJ, Flannery JT. Medulloblastoma in childhood: An epidemiological study. J Neurosurg, 1984; 61:657–664

41. Provias JP, Becker LE. Cellular and molecular pathology of medulloblastoma. J Neurooncol, 1996; 29:35–43

42. Hubbard JL, Scheithauer BW, Kispert DB et al. Adult cerebellar medulloblastomas: The pathological, radiographic, and clinical disease spectrum. J Neurosurg, 1989; 70:536–544

43. Giordana MT, Cavalla P, Dutto A et al. Is medulloblastoma the same tumor in children and adults? J Neurooncol, 1997; 35:169–176

44. Iijima M, Nakazato Y. Pale islands in medulloblastoma consist of differentiated cells with low growth potential. Pathol Int, 1997; 47:25–30

45. Loda M, Xu X, Pession A et al. Membranous expression of glucose transporter-1 protein (GLUT-1) in embryonal neoplasms of the central nervous system. Neuropathol Appl Neurobiol, 2000; 26:91–97

46. Moss TH. Tumours of the nervous system. An ultrastructural atlas. London: Springer-Verlag, 1986: pp 75–80.

47. Giordana MT, Schiffer P, Schiffer D. Prognostic factors in medulloblastoma. Childs Nerv Syst, 1998; 14:256–262

48. Schiffer D, Cavalla P, Migheli A et al. Apoptosis and cell proliferation in human neuroepithelial tumors. Neurosci Lett, 1995; 195:81–84

49. Di Rocco C, Iannelli A, Papacci F et al. Prognosis of medulloblastoma in infants. Childs Nerv Syst, 1997; 13:388–396

50. Campbell AN, Chan HSL, Becker LE et al. Extracranial metastases in childhood primary intracranial tumors. A report of 21 cases and review of the literature. Cancer, 1984; 53:974–981

51. Fouladi M, Gajjar A, Boyett JM et al. Comparison of CSF cytology and spinal magnetic resonance imaging in the detection of leptomeningeal disease in pediatric medulloblastoma or primitive neuroectodermal tumor. J Clin Oncol, 1999; 17:3234–3237

52. Schofield D, West DC, Anthony DC et al. Correlation of loss of heterozygosity at chromosome 9q with histological subtype in medulloblastomas. Am J Pathol, 1995; 146:472–480

53. Raffel C, Jenkins RB, Frederick L et al. Sporadic medulloblastomas contain PTCH mutations. Cancer Res, 1997; 57:842–845

54. Pietsch T, Waha A, Koch A et al. Medulloblastomas of the desmoplastic variant carry mutations of the human homologue of Drosophila patched. Cancer Res, 1997; 57:2085–2088

55. Zurawel RH, Allen C, Chiappa S et al. Analysis of PTCH/SMO/SHH pathway genes in medulloblastoma. Genes Chromosomes Cancer, 2000; 27:44–51

56. Reifenberger J, Wolter M, Weber RG et al. Missense mutations in SMOH in sporadic basal cell carcinomas of the skin and primitive neuroectodermal tumors of the central nervous system. Cancer Res, 1998; 58:1798–1803

57. Zurawel RH, Chiappa SA, Allen C et al. Sporadic medulloblastomas contain oncogenic beta-catenin mutations. Cancer Res, 1998; 58:896–899

58. Pomeroy SL, Tamayo P, Gaassenbeek M et al. Prediction of central nervous system embryonal tumour outcome based on gene expression. Nature, 2002; 415:436–442.

59. Walter AW, Mulhern RK, Gajjar A et al. Survival and neurodevelopmental outcome of young children with medulloblastoma at St Jude Children's Research Hospital. J Clin Oncol, 1999; 17:3720–3728
60. Amagasaki K, Yamazaki H, Koizumi H et al. Recurrence of medulloblastoma 19 years after the initial diagnosis. Childs Nerv Syst, 1999; 15:482–485

Histological variants of medulloblastoma

61. Buhren J, Christoph AH, Buslei R et al. Expression of the neurotrophin receptor p75NTR in medulloblastomas is correlated with distinct histological and clinical features: evidence for a medulloblastoma subtype derived from the external granule cell layer. J Neuropathol Exp Neurol, 2000; 59:229–240
62. Giangaspero F, Perilongo G, Fondelli MP et al. Medulloblastoma with extensive nodularity: a variant with favorable prognosis. J Neurosurg, 1999; 91:971–977
63. Rao C, Friedlanger ME, Klein E et al. Medullomyoblastoma in an adult. Cancer, 1990; 65:157–163
64. Chowdhury C, Roy S, Mahapatra AK et al. Medullomyoblastoma. A teratoma. Cancer, 1995; 55:1495–1500
65. Holl T, Kleihues P, Yasargil MG et al. Cerebellar medullomyoblastoma with advanced neuronal differentiation and hamartomatous component. Acta Neuropathol, 1991; 82:408–413
66. Kalimo H, Paljarvi L, Ekfors T et al. Pigmented primitive neuroectodermal tumor with multipotential differentiation in cerebellum (pigmented medullomyoblastoma). A case with light- and electron-microscopic, and immunohistochemical analysis. Pediatr Neurosci, 1987; 13:188–195
67. Bergmann M, Pietsch T, Herms J et al. Medullomyoblastoma: a histological, immunohistochemical, ultrastructural and molecular genetic study. Acta Neuropathol (Berl), 1998; 95:205–212
68. Best PV, A medulloblastoma-like tumour with melanin formation. J Pathol, 1973; 110:109–111
69. Boesel CP, Suhan JP, Sayers MP. Melanotic medulloblastoma. Report of a case with ultrastructural findings. J Neuropathol Exp Neurol, 1978; 37:531–543
70. Jimenez CL, Carpenter BF, Robb IA. Melanotic cerebellar tumor. Ultrastruct Pathol, 1987; 11:5–6

Supratentorial primitive neuroectodermal tumours (PNETs)

71. Rorke LB. Presidential address. The cerebellar medulloblastoma and its relationship to primitive neuroectodermal tumours. J Neuropathol Exp Neurol, 1983; 42:1–15
72. Becker LE, Hinton D. Primitive neuroectodermal tumours of the central nervous system. Human Pathol, 1983; 14:538–550
73. Horten BC, Rubinstein LJ. Primary cerebral neuroblastoma. A clinicopathological study of 35 cases. Brain, 1976; 99:735–756
74. Bailey P, Cushing H. Medulloblastoma cerebelli: a common type of mid-cerebellar glioma of childhood. Arch Neurol Psychiatry, 1925; 14:192–224
75. Bennett JP Jr, Rubinstein LJ. The biological behaviour of primary cerebral neuroblastoma: a reappraisal of the clinical course in a series of 70 cases. Ann Neurol, 1984; 16:21–27
76. McLendon RE, Bentley RC, Parisi JE et al. Malignant supratentorial glial-neuronal neoplasms: report of two cases and review of the literature. Arch Pathol Lab Med, 1997; 121:485–492
77. Hassin GB, Munch-Petersen CJ. Central neurogenic tumours (neuroblastoma and ganglioneuroma). A pathological study of two cases. J Neuropathol Clin Neurol, 1951; 1:63–80
78. Kepes JJ, Belton K, Roessmann U et al. Primitive neuroectodermal tumours of the cauda equina in adults with no detectable primary intracranial neoplasm – three case studies. Clin Neuropathol, 1985; 4:1–11
79. Rutherford GS, Hewlett RH. Atlas of correlative surgical neuropathology and imaging. Dordrecht: Kluwer Academic, 1994
80. Gould VB, Rorke LB Jansson DS et al. Primitive neuroectodermal tumours of the central nervous system express neuroendocrine markers and may express all classes of intermediate filaments. Hum Pathol, 1990; 21:245–252

81. Molenaar WM, Rorke LB, Trojanowski JQ. Neural tumours. In: Calvin RB, Bhan AK, McCluskey RT, eds. Diagnostic immunopatholog, 2nd edn. New York: Raven Press, 1993: pp 651–668
82. Gould VE, Jansson DS, Molenaar WM, et al. Primitive neuroectodermal tumors of the central nervous system. Patterns of expression of neuroendocrine markers, and all classes of intermediate filament proteins. Lab Invest, 1990; 62:498–509
83. Ojeda VJ, Stokes BAR, Lee MA et al. Primary cerebral neuroblastomas. A clinicopathological study of one adolescent and five adult patients. Pathology, 1986; 18:41–49
84. Pigott TJ, Punt JA, Lowe JS et al. The clinical, radiological and histopathological features of cerebral primitive neuroectodermal tumours. Brit J Neurosurg, 1990; 4:287–297
85. Rhodes RH, Cole M, Takaoka Y et al. Intraventricular cerebral neuroblastoma. Analysis of subtypes and comparison with hemispheric neuroblastoma. Arch Pathol Lab Med, 1994; 118:897–911
86. Pruchon E, Chauveinc L, Sabatier L et al. A cytogenetic study of 19 recurrent gliomas. Cancer Genet Cytogenet, 1994; 76:85–92
87. Burnett ME, White EC, Sih S et al. Chromosome arm 17p deletion analysis reveals molecular genetic heterogeneity in supratentorial and infratentorial neuroectodermal tumours of the central nervous system. Cancer Genet Cytogenet, 1997; 97:25–31
88. Horten BC, Rubinstein LJ. Primary cerebral neuroblastoma. A clinicopathological study of 35 cases. Brain, 1976; 99:735–756
89. Albright AL, Wisoff JH, Zeltzer P et al. Prognostic factors in children with supratentorial (nonpineal) neuroectodermal tumours. A neurosurgical perspective from the Childrens Cancer Group. Pediatr Neurosurg, 1995; 22:1–7
90. Rorke LB, Trojanowski JQ, Lee VMY et al. Primitive neuroectodermal tumours of the central nervous system. Brain Pathol, 1997; 7:765–784
91. Geyer JR, Zeltzer PM, Boyett JM et al. Survival of infants with primitive neuroectodermal tumours or malignant ependymomas of the CNS treated with eight drugs in one day: a report from the Childrens Cancer Group. J Clin Oncol, 1994; 12:1607–1615

Polar spongioblastoma

92. Kleihues P, Cavanee WK. Pathology and genetics of tumours of the nervous system. Lyon: IARC, 1997
93. Yagishita S, Kawano N, Oka H et al. Palisades in cerebral astrocytoma simulating the so-called polar spongioblastoma: a histological, immunohistochemical, and electron microscopical study of an adult case. Noshuyo Byori, 1996; 13:21–25

Atypical teratoid-rhabdoid tumours

94. Biggs PJ, Garen PD, Powers JM et al. Malignant rhabdoid tumor of the central nervous system. Hum Pathol, 1987; 18:332–337
95. Burger PC, Yu IT, Tihan T et al. Atypical teratoid/rhabdoid tumor of the central nervous system: A highly malignant tumor of infancy and childhood frequently mistaken for medulloblastoma: A Pediatric Oncology Group study. Am J Surg Pathol, 1998; 22:1083–1092
96. Proust F, Laquerriere A, Constantin B et al. Simultaneous presentation of atypical teratoid-rhabdoid tumor in siblings. J Neurooncol, 1999; 43:63–70
97. Manhoff DT, Rorke LB, Yachnis AT. Primary intracranial atypical teratoid/rhabdoid tumor in a child with Canavan's disease. Pediatr Neurosurg, 1995; 22:214–222
98. Muller M, Hubbard SL, Provias J et al. Malignant rhabdoid tumour of the pineal region. Can J Neurol Sci, 1994; 21:273–277
99. Tamiya T, Nakashima H, Ono Y et al. Spinal atypical teratoid/rhabdoid tumor in an infant. Atypical teratoid-rhabdoid tumour. Pediatr Neurosurg, 2000; 32:145–149
100. Ho DM, Hsu CY, Wong TT et al. Atypical teratoid/rhabdoid tumour of the central nervous sytem: a comparative study with primitive neuroectodermal tumour/medulloblastoma. Acta Neuropathol, 2000; 99:482–488
101. Lu L, Wilkinson EJ, Yachnis AT. CSF cytology of atypical teratoid/rhabdoid tumor of the brain in a two-year old girl. Diagn Cytopathol, 2000; 23:329–332

102. Biegel JA. Genetics of pediatric central nervous system tumors. J Pediatr Hematol Oncol, 1997; 19:492–501

103. Rubio A. 4 year old girl with ring chromosome 22 and brain tumor. Brain Pathol, 1997; 7:1027–1028

104. Versteege I, Sevenet N, Lange J et al. Truncating mutations of hSNF5/INI1 in aggressive paediatric cancer. Nature, 1998; 394:203–206

105. Biegel JA, Zhou JY, Rorke LB et al. Germ-line and acquired mutations of INI1 in atypical teratoid and rhabdoid tumors. Cancer Res, 1999; 59:74–79

106. Hilden JM, Watterson J, Longee DC et al. Central nervous system atypical teratoid tumor/rhabdoid tumor: response to intensive therapy and review of the literature. J Neurooncol, 1998; 40:265

8 Neuronal and mixed neuronal–glial tumours

Tumours containing neurons are relatively uncommon in the nervous system compared to other groups and comprise a wide variety of lesions, including pure neoplasms of central neuronal lineage, mixed tumours, tumours arising from the peripheral paraganglion system and the quasi-hamartomatous Lhermitte–Duclos disease (dysplastic gangliocytoma of cerebellum). The World Health Organisation (WHO) classification recognises the entities shown in Table 8.1 as a subgroup within the larger category of tumours of neuroepithelial tissues.

Table 8.1 Neuronal and mixed neuronal–glial tumours

Ganglioglioma
Gangliocytoma
Anaplastic ganglioglioma
Desmoplastic infantile ganglioglioma/astrocytoma
Dysembryoplastic neuroepithelial tumour
Central neurocytoma and neurocytoma
Cerebellar liponeurocytoma
Paraganglioma
Dysplastic gangliocytoma of cerebellum (Lhermitte–Duclos)

Gangliocytoma, ganglioglioma and anaplastic ganglioglioma

These tumours contain mature neoplastic ganglionic cells, either in combination with neoplastic glial cells (*ganglioglioma*) or alone (*gangliocytoma*). Such lesions can be grouped together as benign ganglion cell tumours. In contrast to the low grade nature of both these entities, *anaplastic ganglioglioma* has an aggressive pattern of growth. A recently described histological variant of ganglioglioma is the *papillary glioneuronal tumour*, distinguished by a distinctive imaging and histological appearance.

Incidence and site

All these lesions are uncommon forms of neuroepithelial tumour, believed to account for just over 1% of all brain tumours.[1] The commonest site for gangliogliomas is the temporal lobe.[2-4] An intraventricular location has also been described[5] and ganglion cell containing tumours can arise in any part of the neuraxis, including the cerebellum,[6-9] brain stem,[10,11] spinal cord[12-16] and cranial nerves, especially optic nerve.[15,17-19] In one case series 84% of the tumours were distributed in the temporal lobes, 10% in the frontal lobes, 2% in the occipital lobes and 4% in the infratentorial compartment.[20] Similar lesions are also described in the pituitary gland and pineal gland,[21-24] and multifocality has also been reported.[25,26]

Clinical features

These tumours may affect patients at any age but most are encountered in the first three decades of life. Clinical signs and symptoms are dependent on the site. Those lesions arising in the cerebral hemispheres most commonly present with seizures, and gangliogliomas of the temporal lobe are particularly associated with a history of chronic temporal lobe epilepsy resistant to treatment.[3-5] By contrast, the tumours arising in the brain stem and cord tend to present with a shorter duration of signs and symptoms relating to mass effect.

Radiology

Ganglionic tumours are typically well circumscribed rounded masses or may occur as a cyst with a mural nodule. Computerised tomography (CT) scans show tumours as solid (50%) or partly cystic (50%). Isodense or hypodense areas with mineralisation are seen in about 40% and there is variable contrast enhancement.[2] Magnetic resonance (MR) scans show lesions to be isointense or hypointense on T1-weighted sequences and hyperintense on T2-weighted sequences with variable enhancement seen in about 40%.[2,8,27] The finding of decreased or normal positron emission tomography or single photon emission computerised tomography (SPECT) activity in ganglioglioma correlates well with low grade; while tumours with increased SPECT activity have been shown to be high grade.[28] Papillary glioneuronal tumours are contrast enhancing lesions seen in periventricular regions of the temporal, parietal, or frontal lobes, often with a cystic component.[29]

Pathology

Macroscopic features

Typically tumours are rubbery, pale, solid lesions that can be gritty on cutting as a result of focal mineralisation. Lesions with a cyst/nodule configuration are also seen (Fig. 8.1). In anaplastic lesions, areas of necrosis and haemorrhage may be present.

Intraoperative diagnosis

The key to a correct intraoperative diagnosis of a ganglion cell neoplasm is awareness of the diagnostic possibility based on clinical and imaging features. In smear preparations a confident diagnosis may not be possible as architectural features revealing the distribution of neuronal cells relative to glial elements is not preserved. Some lesions smear very poorly because of the desmoplastic response encountered. When tumour does smear it is generally in a non-uniform pattern, with close adherence of cells around vessels. It may be easy to see lymphoid cells which run out from dense cellular trails in the preparation (Fig. 8.2). In cases where ganglion cells are plentiful and predominant they will be visible as large voluminous cells with large rounded nuclei, having prominent large nucleoli (Fig. 8.3). When astroglial cells

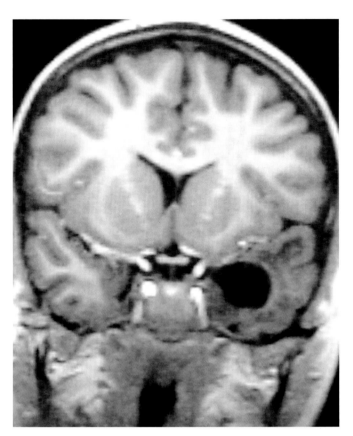

Fig. 8.1 **Ganglioglioma.** Cyst/nodule configuration. MR scan showing a ganglioglioma in the temporal lobe.

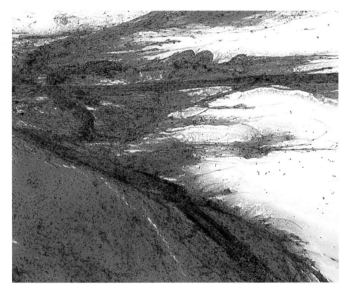

Fig. 8.2 **Ganglioglioma.** At low magnification perivascular lymphoid infiltrates may be prominent. H & E.

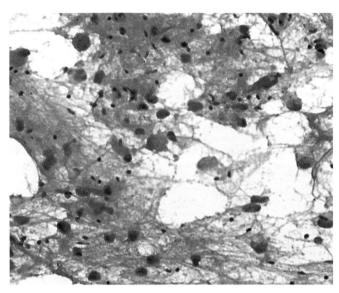

Fig. 8.3 **Ganglioglioma.** Smear preparation. Neuronal and glial cells are visible on close inspection. H & E.

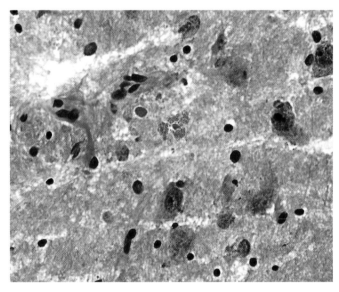

Fig. 8.4 **Ganglioglioma.** Frozen sections may show features of astroglial tumours but the presence of neuronal cells, granular bodies and Rosenthal fibres is usually diagnostic. H & E.

predominate smear appearances can be identical with those seen in pilocytic or fibrillary astrocytomas (see Chapter 4). When small neurocytic cells dominate the picture a lesion may be confused with a neurocytoma or oligodendroglioma, since the two lesions may appear virtually identical on light microscopic examination. Care must be taken not to confuse pleomorphic ganglion cells with pleomorphic astroglial cells, and hence make an inappropriate diagnosis of a high grade astroglial tumour. Using frozen sections, the identification of large cells, consistent with ganglion cells, together with an appropriate stromal background is usually sufficient to establish a correct diagnosis (Fig. 8.4).

Histological features

Gangliocytomas are composed of aggregates and nests of neuronal cells (Figs 8.5 and 8.6) in a background comprised

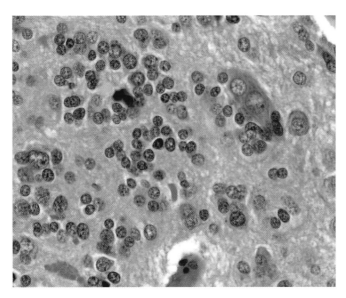

Fig. 8.5 **Gangliocytoma**. Small neuronal cells are shown with rounded nuclei together with larger ganglionic cells, some being binucleate. H & E.

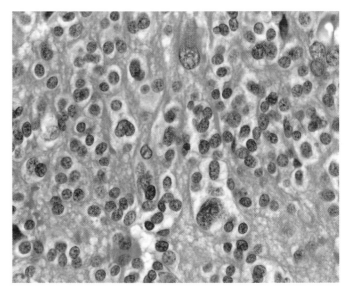

Fig. 8.6 **Gangliocytoma**. Cells in small nests surrounded by pink-staining stroma. H & E.

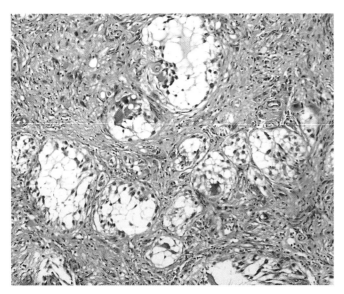

Fig. 8.7 **Ganglioctyoma**. Islands of neuronal cells are set in a glial stroma. H & E.

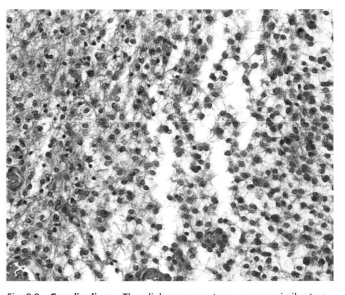

Fig. 8.8 **Ganglioglioma**. The glial component may appear similar to a protoplasmic astrocytoma. H & E.

of neuropil containing benign glial elements, set in a reticulin containing stroma (Fig. 8.7).[30,31] In general cellularity is not high. The glial component of ganglioglioma typically resembles that seen astrocytomas (Figs 8.8 and 8.9). The neoplastic astroglial element may resemble that seen in a pilocytic astrocytoma in many cases (Fig. 8.9) and may contain areas of microcystic change. Large swollen astrocytic cells may be present with nuclear features that resemble those of ganglion cells (Fig. 8.10), making immunohistochemical identification of cellular phenotype important in many cases. The ganglion cells seen in ganglion cell tumours are typically large with multiple

processes and binucleate forms may be seen. Nuclei are large, rounded and appear somewhat hyperchromatic, having large nucleoli (Fig. 8.11). The cells typically show prominent Nissl substance and may have voluminous cytoplasm. In contrast to entrapped background neurones in diffuse astrocytomas, the tumour ganglion cells are usually irregularly distributed, often with clusters of large irregular ganglionic perikarya abutting one another. In some tumours the ganglion cell component is relatively inconspicuous, cells having an elongated, fusiform morphology blending in with surrounding stroma and glial cells. In both gangliocytoma and ganglioglioma, clusters or sheets of smaller

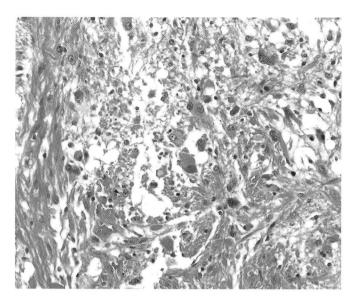

Fig. 8.9 **Ganglioglioma.** The glial component may appear similar to a pilocytic astrocytoma. H & E.

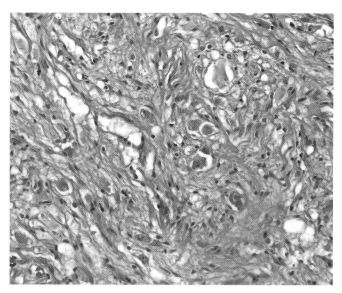

Fig. 8.10 **Ganglioglioma.** Large ganglion-like cells can be seen in gangliogliomas, shown in this area of desmoplasia. Immunochemistry is required to establish their phenotype. H & E.

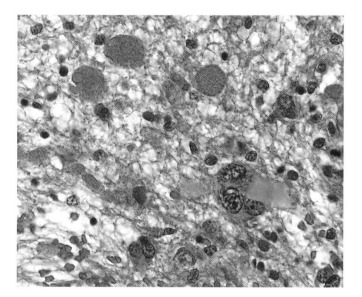

Fig. 8.11 **Ganglioglioma.** Large hyperchromatic binucleate ganglion cells in a ganglioglioma. Note granular eosinophilic bodies. H & E.

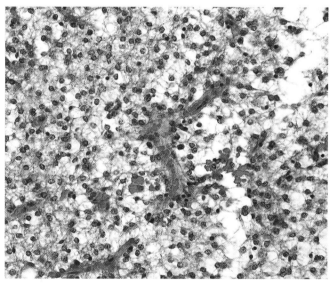

Fig. 8.12 **Ganglioglioma.** Sheets of small neuronal cells in gangliogliomas superficially resemble oligodendrocytes. H & E.

neuronal cells may be a dominant cell type. These may superficially resemble oligodendrocytes, having rounded nuclei and an artefactual perinuclear halo (Fig. 8.12). Immunohistochemistry shows a neuronal phenotype to these cells (see below).

The identification of stromal features is an important part of establishing a diagnosis of ganglioglioma, especially in problematic cases:

• Hyalinised vessels are typically prominent in ganglion cell tumours associated with focal, usually perivascular, lymphocytic infiltration (Figs 8.13 and 8.14).
• In most tumours, reticulin staining outlines an ill-defined lobular pattern on low magnification, with swathes of condensed reticulin surrounding loose islands that contain clusters of ganglion cells. More extensive areas of desmoplasia with collagenisation, devoid of neuronal cells, are seen in some lesions (Fig. 8.15).
• Granular bodies and hyaline bodies are seen in most lesions, forming an important clue to diagnosis in small biopsy samples where other architectural features are absent (Figs 8.11 and 8.16).

The margins of both gangliocytomas and gangliogliomas are generally well circumscribed; however, it is not

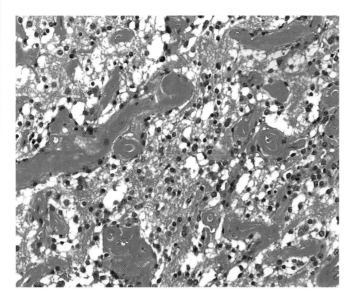

Fig. 8.13 **Ganglioglioma.** Hyalinised vessels are prominent in some ganglion cell tumours. H & E.

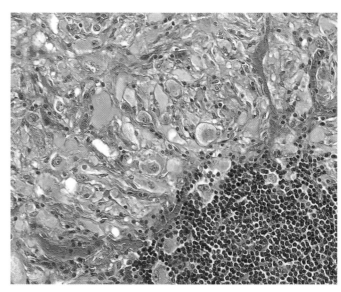

Fig. 8.14 **Ganglioglioma.** Focal lymphoid aggregates are commonly seen. H & E.

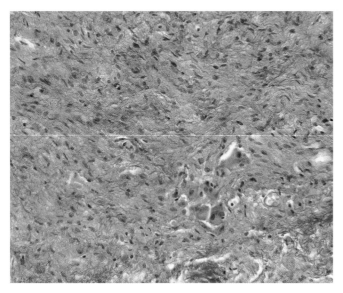

Fig. 8.15 **Ganglioglioma.** This tumour shows extensive areas of desmoplasia with collagenisation and few neuronal cells. Van Gieson.

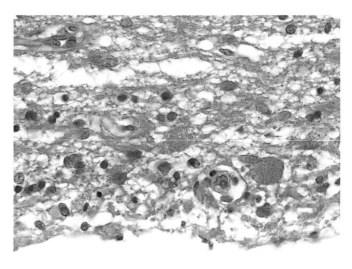

Fig. 8.16 **Ganglioglioma.** Granular bodies are prominent in this sample from the wall of a ganglioglioma cyst. H & E.

infrequent for gangliogliomas to show infiltration in the leptomeninges (Fig. 8.17), a feature that is not associated with malignant behaviour.[32] Unusual features described in some cases include melanin pigmentation[33] and neurofibrillary tangles.[34]

Papillary glioneuronal tumour is a histological variant of ganglioglioma in which there is a pseudopapillary architecture to the lesion. These lesions typically develop in white matter adjacent to the lateral ventricles with a cystic component on imaging. Sheets of small neuronal cells are interspersed with cells showing ganglionic maturation and there are areas of papillary

architecture, in which papillae are covered by plump cuboidal cells and contain hyalinised vessels[29,35,36] (Figs 8.18–8.21).

Anaplastic gangliogliomas are characterised by cellular atypia in the glial component similar to that seen in anaplastic astrocytoma and glioblastoma (see Chapter 4). Very small numbers of mitoses may be seen in benign ganglion cell tumours, but the presence of high numbers of mitoses, marked cellular pleomorphism in the astroglial component, vascular endothelial proliferation or necrosis are all sinister features and indicate that the tumour is anaplastic.

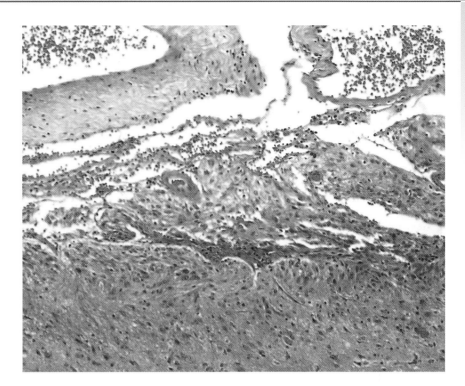

Fig. 8.17 **Ganglioglioma.** This tumour extends into the meninges in this example from a temporal lobe ganglioglioma. H & E.

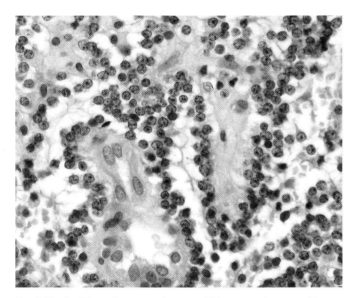

Fig. 8.18 **Papillary glioneuronal tumour.** This tumour has a papillary architecture with rounded cells covering vascular stromal cores. H & E.

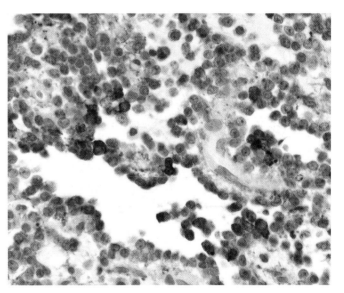

Fig. 8.19 **Papillary glioneuronal tumour.** Synaptophysin immunoreactivity is seen in a proportion of cells.

Immunohistochemistry

The neuronal phenotype of ganglion cells and small round neuronal cells (neurocytes) can be determined by several immunohistochemical stains (Figs 8.22–8.24).[30,37–39] In one large series neuronal cells were positive for synaptophysin (100%), class III beta-tubulin (100%), neurofilament protein (NFP) (90%), and chromogranin-A (86%), S-100 protein (71%) and vimentin (24%).[38] Alpha-synuclein is also expressed in a high proportion of

gangliogliomas, the positive cells being large and resembling dysmorphic neurons.[40,41] Synaptophysin is expressed in neurons in ganglioglial tumours (Fig. 8.22) and detection of surface perikaryal labelling for synaptophysin has been proposed as a way of distinguishing neoplastic neuronal elements from background neurons over-run by glioma cells. However studies have shown that this is also a property of normal neurons[42,43] and therefore we would urge extreme caution in the use of

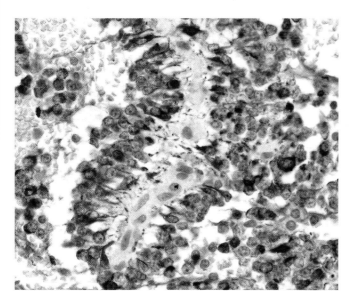

Fig. 8.20 **Papillary glioneuronal tumour.** GFAP expression.

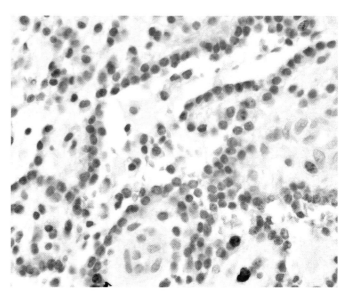

Fig. 8.21 **Papillary glioneuronal tumour.** Cell proliferation markers show a low labelling index with Ki-67/MIB-1.

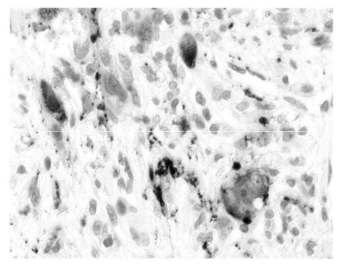

Fig. 8.22 **Ganglicytoma.** Synaptophysin staining is seen in large ganglionic cells as well as smaller neurocytic cells.

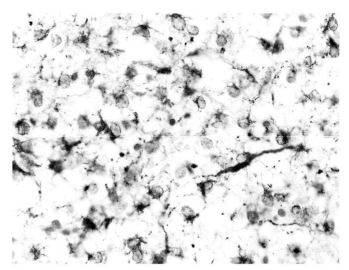

Fig. 8.23 **Ganglioglioma.** GFAP expression in this example is restricted to a few glial processes. In other tumours with a dominant glial component GFAP expression can dominate the picture.

background synaptophysin immunostaining as a method of evaluating a possible tumour ganglion cell component in diffusely infiltrating glial neoplasms. Immuno-reactivity for a variety of neurotransmitter substances has been described but is generally of no diagnostic usefulness.

Glial fibrillary acidic protein (GFAP) immunoreactivity is seen in stromal cells in gangliocytomas and in the neo-plastic glial cells in ganglioglioma (Fig. 8.23). In assessment of gliomas with unidentified large ganglion-like cells, positive GFAP staining is very useful in ascertaining that these are atypical astrocytic cells. In gangliogliomas where ganglion cells are in low density and have adopted an elongated spindle cell profile, negative staining in preparations for GFAP is a useful way of assessing the neuronal cells, revealed in negative contrast against the surrounding glial background.

Electron microscopy

The most useful ultrastructural feature of ganglionic tumours is the presence of dense core neurosecretory granules. These can vary widely in size and are present in neuronal cell processes and, to a lesser extent, in peri-karyal cytoplasm. Smaller, empty synaptic vesicles may also be found in the cell processes and well formed synapse-like structures are also inconsistently reported.[38] In gangliogliomas, a distinct population of astroglial cells

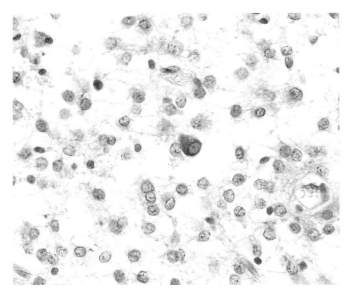

Fig. 8.24 **Ganglioglioma.** Chromogranin-A immunoreactivity can be demonstrated in large neuronal cells and may also be seen in smaller neurocyte-like cells.

can usually be discerned, lacking neurosecretory granules but with processes filled by glial intermediate filaments.

Proliferation indices

In about 70% of cases the Ki-67/MIB-1 labelling index is less than 1%[31] with a range of 0.6–10.5% and a mean of 2.7%. The Ki-67/MIB-1 index is significantly higher in recurrent tumours.[38]

Molecular biology and genetics

No genetic predisposition has been noted for the vast majority of tumours although ganglioglioma has been reported in neurofibromatosis type 1 and 2[45] and Turcot syndrome.[46] Cytogenetic abnormalities have been noted in some small series but appear inconsistent.[47–51] *PTEN* mutations have not been found.[52] In one published series, no tumour showed aberrant expression of p53.[31]

Differential diagnosis

Astroglial tumour with entrapped neurons

Establishing the nature of clusters of neurones in an astroglial neoplasm is one of the most common problems in diagnostic neuropathology. When surgical samples are from the superficial part of an astroglial tumour, neoplastic astrocytes infiltrate around cortical neurons raising the diagnostic possibility of a ganglioglioma. This diagnostic problem is enhanced in stereotactic biopsy samples, where few architectural features may be repre-

sented in the sample. Some features of histological assessment are helpful in resolving this problem:

- If the neurons are regular in size and show a uniform polar organisation, sometimes evident in laminae, then they are most likely to represent benign entrapped cells.
- If the neurons are irregularly distributed in clusters, vary in shape and size, with binucleate forms, and are surrounded by a reticulin rich stroma they are most likely to be neoplastic.
- Satellitosis of tumour ganglion cells by the glial component is not a feature of gangliogliomas but is a well recognised feature in cortex over-run by an infiltrating glioma. It should be noted, however, that gangliogliomas have diffusely infiltrating margins, where their glial cell population may exhibit satellitosis around infiltrated background neurones.
- The presence of hyaline vessels, focal lyphocytic infiltration and granular bodies should be a strong indication that a lesion is a ganglion cell tumour rather than an astroglial tumour with entrapped neurons.

If neoplastic ganglion cells are positively identified, then depending on the cytology of the glial component, a diagnosis of ganglioglioma or anaplastic ganglioglioma should be considered.

Cystic change and fibrillary astrocytoma

Knowing the imaging features of a tumour and the site from which a biopsy sample has been taken are the best safeguard against mistaking part of the cyst wall from a ganglion cell tumour (Fig. 8.25) for an astrocytoma. The cyst wall of a ganglioglioma or gangliocytoma is generally of low to moderate cellularity and composed of astroglial tissue, devoid of ganglion cells. Sparse lymphoid cells are not uncommonly seen in the wall. When a tumour nodule is known to be associated with the cyst it is unwise to attempt a definitive diagnosis based just upon the cyst wall.

Pilocytic astrocytoma

Many gangliogliomas have a dominant component composed of pilocytic pattern astrocytoma, including areas with a microcystic pattern. The danger in making this diagnosis erroneously is highest in tumours from the cerebellum, where pilocytic astrocytoma is an expected lesion, and it is easy to overlook a small component of neoplastic ganglion cells.

Oligodendroglioma/mixed oligoastrocytoma

In small samples the neurocytes in a gangliocytoma or ganglioglioma may resemble oligodendrocytes, suggesting an oligodendroglial component to a tumour (Fig. 8.12). This idea may be reinforced by the presence of

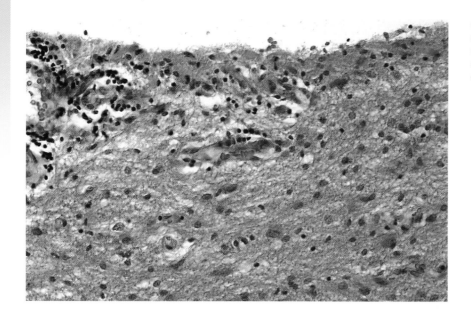

Fig. 8.25 **Ganglioglioma.** Biopsy from the wall of a ganglioglioma showing astroglial cells and absence of neuronal cells. Lymphoid infiltration and granular bodies are important clues to the diagnosis. H & E.

microcalcification, seen frequently in oligodendroglial tumours. The finding of hyaline vessels, focal lymphocytic infiltration and granular bodies should be a strong indication that a lesion is a ganglion cell tumour, reinforced by a neuronal phenotype on immunohistochemical staining.

Meningioangiomatosis

This is a nodular lesion composed of dense collagenous stroma containing vessels with interspersed islands containing cortical ganglionic cells, often associated with neurofibromatosis type 2 (see Chapters 13 and 19). Identification of the distinctive architecture of these lesions, compared to the less well defined lobular architecture seen in gangliogliomas and gangliocytomas is the key to diagnosis.

Pleomorphic xanthoastrocytoma

These tumours may have a cyst with a mural nodule and, usually at the deep interface with adjacent brain, they may show a reticulin rich stroma, hyaline vessels, eosinophilic bodies and large pleomorphic cells that resemble ganglion cells. Immunohistochemistry is helpful in revealing an astroglial origin for the large cells. Some tumours have been described with features of both pleomorphic xanthoastrocytoma (PXA) and ganglioglioma, in which the gliomatous component of the ganglion cell-containing tumour has been PXA.[53–59]

Ependymoma

Papillary glioneuronal tumours must be distinguished from ependymomas. The finding of a papillary lesion adjacent to a ventricle with GFAP positive elements may suggest an ependymoma, however finding immunoreactivity for neuronal markers in cells around the papillae reveals the correct diagnosis.

Therapy and prognosis

In the WHO classification, pure ganglion cell tumours are grade I lesions. Gangliogliomas are graded according to the nature of the glial component, as for astrocytic tumours, and may be grade I or II. Surgical removal is the treatment of choice and is usually curative with complete excision.[30,60–62] Anaplastic gangliogliomas are characterised by a glial component corresponding to anaplastic astrocytoma and are regarded as grade III lesions. Radiotherapy should be considered for these lesions in a manner similar to that for anaplastic astrocytoma.[61] Extracranial spread of tumour has been described rarely.[63]

Desmoplastic infantile ganglioglioma

This is a relatively recently characterised tumour incorporating the previously designated entities of desmoplastic infantile ganglioglioma (DIG), superficial desmoplastic infantile astrocytoma (DIA),[64] superficial cerebral astrocytoma attached to dura and desmoplastic cerebral astrocytoma of infancy. All these lesions are typically large cystic tumours seen in infancy and have a good prognosis following surgical resection.

Incidence and site

Desmoplastic infantile gangliomas are rare tumours and typically present in the first 2 years of life, with isolated cases reported up the age of 25 years.[65–69] They are mainly supratentorial, most commonly arising in the frontoparietal region.

Clinical features

Most cases present with a short history relating to raised intracranial pressure, typically with expanding head circumference and bulging fontanelles, but some cases may present with seizures.[66,70] CT scans show large, up to 15 cm, cystic lesions with a superficial hypodense component that enhances after contrast administration. MR scans show a cystic mass with an isodense periphery that enhances with gadolinium. Surrounding oedema may be present.[71,72]

Pathology

Macroscopic features

The tumour tissue is typically firm, grey, rubbery and attached to dura. Deep portions are softer with cystic areas containing watery fluid. The tumour masses are usually very large at the time of surgical intervention, measuring 8–15 cm in maximum diameter.

Intraoperative diagnosis

These lesions may be a challenge for intraoperative diagnosis. It is most important to keep the diagnosis in mind when confronted with clinical and imaging data indicating a large supratentorial tumour in a patient in the first decade of life. The tissue is characteristically firm in consistency and may not smear well, making a frozen section essential to obtain a diagnosis. If areas are selected that are soft and do smear then there is a chance that small cell areas may be selected, giving a false impression of overall cellularity and suggesting the diagnosis of a small cell malignant tumour (Fig. 8.26).

In cryostat sections the most important observation is the presence of a desmoplastic spindle cell component. In most cases ganglion cells will not be visible on frozen section. The presence of small cell areas and necrosis may lead to a mistaken opinion that the lesion is a high grade astroglial tumour.

Given that complete excision is the most important aspect for achieving a good clinical outcome, a diagnosis of desmoplastic spindle cell tumour is appropriate during an intraoperative consultation, reserving a final diagnosis after wide sampling for conventional histology.

Histological features

Desmoplastic infantile gangliomas exhibit several patterns and wide variations to this tumour are encountered histologically. The background to the tumour usually consists of streams of spindle shaped astrocytes set in a reticulin dense collagenous stroma (Figs 8.27 and 8.28). These areas may show a vague storiform pattern and contain a variable density of thin walled but sometimes ectatic blood vessels. Within this general background several patterns can be seen:

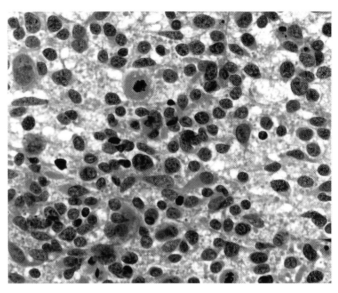

Fig. 8.26 **Desmoplastic infantile ganglioglioma.** This smear shows a small cell area of tumour which in the absence of other information might suggest the diagnosis of a small cell malignant tumour. H & E.

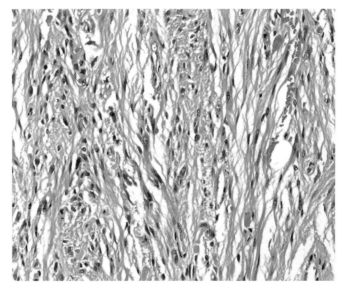

Fig. 8.27 **Desmoplastic infantile ganglioglioma.** The background to the tumour is seen as a spindle cell stroma. H & E.

- There may be cellular areas of plump, gemistocytic astrocytes (Fig. 8.29) or pleomorphic astrocytes (Fig. 8.30).
- Ganglion cells are arranged as scattered clusters and single cells. Some of these are large, typical ganglion cells recognisable on haematoxylin and eosin (H & E) staining with a large round nucleus and prominent nucleolus, voluminous basophilic cytoplasm and cell processes (Fig. 8.31). Other ganglion cells appear atypical and multinucleate.
- Small polygonal neuronal cells may be seen, arranged in groups and cords of cells.

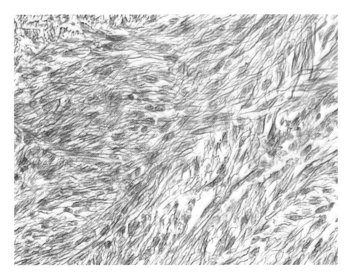

Fig. 8.28 **Desmoplastic infantile ganglioglioma.** Dense pericellular reticulin network.

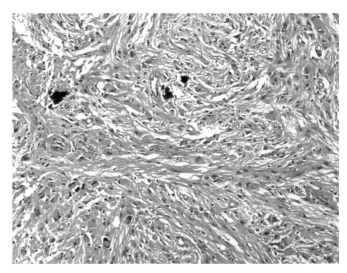

Fig. 8.29 **Desmoplastic infantile ganglioglioma.** Cellular areas of plump gemistocytic astrocytes. H & E.

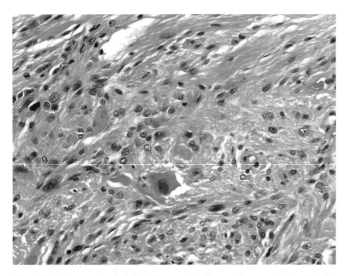

Fig. 8.30 **Desmoplastic infantile ganglioglioma.** Pleomorphism. H & E.

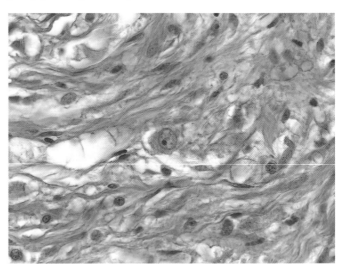

Fig. 8.31 **Desmoplastic infantile ganglioglioma.** A typical ganglion cell is seen in the centre of the field. H & E.

- Clusters, islands or sheets of primitive small cells are often present (Fig. 8.32), with rounded basophilic nuclei resembling neuroblasts in which numbers of mitoses may be seen.
- Tumour permeation in leptomeninges and down the Virchow–Robin spaces may be present.
- In a small proportion of tumours, areas of necrosis (Fig. 8.32) and focal vascular endothelial proliferation have been noted.

When not obvious histologically, a search for ganglion cells using immunohistochemical techniques is mandatory (see below). The extent of astroglial maturation should also be assessed using immunohistochemistry for GFAP. In the absence of ganglion cells and with confirmed astroglial differentiation in spindle cells, use of the terms desmoplastic neuroepithelial tumour or DIA is appro-

priate. In the presence of a defined gangion cell or polygonal neuronal component, either seen on H & E staining or defined by immunohistochemistry, the terms desmoplastic neuroepithelial tumour or DIG should be used.

Immunohistochemistry

Immunohistochemical staining is an important part of tumour assessment and differential diagnosis. As might be expected from the complex histological phenotype, immunohistochemistry exhibits heterogeneity in different tumour areas. GFAP is expressed by spindle shaped astrocytes (Fig. 8.33) and any clusters of plump astroglial cells. However, many spindle cells do not express GFAP and only express vimentin, suggesting a fibroblastic phenotype. Ganglion cells and polygonal neuronal cells may show synaptophysin, neurofilament protein and

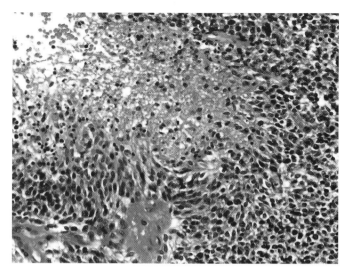

Fig. 8.32 **Desmoplastic infantile ganglioglioma.** Sheets of small primitive cells with evidence of necrosis. H & E.

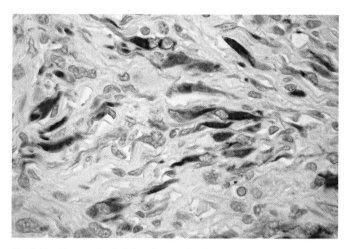

Fig. 8.33 **Desmoplastic infantile ganglioglioma.** GFAP is expressed by spindle shaped astrocytes. Immunocytochemical staining for GFAP.

tubulin immunoreactivity even when the nature of such cells is not obvious on H & E staining.

Electron microscopy

Ultrastructural examination shows external lamina around tumour cells in desmoplastic spindle cell areas and dense core neurosecretory granules may help identify ganglion cells. In practice ultrastructural examination does not usually play a useful part in establishing a diagnosis.

Cell proliferation and histogenesis

Based on the superficial location of this lesion and the presence of desmoplasia, a derivation from subpial astrocytes has been postulated, relating these lesions to pleomorphic xanthoastrocytoma. Studies using cell pro-liferation markers such as Ki-67/MIB-1 show focally high labelling indices.

Molecular biology

There are only limited studies on cytogenetic abnormalities in these uncommon lesions, and no general pattern has emerged.[73] However, molecular genetic analysis has sug-gested that the mutations common in other forms of astrocytoma are not seen in desmoplastic infantile tumours.[48]

Differential diagnosis

Neuroblastoma

The presence of a prominent small cell neuroblast-like component may suggest the diagnosis of a neuroblastoma or primitive neuroectodermal tumour. Indeed, several lesions now recognised to be DIG were originally diag-nosed as neuroblastomatous. The presence of such small cell areas must always be interpreted in the light of other regions in the tumour.

Pleomorphic xanthoastrocytoma

A cyst/tumour configuration with a superficial desmo-plastic component are also features of pleomorphic xanthoastrocytoma. An important distinction is that PXA does not have prominent neuronal elements or the finely elongated cells characteristic of these lesions. In addition, DIGs do not show markedly pleomorphic lipidised tumour giant cells and the presence of such components should suggest the diagnosis of PXA.

Meningioma

If the superficial desmoplastic element of a tumour is sampled then there can be striking resemblance on H & E staining to fibroblastic meningioma. Immunohistochemical assessment for GFAP and neuronal markers will gener-ally reveal elements that are not seen in meningiomas, allowing a correct diagnosis to be made. Although meningiomas are uncommon in infancy and childhood, an immunohistochemical assessment should be made in lesions that have a spindle cell pattern to avoid misdiagnosis.

Mesenchymal tumours

Several spindle cell mesenchymal tumours can arise in relation to the meninges and may be confused with the desmoplastic component of a DIG or DIA. *Solitary fibrous tumours* can be recognised by immunoreactivity for CD34. Immunostaining for GFAP and a neuronal marker such as synaptophysin should be part of assessment of all spindle cell lesions in relation to the meninges such that a correct diagnosis may be made. *True sarcomas* of the meninges may be seen and are characterised by cellular pleomorphism, hyperchromatism and a high cell proliferation rate, none of which is characteristic of the desmoplastic component of DIA or DIG.

Malignant glioma and gliosarcoma

Spindle cell gliomas are well recognised in adults, especially when there is meningeal involvement, and they may also be seen in childhood.[74] Such lesions will show GFAP immunoreactivity in neoplastic spindle cells but will not show a neuronal element. Pronounced nuclear pleomorphism, hyperchromatism and a high mitotic rate are generally seen in a malignant spindle cell astroglial tumour.

Therapy and prognosis

In the WHO classification DIA and DIG are grade I lesions. In the small number of tumours documented, the outcome appears favourable provided that complete excision is achieved.[70,75] Given that the surgery has been meticulous in this respect, the presence of a prominent small cell component, frequent mitoses and necrosis do not appear to be related to a worse clinical outcome.

Dysembryoplastic neuroepithelial tumour

Dysembryoplastic neuroepithelial tumours (DNTs) are low grade lesions composed of a mixture of glial and neuronal cells, typically arising in cortical regions in children and younger adults, and strongly associated with epilepsy.[76] The architectural and histological aspects of these lesions has led to past debate on whether they are hamartomatous overgrowths rather than true neoplasms. Two main forms are described, termed complex and simple. Continued debate surrounds a proposal for a third non-specific form of DNT.[77]

Incidence and site

DNTs exhibit a male dominance and present mainly in the second and third decades, although examples in later life are described.[78] Most lesions are encountered in the medial temporal lobe but they may be seen in any cortical area. Uncommonly, examples have been described in the basal ganglia[79] and cerebellum[80,81] and septum pellucidum.[82]

Clinical features

Most examples of DNTs are encountered in the management of epilepsy in children and young adults, typically where there is a longstanding history of complex partial seizures refractory to drug treatment. In this context they are diagnosed both radiologically and subsequently in the laboratory in samples removed during epilepsy

surgery.[4,5,83] Features of mass effect are very rare. Intra-lesional haemorrhage has been described in a few cases.[84]

Radiology

Radiological imaging plays an important role in diagnosis. Typical lesions show a ribbon-like area of abnormal intracortical signal which is frequently multinodular (Fig. 8.34). The affected cortical regions appear distorted and may appear thickened. On CT scanning, the lesions are usually hypodense or isodense and may show mineralisation. MR imaging shows hyperintense signal on T2-weighted sequences and a hypointense signal on T1-weighted sequences. Contrast enhancement is generally not a feature but focal enhancement may be seen in about 30% of cases. Involvement of underlying white matter is commonly seen in lesions in the temporal lobes. DNTs do not show radiological evidence of mass effect, except in uncommon examples associated with large cysts, and are not associated with perilesional oedema, an aspect that helps in discrimination between DNT and other glial tumours.[85–88]

Pathology

Macroscopic features

When seen in surgical samples, the affected cortex appears thickened and the line of demarcation with underlying white matter is usually indistinct. The lesion is typically

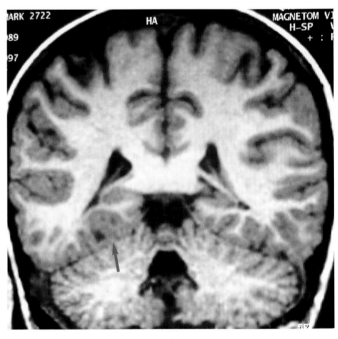

Fig. 8.34 **Dysembryoplastic neuroepithelial tumour.** MR imaging flair sequence showing a ribbon-like nodular intracortical abnormality in the hippocampus and parahippocampal gyrus in which small cystic foci are evident (arrow).

semitranslucent and grey in colour with a soft gelatinous texture. Small microcystic foci may be seen, as may ill-defined nodular areas of firmer, white tissue.

Intraoperative diagnosis

It is uncommon to be required to give an intraoperative opinion on a lesion that subsequently turns out to be a DNT and, even when asked, smear preparations and frozen sections may not allow a confident diagnosis to be established. However, it is generally easy to establish that the lesion is a low grade glioma, and this is usually enough to plan immediate surgical management. The combination of the following features are important clues to a more specific diagnosis:

* Age in first three decades of life.
* Dominant clinical feature of partial seizures.
* Imaging showing an intracortical lesion with absence of mass effect and oedema.

In the presence of the above features a smear preparation that shows a combination of oligodendroglial cells and neurons, or a frozen section which is fortunate enough to include a specific glioneuronal component may be enough to suggest the diagnosis of DNT. In many instances, however, discrimination from a low grade oligodendroglioma may be impossible in smear preparations or frozen sections. Other lesions where only a glial focus is sampled may give an appearance identical to a low grade astrocytoma with pilocytic cells and Rosenthal fibres. Even where a diagnosis of DNT seems most likely from the clinical and radiological features, a report of 'low grade glial or glioneuronal lesion' is usually most appropriate

in these circumstances, waiting on paraffin embedded sections to establish a definitive diagnosis.

Histological features

At a low magnification DNTs most often appear as a multinodular lesion expanding an abnormal cortical layer and pushing down into white matter (Fig. 8.35).[78,89,90] At higher magnifications, the tumours are defined by the presence of a *specific glioneuronal component* (Fig. 8.36). In large samples of well orientated material this component is seen as ribbons of axons, generally arranged around long thin walled vessels, which are coated on each side by a layer of small cells resembling oligodendroglia. These ribbons tend to be aligned perpendicular to the cortical surface and demarcate pale-staining zones of looser texture that contain isolated, mature large neurones and scattered, small stellate astrocytes (Fig. 8.37). The neuronal cells and astrocytes commonly appear to 'float' in pale-staining bubbly eosinophilic proteinaceous material or mucinous material that stains positively with Alcian blue. The specific glioneuronal component may appear as long columns in between the parallel ribbons of axons and oligodendroglial cells. Alternatively, there may be irregularly shaped islands and interconnected sinusoidal cords rimmed by the oligodendroglial cells. In samples removed piecemeal, an obvious orientation with respect to a cortical surface may not be evident.

The simple form of DNT is composed only of areas recognised as the specific glioneuronal component.

The complex form of DNT is composed of areas recognised as the specific glioneuronal component in addition to adjacent areas of cortical dysplasia and glial foci.

Fig. 8.35 **Dysembryoplastic neuroepithelial tumour.** At a low magnification DNTs often appear as multiple nodules of loose textured material expanding an abnormal cortical layer. H & E.

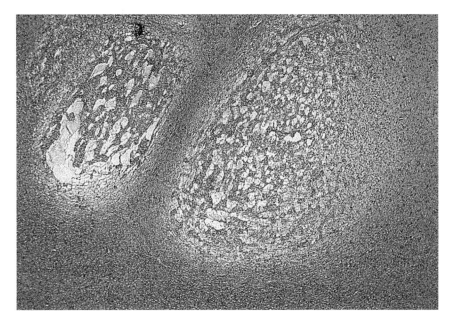

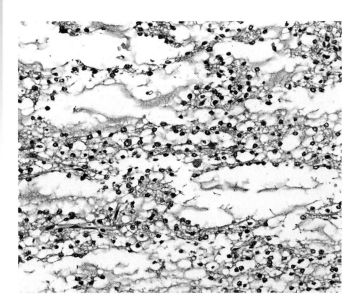

Fig. 8.36 **Dysembryoplastic neuroepithelial tumour.** The specific glioneuronal component is seen as ribbons of oligodendroglial cells lining cystic spaces arranged around long thin walled vessels. H & E.

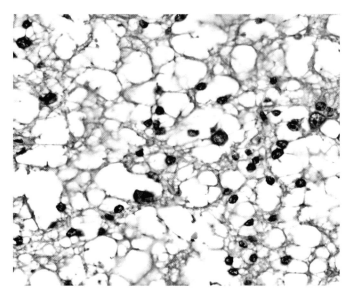

Fig. 8.37 **Dysembryoplastic neuroepithelial tumour.** Pale-stained zones that contain isolated, mature large neurons and scattered, small stellate astrocytes. H & E.

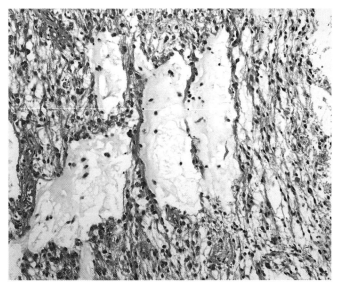

Fig. 8.38 **Dysembryoplastic neuroepithelial tumour.** Astroglial foci, often with a microcystic morphology are also present within lesions. H & E.

- Cortical dysplasia is characterised by histoarchitectural disorganisation. It is often seen at the margins between the main lesion and adjacent normal cortex.
- Glial foci are composed of astroglial and/or oligodendroglial cells of highly variable appearance both within and between cases (Fig. 8.38). In most cases the foci can be seen at low magnification as distinct, generally multiple, rounded nodules within the lesion. In other cases they are more diffuse and lack a rounded, nodular architecture. Histologically these areas can resemble low grade astrocytoma, pilocytic astrocytoma, or low grade oligodendroglioma. Features that may cause concern in glial foci, but are innocent, include nuclear pleomorphism, mitoses or vascular endothelial proliferation.

There may be a rich vascular supply within a DNT, with areas histologically resembling an angiomatous lesion. Hyalinisation of vessels may be seen. In some lesions mineralisation of the tumour vascular network is prominent. Melanin pigment has also been described.[91]

Immunohistochemistry

Neurons within DNTs immunostain for classical neuronal markers such as synaptophysin or chromogranin A. These antibodies are also reported to stain a proportion of smaller cells with rounded nuclei that resemble oligodendroglia. Glial elements stain with GFAP.[90,92–94] Oligodendroglial elements have been reported to stain with markers of oligodendroglia.[95]

Electron microscopy

Ultrastructural studies have shown features confirming the nature of the mixed neuronal and glial elements.[92] However, there is little place for ultrastructural examination in routine diagnosis.

Proliferation indices

Cell proliferation studies have shown variable labelling indices, generally reflecting a low proliferative potential.[86,90,93].

Differential diagnosis

Ganglioglioma

Areas within a ganglioglioma may resemble the specific glioneuronal component in a DNT, especially if foci of microcystic change are seen. However, the neurones in DNTs are uniform, small rounded or pyramidal cells and do not show the atypical cytological features and large size of ganglion cells in gangliogliomas and gangliocytomas. While granular bodies may be seen in a DNT, the presence of focal lymphocytic infiltration is again most suggestive of a ganglion cell-containing tumour. As a word of caution when addressing the distinction between DNTs and gangliogliomas/cytomas, it should be noted that lesions have been described as composite DNT and ganglioglioma.[96,97]

Oligodendroglioma

The presence of microcystic change in an oligodendroglioma may give an appearance that resembles the specific glioneuronal component of a DNT, especially in small or poorly orientated tissue samples. This possibility may be strengthened if cortical neurones are entrapped in oligodendroglial tumour. This differential diagnosis is also discussed from the perspective of oligodendroglioma in Chapter 5. The following features should help in differential diagnosis:

- If the neurons are regular in size and show a uniform polar organisation, sometimes evident in laminae, then they are most likely to represent benign entrapped cells.
- Uniform satellitism of neuronal cells by the oligodendroglial cells is not a feature of DNT but is a well recognised feature of cortex infiltrated by oligodendroglioma. In compact areas of DNT a proportion of neurons may have closely apposed oligodendroglial cells but most do not.
- Subpial condensation of tumour growth is a particular feature of oligodendroglioma.
- Diffuse white matter involvement argues for a diagnosis of oligodendroglioma. DNTs tend to be much better circumscribed tumours.

If clinical features include age in first three decades and partial seizures as the dominant symptom, and if imaging shows an intracortical lesion with absence of mass effect and oedema then, even when the histological features suggest an oligodendroglioma, the diagnosis of DNT should be considered. If the biopsy sample is small and may not represent the whole lesion, cautious wording in a report may be appropriate, i.e. making a diagnosis of possible oligodendroglioma but also stating that the glial component of a DNT cannot be excluded. We do not advocate making the diagnosis of a non-specific form of DNT in the absence of clear histological evidence of the specific glioneuronal component.

Therapy and prognosis

These lesions are low grade and studies have shown absence of progression even after partial surgical resection. Tumours that are completely resected have a good chance of cure with respect to severity of epilepsy, especially where they are resected en bloc as part of a partial temporal lobectomy specimen. One case report has suggested malignant transformation can occur, but the evidence for this remains anecdotal.[98]

Central neurocytoma

These tumours are composed of medium sized round neuronal cells and generally have a good prognosis, corresponding to a grade I lesion. Historically many such lesions were regarded as intraventricular oligodendrogliomas or ependymomas until detailed immunocytochemical clarification of their neuronal phenotype was established. Although the term 'central' neurocytoma is still used by the WHO classification, these tumours are now well described outside their original central location in the midline of the cerebral ventricular system (see below), and there is a case for using the abbreviated title 'neurocytoma' in such circumstances.

Incidence and site

Central neurocytomas have been found to constitute less than 1% of all intracranial tumours[99] and affect both males and female equally. They occur at any age up to the seventh decade with a peak in the third decade.[99–107] The majority of cases have been described in a midline site, straddling the lateral and third ventricles, often in relation to the foramen of Munro. However, cases with no ventricular connection are now well documented.[108] Such extraventicular neurocytomas often contain ganglion cells and their relationship to other forms of neuronal or glial-neuronal tumour is debatable.[109–118] Neuropathologists are sometimes shown tumours from outside the nervous system and it is of interest to note the presence of a neurocytoma reported in an ovarian teratoma.[119]

Clinical features

Most patients present with clinical features of raised intracranial pressure, reflecting the central site of most lesions with blockage of cerebrospinal fluid (CSF) flow often leading to obstructive hydrocephalus. Acute presentation with haemorrhage is also well described.[120–123]

CT scans show either isodense or mildly hyperdense lesions, with strong, generally uniform contrast enhancement. Mineralisation may be present and cystic change has been reported. MR scans show high signal on both T1- and T2-weighted sequences, again with strong enhancement after administration of contrast media (Fig. 8.39).[124]

Pathology

Macroscopic features

The tumour tissue is usually firm with a colour similar to grey matter. There may be a grittiness when cutting the specimen, reflecting focal mineralisation.

Intraoperative diagnosis

A diagnosis of neurocytoma should initially be suggested by imaging and clinical features, especially when the tumour has a typical, central ventricular location. For neurocytomas that arise in extraventricular sites, the intraoperative diagnosis may be more challenging. Neurocytomas smear easily, producing monotonous discohesive cellular sheets of uniform, rounded nuclei set in a granular background matrix material (Figs 8.40 and 8.41). When smearing, a gritty texture may be evident caused by mineralisation in the tumour. Cytoplasm is generally not seen around most nuclei and cell borders are often poorly defined. The nuclei have a finely stippled chromatin pattern in which small inconspicuous nucleoli may be seen. Blood vessels are seen as long, thin walled

structures and foci of mineralisation may also be visible in the smears.

In frozen sections the dominant feature is uniform sheets of cells with rounded nuclei. Ill-defined rosettes or areas of finely filamentous neuropil may be evident. With this appearance and a typical central location, the diagnosis can usually be made with some confidence, since the major cytological differential diagnosis lies with oligodendrogliomas, which are most unlikely at this site.

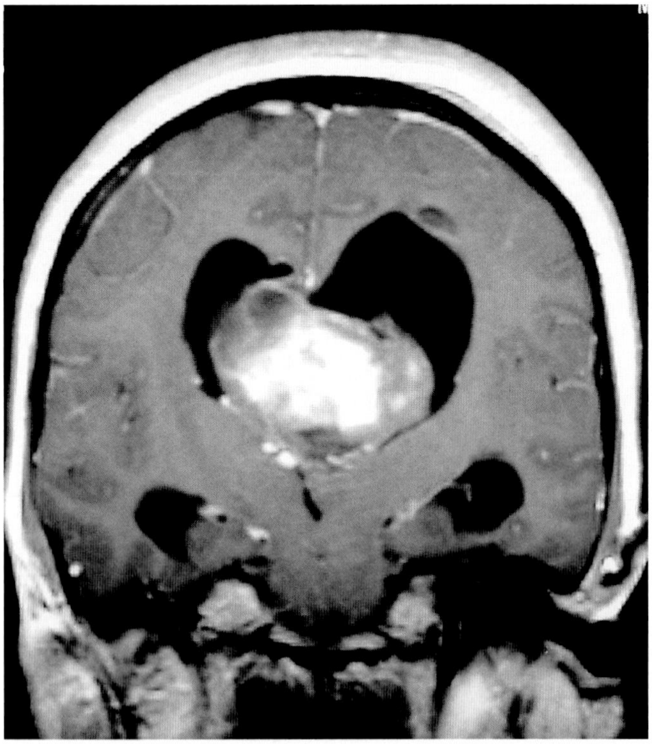

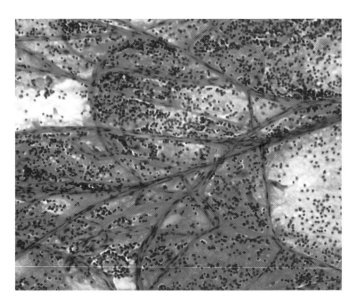

Fig. 8.40 **Central neurocytoma.** Smear preparation. At low magnification long thin capillary sized vessels are generally prominent. H & E.

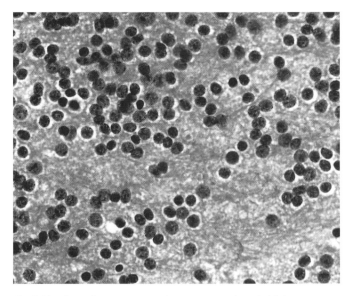

Fig. 8.41 **Central neurocytoma.** Smear preparation. At higher magnification neurocytoma shows monotonous sheets of uniform rounded nuclei set in a granular background material. H & E.

Fig. 8.39 **Central neurocytoma.** MR scans show high signal on both T1- and T2-weighted sequences with strong enhancement.

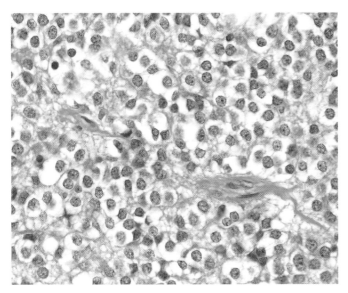

Fig. 8.42 **Central neurocytoma.** Neurocytomas appear virtually identical to oligodendrogliomas in routine preparations. H & E.

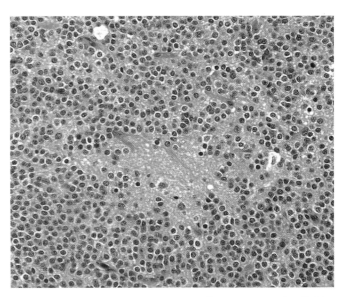

Fig. 8.43 **Central neurocytoma.** Tumour cells are set in an identifiable pink-stained neuropil. H & E.

Histological features

Neurocytomas are composed of uniform, medium sized cells with rounded nuclei and small amounts of cytoplasm.[99] In H & E stained sections they appear virtually identical to the cells in oligodendrogliomas, including the presence of artefactual cytoplasmic vacuolation in fixed tissue leading to a nuclear halo or 'fried egg' appearance (Fig. 8.42). The cells are generally closely apposed but may also be set in an identifiable finely filamentous stroma. This background stroma has a delicate, neuropil-like quality often forming ill-defined solid rosettes or fibrillary, nuclear free zones (Figs 8.43 and 8.44). Tumour cell nuclei are generally rounded, and in well fixed material the chromatin has a finely stippled appearance with small inconspicuous nucleoli.

In a small proportion of tumours isolated cells have a more ganglionic nuclear appearance with a prominent nucleolus, and sometimes there may also be a hint of a basophilic Nissl substance (Fig. 8.45). Tumour blood vessels are typically long, thin walled, straight capillary sized vessels (Fig. 8.46). In some areas perivascular pseudorosettes can be seen. Uncommonly, foci of vascular endothelial proliferation may be present. Mineralisation is commonly found in neurocytomas in the form of small calcospherites.

Mitoses, nuclear pleomorphism or hyperchromatism are generally not seen in neurocytomas. Some tumours have been reported with significant mitotic activity, vascular proliferation and necrosis, and these have been termed atypical neurocytomas.[125–127] However, it should be noted that histological atypia alone has not been shown to correlate well with adverse outcome whilst the

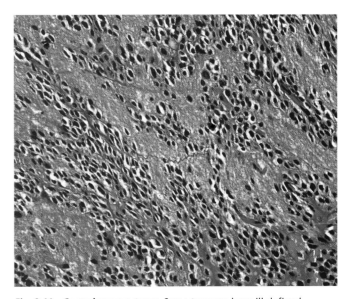

Fig. 8.44 **Central neurocytoma.** Some tumours have ill-defined rosettes or fibrillary, nuclear free zones. H & E.

proliferation potential of central neurocytomas has been suggested as a more reliable predictor of behaviour. As a result, the term proliferating neurocytoma has been proposed for tumours with high mitotic activity.[128]

Immunohistochemistry

Immunohistochemistry shows strong positivity for synaptic markers such as synaptophysin in the neuropil of the tumour (Fig. 8.47).[104,129] The tumour cells express cytoskeletal elements characteristic of neurones, such as class III beta-tubulin and microtubule associated protein-2 (MAP-2) and neurofilament protein. GFAP immuno-

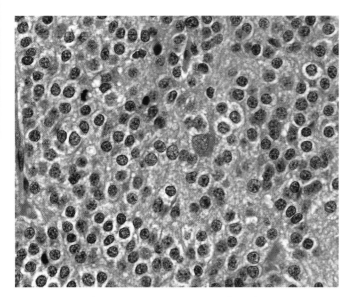

Fig. 8.45   **Central neurocytoma.** Ganglionic cells can be seen in some neurocytomas. H & E.

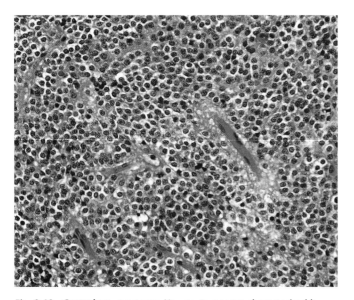

Fig. 8.46   **Central neurocytoma.** Neurocytomas are characterised by long thin capillary sized vessels. H & E.

staining usually detects only a few astroglial cells within the tumour, which are interpreted as being reactive stromal cells (Fig. 8.48).[130] Alpha-synuclein immunoreactivity has recently been described in neurocytomas in one series[41] but not in another.[40] In some studies neoplastic cells in neurocytomas have been shown to express both synaptophysin as well as GFAP.[131] An unusual case of cerebellar neurocytoma with rhabdomyomatous differentiation has also been described.[132]

Electron microscopy

Ultrastructural examination shows cell processes which contain microtubules and both dense core and clear neuro-

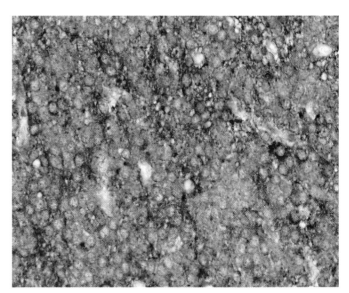

Fig. 8.47   **Central neurocytoma.** Strong positivity for synaptophysin seen in both cells and the neuropil of the tumour.

secretory granules (Fig. 8.49). Cell contacts with features of synapses can also be seen.[104,105,129]

Proliferation indices

Cell proliferation studies have generally shown low labelling fractions using Ki-67/MIB-1 antibodies.[133,134] As alluded to above, however, a significant proportion of tumours have shown labelling indices in excess of 2%, and these have been associated with a less favourable clinical outcome.[127,135] Increased labelling has also been seen in tumour recurrences compared to original excision samples,[136] strengthening the evidence that the proliferation potential of central neurocytomas is a useful predictor of clinical outcome.[137]

Molecular biology

Only limited studies have been performed on cytogenetic and molecular genetic aspects of neurocytoma with no consistent results.[138] Gain of chromosome 7 has been shown in three of nine neurocytomas studied in one series.[139] Recurrent genetic changes on chromosomes 2p, 10q and 18q in central neurocytomas have been shown using fluorescent in situ hybridisation in another study.[140] Despite a superficial morphological resemblance, central neurocytomas are genetically distinct from oligodendrogliomas, and chromosomes 1p and 19q probably do not appear to play a role in their pathogenesis.[141] No evidence of *TP53* mutations[142] amplification of *EGFR*[141] or *MYCN* amplification[143] have been seen in limited studies, although one tumour showed amplification of *MYCN* in another series suggesting it may occur as a rare event.[141]

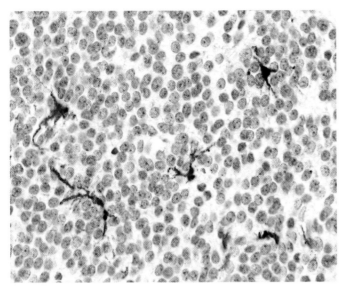

Fig. 8.48 **Central neurocytoma.** GFAP expression is limited to stromal astrocytes.

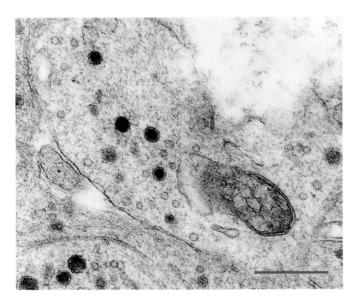

Fig. 8.49 **Central neurocytoma.** Cell processes which contain microtubules and both dense core and clear neurosecretory granules Electron micrograph. Bar = 1 µm.

Histogenesis

The histogenesis of neurocytomas is uncertain. They have been suggested to be derived from multipotential progenitor cells, as well as from cells committed to a neuronal lineage.[144,147] The tumour cells have been shown to have physiological properties consistent with neurons.[148]

Differential diagnosis

Oligodendroglioma

Many examples of central neurocytoma have been discovered in review of cases originally diagnosed as intraventricular oligodendroglioma, since the two lesions may appear virtually identical on light microscopic examination. The nuclei of oligodendrogliomas, however, tend to have a less finely stippled chromatin pattern than those seen in neurocytomas. The background fibrillarity in oligodendrogliomas is coarse in contrast to the delicate, neuropil-like quality in neurocytomas. The best method of distinguishing neurocytomas from oligodendrogliomas, however, is to perform immunohistochemistry for neuronal markers such as synaptophysin. Even so, interpretation of samples from the less cellular infiltrating edge of a tumour may still be problematic and it is important not to be mislead by synaptophysin immunostaining of tumour-infiltrated background neuropil. Ultrastructural examination is often useful in the differential diagnosis of neurocytoma, again provided that cellular areas of tumour are examined and not infiltrated neuropil at the tumour margins.

Clear cell ependymoma

Clear cell ependymoma has been described in sites frequented by more classical ependymomas, including a ventricular or periventricular location. On light microscopic examination, especially in small biopsy samples, there can be great similarity with a neurocytoma, including the presence of nuclear free zones around vessels.[149] The possibility of a clear cell ependymoma should be prompted both by histology as well as the location of the lesion. Ependymomas lack synaptophysin immunoreactivity and will variably express GFAP, which also raises a differential diagnosis with oligodendroglioma. Ultrastructural examination is useful in establishing a diagnosis of ependymoma and can also demonstrate neuronal features if the lesion is a neurocytoma.

Pituitary adenoma

In some instances a pituitary adenoma may grow up into the third ventricle and cytologically there can be a close resemblence to a neurocytoma. In practice this is hardly ever a diagnostic problem, since preoperative imaging will have demonstrated the intrasellar origin of adenomas extending into the third ventricle.

Dysembryoplastic neuroepithelial tumour

In small biopsy samples the round cell element in a DNT may raise the possibility of a neurocytoma. While imaging features and anatomic site are the main features that would favour a DNT rather than a neurocytoma, non-central forms of neurocytoma have been described, as have DNTs in non-classical locations. Histologically, neurocytomas are not described either as multinodular or primarily intracortical, both features which are highly suggestive of DNT.

Clear cell meningioma

Meningiomas may grow in an intraventricular location and clear cell areas in a meningioma may lend histological similarity to a neurocytoma, or, indeed, oligodendroglioma (see above). Immunohistochemical investigation is usually reliable in helping to make the distinction between clear cell meningioma and neurocytoma.

Primitive neuroectodermal tumour (PNET)

Some neurocytomas have a significant mitotic activity and microvascular proliferation. When a neuronal phenotype is confirmed using immunohistochemistry and electron microscopy, the possibility of a neuronally differentiated PNET arises. PNETs generally have little light microscopic evidence of a neuropil and their nuclei are small and hyperchromatic, lacking perinuclear halos.

Therapy and prognosis

Complete surgical excision is the mainstay of therapy, but radiotherapy has also been reported to be useful in cases of subtotal excision.[107,150] A favourable response to chemotherapy has also been described.[151,152] Many central neurocytomas originally diagnosed as intraventricular oligodendrogliomas were inadvertently treated with both surgery and radiotherapy, although given the correct diagnosis in such cases, the role of radiotherapy in neurocytomas must remain uncertain.

In most cases neurocytomas have a generally good prognosis and are classed as grade II lesions in the WHO classification. The presence of bland histology or the identification of atypical features such as vascular proliferation are not entirely reliable as predictors of clinical behaviour. In particular, some tumours with bland histology have been reported to recur or disseminate[153–155] and ganglionic maturation has been seen in a case of tumour recurrence.[156] Conversely some studies have suggested that cases with atypical features do not behave differently from those with bland histology,[155,157] whilst others suggest that cases with a high proliferation labelling index are associated with a poor outcome with recurrence.[127,137,158]

Cerebellar liponeurocytoma

These tumours are characterised histologically by a mixture of mature neurocytic and neuronal cells intermixed with areas having the appearance of mature adipose tissue. They were originally described as 'lipomatous medulloblastomas'[159–161] but in contrast to medulloblastomas they are seen in adult life and have a good prognosis. Other terminology used in the past includes:

- Lipomatous glioneurocytoma.[162]
- Lipidised mature neuroectodermal tumour of the cerebellum.[163]
- Medullocytoma.[164]
- Neurolipocytoma.[165]

The term cerebellar liponeurocytoma has recently been agreed for this entity and is used in the latest WHO classification.

Incidence and site

Cerebellar liponeurocytomas are extremely rare tumours, but no precise incidence statistics are available. All the reported examples have arisen in the cerebellum. They have been described in both the vermis and the cerebellar hemispheres, and may also present as lesions growing out into the cerebellopontine angle.

Clinical features

Patients typically present in the fifth decade with clinical features of a mass lesion in the posterior fossa. Radiologically, the adipose component may cause focal high signal on T1-weighted MR sequences.

Pathology

Macroscopic features

No reliable information is available on the macroscopic appearances of these tumours, given their rarity and recent recognition as a tumour entity.

Intraoperative diagnosis

Few case studies have been reported on the intraoperative diagnosis in these lesions. There is clearly the potential for confusion with a medulloblastoma, given the site of the tumour and known occurrence of medulloblastoma in adults. In smear preparations, the most useful distinguishing features of liponeurocytomas are the absence of mitoses and nuclear atypia, but if a lipoid component is visible this should allow a firm diagnosis (Fig. 8.50).

Histological features

Histologically, the tumour has two components:

1. *The neuronal/neurocytic component* is composed of sheets of uniform cells with rounded nuclei and sparse, often vacuolated cytoplasm (Figs 8.51 and 8.52). In many cases the cells have an oligodendroglial-like appearance. Mitoses are not seen and features such as necrosis or vascular proliferation are not usually present, although have been described in recurrent lesions.

2. *The adipose component* is seen as either single or clustered clear, rounded spaces where fat has been removed during processing (Figs 8.51 and 8.52). In this respect the adipose areas resemble mature adipose tissue. Neuronal cells surround many of these fat containing spaces. The cells containing fat vacuoles have been characterised as both neuronal and glial, suggesting that the accumulation develops from lipomatous maturation in neoplastic cells.

Immunohistochemistry

Immunochemical staining shows strong expression of neuronal antigens (synaptophysin and MAP-2) in the cellular sheets as well as in cells surrounding and enclosing fat vacuoles. Focal GFAP staining is also seen in a proportion of cells in the tumour in most cases.

Electron microscopy

Ultrastructural investigation shows microtubule-rich cell processes suggestive of neurites as well as both dense core and clear cell vesicles. Infrequent synaptic structures may also be seen.

Molecular biology and histogenesis

There have been no conclusive reports of cell biology or genetics in these rare lesions. Immunochemical detection of neuronal or glial proteins in cells containing fat vacuoles suggests a transformation in neoplastic cells rather than incorporation of a reactive 'stromal' population of benign adipocytes in the tumour.[161]

Differential diagnosis

Medulloblastoma

The cellular areas may appear to represent a medulloblastoma, especially in small biopsy samples. This impression can be reinforced in areas of tumour that have few areas of fat vacuolation. In contrast to medulloblastoma, cells in liponeurocytoma have rounded rather than carrot shaped or elliptical nuclei, mitoses are not seen and apoptotic bodies are not generally identifiable.

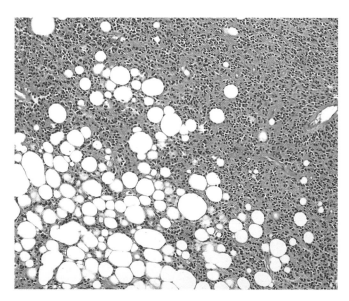

Fig. 8.51 **Cerebellar liponeurocytoma.** The neuronal/neurocytic component is seen as sheets of uniform cells with rounded nuclei with the adipose component visible as either single or clustered clear rounded spaces. H & E.

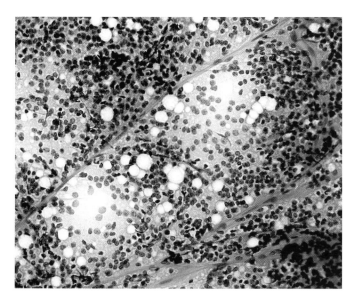

Fig. 8.50 **Cerebellar liponeurocytoma.** Areas of lipid vacuolation can be recognised in smear preparations against a background of rounded oligodendroglial-like cells. Toluidine blue.

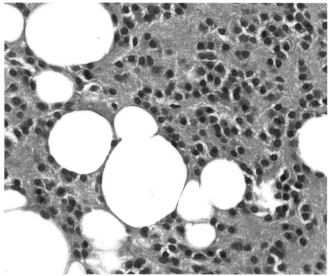

Fig. 8.52 **Cerebellar liponeurocytoma.** Higher magnification. H & E.

Therapy and prognosis

In the limited number of cases described, these tumours have a good prognosis following surgical resection. They correspond to grade II lesion in the WHO classification.

Paraganglioma

Paragangliomas are neuroendocrine tumours arising from neural crest cells associated with autonomic paraganglia throughout the body. They are typified by a mixture of neuroendocrine cells and sustentacular support cells. Outside the adrenal gland, paragangliomas occur at a variety of systemic sites, but when encountered within the central nemous system (CNS), they are almost all confined to the region of the cauda equina. They may also invade the cranial cavity as local extensions from the skull base.

Incidence and site

Paragangliomas of the CNS are generally seen after the first decade with a peak incidence in the sixth decade.[166] They usually occur as intradural lesions in the region of the cauda equina.[167–170] They are much less common at other levels of the spinal cord.[171] CNS paragangliomas may also be encountered as intracranial extensions of skull base tumours, particularly those with a jugulotympanic origin.[172]

Clinical features

The cauda equina tumours typically present as slowly expansile lesions causing lower back pain or clinical features of disturbed lower spinal nerve root function.[170] Some of the spinal tumours present with raised intracranial pressure.[131–175] Those lesions extending into the cranial cavity from the skull base typically present with hearing disturbance, audible bruits and, with more extensive tumours, multiple cranial nerve palsies.

Radiology

On imaging paragangliomas appear as isodense but enhancing masses on CT scanning. MR imaging shows them to be isodense or hypodense lesions on T1-weighted sequences but hyperintense on T2-weighted sequences. Discrimination from other lesions in the cauda equina region is often difficult.[176] However, like some other neuroendocrine tumours, paragangliomas express somatostatin type 2 receptors and can be imaged using octreotide, a somatostatin analogue that is coupled to a radioisotope. This method has been suggested to have an accuracy of 90%, a sensitivity of 94% and a specificity of 75%[177]

Pathology

Macroscopic features

Paragangliomas of the cauda equina are generally egg shaped or sausage shaped, encapsulated, dark red tumours attached to the filum terminale or a nerve root. Most are 3–4 cm in length and 1–2 cm in diameter. On the cut surface, the fixed tumour tissue is soft and dark grey–brown in colour.

Intraoperative diagnosis

When lesions are small and easily removed, complete neurosurgical excision is generally achieved, the pathologist receiving the entire tumour. Less commonly large tumours may be biopsied to ascertain their nature and plan further local surgical managament. Paragangliomas generally do not smear well and a frozen section is frequently required for intraoperative diagnosis (Figs 8.53 and 8.54). The characteristic packeted or alveolar architecture of a paraganglioma is usually apparent in frozen sections, with uniform rounded cells and prominent zellballen (see below).

Histological features

The most dominant aspect of the histology of paragangliomas are well formed nests and lobules (termed zellballen; Fig. 8.55) composed of uniform, polygonal *chief cells*. These cells have finely granular pink-stained cytoplasm with rounded nuclei (Fig. 8.56). Cytoplasmic argyrophil granules can be seen in chief cells using staining with the Grimelius technique. Around these nests are thin walled capillary sized blood vessels forming a rich and arborising network (Fig. 8.57). Less well defined are inconspicuous sustentacular cells which are mainly detected as rows of an elongated nuclei around the periphery of the chief cell nests. Mitoses are generally not seen but may be present in low density. As with many neuroendocrine tumours variation in nuclear size with hyperchromatic nuclei may be seen, but is of no prognostic importance. Hyalinised vessels and stromal hyalinisation are commonly present (Figs 8.58 and 8.59).

In some tumours, and especially those from the cauda equina, chief cells are arranged in cords and ribbons separated by capillary blood vessels (Figs 8.60 and 8.61). This more epithelial, ribbon-like pattern can simulate that seen in a myxopapillary ependymoma. Chief cells may show clear cell cytoplasm, oncocytic change or melanin pigmentation. Single cells and clusters of cells with ganglion cell maturation may also be seen, when the diagnostic term gangliocytic paraganglioma is appropriate.[178]

A tumour with both ependymal and paragangliomatous features has been described.[179] Oncocytic change has also been reported in a lesion in the filum terminale.[180]

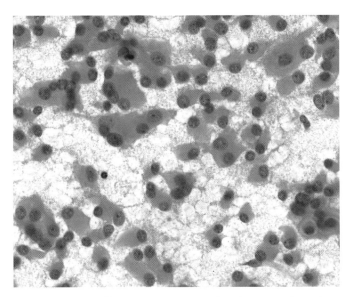

Fig. 8.53 **Paraganglioma.** In smear preparations from a cauda equina lesion the picture is dominated by epithelial pattern chief cells with large rounded nuclei and bright pink-staining cytoplasm. H & E.

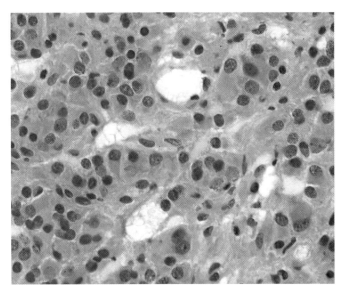

Fig. 8.54 **Paraganglioma.** In frozen sections sheets and ribbons of large epithelial cells would raise problems in distinction from a myxopapillary ependymoma. H & E.

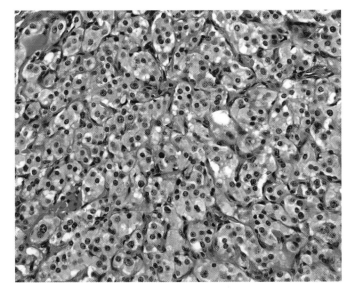

Fig. 8.55 **Paraganglioma.** Paragangliomas are formed of well formed nests and lobules (termed zellballen). H & E.

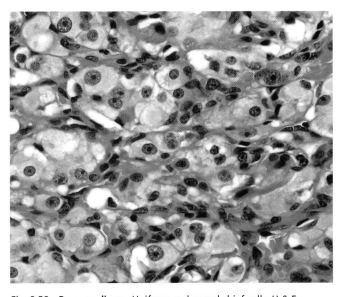

Fig. 8.56 **Paraganglioma.** Uniform, polygonal chief cells. H & E.

Immunohistochemistry

Chief cells are immunoreactive for neurone-specific enolase, synaptophysin, chromogranin-A, and neurofilament protein reflecting neuroendocrine differentiation[181] (Figs 8.62–8.67). Cytokeratin expression is seen, often as a paranuclear accumulation in lesions from the cauda equina[182,183] but is not frequent in paragangliomas from other head (Fig. 8.65) and neck sites.[184,185] S-100 staining highlights sustentacular cells as long processes running around nests of chief cells (Fig. 8.67). Sustentacular cells may also show GFAP immunoreactivity.[186]

Electron microscopy

Electron microscopic examination shows large dense core granules in chief cells, which are connected by adherens type cellular junctions.[186] Fibrous bodies, corresponding to intermediate filament aggregates are seen in paragangliomas of the filum terminale.[187]

Proliferation indices

Head and neck paragangliomas have been shown to have a median growth rate of 1.0 mm/year and a median tumour doubling time of 4.2 years.[188] Ki-67/MIB-1 labelling indices of around 2% have been described.[189]

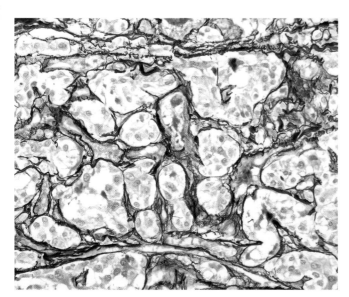

Fig. 8.57 **Paraganglioma.** The nested architecture is emphasised on reticulin staining.

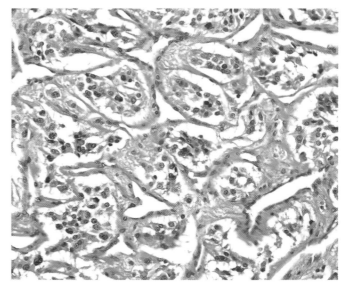

Fig. 8.58 **Paraganglioma.** Many paragangliomas show stromal hyalinisation. H & E.

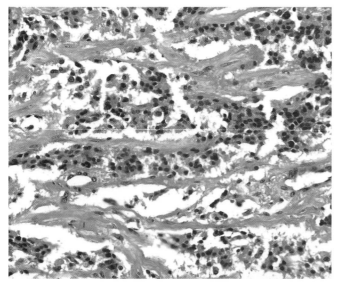

Fig. 8.59 **Paraganglioma.** In small biopsy samples such hyalinisation and low cellularity may obscure the diagnostic zellballen pattern. H & E.

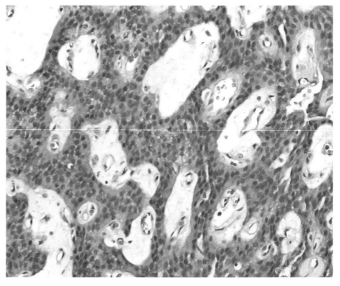

Fig. 8.60 **Paraganglioma.** A ribbon-like pattern is characteristically seen in examples from the cauda equina. H & E.

Molecular biology and genetics

There are no known genetic predispositions to development of paragangliomas of the cauda equina. However, about 9% of head and neck paragangliomas have been linked to genes on chromosome 11,[190,191] one being characterised as a mutation in the *SDHD* gene, a mitochondrial complex II gene on chromosome 11q23.[192]

Differential diagnosis

The main differential diagnosis is at the clinical and macroscopic level with tumours known to occur in the region of the filum terminale, mainly *myxopapillary ependymoma* and *Schwannoma*. Histologically, Schwannomas can usually be easily distinguished, but confusion with myxopapillary ependymomas may arise with paragangliomas that lack the typical packeted architecture with zellballen and are composed of ribbon-like arrangements of epithelial cells with hyalinised stroma and vessels. Immunochemical staining for neuroendocrine markers is the simplest and most reliable way to establish the diagnosis when there is any doubt.

Therapy and prognosis

Local surgical excision is generally curative for paragangliomas of the cauda equina region, with a small rate

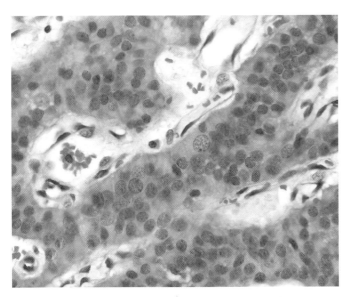

Fig. 8.61 **Paraganglioma.** Carcinoid tumour-like neuroendocrine features are seen on high magnification. H & E.

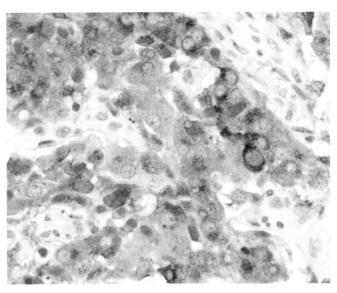

Fig. 8.62 **Paraganglioma.** Paraganglioma showing expression, in chief cells of the neuronal marker chromogranin-A.

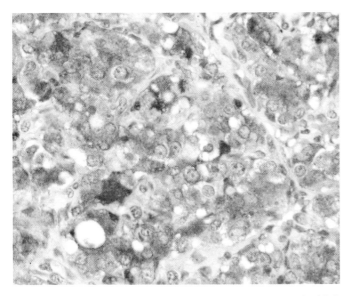

Fig. 8.63 **Paraganglioma.** Paraganglioma showing expression, in chief cells of the neuronal marker synaptophysin.

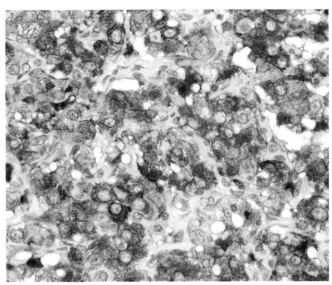

Fig. 8.64 **Paraganglioma.** Paraganglioma showing expression, in chief cells, of the neuronal marker neuron specific enolase.

of local recurrence. When it is only possible to perform a subtotal resection, the tumours may recur and irradiation is indicated.[170] The presence of S-100 positive sustentacular cells has been suggested as a criterion possibly to exclude malignancy in individual cases.[193] Paragangliomas extending into the cranial cavity from the skull base (see Chapter 18) are usually much more difficult to excise and are therefore more prone to local recurrence. Frankly malignant behaviour in head and neck paragangliomas has also been described,[194–196] as has metastasis from cauda equina lesions.[197]

Dysplastic gangliocytoma of cerebellum (Lhermitte–Duclos disease)

This enigmatic condition affecting the cerebellum was first described in 1920 by Lhermitte and Duclos[198] and combines features of congenital malformation, hamartomatous overgrowth and true neoplasm. It is intimately associated with Cowden syndrome, a hereditary disorder caused by a germline mutation in the *PTEN* tumour suppressor gene on chromosome 10q23, which is fully described in Chapter 19. Patients with Cowden syndrome are predisposed to the development of mucocutaneous hamartomas and a variety of systemic tumours during adult life.[199] Up to one-half of

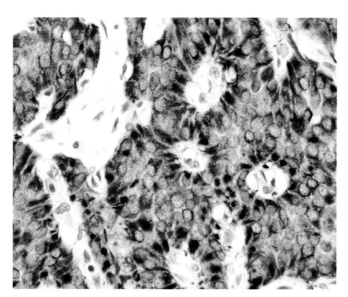

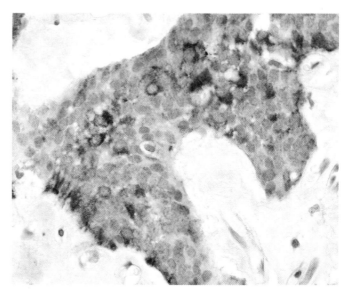

Fig. 8.65 **Paraganglioma.** Cytokeratin staining can be seen in ribbon pattern tumours from the cauda equina.

Fig. 8.66 **Paraganglioma.** Confirmation of the neuroendocrine pattern with synaptophysin.

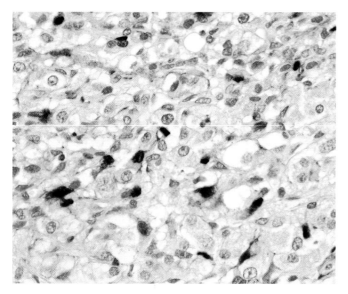

Fig. 8.67 **Paraganglioma.** Sustentacular cells stain with S-100 and are seen around the nests of chief cells.

all cerebellar dysplastic gangliocytomas arise in patients who have, or later develop, typical clinical features of Cowden syndrome[200] and apparently isolated cerebellar lesions are currently thought to represent part of the phenotypic spectrum of the disorder.[201,202]

Incidence and site

Dysplastic gangliocytomas of the cerebellum usually present during the second or third decade of life, with a preponderance of males.[203] Occasional congenital cases have been reported, presenting in the neonatal period.[204] The disorder is exceedingly rare, with only 72 reported

cases found by a review in 1994.[200] The lesion is usually confined to part of one or other cerebellar hemisphere.

Clinical features

Many cases present clinically with a cerebellar syndrome, predominantly ataxic in nature, sometimes with an antecedant history of mild mental retardation and/or seizures.[205] In some instances there is a more acute presentation with clinical features of raised intracranial pressure due to obstructive hydrocephalus. The mean duration of symptoms prior to diagnosis is 40 months[200] and the average age at diagnosis 34 years, ranging from birth to 74 years.[206] It is important to note that early presentations may preceed other manifestations of Cowden syndrome by many years (see prognosis, below).

Radiology

Radiological scans typically show focal distortion of one cerebellar hemisphere with enlargement of the cerebellar folia clearly visible in MR images.[207] The abnormal area is hyperintense in T2-weighted MR images but there is no enhancement following administration of gadolinium.[204]

Pathology

Macroscopic features

Externally, the affected cerebellar hemisphere shows a localised area of expansion, proud to the surrounding pial surface, with obvious expansion of the folia. On cut section, the area of expanded folia appears moderately well defined and extends down to the junction with white matter (Fig. 8.68). In post-mortem specimens, considerable compression and distortion of the surrounding, unaffected, cerebellar hemisphere may be apparent.

Histological features

At the junction with expanded folia, normal cerebellar cortex merges relatively abruptly with greatly thickened, abnormal architecture (Fig. 8.69). There is an inverted arrangement, with a thick outer plexus of myelinated white matter, sometimes divided into a horizontally orientated outer zone and a radially arranged inner one. Beneath this lies a broad layer of grey matter containing sheets of large, randomly arranged dysplastic ganglion cells, sometimes resembling bizarre Purkinje cells (Fig. 8.70). These are interspersed with a variable population of much smaller neuronal cells with hyperchromatic, dot-like nuclei.

Immunocytochemistry

As might be expected, the abnormal grey matter layer shows widespread expression of pan-neuronal antigens, including neuron specific enolase and synaptophysin. However, only very few of the large dysplastic ganglion cells immunostain with antibodies to Purkinje cell antigens, such as Leu4, PEP19 and calbindin, bringing in to question their relationship with normal Purkinje neurons.[208,209]

Proliferation indices and grading

Dysplastic cerebellar gangliocytomas are listed as grade I lesions in the WHO classification. They appear to be biologically indolent lesions, and immunocytochemical studies of cell proliferation markers have shown low or absent activity.[208]

Histogenesis

It is still unclear whether dysplastic cerebellar gangliocytomas are hamartomatous or truly neoplastic lesions. It is often assumed that the larger ganglionic cells are dysplastic Purkinje cells, despite their immunocytochemical profile (see above) and that the smaller neuronal cells are similarly derived from granular layer neurons.[208] Ultrastructural and Golgi studies have lent support to the latter proposal, showing features of abnormal granular

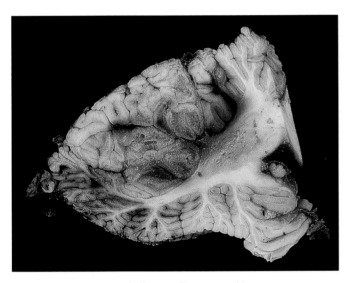

Fig. 8.68 **Dysplastic cerebellar gangliocytoma.** This post-mortem specimen shows a moderately well circumscribed area of expanded cortical folia in the superior part of the cerebellar hemisphere, with compression of adjacent cerebellar tissue. The haemorrhage relates to biopsy surgery performed prior to death.

Fig. 8.69 **Dysplastic cerebellar gangliocytoma.** The expanded folia show an inverted architecture with a thick outer plexus of myelinated fibres covering a broad zone of abnormal grey matter. A relatively abrupt transition with normal cerebellar cortex is seen to the left of the figure with a normal folium immediately above. Luxol fast blue/cresyl violet.

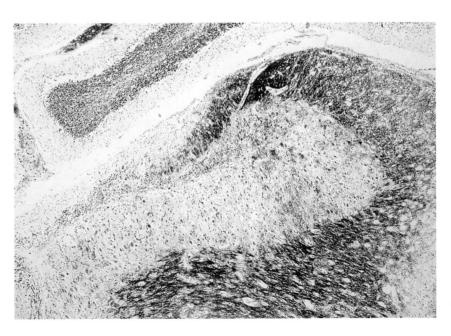

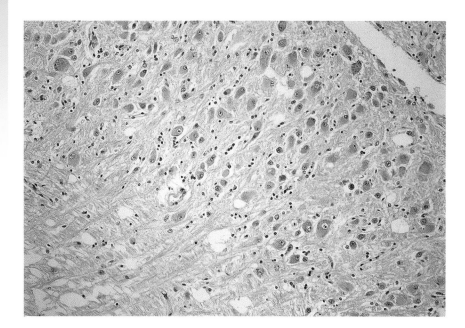

Fig. 8.70 **Dysplastic cerebellar gangliocytoma.** The deeper layer of abnormal grey matter contains sheets of large, randomly arranged, dysplastic ganglion cells interspersed with the dot-like nuclei of much smaller neuronal cells. H & E.

neurons with aberrantly myelinated axons.[210–212] Against this must be set the neoplastic behaviour of those cases which have grown and recurred after surgical excision[213] and the examples presenting in adults with previously normal radiology.[208]

Differential diagnosis

In surgical biopsy specimens, the main differential diagnosis is that of non-dysplastic *gangliocytoma* or *ganglioglioma* arising in the cerebellum. The major deciding factor here will be the architecture of the dysplastic lesion and, if the specimen permits, the relationship with adjacent non-dysplastic cerebellar cortex. Where a particularly fragmented surgical specimen causes uncertainty, the distinctive appearance of a preoperative MR scan will usually resolve the problem.

Treatment and prognosis

Subtotal surgical debulking is the usual treatment in cases with raised intracranial pressure due to obstructive hydrocephalus and usually provides lasting relief of presenting symptoms, with no evidence of subsequent tumour progression. There have been occasional reports of clinical recurrence after surgical excision[213] but subtotal excision of the recurrent tumour has again been effective.[214] Some authors have advocated simple decompressive duroplasty rather than surgical removal of the lesion.[215] In view of the relationship with Cowden syndrome, it is important to screen all patients presenting with cerebellar dysplastic gangliocytomas for systemic manifestations of the syndrome, especially breast and pelvic cancers.[200] Even in apparently islolated cases, long term follow up is essential because of the risk of systemic malignancies developing later in life.[201]

REFERENCES

Gangliocytoma, ganglioglioma and anaplastic ganglioglioma

1. Zhu JJ, Leon SP, Folkerth RD et al. Evidence for clonal origin of neoplastic neuronal and glial cells in gangliogliomas. Am Pathol, 1997; 151:565–571
2. Smith NM, Carli MM, Hanieh A et al. Gangliogliomas in childhood. Childs Nerv Syst, 1992; 8:258–262
3. Wolf HK, Wiestler OD. Surgical pathology of chronic epileptic seizure disorders. Brain Pathol, 1993; 3:371–380
4. Wolf HK, Campos MG, Zentner J et al. Surgical pathology of temporal lobe epilepsy. Experience with 216 cases. J Neuropathol Exp Neurol, 1993; 52:499–506
5. Majos C, Aguilera C, Ferrer I et al. Intraventricular ganglioglioma: case report. Neuroradiology, 1998; 40:377–379
6. Mizuno J, Nishio S, Barrow DL et al. Ganglioglioma of the cerebellum: case report. Neurosurgery, 1988; 21:584–588
7. Blatt GL, Ahuja A, Miller LL et al. Cerebellomedullary ganglioglioma: CT and MR findings. AJNR. Am J Neuroradiol, 1995; 16:790–792
8. Furie DM, Felsberg GJ, Tien RD et al. MRI of gangliocytoma of cerebellum and spinal cord. J Comput Assist Tomogr, 1993; 17:488–491
9. Jay V, Greenberg M. Unusual cerebellar ganglioglioma with marked cytologic atypia. Pediatr Pathol Lab Med, 1997; 17:105–114
10. Karamitopoulou E, Perentes E, Probst A, et al. Ganglioglioma of the brain stem: neurological dysfunction of 16-year duration. Clin Neuropath, 1995; 14:162–168
11. Garcia CA, McGarry PA, Collada M. Ganglioglioma of the brain stem. Case report. J Neurosurg, 1984; 60:431–434
12. Miller G, Towfighi J, Page RB. Spinal cord ganglioglioma presenting as hydrocephalus. J Neurooncol, 1990; 9:147–152
13. Constantini S, Houten J, Miller DC et al. Intramedullary spinal cord tumors in children under the age of 3 years. J Neurosurg, 1996; 85:1036–1043
14. Albright L, Byrd RP. Ganglioglioma of the entire spinal cord. Childs Brain, 1980; 6:274–280
15. Bergin DJ, Johnson TE, Spencer WH et al. Ganglioglioma of the optic nerve. Am J Ophthalmol, 1988; 105:146–149
16. Hamburger C, Buttner A, Weis S. Ganglioglioma of the spinal cord: report of two rare cases and review of the literature. Neurosurgery, 1997; 41:1410–1415; discussion 1415–1416
17. Harmon HL, Gossman MD, Buchino JJ et al. Orbital ganglioglioma arising from ectopic neural tissue. Am J Ophthalmol, 2000; 129:109–111
18. Athale S, Hallet KK, Jinkins JR. Ganglioglioma of the trigeminal nerve: MRI. Neuroradiology, 1999; 41:576–578

19. Chilton J, Caughron MR, Kepes JJ. Ganglioglioma of the optic chiasm: case report and review of the literature. Neurosurgery, 1990; 26:1042–1045

20. Zentner J, Wolf HK, Ostertun B et al. Gangliogliomas: clinical, radiological, and histopathological findings in 51 patients. J Neurol Neurosurg Psychiatry, 1994; 57:1497–1502

21. Faillot T, Sichez JP, Capelle L et al. Ganglioglioma of the pineal region: case report and review of the literature. Surg Neurol, 1998; 49:104–107; discussion 107–108

22. Hunt SJ, Johnson PC. Melanotic ganglioglioma of the pineal region. Acta Neuropathol, 1989; 79:222–225

23. Packer RJ, Sutton LN, Rosenstock JG et al. Pineal region tumors of childhood. Pediatrics, 1984; 74:97–102

24. Tokoro K, Chiba Y, Ohtani T et al. Pineal ganglioglioma in a patient with familial basal ganglia calcification and elevated serum alpha-fetoprotein: case report. Neurosurgery, 1993; 33:506–511; discussion 511

25. Yamamoto T, Komori T, Shibata N et al. Multifocal neurocytoma/gangliocytoma with extensive leptomeningeal dissemination in the brain and spinal cord. Am J Surg Pathol, 1996; 20:363–370

26. al-Sarraj ST. Multifocal neurocytoma/ganglioglioma. Am J Surg Pathol, 1997; 21:258–259

27. Patel U, Pinto RS, Miller DC et al. MR of spinal cord ganglioglioma. AJNR. Am J Neuroradiol, 1998; 19:879–887

28. Kincaid PK, El-Saden SM, Park SH, et al. Cerebral gangliogliomas: preoperative grading using FDG-PET and 201T1-SPECT. AJNR. Am J Neuroradiol, 1998; 19:801–806

29. Komori T, Scheithauer BW, Anthony DC et al. Papillary glioneuronal tumor: a new variant of mixed neuronal-glial neoplasm. Am J Surg Pathol, 1998; 22:1171–1183

30. Miller DC, Lang FF, Epstein FJ. Central nervous system gangliogliomas. Part 1: Pathology. J Neurosurg, 1993; 79:859–866

31. Wolf HK, Muller MB, Spanle M et al. Ganglioglioma: a detailed histopathological and immunohistochemical analysis of 61 cases. Acta Neuropathol, 1994; 88:166–173

32. Chintagumpala MM, Armstrong D, Miki S et al. Mixed neuronal-glial tumors (gangliogliomas) in children. Ped Neurosurg, 1996; 24:306–313

33. Soffer D, Lach B, Constantini S. Melanotic cerebral ganglioglioma: evidence for melanogenesis in neoplastic astrocytes. Acta Neuropathol, 1992; 83:315–323

34. Soffer D, Umansky F, Goldman JE. Ganglioglioma with neurofibrillary tangles (NFTs): neoplastic NFTs share antigenic determinants with NFTs of Alzheimer's disease. Acta Neuropathol, 1995; 89:451–453

35. Kim DH, Suh YL. Pseudopapillary neurocytoma of temporal lobe with glial differentiation. Acta Neuropathol, 1997; 94:187–191

36. Bouvier-Labit C, Daniel L, Dufour H et al. Papillary glioneuronal tumour: clinicopathological and biochemical study of one case with 7-year follow up. Acta Neuropathol, 2000; 99:321–326

37. Smith TW, Nikulasson S, De Girolami U et al. Immunohistochemistry of synapsin I and synaptophysin in human nervous system and neuroendocrine tumors. Applications in diagnostic neuro-oncology. Clin Neuropathol, 1993; 12:335–342

38. Hirose T, Scheithauer BW, Lopes MB et al. Ganglioglioma: an ultrastructural and immunohistochemical study. Cancer, 1997; 79:989–1003

39. Diepholder HM, Schwechheimer K, Mohadjer M et al. A clinicopathologic and immunomorphologic study of 13 cases of ganglioglioma. Cancer, 1991; 68:2192–2201

40. Raghavan R, White CL, Rogers B et al. Alpha-synuclein expression in central nervous system tumors showing neuronal or mixed neuronal/glial differentiation. J Neuropathol Exp Neurol, 2000; 59:490–494

41. Kawashima M, Suzuki SO, Doh-ura K et al. alpha-Synuclein is expressed in a variety of brain tumors showing neuronal differentiation. Acta Neuropathol, 2000; 99:154–160

42. Zhang PJ, Rosenblum MK. Synaptophysin expression in the human spinal cord. Diagnostic implications of an immunohistochemical study. Am J Surg Pathol, 1996; 20:273–276

43. Quinn B. Synaptophysin staining in normal brain: importance for diagnosis of ganglioglioma. Am J Surg Pathol, 1998; 22:550–556

44. Parizel PM, Martin JJ, Van Vyve M et al. Cerebral ganglioglioma and neurofibromatosis type I. Case report and review of the literature. Neuroradiology, 1991; 33:357–359

45. Sawin PD, Theodore N, Rekate HL. Spinal cord ganglioglioma in a child with neurofibromatosis type 2. Case report and literature review. J Neurosurg, 1999; 90:231–233

46. Tamiya T, Hamazaki S, Ono Y et al. Ganglioglioma in a patient with Turcot syndrome. Case report. J Neurosurg, 2000; 92:170–175

47. Neumann E, Kalousek DK, Norman MG et al. Cytogenetic analysis of 109 pediatric central nervous system tumors. Cancer Genet Cytogenet, 1993; 71:40–49

48. Vagner-Capodano AM, Gentet JC, Gambarelli D et al. Cytogenetic studies in 45 pediatric brain tumors [published erratum appears in Pediatr Hematol Oncol 1993 Jan–Mar;10(1):117]. Pediatr Hematol Oncol, 1992; 9:223–235

49. Orellana C, Hernandez-Marti M, Martinez F et al. Pediatric brain tumors: loss of heterozygosity at 17p and TP53 gene mutations. Cancer Genet Cytogenet, 1998; 102:93–99

50. Bhattacharjee MB, Armstrong DD, Vogel H et al. Cytogenetic analysis of 120 primary pediatric brain tumors and literature review. Cancer Genet Cytogenet, 1997; 97:39–53

51. Jay V, Squire J, Blaser S et al. Intracranial and spinal metastases from a ganglioglioma with unsual cytogenetic abnormalities in a patient with complex partial seizures. Childs Nerv Syst, 1997; 13:550–555

52. Duerr EM, Rollbrocker B, Hayashi Y et al. PTEN mutations in gliomas and glioneuronal tumors. Oncogene, 1998; 16:2259–2264

53. Furuta A, Takahashi H, Ikuta F et al. Temporal lobe tumor demonstrating ganglioglioma and pleomorphic xanthoastrocytoma components. Case report. J Neurosurg, 1992; 77:143–147

54. Kordek R, Biernat W, Sapieja W et al. Pleomorphic xanthoastrocytoma with a gangliomatous component: an immunohistochemical and ultrastructural study. Acta Neuropathol, 1995; 89:194–197

55. Kros JM, Vecht CJ, Stefanko SZ. The pleomorphic xanthoastrocytoma and its differential diagnosis: a study of five cases. Hum Pathol, 1991; 22:1128–1135

56. Lindboe CF, Cappelen J, Kepes JJ. Pleomorphic xanthoastrocytoma as a component of a cerebellar ganglioglioma: case report. Neurosurgery, 1992; 31:353–355

57. Perry A, Giannini C, Scheithauer BW et al. Composite pleomorphic xanthoastrocytoma and ganglioglioma: report of four cases and review of the literature. Am J Surg Pathol, 1997; 21:763–771

58. Powell SZ, Yachnis AT, Rorke LB et al. Divergent differentiation in pleomorphic xanthoastrocytoma. Evidence for a neuronal element and possible relationship to ganglion cell tumors. Am J Surg Pathol, 1996; 20:80–85

59. Vajtai I, Varga Z, Aguzzi A. Pleomorphic xanthoastrocytoma with gangliogliomatous component. Pathol Res Pract, 1997; 193:617–621

60. Johnson JHJ, Hariharan S, Berman J et al. Clinical outcome of pediatric gangliogliomas: ninety-nine cases over 20 years. Pediatr Neurosurg, 1997; 27:203–207

61. Lang FF, Epstein FJ, Ransohoff J, et al. Central nervous system gangliogliomas. Part 2: Clinical outcome. J Neurosurg, 1993; 79:867–873

62. Rumana CS, Valadka AB, Contact CF. Prognostic factors in supratentorial ganglioglioma. Acta Neurochir, 1999; 141:63–68; discussion 68–69

63. Araki M, Fan J, Haraoka S et al. Extracranial metastasis of anaplastic ganglioglioma through a ventriculoperitoneal shunt: a case report. Pathol Int, 1999; 49:258–263

Desmoplastic infantile ganglioma

64. Louis DN, von Deimling A, Dickersin GR et al. Desmoplastic cerebral astrocytomas of infancy: a histopathologic, immunohistochemical, ultrastructural, and molecular genetic study. Hum Pathol, 1992; 23:1402–1409

65. VandenBerg SR. Desmoplastic infantile ganglioglioma and desmoplastic cerebral astrocytoma of infancy. Brain Pathol, 1993; 3:275–281

66. VandenBerg SR, May EE, Rubinstein LJ et al. Desmoplastic supratentorial neuroepithelial tumors of infancy with divergent differentiation potential (desmoplastic infantile gangliogliomas). Report on 11 cases of a distinctive embryonal tumor with favorable prognosis. J Neurosurg, 1987; 66:58–71

67. Paulus W, Schlote W, Perentes E et al. Desmoplastic supratentorial neuroepithelial tumours of infancy. Histopathology, 1992; 21:43–49

68. Kuchelmeister K, Bergmann M, von Wild K et al. Desmoplastic ganglioglioma: report of two non-infantile cases. Acta Neuropathol, 1993; 85:199–204

69. Galatioto S, Gullotta F. Desmoplastic non-infantile ganglioglioma. J Neurosurg Sci, 1996; 40:235–238

70. Duffner PK, Burger PC, Cohen ME et al. Desmoplastic infantile gangliogliomas: an approach to therapy. Neurosurgery, 1994; 34:583–589; discussion 589

71. Tenreiro-Picon OR, Kamath SV, Knorr JR et al. Desmoplastic infantile ganglioglioma: CT and MRI features. Pediatr Radiol, 1995; 25:540–543

72. Sperner J, Gottschalk J, Neumann K et al. Clinical, radiological and histological findings in desmoplastic infantile ganglioglioma. Childs Nerv Syst, 1994; 10:458–462; discussion 462–463

73. Park JP, Dossu JR, Rhodes CH. Telomere associations in desmoplastic infantile ganglioglioma. Cancer Genet Cytogenet, 1996; 92:4–7

74. al-Sarraj ST, Bridges LR. Desmoplastic cerebral glioblastoma of infancy. Br J Neurosurg, 1996; 10:215–219

75. Mallucci C, Lellouch-Tubiana A, Salazar C et al. The management of desmoplastic neuroepithelial tumours in childhood. Childs Nerv Syst, 2000; 16:8–14

Dysembryoplastic neuroepithelial tumour

76. Daumas-Duport C, Scheithauer BW, Chodkiewicz JP et al. Dysembryoplastic neuroepithelial tumor: a surgically curable tumor of young patients with intractable partial seizures. Report of thirty-nine cases. Neurosurgery, 1988; 23:545–556

77. Daumas-Duport C, Varlet P, Bacha S et al. Dysembryoplastic neuroepithelial tumors: nonspecific histological forms – a study of 40 cases. J Neurooncol, 1999; 41:267–280

78. Gottschalk J, Korves M, Skotzek-Konrad B et al. Dysembryoplastic neuroepithelial micro-tumor in a 75-year-old patient with long-standing epilepsy. Clin Neuropathol, 1993; 12:175–178

79. Cervera-Pierot P, Varlet P, Chodkiewicz JP et al. Dysembryoplastic neuroepithelial tumors located in the caudate nucleus area: report of four cases. Neurosurgery, 1997; 40:1065–1069; discussion 1069–1070

80. Kuchelmeister K, Demirel T, Schlorer E et al. Dysembryoplastic neuroepithelial tumour of the cerebellum. Acta Neuropathol, 1995; 89:385–390

81. Yasha TC, Mohanty A, Radhesh S et al. Infratentorial dysembryoplastic neuroepithelial tumor (DNT) associated with Arnold-Chiari malformation. Clin Neuropathol, 1998; 17:305–310

82. Baisden BL, Brat DJ, Melhem ER et al. Dysembryoplastic neuroepithelial tumor-like neoplasm of the septum pellucidum: a lesion often misdiagnosed as glioma: report of 10 cases. Am J Surg Pathol, 2001; 25:494–499

83. Daumas-Duport C. Dysembryoplastic neuroepithelial tumours. Brain Pathol, 1993; 3:283–295

84. Thom M, Gomez-Anson B, Revesz T et al. Spontaneous intralesional haemorrhage in dysembryoplastic neuroepithelial tumours: a series of five cases. J Neurol Neurosurg Psychiatry, 1999; 67:97–101

85. Koeller KK, Dillon WP. Dysembryoplastic neuroepithelial tumors: MR appearance. AJNR. Am J Neuroradiol, 1992; 13:1319–1325

86. Raymond AA, Halpin SF, Alsanjari N et al. Dysembryoplastic neuroepithelial tumor. Features in 16 patients. Brain, 1994; 117:461–475

87. Kuroiwa T, Bergey GK, Rothman MI et al. Radiologic appearance of the dysembryoplastic neuroepithelial tumor. Radiology, 1995; 197:233–238

88. Kuroiwa T, Kishikawa T, Kato A et al. Dysembryoplastic neuroepithelial tumors: MR findings. J Comput Assist Tomogr, 1994; 18:352–356

89. Leung SY, Gwi E, Ng HK et al. Dysembryoplastic neuroepithelial tumor. A tumor with small neuronal cells resembling oligodendroglioma. Am J Surg Pathol, 1994; 18:604–614

90. Prayson RA, Morris HH, Estes ML et al. Dysembryoplastic neuroepithelial tumor: a clinicopathologic and immunohistochemical study of 11 tumors including MIB1 immunoreactivity. Clin Neuropathol, 1996; 15:47–53

91. Elizabeth J, Bhaskara RM, Radhakrishnan VV et al. Melanotic differentiation in dysembryoplastic neuroepithelial tumor. Clin Neuropathol, 2000; 19:38–40

92. Hirose T, Scheithauer BW, Lopes MB et al. Dysembryoplastic neuroepithelial tumor (DNT): an immunohistochemical and ultrastructural study. J Neuropathol Exp Neurol, 1994; 53:184–195

93. Wolf HK, Buslei R, Blumcke I et al. Neural antigens in oligodendrogliomas and dysembryoplastic neuroepithelial tumors. Acta Neuropathol, 1997; 94:436–443

94. Honavar M, Janota I, Polkey CE. Histological heterogeneity of dysembryoplastic neuroepithelial tumour: identification and differential diagnosis in a series of 74 cases. Histopathology, 1999; 34:342–356

95. Gyure KA, Sandberg GD, Prayson RA et al. Dysembryoplastic neuroepithelial tumor: an immunohistochemical study with myelin oligodendrocyte glycoprotein. Arch Pathol Lab Med, 2000; 124:123–126

96. Hirose T, Scheithauer BW. Mixed dysembryoplastic neuroepithelial tumor and ganglioglioma. Acta Neuropathol, 1998; 95:649–654

97. Prayson RA, Composite ganglioglioma and dysembryoplastic neuroepithelial tumor. Arch Pathol Lab Med, 1999; 123:247–250

98. Hammond RR, Duggal N, Woulfe JM et al. Malignant transformation of a dysembryoplastic neuroepithelial tumor. Case report. J Neurosurg, 2000; 92:722–725

Central neurocytoma

99. Hassoun J, Soylemezoglu F, Gambarelli D et al. Central neurocytoma: a synopsis of clinical and histological features. Brain Pathol, 1993; 3:297–306

100. Hassoun J, Gambarelli D, Grisoli F et al. Central neurocytoma. An electron-microscopic study of two cases. Acta Neuropathol, 1982; 56:151–156

101. Townsend JJ, Seaman JP. Central neurocytoma – a rare benign intraventricular tumor. Acta Neuropathol, 1986; 71:167–170

102. Nishio S, Tashima T, Takeshita I et al. Intraventricular neurocytoma: clinicopathological features of six cases. J Neurosurg, 1988; 68:665–670

103. Louis DN, Swearingen B, Linggood RM et al. Central nervous system neurocytoma and neuroblastoma in adults – report of eight cases. J Neurooncol, 1990; 9:231–238

104. von Deimling A, Janzer R, Kleihues P et al. Patterns of differentiation in central neurocytoma. An immunohistochemical study of eleven biopsies. Acta Neuropathol, 1990; 79:473–479

105. Barbosa MD, Balsitis M, Jaspan T et al. Intraventricular neurocytoma: a clinical and pathological study of three cases and review of the literature. Neurosurgery, 1990; 26:1045–1054

106. von Deimling A, Kleihues P, Saremaslani P et al. Histogenesis and differentiation potential of central neurocytomas. Lab Invest, 1991; 64:585–591

107. Schild SE, Scheithauer BW, Haddock MG et al. Central neurocytomas. Cancer, 1997; 79:790–795

108. Brat DJ, Scheithauer BW, Eberhart CG, Burger PC. Extraventricular neurocytomas: pathological features and clinical outcome. Am J Surg Pathol, 2001; 25:1252–1260

109. Coca S, Moreno M, Martos JA et al. Neurocytoma of spinal cord. Acta Neuropathol, 1994; 87:537–540

110. Tatter SB, Borges LF, Louis DN. Central neurocytomas of the cervical spinal cord. Report of two cases [published erratum appears in J Neurosurg 1995 Apr; 82:706]. J Neurosurg, 1994; 81:288–293

111. Soontornniyomkij V, Schelper RI. Pontine neurocytoma. J Clin Pathol, 1996; 49:764–765

112. Giangaspero F, Cenacchi G, Losi L et al. Extraventricular neoplasms with neurocytoma features. A clinicopathological study of 11 cases. Am J Surg Pathol, 1997; 21:206–212

113. Funato H, Inoshita N, Okeda R et al. Cystic ganglioneurocytoma outside the ventricular region. Acta Neuropathol, 1997; 94:95–98

114. Enam SA, Rosenblum ML, Ho KL. Neurocytoma in the cerebellum. Case report. J Neurosurg, 1997; 87:100–102

115. Brandis A, Heyer R, Hori A et al. Cerebellar neurocytoma in an infant: an important differential diagnosis from cerebellar neuroblastoma and medulloblastoma? Neuropediatrics, 1997; 28:235–238

116. Tortori-Donati P, Fondelli MP, Rossi A et al. Extraventricular neurocytoma with ganglionic differentiation associated with complex partial seizures. AJNR. Am J Neuroradiol, 1999; 20:724–727

117. Stephan CL, Kepes JJ, Arnold P et al. Neurocytoma of the cauda equina. Case report. J Neurosurg, 1999; 90:247–251

118. Nishio S, Takeshita I, Kaneko Y et al. Cerebral neurocytoma. A new subset of benign neuronal tumors of the cerebrum. Cancer, 1992; 70:529–537

119. Hirschowitz L, Ansari A, Cahill DJ et al. Central neurocytoma arising within a mature cystic teratoma of the ovary. Int J Gynecol Pathol, 1997; 16:176–179

120. Okamura A, Goto S, Sato K et al. Central neurocytoma with hemorrhagic onset. Surg Neurol, 1995; 43:252–255

121. Taylor CL, Cohen ML, Cohen AR. Neurocytoma presenting with intraparenchymal cerebral hemorrhage. Pediatr Neurosurg, 1998; 29:92–95

122. Balko MG, Schultz DL. Sudden death due to a central neurocytoma. Am J Forensic Med Pathol, 1999; 20:180–183

123. Smoker WR, Townsend JJ, Reichman MV. Neurocytoma accompanied by intraventricular hemorrhage: case report and literature review. AJNR. Am J Neuroradiol, 1991; 12:765–770

124. McConachie NS, Worthington BS, Cornford EJ et al. Review article: computerised tomography and magnetic resonance in the diagnosis of intraventricular cerebral masses. Br J Radiol, 1994; 67:223–243

125. Yasargil MG, von Ammon K, von Deimling A et al. Central neurocytoma: histopathological variants and therapeutic approaches. J Neurosurg, 1992; 76:32–37

126. Mrak RE. Malignant neurocytic tumor. Hum Pathol, 1994; 25:747–752

127. Soylemezoglu F, Scheithauer BW, Esteve J et al. Atypical central neurocytoma. J Neuropathol Exp Neurol, 1997; 56:551–556

128. Mackenzie IR. Central neurocytoma: histologic atypia, proliferation potential, and clinical outcome. Cancer, 1999; 85:1606–1610

129. Kubota T, Hayashi M, Kawano H et al. Central neurocytoma: immunohistochemical and ultrastructural study. Acta Neuropathol, 1991; 81:418–427

130. Hessler RB, Lopes MB, Frankfurter A et al. Cytoskeletal immunohistochemistry of central neurocytomas. Am J Surg Pathol, 1992; 16:1031–1038

131. Tsuchida T, Matsumoto M, Shirayama Y et al. Neuronal and glial characteristics of central neurocytoma: electron microscopical analysis of two cases. Acta Neuropathol, 1996; 91:573–577

132. Pal L, Santosh V, Gayathri N et al. Neurocytoma/rhabdomyoma (myoneurocytoma) of the cerebellum. Acta Neuropathol, 1998; 95:318–323

133. Robbins P, Segal A, Narula S et al. Central neurocytoma. A clinicopathological, immunohistochemical and ultrastructural study of 7 cases. Pathol Res Pract, 1995; 191:100–111

134. Kim DG, Kim JS, Chi JG et al. Central neurocytoma: proliferative potential and biological behavior. J Neurosurg, 1996; 84:742–747

135. Fujimaki T, Matsuno A, Sasaki T et al. Proliferative activity of central neurocytoma: measurement of tumor volume doubling time, MIB-1 staining index and bromodeoxyuridine labeling index. J Neurooncol, 1997; 32:103–109

136. Christov C, Adle-Biassette H, Le Guerinel C. Recurrent central neurocytoma with marked increase in MIB-1 labelling index. Br J Neurosurg, 1999; 13:496–499

137. Ashkan K, Casey AT, D'Arrigo C et al. Benign central neurocytoma. Cancer, 2000; 89:1111–1120

138. Cerda-Nicolas M, Lopez-Gines C, Peydro-Olaya A et al. Central neurocytoma: a cytogenetic case study. Cancer Genet Cytogenet, 1993; 65:173–174

139. Taruscio D, Danesi R, Montaldi A et al. Nonrandom gain of chromosome 7 in central neurocytoma: a chromosomal analysis and fluorescence in situ hybridization study. Virchows Arch, 1997; 430:47–51

140. Yin XL, Pang JC, Hui AB et al. Detection of chromosomal imbalances in central neurocytomas by using comparative genomic hybridization. J Neurosurg, 2000; 93:77–81

141. Tong CY, Ng HK, Pang JC et al. Central neurocytomas are genetically distinct from oligodendrogliomas and neuroblastomas. Histopathology, 2000; 37:160–165

142. Nozaki M, Tada M, Matsumoto R et al. Rare occurrence of inactivating p53 gene mutations in primary non-astrocytic tumors of the central nervous system: reappraisal by yeast functional assay. Acta Neuropathol, 1998; 95:291–296

143. Jay V, Edwards V, Hoving E et al. Central neurocytoma: morphological, flow cytometric, polymerase chain reaction, fluorescence in situ hybridization, and karyotypic analyses. Case report. J Neurosurg, 1999; 90:348–354

144. Westphal M, Stavrou D, Nausch H et al. Human neurocytoma cells in culture show characteristics of astroglial differentiation. J Neurosci Res, 1994; 38:698–704

145. Valdueza JM, Westphal M, Vortmeyer A et al. Central neurocytoma: clinical, immunohistologic, and biologic findings of a human neuroglial progenitor tumor. Surg Neurol, 1996; 45:49–56

146. Ishiuchi S, Tamura M. Central neurocytoma: an immunohistochemical, ultrastructural and cell culture study. Acta Neuropathol, 1997; 94:425–435

147. Westphal M, Meissner H, Matschke J et al. Tissue culture of human neurocytomas induces the expression of glial fibrillary acidic protein. J Neurocytol, 1998; 27:805–816

148. Patt S, Schmidt H, Labrakakis C et al. Human central neurocytoma cells show neuronal physiological properties in vitro. Acta Neuropathol, 1996; 91:209–214

149. Min KW, Scheithauer BW. Clear cell ependymoma: a mimic of oligodendroglioma: clinicopathologic and ultrastructural considerations. Am J Surg Pathol, 1997; 21:820–826

150. Kim DG, Paek SH, Kim IH et al. Central neurocytoma: the role of radiation therapy and long term outcome. Cancer, 1997; 79:1995–2002

151. Dodds D, Nonis J, Mehta M et al. Central neurocytoma: a clinical study of response to chemotherapy. J Neurooncol, 1997; 34:279–283

152. Brandes AA, Amista P, Gardiman M et al. Chemotherapy in patients with recurrent and progressive central neurocytoma. Cancer, 2000; 88:169–174

153. Tomura N, Hirano H, Watanabe O et al. Central neurocytoma with clinically malignant behavior. AJNR. Am J Neuroradiol, 1997; 18:1175–1178

154. Eng DY, DeMonte F, Ginsberg L et al. Craniospinal dissemination of central neurocytoma. Report of two cases. J Neurosurg, 1997; 86:547–552

155. Sgouros S, Carey M, Aluwihare N et al. Central neurocytoma: a correlative clinicopathologic and radiologic analysis. Surg Neurol, 1998; 49:197–204

156. Schweitzer JB, Davies KG. Differentiating central neurocytoma. Case report. J Neurosurg, 1997; 86:543–546

157. Sharma MC, Rathore A, Karak AK et al. A study of proliferative markers in central neurocytoma. Pathology, 1998; 30:355–359

158. Wharton SB, Antoun NM, Macfarlane R et al. The natural history of a recurrent central neurocytoma-like tumor [published erratum appears in Clin Neuropathol 1998 Jul–Aug; 17:236]. Clin Neuropathol, 1998; 17:136–140

Cerebellar liponeurocytoma

159. Budka H, Chimelli L. Lipomatous medulloblastoma in adults: a new tumor type with possible favorable prognosis. Hum Pathol, 1994; 25:730–731

160. Orlandi A, Marino B, Brunori M et al. Lipomatous medulloblastoma. Clin Neuropathol, 1997; 16:175–179

161. Soylemezoglu F, Soffer D, Onol B et al. Lipomatous medulloblastoma in adults. A distinct clinicopathological entity. Am J Surg Pathol, 1996; 20:413–418

162. Alleyne CHJ, Hunter S, Olson JJ et al. Lipomatous glioneurocytoma of the posterior fossa with divergent differentiation: case report. Neurosurgery, 1998; 42:639–643

163. Gonzalez-Campora R, Weller RO. Lipidized mature neuroectodermal tumour of the cerebellum with myoid differentiation. Neuropathol Appl Neurobiol, 1998; 24:397–402

164. Min KW. Medullocytoma and glioneurocytoma: related tumours? Am J Surg Pathol, 1997; 21:615–616

165. Ellison DW, Zygmunt SC, Weller RO. Neurocytoma/lipoma (neurolipocytoma) of the cerebellum. Neuropathol Appl Neurobiol, 1993; 19:95–98

Paraganglioma

166. Lack E. Tumors of the adrenal gland and extra-adrenal paraganglia. Washington, DC: Armed Forces Institute of Pathology, 1997

167. Lipper S, Decker RE. Paraganglioma of the cauda equina. A histologic, immunohistochemical, and ultrastructural study and review of the literature. Surg Neurol, 1984; 22:415–420

168. Pigott TJ, Lowe JS, Morrell K et al. Paraganglioma of the cauda equina. Report of three cases. J Neurosurg, 1990; 73:455–458

169. Raftopoulos C, Flament-Durand J, Brucher JM et al. Paraganglioma of the cauda equina. Report of 2 cases and review of 59 cases from the literature. Clin Neurol Neurosurg, 1990; 92:263–270

170. Sonneland PR, Scheithauer BW, LeChago J et al. Paraganglioma of the cauda equina region. Clinicopathologic study of 31 cases with special reference to immunocytology and ultrastructure. Cancer, 1986; 58:1720–1735

171. Moran CA, Rush W, Mena H. Primary spinal paragangliomas: a clinicopathological and immunohistochemical study of 30 cases. Histopathology, 1997; 31:167–173

172. Hodge KM, Byers RM, Peters LJ. Paragangliomas of the head and neck. Arch Otolaryngol Head Neck Surg, 1988; 114:872–877

173. Haslbeck KM, Eberhardt KE, Nissen U et al. Intracranial hypertension as a clinical manifestation of cauda equina paraganglioma. Neurology, 1999; 52:1297–1298

174. Ashkenazi E, Onesti ST, Kader A et al. Paraganglioma of the filum terminale: case report and literature review. J Spinal Disord, 1998; 11:540–542

175. Paleologos TS, Gouliamos AD, Kourousis DD et al. Paraganglioma of the cauda equina: a case presenting features of increased intracranial pressure. J Spinal Disord, 1998; 11:362–365

176. Boukobza M, Foncin JF, Dowling-Carter D. Paraganglioma of the cauda equina: magnetic resonance imaging. Neuroradiology, 1993; 35:459–460

177. Telischi FF, Bustillo A, Whiteman ML et al. Octreotide scintigraphy for the detection of paragangliomas. Arch Otolaryngol Head Neck Surg, 2000; 122:358–362

178. Djindjian M, Ayache P, Brugiers P et al. Giant gangliocytic paraganglioma of the filum terminale. Case report. J Neurosurg, 1990; 73:459–461

179. Caccamo DV, Ho KL, Garcia JH. Cauda equina tumor with ependymal and paraganglionic differentiation. Hum Pathol, 1992; 23:835–838

180. Gaffney EF, Doorly T, Dinn JJ. Aggressive oncocytic neuroendocrine tumour ('oncocytic paraganglioma') of the cauda equina. Histopathology, 1986; 10:311–319

181. Milroy CM, Ferlito A. Immunohistochemical markers in the diagnosis of neuroendocrine neoplasms of the head and neck. Ann Otol, Rhinol Laryngol, 1995; 104:413–418

182. Labrousse F, Leboutet MJ, Petit B et al. Cytokeratin expression in paragangliomas of the cauda equina. Clin Neuropathol, 1999; 18:208–213

183. Orrell JM, Hales SA. Paragangliomas of the cauda equina have a distinctive cytokeratin immunophenotype. Histopathology, 1992; 21:479–481

184. Johnson TL, Zarbo RJ, Lloyd RV et al. Paragangliomas of the head and neck: immunohistochemical neuroendocrine and intermediate filament typing. Mod Pathol, 1988; 1:216–223

185. Chetty R, Pillay P, Jaichand V. Cytokeratin expression in adrenal phaeochromocytomas and extra-adrenal paragangliomas. J Clin Pathol, 1998; 51:477–478

186. Hirose T, Sano T, Mori K et al. Paraganglioma of the cauda equina: an ultrastructural and immunohistochemical study of two cases. Ultrastruct Pathol 1988; 12:235–243

187. Ironside JW, Royds JA, Taylor CB et al. Paraganglioma of the cauda equina: a histological, ultrastructural and immunocytochemical study of two cases with a review of the literature. J Pathol, 1985; 145:195–201

188. Jansen JC, van den Berg R, Kuiper A et al. Estimation of growth rate in patients with head and neck paragangliomas influences the treatment proposal. Cancer, 2000; 88:2811–2816

189. Karamitopoulou E, Perentes E, Diamantis I et al. Ki-67 immunoreactivity in human central nervous system tumors: a study with MIB 1 monoclonal antibody on archival material. Acta Neuropathol, 1994; 87:47–54

190. Niemann S, Steinberger D, Muller U. PGL3, a third, not maternally imprinted locus in autosomal dominant paraganglioma. Neurogenetics, 1999; 2:167–170

191. Lemaire M, Persu A, Hainaut P et al. Hereditary paraganglioma. J Int Med, 1999; 246:113–116

192. Baysal BE, Ferrell RE, Willett-Brozick JE et al. Mutations in SDHD, a mitochondrial complex II gene, in hereditary paraganglioma. Science, 2000; 287:848–851

193. Achilles E, Padberg BC, Holl K et al. Immunocytochemistry of paragangliomas–value of staining for S-100 protein and glial fibrillary acid protein in diagnosis and prognosis. Histopathology, 1991; 18:453–458

194. Johnstone PA, Foss RD, Desilets DJ. Malignant jugulotympanic paraganglioma. Arch Pathol Lab Med, 1990; 114:976–979

195. Lack EE, Cubilla AL, Woodruff JM. Paragangliomas of the head and neck region. A pathologic study of tumours from 71 patients. Hum Pathol, 1979; 10:191–218

196. Sharma HS, Madhavan M, Othman NH et al. Malignant paraganglioma of frontoethmoidal region. Auris Nasus Larynx, 1999; 26:487–493

197. Roche PH, Figarella-Branger D, Regis J et al. Cauda equina paraganglioma with subsequent intracranial and intraspinal metastases. Acta Neurochir, 1996; 138:475–479

Dysplastic gangliocytoma of cerebellum (Lhermitte–Duclos disease)

198. Lhermitte J, Duclos G. Sur un ganglioneurome diffus du coertex du cervelet. Bull Assoc Fran Etude Cancer, 1920; 9:99–107

199. Louis DN, von Deimling A. Hereditary tumour syndromes of the nervous system: Overview and rare syndromes. Brain Pathol, 1995; 5:145–151

200. Vinchion M, Blond S, Lejeune JP et al. Association of Lhermitte-Duclos and Cowden disease: report of a new case and review of the literature. J Neurol Neurosurg Psychiatry, 1994; 57:699–704

201. Vital A, Vital C, Martin N et al. Lhermitte-Duclos type cerebellum hamartoma and Cowden disease. Clin Neuropathol, 1994; 13:229–231

202. Padberg GW, Schot JD, Vielvoye GJ et al. Lhermitte-Duclos disease and Cowden disease: a single phakomatosis. Ann Neurol, 1991; 29:517–523

203. Russell DS, Rubinstein LJ. In: Pathology of tumours of the nervous system, 5th edn. London: Edward Arnold, 1989: pp 302–304

204. Verdu A, Garde T, Madero S. Lhermitte-Duclos disease in a ten year old child: clinical follow-up and neuroimaging data from birth. Rev Neurol, 1998; 27:597–600

205. Eng C, Murday V, Seal S et al. Cowden syndrome and Lhermitte-Duclos disease in a single family: a single genetic syndrome with pleiotrophy? J Med Genet, 1994; 31:458–461

206. Ambler M, Pogacar S, Sidman R. Lhermitte-Duclos disease (granular cell hypertrophy of the cerebellum) pathological analysis of the first familial cases. J Neuropath Exp Neurol, 1969; 28:622–647

207. Milbouw G, Born JD, Martin D et al. Clinical and radiological aspects of dysplastic gangliocytoma (Lhermitte-Duclos disease): a report of two cases with review of the literature. Neurosurgery, 1988; 22:124–128

208. Hair LS, Symmans F, Powers JM et al. Immunohistochemistry and proliferative activity in Lhermitte-Duclos disease. Acta Neuropathol, 1992; 84:570–573

209. Shiurba RA, Buffinger NS, Spencer EM et al. Basic fibroblast growth factor and somatomedin C in human medulloepithelioma. Cancer, 1991; 68:798–808

210. Pritchett PS, King TI. Dysplastic ganglioma of the cerebellum – an ultrastructural study. Acta Neuropathol 1978; 42:1–5

211. Ferrer I, Isamet F, Acebes J. A golgi and electron microscopic study of a dysplastic gangliocytoma of the cerebellum. Acta Neuropathol, 1979; 47:163–165

212. Reznik M, Schoenen J. Lhermitte-Duclos disease. Acta Neuropathol, 1983; 59:88–94

213. Marano SR, Johnson PC, Spetzler RF. Recurrent Lhermitte–Duclos disease in a child. Case report. J Neurosurg, 1988; 69:599–603

214. Hashimoto H, Iida J, Nishi N et al. Recurrent Lhermitte–Duclos disease – case report. Neuro Med Chir (Tokyo), 1997; 37:692–696

215. Tuli S, Provias JP, Bernstein M. Lhermitte-Duclos disease: literature review and novel treatment strategy. Can J Neurol Sci, 1997; 24:155–160

9 Pineal parenchymal tumours

A wide variety of tumour types may occur in the pineal region, but for practical purposes it is convenient to divide them into the following broad categories:

- Teratomas, including germinomas.
- Pineal parenchymal tumours.
- Glial and miscellaneous tumours.
- Cysts.

The World Health Organisation (WHO) classifies pineal germinomas with other germ cell neoplasms and these are described in Chapter 10. Primary neoplasms of the pineal parenchyma are subdivided by the WHO as follows:

- Pineocytomas.
- Pineoblastomas.
- Pineal parenchymal tumours of intermediate differentiation.

All these are discussed below, although the tumours showing intermediate differention are incorporated into the section covering pineoblastoma in this account. The chapter also includes a description of primary glial neoplasms of the pineal gland and a summary of other tumours which may occur in the pineal region. Pineal cysts are described together with other types of nervous system cyst in Chapter 17.

Finally, it should be noted that the term 'pinealoma' frequently appears in the older literature, variously referring to both germinomas of the pineal region and primary pineal parenchymal tumours.[1,2] The importance of distinguishing between the two types of lesion is now clearly understood and the use of this term has been abandoned in more recent accounts.

Pineocytoma

Pineocytomas are distinguished from the more primitive pineoblastomas by their greater degree of differentiation and relatively benign clinical course. They have been sub-classified according to histological evidence of neuronal, astrocytic or divergent differentiation.[2,3] In prognostic terms, however, the most significant subdivision relates to the presence or absence of large 'pineocytomatous' rosettes[4] (Table 9.1). These structures have been variously interpreted as evidence of neuronal differentiation[2,5] or simply of pineocytic specialisation,[4] and their occurrence nearly always heralds a slower growth rate and better clinical outcome.[4,6] Conversely, tumours lacking the rosettes are associated with a much more malignant biological behaviour.[4,7] It has been argued that pineo-cytomatous rosettes are indispensable for the diagnosis of pineocytoma and where they are not seen, the tumour should be classed with the more primitive pineo-blastomas.[4] Despite this, there appears to be a distinct group of non-rosette bearing lesions which lack any

Table 9.1 Histological subtypes of pineocytoma

Pineocytomatous rosettes
  No other differentiation
  Focal differentiation
    Ganglionic
    Astrocytic
    Gangliogliomatous

Papillary, no rosettes
  Undifferentiated
  Focal astrocytic differentiation

features of a primitive neuroectodermal tumour and these tumours are probably best considered as malignant variants of typical pineocytoma, as in this account.[5,7]

Incidence

Taken together, primary tumours of pinealocytes account for about a quarter of all pineal region tumours[8,9] and the largest published series of primary parenchymal neoplasms suggests that just over one-half of these are pineocytomas.[5] More specifically, pineocytomas have been estimated as accounting for anything between 8 and 13% of all tumours in the pineal region[10–12] and about 1.3% of all intracranial tumours.[13] Pineocytomas are most common in later adult life,[5,14] and this is particularly so for the lesions containing pineocytomatous rosettes.[2,4] The malignant, non-rosette bearing tumours occur more often in children,[10,15] but still account for less than 0.25% of all paediatric brain tumours.[16] Most series of pineo-cytomas have indicated a slight preponderance of males over females.[2,4,12]

Aetiology

Pineocytomas arise from primary neuroepithelial cells of the mature pineal gland, the so-called pinealocytes,[5] with which they share a number of specific cytological features, including club ended argyrophilic cell processes abutting onto vascular basement membranes.[17,18] Although normal adult human pinealocytes have a purely neuro-secretory function, pineocytoma cells may also show ultrastructural evidence of photoreceptor differen-tiation,[2,19] similar to that found both in the pinealocytes of other mammalian species[19,20] and in the photosensory pineal organ of lower order vertebrates.[21] This suggests that the pineal neuroepithelial cells giving rise to pineocytomas in man are phylogenetically related to the photosensory pineal cells of submammalian species.[2,21] Pineocytomas may be produced experimentally by the intracerebral inoculation of newborn hamsters with the JC human papovavirus strain and such experimental tumours again show ultrastructural evidence of their photosensory cell phylogenetic lineage.[21] Cytogenetic information on pineocytomas is very scanty, and the few reported human cell lines have shown simultaneous but inconsistent alterations or losses of several different chromosomes.[22,23]

Clinical features

Headache, vomiting and other evidence of raised intracranial pressure are the most common presenting complaints, resulting from hydrocephalus due to aqueduct compression.[8,9] Preceding this, there is often a much longer history of cerebellar or eye movement disorder, and such symptoms may date back several years in some adult cases.[2,4] Parinaud syndrome is characteristic of pineal region tumours and consists of paralysis of vertical conjugate eye movements, sometimes with selective loss of pupillary reaction to light. It is caused by local pressure on the quadrigeminal plate area.[9] Local compressive effects may also result in third nerve palsies and cerebellar disturbances, including ataxia, tremor, nystagmus and vertigo.[8,9] Less commonly there may be visual field disturbances, sensory or extrapyramidal disorders relating to thalamic distortion, or evidence of hypothalamic disturbance.[8] In contrast to some germ cell tumours of the pineal region, serum and cerebrospinal fluid (CSF) levels of human chorionic gonadotropin and alpha-fetoprotein are never raised.[8]

Radiology

There are no specific radiological features distinguishing pineocytomas from most other pineal region tumours.[24,25] Computerised tomography (CT) typically shows a well demarcated isodense or hyperdense pineal mass,[12,26] usually associated with dilated lateral and third ventricles.[8] There is frequently evidence of tumour calcification, which can be massive[12,14,17] and the lesions show marked, homogeneous signal enhancement after injection of contrast media.[12,26] The anatomical extent of pineal region tumours is probably best demonstrated by magnetic resonance imaging (MRI) (Fig. 9.1), which may in some cases identify pineocytomas not demonstrated by CT.[8,27] Pineocytomas are usually hypodense compared with brain on T1-weighted MR images, hyperdense using T2-weighting and again show uniform contrast enhancement.[26] Angiography may be useful in helping to exclude pineal region vascular malformations or meningiomas.[8,9]

Pathology

Macroscopic features

Most pineocytomas are well-defined tumours which compress surrounding structures without evidence of local infiltration. They frequently project into the third ventricle and may sometimes form a cast-like mass filling the posterior part of the dilated ventricular cavity (Fig. 9.2). The pineal gland is usually entirely destroyed and cannot be separately identified even at autopsy, although in rare cases it may remain visible or even become enlarged. The cut surface of the tumour is characteristically pale and greyish with a lobulated appearance. It is frequently gritty in texture due to mineralisation, and older lesions may be massively calcified. Focal haemorrhages and cysts can be present on sectioning but gross evidence of necrosis is not usually seen.

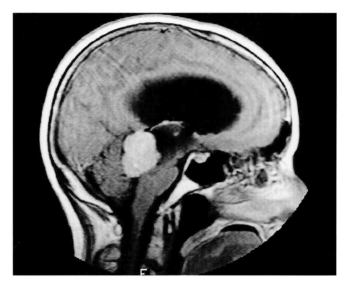

Fig. 9.1 **Pineocytoma.** Sagittal T1-weighted MRI scan of a pineocytoma. The tumour is enhancing after administration of contrast and there is obstructive enlargement of the lateral ventricles.

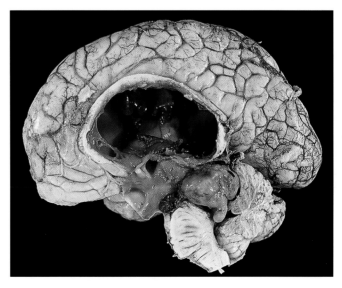

Fig. 9.2 **Pineocytoma.** The tumour forms a cast-like mass, filling the posterior part of the enlarged third ventricle and extending down the dilated aqueduct into the fourth ventricle.

Intraoperative diagnosis

Smear preparations show cells with indistinct cytoplasm and quite uniform, small, rounded nuclei containing coarsely clumped chromatin. There is a network of delicate, branching, thin walled blood vessels to which the cells cling in a loose papillary fashion like that seen in astrocytomas, but there is no sense of the organised perivascular cuffing typical of ependymomas (Fig. 9.3). A large proportion of cells smear out in sheets away from the vessels, but even here the scanty perinuclear cytoplasm remains indistinct. There is a finely filamentous background stroma which is often a prominent feature. In some cases, there may be numerous separate islands of this filamentous material, not associated with vessels and containing isolated aggregates of cell nuclei. Rosettes are not usually seen on smear preparations. The appearances can be similar to those of oligodendroglioma smears, and knowledge of the specific site of the lesion is clearly important. Frozen sections may be helpful in showing the large pineocytomatous rosettes, although care should be taken not to confuse these with ependymal perivascular pseudorosettes (see Chapter 6).

Histological features

The tumour cells are small and quite uniform in shape, with rounded, darkly staining nuclei and coarsely clumped chromatin. Their cytoplasm is usually scanty and ill-defined, but single, polar, cytoplasmic processes may be apparent in some cells. These processes are similar to those of normal pinealocytes and are the fundamental diagnostic hallmark of pineocytomas (Fig. 9.4). They are most clearly seen using specific silver carbonate techniques on either frozen or paraffin sections.[28] They

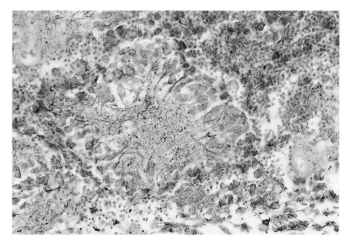

Fig. 9.4 **Pineocytoma**. Radially orientated argyrophilic cell processes can be seen in this pineocytomatous rosette. Silver impregnation.

have distinctive club shaped terminations and may either be randomly arranged or orientated towards blood vessels.

In terms of architecture, most adult pineocytomas consist of sheets of tumour cell nuclei embedded in a finely filamentous stroma and forming numerous pineocytomatous rosettes (Fig. 9.5). These rosettes consist of large, anucleate areas of eosinophilic, filamentous stroma, sometimes several hundred microns across and surrounded by quite closely packed cell nuclei. Club ended argyrophilic processes can nearly always be demonstrated in the central area (Fig. 9.4), but the polar outline of the cells is not usually apparent on routine stains. The thin walled vessels present in the tumour are not related to the rosettes, and there is little evidence of a perivascular orientation of tumour cells in this type of

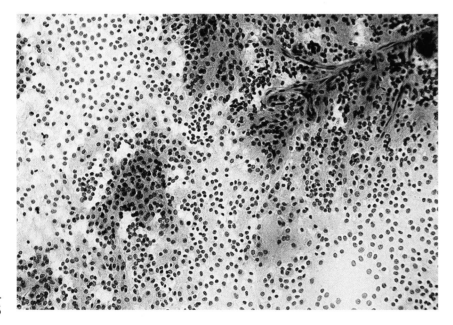

Fig. 9.3 **Pineocytoma**. Smear preparation. The small, uniform cell nuclei smear out from blood vessels and are embedded in islands of finely fibrillar background material. Toluidine blue.

Fig. 9.5 **Pineocytoma**. Sheets of closely packed, small, rounded nuclei are interrupted by irregular pineocytomatous rosettes. H & E.

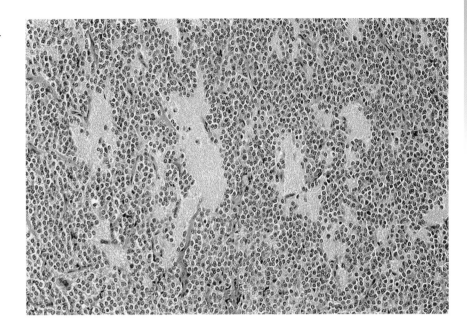

pineocytoma. Some authorities have regarded the large rosettes as evidence of pineocytomatous specialisation[4] whilst others consider them to represent neuronal differentiation.[2,5] Mitoses are usually very uncommon in rosette-forming pineocytomas, and there is frequently overt evidence of ganglionic differentiation in the form of large, pleomorphic ganglion cells. These contain cresyl violet-stained Nissl granules and have multiple neuritic processes, visible using standard silver impregnations. In some adult pineocytomas, astrocytic elements are limited to reactive cells and processes around the margins of the tumour, but other cases may show evidence of a more extensive astrocytic component.[2,4,29] This typically consists of areas with pleomorphic astrocytic cells, coarse phosphotungstic acid haematoxylin (PTAH)-staining fibrillar processes, Rosenthal fibres, and sometimes microcysts (Fig. 9.6). Such appearances have been interpreted as astrocytic differentiation[5,29] although distinction from entrapped, reactive pineal gland astrocytes is not always clear. Where astrocytic and ganglionic differentiation are present in the same tumour, the appearances can be indistinguishable from gangliogliomas occuring elsewhere in the central nervous system (Chapter 8).[4,30] The slow growing adult type pineocytomas often become heavily calcified, and some very longstanding examples may be almost entirely replaced by confluent areas of mineralisation surrounded by intense astrocytic gliosis (Fig. 9.7).

The largest published series of pineocytomas has suggested that tumours showing pineocytomatous rosettes, regardless of other differentiating features, account for approximately three-quarters of all cases.[5] The remaining cases are typically from a younger age group[10,15] and

lack rosettes. They have a papillary architecture, with cells clinging to a fine, branching vascular network (Fig. 9.8). The club ended, argyrophylic cell processes are directed towards the vessel walls, producing an appearance of perivascular pseudorosettes in cross-section, or linear palisades in longitudinal orientation. Between the vascular septa, the cells are more loosely arranged and this may give a lobulated or nested appearance to the tumour in some cases. Mitoses are more often present in this type of pineocytoma and there is frequently diffuse infiltration of local structures or metastatic spread in the CSF pathways.[7,10] Very occasionally, astrocytic differentiation of low or high grade cytology has also been described in these cases,[5] although the difficulty of distinguishing this from entrapped reactive astrocytic elements of the normal gland must again be emphasised.

Immunocytochemistry

In typical rosette forming pineocytomas, a proportion of tumour cells usually stain positively with antibodies to neuron specific enolase (NSE).[31] More widespread NSE immunoreactivity is present when there is histological evidence of ganglionic differentiation.[32,33] Some cases may also show positive staining using antibodies to neurofilament protein and synaptophysin, especially in the central areas of large pineocytomatous rosettes[34] (Fig. 9.9). Under normal circumstances, pineocytoma cells themselves are unstained using antibodies to glial fibrillary acidic protein (GFAP),[32] but most tumours contain variable numbers of positive staining cell bodies and processes because of entrapped reactive astrocytic cells derived from the normal gland.[33] This is especially

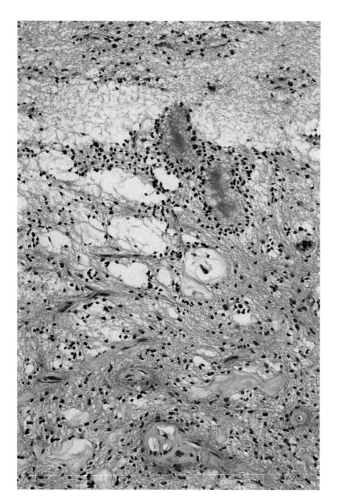

Fig. 9.6 **Pineocytoma**. There is evidence of astrocytic differentiation, with coarse fibrillary processes and microcystic spaces. Two pineocytomatous rosettes are also present towards the top of the field. H & E.

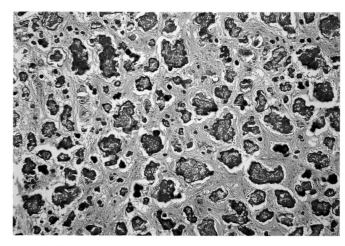

Fig. 9.7 **Pineocytoma**. The tumour in this longstanding example has been largely replaced by numerous calcified bodies embedded in a gliotic background. H & E.

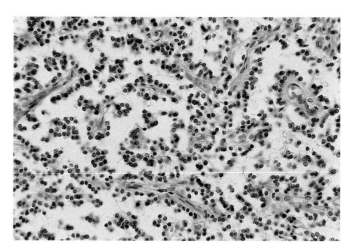

Fig. 9.8 **Pineocytoma**. This childhood example shows a papillary pattern, with tumour cells clinging to branching capillary blood vessels. Despite the uniform cytology, the lesion was widely disseminated in the CSF pathways. H & E.

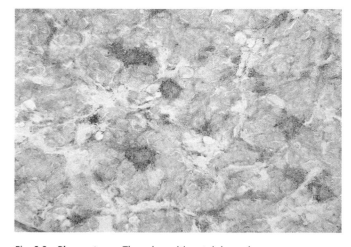

Fig. 9.9 **Pineocytoma**. There is positive staining using immunocytochemistry for synaptophysin, particularly in the centre of pineocytomatous rosettes.

marked near tumour margins and in longer-standing lesions (Fig. 9.10). In areas of tumour showing histological evidence of astrocytic differentiation, GFAP immunoreactivity may also be seen in obviously malignant cells with atypical cytological features.[2,5] All pineal parenchymal tumours, including pineocytomas, have been found to show immunocytochemical expression of both chromogranin-A and alpha-B crystallin.[35] A proportion of pineocytomas also contain scattered cells which react with antibodies to retinal S-antigen, and this is felt to represent further evidence of the evolutionary derivation of human pineocytes from the pineal photoreceptor cells of lower vertebrate species.[36,37] Immunoreactivity for retinal S-antigen is also found in several primitive neuroectodermal tumours, however, and cannot be regarded as a specific feature of pineocytomas.[37-39] In contrast to pineal germinomas, pineocytomas do not show immunoreactivity for placental alkaline phosphatase (PLAP).[40]

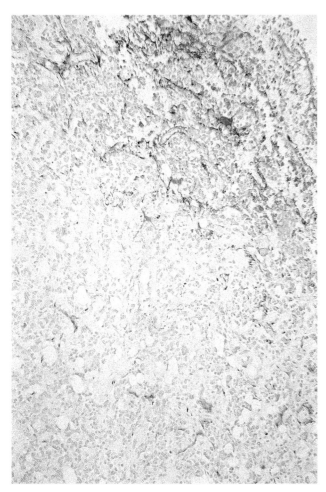

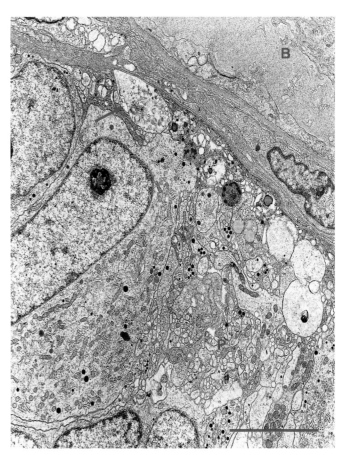

Fig. 9.10 **Pineocytoma**. Reactive astrocytic cell processes are entrapped within the tumour, especially towards the margin of the lesion at the top of this field. Immunocytochemistry for GFAP.

Fig. 9.11 **Pineocytoma**. The tumour cell perikarya are separated by numerous fine interlacing processes (P). These are closely applied to the outer basement membrane around a blood vessel (B), where they form bulb-like expansions (arrow). Electron micrograph. Bar = 4 μm.

Electron microscopy

Ultrastructurally, pineocytomas typically consist of separate groups of cell perikarya widely separated by numerous fine interlacing processes[18,31] (Fig. 9.11). The cell cytoplasm usually contains abundant neurosecretory dense core vesicles, which are larger than those found in central neuroblastomas and may be up to 300 nm in external diameter (Fig. 9.12). The fine cytoplasmic processes are the ultrastructural equivalent of the club ended argyrophilic processes seen at light microscope level. They are electron lucent and contain longitudinally orientated 20 nm microtubles. They are closely applied to the outer basement membrane of blood vessels, where they often can be seen to form bulb-like expansions[17,18] (Fig. 9.11). Astrocytic cell processes filled with intermediate glial filaments are also usually present, and in most cases are probably derived from incorporated pineal gland astrocytes. Many typical, rosette-bearing pineocytomas show specific evidence of neuronal differentiation at ultrastructural level, which has prompted suggestions that the rosettes themselves may be a neuroblastic feature.[5] For example, there are often abundant 40–60 nm diameter clear synaptic vesicles in these tumours, sometimes aggregated around desmosome-like membrane thickenings to form synaptic complexes[2,19,31] (Fig. 9.12). In some cases there may also be evidence of photoreceptor specialisation, normally only seen in the pineal glands of lower order mammals and the pineal photoreceptor organs of non-mammalian species. Structures associated with photosensory function include vesicle crowned lamellae (synaptic ribbons), microtubular sheaves and bulb ended cilia with a 9 + 0 axial skeleton (see Chapter 2).[2,17,19] Fully formed retinal fleurettes, like those found in some pineoblastomas and experimentally induced animal pineocytomas are not a feature of well differentiated human pineocytomas.

Melatonin production

Parenchymal cells of the human pineal gland are responsible for the production and secretion of melatonin[41] and there have been several reports of raised serum hormone levels in association with pineocytomas,

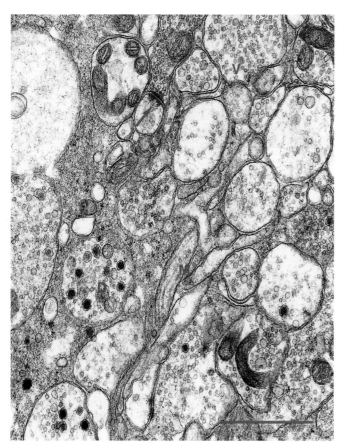

Fig. 9.12 **Pineocytoma**. The fine cytoplasmic processes contain 20 nm microtubules (M) and neurosecretory dense core vesicles (D). Neuronal differentiation is suggested by numerous small synaptic vesicles (V) and synaptic structures (arrow). Electron micrograph. Bar = 1 μm.

suggesting possible hormone production by the tumour.[42] The melanin synthesising enzyme hydroxy-O-methyl transferase has been found in homogenates of experimental hamster pineocytoma tissue,[43] but there is no similar biological evidence that human pineocytomas have the capacity to produce the hormone.[5] Moreover, raised serum levels have been reported in conjunction with many tumours of the pineal region, including non-parenchymal types such as germinomas,[42,44] and in some cases of pineocytoma melatonin levels have been abnormally low or simply lacked a circadian variation.[41] This suggests non-specific mechanical interference with the normal pineal regulatory mechanism rather than tumour hormone production, and serum melatonin estimation is therefore unlikely to be helpful in the clinical diagnosis of pineal region tumours.[41,45]

Differential diagnosis

Germinoma

This is the commonest tumour of the pineal region and its marked sensitivity to irradiation means that distinction from pineocytoma is of great therapeutic importance. Typical adult type pineocytomas are usually easily identified by the presence of large pineocytomatous rosettes, but papillary, non-rosette forming tumours may show a pseudolobular pattern which is less easy to distinguish from germinoma. In contrast to such pineocytomas, germinomas lack a distinct perivascular orientation of tumour cells and do not show argyrophilic club ended processes on appropriate silver carbonate staining. They also usually contain prominent aggregates of typical small lymphocytes. The tumour cells are larger than those of pineocytoma, with clear cytoplasm and better defined cytoplasmic margins. In addition, many germinomas stain immunocytochemically for PLAP, not found in pineocytomas.

Astrocytoma

Astrocytomas may arise primarily in the pineal gland and need to be distinguished from pineocytomas containing prominent reactive astrocytic elements or showing true astrocytic differentiation. GFAP immunocytochemistry is not likely to be useful in this context, but immunoreactivity for NSE, synaptophysin or retinal S-antigen may help to identify positively the pineocytic nature of the tumour in some cases. Other features which may be useful in distinguishing a primary pineocytoma include the presence of large pineocytomatous rosettes, unequivocal ganglion cells or club ended, argyrophilic cell processes.

Ependymoma

Third ventricular ependymomas may involve the pineal region and care must be taken not to confuse the histological appearances of ependymoma pseudorosettes and pineocytomatous rosettes. In contrast to pineocytomatous rosettes, the pseudorosettes of ependymoma are perivascular structures and have an obviously radial gliofibrillary architecture on routine stains. In cross-cut examples, the central blood vessel may not be visible in the plane of section, but the anucleate zone of fibrillary material lacks the argyrophilic club-ended processes of pineocytomas and is positively stained with PTAH or antibodies to GFAP. Blepharoplasts may also be useful in identifying ependymoma, but tubular rosettes should be interpreted with caution, because similar structures may occur as a result of photoreceptor differentiation in tumours with mixed pineocytoma and pineoblastoma areas (see below).

Astroblastoma

Although very rare tumours, these have been reported in the pineal region[55] and show a similar perivascular architecture to the non-rosette forming pineocytomas of papillary pattern. In astroblastomas, the centrally directed cell processes are usually broader than those of pineocytomas and do not stain with appropriate silver carbonate methods. Immunocytochemical staining for GFAP is not always helpful because pineocytomas often contain positively stained astrocytic elements. Immunoreactivity for NSE or retinal S-antigen may not be present in non-rosette forming pineocytomas and again cannot be relied on in this context.

Central neurocytoma

These tumours usually arise in the anterior septal area, but if large they may also extend posteriorly to involve the pineal region. They can show a superficial histological resemblance to non-rosette forming pineocytomas and the two entities may and be difficult to distinguish in a small biopsy sample. The cells of central neurocytoma have uniform small rounded nuclei similar to those of pineocytomas, but often show oligodendroglial-like cytoplasmic clearing. Although they usually have a similar branching meshwork of delicate blood vessels, they do not show the perivascular orientation of cells seen in papillary pineocytomas and also lack club ended argyrophilic processes. The large rosettes of typical pineocytomas are again not seen in neurocytomas. Immunocytochemical expression of NSE and synaptophysin may be found in either tumour, although it is a more constant and widespread feature of neurocytomas.

Therapy

Obtaining a firm histological diagnosis is an essential part of treatment for pineocytomas because of the diversity of tumour types occurring in the pineal region and their different responses to therapy.[8,24,46] Some authorities advocate using a stereotactic biopsy in the first instance, on the grounds that if the lesion turns out to be a germinoma it can be treated by radiation alone and open surgery can often be avoided.[8,47,48] However, the mortality associated with surgery in the pineal region has fallen dramatically in recent years[16,46,49] and an initial open surgical approach is now also a reasonable option.[26,50] In either case, the definitive treatment of choice for pineocytomas is surgical excision, which should be as complete as possible.[16,51] CSF shunting may be needed if only partial excision is possible and there is persisting mass effect.[26] The role of postoperative radiotherapy is still rather controversial, and there are some suggestions that typical rosette-bearing pineocytomas may not be sufficiently radiosensitive to warrant giving therapy.[4,6] Especially where only partial excision has been possible, however, local tumour bed irradiation is often advocated,[8,52] together with craniospinal axis therapy if there is evidence of CSF dissemination at surgery.[53] For childhood tumours, axis irradiation or chemotherapy should be considered

wherever possible because of the greater risk of CSF seeding,[10,14] particularly if the biopsy shows a papillary tumour pattern without pineocytomatous rosettes.[2,6]

Prognosis

The prognosis of pineocytomas is directly releated to their histological subtype, with the presence or absence of pineocytomatous rosettes as the most important determinant of survival.[5,6] Typical, rosette-forming tumours are usually slow growing, circumscribed tumours which compress rather than infiltrate adjacent structures,[4,11] and are much less likely to disseminate in the CSF pathways than the more primitive pineoblastomas.[4,13] For these tumours, survival after surgical debulking and radiotherapy is usually at least 4 years from the time of operation.[2,51] One large series has published 3- and 5-years survivals of 100% and 67% respectively,[54] and there are reports of cases remaining disease free for as long as 13[4,14] or even 29 years.[53] Surgical mortality is quoted as less than 5%[46,50] and death is usually related to complications of local recurrence rather than CSF dissemination.[53] Papillary tumours lacking either pineocytomatous rosettes or evidence of astrocytic and ganglionic differentiation have a much poorer prognosis than other subtypes of pineocytoma and are associated with a high rate of CSF dissemination, especially in children.[10,14] Local recurrences are usual within 2 years of surgery[46] and most reported cases are dead from tumour recurrence or dissemination well within that time.[2,7] Lastly are a group of pineocytomas which lack pineocytomatous rosettes but show evidence of astrocytic differentiation.[2] These are too seldom reported for generalised prognostic comment, but survival is probably dependent on the malignant grade of the astrocytic component of the tumour.[5,6]

Pineoblastoma

Pineoblastomas are primitive tumours of primary pineal parenchymal origin which lack the degree of differentiation normally seen in pineocytomas and are associated with a highly malignant biological behaviour. In many respects pineoblastomas resemble other primitive neuroectodermal tumours of the CNS, including neuroblastomas and medulloblastomas, and some authorities favour a unifying classification for all such tumours.[55,56] More usually, however, pineoblastomas are grouped together with pineocytomas in view of their differentiating capacity and specialised site.[57] Another reason for classifying pineoblastomas alongside pineocytomas is the occurrence of transitional or mixed lesions, with areas typical of both types of tumour.[5] Such tumours appear as a separate subgroup of primary pineal tumours in the WHO classification, designated as 'pineal parenchymal tumours of intermediate differentiation'. In practical terms, however, these lesions are probably best regarded as pineoblastomas exhibiting focal pineocytic differentiation, since their behaviour is almost inevitably that of the more primitive tumour type.[15] Pineoblastomas have also been subclassified according to their evidence of differentiating activity, whether pineocytic, retinoblastic or neuronal[2,5] (Table 9.2), but this is again of little prognostic significance and a highly malignant growth pattern is the rule in all cases.[15]

Incidence

Like pineocytomas, pineoblastomas are very rare tumours and calculation of their incidence can only be based on a small series of published reports. They have been variously reported as accounting for between 1 and 2% of all intracranial tumours[14,16] and between 8 and 15% of all tumours occurring in the pineal region.[11,12] Their incidence is probably quite similar to that of pineocytomas, although one large series of primary parenchymal tumours has shown a slight preponderance of pineocytoma over pineoblastoma.[5] Pineoblastomas are typically tumours of younger age groups, with a peak incidence in the first decade of life.[2] Exceptionally, cases presenting up to the early 50s have been reported.[4] Larger series suggest a slight preponderance of male patients,[4,5] although some studies have not substantiated this.[16]

Aetiology

Pineoblastomas and pineocytomas share a common origin in the primary neuroepithelial cells of the pineal gland, and typical pineocytic club ended processes can be demonstrated both histologically and ultrastructurally in a significant proportion of pineoblastomas.[2,58] Rarer examples which contain larger areas of histologically typical pineocytoma also help to confirm the pineal parenchymal origin of pineoblastomas.[5] In addition, pineoblastomas frequently demonstrate the photosensory cell evolutionary lineage of human pinealocytes, with ultrastructural evidence of photoreceptor differentiation similar to that found both in the photosensory pineal organ of submammalian species[20,59] and in the developing human fetal gland.[2,59] This is frequently more marked than in pineocytomas and some cases show frank retinoblastomatous differentiation, including the presence of typical retinoblastic fleurettes.[2,60] Rarely, pineoblastomas arise in cases of familial or sporadic bilateral retinoblastoma, producing a syndrome referred to as 'trilateral retinoblastoma'.[61,62] The retinoblastoma gene *RB1* on chromosome 13q14 is a well researched tumour suppressor gene which has been implicated in the development of a variety of human malignancies both within and outside the CNS.[63] Familial retinoblastomas occur when a second, somatic mutation arises in individuals already carrying a germline defect, whilst sporadic cases require somatic mutations on both copies of the chromosome.[64,65] Cases of trilateral retinoblastoma therefore suggest that mutation of the retinoblastoma gene confers neoplastic susceptibility on all cell lines of photoreceptor lineage, including those in the pineal gland.[66,67] Pineoblastomas not associated with bilateral retinoblastomas may also have a genetic predisposition, as suggested by the occurrence of familial[68,69] and congenital[70] examples of the tumour. However, cytogenetic information on isolated pineoblastomas is sparse and anecdotal at present. There have been reports of an interstitial deletion of chromosome 11q[71] and an isochromosome 17q[72] in two separate human culture lines, but an entirely normal karyotype has also been described in a third, unrelated line[73] and no consistent pattern is emerging.

Clinical features

Pineoblastomas usually present with signs and symptoms characteristic of all pineal region tumours, although the antecedant history is typically shorter than that of pineocytomas, with a mean duration of about 6 months.[3,4] The commonest presentation is that of acute hydrocephalus due to mechanical obstruction of the aqueduct.[8,9] Focal interference with oculomotor pathways may produce Parinaud syndrome of selective vertical gaze palsy, a characteristic feature of pineal region space occupying lesions.[9] The relatively rapid growth and infiltrative nature of pineoblastomas means that a wide range of adjacent anatomical structures may also be affected by the tumour, and clinical evidence of thalamic, hypothalamic or cerebellar disturbances is not uncommon.[8,9] In addition, there may be visual field defects, nystagmus and specific cranial nerve palsies, especially involving the third cranial nerves.

Radiology

Pineoblastomas are typically isodense or slightly hyperdense to brain on CT scans[12] and are almost invariably associated with obstructive hydrocephalus by the time of presentation. They less often show calcification than

Table 9.2 Histological subtypes of pineoblastoma

Undifferentiated

Focal differentiation
Retinoblastic
Ganglionic
Astrocytic
Pineocytic*

*Designated as 'Pineal parenchymal tumours of intermediate differentiation' in the WHO classification

pineocytomas[12] and tend to be poorly marginated owing to their infiltrative growth pattern.[8] There is usually significant enhancement of the tumour after giving intravenous contrast media, which may reveal central lucencies in some cases, a feature not described in pineocytomas.[12] Despite this, CT is not generally felt reliable as a method of distinguishing between different types of tumour occurring in the pineal region.[24,25] MRI, however, is a particularly sensitive method of defining the limits of tumours in this region and in some cases may be useful in helping to distinguish between primary pineal parenchymal tumours from germ cell or teratoid tumours occurring at the same site.[74,75] Like pineocytomas, the MRI signal of pineoblastomas is hypo- or isointense in T1-weighted images and hyperintense with T2-weighting, but it is more likely to be heterogeneous, especially after contrast enhancement.

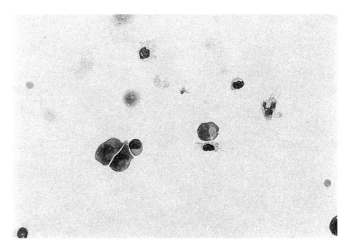

Fig. 9.13 **Pineoblastoma**. Cytospin preparation from a patient with dissemination of tumour cells in the CSF. Giemsa.

Pathology

Macroscopic features

Pineoblastomas replace and destroy the pineal gland, which is not usually identifiable macroscopically. They commonly bulge into the posterior part of the third ventricle and cause compression of the midbrain tectum and aqueduct. There is nearly always a resulting obstructive hydrocephalus involving the lateral and third ventricles. Although relatively circumscribed over their ventricular surfaces, pineoblastomas are often less well defined lesions than pineocytomas on naked eye examination, with evidence of diffuse infiltration of local structures at the tumour margins. Cut section typically reveals a soft, pinkish-grey tumour with a gelatinous texture, and calcification is not usually apparent. There are frequently areas of focal haemorrhage and necrosis, and there may also be well defined cystic spaces. Nearly all cases coming to autopsy show evidence of widespread spread in the CSF pathways (Fig. 9.13), and multiple tumour nodules are frequently apparent over both the cranial and spinal pial surfaces in such cases.

Intraoperative diagnosis

Using smear preparations, pineoblastomas have an appearance which is usually indistinguishable from that of other primitive neuroectodermal tumours, and knowledge of the precise location and extent of the lesion is essential for intraoperative diagnosis. The smears are typically very cellular, forming a uniform monolayer of thinly spread tumour cells with little tendency to adhere to blood vessels (Fig. 9.14). Where they are evenly spread, the cell nuclei appear larger than they do in paraffin sections. They are polygonal in outline and show prominent nuclear moulding, unlike lymphoid neoplasms. Mitoses are frequently encountered, but nuclear

pleomorphism is not usually a prominent feature. There is only scantly, indistinct perinuclear cytoplasm, and the nuclei are typically set in a very fine, sparse fibrillary background. Rosettes are not usually apparent on smear preparations. Frozen sections may reveal tubular rosettes in some cases but are otherwise unlikely to help in the distinction from other primitive neoplasms, such as transtentorial extension from a medulloblastoma.

Histological features

Pineoblastomas are highly cellular, primitive tumours, which in most cases are histologically similar to medulloblastomas and other primitive neuroectodermal neoplasms. The cells are relatively small and are closely packed together in monotonous sheets (Fig. 9.15). The cell nuclei are small, rounded and dark staining with a coarse chromatin pattern. There are frequent mitoses. Perinuclear cytoplasm is extremely scanty and indistinct, but there is usually a sparse, eosinophilic fibrillary background, and in some cases there may be solid, Homer Wright rosettes like those seen in medulloblastomas (Fig. 9.16). Focal areas of necrosis are often present (Fig. 9.16). Blood vessels are mainly thin walled, and there is usually little suggestion of a perivascular orientation of cells like that seen in papillary pineocytomas. With a modified Hortega silver carbonate stain[28] coarse argyrophilic cell processes can be found around vessels in a significant proportion of cases,[2] but these are usually much less numerous than in pineocytomas and can lack the typical club ended expansions. In occasional examples, undifferentiated pineoblastoma tissue may blend with focal areas of typical papillary pattern pineocytoma, and some otherwise primitive looking tumours may contain unexpectedly large numbers of club ended pineocytic cell processes. Such mixed or transitional appearances have been interpreted

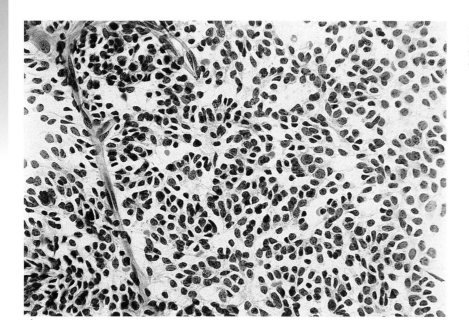

Fig. 9.14 **Pineoblastoma**. Smear preparation. Pleomorphic, moulded cell nuclei form a diffuse sheet, with little tendency to cling to blood vessels. Toluidine blue × 100.

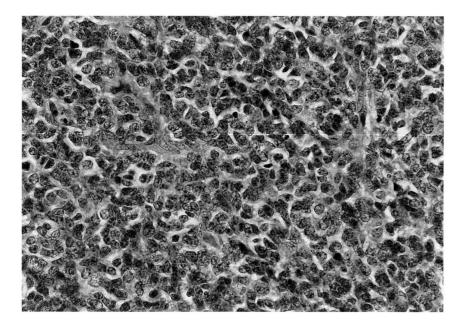

Fig. 9.15 **Pineoblastoma**. Cells with small, rounded nuclei and indistinct cytoplasm are closely packed in monotonous sheets. The histological appearances are similar to those of other primitive neuroectodermal tumours. H & E.

as pineocytomatous differentiation occurring in a pineoblastoma, in a fashion analogous to the maturation seen in some peripheral neuroblastomas.[5] The WHO classification designates these lesions as 'primary pineal parenchymal tumours of intermediate differentiation'. Very rarely, a lobular pattern has also been described in pineoblastomas, with smaller, more primitive cells at the periphery of the lobules, grading into larger cells mixed with blood vessels towards their centres.[2] This corresponds to the 'pale island' pattern of maturation seen in some medulloblastomas, and it is important to avoid confusion with the lobulated architecture of pineal germinomas, in which the smaller

cells are an entirely separate population of typical mature lymphocytes.

In contrast to pineocytomas, evidence of photoreceptor or retinoblastic differentiation may be apparent at light microscope level in some pineoblastomas. This usually takes the form of tubular ('Flexner–Wintersteiner') rosettes,[4,76] but occasionally there may be fleurettes composed of fan shaped sheaves of bulbous cytoplasmic processes protruding into a lumen, identical to those seen in retinoblastomas.[2,60] Pineoblastomas show histological evidence of astrocytic and ganglionic differentiation much less frequently than pineocytomas, but there have been very occasional reports of examples showing

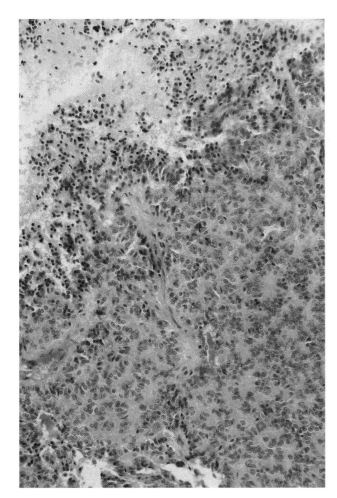

Fig. 9.16 **Pineoblastoma**. The tumour is forming numerous Homer Wright rosettes. An area of necrosis is present towards the top of the field. H & E.

bizzare, obviously neoplastic astrocytic cells, either in isolation or in conjunction with mature, Nissl-bearing ganglion cells.[77] It should be emphasised, however, that the vast majority of pineoblastomas appear uniformly primitive. Tumour seedlings in the CSF are also usually primitive in appearance, even when there is evidence of differentiating activity in the primary pineal tumour. Melanin pigment has been described in pineoblastomas, as in other primitive neuroectodermal tumours,[78] in this case possibly reflecting the transient melanin forming stage of the developing human fetal pineal gland.[5]

Immunocytochemistry

Pineoblastoma cells are unstained with antibodies to GFAP,[2,79] but there are usually positive staining reactive astrocytic elements near the more diffusely infiltrating margins of the tumour[2] and sometimes also trapped in deeper, more solid areas.[2,80] Like pineocytomas, a proportion of pineoblastomas contain occasional cells staining positively with antibodies to retinal S-antigen,

both in sporadic cases and those occurring in conjunction with ocular retinoblastomas.[37,81] The S-antigen immunostaining is usually seen in cells forming tubular, Flexner–Wintersteiner rosettes or retinoblastic fleurettes.[5] Such immunocytochemical evidence of photoreceptor differentiation again emphasises the evolutionary lineage of human pinealocytes from the photoreceptor cells of the pineal organs in lower order vertebrate species.[2,5] Pineoblastomas have recently been reported to express the alpha-subunit of S-100 protein, although there is no staining with the more usual antibodies directed at the beta-subunit.[82] Immunocytochemical expression of neuronal antigens such as neuron specific enolase and neurofilament protein have only seldom been reported in pineoblastomas,[83] and in distinction from pineal germinomas, they are not stained with antibodies to placental alkaline phosphatase.[40]

Electron microscopy

Most cases of pineoblastoma have a predominantly primitive ultrastructural appearance, with closely packed, pleomorphic tumour cells, occasionally separated by scanty cytoplasmic processes containing 20 nm microtubules.[18,19] The cell nuclei are often irregularly indented and the scanty rims of perinuclear cytoplasm contain mostly polyribosomes. Scattered dense core vesicles may be found in the perinuclear cytoplasm or cell processes, but they are very infrequent compared to the vesicles seen in pineocytomas. There may also be filament filled astrocytic processes coursing through the tumour, almost certainly derived from non-neoplastic astrocytes of the pineal gland. Despite the predominantly primitive appearance, many cases show at least some ultrastructural evidence of photoreceptor differentiation, usually in the form of synaptic ribbons (vesicle crowned lamellae), microtubular sheaves or bulb ended cilia with a 9+0 axial skeleton[18,58,59] (Fig. 9.17). These structures are similar to those found in the pineal glands of other mammalian species and human fetuses,[60,84,85] and also in the pineal photoreceptor organs of lower order vertebrates.[20,59] Retinoblastic fleurettes may also be found on ultrastructural examination, with clusters of bulb ended cytoplasmic protrusions projecting into intercellular lumina.[59] Annulate lamellae and concentric whorls of smooth endoplasmic reticulum have also been described in pineoblastomas, although these are less specifically associated with a photosensory derivation.[59]

Differential diagnosis

Medulloblastoma and other primitive neuroectodermal tumours

The distinction of pineoblastomas from other primitive neuroectodermal tumours relies heavily on specific knowledge of the primary site of the lesion, and where a

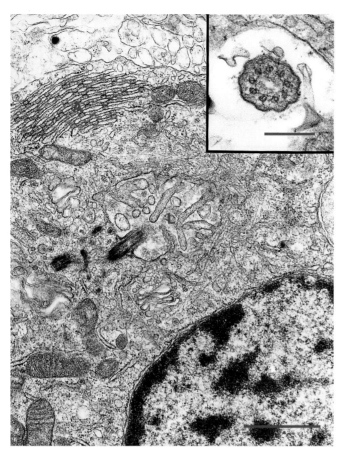

Fig. 9.17 **Pineoblastoma.** There is ultrastructural evidence of photoreceptor differentiation, with cilia protruding into an intracytoplasmic lumen (L) and annulate lamellae (A). Electron micrograph. Bar = 1 μm. Inset: The cilia have a neuronal configuration, with a 9 + 0 axial skelton. Bar = 0.25 μm.

large tumour breaches the tentorium the possibility of medulloblastoma invading the pineal region may need to be considered. The basic histological features of both tumours are very similar, but evidence of pineo-cytomatous differentiation, such as blunt ended argyrophilic processes can help to identify positively a pineoblastoma. In addition, a proportion of otherwise entirely primitive pineoblastomas show evidence of photoreceptor differentiation, and features such as tubular rosettes or cells staining with antibodies to retinal S-antigen provide strong evidence of a pineal origin for the tumour. When the primary site is clinically obscure and the biopsy is from a CSF seeding, the differential diagnosis must include all forms of primitive neuro-ectodermal tumour, including central neuroblastoma, and a precise diagnosis may not be possible. Features of pineocytomatous or photoreceptor differentiation are again worth looking for, but it must be remembered that differentiating features are rarely seen in the metastases of primitive neuroectodermal tumours, even when they are present in the tumour at its primary site.

Metastatic carcinoma

Systemic metastases to the pineal region are rare but well described, and a solitary metastasis from an undisclosed, poorly differentiated small cell carcinoma may mimic a pineoblastoma both clinically and histologically.[86,87] Evidence of pineocytic or retinoblastic differentiation may again be useful, but the quickest and surest way of identifying a metastatic carcinoma is with immunocyto-chemistry for epithelial antigens such as cytokeratin or epithelial membrane antigen. Expression of neuron-specific enolase should not be relied on, since it is found in small cell carcinomas of the bronchus as well as some cases of pineoblastoma.

Therapy

The most important factor influencing the treatment and prognosis of pineoblastomas is their very marked tendency to disseminate in the CSF pathways.[26] This occurs clinically in well over half of cases[4,16] and the seeding rate has been 100% in post-mortem series.[2,5] In addition, pineoblastomas often widely infiltrate neural structures in the adjacent midbrain, thalamus and hypothalamus[4,11] and may even extend to involve dura and skull bone.[76] Pressure on the aqueduct produces an obstructive hydrocephalus, and this is an almost in-variable complication of pineoblastoma, in common with other pineal tumours.[9] Rarely, the clinical course may also be complicated by systemic metastases, which have been reported both in lung and lymph nodes[76] and also in the abdominal cavity as a result of ventriculoperitoneal CSF shunting.[88]

Effective treatment of any pineal region tumour is dependent on achieving a firm histological diagnosis, because of the wide spectrum of tumours occurring at this site and their varying response to different forms of therapy.[8,24] A tissue diagnosis may be obtained by an initial stereotactic or ventriculoscopic biopsy[47,48] or at primary craniotomy. With more recent advances in operative technology, open surgery to the pineal region is associated with relatively low operative mortality rates[16,46] and surgical debulking is often now performed as the primary procedure, especially if there is urgency to relieve obstructive hydrocephalus.[8] In some cases com-plete local excision may be possible[49] but local tumour infiltration usually prevents this.[4,11] Pineoblastomas are relatively radiosensitive tumours[89] and postoperative radiotherapy is an important part of treatment which undoubtedly prolongs survival over surgery alone.[4,89] In view of the frequency of CSF seeding, most authorities advocate irradiation of the entire neuraxis in older children, even if there is no evidence of tumour dissemination at the time of surgery.[6,8,16] The effects of irradiation appear to be enhanced when combined with chemotherapy[90] but use of postoperative chemotherapy alone has not been found of value in infants under 18 months of age.[90,91] Follow-up should include regular radiological and cytological screening for evidence of subclinical spread in the CSF pathways.[92] The problem of tumour dissemination in the CSF has also been tackled using intrathecal administration of radiolabelled tumour antibodies, with one reported case showing prolonged remission.[93]

Prognosis

Despite advances in treatment, the prognosis in cases of pineoblastoma has remained much less favourable than for pineal germinomas or well differentiated, rosette forming pineocytomas.[8,94] Although surgically related deaths are now uncommon,[46] many cases succumb from the effects of local tumour spread or CSF dissemination quite early in the postoperative course,[16] and survival beyond 2 years is uncommon.[2,92] The prognosis is highly dependent on the extent of disease at diagnosis, with much shorter median survival times in cases showing evidence of spinal seeding at presentation.[95] Adults without evidence of seeding at diagnosis appear to have the greatest chance of longer term survival.[95] It is also perhaps significant that most pineoblastoma patients alive more than 2 years postoperatively have received both neuraxis irradiation and chemotherapy.[14,96,97]

Glial and miscellaneous tumours of the pineal region

Glial tumours of the pineal region have a similar incidence to that of the primary neuroepithelial pineal tumours, and account for between 20 and 30% of pineal neoplasms in most large series.[12,98] Pineal gliomas are most commonly of astrocytic type[13] and vary in malignant grade from juvenile pilocytic lesions[99] to glioblastomas.[11,16] Most of the astrocytic tumours are assumed to arise primarily within the pineal gland from the astrocytes which form a normal part of the gland structure.[80] Some smaller tumours may be entirely confined within the boundaries of an intact pineal gland,[100] but in most cases the lesions are much more extensive, with complete destruction of the gland and spread to adjacent structures.[99,102] Where pineal tissue is still identifiable, care must be taken not to confuse the lesion with focal astrocytic differentiation occurring within a pineocytoma.[2,29] *Gangliogliomas* have been reported in the pineal region, and in some cases these have been interpreted as pineocytomas transformed by extensive, divergent, astrocytic and neuronal differentiation.[3,30] *Ependymomas* may also replace the pineal gland, although they occur rather less frequently than astrocytic tumours at this site.[11] In most cases they are unlikely to have arisen

Table 9.3 Pineal region tumours and tumour-like conditions

Pineal parenchymal origin
  Pineocytoma
  Pineoblastoma
  Astrocytoma
  Glioblastoma

Non-parenchymal origin
  Germ cell tumours and teratomas
  Ependymoma
  Metastases
  Meningioma
  Vascular malformations
  Pineal cyst
  Dermoid/epidermoid cyst

within the gland itself, and have probably taken origin from the ependymal lining of the adjacent posterior third ventricle. *Astroblastomas* may also arise in the pineal region,[101] but older reports of oligodendroglioma[11] have probably arisen from misdiagnosed *central neurocytoma* spreading back from the anterior septal region.

In addition to germ cell neoplasms, primary pineal parenchymal tumours and gliomas, a number of other tumour types may be encountered in the pineal region, and these must be remembered when considering the differential diagnosis of lesions at this site (Table 9.3). *Metastases* to the pineal gland are rare compared with those in other intracranial sites[103] but a solitary pineal metastasis can be the presenting feature in patients with an undisclosed systemic primary tumour.[86,104] Primary tumours described in association with solitary pineal metastases have included lesions as diverse as gastric carcinoma[105] and hepatic angiosarcoma,[104] but the most commonly reported primary lesions have been carcinomas of the lung,[106,107] especially those of small cell undifferentiated type.[86,87] *Meningiomas* may also occupy the pineal region, and in one study accounted for 8 of 60 tumours at this site.[12] They may take origin from the leptomeninges adjacent to the pineal gland,[101] but some cases arise from the tela choroidea of the third ventricle, and are entirely deep seated without dural attachment.[108] Less common types of tumour which may present as pineal space occupying lesions include *angiomatous malformations*,[13,109] *haemangiopericytomas*, *paragangliomas*, *craniopharyngiomas*, *dermoid* and *epidermoid cysts* and *lipomas*.[13] *Pineal cysts* also need to be considered in this context and are described separately in Chapter 17.

REFERENCES

1. Russell DS. The pinealoma, its relationship to teratoma. J Pathol Bacteriol, 1944; 56:145–150
2. Herrick MK, Rubinstein LJ. The cytological differentiating potential of pineal parenchymal neoplasms (true pinealomas). A clinicopathologic study of 28 tumors. Brain, 1979; 102:289–320

3. Horrax G, Bailey P. Pineal pathology. Further studies. Arch Neurol, 1928; 19:394–414

4. Borit A, Blackwood W, Mair WGP. The separation of pineocytoma from pineoblastoma. Cancer, 1980; 45:1408–1418

5. Russell DS, Rubinstein LJ. Pathology of tumours of the nervous system, 5th Edn. London: Edward Arnold, 1989: pp 380–394

6. Rubinstein LJ. Cytogenesis and differentiation of pineal neoplasms. Hum Pathol, 1981; 12:441–448

7. Trojonowski JQ, Tascos NA, Rorke LB. Malignant pineocytoma with prominent papillary features. Cancer, 1982; 50:1789–1793

8. Sawaya R, Hawley DK, Tobler WD et al. Pineal and third ventricular tumours. In: Youmans, JR, ed. Neurological surgery, 3rd edn. Philadelphia: Saunders, 1990: pp 3171–3203

9. Smith RA, Estridge MN. Pineal tumours. In: Vinken PJ, Bruyn GW, eds. Handbook of clinical neurology, vol. 17. Tumours of the brain and skull, Part II. New York: Elsevier, 1974: pp 648–665

10. D'Andrea AD, Packer RJ, Rorke LB et al. Pineocytomas of childhood. A reappraisal of natural history and response to therapy. Cancer, 1987; 59:1353–1357

11. Degirolami U, Schmidek H. Clinicopathological study of 53 tumours of the pineal region. J Neurosurg 1973; 39:455–462

12. Ganti SR, Hilal SK, Stein BM et al. CT of pineal region tumours. Am J Neurol Radiol, 1986; 7:97–104

13. Packer RJ, Sutton LN, Rosenstock JG et al. Pineal region tumours of childhood. Pediatrics, 1984; 74:97–102

14. Scheithauer BW. Neuropathology of pineal region tumors. Clin Neurosurg, 1985; 31:351–383

15. Rubinstein LJ. Atlas of tumour pathology, Fascicle 6, 2nd series. Supplement: Tumours of the central nervous system. Washington: Armed Forces Institute of Pathology, 1982: pp S15–S20

16. Hoffman HJ, Yoshida M, Becker LE et al. Experience with pineal region tumours in childhood. Neurol Res, 1984; 6:107–112

17. Nielsen SL, Wilson CB. Ultrastructure of a 'pineocytoma'. J Neuropathol Exp Neurol, 1975; 34:148–158

18. Moss TH. Tumours of the nervous system. An ultrastructural atlas. London: Springer, 1986: pp 57–65

19. Hassoun J, Gambarelli D, Peragut JC et al. Specific ultrastructural markers of human pinealomas. Acta Neuropathol (Berl), 1983; 62:31–40

20. Vourath L. Synaptic ribbons of a mammalian pineal gland. Circadian changes. Z Zellforsch, 1973; 145:171–183

21. Varakis J, Zurhein GM. Experimental pineocytoma of the syrian hamster induced by a human papovirus (JC). A light and electron microscopic study. Acta Neuropathol (Berl), 1976; 35:243–264

22. Bello MJ, Rey JA, de Campos JM et al. Chromosomal abnormalities in a pineocytoma. Cancer Genet Cytogenet, 1993; 71:185–186

23. Rainho CA, Roggatto SR, de Moraes LC et al. Cytogenetic study of a pineocytoma. Cancer Genet Cytogenet, 1992; 64:127–132

24. Chang T, Teng MM, Guo WY et al. CT of pineal tumors and intracranial germ-cell tumors. Am J Roentgenol, 1989; 153:1269–1274

25. Weisberg LA. Clinical and computerised tomographic correlations of pineal neoplasms. Comput Radiol, 1984; 8:285–292

26. Harsh GR, Wilson CB. Neuroepithelial tumours of the adult brain. In: Youmans JR, ed. Neurological surgery, 3rd edn. Philadelphia: Saunders, 1990: pp 3040–3136

27. Tracy PT, Hanigan WC, Kalyan-Raman UP. Radiological and pathological findings in three cases of childhood pineocytomas. Childs Nerv Syst, 1986; 2:297–300

28. Degirolami U, Zvaigne O. Modification of the Achucarro-Hortega pineal stain for paraffin embedded formalin-fixed tissue. Stain Technology, 1973; 48:48–50

29. Borit A, Blackwood W. Pineocytoma with astrocytomatous differentiation. J Neuropathol Exp Neurol, 1979; 38:253–258

30. Rubinstein LJ, Okazaki H. Gangliogliomatous differentiation in a pineocytoma. J Pathol, 1970; 102:27–32

31. Fukushima T, Tomonaga M, Sawada T et al. Pineocytoma with neuronal differentiation – case report. Neurol Med Chir (Tokyo), 1990; 30:63–68

32. Collins VP. Pineocytoma with neuronal differentiation demonstrated immunocytochemically. A case report. Acta Pathol Microbiol Immunol Scand (A), 1987; 95:113–117

33. Okeda R, Song SJ, Nakajima T et al. Pineocytoma. Observation of an autopsy case by electron microscopy and cell markers. Acta Pathol (Jpn), 1984; 34:911–918

34. Jouvet A, Fevre-Montange M, Besancon R et al. Structural and ultrastructural characteristics of human pineal gland and pineal parenchymal tumours. Acta Neuropathol (Berl), 1994; 88:334–348

35. Numoto RT. Pineal parenchynal tumours: cell differentiation and prognosis. J Cancer Res Clin Oncol, 1994; 120:683–690

36. Korf HW, Klein DC, Zigler JS et al. S-antigen-like immunoreactivity in a human pineocytoma. Acta Neuropathol (Berl), 1986; 69:165–167

37. Perentes E, Rubinstein LJ, Herman MM et al. S-antigen immunoreactivity in human pineal glands and pineal parenchymal tumors. A monoclonal antibody study. Acta Neuropathol (Berl), 1986; 71:224–227

38. Bonnin JM, Perentes E. Retinal S-antigen immunoreactivity in medulloblastomas. Acta Neuropathol (Berl), 1988; 76:204–207

39. Korf HW, Czerwionka M, Reiner J et al. Immunocytochemical evidence of molecular photoreceptor markers in cerebellar medulloblastomas. Cancer, 1987; 60:1763–1766

40. Shinoda J, Miwa Y, Sakai N et al. Immunohistochemical study of placental alkaline phosphatase in primary intracranial germ-cell tumors. J Neurosurg, 1985; 63:733–739

41. Vorkapic P, Waldhauser F, Bruckner R et al. Serum melatonin levels: A new neurodiagnostic tool in pineal region tumors? Neurosurgery, 1987; 21:817–824

42. Miles A, Tidmarsh SF, Philbrick D et al. Diagnostic potential of melatonin analysis in pineal tumours. N Engl J Med, 1985; 313:329–330

43. Quay WB. Experimental and spontaneous pineal tunours: Findings relating to endocrine and oncogenic factors and mechanisms. J Neural Transm, 1980; 48:9–23

44. Tapp E. Melatonin as a tumour marker in a patient with pineal tumour. Br Med J, 1978; 2:636

45. Fetell MR, Stein BM. Neuroendocrine aspects of pineal tumors. Neurol Clin, 1986; 4:877–905

46. Neuwelt EA. An update on the surgical treatment of malignant pineal region tumors. Clin Neurosurg, 1985; 32:397–428

47. Pluchino F, Broggi G, Fornari M et al. Surgical approach to pineal tumours. Acta Neurochir (Wien), 1989; 96:26–31

48. Conway LW. Stereotaxic diagnosis and treatment of intracranial tumors including an initial experience with cryosurgery for pinealomas. J Neurosurg, 1973; 38:453–460

49. Neuwelt EA, Glasberg M, Frankel E et al. Malignant pineal region tumours. J Neurosurg, 1979; 51:597–605

50. Rout D, Sharma A, Raddhakrishnan VV et al. Exploration of the pineal region: Observations and results. Surg Neurol, 1984; 21:135–140

51. Jamieson KG. Excision of pineal tumours. J Neurosurg, 1971; 35:550–553

52. Sakoda K, Uozumi T, Kawamoto K et al. Responses of pineocytoma to radiation therapy and chemotherapy – report of two cases. Neurol Med Chir (Tokyo), 1989; 29:825–829

53. Disclafani A, Hudgins RJ, Edwards MS et al. Pineocytomas. Cancer, 1989; 63:302–304

54. Schild SE, Scheithauer BW, Schomberg PJ et al. Pineal parenchhymal tumours. Clinical, pathologic, and therapeutic aspects. Cancer, 1993; 72:870–880

55. Becker LE, Hinton D. Primitive neuroectodermal tumors of the central nervous system. Hum Pathol, 1983; 14:538–550

56. Rorke LB. The cerebellar medulloblastoma and its relationship to primitive neuroectodermal tumors. J Neuropathol Exp Neurol, 1983; 42:1–15

57. Rubinstein LJ. Embryonal central neuroepithelial tumors and their differentiating potential. A cytogenetic view of a complex neuro-oncological problem. J Neurosurg, 1985; 62:795–805

58. Markesbery WR, Haugh RM, Young AB. Ultrastructure of pineal parenchymal neoplasms. Acta Neuropathol (Berl), 1981; 55:143–149

59. Kune KT, Damjanov I, Katz SM et al. Pineoblastoma: An electron microscopic study. Cancer, 1979; 44:1692–1699

60. Stefanko SZ, Manschot WA. Pineoblastoma with retinoblastomatous differentiation. Brain, 1979; 102:321–332

61. Blach LE, McCormick B, Abramson DH et al. Trilateral retinoblastoma – incidence and outcome: a decade of experience. Int J Radiat Oncol Biol Phys, 1994; 29:729–733

62. De Potter P, Shields CL, Shields JA. Clinical variations of trilateral retinoblastoma: a report of 13 cases. J Pediatr Ophthalmol Strabismus, 1994; 31:26–31

63. Lin SC, Skapek SX, Lee EY. Genes in the RB pathway and their knockout in mice. Sem Cancer Biol 1996; 7:279–289

64. Lohmann DR, Brandt B, Hopping W et al. The spectrum of RB1 germ-line mutations in hereditary retinoblastoma. Am J Hum Genet, 1996; 58:940–949

65. Loohmann DR, Brandt B, Passarge E et al. Molecular genetics and diagnosis of retinoblastoma. Significance for ophthalmological practice. Ophthalmologe, 1997; 94:263–267

66. Kingston JE, Plowman PN, Hungerford JL. Ectopic intracranial retinoblastoma in childhood. Opthalmol 1985; 69:742–748

67. Johnson DL, Chandra R, Fisher WS et al. Trilateral retinoblastoma: Ocular and pineal retinoblastomas. J Neurosurg, 1985; 63:367–370

68. Peyster RG, Ginsberg F, Hoover ED. Computerised tomography of familial pineoblastoma. J Comput Assist Tomogr, 1986; 10:32–33

69. Lesnick JE, Chayt KJ, Bruce DA et al. Familial pineoblastoma. Report of two cases. J Neurosurg, 1985; 62:930–932

70. Lilue RE, Jequier S, O'Gorman AM. Congenital pineoblastoma in the newborn: Ultrasound evaluation. Radiology, 1985; 154:363–365

71. Sreekantaiah C, Jockin H, Brecher ML et al. Interstitial deletion of chromosome 11q in a pineoblastoma. Cancer Genet Cytogenet, 1989; 39:125–131

72. Kees UR, Biegel JA, Ford J et al. Enhanced MYCN expression and isochromosome 17q in pineoblastoma cell lines. Genes Chromosomes Cancer, 1994; 9:129–135

73. Jennings MT, Jennings DL, Ebrahim SAD et al. *In vitro* karyotypic and immunophenotypic characterisation of primitive neuroectodermal tumours: similarities to malignant gliomas. Europ J Cancer, 1992; 28A:762–766

74. Tien RD, Barkovich AJ, Edwards MS. MR imaging of pineal tumors. Am J Roentgenol, 1990; 155:143–151

75. Kilgore DP, Strother CM, Starshak RJ et al. Pineal germinoma: MR imaging. Radiology, 1986; 158:435–438

76. Banerjee AK, Kak VK. Pineoblastoma with spontaneous intra- and extracranial metastasis. J Pathol, 1974; 114:9–12

77. Sobel RA, Trice JE, Nielson SL et al. Pineoblastoma with ganglionic and glial differentiation. Report of two cases. Acta Neuropathol (Berl), 1981; 55:243–246

78. Best PV. A medulloblastoma-like tumour with melanin formation. J Pathol, 1973; 110:109–111

79. Schindler E, Gullotta F. Glial fibrillary acidic protein in medulloblastomas and other embryonic CNS tumours of children. Virchows Arch (A) 1983; 398:263–275

80. Papasozomenos S, Shapiro S. Pineal astrocytoma: Report of a case, confined to the epiphysis, with immunocytochemical and electron microscopic studies. Cancer, 1981; 47:99–103

81. Rodrigues MM, Bardenstein DS, Donoso LA et al. An immunohistopathologic study of trilateral retinoblastoma. Am J Ophthalmol, 1987; 103:776–781

82. Hayashi K, Hoshida Y, Horie Y et al. Immunohistochemical study on the distribution of alpha and beta subunits of S-100 protein in brain tumours. Acta Neuropathol (Berl), 1991; 81:657–663

83. Okuda Y, Taomoto K, Saya H et al. Pineoblastoma with neuronal differentiation–immunohistochemical and immunocytochemical studies. J Neurooncol, 1988; 6:193–198

84. Wartenberg H. The mammalian pineal organ: Electron microscopic studies on the fine structure of pinealocytes, glial cells and on the perivascular component. Z Zellforsch, 1968; 86:74–97

85. Lin HS. Transformation of centrioles in pinealocytes of adult guinea pigs. J Neurocytol, 1972; 1:61–68

86. Kashiwagi S, Hatano M, Yokoyama T. Metastatic small cell carcinoma to the pineal body: Case report. Neurosurgery, 1989; 25:810–813

87. Toner GC, Pike J, Schwarz MA. The blood-brain barrier and response of CNS metastases to chemotherapy. J Neurooncol, 1989; 7:21–24

88. Pfletschinger J, Olive D, Czorny A et al. Peritoneal metastasis of a pineoblastoma in a patient with a ventriculo-peritoneal shunt. Pediatrie, 1986; 41:231–236

89. Bloom HJG. Intracranial tumours: Response and resistance to therapeutic endeavours, 1970-1980. Int J Radiat Oncol Biol Phys, 1982; 8:1083–1113

90. Jakacki RI, Zeltzer PM, Boyett JM et al. Survival and prognostic factors following radiation and/or chemotherapy for primitive neuroectodermal tumors of the pineal region in infants and children: a report of the Childrens Cancer Group. J Clin Oncol, 1995; 13:1377–1383

91. Geyer JR, Zeltzer PM, Boyett JM et al. Survival of infants with primitive neuroectodermal tumors or malignant ependymomas of the CNS treated with eight drugs in 1 day: a report from the Childrens Cancer Group. J Clin Oncol, 1994; 12:1607–1615

92. Kun LE, D'Souza B, Tefft M. The value of surveillance testing in childhood brain tumors. Cancer, 1985; 56(suppl):1818–1823

93. Coakham HB, Richardson, RB, Davies AG et al. Neoplastic meningitis from a pineal tumour treated by antibody-guided irradiation via the intrathecal route. Br J Neurosurg, 1988; 2:199–209

94. Levin CV, Rutherfoord GS. Pineal tumours at Groote Schuur Hospital. 1976–1984 S Afr Med J, 1985; 68:33–35

95. Chang SM, Lillis-Hearnr PK, Larson DA et al. Pineoblastoma in adults. Neurosurgery, 1995; 37:383–390

96. Kovnar EH, Kellie SJ, Horowitz ME et al. Preirradiation cisplatin and etoposide in the treatment of high-risk medulloblastoma and other malignant embryonal tumors of the central nervous system: A phase II study. J Clin Oncol, 1990; 8:330–336

97. Allen JC, Helson L, Jerob B. Pre-radiation chemotherapy for newly diagnosed childhood brain tumors. A modified phase II trial. Cancer, 1983; 52:2001–2006

98. Stein BM. Operative approaches to midline tumors. Acta Neurochir Suppl(Wien), 1985; 35:42–49

99. Degirolami U, Armbrustmacher VW. Juvenile pilocytic astrocytoma of the pineal region. Cancer, 1982; 50:1185–1188

100. Benjamin JC, Furneaux CE, Scholtz CL. Pineal astrocytoma. Surg Neurol, 1985; 23:139–142

101. Zeitlin H. Tumours in the region of the pineal body: Clinicopathologic report of 3 cases. Arch Neurol Psychiatry, 1935; 34:567–586

102. Norbut AM, Mendolow H. Primary glioblastoma multiforme of the pineal region with leptomeningeal metastases: A case report. Cancer, 1981; 47:592–596

103. Ortega P, Malumud N, Shimkin MG. Metastasis to the pineal body. Arch Pathol, 1951; 52:518–528

104. Seto H, Matsukado Y, Kuratsu J et al. Angiosarcoma of the liver and pineal region. No Shinkei Geka, 1988; 16:409–413

105. Yanamoto H, Kakita K, Fukuma S. Pineal metastasis – a case report and a review of literature. No Shinkei Geka, 1987; 15:1329–1334

106. Halpert B, Erickson EE, Fields WS. Intracranial involvement from carcinoma of the lung. Arch Pathol, 1960; 69:93–103

107. Tomita T, Wetzel N. Metastasis to the midbrain. Report of two cases. J Neurooncol, 1984; 2:73–77

108. Roda JM, Perez-Higueras A, Oliver B et al. Pineal region meningiomas without dural attachment. Surg Neurol, 1982; 17:147–151

109. Hubschmann O, Kasoff S, Doniger D et al. Cavernous haemangioma in the pineal body. Surg Neurol, 1976; 6:349–351

10 Germ cell tumours

Germ cell tumours in the central nervous system (CNS) arise most often in the region of the pineal gland, where as a group they occur at a higher frequency than primary pineal parenchymal tumours.[1–3] As noted above, it should be recalled that many of the descriptions of 'pinealoma' in the past have included examples of what would now be classified as a germinoma; the World Health Organisation (WHO) classification for tumours of the CNS clearly recognises the separation of this group of tumours from primary parenchymal tumours of the pineal gland.[4] Germ cell tumours in the CNS may also arise in the region of the hypothalamus (in the older literature these are occasionally referred to as 'ectopic pinealomas')[5–7] and more rarely in other midline structures including the spinal cord,[8–10] but very occasional examples have been described in other locations,[11] including the basal ganglia and thalamus.[12–14] The classification adopted by the WHO for germ cell tumours in the CNS is identical to those for germ cell tumours arising in the testis[15] (see Table 10.1); these entities are discussed below. Dermoid and epidermoid cysts and related lesions are discussed in Chapter 17, and atypical teratoid/rhabdoid tumours are described in Chapter 7.

Incidence

Germ cell tumours arising in the CNS are rare, accounting for around 0.5% of intracranial tumours in Europe and North America.[1,2,7,16–19] A much higher incidence of 4–5% has been described in Japan and Taiwan (comprising both germinomas and teratomas), although the validity of this observation has been questioned because of bias arising from selective case reporting.[20–22] Most intracranial germ cell tumours are germinomas (Table 10.2); these occur most frequently in children between the ages of 10 and 12 years and are extremely uncommon after the age of 35 years.[1,3,18,19,23] Germinomas occur more frequently in males, particularly in the pineal region, whereas in females the region of the hypothalamus is most often involved. Teratomas (both benign and malignant) account for the second

commonest group of germ cell tumours, and occur across a wider age range than germinomas.[1,2,19,24] Benign teratomas occur most often in young children and infants and are the most common form of congenital intracranial tumour.[25,26] Although most of these congenital teratomas occur in females, teratomas in older children show a marked male predominance. Most teratomas occur in children under 10 years of age, but there is a second peak in incidence between the ages of 16 and 18; cases occurring in patients over the age of 40 are extremely uncommon.[2,4,6,18,19] The other three malignant germ cell tumours (choriocarcinoma, yolk sac tumour and embryonal cell carcinoma) all occur more often in male patients, with choriocarcinoma tending to involve younger patients below the age of 10 years, and embryonal cell carcinoma and yolk sac tumour occurring most often in adolescents aged 12–16 years.[1,2,3,7,16–18,22,27–29] As with other germ cell tumours, cases of these three tumour types in patients over the age of 40 years are markedly uncommon. The relative frequencies of CNS germ cell tumours are listed in Table 10.2.

Aetiology

It is widely believed that germ cell tumours in the CNS and other extragonadal sites arise from residual germ cells (usually in the midline structures of the CNS, or in the anterior mediastinum). The presence of residual germ cells at these sites has been generally attributed to a migrational defect, since germ cells become separated from somatic cells in embryogenesis and migrate to the developing gonadal blastema at an early stage.[31] It has also been suggested that germ cells might undergo a secondary migration to the region of the diencephalon, where they may play a role in the subsequent development of the CNS.[32] Another theory suggests that embryonic cells at various stages of development may be involved in the stream of lateral mesoderm at the time of primitive streak formation, and carried into the future cranial area to become misplaced into the brain during neural tube formation.[33]

Table 10.1 WHO histological classification of germ cell tumours (modified for use on CNS tumours)[4,15]

Tumours of one histological type (pure forms)
a. Germinoma
   Variant: germinoma with syncytiotrophoblastic giant cells
b. Embryonal carcinoma
c. Yolk sac tumour
d. Choriocarcinoma
e. Teratoma
   i   Mature teratoma
   ii Immature teratoma
   iii Teratoma with malignant transformation

Tumours of more than one histological type (mixed forms)

Table 10.2 Relative frequencies of germ cell tumours in the CNS[1,3,4,7,18,22,30,68]

Tumour	Frequency (%)
Germinoma	50
Immature teratoma	14
Mature teratoma	6
Teratoma with malignant transformation	4
Embryonal carcinoma	3
Yolk sac tumour	2
Choriocarcinoma	1
Mixed germ cell tumours	20

It has been established that patients with Klinefelter syndrome (47XXY) are at greater risk of developing germ cell tumours in the gonads and elsewhere in the body;[34,35] there is evidence of a generalised defect in the germ cell migration in these patients. Germinomas in the CNS may occur in association with germ cell neoplasms elsewhere in the body[36] and one example of a CNS germinoma has been associated with cryptorchidism.[37] Apart from the association with Klinefelter syndrome, intracranial germinomas have been reported in patients with Down syndrome.[36,38,39] Both germinomas and teratomas have been reported in otherwise apparently normal siblings.[40,41] Occasional germ cell tumours in the brain are associated with haematological malignancies, for example in a recent case report where a suprasellar germinoma was accompanied by mixed lineage acute myeloid leukaemia.[42]

Little is known of the cytogenetics or molecular genetics of germ cell tumours in the CNS. Cytogenetic studies of cerebral germ cell tumours have found isochromosome 12p, which is also found in gonadal and other extragonadal germ cell tumours.[43–45] A recent study using comparative genomic hybridisation in a range of pineal germ cell tumours also found similar chromosomal imbalances to their extracerebral counterparts.[46] One molecular genetic study detected *TP53* mutations by single-strand confirmation polymorphism analysis in 3/5 endodermal sinus tumours and 1/7 CNS germinomas;[47] these findings are broadly comparable with the scanty literature on this topic in gonadal germ cell tumours, although another recent study of seven germinomas and seven other CNS germ cell tumours found no evidence of *TP53* mutations.[48]

Clinical features

The presenting clinical features for germ cell tumours are most conveniently considered in two groups relating to the major sites at which these tumours arise in the CNS: the pineal gland region and the region of the hypothalamus. Pineal region tumours usually present with features relating to:

1. raised intracranial pressure and hydrocephalus;
2. compression of adjacent structures in the brain stem; and
3. endocrine abnormalities.[1,3,22]

Most patients present with headache relating to raised intracranial pressure, which is usually accompanied by hydrocephalus as a consequence of obstruction of the outflow of the third ventricle. Unless relieved, additional symptoms of hydrocephalus will occur including nausea and vomiting, papilloedema and eventually impairment of higher functions. Compression of the brain stem most often leads to disturbances of extraocular movements (Parinaud syndrome) with a prominent paralysis of

upgaze or convergence movements. Compression or invasion of the midbrain involving the periaqueductal grey matter can cause paralysis of downgaze and ptosis. Very occasionally, patients present with hearing disturbances and involvement of the superior cerebellar peduncles can cause ataxia. Endocrine abnormalities are uncommon and may result from the effects of hydrocephalus. However, precocious puberty has been documented on many occasions in association with pineal germ cell tumours.[1,16,22] This may also occur in patients with hypothalamic tumours as a consequence of disturbed pituitary function, but it has been clearly established that in males many cases of precocious puberty are associated with the secretion of ectopic beta-human chorionic gonadotropin (beta-hCG) from syncytiotrophoblastic cells in choriocarcinomas or mixed germ cell tumours.[49] In such patients, the primary tumour usually occurs in the region of the pineal gland, but cases have also occasionally been described with tumours arising in the spinal cord.[8] Pineal region germ cell tumours, particularly choriocarcinomas, can present with a pineal apoplexy as a consequence of extensive haemorrhage into the gland.[1,3] This unusual presentation is not confined to germ cell tumours and may also occur with pineal parenchymal tumours.

Patients with hypothalamic germ cell tumours commonly present with:

1. diabetes insipidus (the most characteristic presenting feature);
2. visual field defects as a result of optic chiasm or optic nerve compression; and
3. other abnormalities of the hypothalamic–pituitary axis.

The latter can result in pan-hypopituitarism, delayed or failure of growth, delayed sexual development or precocious puberty.[5,30,50] The latter feature usually occurs in males, but has occasionally been reported in females; in one recent case report, precocious puberty was associated with diabetes insipidus in an 11-year-old girl with a suprasellar immature teratoma.[51] Large hypothalamic region tumours may also present with hydrocephalus as a consequence of third ventricle or aqueduct obstruction. Hypothalamic germ cell tumours may arise concurrently with similar tumours in the pineal gland; in such instances the clinical features reflect the dual sites of pathology.[1,50] Germinomas have very rarely been reported as a primary intramedullary lesion in the spinal cord, when patients present with progressive paraparesis or complete paraplegia.[8–10] Germ cell tumours in the CNS may be associated with other germ cell tumours at gonadal and extragonadal sites, and an example of a metachronous neurohypophyseal germinoma occurring 8 years after a pineal mature teratoma has recently been reported.[52]

Radiology

Computerised tomography (CT) scans of germinomas show homogeneous isointense or more commonly hyperintense solid tissue masses (in comparison with grey matter), which exhibit variable contrast enhancement.[53,54] Focal calcification may be present both in the tumour itself and in the engulfed or compressed pineal tissue. Magnetic resonance imaging (MRI) scans also show relative hyperintensity in T2-weighted images, but germinomas appear isodense with white matter in T1-weighted sequences.[1,55] Gadolinium studies usually show homogeneous contrast enhancement in germinomas (Fig. 10.1).

In contrast, teratomas exhibit a wide range of radiological appearances which reflect their heterogenous tissue composition.[54] This is particularly true in MRI imaging, which can demonstrate various signal characteristics reflecting cystic elements, soft tissue components and lipid (Fig. 10.2), while focal calcification is best identified on CT scans.[55] Malignant teratomas are particularly prone to haemorrhage and usually invade adjacent structures. Most mature teratomas are well circumscribed and contain areas of low attenuation on CT scans because of their adipose tissue content.

Other types of germ cell tumour often show infiltration of adjacent structures with heterogeneity of signal characteristics on both MRI and CT studies which reflects haemorrhage, particularly in choriocarcinoma. CT and MRI scans are useful for the demonstration of local invasion, cerebrospinal fluid (CSF) metastases (contrast-enhancing nodules along the ventricular lining or subarachnoid space) and hydrocephalus.[53–55]

Germinoma

Pathology

It is convenient to consider the pathology of intracranial germ cell tumours in three groups – germinomas, teratomas, and others (comprising embryonal carcinoma, yolk sac tumour, choriocarcinoma and mixed germ cell tumours). The latter group (with the exception of mixed germ cell tumours) are exceedingly uncommon as single entities and this is reflected in the relative paucity of literature on these neoplasms. Although teratomas exhibit a wide diversity of histological subtypes and biological behaviour, the other two categories can be considered to represent a relatively consistent spectrum of tumour pathology and biology.

Germinomas occur most frequently in the first two decades of life, with males affected around twice as often as females.[2,16,30] Most tumours are located in the region of the pineal gland and although an origin in the supraseller region is relatively uncommon, germinomas may arise in

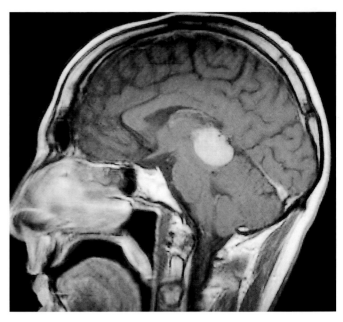

Fig. 10.1 **Germinoma**. Gadolinium-enhanced MRI scan in an 11-year-old boy, showing a homogeneous enhancing pineal germinoma. The tumour indents the posterior wall of the third ventricle. (Courtesy of Dr D Collie, Edinburgh.)

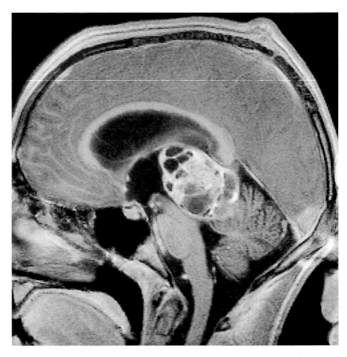

Fig. 10.2 **Mature teratoma**. Gadolinium-enhanced MRI scan of a mature pineal teratoma shows a large multiloculate cystic lesion which is well defined, with areas of variable enhancement. This large tumour is compressing the brain stem and is causing severe obstructive hydrocephalus. (Courtesy of Dr D Collie, Edinburgh.)

the deep grey matter regions of the basal ganglia and thalamus.[12,13] The clinical and radiological features of germinomas are described above.

Macroscopic features

Germinomas have the capacity to infiltrate adjacent brain structures, and often appear as ill-defined masses regardless of the site of origin. Smaller lesions in the pineal gland may occupy the entire gland or may appear partly encapsulated and relatively well circumscribed from the surrounding tissue. The tumours have a soft consistency with a grey–pink cut surface, within which multiple foci of haemorrhage may be present (Fig. 10.3). Cystic change within the substance of the tumour is not uncommon, and may be a consequence of previous haemorrhage.

Extensive infiltration of adjacent structures occurs most often in hypothalamic region tumours, in which the anterior portion of the third ventricle, the pituitary stalk and optic chiasm will all be involved. Pituitary gland invasion is uncommon, although involvement of the stalk may result in compression of the pituitary gland within the sella turcica. In pineal region tumours, the posterior portion of the third ventricle, the cerebral aqueduct and quadrigeminal plate may all be involved and the normal pineal gland structure may be unrecognisable. The few intramedullary spinal cord germinomas reported in the literature have generally arisen in the thoracic cord, with infiltration of both grey and white matter.[8–10] This capacity for local invasion can pose problems during neurosurgery for either biopsy or resection.[1,3]

Intraoperative diagnosis

Germinomas are soft enough for both smear and cryostat preparations to be made for the purposes of intraoperative diagnosis. Smear preparations characteristically exhibit two distinct cell populations: large pleomorphic tumour cells and small lymphocytes, which may be perivascular.[56] The large tumour cells tend to spread away from blood vessels in irregular clusters in a monolayer, with no evidence of a gliofibrillary tumour matrix. The clusters of large tumour cells stand out in contrast to the uniform population of small reactive lymphocytes (Fig. 10.4). Tumour cell nuclei are large and rounded with a prominent single nucleolus. A variable quantity of cytoplasm is present and the cells may appear spheroidal or polygonal. Mitotic activity is usually identifiable within the tumour cell population, but not in the reactive lymphocytes. The reactive lymphocytes may be present around blood vessels but frequently form an irregular admixture with the larger tumour cells throughout the smear. Occasional germinomas contain syncytiotrophoblastic giant cells, which are readily identifiable in smear preparations because of their large size, irregular shape and nuclei. There may be evidence of both recent and previous haemorrhage within the smear preparation, and larger tumours may contain foci of necrosis. Mixed germ cells tumours frequently contain germinomatous

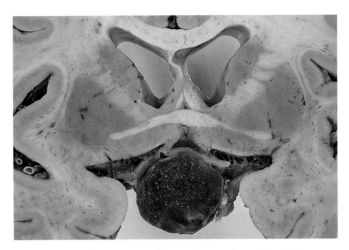

Fig. 10.3 **Germinoma**. Suprasellar germinoma viewed intact at autopsy, comprising a well defined tumour mass with focal haemorrhage and a non-homogeneous cut surface. The patient was a 14-year-old male who had previously received cranial irradiation for treatment of this lesion.

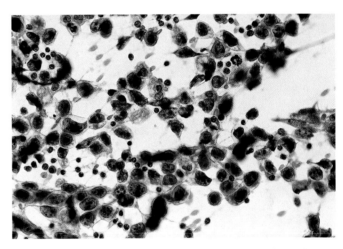

Fig. 10.4 **Germinoma**. A smear preparation from a pineal germinoma. The smear shows a characteristic dual population of large tumour cells with eosinophilic cytoplasm and well defined nuclei, along with smaller lymphocytes. H & E.

tissue; other germ cell tumour elements should be actively searched for in smear preparations containing germinoma tissue.

Cryostat sections of germinomas will also illustrate clearly the two distinct cell types within the tumour (Fig. 10.5), although it should be noted that the large tumour cells are particularly susceptible to crush artefact. The large tumour cells are arranged in solid sheets, within which irregular aggregates of lymphocytes are present. Small foci of calcification may also be identified, which can lead to diagnostic confusion with normal pineal structures or other types of tumour, particularly oligodendroglioma. In some tumours, the population of lymphocytes may be of sufficient focal density to raise the possibility of an inflammatory process; however,

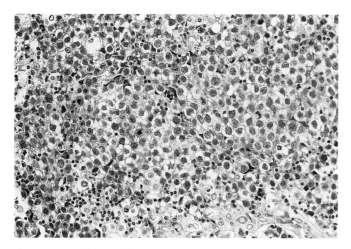

Fig. 10.5 **Germinoma**. This cryostat section shows large tumour cells with well defined cell margins, rounded nuclei with prominent nucleoli and a patchy lymphocytic infiltrate are shown. The tumour cell cytoplasm is paler than in paraffin sections. H & E.

close inspection usually reveals the characteristic large pleomorphic tumour cells with a large single nucleolus within the rounded nucleus.

Histological features

The histological features of germinomas show no particular variation in relation to the anatomical site of occurrence within the CNS. The intracranial germ cell tumours show similar histological, cytological and immunocytochemical features to the seminoma of the testis and the dysgerminoma of the ovary.[29,57,58] In larger specimens, the tumour architecture frequently exhibits a

lobular arrangement, where irregular aggregates of tumour cells and lymphocytes are divided by fibrovascular connective tissue septae (Fig. 10.6). The vascular endothelium within germinomas usually consists of small capillary channels of relatively uniform calibre, which are often surrounded by connective tissue and may show evidence of recent or previous haemorrhage.

The population of tumour cells is clearly distinguishable from the small reactive lymphocytes in paraffin sections, as in smear preparations. In paraffin sections, the large tumour cells usually exhibit a well defined cell margin around the polygonal or ovoid periphery (Figs 10.7 and 10.8); the cytoplasm usually appears more vacuolated than smear preparations, often giving a 'clear cell' appearance. This probably results from fixation artefact and this appearance is not seen in all cells within the tumour. Elsewhere, the cytoplasm is faintly eosinophilic and many tumour cells will give a strong positive reaction with a periodic acid–Schiff (PAS) stain (Fig. 10.9), unless prolonged fixation has occurred, when the PAS positivity will be significantly reduced or even abolished. The tumour cell nuclei are variable in size but usually have a rounded outline and contain a prominent single nucleolus. Other smaller nucleoli are occasionally present, and although the nuclei are pleomorphic the presence of multinucleate tumour cells should raise the suspicion of a trophoblastic element that should be investigated further by immunocytochemistry[49,57] (Table 10.3). Mitotic figures are frequently identified within the tumour cell population, and necrosis is not uncommon in large tumours. Necrosis will also occur as a consequence of tumour irradiation, which may be accompanied by reactive glial proliferation, particularly at the tumour margin.

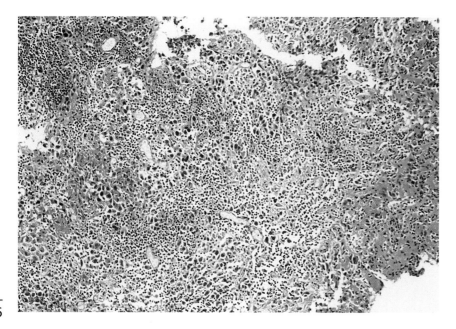

Fig. 10.6 **Germinoma**. Solid sheets of large eosinophilic tumour cells with a patchy lymphocytic infiltrate are characteristic. The pleomorphic nuclei in the tumour cell population are evident at low magnification. H & E.

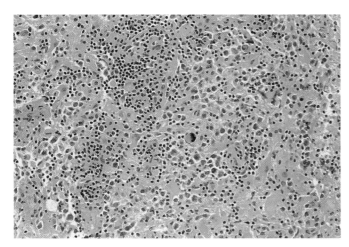

Fig. 10.7 **Germinoma**. The prominent nuclear pleomorphism in some germinomas can give rise to concerns that other germ-cell tumour elements may be present. This can be resolved on immunocytochemistry (see Table 10.3). H & E.

The lymphocytic infiltrate within germinomas consists predominantly of T-lymphocytes (Fig. 10.10), although occasional plasmacytoid cells and B-lymphocytes may also be identified.[59–61] Macrophages are usually present only in very small numbers but occasionally multinucleate foreign body-type giant cells are found, analogous to those occurring in the granulomatous reaction first described in testicular seminomas. This feature can lead to diagnostic difficulties if the possibility of a germinoma is not considered and the appropriate immunocytochemical investigations undertaken[62] (Fig. 10.11). As noted above, the presence of multinucleate giant cells should raise the suspicion of focal syncytiotrophoblastic differentiation and requires the appropriate immunocytochemical investigation (Table 10.3). In some cases of germinoma, the lymphocytic infiltrate may be sufficiently marked to raise the suspicion of a reactive

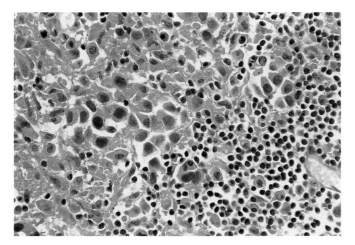

Fig. 10.8 **Germinoma**. The large tumour cells in germinomas contain abundant eosinophilic cytoplasm, often with an eccentric nucleus and areas of cohesive architecture which can mimic metastatic carcinoma. The population of small lymphocytes in contrast is uniform in terms of its nuclear morphology. H & E.

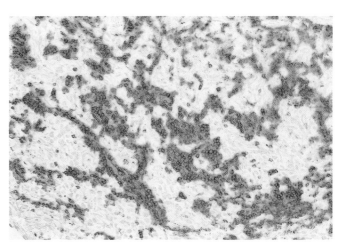

Fig. 10.10 **Germinoma**. Immunocytochemistry for CD3 demonstrates that the population of small lymphocytes within this germinoma is composed of T-cells.

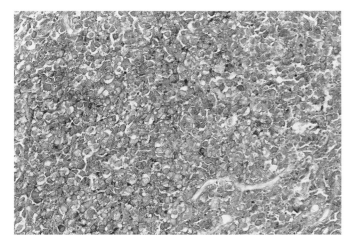

Fig. 10.9 **Germinoma**. A PAS stain shows strong cytoplasmic positivity within the tumour cells.

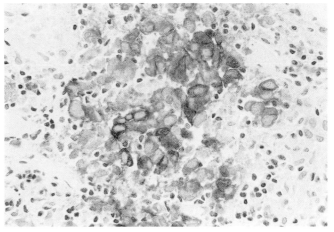

Fig. 10.11 **Germinoma**. Immunocytochemistry for PLAP. Strong cytoplasmic positivity is shown within most of the large tumour cells, although the intensity of the reaction is somewhat variable. The small lymphocytes are unstained.

inflammatory process or a primary CNS lymphoma. These difficulties can be resolved by a careful search for neoplastic cells within the lymphoid cell population and the use of immunocytochemistry for lymphoid cell subpopulations (see Chapter 11).

Since the presence of other germ cell elements within otherwise 'pure' germinomas is of adverse prognostic significance, it is essential to undertake sufficient tissue sampling both in terms of tissue blocks and levels throughout the block to ensure that no other germ cell elements are present. Most mixed germ cell tumours contain a substantial proportion of germinoma tissue; the identification of other germ cell elements is considerably facilitated by immunocytochemistry (see Table 10.3 and below).

Immunocytochemistry

Immunocytochemical investigations are invaluable in the diagnosis of intracranial germ cell tumours, particularly for the identification of elements of choriocarcinoma, yolk sac tumour or embryonal carcinoma (Table 10.3) in mixed germ cell tumours.[4,6,29,30,57,58,61] In pure germinomas, immunocytochemistry for placental alkaline phosphatase (PLAP) will give a positive reaction in a membranous distribution, with occasional cells also showing focal cytoplasmic positivity (Fig. 10.11). Focal positivity for PLAP may also be encountered in other germ cell tumours, but pure germinomas exhibit a negative reaction for alpha-fetoprotein (AFP), beta-hCG and human placental lactogen (hPL). Occasional apparently typical germinomas can show patchy positivity on immunocytochemistry for cytokeratins.[63] It is important to recognise that this is not confined to intracranial germ cell tumours and appears to be of no apparent clinical significance. The large tumour cells may also give a positive reaction on immunocytochemistry for vimentin, but this is seldom of practical use in differential diagnosis.

The lymphocytic infiltrate in germinomas will give positive staining reaction on immunocytochemistry for

CD45 and pan T-cell markers such as CD3 (Fig. 10.10), whereas only a minority of cells will react to B-cell markers such as CD20.[59–61] As mentioned above, macrophages and even occasional foreign body giant cells can be identified in tumours which contain foci of granulomatous information. In these cases, the multinucleate giant cells will give a negative reaction for beta-hCG, but a positive reaction for CD68 and other macrophage epitopes.

Electron microscopy

Relatively few detailed ultrastructural studies have been performed on intracranial germinomas, and those in the literature indicate that they exhibit similar features to testicular seminomas.[57] In particular, glycogen is abundant in the cytoplasm, which also contains conspicuous rough endoplasmic reticulum and Golgi apparatus. Intermediate filament bundles may also be identified and several types of cell junctions occur, including desmosomes.[64]

Differential diagnosis

Germinomas have in the past been confused with *pineal parenchymal neoplasms* and since the identification of pure germinomas is of major clinical and prognostic significance it is important to establish a clear differential diagnosis between these entities. In most cases, recognition of a germinoma from a *pineocytoma* is not difficult in view of the characteristic dual population of the large tumour cells and small reactive lymphocytes in the germinoma. Typical adult type pineocytomas usually contain large rosettes, but some tumours may exhibit a more solid growth pattern which is more difficult to distinguish from germinoma. The perivascular orientation of tumour cells in pineocytomas is characteristic and the tumour cells are in general smaller than the large tumour cells in germinoma. *Pineal parenchymal tumours of intermediate differentiation* usually contain a mixed population of tumour cells of varying size, which are more likely to be confused with a germinoma, particularly if the pineal rosettes are absent. Immunocytochemistry greatly facilitates differential diagnosis, since immunoreactivity for PLAP does not occur in pineocytomas, which in addition are unlikely to exhibit PAS positivity.

The distinction between germinomas and *other CNS germ cell tumours* is discussed below in terms of morphology and immunocytochemistry (Table 10.3). *Metastatic germ cell tumours* can be confused with primary CNS tumours, although the sites of occurrence are wider, and multiple lesions may be present; a full clinical history is essential to exlude this possibility.

Germinomas may be confused at intraoperative diagnosis with *oligodendroglioma* in view of the population of round cells with a centrally located nucleus and the

Table 10.3 Immunocytochemistry in CNS germ cell tumours[4,6,29,30,57,58,63]

Tumour	PLAP	beta-hCG	AFP	hPL	Cytokeratins	EMA
Germinoma	+	+[a]	–	–	+[c]/–	–
Teratoma	–	–	+[b]/–	–	+[c]	+/–
Embryonal carcinoma	+	–	–	–	+	–
Yolk sac tumour	+/–	–	+	–	+	–
Choriocarcinoma	+/–	+	–	+	+[d]	+/–

a = germinoma with syncytiotrophoblastic giant cells; b = glandular enteric tissues; c = epithelial tissues; d = syncytiotrophoblast

AFP, alpha-fetoprotein; β-hCG, beta-human chorionic gonadotropin; EMA, epithelial membrane antigen; hPL, human placental lactogen; PLAP, placental alkaline phosphatase.

absence of a gliofibrillary matrix. In addition, the finely branching vascular pattern and focal calcification present in germinomas may also cause diagnostic confusion. In paraffin sections, the differences are usually more evident, since the tumour cells of oligodendroglioma are smaller than those of germinoma, and occur without a characteristic lymphocytic infiltrate. Immunocytochemistry will facilitate differential diagnosis in paraffin sections, since oligodendrogliomas do not express PLAP and are not PAS positive.

Central neurocytoma occurs most frequently in the vicinity of the ventricular system and although it is uncommon for central neurocytomas to occur around the third ventricle, this can cause confusion with germinomas in view of the relatively uniform population of small rounded non-process forming cells in both tumours. The tumour cells in germinomas are larger than those in central neurocytomas and contain more abundant cytoplasm with a prominent centrally located nucleolus. As above, immunocytochemistry will facilitate differential diagnosis since central neurocytomas do not express PLAP and germinomas do not express synaptophysin or other neuronal proteins.

Germinomas may be confused with *malignant lymphomas* (particularly at intraoperative diagnosis) if there is an extensive population of reactive lymphocytes within the tumour, since these can mask the underlying population of large tumour cells. However, close inspection will reveal that the reactive lymphocytes and germinomas have a less marked perivascular distribution than the tumour cells in malignant lymphomas, which also contain a wide variety of nuclear morphology and exhibit mitotic and activity and invasion of the blood vessel wall. The neoplastic cells in germinomas are larger than those in most malignant lymphomas and, in contrast, exhibit a relatively uniform appearance. Immunocytochemistry can aid differential diagnosis by using the appropriate antibodies to lymphoid cells (see Chapter 11) and PLAP.

Pituitary adenomas or carcinomas may be confused with germinomas which arise in the region of the hypothalamus. The dual cell population characteristic of germinomas is not encountered in pituitary adenomas which are usually more vascular than germinomas and exhibit a wider range of nuclear morphology. Immunocytochemistry will also resolve this possibility since germinomas do not react with antibodies to anterior pituitary hormones or neuroendocrine proteins such as chromogranin.

The large tumour cells in germinomas may be confused with those in *malignant melanoma* since both tumours contain cells which frequently exhibit a rounded outline with a prominent cell margin, a large nucleus with a prominent single nucleolus and relatively abundant eosinophilic cytoplasm. However, the tumour cells in malignant melanoma are frequently larger than in germinomas and usually (but not always) contain visible melanin pigment. Mitotic activity in malignant melanoma is usually more marked than in germinoma and there is not a conspicuous lymphocytic infiltrate in most metastatic melanoma deposits. Immunocytochemistry can also resolve this potential difficulty, since malignant melanomas do not express PLAP and germinomas do not express HMB45, S-100 protein or neuron specific enolase. Electron microscopy will also allow a clear distinction between these tumours, with premelanosomes and melanosomes present in malignant melanoma, but not germinoma cells.

The large tumour cells in germinomas may also be confused with *metastatic carcinoma*, particularly if there is evidence of necrosis. The solid or lobulated growth pattern characteristic of germinomas may also be encountered in metastatic carcinomas, but the clearly defined cell margins in germinomas and the relative uniformity of the nuclei are aids to differential diagnosis. As above, immunocytochemistry is invaluable in clarifying this differential diagnosis, since metastatic carcinomas do not express PLAP or other germ cell markers. As noted above, germinomas may focally express cytokeratins (and occasionally epithelial membrane antigen) but this does not occur in such a widespread distribution as in most metastatic carcinomas. The PAS positivity which is characteristic of germinomas should not be confused with that occurring in metastatic adenocarcinomas. The differential diagnosis for germinomas is summarised in Table 10.4.

Therapy

The diagnosis of germinomas and other intracranial germ cell tumours has been greatly facilitated by the use of stereotactic neurosurgical biopsy,[1,3] accompanied by CSF studies of the germ cell markers AFP, beta-hCG and PLAP.[18,22,28,65] Advances in neuroradiology have also allowed the easy detection and delineation of intracranial germinomas at all sites in the neuroaxis. Since germinomas are sensitive to irradiation,[66,67] many neurosurgeons will prefer to perform a stereotactic biopsy without further neurosurgical exploration. However, tumour resection may be achievable for both pineal and hypothalamic tumours; surgical complications may include extraocular movement abnormalities, ataxia and altered mental status for pineal region tumours, and visual disturbance and endocrine abnormalities from hypothalamic tumours.[1,3] Germinomas are markedly sensitive to irradiation, which is frequently curative.[67,68] Surgery followed by irradiation of 5000 cGy have been accompanied by 10-year survivals of at least 70%, with recent series reporting 10-year survival at around 90% and 20-year survival at 80%.[3,67,68] However, long term complications of radiotherapy may

Table 10.4 Differential diagnosis of CNS germ cell tumours

Tumour	Differential diagnosis
Germinoma	Other CNS germ cell tumours
	Pineocytoma
	Pituitary adenoma
	Oligodendroglioma
	Central neurocytoma
	Lymphoma
	Metastatic malignant melanoma
	Metastatic carcinoma
	Metastatic seminoma / dysgerminoma
Mature teratoma	Dermoid cyst
	Epidermoid cyst
	Craniopharyngioma
	Rathke's cleft cyst
	Ganglioglioma
	Brain heterotopia
	Metastatic carcinoma
	Metastatic sarcoma
	Other CNS germ cell tumours
Immature teratoma	Other CNS germ cell tumours
	Metastatic teratoma
	Medulloepithelioma
	Neuroblastoma
	PNET
	Ependymoblastoma
	Pineoblastoma
	Metastatic neuroblastoma
Teratoma with malignant transformation	Other CNS germ cell tumours
	Metastatic teratoma
	Metastatic carcinoma
	Metastatic sarcoma
	Gliomas – astrocytoma, oligodendroglioma, ependymoma
Mixed germ cell tumour	Other CNS germ cell tumours
	Metastatic germ cell tumours
	Metastatic carcinoma
	Metastatic sarcoma
	Metastatic neuroblastoma
Embryonal carcinoma	Other CNS germ cell tumours
	Metastatic germ cell tumours
	Metastatic carcinoma
	Metastatic melanoma
Yolk sac tumour	Other CNS germ cell tumours
	Metastatic germ cell tumours
	Metastatic carcinoma
Choriocarcinoma	Other CNS germ cell tumours
	Metastatic germ cell tumours
	Glioblastoma

PNET, primary neuroectodermal tumour
CNS, central nervous system

occur including cognitive deficits, endocrine abnormalities and, less commonly, radiation induced necrosis. These delayed complications are likely to be identifiable should they occur in patients with germinomas because of their prolonged survival. Recurrence of germinomas has been reported following irradiation at all primary sites in the CNS.[69] Trials of chemotherapy as a main treatment for germinomas and other intracranial germ cell tumours are currently under way.[70–72]

Prognosis

The prognosis of all intracranial germ cell tumours is greatly influenced by the histological subtype,[73] which places a high priority on the neuropathologist concerned with the diagnosis of intracranial tumours accurately to identify and categorise the different varieties of intracranial germ cell tumours. The prognostic significance of occasional syncytiotrophoblastic giant cells in monomorphic germ cell tumours other than choriocarcinomas remains uncertain, although earlier reports have suggested that even small numbers of these cells in germinomas may adversely influence survival.[4,72] Germinomas have the capacity to infiltrate the ventricular system and the spinal meninges; the incidence of CSF spread has been widely variable in the literature (52% in a recent study).[74] Accordingly, it has been suggested that prophylactic craniospinal irradiation should be considered as part of a management regime. Systemic metastases from intracranial germinomas have also been reported, some of which have occurred as intra-abdominal metastases via a ventriculoperitoneal shunt.[75–77] Recurrence of the tumour locally or tumour metastasis is of adverse prognostic significance,[18] although chemotherapy has been shown to be effective in CNS germinoma even after distant blood borne metastases.[22,73] A recent review has reported a 5-year survival of 96% for pure germinomas;[73] this is likely to continue to improve as more efficient ways of delivering radiation therapy into small volumes of the CNS become available.

Teratoma

Teratomas comprise an irregular and often bizarre admixture of ectodermal, endodermal and mesodermal tissues. The spectrum of differentiation, however, varies enormously from case to case; this is reflected in the earlier terminology for these lesions, which comprise a wide range of terms now considered obsolete (see Ref. 78 for review). Teratomas are classified according to the degree of differentiation in the three major components as mature, immature or teratomas with malignant areas.[15] This section is concerned with teratomas arising in the brain and in the region of the spinal cord; sacrococcygeal region teratomas are discussed below.

Incidence and site

As mentioned above, teratomas are rare and occur predominantly within the first two decades of life.[1,3,30,79] The commonest sites for these tumours are in the pineal gland and the suprasellar regions; occasional tumours have been described in the posterior fossa and basal ganglia.[2,4,18,80,81] Intracranial teratomas are one of the commonest forms of congenital brain tumours, most of which at this age occur in females.[25,26,30] Some congenital tumours can reach an enormous size and occasionally result in severe complications during delivery.[82] Reported series of pineal teratomas suggest a male predominance, with onset at an earlier age than pineal region germinomas.[24,83]

Pathology

Macroscopic features

The structure, growth pattern and macroscopic features of teratomas reflect their individual tissue constituents, and (as might be expected) this varies enormously from case to case. However, a few general principles can be applied; most mature teratomas are well defined apparently encapsulated lesions which grow by expansion and compression of the adjacent structures. Many are cystic and on cross section contain abundant keratin, cartilage, hair, bone and (vary rarely) teeth.[84] Leakage of the cyst contents can result in a foreign body giant cell reaction in the adjacent tissues, which makes neurosurgical resection difficult, even with an apparently well encapsulated lesion. In contrast, immature teratomas and teratomas with malignant areas invade and infiltrate adjacent structures, with a less well defined tumour margin. The cut surfaces of these tumours do not always exhibit the well defined structures present in the mature teratomas and frequently contain multiple areas of haemorrhage and necrosis (Fig. 10.12). A remarkable example of an intracranial teratoma containing multiple fetuses has been recorded.[85]

Cryostat sections and smear preparations

Mature teratomas are frequently composed of solid tissue elements which do not smear easily. In all teratomas, smear preparations often contain a mixture of different cell types, in which epithelial and glial tissues may be present. However, the diagnosis of teratoma is often better made on cryostat sections, when the nature of the multiple constituent tissue types and their relationship to each other can be readily appreciated (Fig. 10.13). Immature tissue elements are better recognised in cryostat sections than smear preparations, where they may be mistaken for malignant neuroepithelial tissue (Figs 10.14 and 10.15). Sampling of the lesions for intraoperative diagnosis is important and extensively haemorrhagic or necrotic tissues best avoided. Likewise, the tumour capsule or margin may exhibit a wide range of reactive changes including astrocytosis, chronic inflammation and a foreign-body giant cell reaction to

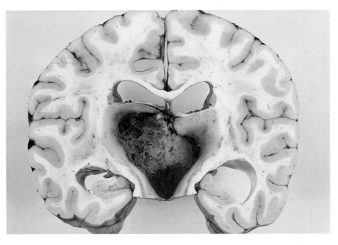

Fig. 10.12 **Malignant teratoma.** This tumour arose in the pineal region and invaded the thalamus and third ventricle. The patient was an 8-year-old boy who had been treated with radiotherapy and chemotherapy, which was followed by a massive tumour recurrence and haemorrhage.

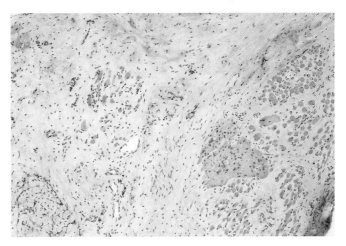

Fig. 10.13 **Mature teratoma.** Cryostat section. An irregular admixture of mature neural, skeletal muscle and connective tissue elements are shown including prominent blood vessels. H & E.

leaked keratin and its breakdown products. This can give a misleading appearance at intraoperative diagnosis and tissue sampling from viable areas towards the periphery of the tumour is to be recommended.

Microscopic features

Mature teratoma Mature teratomas are readily identifiable as they contain a bizarre mixture of tissue elements that show no evidence of malignancy.[15,79] In particular, mitotic activity is inconspicuous, and necrosis is usually absent. Most examples are cystic, with multiple irregular cavities lined by respiratory or enteric-type epithelium (Fig. 10.16). Occasional structures resembling the gut can be formed with mucosa and a muscular coat

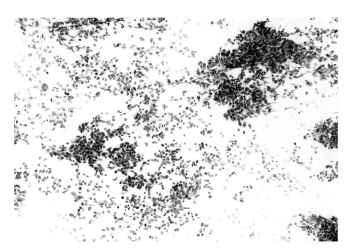

Fig. 10.14 **Immature teratoma**. Smear preparation. A population of poorly differentiated small anaplastic cells are shown which can be confused with PNET, cerebral neuroblastoma and metastatic lesions. Toluidine blue.

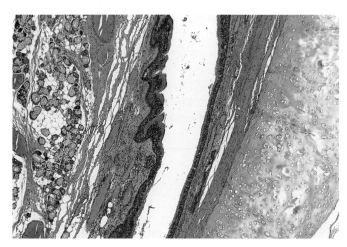

Fig. 10.16 **Mature teratoma**. Enteric epithelium (centre) is often a prominent feature in mature teratomas. In this case an admixture with cartilage and salivary tissue is shown. H & E.

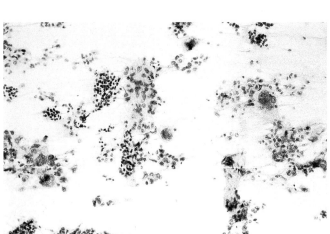

Fig. 10.15 **Teratoma with malignant transformation**. Smear preparation showing a mixed population of small primitive tumour cells and larger pleomorphic cells with abundant cytoplasm, superficially resembling glioblastoma are shown. Toluidine blue.

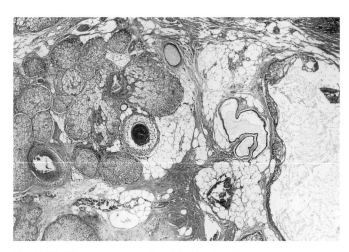

Fig. 10.17 **Mature teratoma**. Paraffin histology in a mature teratoma. A bizarre admixture of tissues is depicted, often including large cystic structures lined by respiratory epithelium, nerve fibres, pilosebaceous structures and adipose tissue. Care must be taken to differentiate the lesion from a dermoid cyst if neuroectodermal tissue is not prominent. H & E.

which is often incomplete. Solid or cystic foci of squamous epithelium may also be present; the cysts are usually distended with keratin. Mesodermal components usually comprise striated or smooth muscle, cartilage, bone and fat (Fig. 10.17). Hair shaft structures may be abundant, and some of the cysts may contain hair strands in addition to keratin produced by the lining squamous epithelium. Ectodermal tissue components include skin, choroid plexus and neuroepithelial tissues which can include both glial and neuronal components.

Teratomas with malignant transformation This group of tumours also comprises 'adult-type' tissue elements, similar to those seen in the mature teratoma.[15,79] However, in this category of tumour at least one of the constituent elements undergoes malignant transformation.

This most often occurs in the mesenchymal tissue, resulting in a rhabdomyosarcoma (Fig. 10.18) or other forms of sarcoma,[86] or less commonly in the epithelial tissues resulting in a carcinoma (often an adenocarcinoma) (Fig. 10.19) or, rarely, a carcinoid tumour.[87,88] The nature of the malignant component can be further investigated by appropriate techniques, including immunocytochemistry and electron microscopy as for the corresponding form of malignancy arising at the appropriate site in the body. In this group of tumours (and to a lesser extent in mature teratomas) the presence of glandular enteric epithelium can result in elevated levels of AFP in the CSF, which should not be interpreted as indicative of malignant germ cell elements or yolk sac tumour.

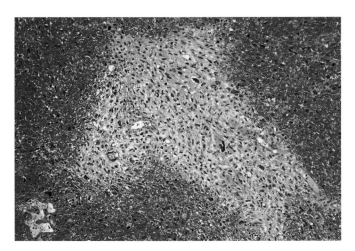

Fig. 10.18 **Teratoma with malignant transformation.** Rhabdomyosarcoma arising in a teratoma with widespread haemorrhage. Strap cells are present, which give a strong positive reaction on immunocytochemistry for desmin. H & E.

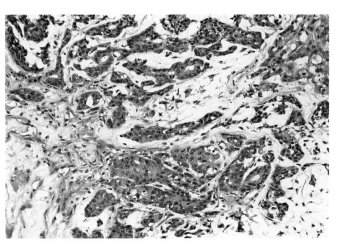

Fig. 10.19 **Teratoma with malignant transformation.** Adenocarcinoma arising in a teratoma, surrounded by cartilaginous tissue. H & E.

Fig. 10.20 **Immature teratoma.** Primitive neuroectodermal tissue forms characteristic tubular structures, admixed with cystic tissue lined by epithelium. H & E.

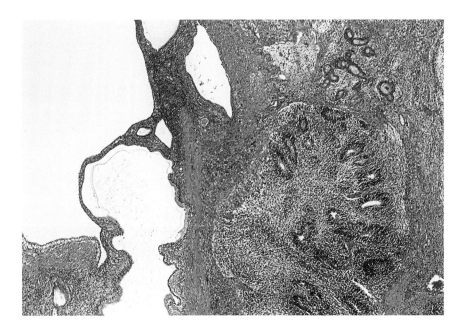

Immature teratoma This group of tumours constitutes the majority of teratomas arising within the CNS.[65,79,83] The immature tissue component frequently comprises primitive embryonic mesenchymal tissue or neuroectodermal tissue which may contain rosettes and canalicular structures which are reminiscent of the developing neural tube and resemble ependymoblastic rosettes (see Chapter 7) (Fig. 10.20). The immature neuroepithelial structures can include structures resembling medulloepithelioma, neuroblastoma, ependymoblastoma, retinoblastoma or melanotic neuroepithelial tissue. Most immature teratomas also contain mature tissue elements, and the immature tissue component can represent only a small component of the tumour. It is therefore essential when sampling and examining a teratoma to ensure that enough representative material has been examined in order to be certain that a small focus of immature tissue has not been overlooked, as this will undoubtedly influence the diagnosis and treatment of the patient.

Differential diagnosis

Well differentiated teratomas may be confused with *epidermoid or dermoid cysts*; the identification of neuroectodermal and other forms of mesenchymal tissue is obviously of major diagnostic importance. Confusion with other forms of suprasellar cyst can also be made including *Rathke's cleft cyst* and *craniopharyngioma* (particularly the squamous papillary type); this can be resolved by the identification of neuroectodermal tissue both histologically and by immunocytochemistry as appropriate. Mature teratomas containing a predominance of neuroepithelial tissue with mature glial and neuronal elements can be confused with a *brain heterotopia*, a *hypothalamic hamartoma* or a well differentiated *ganglioglioma*. In such cases, careful inspection for the mesodermal and endodermal components will ensure the appropriate diagnosis of mature teratoma.

Teratoma with malignant areas can be confused with metastatic tumours including *metastatic sarcomas and carcinomas*. However, the identification of neuroectodermal and mesodermal components as part of the lesion will ensure an appropriate diagnosis. Because of the bizarre admixture of tissues and teratomas it is important to is important to study carefully the nature of the constituent cells in order that a bizarre arrangement of gland-like structures is not mistakenly diagnosed as an infiltrating *adenocarcinoma*, or that a predominance of irregularly arranged muscle fibres is not mistaken for a *rhabdomyosarcoma*. A malignant glial component can be confused with an intrinsic *glioma*, but careful inspection will usually reveal the characteristic admixture of cell types.

The identification of primitive neuroepithelial tissue in immature teratomas requires careful assessment of the cytological features, in which nuclear pleomorphism and mitotic activity are readily identifiable. In particular, careful differentiation from *immature normal CNS elements*, including the external granular cell layer of the cerebellum and residual cerebral periventricular germinal matrix, is essential for diagnosis. Although this is a particular problem in congenital and infantile tumours, immature normal CNS elements do not exhibit the cytological and nuclear pleomorphism characteristic of immature teratomas. Immature teratomas can also be mistaken for forms of CNS embryonal tumours including *medulloepithelioma, neuroblastoma, PNET, ependymoblastoma, pineoblastoma and neuroblastoma*. The characteristic glandular and canalicular-like structures within the primitive neuroectoderm is usually sufficient to ensure accurate diagnosis, and the identification of other immature elements, e.g. cartilage, or the presence of other mature tissue elements in the lesion will avoid this potential difficulty. This in turn is dependent on accurate tissue sampling and a close inspection and identification of the constituent cell types within the lesion, and by immunocytochemistry for PLAP (Table 10.3). The differential diagnosis for CNS teratomas is summarised in Table 10.4.

Therapy and prognosis

Recent developments in the neurosurgical approaches to pineal and hypothalamic region tumours have enabled resection (either partial or complete) of teratomas, but in many cases surgery is confined to stereotactic biopsy.[3] The influence of surgery on outcome is dependent on the histological diagnosis of the subtype of teratoma, since immature teratomas and teratomas with malignant areas are better treated by a gross total surgical resection.[1,3] Radiation therapy is particularly important in the treatment of germ cell tumours, although the responses to treatment in teratomas are not as high as in germinomas.[19,73] Chemotherapy for germ cell tumours in the CNS has been based upon successful treatments for corresponding tumours arising in the testis and most nongerminomatous tumours are treated with chemotherapy prior to irradiation. However, there is no consensus on the optimal time of administration of chemotherapy, or of the best combination of drugs although the combination of chemotherapy including cisplatin and etoposide has resulted in improved response rates.[73]

Mature teratomas are generally associated with good 5- and 10-year survival rates of over 90%, but in malignant teratomas the survival rate is much lower and most patients rarely live beyond 2 years following diagnosis.[1,70,73] This is likely to improve following recent advances in chemotherapy. Interestingly, some immature teratomas have been shown to undergo differentiation and maturation following treatment, but it is not certain as to whether this is a consequence of the treatment itself or is part of the natural biology of this intriguing group of neoplasms.[89] The 'growing teratoma' syndrome is a recognised complication of non-germinomatous germ cell tumours, when a residual mature teratoma component continues to enlarge after chemotherapy.[90]

Spinal teratomas

The commonest form of teratoma to occur in the region of the spine is the sacrococcygeal teratoma (see below), which usually does not involve the spinal cord. Other teratomas are uncommon in the region of the spine although occasional cases have been described, including one in which a carcinoid tumour arose within a recurrent teratoma.[88]

Other germ cell tumours

The remaining categories of germ cell tumours (choriocarcinoma, yolk sac tumour and embryonal cell carcinoma) can be conveniently grouped together for purposes of discussion, since they are all extremely rare as 'pure' entities and tend to behave in a similar aggressive fashion which is associated with a poor clinical outcome.[73] The tumours all exhibit malignant behaviour and cannot be distinguished reliably on clinical grounds, although the use of biochemical analysis of the CSF may give an indication of the predominant tissue component in yolk sac tumours (AFP) and choriocarcinoma (beta-hCG and hPL). These tumours can arise at either the pineal or suprasellar sites and are ill-defined invasive lesions which have a propensity to spread via the CSF. Haemorrhage is common within all three tumour categories, particularly choriocarcinoma. As in other rapidly growing malignant germ cell tumours, foci of necrosis are characteristically present.

Embryonal carcinoma

This neoplasm is composed of large cells with abundant cytoplasm and ill-defined borders which can grow in solid sheets, cords or gland-like structures with poorly developed papillae[4,15] (Fig. 10.21). The cells contain a variable quantity of eosinophilic or clear cytoplasm and have large rounded clear vesicular nuclei with prominent nucleolus; nuclear 'crowding' is common. Mitotic activity is usually widespread and multiple foci of necrosis and haemorrhage may occur[91,92] (Fig. 10.22). The stroma is variable, and can include solid areas which may give rise to the suspicion that the tumour is a teratoma. The tumour cells exhibit positive immunocytochemical staining with antibodies to PLAP and cytokeratins, a combination which distinguishes them from most other germ cell tumours. Immunocytochemistry for epithelial membrane antigen (EMA) and beta-hCG is negative, and for AFP and hPL is positive only in occasional cells (Table 10.3).

Yolk sac tumour

This neoplasm is composed of small primitive cells set in a loose matrix. These vary from elongated spindle cells to columnar cells, and contain relatively uniform rounded nuclei. The tumour cells can be arranged in a wide variety of patterns, including solid, cystic or papillary structures[4,15] (Fig. 10.23). Typically, the tumour cells form sinusoidal channels around Schiller–Duval bodies, composed of fibrovascular projections covered by papillary collections of tumour cells (Fig. 10.24). Eosinophilic, PAS positive hyaline globular structures are a characteristic feature which can be identified most often within the stroma, but are also present in some tumour cells. These structures exhibit strong immunoreactivity for AFP, which also will stain the cytoplasm of some tumour cells, facilitating differential diagnosis from other germ cell

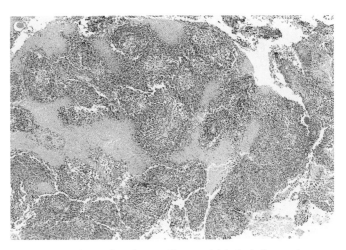

Fig. 10.22 **Embryonal carcinoma**. These multiple foci of necrosis resemble glioblastoma at low-power magnification. H & E.

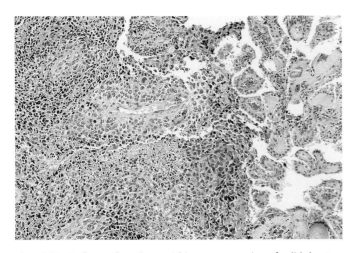

Fig. 10.21 **Embryonal carcinoma**. This tumour consists of solid sheets of large pale-staining cells with poorly defined margins, invading the wall of the third ventricle and choroid plexus. H & E.

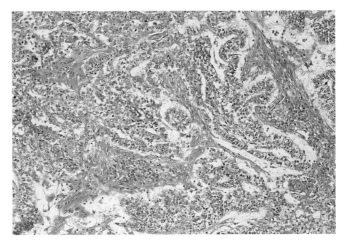

Fig. 10.23 **Yolk sac tumour**. This tumour comprises delicate stands of pale-staining cells, often with a pseudopapillary structure. H & E.

tumours[93–95] (Fig. 10.25). Necrosis is less frequently observed in yolk sac tumours than in embryonal carcinoma or choriocarcinoma, but mitotic activity is usually readily identifiable.

Choriocarcinoma

This extremely rare form of germ cell tumour is identifiable histologically by the presence of both syncytio- and cytotrophoblastic elements.[4,15] However, it should be remembered that occasional syncytiotrophoblastic cells can occur within otherwise typical germinomas (and occasionally in embryonal carcinomas and yolk sac tumours) and these will exhibit an identical immunophenotype.[49] The giant cells frequently contain irregular clusters of nuclei arising in large sheet-like aggregates of cells containing abundant glassy cytoplasm

which is frequently eosinophilic. The cytotrophoblastic component may comprise the bulk of the tumour. This contains uniform cells with a single vesicular nucleus and pale-staining cytoplasm which form cohesive solid sheets. Irregular vascular channels are characteristically present in choriocarcinomas and these can form large sinusoidal dilatations, frequently accompanied by extensive haemorrhage and necrosis[96–98] (Fig. 10.26). The syncytiotrophoblastic elements characteristically comprise large multinucleate giant cells which exhibit strong staining on immunocytochemistry for beta-hCG and hPL, the latter allowing a clear differentiation from most other germ cell tumours[96–99] (Fig. 10.27).

Differential diagnosis

The differential diagnosis for embryonal carcinoma, yolk sac tumour and choriocarcinoma includes *other CNS germ*

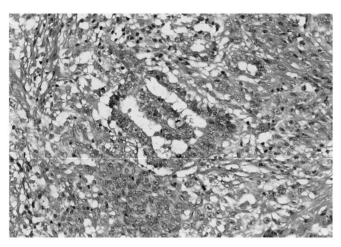

Fig. 10.24 **Yolk sac tumour**. A Schiller–Duval body (centre) can be seen. This is a characteristic histological feature in yolk sac tumours. H & E.

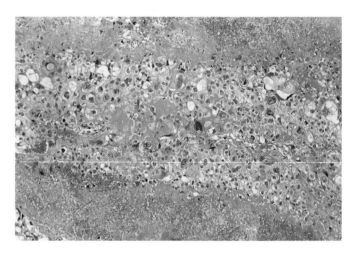

Fig. 10.26 **Choriocarcinoma**. Choriocarcinomas are often extensively haemorrhagic, which requires a careful search for the characteristic syncytio- and cytotrophoblastic cells. H & E.

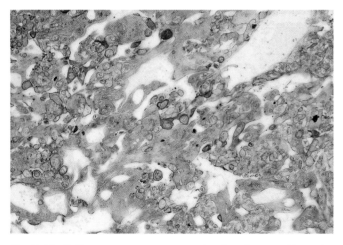

Fig. 10.25 **Yolk sac tumour**. Immunocytochemistry for AFP. This results in an intense positive reaction within the eosinophilic droplets in a yolk sac tumour, with a more variable pattern of positivity in the tumour cells.

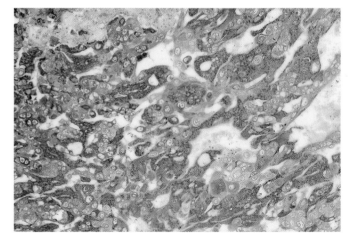

Fig. 10.27 **Choriocarcinoma**. Immunocytochemistry for beta-hCG gives a strong positive reaction in the syncytiotrophoblastic elements.

cell tumours. Adequate sampling for histology, careful attention to morphology (as described above) and immunocytochemistry will help resolve most difficulties; the opinion of an expert on germ cell tumours arising elsewhere in the body will be helpful. *Metastatic germ cell tumours* should also be considered in the differential diagnosis; metastatic tumours are frequently multiple and widely distributed in the CNS, and a relevant clinical history is essential. *Metastatic carcinoma* can be confused with embryonal carcinoma, and occasionally with yolk sac tumour; immunocytochemistry and relevant clinical data will help clarify this difficulty. The large nuclei and prominent nucleoli of embryonal carcinoma may be confused with *malignant melanoma*, but the growth pattern of the tumour usually allows a clear distinction to be made, which can be further reinforced by immunocytochemistry (Table 10.3). Choriocarcinoma may be confused with *other neoplasms containing mutinucleate giant cells*, including *glioblastoma*, but immunocytochemistry will demonstrate the diagnostic immunophenotype for this rare neoplasm. The differential diagnosis for these rare neoplasms is summarised in Table 10.4.

Therapy and prognosis

The prognosis for patients with choriocarcinoma, embryonal carcinoma and yolk sac tumour in the CNS is poor with most patients being dead within 2 years of diagnosis, despite treatment with radiotherapy and chemotherapy.[2,17,18,73] In addition to extensive local invasion, these tumours can metastatise through the CSF pathway to the spinal leptomeninges and both blood-borne spread to the lung and bone and ventriculo-peritoneal shunt related metastases have been recorded.[7,27,92,100]

Mixed germ cell tumours

Mixed germ cell tumours account for a significant proportion of CNS germ cell tumours (see Table 10.2) and this possibility should always be borne in mind when a germ cell tumour of the CNS is under histological investigation. This requires adequate histological sampling and immunocytochemistry in order to ensure that germ cell elements other than the predominant histological type can be excluded. It should also be noted that the presence of beta-hCG-positive giant cells in germinomas may be of adverse significance in terms of prognosis and response to treatment (see above). In most mixed germ cell tumours there is an admixture of germinoma, immature teratoma and other germ cell tumour elements (Figs 10.28 and 10.29). The identification of these different histological tumour types is of major significance in determining prognosis (particularly in

tumours with predominant features of germinoma or mature teratoma), since very poor survival rates are reported in malignant mixed germ cell tumours (most patients are dead within 1 year of diagnosis).[7,18,73]

Sacrococcygeal teratoma

Teratomas involving the sacrococcygeal region occur at a frequency of around 1 in 40 000 live births, and usually present during the neonatal period of life with an enlarging deformity that can reach enormous proportions if untreated.[101,102] Far fewer present in childhood and early adulthood with pain and structural disruption of the vertebrae and compression of the spinal cord, bowel, bladder and sciatic nerves.[103] Most of these lesions occur in females and are not associated with germ cell tumours

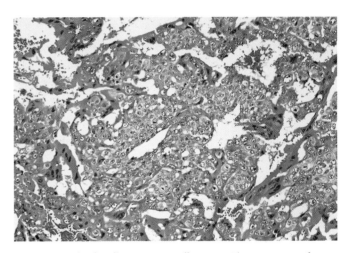

Fig. 10.28 **Mixed malignant germ cell tumour.** These tumours often contain embryonal carcinoma, with cords of pale-staining cells, and sheets of syncytiotrophoblastic elements which are more intensely eosinophilic. H & E.

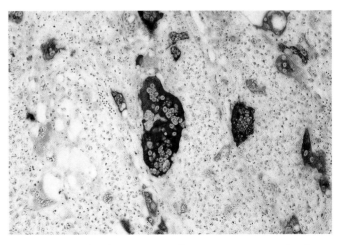

Fig. 10.29 **Mixed malignant germ cell tumour.** Immunocytochemistry for beta-hCG. Strong cytoplasmic staining is shown in syncytiotrophoblastic elements.

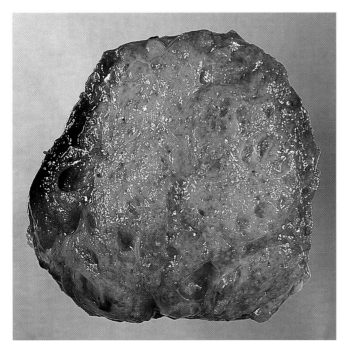

Fig. 10.30 **Sacrococcygeal teratoma**. This large sacrococcygeal teratoma is a well defined lobulated mass. It comprises large quantities of adipose tissue with cystic and haemorrhagic areas. This case was resected from a 9-day-old girl, following prenatal detection by ultrasound. (Courtesy of Dr J Keeling, Edinburgh.)

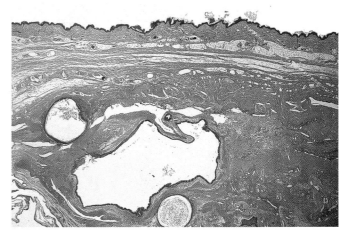

Fig. 10.31 **Sacrococcygeal teratoma**. Histology of the specimen in Fig. 10.30. This shows an irregular mixture of mature glandular, neural and connective tissue elements in the subcutaneous tissue. H & E.

in other areas of the body. The presacral and coccygeal regions are most often involved by a progressively enlarging partly-encapsulated mass which protrudes into the soft tissue and muscle of the lumbar and gluteal regions (Fig. 10.30). Intradural extension is an uncommon occurrence. On macroscopic examination, the tumour usually contains a large quantity of fatty tissue, with both solid and cystic areas. Focal haemorrhage is usually present, but necrosis is uncommon. Histological examination reveals that most cases are examples of mature teratomas with the usual bizarre admixture of tissues derived from all three cell layers[101] (Fig. 10.31). Some sacrococcygeal teratomas contain immature tissue, usually immature neuroectodermal tissue, but this does not appear to alter the prognosis substantially.[102] Complete excision is usually curative for both benign and malignant non-metastatic lesions, and should be accompanied by removal of the coccyx in order to avoid recurrence from any residual teratomatous tissue.[104] A small number of tumours (less than 5%) contain malignant elements, which can result in local recurrence or metastases.[102] Survival for patients with malignant metastatic teratomas is excellent with current chemotherapeutic regimes. Diagnosis of sacrococcygeal teratoma in utero is now possible, and fetal surgery has been proposed in selected cases.[105]

REFERENCES

1. Bruce DA, Schut L, Sutton LN. Pineal tumours. In: McLaurin RL, Venes JL, Schut L, Epstein F, eds. Pediatric neurosurgery. Philadelphia: W B Saunders, 1989: pp 409–416
2. Bruce JN. Pineal tumors. Neurosurg Clin N Am, 1990; 1:123–138
3. Edwards MBS, Baumgartner JE. Pineal region tumors. In: Cheek WR, Marlin AE, McLone DG et al. eds. Pediatric neurosurgery. Philadelphia: W B Saunders, 1994: pp 429–436
4. Kleihues P, Cavanee WK, eds. World Health Organization classification of tumours. Pathology and genetics of tumours of the nervous system. IARC Press, Lyon, 2000
5. Ghatak NR, Hirano A, Zimmerman HM. Intrasellar germinomas: a form of ectopic pinealoma. J Neurosurg, 1969; 31:670–675
6. Schild SE, Scheithauer BW, Haddock MG et al. Histologically confirmed pineal tumors and other germ cell tumors of the brain. Cancer, 1996; 78:2564–2571
7. Jennings MT, Gelman R, Hochberg F. Intracranial germ cell tumors: natural history and pathogenesis. J Neurosurg, 1985; 63:155–167
8. Hisa S, Morinaga S, Kobayashi Y et al. Intramedullary spinal cord germinoma producing HCG and precocious puberty in a boy. Cancer, 1985; 55:2845–2849
9. Itoh Y, Mineura K, Sasajima H et al. Intramedullary spinal cord germinoma: case report and review of the literature. Neurosurgery, 1996; 38:187–190
10. Matsuyama Y, Nagasaka T, Mimatsu K et al. Intramedullary spinal cord germinoma. Spine, 1995; 20:2338–2340
11. Masuzawa T, Shimabukuro H, Nakahara N et al. Germ cell tumors (germinoma and yolk sac tumor) in unusual sites in the brain. Clin Neuropathol, 1986; 5:190–202
12. Higano S, Takahashi S, Ishii K et al. Germinoma originating in the basal ganglia and thalamus: MR and CT evaluation. Am J Neuroradiol, 1994; 15:1435–1441
13. Kobayashi T, Kageyama N, Kida Y et al. Unilateral germinomas involving the basal ganglia and thalamus. J Neurosurg, 1981; 55:55–62
14. Tamaki N, Lin T, Shirataki K. Germ cell tumors of the thalamus and the basal ganglia. Childs Nerv Syst, 1990; 3–7
15. Mostofi FK, Sesterhenn IA. Histological typing of testis tumours. Berlin: Springer-Verlag, 1998
16. Dearnaley DP, A'Hern RP, Whittaker S et al. Pineal and CNS germ cell tumours: Royal Marsden Hospital experience 1962–1987. Int J Radiat Oncol Biol Phys, 1990; 18:773–781
17. Donat JF, Okazaki H, Gomez MR et al. Pineal tumors. A 53-year experience. Arch Neurol, 1978; 35:736–740
18. Hoffman HJ, Otsubo H, Hendrick EB et al. Intracranial germ cell tumors in children. J Neurosurg, 1991; 545–551

19. Hoffman HJ, Yoshida M, Becker LE et al. Pineal region tumors in childhood. Experience at the Hospital for Sick Children. Pediatr Neurosurg, 1994; 21:91–104
20. Brain Tumor Registry Committee. A statistical study of brain tumors in Japan: general features. Jpn J Clin Oncol, 1987; 17:19–28
21. Koide O, Watanabe Y, Sato K. A pathological survey of intracranial germinoma and pinealoma in Japan. Cancer, 1980; 45:2119–2130
22. Matsutani M, Sano K, Takakura K et al. Primary intracranial germ cell tumors: a clinical analysis of 153 histologically verified cases. J Neurosurg, 1997; 86:446–455
23. Horowitz MB, Hall WA. Central nervous system germinomas. A review. Arch Neurol, 1991; 48:652–657
24. Jellinger K. Primary intracranial germ cell tumors. Acta Neuropathol, 1973; 25:291–306
25. Ferreira J, Eviatar L, Schneider S et al. Prenatal diagnosis of intracranial teratoma. Ped Neurosurg, 1993; 19:84–88
26. Greenhouse AH, Neubuerger KT. Intracranial teratoma of the newborn. Arch Neurol, 1960; 3:718–724
27. Bamberg M, Metz K, Alberti W et al. Endodermal sinus tumor of the pineal region. Metastases through a ventriculoperitoneal shunt. Cancer, 1984; 54:903–906
28. Ho DM, Liu H-C. Primary intracranial germ cell tumor. Pathologic study of 51 patients. Cancer, 1992; 70:1577–1584
29. Bjornsson J, Scheithauer BW, Okazaki H et al. Intracranial germ cell tumors: pathobiological and immunohistochemical aspects of 70 cases. J Neuropathol Exp Neurol, 1985; 44:32–46
30. Rueda-Pedraza ME, Heifetz SA, Sesterhenn IA et al. Primary intracranial germ cell tumors in the first two decades of life. A clinical, light-microscopic and immunohistochemical analysis of 54 cases. Perspect Ped Pathol, 1987; 10:160–207
31. Rosai J, Parkash V, Reuter VE. The origin of mediastinal germ cell tumors in man. Int J Surg Pathol, 1994; 2:73–78
32. Friedman NB, Van de Velde RL. Germ cell tumors in man, pleiotropic mice and continuity of germplasm and somatoplasm. Hum Pathol, 1981; 12:772–776
33. Sano K. Pathogenesis of intracranial germ cell tumors reconsidered. J Neurosurg, 1999; 90:258–264
34. Ahagon A, Yoshida Y, Kusuno et al. Suprasellar germinoma in association with Klinefelter's syndrome. J Neurosurg, 1983; 58:136–138
35. Arens R, Marcus D, Engelberg S et al. Cerebral germinomas and Klinefelter syndrome. A review. Cancer, 1988; 61:1228–1231
36. Hashimoto T, Sasagawa I, Ishigooka M et al. Down's syndrome associated with intracranial germinoma and testicular embryonal carcinoma. Urol Int, 1995; 55:120–122
37. Laing RW, Brada M. Intracranial germ cell tumour in association with cryptorchidism. Clin Oncol, 1992; 4:269–270
38. Fujita T, Yamada K, Saitoh H et al. Intracranial germinomas and Down's syndrome – case report. Neurol Med Chir (Tokyo), 1992; 32:163–165
39. Tanabe M, Mizushima M, Anno Y et al. Intracranial germinoma with Down's syndrome: a case report and review of the literature. Surg Neurol, 1997; 47:28–31
40. Aoyama I, Kondo A, Ogawa H et al. Germinoma in siblings: case reports. Surg Neuro, 1994; 41:313–317
41. Wakai S, Segawa H, Kitahara S et al. Teratoma in the pineal region in two brothers. Case reports. J Neurosurg, 1980; 53:239–243
42. Krywicki R, Bowen K, Anderson L et al. Mixed-lineage acute myeloid leukemia associated with a suprasellar dysgerminoma. Am J Clin Oncol, 1995; 18:83–86
43. Dal Chin P, Dei Tos AP, Qi H et al. Immature teratoma of the pineal gland with isochromosome 12p. Acta Neuropathol, 1998; 95:107–110
44. de Bruin TW, Slater RM, Defferrari R et al. Isochromosome 12p-positive pineal germ cell tumor. Cancer Res, 1994; 54:1542–1544
45. Suijkerbuijk JW, Looijenga L, de Jong B et al. Verification of isochromosome 12p and identification of other chromosome 12 aberrations in gonadal and extragonadal human germ cell tumors by bicolor double fluorescence *in situ* hybridization. Cancer Gen Cytogenet, 1992; 63:8–16
46. Rickert CH, Simon R, Bergmann M et al. Comparative genomic hybridization in pineal germ cell tumors. J Neuropathol Exp Neurol, 2000; 59:815–821

47. Feng X, Zhang S, Ichikawa T et al. Intracranial germ cell tumors: detection of p53 gene mutations by single-strand conformation polymorphism analysis. Jpn J Cancer Res, 1995; 86:555–561
48. Nozaki M, Tada M, Matsumoto R et al. Rare occurrence of inactivating p53 gene mutations in primary non-astrocytic tumors of the central nervous system: reappraisal by yeast function assay. Acta Neuropathol, 1998; 95:291–296
49. Aguzzi A, Hedinger CE, Kleihues P et al. Intracranial mixed germ cell tumor with syncytiotrophoblastic giant cells and precocious puberty. Acta Neuropathol, 1988; 75:427–431
50. Legido A, Packer RJ, Sutton LN et al. Suprasellar germinomas in childhood. A reappraisal. Cancer, 1989; 63:340–344
51. O'Marcaigh AS, Ledger GA, Roche PC et al. Aromatase expression in human germinomas with possible biological effects. J Clin Endocrinol Metab, 1995; 80:3763–3766
52. Ikeda J, Sawamura Y, Kato T et al. Metachronous neurohypophyseal germinoma occurring 8 years after total resection of pineal mature teratoma. Surg Neurol, 1995; 49:205–208
53. Chang T, Teng MM-H, Guo W-Y et al. CT of pineal tumors and intracranial germ-cell tumors. Am J Neuroradiol, 1989; 10:1039–1044
54. Fujimaki T, Matsutani M, Funada et al. CT and MRI features of intracranial germ cell tumors. J Neurooncol, 1994; 19:217–226
55. Sumida M, Oosumi T, Kiya K et al. MRI of intracranial germ cell tumours. Neuroradiology, 1995; 37:32–37
56. Ng HK. Cytological diagnosis of intracranial germinomas in smear preparations. Acta Cyto, 1995; 39:693–697
57. Felix I, Becker LE. Intracranial germ cell tumors in children: an immunohistochemical and electron microscopic study. Pediatr Neurosurg, 1990; 16:156–162
58. Bentley AJ, Parkinson MC, Harding BN et al. A comparative morphological and immunohistochemical study of testicular seminomas and intracranial germinomas. Histopathology, 1990; 17:443–449
59. Paine JT, Handa H, Yamasaki T et al. Suprasellar germinoma with shunt metastasis: report of a case with an immunohistochemical characterisation of the lymphocyte subpopulations. Surg Neurol, 1986; 25:55–61
60. Saito T, Tanaka R, Kouno M et al. Tumor-infiltrating lymphocytes and histocompatability antigens in primary intracranial germinomas. J Neurosurg, 1989; 70:81–85
61. Wei Y-Q, Hang Z-B, Liu K-F. *In situ* observation of inflammatory cell-tumor cell interaction in human seminomas (germinomas): light, electron microscopic, and immunohistochemical study. Hum Pathol, 1992; 23:421–428
62. Kraichoke S, Cosgrove M, Chandrasoma PT. Granulomatous inflammation in pineal germinoma: a cause of diagnostic failure at stereotaxic brain biopsy. Am J Surg Pathol, 1988; 12:655–660
63. Nakagawa Y, Perentes E, Ross GW et al. Immunohistochemical differences between intracranial germinomas and their gonadal equivalents. An immunoperoxidase study of germ cell tumours with epithelial membrane antigen, cytokeratin and vimentin. J Pathol, 1988; 156:67–72
64. Min K-W, Scheithauer BW. Pineal germinomas and testicular seminoma: a comparative ultrastructural study with special references to early carcinomatous transformation. Ultrastruct Pathol, 1998; 14:483–496
65. Matsutani M, Takakura K, Sano K. Primary intracranial germ cell tumors: pathology and treatment. Prog Exp Tumor Res, 1987; 30:307–312
66. Jenkin RD, Simpson WJ, Keen CW. Pineal and suprasellar germinomas. Results of radiation treatment. J Neurosurg, 1978; 48:99–107
67. Sung Dl, Harisiadis L, Chang CH. Midline pineal tumors and suprasellar germinomas: highly curable by irradiation. Radiology, 1998; 128:745–751
68. Sawamura Y, Ikeda J, Shirato H et al. Germ cell tumours of the central nervous system: treatment consideration based on 111 cases and their long-term clinical outcomes. Euro J Cancer, 1998; 34:104–110
69. Ono N, Isobe I, Uki J et al. Recurrence of primary intracranial germinomas after complete response with radiotherapy: recurrence patterns and therapy. Neurosurgery, 1994; 35:615–621
70. Balmaceda C, Heller G, Rosenblum M et al. Chemotherapy without irradiation – a novel approach for newly diagnosed CNS germ cell tumors: results of an international cooperative trial. The First

International Central Nervous System Germ Cell Tumor Study. J Clin Oncol, 1996; 14:2908–2915

71. Matsutani M, Ushio Y, Abe H et al. Combined chemotherapy and radiation therapy for central nervous system germ cell tumors: preliminary results of a phase II study of the Japanese Pediatric Brain Tumor Study Group. Neurosurg Focus, 1998; 5:1–5

72. Uematsu T, Tsuura Y, Miyamoto K et al. The recurrence of primary intracranial germinomas. Special reference to germinoma with syncytiotrophoblastic giant cells. J Neurooncol, 1992; 13:247–256

73. Brandes AA, Pasetto LM, Monfardini S. The treatment of cranial germ cell tumours. Cancer Treat Rev, 2000; 26:233–242

74. Shibamoto Y, Oda Y, Yamashita J et al. The role of cerebrospinal fluid cytology in radiotherapy planning for intracranial germinoma. Int J Radiat Oncol Biol Phys, 1994; 30:1089–1094

75. Balsatis M, Rothwell I, Pifott TJD. Systemic metastasis from primary intracranial germinoma: a case report and literature review. Br J Neurosurg, 1989; 3:717–723

76. Borden S, Weber AL, Toch R et al. Pineal germinoma. Long-term survival despite hematogenous metastases. Arch Dis Child, 1973; 126:214–216

77. Gay JC, Janco RL, Lukens JN. Systemic metastases in primary intracranial germinoma. Case report and literature review. Cancer, 1985; 55:2688–2690

78. Zülch KJ. Brain tumors: Their biology and pathology. Berlin: Springer Verlag, 1986

79. Gonzalez-Crussi F. Extragonadal teratomas. 2nd series, fascicle 18. In: Atlas of tumor pathology. Washington, DC: Armed Forces Institute of Pathology, 1999

80. Drapkin AJ, Rose WS, Pellmar MB. Mature teratoma in the fourth ventricle of an adult: case report and review of the literature. Neurosurgery, 1987; 21:404–410

81. Heifetz SA, Cushing B, Giller R et al. Immature teratomas in children: pathologic considerations. Am J Surg Pathol, 1998; 22:1115–1124

82. Washburne JF, Magann EF, Chauhan SP et al. Massive congenital intracranial teratoma with skull rupture at delivery. Am J Gynecol, 1995; 173:226–228

83. Herrmann HD, Westphal M, Winkler K et al. Treatment of nongerminomatous germ-cell tumors of the pineal region. Neurosurgery, 1994; 34:524–529

84. Bochner SJ, Scarff JE. Teratoma of the pineal body. Classification of the embryonal tumors of the pineal body; report of a case of teratoma of the pineal body presenting formed teeth. Arch Surg, 1938; 36:303–329

85. Naudin ten Cate LN, Vermeij-Keers C, Smit DA et al. Intracranial teratoma with multiple fetuses. Pre- and post-natal appearance. Hum Pathol, 1995; 26:804–807

86. Preissig SH, Smith MT, Huntington HW. Rhabdomyosarcoma arising in a pineal teratoma. Cancer, 1979; 44:281–284

87. Freilich RJ, Thompson SJ, Walker RW et al. Adenocarcinomatous transformation of intracranial germ cell tumors. Am J Surg Pathol, 1995; 19:537–544

88. Ironside JW, Jefferson AA, Royds JA et al. Carcinoid tumour arising in a recurrent intradural spinal teratoma. Neuropathol Appl Neurobiol, 1984; 10:479–489

89. Shaffrey ME, Lanzino G, Lopes MB et al. Maturation of intracranial immature teratomas. Report of two cases. J Neurosurg, 1996; 85:672–676

90. O'Callaghan AM, Katapodis O, Ellison DW et al. The growing teratoma syndrome in a nongerminomatous germ cell tumor of the pineal gland: a case report and review. Cancer, 1997; 80:942–947

91. Koeleveld RF, Cohen AR. Primary embryonal-cell carcinoma of the parietal lobe. J Neurosurg, 1991; 75:468–471

92. Packer RJ, Sutton LN, Rorke LB et al. Intracranial embryonal cell carcinoma. Cancer, 1984; 54:520–524

93. Eberts TJ, Ransburg RC. Primary intracranial endodermal sinus tumor. J Neurosurg, 1979; 50:246–252

94. Kirikae M, Arai H, Hidaka T et al. Pineal yolk sac tumor in a 65-year old man. Surg Neurol, 1994; 42:253–258

95. Kirkove CS, Brown AP, Symon L. Successful treatment of a pineal endodermal sinus tumor. J Neurosurg, 1991; 74:832–836

96. Furukawa F, Haebara H, Hamashima Y. Primary intracranial choriocarcinoma arising from the pituitary fossa. Report of an autopsy case with literature review. Acta Pathol Jpn, 1986; 36:773–781

97. Jones WB, Wagner-Reiss KM, Lewis JL Jr. Intracranial choriocarcinoma. Gynecol Oncol, 1990; 38:234–243

98. Page R, Doshi B, Sharr MM. Primary intracranial choriocarcinoma. J Neurol Neurosurg Psychiatry, 1986; 49:93–95

99. Bjornsson J, Scheithauer BW, Leech RW. Primary intracranial choriocarcinoma: a case report. Clin Neuropathol, 1986; 5:242–245

100. Borit A. Embryonal carcinoma of the pineal region. J Pathol, 1969; 97:165–172

101. Uchiyama M, Iwafuchi M, Naitoh M et al. Sacrococcygeal teratoma: a series of 19 cases with long-term follow-up. Eur J Pediatr Res, 1999; 9:158–162

102. Rescorla FJ, Sawin RS, Coran AG et al. Long-term outcome for infants and children with sacrococcygeal teratoma: a report from the Childrens Cancer Group. J Pediatr Surg, 1998; 33:171–176

103. Ng EW, Porcu P, Loehrer PJ Sr. Sacrococcygeal teratoma in adults: case reports and a review of the literature. Cancer, 1999; 86:1198–1202

104. Ribeiro PR, Guys JM, Lena G. Sacrococcygeal teratoma with an intradural and extramedullary extension in a neonate: case report. Neurosurgery, 1999; 44:398–400

105. Chisholm CA, Heider AL, Kuller JA et al. Prenatal diagnosis and perinatal management of fetal sacrococcygeal teratoma. Am J Perinatol, 1998; 15:503–505

11 Lymphoreticular neoplasms

The central nervous system (CNS) can be involved by a variety of lymphoid neoplasms occurring either as primary lesions, secondary deposits or extensions from adjacent tumours. Primary lymphoid tumours have been recognised to occur in the CNS for many years, but in earlier decades there was considerable confusion as to whether these tumours were of microglial origin or part of the peripheral lymphoid tumours known at the time as reticulum cell sarcomas. These difficulties were partly resolved in 1974, when a symposium in Vienna helped set these CNS tumours within the context of peripheral lymphoid tumours.[1] Since then, despite several changes in the categorisation and nomenclature of lymphoid neoplasms, a classification has been recently agreed which is applicable to all lymphoid neoplasms (the REAL classification: Revised European–American Classification of Lymphoid Neoplasms).[2] As our understanding of the cell biology and molecular genetics of lymphoid neoplasms increases, it is unlikely that this classification will remain unaltered;[3] at present, it serves as a satisfactory framework within which to categorise these tumours. Apart from primary lymphomas, the CNS can also be involved by a range of other lymphoid tumours including Hodgkin's disease, leukaemias, plasma cell neoplasms and histiocytoses and secondary lymphoid tumours. This chapter will consider each of these entities in turn, commencing with the primary CNS lymphomas.

Primary CNS lymphoma

Incidence

The incidence of primary CNS lymphoma has increased markedly over recent years.[4] Prior to the 1980s, these were considered to be rare tumours, accounting for less than 1% of all brain tumours and less than 2% of malignant lymphomas from all body sites.[1] Subsequently, a marked increase in incidence has been reported in most neuropathological series, involving both immunocompetent and immunodeficient patients.[5–8] This trend is not, however, universal.[9] The increasing incidence is explicable on several counts, including improved investigation of patients (with the increasing using of stereotactic brain biopsies for deep-seated lesions), increased clinical and neuropathological diagnostic awareness, the more widespread use of immunocytochemistry, and the growing number of immunosuppressed individuals who are at increased risk of developing these tumours.[10–12] This is particularly relevant in relation to the AIDS pandemic; it has been estimated that up to 12% of AIDS patients may develop a primary CNS lymphoma, particularly during the terminal stages of the disease.[10,11] The incidence of this tumour in AIDS patients is approximately 3600 times higher than in the general population, with an estimated incidence of 4.7 per 1000 person-years.[10] New AIDS treatment regimes which reduce viral load and prolong survival may reduce this figure. Other immunodeficiency syndromes have contributed to this increase in primary CNS lymphomas, including patients with congenital immunodeficiencies whose survival times have improved in recent years, and increasing numbers of patients with organ transplants; numerous other secondary causes of immunodeficiency are associated with primary CNS lymphoma[7,13–18] (Table 11.1).

Site

CNS lymphoma is considered primary if the patient in question presents with a neurological complaint which is proven to be due to lymphoma on a CNS tissue diagnosis, and there is no evidence of lymphoma in any other site except the brain, leptomeninges, spinal cord or eye at the time of presentation.[19] Lymphomas primarily involving adjacent structures including the epidural space, orbit, skull or vertebral column are therefore not considered within the group of primary CNS lymphomas.

Aetiology

Most recent studies have found an almost constant association between Epstein–Barr virus (EBV) infection and primary CNS lymphoma in immunodeficient patients (see Refs 7 and 20 for reviews). In many of the inherited conditions resulting in immunodeficiency, there is also an association with primary systemic lymphomas. Primary CNS lymphoma occurs as a second malignancy in around 8% of cases, after a latent period of 5–15 years in patients with systemic Hodgkin's disease, leukaemia and adenocarcinomas of the colon, thyroid and breast.[21] Primary

Table 11.1 Predisposing factors for primary CNS lymphoma[7,11,13–21,26]

Congenital or inherited immunodeficiency	Acquired immunodeficiency	Malignancy
Wiskott–Aldrich syndrome	AIDS	Hodgkin's disease
X-linked lymphoproliferative syndrome	Post-transplantation immunosuppression	Non-Hodgkin's lymphoma
IgA deficiency	Immunological disorders – sarcoidosis, Sjogren syndrome, rheumatoid arthritis, systemic lupus erythematosus, idiopathic thrombocytopenic purpura, vasculitis, localised angiitis of the CNS	Chronic lymphocytic leukaemia
		Colonic carcinoma
		Thyroid carcinoma
		Breast carcinoma

CNS lymphoma has also been associated with meningiomas[22] and a low grade astrocytoma in a child,[23] possibly representing no more than a fortuitous occurrence.

Clinical features

Primary CNS lymphoma can occur at all ages, but has a peak incidence in immunocompetent patients in the sixth and seventh decades of life, with a slight male predominance.[5,24,25] In immunodeficient patients this age distribution is markedly altered, with a small peak occurring beneath the age of 10 years in individuals with congenital immunodeficiencies,[20,26] followed then by a larger peak in the fourth decade of life in individuals who are transplant recipients[16,17] and those suffering from AIDS.[8,10,11,16] The vast majority of the latter cohort (greater than 90%) are males; a male predominance also occurs in individuals with inherited immunodeficiency syndromes. Although most cases of primary CNS lymphomas in AIDS arise in adults, there have been occasional reports in children under 3 years of age,[27,28] representing the youngest cases in the literature. T-cell lymphomas (including Ki-1 anaplastic lymphomas) occur rarely as primary CNS lymphomas in immunocompetent patients, although occasional cases have been described in individuals with AIDS.[29–32] The age at onset in non-immunocompromised patients is younger than for patients with B-cell tumours.

Although no specific pattern of clinical features relates to primary CNS lymphoma, there is a characteristic disease pattern which reflects the sites of anatomical predilection for this tumour, with prominent frontal lobe signs and symptoms including personality change, memory loss and neuropsychiatric symptoms.[5,19,25] Other common features at presentation include cerebellar signs and symptoms, motor dysfunction, headache and visual changes, with seizures occurring in around 10% of patients. Many tumours are multifocal, and this is reflected in the clinical manifestations of the underlying disease. Ocular involvement can occur in up to 20% of patients, and may be readily identified on slit-lamp examination.[33] There appears to be no striking difference between the clinical features of the disease in immunocompetent and immuno-suppressed patients.[10,24,25] Occasional cases present with unusual clinical features including cranial neuropathy, diabetes insipidus and narcolepsy; it has been suggested that this group of tumours is the most common cause of tumour-induced central neurogenic hyperventilation.[34]

In contrast, patients with secondary lymphoma in the nervous system usually present with non-specific features of raised intracranial pressure and a range of non-specific neurological abnormalities (see Chapter 12). The lengthy latent period for CNS lymphoma to occur as a second malignancy has been noted above; in contrast, transplantation-associated lymphomas occur most fre-

quently 1–2 years after transplantation[16,17] and AIDS-associated lymphomas are most commonly seen in the final stages of the full-blown syndrome.[10,11]

A small subset of patients with primary CNS lymphomas present with non-specific neurological symptoms and signs, and on neuroradiological investigations have a transient contrast-enhancing lesion which recedes spontaneously or on treatment with corticosteroids.[35,36] These sentinel lesions are followed after several months by a new set of signs and symptoms which relate to a B-cell primary CNS lymphoma; the pathological diagnosis of sentinel lesions is discussed in detail below.

Radiology

In computerised tomography (CT) scans, primary CNS lymphomas appear as hyperdense masses in the brain, often with a bilateral and symmetrical pattern of contrast enhancement, particularly in the subependymal region of the cerebral white matter (Fig. 11.1).[37–39] Magnetic resonance imaging (MRI) is the investigation of choice for primary CNS lymphomas, in which the lesions are usually hypointense to isointense on T1-weighted images and isointense to hyperintense on T2-weighted imaging.[39,40] The tumours exhibit homogeneous or solid enhancement following the intravenous administration of gadolinium

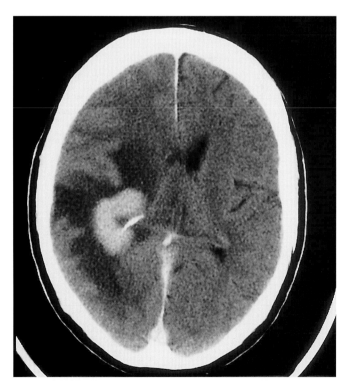

Fig. 11.1 **Cerebral lymphoma.** Contrast-enhanced CT scan. The scan shows a characteristic periventricular location around the trigone of the lateral ventricle. There is a considerable degree of oedema in the surrounding white matter. (Courtesy of Dr D Collie, Edinburgh.)

as a contrast agent (Fig. 11.2). Most lesions are associated with mild to moderate oedema and multifocal deposits are observed in around 50% of cases.[40] On MRI scans, the tumour deposits are frequently large, with most measuring greater than 2 cm in diameter, but the mass effects may be relatively small as the degree of tumour-associated oedema is not as great as in gliomas or metastatic carcinoma.[39,40]

Most CNS lymphomas arise in the periventricular white matter and involve the corpus callosum, thalamus or basal ganglia.[41] The frontal white matter is the most commonly involved site, and tumours may exhibit a 'butterfly' appearance with bilateral symmetrical high signal foci in the frontal lobes and corpus callosum (Fig. 11.2). Ring enhancing lesions in immunocompromised patients (particularly in AIDS) may be difficult to distinguish from non-neoplastic infectious processes, particularly toxoplasmosis.[5,24,40] As well as parenchymal deposits, primary nervous system lymphomas may present as irregular foci of infiltration in the meninges,[40–42] visible as hyperintense deposits, the smallest of which can be missed even in contrast-enhanced MRI scans. The use of corticosteroids will reduce brain oedema and can alter the tumour enhancement or cause a temporary disappearance (in radiological terms) of the lesion, which is sometimes referred to as a 'ghost' tumour.[43]

Pathology

Macroscopic features

Most primary CNS lymphomas occur as deep seated tumour masses in the white matter adjacent to the ventricular system, causing irregular expansion of the white matter or involvement of the basal ganglia and thalamus.[5,11,24,25] The larger tumours may contain foci of haemorrhage or necrosis, resembling an infarct or a glioblastoma, particularly in AIDS. On sectioning the brain, the tumours may exhibit a white–tan or grey discolouration in relation to the adjacent neuropil, resembling 'fish flesh' (Fig. 11.3). The tumour margins are poorly defined, even in lesions which appear well delineated on MRI scans. The degree of oedema and mass effect is often surprisingly restricted in relation to the size of the tumour. Multiple tumour sites are not uncommon,[11,25] and some of the larger hemispheric tumours can exhibit a symmetrical pattern of involvement in the subcortical white matter of both hemispheres, usually involving the corpus callosum. Occasional lymphomas will widely infiltrate the cerebral hemispheres, producing variable expansion of grey and white matter structures without a single tumour mass; this pattern of growth is referred to as lymphomatosis cerebri.[44] In AIDS, the tumour deposits are usually large and necrotic (Fig. 11.4) and often occur in association with other pathologies including progressive multifocal leucoencephalopathy, toxoplasmosis and a wide range of bacterial, fungal and viral infections.[10,11,24] Macroscopic differential diagnosis of primary CNS lymphomas in AIDS is complicated by their resemblance to treated toxoplasma lesions. Cerebellar lymphomas occur most often as ill-defined masses in the white matter, either as solitary tumours or in association with supratentorial lesions.[11,19] Lymphomas arising in the spinal cord are remarkably

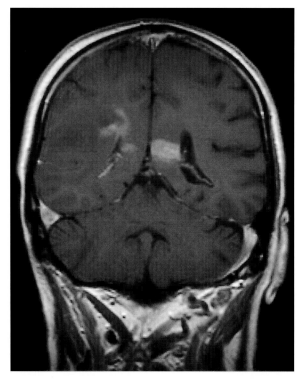

Fig. 11.2 **Cerebral lymphoma**. T1-weighted MRI scan after gadolinium administration. Bilateral involvement of the central white matter is shown. (Courtesy of Dr D Collie, Edinburgh.)

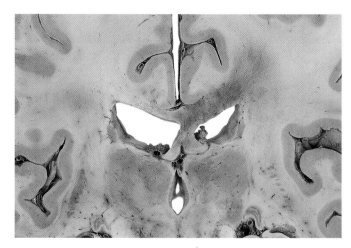

Fig. 11.3 **Cerebral lymphoma**. Diffuse infiltration and expansion of the corpus callosum and central white matter bilaterally in an immunocompetent patient are shown. This pattern can mimic glioblastoma both on macroscopic inspection and on neuroradiology.

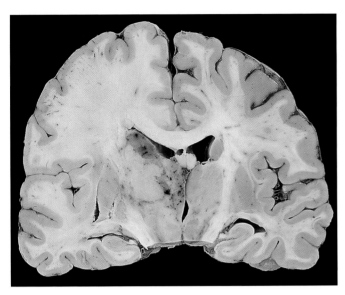

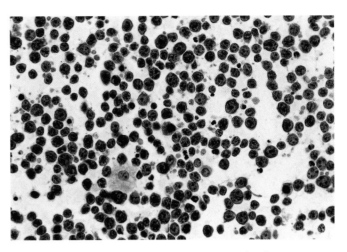

Fig. 11.5 **Cerebral lymphoma**. Smear preparation showing a non-cohesive population of malignant cells without a gliofibrillary matrix. The tumour cells have pleomorphic nuclei and prominent nucleoli; mitoses are easily identified. Toluidine blue.

Fig. 11.4 **Cerebral lymphoma**. The patient was a 36-year-old male with AIDS. The large necrotic tumour is centred in the basal ganglia on the left, but infiltrates widely. Multiple secondary infections were also detected on histology. (Courtesy of Professor J Bell, Edinburgh.)

uncommon; these lesions cause localised expansion and swelling of the cord, and on cross section resemble their cerebral counterparts.[45,46] T-cell lymphomas occur in the CNS as either solitary or multiple lesions; there is a tendency for these tumours to occur in the posterior fossa or in the leptomeninges.[47,48]

Primary B- and T-cell CNS lymphomas can rarely arise in the meninges without extensive CNS parenchymal involvement.[49,50] In the dura mater, the tumours may occur as solitary deposits which superficially resemble meningiomas, but invade the adjacent parenchyma.[51,52] A more diffuse pattern of infiltration may occur, with widespread thickening of the leptomeninges and small tumour nodules in the subarachnoid space or on cranial and spinal nerves, which can resemble carcinomatous meningitis on MRI scans or naked-eye inspection.[50,53]

Intraoperative diagnosis

In view of the association with AIDS, particular care must be taken to establish whether a patient with a suspected CNS lymphoma is at risk of or infected with HIV before intraoperative diagnosis is planned. Given the appropriate facilities, it is still possible to perform intraoperative diagnostic procedures on unfixed tissue with due care for the health and safety of all staff involved, bearing in mind that other pathogens may also be present in the tissue under investigation.

Smear preparations of primary CNS lymphomas are particularly valuable for intraoperative diagnosis, since the tumours usually smear well, and the nuclear mor-

phology is superior to that in cryostat sections. Touch and imprint preparations can also be made, but these offer few advantages over smear preparations. The morphology of the tumour cell nuclei is best observed in smears stained with toluidine blue (Fig. 11.5), which will also demonstrate the characteristic relationship of the tumour cells to the vascular endothelium. The tumour cells spread away from the blood vessels in a non-cohesive monolayer, without a gliofibrillary matrix. The vascular endothelium is abnormal and may appear thickened, with mononuclear cells closely surrounding the endothelium. These mononuclear cells comprise both tumour cells and reactive T-cells, which can be identified by their relatively small size and uniform nuclei. Most CNS lymphomas contain large cells of B-cell origin, particularly immunoblast-like cells, which can be recognised by their large irregular nucleus and prominent nucleolus. Haemorrhage and necrosis may be present, particularly in tumours from patients with AIDS, in whom other pathologies may coexist, e.g. cytomegalovirus (CMV) infection, toxoplasmosis, or giant cell encephalitis.

Cryostat sections of primary CNS lymphomas are useful in demonstrating the relationship of the tumour cells to the vascular endothelium (Fig. 11.6), and the expansion of the blood vessel wall by tumour cells. Nuclear morphology is less distinct than in smear preparations; the perivascular accumulation of tumour cells and reactive T-cells can be mistaken for the perivascular cuffing characteristic of viral encephalitis or multiple sclerosis, but the nuclear features in smear preparations will help resolve this difficulty. Cryostat sections will also demonstrate astrocytosis at the tumour margins, necrosis and the multiple pathologies in AIDS, particularly toxoplasmosis.

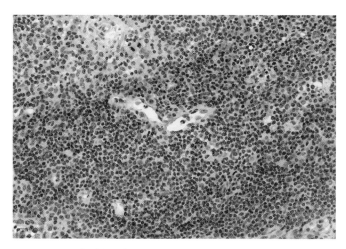

Fig. 11.6 **Cerebral lymphoma**. Cryostat section shows diffuse infiltration of the white matter by a densely cellular tumour population. H & E.

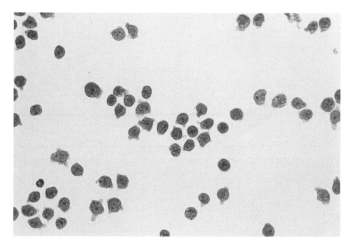

Fig. 11.7 **Cerebral lymphoma**. CSF cytology in malignant lymphoma often contains large numbers of tumour cells, in this case with multiple prominent nucleoli in the pleomorphic nuclei. H & E.

Microscopic features

CSF cytology Examination of the CSF can be of diagnostic value in 20–30% of primary CNS lymphomas.[54] The presence of tumour cells in the CSF is not always associated with a high cell count, and diagnosis depends on the morphology of the tumour cell population. Most cases of primary CNS lymphoma contain numerous immunoblastic and centroblastic cells (Fig. 11.7), with mitotic figures in the abnormal lymphoid cell population. Reactive conditions involving mononuclear cells in the CSF can cause diagnostic problems, as the nuclear morphology in the reactive cells can appear similar to those in low grade CNS lymphomas, and mitotic figures are occasionally present in reactive mononuclear cells. However, a clear distinction is usually possible on immunocytochemistry using lymphocyte subset specific antibodies[55] between primary CNS lymphoma (Fig. 11.8) and reactive conditions in which increased numbers of mononuclear cells are present. Flow cytometry may also be used to characterise the tumour cells.[56] As in other neoplastic conditions involving the subarachnoid space, multiple samples may be required for diagnostic confirmation if a biopsy is not contemplated. It is also possible to apply molecular genetic techniques to CSF samples for diagnostic purposes.[57]

Microscopic features of CNS lymphomas Primary CNS lymphomas exhibit a characteristic angiocentric pattern of tumour infiltration, with blood vessels surrounded by a collar of neoplastic cells which infiltrate the perivascular space, usually for much further than the macroscopic limits of the tumour would indicate.[5,11,25] (Fig. 11.9). The affected blood vessels do not exhibit endothelial hyperplasia, but the reticulin network around the tumour is expanded (Fig. 11.10), with reticulin fibres separating the tumour cells into small clusters. Endothelial cell apoptosis has recently been

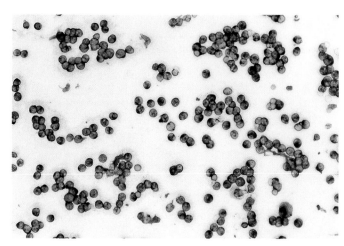

Fig. 11.8 **Cerebral lymphoma**. Immunocytochemistry for CD20 shows strong positivity in the malignant cell population in the CSF, indicating a B-cell lymphoma (same case as Fig. 11.7).

identified by electron microscopy in a study of 24 primary CNS B-cell lymphomas.[58] Invasion of the lumen of the blood vessels and vascular occlusion is exceptional. Parenchymal infiltration is variable throughout the tumour and may occur in a multicentric fashion, with irregular groups of tumour cells infiltrating the oedematous brain in single lines or small groups. Towards the infiltrating edge of the tumour there is usually an astrocytic reaction which occasionally can be pronounced; this can cause diagnostic difficulties and lead to potential error if the infiltrating margin of the tumour alone is sampled.

The cytological features of primary CNS lymphomas are variable; most are high grade B-cell tumours, in which there is a predominant population of large immunoblastic cells with abundant cytoplasm, an irregular nucleus and a single prominent nucleolus[59] (Fig. 11.11). In other tumours, a population of centroblastic cells may predominate, which are smaller in size than immunoblasts,

Fig. 11.9 **Cerebral lymphoma**. Low power examination usually reveals a perivascular accumulation of tumour cells with extensive parenchymal infiltration. H & E.

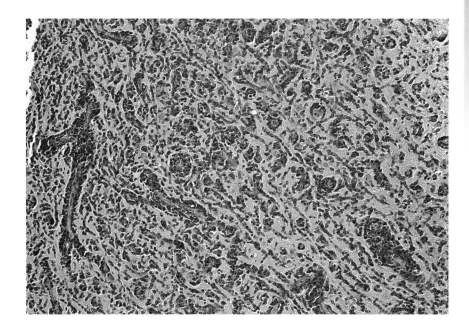

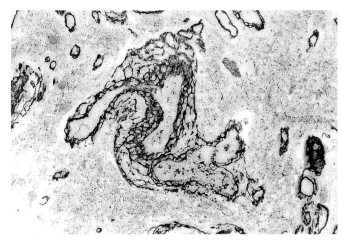

Fig. 11.10 **Cerebral lymphoma**. A reticulin stain demonstrates the characteristic expansion of the reticulin framework around blood vessels which is typical of this tumour (and other extranodal lymphomas).

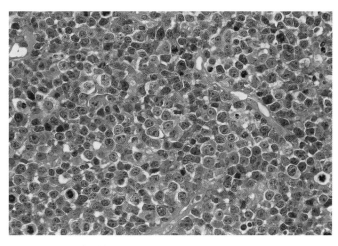

Fig. 11.11 **Cerebral lymphoma**. High power examination shows a high grade tumour composed predominantly of immunoblasts and centroblast-like cells. H & E.

but contain multiple nucleoli.[5,11,25,39] Lymphoplasmacytoid cells may also be encountered, usually as part of a mixed tumour cell population, since low grade tumours with this cell type as a predominant form are rare.[5] However, lymphoplasmacytoid cells may occur as part of a mixed population including centrocytic cells in tumours considered as intermediate grade lymphomas[5] (Fig. 11.12). In patients with AIDS, large cell Burkitt-type B-cell tumours may occur (Fig. 11.13), where the background population of large tumour cells is studded by macrophages, giving a 'starry sky' appearance.[27] The great majority of primary CNS lymphomas are B-cell tumours which express pan-B-cell markers such as CD20[10,25] (Fig. 11.14); many tumour cells do not express the pan-leukocyte antigen CD45,

which cannot therefore be relied upon as a single tumour 'marker'. Most tumours will also express cytoplasmic or surface immunoglobulins in a monoclonal form, the most frequent of which is IgM kappa. Reactive T-lymphocytes can be seen in any of the primary B-cell lymphomas[60] and are often present as a population of relatively uniform small cells around blood vessels, most of which are CD3 positive on immunocytochemistry (Fig. 11.15). In some tumours (either focally or diffusely) this population of reactive T-cells can predominate over the neoplastic B-cells, as in a 'T-cell rich B-cell lymphoma'. These reactive cells can cause diagnostic confusion, particularly if they occur in large numbers within small biopsy specimens. Molecular genetic studies to identify clonal alterations in

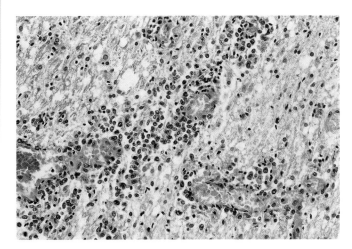

Fig. 11.12 Cerebral lymphoma. This intermediate grade cerebral lymphoma in an immunocompetent patient contains a relatively uniform population of lymphoplasmacytoid and centrocytic tumour cells, without necrosis. H & E.

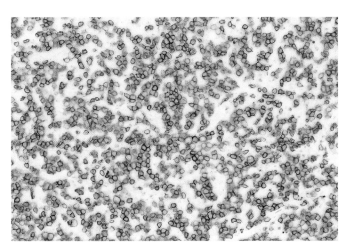

Fig. 11.14 Cerebral lymphoma. Immunocytochemistry for CD20 shows strong positivity in most primary cerebral lymphomas, confirming their B-cell lineage.

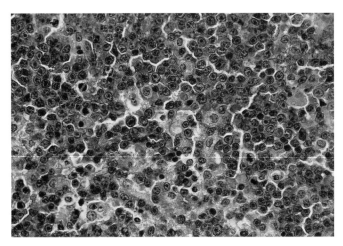

Fig. 11.13 Cerebral lymphoma. High grade B-cell lymphomas in patients with AIDS can exhibit a Burkitt-like morphology, with necrosis and macrophage infiltration. H & E.

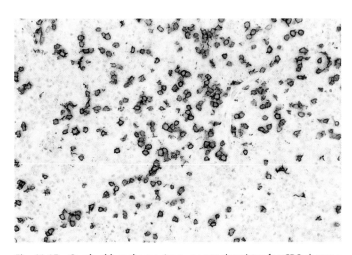

Fig. 11.15 Cerebral lymphoma. Immunocytochemistry for CD3 shows a high percentage of reactive T-cells within this malignant lymphoma.

the B-cell immunoglobulin gene (and a corresponding absence of monoclonality in the T-cell receptor gene) are helpful in clarifying the diagnosis[61,62] in such cases.

Primary T-cell lymphomas in the CNS are rare; they usually contain a population of small lymphoid cells with scanty cytoplasm and a prominent cleaved nucleus[47,48] (Figs 11.16 and 11.17). An important subset of T-cell lymphomas is the anaplastic large cell tumours, which may be mistaken for high grade B-cell tumours if the appropriate investigations are not performed.[29–31] A suggested schema for the investigation and diagnosis of primary CNS lymphoma is summarised in Table 11.2. Biopsies taken from patients with primary CNS lymphomas after the administration of corticosteroids can exhibit a marked astrocytic gliosis accompanied by an infiltrate of reactive T-lymphocytes and macrophages[35,36] (Fig. 11.18). This can cause diagnostic difficulties, particularly if the tumour cell population is sparse in relation to the reactive cells (see below under differential diagnosis).

The histological subtypes of CNS lymphomas arising in the posterior fossa and spinal cord resemble those for primary brain lymphomas.[45,46,48] In contrast, a subset of primary lymphomas arising in the cranial dura has recently been described, which bears a resemblance to the B-cell lymphomas arising in mucosa-associated lymphoid tissues (MALT) elsewhere in the body.[51,52] These tumours consist of a diffuse infiltrate of small lymphoplasmacytoid cells, with a variable admixture of centrocytic cells. They occur predominantly in adult immunocompetent females, and have an indolent growth rate with a favourable response to treatment. Other leptomeningeal lymphomas resemble their intraparenchymal counterparts in terms of growth and response to treatment, particularly in patients with AIDS.[50]

Fig. 11.16 **Cerebral lymphoma**. A primary T-cell lymphoma in the brain is composed of small tumour cells with scanty cytoplasm and an irregular 'cleaved' nucleus. H & E.

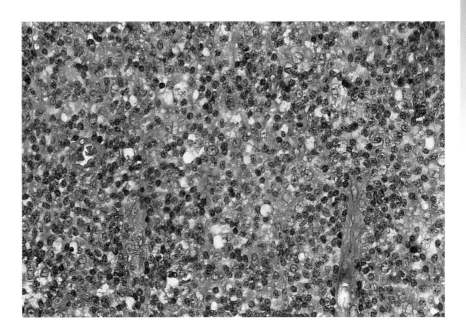

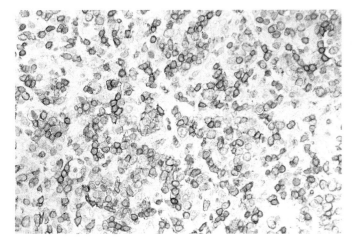

Fig. 11.17 **Cerebral lymphoma**. Immunocytochemistry in a primary T-cell lymphoma shows widespread positivity for CD3 (same case as Fig. 11.16).

Table 11.2 Suggested investigations for primary CNS lymphomas

Intraoperative diagnosis	Differential diagnosis
Smear preparation	GFAP
Toluidine blue, haematoxylin and eosin,	Synaptophysin
Giemsa	Cytokeratins
	EMA
Cryostat sections	Antibodies and stains for microorganisms
Haematoxylin and eosin	
Paraffin histology	
Routine stains	
Haematoxylin and eosin	
Reticulin	
Immunocytochemistry	
B-cell markers CD20, CD79a	
T-cell markers CD3, CD45RO	
Immunoglobulins and light chains	
Specialised investigations	
PCR for immunoglobulin and T-cell receptor gene rearrangements	
EBV EBER, EBNA, LMPs (see Table 11.5)	
Oncoproteins bcl-2, p53, c-myc	

EBER, Epstein–Barr virus non-polyadenylated RNAs; EBNA Epstein–Barr virus nuclear antigen; EBV, Epstein–Barr virus; EMA, epithelial membrane antigen; GFAP, glial fibrillary acidic protein; LMP, latent membrane protein; PCR, polymerase chain reaction.

As discussed previously, the application of morphological and immunophenotypic classification systems based on systemic nodal lymphomas to primary CNS lymphomas is difficult and in the REAL classification system (Table 11.3) the majority of such tumours would be classified as diffuse large B-cell lymphomas.[59] These tumours exhibit widespread mitotic activity and a high labelling index with Ki-67/MIB-1.[63] Allowing for changes in nomenclature in the past few decades, it is possible to summarise an approximate categorisation of subtypes of primary CNS lymphoma in AIDS and non-AIDS patients using the REAL classification (Table 11.4). Low grade tumours including lymphocytic, lymphoplasmacytoid and plasmacytoid lymphomas are infrequently reported.[5] True histiocytic lymphomas occur

very rarely as primary CNS tumours; these often contain a prominent inflammatory component, which can hinder diagnosis.[64]

Analysis of survival data based on histological subclassification in CNS lymphomas has not yielded much helpful information relating to the subclassification of high grade large cell tumours, and although occasional

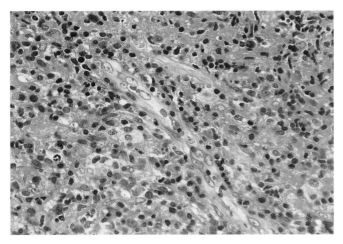

Fig. 11.18 Cerebral lymphoma. Corticosteroid therapy can modify the cytological features of primary cerebral lymphoma. In this biopsy the lymphoma contains large numbers of foamy macrophages, suggestive of a demyelinating or infectious process. H & E.

reports claiming a better prognosis of patients with low grade tumours have been published, the findings are inconsistent.[5,24,25] In view of this, it has been suggested that primary CNS lymphoma subtyping has to be considered as having little clinical relevance at present.

Molecular biology

Relatively few cytogenetic studies have been performed on primary CNS lymphomas, but there are reports of clonal abnormalities in chromosomes 1, 6, 7 and 14, in addition to translocations similar to those reported in nodal B-cell lymphoma.[65] A recent study employed a comparative genomic hybridisation technique to identify chromosomal abnormalities in a series of primary CNS lymphomas. The findings demonstrated losses on chromosome 6q, with gains on chromosomes 12q, 18q and 22q in most tumours; further studies are required to establish the significance of these findings. Molecular genetic studies to identify immunoglobulin gene rearrangements in primary CNS lymphomas have indicated that most B-cell tumours are derived from highly mutated germinal centre B-cells, but futher work is required to clarify the molecular pathogenesis of these tumours.[61,66] Other molecular genetic abnormalities have not been extensively studied in primary CNS lymphomas, but *CDKN2A* inactivation appears to represent an important molecular mechanism. In contrast, mutations of *TP53* and alterations of *BCL-2* appear to be of minor significance.[67]

Molecular genetic studies have also been employed to investigate the role of the EBV in the pathogenesis of primary CNS lymphomas. EBV is a transforming human herpesvirus (HHV) which is associated with an

Table 11.3 REAL classification of lymphoid neoplasms[2]

B-cell neoplasms	T-cell and putative NK-cell neoplasms	Hodgkin's disease
I. Precursor B-cell neoplasm 1. Precursor B-lymphoblastic leukaemia / lymphoma	*I. Precursor T-cell neoplasm* 1. Precursor T-lymphoblastic lymphoma / leukaemia	I. *Lymphocyte predominance* II. *Nodular sclerosis* III. *Mixed cellularity* IV. *Lymphocyte depletion* V. *Provisional entity: lymphocyte-rich classical Hodgkin's disease*
II. Peripheral B-cell neoplasms 1. B-cell chronic lymphocytic leukaemia / prolymphocytic leukaemia / small lymphocytic lymphoma 2. Lymphoplasmacytoid lymphoma / immunocytoma 3. Mantle cell lymphoma 4. Follicle centre cell lymphoma, follicular (provisional cytological grades: I small cell, II mixed small and large cell, III large cell) 5. Marginal zone B-cell lymphoma, extranodal (MALT-type ± monocytoid B-cells); provisional subtype: nodal (± monocytoid B-cells) 6. Provisional entity: splenic marginal zone lymphoma (± villous lymphocytes) 7. Hairy cell leukaemia 8. Plasmacytoma / plasma cell myeloma 9. Diffuse large B-cell lymphoma; subtype: primary mediastinal (thymic) B-cell lymphoma 10. Burkitt's lymphoma 11. Provisional entity: high-grade B-cell lymphoma, Burkitt-like	*II. Peripheral T-cell and NK-cell neoplasms* 1. T-cell chronic lymphocytic leukaemia / lymphoma 2. Large granular lymphocyte leukaemia: T-cell type; NK-cell type 3. Mycosis fungoides / Seazary syndrome 4. Peripheral T-cell lymphomas, unspecified; provisional cytological categories: medium-sized cell, mixed medium and large cell, large cell, lymphoepitheliod cell. Provisional subtypes: hepatosplenic γδ T-cell lymphoma; subcutaneous panniculitic T-cell lymphoma 5. Angioimmunoblastic T-cell lymphoma 6. Angiocentric lymphoma 7. Intestinal T-cell lymphoma (± enteropathy-associated) 8. Adult T-cell lymphoma / leukaemia 9. Anaplastic large cell lymphoma, CD30+, T-cell and null-cell types 10. Provisional entity: anaplastic large-cell lymphoma, Hodgkin-like	

MALT, mucosa-associated lymphoid tissues; NK, natural killer; REAL, Revised European–American Classification of Lymphoid Neoplasms.

Table 11.4 Reported incidence of subtypes of primary CNS lymphoma (REAL classification) (based on other classifications in references).[1,5,-7,10,19,2,2,47,59]

Non-AIDS cases		AIDS cases	
Diffuse follicle centre cell lymphoma grade III	40%	Diffuse large B-cell lymphoma	65%
Diffuse large B-cell lymphoma	20%	Diffuse follicle centre cell lymphoma grade III	20%
Diffuse follicle centre cell lymphoma grade I–II	10%	Diffuse follicle centre cell lymphoma grade I–II	5%
Diffuse small lymphocytic and lymphoplasmacytoid		Diffuse small lymphocytic and lymphoplasmacytoid	
lymphoma	10%	lymphoma	<5%
Peripheral T-cell lymphoma	<1%	High grade B-cell lymphoma, Burkitt-like	<5%
		Peripheral T-cell lymphoma	<5%

REAL, Revised European–American Classification of Lymphoid Neoplasms.

increasing number of malignancies as defined by the detection of viral nucleic acids and gene products in tumour cells. EBV DNA sequences have been consistently found in AIDS-related primary CNS lymphomas as well as lymphomas occurring in other immunocompromised hosts (see Ref. 7 for review). In addition to EBV DNA, six virus-encoded nuclear antigens have been identified, and several latent membrane proteins and abundant non-polyadenylated nuclear RNAs (EPER1 and EPER2) have also been demonstrated in tumour cells. Most AIDS-related lymphomas appear to express EBNA2, LMP and EPER (latency pattern III – see Table 11.5), similar to B-cells which have been transformed by EBV into lymphoblastoid cell lines in vitro.[68] PCR assays for EBV DNA in cerebrospinal fluid (CSF) have been claimed to be highly specific and sensitive for the detection of primary CNS lymphomas in AIDS patients.[57] Another virus which has been implicated in the pathogenesis of these tumours is HHV-8,[69] although a recent comprehensive study concluded that infection with this virus is not a feature of primary CNS lymphomas in patients with AIDS.[70]

Differential diagnosis

The histological differential diagnosis of primary CNS lymphoma is listed in Table 11.6. Perhaps the commonest clinical and radiological differential diagnosis (particularly in immunocompetent patients) is *glioblastoma*. Fortunately, this difficulty is usually easy to resolve at intraoperative diagnosis, since lymphomas lack the vascular endothelial proliferation, gliofibrillary matrix and marked nuclear pleomorphism that characterises glioblastomas in smear preparations. These features may not be so evident in tumours which are markedly necrotic, in which case diagnosis may be deferred until paraffin sections are available, although a careful inspection of the smears and cryostat sections usually identifies the characteristic perivascular orientation of the tumour cells in primary CNS lymphoma. Confusion might also arise in cytological terms in smear preparations with *oligodendroglioma*, but the relative uniformity of the nuclei, the delicately

Table 11.5 EBV latency in virus-associated lymphomas[7,68]

Latency	EBER	EBNA	LMP	Lymphoma
I	+	1	–	Burkitt's lymphoma
II	+	1	1 and 2	Hodgkin's disease T-cell non-Hodgkin's lymphoma
III	+	1, 2,3A,3B	1 and 2	Post-transplantation Lymphoproliferative disorders Primary CNS Lymphoma in AIDS

EBER, Epstein–Barr virus non-polyadenylated RNAs; EBNA, Epstein–Barr virus nuclear antigen; EBV, Epstein–Barr virus; LMP, latent membrane protein.

branching blood vessels and focal calcification all help distinguish these tumours from primary CNS lymphoma. Immunocytochemistry for glial fibrillary acidic protein (GFAP) and lymphoid cell markers will also help resolve any morphological diagnostic difficulties with glioblastoma and oligodendroglioma.

Primary CNS lymphomas may also be confused with *malignant embryonal tumours* arising in the CNS, including *medulloblastoma, ependymoblastoma, neuroblastoma, pineoblastoma* and *primary neuroectodermal tumour*, particularly when necrosis is present. Both tumour categories contain populations of small neoplastic cells with a high mitotic rate and evidence of apoptosis, but close attention to the nuclear morphology and the relationship of the tumour cells to blood vessels can help resolve this problem at intraoperative diagnosis. Paraffin section histology and immunocytochemistry will provide definitive information, since B- and T-cell lymphoid cell markers are not widely expressed in primary embryonal CNS neoplasms.

Other intrinsic CNS neoplasms containing populations of reactive T-cells can be mistaken for primary CNS lymphomas, particularly *germinomas* and *gangliogliomas*. The relationship of the tumour cells to blood vessels and the nuclear morphology of CNS lymphomas are usually sufficient to allow an accurate intraoperative diagnosis, but immunocytochemistry on paraffin sections will be conclusive, since lymphomas do not express placental

Table 11.6 Differential diagnosis of primary CNS lymphoma

Intraparenchymal	Subarachnoid
Lymphoproliferative lesions	Reactive lymphocytosis in CSF
Metastatic non-Hodgkin's lymphoma	Chronic meningitis
	Tuberculosis
Metastatic leukaemia	Metastatic lymphoma / leukaemia
Hodgkin's disease	Metastatic melanoma
Other lymphomas – lymphomatoid granulomatosis, angiotrophic large cell lymphoma	Metastatic small cell carcinoma
	Metastatic PNET / medulloblastoma
Gliomas	
Astrocytoma (at lesion margin)	
Oligodendroglioma	
Glioblastoma	
Ganglioglioma	
Embryonal tumours	
PNET / medulloblastoma	
Neuroblastoma	
Pineoblastoma	
Ependymoblastoma	
Other tumours	
Pituitary adenoma	
Germinoma	
Lymphoplasmacytoid-rich meningioma	
Metastatic small cell carcinoma	
Melanoma (primary or metastatic)	
Non-neoplastic lesions	
Viral encephalitis	
Multiple sclerosis	
Postinfectious encephalitis	
Progressive multifocal leukoencephalopathy	
CMV encephalitis	
Toxoplasmosis	

CSF, cerebrospinal fluid, PNET, primary neuroectodermal tumour

alkaline phosphatase (PLAP) or other germ cell 'markers', synaptophysin, neurofilament protein or GFAP. *Pituitary adenomas* may be confused with primary CNS lymphoma at intraoperative diagnosis, but the absence of cellular cohesion, the perivascular orientation of the tumour cells and the high mitotic rate and apoptosis in primary CNS lymphomas usually allow a clear distinction, which can be reinforced on immunocytochemistry for lymphoid cell antigens and pituitary hormones, and by electron microscopy.

Primary CNS lymphoma may be confused with *metastatic small cell carcinoma* at intraoperative diagnosis, since both tumours contain small neoplastic cells with a high mitotic rate and apoptotic cells. The cellular cohesion, nuclear 'moulding' and lack of perivascular tumour cell orientation allow the metastatic small cell carcinoma to be distinguished from the lymphoma, and this distinction is further reinforced on paraffin section histology

and immunocytochemistry for lymphoid cell surface antigens, and cytokeratins, epithelial membrane antigen, neurone specific enolase, chromogranin and synaptophysin in the small cell carcinoma. It should be noted in passing that the inexperienced observer may also confuse the *small granular neurones of the cerebellar cortex* with either a metastatic small cell carcinoma or a lymphoma; the nuclear uniformity, lack of cellular cohesion and anatomical relationship of granular neurones to other cerebellar cortical neurones will resolve the problem, which is unlikely to recur with experience.

It is also unlikely that primary CNS lymphoma would ever be confused with one of the commoner subtypes of *meningioma* either at intraoperative diagnosis or on examination of paraffin sections, although this difficulty may occasionally arise in clinical and neuroradiological terms. The characteristic arachnoidal morphology and the presence of sheets and whorls of tumour cells with psammoma bodies are characteristic of meningiomas, but are never encountered in lymphomas. However, the lymphoplasmacyte-rich meningioma may cause diagnostic difficulties, since it contains dense follicular aggregates and infiltrates of small lymphoplasmacytoid cells.[71] The differential diagnosis in such a case would include a primary dural MALToma, and other lymphoid lesions such as Castleman's disease. Immunocytochemical studies to identify the meningothelial component in these lesions will aid diagnosis.[71]

A more problematic differential diagnosis exists between *other types of lymphoma* including *secondary lymphoma in the CNS, Hodgkin's disease, lymphomatoid granulomatosis* and *angiotrophic large cell lymphoma*. Often it is not possible to resolve this difficulty, much of which is dependent on relevant clinical information and accurate disease staging. A distinction between a primary non-Hodgkin's lymphoma and Hodgkin's disease in the CNS can be problematic, although the latter is extremely uncommon and these difficulties can often be resolved only on immunocytochemical or molecular genetic studies. Occasionally a difficulty may be encountered in confusing a *reactive process* with a primary CNS lymphoma, particularly disorders in which perivascular lymphocytic cuffing occurs including *viral or postinfectious encephalitis, multiple sclerosis* and *progressive multifocal leuco-encephalopathy*. These difficulties can often be resolved by close inspection of the nuclear features of the perivascular lymphoid cells, and immunocytochemistry is useful in confirming their polymorphous composition. It should be borne in mind that patients with immunodeficiency, particularly AIDS patients, can suffer from multiple pathological processes in the brain including *toxoplasmosis, CMV encephalitis* and *progressive multifocal leuco-encephalopathy*, as well as a concurrent primary CNS lymphoma. This differential diagnosis requires extensive investigation by a wide range of immunocytochemical and, if necessary, molecular genetic techniques.

Another difficult diagnostic situation can arise in patients with *sentinel lesions*, particularly after treatment with corticosteroids. These may exhibit a range of histological features, including active demyelination with axonal sparing, an inflammatory infiltrate comprising mainly T-cells and macrophages with few B-cells and no cytological evidence of malignancy.[35,36] Sentinel lesions may represent a host immune reaction against the neoplasm, although the mechanism of involution is unknown. Follow-up biopsies on such cases have found unequivocal evidence of primary CNS B-cell lymphoma, usually of diffuse large cell or immunoblastic subtypes. Biopsies taken from patients with *primary CNS lymphoma following corticosteroid therapy* can also cause diagnostic difficulties, since there is usually a predominance of reactive T-cells and macrophages with reactive astrocytes and relatively few tumour cells. Even with an adequate clinical history, it can be impossible to arrive at a diagnosis under these circumstances and rebiopsy may be required at a later date (once corticosteroid therapy has been discontinued) in order to obtain more representative material.

Therapy and prognosis

It is accepted that the histological grading of primary CNS lymphomas is not always of prognostic significance and clinical parameters are more important, particularly the presence of coexisting immunodeficiency, and especially in patients with AIDS.[15,39] Favourable prognostic factors have included single lesions with an absence of meningeal infiltration at a relatively young age and a preoperative Karnofsky score of over 70.[72–74] The standard treatment for primary CNS lymphoma is whole brain irradiation, but although complete disease remission is achieved, relapse is common and median survival is around 1 year.[75] Current treatment regimes usually include radiotherapy and corticosteroid therapy with pre- or postradiation chemotherapy. There has been no consensus on the most appropriate drugs to use; most regimes favour combination chemotherapy.[76,77] Patients with AIDS have a very poor prognosis with a median survival of only 2–6 months with a primary CNS lymphoma, although selected patients without other extensive disease may survive for longer when treated with multimodal therapy.[39,72,73] Immunosuppressed patients with primary CNS lymphoma usually benefit from a reduction in their immunosuppressive therapy, with tumour shrinkage noted on reduction of immunosupression. Most deaths in primary CNS lymphomas occur as a consequence of tumour recurrence, but in patients with AIDS the existence of other intracranial and systemic pathologies are also of major prognostic significance. Tumour recurrences are usually confined to the CNS, but may occur in areas other than those involved by the primary lesion, involving the spinal cord, meninges or eye. Up to 10% of patients have been reported with metastatic disease outside the CNS at autopsy; this usually involves extranodal sites, including the lungs.[78]

Post-transplant lymphoproliferative disorders

The association between primary CNS lymphoma and immunosuppression was first described in patients who had undergone renal transplantation. Since then, this complication has arisen in various other types of organ transplantation and in the largest group (the renal transplant patients) the incidence of this tumour is increased up to 50 times compared with an age and sex matched control population.[16–18,79] The frequency of these post-transplantation tumours relates to the degree of immunosuppression required to prevent rejection and to the organ type. Primary CNS lymphoma accounts for around 25% of all transplantation associated lymphomas. In recent years, the use of cyclosporin A into post-transplant treatment regimes has significantly reduced the incidence of both systemic and cerebral lymphoma as a post-transplantation complication.[80]

EBV is thought to be critical in the pathogenesis of this complication. Iatrogenic immunosuppression in transplant recipients results in impaired T-cell immunity, which facilitates the outgrowth of EBV-infected B-cells.[7,81,82] Most examples of post-transplant lymphoproliferative disorders express EBV latency III viral proteins (see above) and may regress when T-cell immunity is restored by the withdrawal of immunosuppression.[81] These disorders can be divided into three main groups on the basis of morphology, clonality, EBV status and oncogene expression (Table 11.7); multiple forms may occur within a single patient at different sites in the body.[82,83] The commonest group, 'polymorphic post-transplant lymphoproliferative disorder' (Figs 11.19 and 11.20), responds variably to the withdrawal of immunosuppression, but the post-transplant lymphoproliferative disease–malignant lymphoma immunoblastic group behaves in an overtly malignant fashion, often with a poor response to therapeutic intervention and short survival times.[81–83]

CNS involvement in other types of lymphoproliferative disorders

Other neoplastic lymphoproliferative disorders involving the CNS are listed in Table 11.8.

Angiofollicular lymph node hyperplasia

This disorder (also known as Castleman's disease) is an uncommon disorder which most often occurs in systemic

Table 11.7 Post-transplantation lymphoproliferative syndrome subtypes[81–83]

Subtype	Sites	B-cell clonality	EBV status	Oncogene status
Plasmacytic hyperplasia	Lymph nodes, oropharynx	Polyclonal	Multiple EBV infectious events	No abnormalities
Polymorphic lymphoproliferative diseases	Lymph nodes, lung, gut	Monoclonal	Single form of EBV	No abnormalities
Malignant lymphoma, multiple myeloma	Widespread	Monoclonal	Single form of EBV	*c-myc, ras, p53* abnormalities

EBV, Epstein–Barr virus.

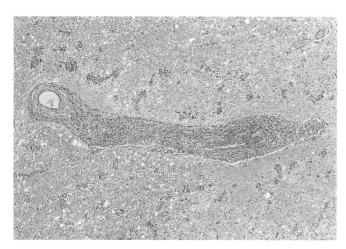

Fig. 11.19 **Post-transplant lymphoproliferative syndrome**. The patient was a renal transplant recipient. A perivascular aggregate of lymphoplasmacytoid and centroblastic cells is shown. H & E.

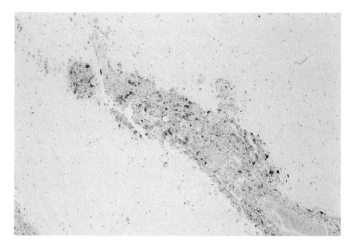

Fig. 11.20 **Post-transplant lymphoproliferative syndrome**. Immunocytochemistry for the Epstein–Barr virus latent membrane protein shows variable positivity within the lymphoid cell population (same case as Fig. 11.19).

Table 11.8 Other neoplastic lymphoproliferative disorders involving the CNS

Brain and spinal cord	Meninges, epidural space and bone
Angiotrophic large cell lymphoma	Angiofollicular lymph node hyperplasia
Burkitt's lymphoma	
Hodgkin's disease	Hodgkin's disease
Leukaemia – acute and chronic	Leukaemia – acute and chronic
Lymphomatoid granulomatosis	Multiple myeloma
Mycosis fungoides	Plasmacytoma
Richter syndrome	
Waldenstrom's macroglobulinaemia	

lymph nodes but can arise in extranodal sites, including the dura mater and subcutaneous tissue of the scalp.[84–86] Involvement of the CNS is extremely uncommon, and usually occurs as a focal tumour-like mass which on histological examination shows the characteristic feature of this disease with proliferations of lymphoid cells and plasma cells and focal areas of germinal centre formation (Fig. 11.21).

Angiotrophic (intravascular) large cell lymphoma

This unusual disorder is an intravascular lympho-proliferative disorder, but has a predilection for the CNS. There has been considerable debate in the past on the origin of the characteristic large malignant intravascular cells, but these have been conclusively shown to be of lymphoid origin and predominantly B-cell neoplasms.[87] Occasional cases of T-cell intravascular large cell lymphoma have been reported, one of which was associated with EBV infection.[88] The disorder is often multifocal, and frequently involves the skin in addition to the CNS. Neurological symptoms may be the only manifestation of the disease and some of these disorders appear to be truly restricted to the CNS.[89] CNS involvement can be widespread and the entire neuroaxis can be involved. This is reflected in the clinical symptomatology, which can range from acute or chronic encephalopathy, progressive dementia, cranial neuropathies and a cauda equina syndrome. The clinical abnormalities appear to result from ischaemic damage to the CNS as a consequence of vascular occlusion by the large neoplastic cells which are occasionally attached to the vessel wall (Figs 11.22 and

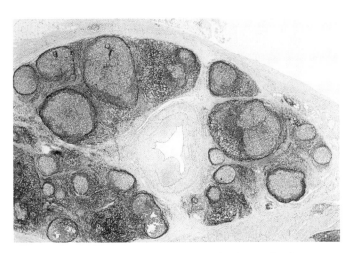

Fig. 11.21 **Castleman's disease**. In this case the disease (hyaline variant) involves the cranial meninges, centred around a large vessel. H & E.

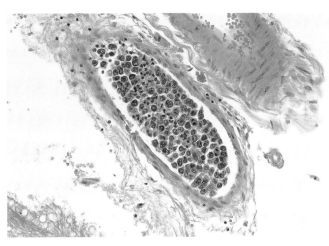

Fig. 11.22 **Intravascular B-cell lymphoma**. A blood vessel in the meninges is filled with large pleomorphic tumour cells. H & E.

11.23). Focal extravascular spread has been reported occasionally, with the formation of perivascular tumour masses.[87] Reduced expression of beta-2 integrins on the tumour cells may contribute to the relatively low frequency of extravascular spread.[90] The prognosis for this condition is poor, with a median survival of only 9.5 months; however, the use of cranial irradiation and combined chemotherapy may be expected to improve this dismal outlook.[87,89]

Hodgkin's disease

Intracranial involvement in Hodgkin's disease is uncommon, and some of the earlier reports in the literature which claim to represent examples of this entity are questionable in terms of their morphological and immunophenotypic characterisation. Most cases of Hodgkin's disease in the CNS are an example of an involvement by systemic disease as dural metastases, which form lobulated circumscribed masses resembling a meningioma. Involvement of the parenchyma is extremely uncommon under these circumstances, although direct invasion from an adjacent dural mass may occur. Diffuse involvement of the subarachnoid space has also been described, but is exceptional. Involvement of the spinal canal has also been described in Hodgkin's disease, usually in the context of widespread disease dissemination or relapse. Most cases present with epidural infiltration, which may be multifocal. The thoracic portion of the epidural space is most commonly involved, followed by the lumbar. This is usually associated with involvement of the adjacent vertebral bodies or by direct extension of masses from the retroperitoneal space or posterior mediastinum.

The clinical features of Hodgkin's disease in the brain relate to the extent and site of the intracranial deposits

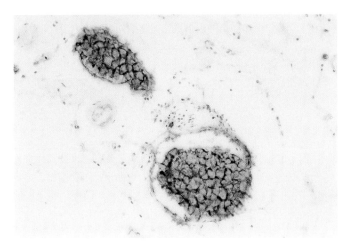

Fig. 11.23 **Intravascular lymphoma**. The tumour cells in malignant intravascular lymphoma stain strongly on immunocytochemistry for CD20 within vessels in a spinal nerve root (same case as Fig. 11.22).

and the associated skeletal involvement. Primary Hodgkin's disease in the brain is very rare; the diagnosis is critically dependent on the identification of Reed-Sternberg cells within the lymphoid population which are immunoreactive to CD30 and CD15, but usually exhibit a negative staining reaction with CD45.[91–93] The accompanying non-neoplastic cells (lymphocytes, plasma cells, eosinophils and histiocytes) are variable in the intraparenchymal primary disease. The histological subtypes of systemic Hodgkin's disease that have been most often reported with CNS involvement are nodular sclerosis and mixed cellularity types; involvement by lymphocyte predominant Hodgkin's disease has apparently never been recorded. Hodgkin's disease has only very rarely presented with spinal cord compression from an epidural deposit (Figs 11.24 and 11.25); spinal cord compression may occur in up to 5% of patients with advanced systemic Hodgkin's disease.[94]

Lymphomatoid granulomatosis

This rare disorder exhibits many clinical and pathological similarities to angiocentric T/NK cell lymphoma, and was formerly included within the group of T-cell lymphoproliferative disorders.[95] Recent studies have indicated that lymphomatoid granulomatosis is a B-cell lymphoma associated with EBV infection, and accompanied by a florid T-cell reaction.[96] EBV nucleic acids are present in clonal form within B-cells in this disease. Extranodal presentation is common, mostly involving the lungs and skin, but the CNS can be involved in up to 20% of cases and some patients may present with CNS manifestations.[97,98] These are extremely variable depending on the site and size of the intra-parenchymal lesions (Fig. 11.26); focal neurological deficits are the commonest clinical abnormalities, although dementia has been described in one case with a diffusely infiltrative disease process.

CNS involvement is characterised by a perivascular polymorphous infiltrate comprising numerous T-lymphocytes (Fig. 11.27), plasma cells and histiocytes in addition to large transformed immunoblasts.[96] These are of B-cell origin and exhibit marked cytological atypia, with expression of CD20 and CD79a. T-lymphocytes can invade endothelium, resulting in vascular necrosis and haemorrhage. EBV may mediate the vascular damage

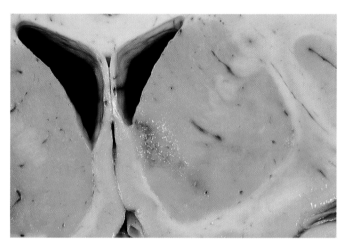

Fig. 11.26 **Lymphomatoid granulomatosis**. A solitary tumour deposit is visible in the caudate nucleus.

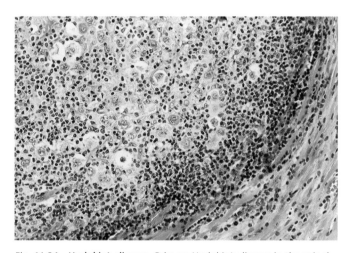

Fig. 11.24 **Hodgkin's disease**. Primary Hodgkin's disease in the spinal epidural space. A nodular sclerosing histology and a large number of Reed–Sternberg cells are seen. H & E.

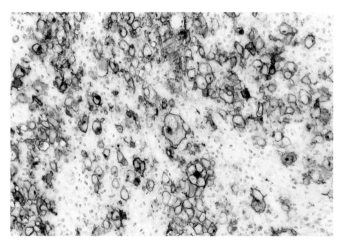

Fig. 11.25 **Hodgkin's disease**. Immunocytochemistry for CD30 shows strong cytoplasmic and membranous staining of the Reed–Sternberg cell population in Hodgkin's disease (same case as Fig. 11.24).

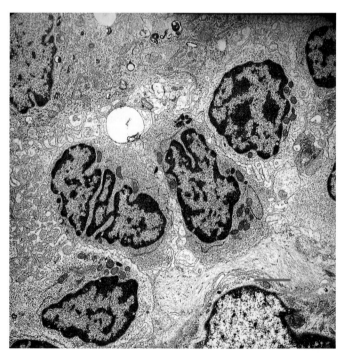

Fig. 11.27 **Lymphomatoid granulomatosis**. Electron microscopy. A population of reactive T-lymphocytes around a blood vessel is shown. Bar = 5 μm.

associated with this disease, possibly involving chemokines IP-10 and Mig.[96] Some cases of lymphomatoid granulomatosis regress spontaneously, but most patients require treatment and CNS involvement will now receive irradiation and combination chemotherapy.[97–100] The lesions of lymphomatoid granulomatosis can be graded histologically into three groups, depending on the number of EBV-positive B-cells. When these are absent or infrequent (grades 1 and 2), treatment by immunomodulation is satisfactory, but grade 3 lesions with numerous EBV positive cells require to be treated as malignant lymphomas.[96]

Mycosis fungoides

This rare systemic T-cell lymphoma most often involves the skin, but is capable of dissemination to other organs including the CNS. CNS involvement usually takes place in the later stages of the disease after the appearance of the skin lesions, and may occur in up to 15% of all cases.[101] The eye may also be involved, often at a rather higher frequency in most reported series; intraocular involvement can be diagnosed cytologically by vitreous biopsy. CNS involvement most often occurs as a meningeal infiltration, but perivascular, solitary and diffuse intraparenchymal deposits have also been described.[102,103] Treatment with cranial irradiation and chemotherapy may have a palliative effect, but long term survival has not been reported in the context of CNS involvement in this disorder.[101,104]

Richter syndrome

This unusual and rare condition is the manifestation of high grade large cell lymphoma in a patient with chronic lymphocytic leukaemia. The clinical manifestations of the disease occur most commonly in systemic lymph nodes, but brain involvement with the large cell lymphoma has been reported in occasional cases.[105] The development of lymphoma suggests transformation from the original lymphocytic clone, but the mechanisms underlying this transformation are uncertain.

Waldenstrom's macroglobulinaemia

Waldenstrom's macroglobulinaemia is a lymphoplasmacytoid B-cell lymphoma which secretes lgM lambda (sometimes referred to as an immunocytoma in the earlier literature). CNS involvement is uncommon, but encephalopathies have been described in association with diffuse infiltration of the brain parenchyma (Bing–Neel syndrome).[106] These have been treated successfully by irradiation after brain biopsy for diagnostic con-

firmation, when numerous lymphoplasmacytoid cells (with Russell bodies and Duchter bodies) stained positively for lgM and lambda light chain.

Spinal epidural lymphoma

Systemic lymphomas can present as spinal epidural masses, without accompanying lymph node involvement. This presentation is unusual, and there are few data on the incidence of this phenomenon; most recent reviews are concerned with only relatively small numbers of cases. Spinal epidural lymphoma can present over a wide age range (11–87 years in one recent series),[107] with a mean age of onset in the sixth decade.[108–113] Most patients present with lumboradicular pain, leg weakness or progressive paraparesis and undergo decompressive laminectomy when an epidural mass is demonstrated by conventional or CT myelography.[113] On MRI scans, these tumours are isodense with the spinal cord on T1-weighted images and hyperintense on proton density or T2-weighted images.[114] Most tumours are located in the thoracic region (Fig. 11.28), extending over several segments, and may infiltrate the adjacent vertebral body to cause vertebral collapse. Extension through the intervertebral foramina is common, resulting in a paravertebral soft tissue mass. Invasion of the vertebral body may occur and the intervetebral disc may also be involved, in contrast to metastatic carcinomas.

Histological studies have inevitably employed a range of lymphoma classifications, but there is general agreement that most tumours are high grade B-cell lymphomas (predominantly diffuse large B-cell lymphomas), but intermediate and low grade tumours are not uncommon (Fig. 11.29); T-cell lymphomas account for around 10% of cases.[107–112] The differential diagnosis (Table 11.9) includes *metastatic carcinoma*, paravertebral *Ewing's sarcoma*, *plasmacytoma/myeloma*; and *chronic inflammation* (including *tuberculosis*), *osteomyelitis*, or *bone abscess* when the vertebral body is involved; immunocytochemistry is helpful in resolving these problems. The possibility of *secondary systemic lymphoma* can be resolved when additional clinical data (particularly disease staging) become available after the initial diagnosis. Patients are usually treated by decompressive laminectomy with subsequent radiotherapy, chemotherapy, or both. Because of the relatively small number of reported series, the prognostic significance of tumour type and grade is uncertain; similar difficulties exist with the therapeutic assessment of radiation or chemotherapy. Most series report survival times ranging from a few weeks to several years, but it is likely that these figures are substantially influenced by the age and neurological status of the patients prior to surgery.[107–111] Further prospective studies are required to assess the optimal therapeutic regimes for these uncommon tumours.

Table 11.9 Differential diagnosis of spinal epidural non-Hodgkin lymphoma

Reactive conditions	Other lymphoproliferative disorders	Other neoplasms
Chronic osteomyelitis	Systemic non-Hodgkin's lymphoma	Metastatic small cell carcinoma
Paraspinal abscess	Hodgkin's disease	Ewing's sarcoma
Tuberculosis	Plasmacytoma	Metastatic neuroblastoma
	Multiple myeloma	
	Leukaemia – acute or chronic	

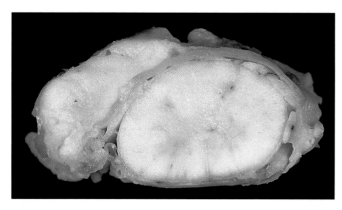

Fig. 11.28 **Spinal epidural lymphoma**. There is spinal cord compression by thoracic epidural space, with infiltration of the dura.

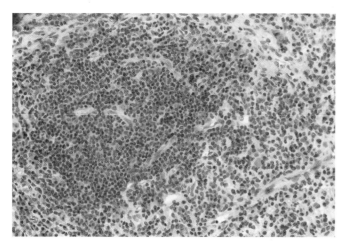

Fig. 11.29 **Spinal epidural lymphoma**. Cryostat section in a low grade primary spinal epidural lymphoma shows infiltration of the dura mater at the margins of the tumour. H & E.

Plasma cell tumours

Three major categories of plasma cell tumours are recognised; multiple myeloma, solitary plasmacytoma of bone and solitary extramedullary plasmacytoma. These tumours are composed of monoclonal populations of plasma cells which express immunoglobulin light and heavy chains, which are readily detectable by immunocytochemical techniques. The relationship between these three disorders is unclear and it appears that many cases of solitary plasmacytoma of bone represent a disorder which will eventually progress to multiple myeloma. All

three categories of tumours can involve the CNS, usually by causing spinal cord compression.

Multiple myeloma

This malignant plasma cell tumour can involve the skull and vertebral column, with erosion of the bone and the formation of an epidural mass which can penetrate the dura and occasionally infiltrate the leptomeninges. Most cases present in late adult life, with a median age of onset around 64 years. Bone pain involving the back is the most common presenting symptom.[115] Skull involvement is common, with multiple lytic deposits in advanced cases (giving the appearances of a 'pepperpot skull' on plain X-ray films); the extramedullary soft tissues including the orbit can also be involved. Compression of the skull and skull base can result in cranial nerve palsies and the comparable process in the vertebral bodies and spinal dura can result in spinal cord compression and paraplegia, particularly in the thoracic region[116] (Fig. 11.30). This usually occurs from a tumour extending from the vertebral mass, without dural penetration.

Most cases are accompanied by the production of a monoclonal immunoglobulin (IgG in 60%, IgA in 20–25% and in 15–20% of cases free immunoglobulin light chains are produced) which can be detected in the serum and urine, or both.[115] Biopsies of the paraspinal or vertebral masses show a population of neoplastic plasma cells which vary in appearance from mature cells to immature cells with a blast-like appearance. Binucleate cells may be present (Fig. 11.31), and mitotic activity is easily detected. Some tumour cells contain rounded intracytoplasmic inclusions known as Russell bodies, which are related to immunoglobulin production (particularly kappa light chains), and intranuclear Duchter bodies. Immunocytochemistry for immunoglobulin light and heavy chains is essential for adequate investigation and diagnosis. Many myelomas do not express pan B-cell antigens, e.g. CD20 or CD79a, but anaplastic evolution of myeloma may occur, resulting in histological and immunophenotypic features resembling B-cell immunoblastic lymphoma.[115,117] The differential diagnosis of multiple myeloma is discussed below. The clinical diagnostic criteria for multiple myeloma are summarised in Table 11.10. Standard treatment for multiple myeloma for several decades has involved the use of melphalan and prednisolone, although resistance to these drugs has been reported in recurrent

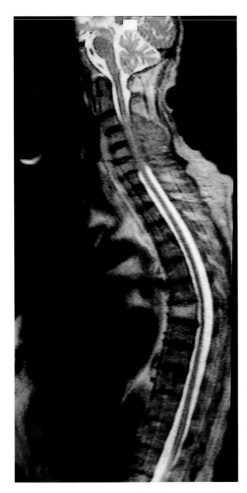

Fig. 11.30 **Multiple myeloma**. T2-weighted MR image of the spine. A cervical soft tissue mass with epidural cord compression and obliteration of the CSF space are shown. The tumour also involves several vertebral bodies, but the intervertebral discs are spared. (Courtesy of Dr D Collie, Edinburgh.)

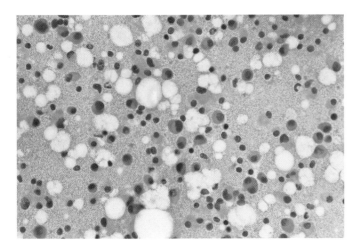

Fig. 11.31 **Multiple myeloma**. Smear preparations in multiple myeloma contain a population of non-cohesive malignant plasmacytoid cells, including binucleate cells. H & E.

Table 11.10   Clinical criteria for the diagnosis of multiple myeloma[115]

Plasmacytoma / myeloma on tissue biopsy, or > 10% plasma cells in a bone marrow biopsy

Clinical features of myeloma:
Bone pain and pathological fracture
Anaemia and marrow failure
Infection due to immunoparesis and marrow failure
Renal impairment

At least one of:
Serum M band (IgG>30 g/l; IgA>20 g/l)
Urine M band (Bence Jones proteinuria)
Osteolytic lesions detected on skeletal survey

or progressive tumours, which usually requires the use of combination chemotherapy;[115,117] the median survival for patients with multiple myeloma is around 3 years. Myeloma may also occur rarely as a meningeal tumour,[118,119] which may resemble a meningioma on radiology and macroscopic examination.

Solitary plasmacytoma

These unusual neoplasms occur in the airways, lymph nodes or the spleen, but may involve the dura mater of the spinal cord and, very occasionally, the intracranial dura around the skull base.[120–122] Plasmacytomas occur more often in females than in males, with a disease onset most often in the sixth decade of life. The spinal cord examples occur most often in the region of the mid-thoracic vertebrae and present with clinical features and radiological findings similar to meningiomas. These lesions form nodular or plaque-like dural masses which may infiltrate the spinal parenchyma.[121] The neoplastic plasma cells can vary from well differentiated to immature cells (Fig. 11.32). The monoclonal nature of the plasma cell population is readily demonstrable on immunocytochemistry for immunoglobulin light and heavy chains, but most plasmacytomas do not express pan B-cell antigens. Amyloid depostion is a well recognised feature of these tumours, and was reported in 25% of cases in one series. Around 50% of cases have a detectable monoclonal antibody in the serum and urine, which in most cases is IgG kappa. Approximately one-third of patients with a solitary plasmacytoma will go on to develop multiple myeloma; this appears to occur more frequently in cases presenting with predominant bone marrow involvement.[121]

Differential diagnosis of plasma cell neoplasms

A distinction between multiple myeloma and plasmacytoma is not always possible on histological grounds alone (unless multiple lesions have been sampled); detailed radiological screening and disease staging is required for accurate classification. The differential

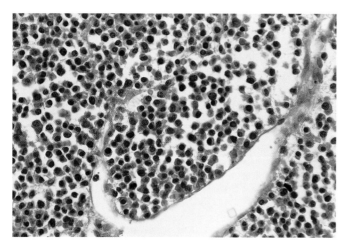

Fig. 11.32 **Plasmacytoma**. Solitary plasmacytoma with a population of well differentiated neoplastic plasma cells surrounding a thin-walled blood vessel in the spinal meninges. H & E.

diagnosis of multiple myeloma and plasmacytoma is listed in Table 11.11. It includes *chronic inflammatory disorders*, particularly *plasma cell granuloma* (see below), and *chronic osteomyelitis* and *abscesses* in bone. The reactive conditions can be distinguished from plasma cell tumours by the use of immunocytochemistry for immunoglobulin light and heavy chains. Antibodies to kappa and lambda light chains do not always give satisfactory results on paraffin embedded material (particularly if this contains bone and has undergone decalcification), and other techniques, including in situ hybridisation for kappa and lambda chains, or molecular genetic techniques to study immunoglobulin gene rearrangements, may be required. The opinion of an expert in the diagnosis of lymphoreticular tumours is always helpful in difficult cases. *Lymphoplasmacytoid lymphomas* may be difficult to distinguish on morphological grounds from plasma cell tumours, although these forms of lymphoma seldom involve the spinal epidural space, vertebral column or skull. IgM production is characteristic of lymphoplasmacytoid lymphomas, but is less common in plasma cell tumours. Other lymphoid neoplasms, particularly *high grade diffuse large B-cell lymphomas*, may be difficult to distinguish

from anaplastic plasma cell tumours when there is a predominant population of immunoblastic tumour cells. Most malignant B-cell lymphomas of this type involve the lymph nodes, and the tumour cells usually express pan B-cell antigens, in contrast to plasma cell tumours. Plasma cell tumours are unlikely to be mistaken for *metastatic carcinoma* on morphological grounds, but it should be recalled that neoplastic cells which resemble mature plasma cells can express epithelial membrane antigen on the cell surface (as do their non-neoplastic counterparts). Spinal plasmacytomas may be confused with meningiomas on radiological examination, but this differential diagnosis seldom poses a problem in histological or immunocytochemical terms, although occasional meningiomas can contain a dense infiltrate of mature plasma cells and lymphocytes (*lymphoplasmacytoid rich meningiomas*). Paravertebral Ewing's sarcoma is included in the histological differential diagnosis, although it occurs at a younger age than most cases of myeloma and plasmacytoma; this possiblity is easily resolved on immunocytochemistry for B-cells, immunoglobulins and light chains, while most cases of Ewing's sarcoma express MIC2, a marker of peripheral primitive neuroectodermal tumours.

Plasma cell granuloma

This is a benign inflammatory condition which most often involves the lungs, but rare examples have been reported in the CNS, mostly involving the meninges (usually as a localised mass in the dura mater).[123] Other intracranial sites have been reported, including the pituitary stalk, and a rare intracerebral case has been reported.[124] Histologically, these lesions contain mature plasma cells with varying numbers of lymphocytes, neutrophil polymorphs, eosinophils and histiocytes within a collagenous stroma. Many previous cases have been reported as inflammatory pseudotumours; some confusion appears to exist in the older literature between plasma cell granulomas in the dura mater, lymphoplasmacytoid meningiomas and cases of histiocytosis.

Table 11.11 Differential diagnosis of plasmacytoma / multiple myeloma

Reactive conditions	Other lymphoproliferative disorders	Other neoplasms
Chronic osteomyelitis	B-cell lymphoplasmacytoid lymphoma / immunocytoma	Metastatic small cell carcinoma
Paraspinal abscess		Lymphoplasmacytoid rich meningioma
Tuberculosis	B-cell chronic lymphocytic leukaemia / prolymphocytic leukaemia / small lymphocytic lymphoma	
Plasma cell granuloma		Ewing's sarcoma
	Diffuse large B-cell lymphoma	
	Hodgkin's disease	

Acute and chronic leukaemia

CNS involvement in acute leukaemias (particularly acute lymphoblastic leukaemia) usually takes the form of diffuse leptomeningeal infiltration (Fig. 11.33). This occurred most frequently in the past as CNS relapse in young patients with controlled systemic disease, but since the development of successful regimes for CNS prophylaxis, this complication is now extremely uncommon.[125] Long term survivors of childhood leukaemia are at increased risk of developing second malignancies, of which around 50% are CNS tumours, mostly gliomas.[126,127] The risk of developing a CNS tumour under these circumstances is highest in children who received cranial irradiation under the age of 5 years as part of CNS prophylaxis.[126]

Meningeal leukaemia may occur in adults with either acute myeloid leukaemia or chronic myeloid leukaemia.[128] Chronic lymphocytic leukaemia may involve the CNS in up to 50% of patients, sometimes producing intracerebral haemorrhage or infarction if the white cell count is markedly elevated.[129] Cerebrovascular complications may also occur in acute leukaemia and in blast cell crisis in other forms of chronic leukaemia.[129] Rarer complications of chronic lymphocytic leukaemia include confusional state, meningitis with isolated cranial nerve palsies, optic neuropathy and cerebellar dysfunction.[130] CNS involvement in leukaemia is often detectable on CSF cytology,[128,130] when large numbers of blast cells may be present, but immunocytochemistry and flow cytometry on multiple samples may be required to differentiate blast cells from reactive lymphocytes if the latter predominate.[131]

Circumscribed destructive cranial, spinal dural or intracerebral masses (formerly referred to as chloromas, or granulocytic sarcomas) in patients with acute or chronic myeloid leukaemia are now uncommon, although they may occur at disease onset before blood and bone marrow abnormalities are detected, or as the first evidence of CNS relapse following successful disease control.[132,133] Most of these lesions show no evidence of myelocytic differentiation, and require immunocytochemical studies to confirm the disease phenotype.

Histiocytic disorders

Histiocytic tumours

This group of lesions includes both benign and neoplastic conditions which have been recently classified into three main groups:[134]

1. Langerhans cell histiocytosis.
2. Non-Langerhans cell histiocytosis.
3. Malignant histiocytosis.

Previous terminology for Langerhans cell histiocytosis includes histiocytosis X (comprising eosinophilic granuloma, Hand–Schüller–Christian disease and

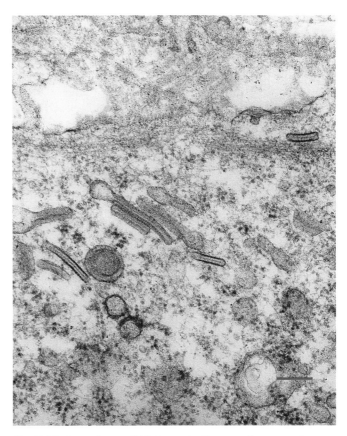

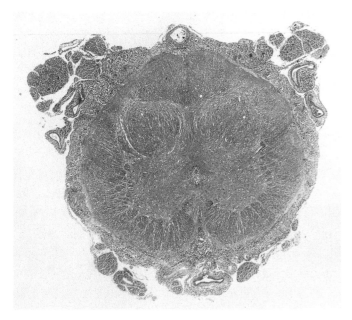

Fig. 11.33　**Leukaemia**. Widespread infiltration of the spinal subarachnoid space, nerve roots and early parenchymal invasion in a patient with acute myeloid leukaemia. H & E.

Fig. 11.34　**Langerhans cell histiocytosis**. Electron microscopy of a Langerhans cell histiocyte shows a characteristic Birbeck granule (centre). Bar = 0.5 μm.

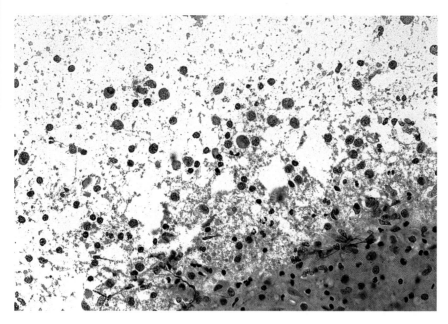

Fig. 11.35 **Langerhans cell histiocytosis.** Smear preparation in Langerhans cell histiocytosis. A mixed population of cells is shown in which histiocytes, macrophages and plasma cells are conspicuous. H & E.

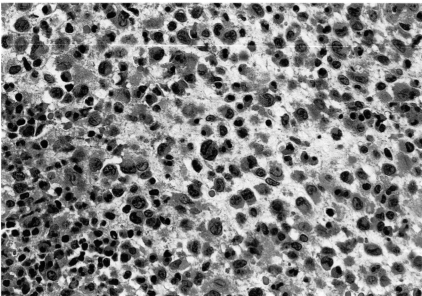

Fig. 11.36 **Langerhans cell histiocytosis.** Paraffin histology shows large numbers of histiocytes, macrophages, plasma cells and eosinophils. H & E.

Letterer–Siwe disease). The diagnosis of these conditions is based upon the recognition of the Langerhans cell, which is a histiocytic dendritic cell which expresses CD1A and contains cytoplasmic Birbeck granules which are identifiable on electron microscopy (Fig. 11.34). The non-Langerhans cell histiocytosis shows macrophage differentiation and does not express CD1A or contain Birbeck granules.[134]

Langerhans cell disorders are the commonest examples of this group and typically occur in children (median age at onset is 10 years), but presentations in adults up to the age of 70 years have been reported.[135,136] Involvement of the cranium is frequent (see Chapter 18), with skull base and orbital involvement accompanied by exophthalms and diabetes insipidus.[137] However, single or multiple foci of infiltration may occur in the parenchyma involving the hypothalamus, infundibulum, optic chiasm, choroid plexus and cerebral hemispheres.[138] The commonest neurological signs and symptoms are diabetes insipidus with other evidence of hypothalamic and pituitary dysfunction, cranial nerve palsies, visual disturbances and ataxia. Neuroimaging can demonstrate extraparenchymal solid masses or multiple lesions in the grey or white matter, and thickening of the pituitary stalk.[136,138,139] On macroscopic examination, or at surgery, the intracranial lesions are often yellow–white and may appear as discrete dual nodules or granular infiltrates; choroid plexus involvement is exceptional, resulting in an intraventricular mass.[140]

Fig. 11.37 **Intracerebral Rosai–Dorfman disease**. This typical lesion contains a mixture of lymphocytes, plasma cells and occasional multinucleate cells which exhibit emperipolesis. H & E.

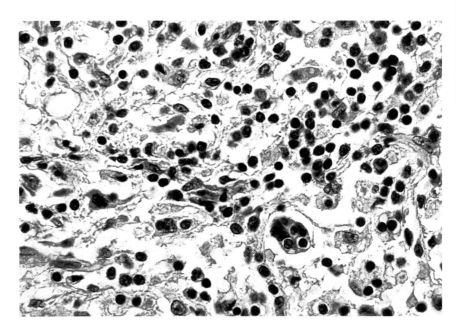

The histological features of Langerhans cell histiocytosis include large numbers of Langerhans cell histiocytes, macrophages, plasma cells, lymphocytes and variable numbers of eosinophils[135,138,139] (Figs 11.35 and 11.36). The Langerhans cell contains abundant cytoplasm, with an ovoid or renoform nucleus which often appears cleaved. Touton giant cells are present and aggregates of eosinophils may also occur. Langerhans cells consistently express S-100 protein, vimentin, human leucocyte antigen (HLA)-DR, beta-2 microglobulin and CD1A with variable CD68 expression.[134,138,139] Non-Langerhans cell macrophages are usually S-100 negative and CD1A negative, but will express CD68 and CD45.

The aetiology of this condition is poorly understood, and controversy exists as to whether it is truly a malignant process.[141] Multifocal disease in monozygotic twins has been described, indicating a genetic basis in at least some cases.[142] The genes responsible for these disorders are unknown. Survival rates in Langerhans cell histiocytosis are good, with over 70% of patients surviving for 20 years but event-free survival at 15 years is only 30%.[136] Unifocal disease may spontaneously regress or require only surgical resection (particularly for single skull lesions), but multisystemic disease requires treatment with combination chemotherapy and carries a higher mortality.[135–137]

CNS involvement can also occur in non-Langerhans histiocytosis; in Erdheim–Chester disease, the characteristic xanthogranulomas have occasionally been reported in the brain,[143–145] usually causing progressive cerebellar symptoms and signs, or diabetes insipidus if the hypothalamus is involved. The lesions are charcteristically composed of Touton-like giant cells, with a variable number of lymphocytes and eosinophils, and relatively scanty fibrosis.[143] A recent study of clonality in Erdheim–Chester disease has indicated that it is a monoclonal proliferative disorder, consistent with a neoplasm.[146]

Intracranial involvement in Rosai–Dorfman disease is uncommon. Most lesions are dura-based and resemble meningiomas on neuroradiology.[147] They are composed of solid sheets of histiocytes (with occasional plasma cells and lymphocytes) within a fibrous stroma.[148] The histiocytic cells may appear vacuolated and contain lymphocytes and plasma cells within their cytoplasm, a phenomenon known as emperipoplesis (Fig. 11.37). Treatment by surgical excision usually carries a good outcome.[147,149]

Malignant haemophagocytic lymphohistiocytosis syndrome

CNS involvement is common in the malignant haemophagocytic lymphohistiocytosis syndrome, with multifocal deposits of non-malignant macrophages (with haemophagocytosis) and lymphocytes in the brain and meninges.[150–152] Some of the larger deposits may become necrotic. Progress in cytokine research has indicated that this disorder occurs as a consequence of uncontrolled, dysregulated immune reactivity caused by a number of underlying conditions: familial disorders, EBV-associated disorders and in association with life-threatening infection in infancy.[153] This very rare disorder is associated with a poor prognosis and is usually fatal unless bone marrow transplantation is performed.[150]

Choroid plexus xanthogranulomas

These lesions are common incidental findings in autopsies (up to 70% of cases). They are intraventricular nodular grey masses which are partly cystic with a granular cut surface which often contains yellow foci relating to accumulation of cholesterol in cholesterol clefts associated with foreign body giant cells, foamy histiocytes and chronic inflammatory infiltrates with plasma cells and lymphocytes.[154] These should be considered as part of the ageing process and should not be confused with xanthomas composed entirely of foamy histiocytes in the choroid plexus which are associated with hypercholesterolaemia, or with histiocytosis.[154] Exceptional cases of choroid plexus xanthogranuloma can present clinically as a symptomatic third ventricle lesion, mimicking a colloid cyst.[155]

REFERENCES

1. Jellinger K, Radaskiewicz TH, Slowik F. Primary malignant lymphomas of the central nervous system in man. Acta Neuropathol (Berl), 1975; (Suppl VI):95–102
2. Harris NL, Jaffe ES, Stein H et al. A revised European-American classification of lymphoid neoplasms: a proposal from the International Lymphoma Study Group. Blood, 1994; 84:1361–1392
3. Paulus W. Classification, pathogenesis and molecular pathology of primary CNS lymphomas. J Neurooncol, 1999; 43:203–208

Primary CNS lymphoma

4. Schabet M. Epidemiology of primary CNS lymphoma. J Neurooncol, 1999; 43:199–201
5. Miller DC, Hochberg FH, Harris NL et al. Pathology with clinical correlations of primary central nervous system non-Hodgkin's lymphoma. The Massachusettes General Hospital experience. Cancer, 1994; 74:1383–1397
6. Ciacci JD, Tellez C, VonRoenn J et al. Lymphoma of the central nervous system in AIDS. Semin Neurol, 1999; 19:213–221
7. Morgello S. Pathogenesis and classification of primary central nervous system lymphoma: an update. Brain Pathol, 1995; 5:383–393
8. Cote TR, Manns A, Hardy CR et al. Epidemiology of brain lymphoma among people with or without acquired immunodeficiency syndrome. AIDS/Cancer Study Group. J Nat Cancer Inst, 1996; 88:675–679
9. Corn BW, Marcus SM, Topham A et al. Will primary central nervous system lymphoma be the most frequent brain tumor daignosed in the year 2000? Cancer, 1997; 79:2409–2413
10. Camilleri-Broet S, Davi F, Feuillard J et al. AIDS-related primary lymphomas: histopathologic and immunohistochemical study of 51 cases. The French study group for HIV-associated tumours. Hum Pathol, 1997; 28:367–374
11. Morgello S, Petito CK, Mouradian JA. Central nervous system lymphoma in the acquired immunodeficiency syndrome. Clin Neuropathol, 1990; 9:205–215
12. Chappell ET, Guthrie BL, Orenstein J. The role of stereotactic biopsy in the management of HIV-related focal brain lesions. Neurosurgery, 1992; 30:825–829
13. Bale JF Jr, Wilson JF, Hill HR. Fatal histiocytic lymphoma of the brain associated with hyperimmunoglobulinemia-E and recurrent infections. Cancer, 1977; 39:2386–2390
14. Brand MM, Marrinkovich VA. Primary malignant reticulosis of the brain in Wiskott-Aldrich syndrome. Report of a case. Arch Dis Child, 1969; 44:536–542
15. Hutter JJ Jr, Jones JF. Results of a thymic epithelial transplant in a child with Wiskott-Aldrich syndrome and central nervous system lymphoma. Clin Immunol Immunopathol, 1981; 18:121–125
16. Martinez AJ. The neuropathology of organ transplantation: comparison and contrast in 500 patients. Pathol Res Prac, 1998; 194:473–486
17. Locker J, Nalesnik M. Molecular genetic analysis of lymphoid tumours arising after organ transplantation. Am J Pathol, 1989; 135:977–987
18. Schober R, Herman MM. Neuropathology of cardiac transplantation. Survey of 31 cases. Lancet 1973; i:962–967
19. Hochberg FH, Miller DC. Primary central nervous system lymphoma. J Neurosurg, 1988; 68:835–853
20. Okano M, Gross TG. A review of Epstein-Barr virus infection in patients with immunodeficiency disorders. Am J Med Sci, 2000; 319:392–396
21. Reni M, Ferreri AJ, Zoldan MC et al. Primary brain lymphomas in patients with a prior or concomitant malignancy. J Neurooncol, 1997; 32:135–142
22. Slowik F, Jellinger K. Association of primary cerebral lymphoma with meningioma: report of two cases. Clin Neuropathol, 1990; 9:69–73
23. Giromini D, Peiffer J, Tzonos T. Occurrence of a primary Burkitt-type lymphoma of the central nervous system in an astrocytoma patient. A case report. Acta Neuropathol, 1981; 54:165–167
24. Herrlinger U, Schabet M, Bitzer M et al. Primary central nervous system lymphoma: from clinical presentation to diagnosis. J Neurooncol, 1999; 43:219–226
25. Tomlinson FH, Kurtin PJ, Suman VJ et al. Primary intracerebral malignant lymphomas: a clinicopathological study of 89 patients. J Neurosurg, 1995; 82:558–566
26. Joncas JH, Russo P, Brochu P et al. Epstein-Barr virus polymorphic B-cell lymphoma associated with leukemia and with congenital immunodeficiencies. J Clin Oncol, 1990; 8:378–384
27. Rodriguez MM, Delgado PI, Petito CK. Epstein-Barr virus-associated primary central nervous system lymphoma in a child with the acquired immunodeficiency syndrome. A case report and review of the literature. Archiv Pathol Lab Med, 1997; 121:1287–1291
28. Del Mistro A, Laverda A, Calabrese F et al. Primary lymphoma of the central nervous system in 2 children with acquired immune deficiency syndrome. Am J Clin Pathol, 1990; 94:722–728
29. Kawamura T, Inamura T, Ikezaki K et al. Primary Ki-1 lymphoma in the central nervous system. J Clin Neurosci 2001; 8:574–577
30. Abdulkader I, Cameselle-Teijeiro J, Fraga M et al. Primary anaplastic large cell lymphoma of the central nervous system. Hum Pathol, 1999; 30:978–981
31. Buxton N, Punt J, Hewitt M. Primary Ki-1-positive T-cell lymphoma of the brain in a child. Pediatr Neurosurg, 1998; 29:250–252
32. Bindal AK, Blisard KS, Melin-Aldama H et al. Primary T-cell lymphoma of the brain in acquired immune deficiency syndrome: case report. J Neurooncol, 1997; 31:267–271
33. Herrlinger U. Primary CNS lymphoma: findings outside the brain. J Neurooncol, 1999; 43:227–230
34. Pauzner R, Mouallem M, Sadej M et al. High incidence of primary cerebral lymphoma in tumor-induced central neurogenic hyperventilation. Arch Neurol, 1989; 46:510–512
35. Alderson L, Fetell MR, Sisti M et al. Sentinel lesions of primary CNS lymphoma. J Neurol Neurosurg Psychiatry, 1996; 60:102–105
36. Brecher K, Hochberg FH, Louis DN et al. Case report of unusual leukoencephalopathy preceding primary CNS lymphoma. J Neurol Neurosurg Psychiatry, 1998; 65:917–920
37. Holtas S, Nyman U, Cronqvist S. Computer tomography of malignant lymphoma of the brain. Neuroradiology, 1984; 26:33–38
38. Jack CR Jr, Reese DF, Scheithauer BW. Radiographic findings in 32 cases of primary CNS lymphoma. Am J Roentgenol, 1986; 146:271–276
39. Iglesias-Rozas JR, Bantz B, Adler T et al. Cerebral lymphoma in AIDS. Clinical, radiological, neuropathological and immunopathological study. Clin Neuropathol, 1991; 10:65–72
40. Johnson BA, Fram EK, Johnson PC et al. The variable MR appearance of primary lymphoma of the central nervous system: comparison with histopathologic features. Am J Neuroradiol, 1997; 18:563–572
41. Roman-Goldstein SM, Goldman DL, Howieson J et al. MR of primary CNS lymphoma in immunologically normal patients. Am J Neuroradiol, 1992; 13:1207–1213
42. Lanfermann H, Heindel W, Schaper J et al. CT and MR imaging in primary cerebral non-Hodgkin's lymphoma. Acta Radiol, 1997; 38:259–267
43. Vaquero J, Martinez R, Rossi E et al. Primary cerebral lymphoma: the 'ghost tumor'. J Neurosurg, 1984; 60:174–176
44. Bakshi R, Massiotta JC, Mischel PS et al. Lymphomatosis cerebri presenting as a rapidly progressive dementia: clinical, neuroimaging and pathologic findings. Dement Geriatr Cogn Disord, 1999; 10:152–157

45. Scild SE, Wharen REJ, Menke DM et al. Primary lymphoma of the spinal cord. Mayo Clin Proc, 1995; 70:256–260

46. Nelson KD, Binkovitz LA, Lyons MK. Primary lymphoma of the spinal cord. Mayo Clin Proc, 1993; 68:1097–1098

47. Morgello S, Maiese K, Petito CK. T-cell lymphoma in the CNS: clinical and pathological features. Neurology, 1989; 39:1190–1196

48. McCue MP, Sandrock AW, Lee JM et al. Primary T-cell lymphoma of the brainstem. Neurology, 43:377–381

49. Marsh WL Jr, Stevenson DR, Long HJ III. Primary leptomeningeal presentation of T cell lymphoma. Report of a patient and review of the literature. Cancer, 1983; 51:1125–1131

50. Lachance DH, O'Neill BP, Macdonald DR et al. Primary leptomeningeal lymphoma: report of 9 cases, diagnosis with immunocytochemical analysis, and review of the literature. Neurology, 1991; 41:95–100

51. Kumar S, Kumar D, Kaldjian EP et al. Primary low grade B-cell lymphoma of the dura: a mucosa associated lymphoid tissue-type lymphoma. Am J Surg Pathol, 1997; 21:81–87

52. Kambham N, Chang Y, Matsushima AY. Primary low grade B-cell lymphoma of mucosa-associated lymphoid tissue (MALT) arising in dura. Clin Neuropathol, 1998; 17:311–317

53. Balmaceda C, Gaynor JJ, Sun M et al. Leptomeningeal tumour in primary central nervous system lymphoma: recognition, significance and implications. Ann Neurol, 1995; 38:202–209

54. Bigner SH. Cerebrospinal fluid (CSF) cytology: current status and diagnostic applications. J Neuropathol Exp Neurol, 1992; 51:235–245

55. Lai AP, Wioerzbicki AS, Norman PM. Immunocytochemical diagnosis of primary cerebral non-Hodgkin's lymphoma. J Clin Pathol, 1991; 44:251–253

56. Finn WG, Peterson LC, James C et al. Enhanced detection of malignant lymphoma in cerebrospinal fluid by multiparameter flow cytometry. Am J Clin Pathol, 1998; 110:341–346

57. Cingolani A, De Luca A, Larocca LM et al. Minimally invasive diagnosis of acquired immunodeficiency syndrome-related primary central nervous system lymphoma. J Nat Cancer Inst, 1998; 90:364–369

58. Molnar PP, O Neill BP, Scheithauer BW, Groothuis DR. The blood–brain barrier in primary CNS lymphomas: ultrastructural evidence of endothelial cell death. Neuro-oncol, 1999; 1:89–100

59. Schwechheimer K, Brauss DF, Schwarzkopf G et al. Polymorphous high-grade B cell lymphoma is the predominant type of spontaneous primary cerebral malignant lymphomas. Histological and immunomorphological evaluation of computed tomography-guided stereotactic brain biopsies. Am J Surg Pathol, 1994; 18:931–937

60. Bashir R, Chamberlain M, Ruby E et al. T-cell infiltration of primary CNS lymphoma. Neurology, 1996; 46:440–444

61. Kumanishi T, Washiyama K, Nishiyama A et al. Primary malignant lymphoma of the brain: demonstration of immunoglobulin gene rearrangements in four cases by the Southern blot hybridization technique. Acta Neuropathol, 1989; 79:23–26

62. Lacocca LM, Capello D, Rinelli A et al. The molecular and phenotypic profile of primary central nervous system lymphoma identifies distinct categories of the disease and is consistent with histogenetic derivation from germinal center-related B cells. Blood, 1998; 92:1011–1019

63. Aho R, Haapasalo H, Alanen et al. Proliferative activity and DNA index do not significantly predict survival in primary central nervous system lymphoma J Neuropathol Exp Neurol, 1995; 54:826–832

64. Cheuk W, Walford N, Lou J et al. Primary histiocytic lymphoma of the central nervous system: a neoplasm frequently overshadowed by a prominent inflammatory component. Am J Surg Pathol, 2001; 25:1372–1379

65. Itoyama T, Sadamori N, Tsutsumi K et al. Primary central nervous system lymphomas. Immunophenotypic, virologic, and cytogenetic findings of three patients without immune defects. Cancer, 1994; 73:455–463

66. Montesinos-Rongen M, Kuppers R, Schluter D et al. Primary central nervous system lymphomas are derived from germinal-center B cells and show a preferential usage of the V4-34 gene segment. Am J Pathol, 1999; 155:2077–2086

67. Cobbers JM, Wolter M, Reifenberger J et al. Frequent inactivation of CDKN2A and rare mutation of TP53 in PCNSL. Brain Pathol, 1998; 8:263–276

68. Auperin I, Mikol J, Oksenhendler E et al. Primary central nervous system malignant non-Hodgkin's lymphomas from HIV-infected and non-infected patients: expression of cellular surface proteins and Epstein–Barr viral markers. Neuropathol Appl Neurobiol, 1994; 20:243–252

69. Corboy JR, Garl PJ, Kleinschmidt-DeMasters BK. Human herpesvirus 8 DNA in CNS lymphomas from patients with and without AIDS. Neurology, 1998; 50:335–340

70. Antinori A, Larocca LM, Fassone L et al. HHV-8/KSHV is not associated with AIDS-related primary central nervous system lymphoma. Brain Pathol, 1999; 9:199–208

71. Miklossy J, Kopniczky Z, Uske A et al. A 43 year old male with generalized epileptic seizures. Brain Pathol, 2000; 10:477–478

72. Raex LE, Patel P, Feun L et al. Natural history and prognostic factors for survival in patients with acquired immune deficiency syndrome (AIDS)-related primary central nervous system lymphoma (PCNSL). Crit Rev Oncol, 1998; 9:199–208

73. Nucklos JD, Liu K, Burchette JL et al. Primary central nervous system lymphomas: a 30-year experience at a single institution. Mod Pathol, 1999; 12:1167–1173

74. Corry J, Smith JG, Wirth A et al. Primary central nervous system lymphoma: age and performance status are more important than treatment modality. Int J Radiat Oncol Biol Phys, 1998; 41:615–620

75. Nelson DF. Radiotherapy in the treatment of primary central nervous system lymphoma (PCNSL). J Neurooncol, 1999; 43:241–247

76. Mead GM, Bleehen NM, Gregor A et al. A Medical Research Council randomized trial into patients with primary cerebral non-Hodgkin's lymphoma: cerebral radiotherapy with and without cyclophosphamide, doxorubicin, vincristine, and prednisone chemotherapy. Cancer, 2000; 89:1359–1370

77. Bessell EM, Graus F, Punt JA et al. Primary non-Hodgkin's lymphoma of the CNS treated with BVAM or CHOD/BVAM chemotherapy before radiotherapy. J Clin Oncol, 1996; 14:945–954

78. Brown MT, McClendon RE, Gockerman JP. Primary central nervous system lymphoma with systemic metastasis: case report and review. J Neurooncol, 1995; 23:207–221

79. Miller WT, Siegel SG, Montone KT. Posttransplantation lymphoproliferative disorder: changing manifestations of disease in a renal transplant population. Crit Rev Diagn Imaging, 1997; 38:569–585

80. Boubenider S, Hiesse C, Goupy C et al. Incidence and consequences of post-transplantation lymphoproliferative disorders. J Nephrol, 1997; 10:136–145

81. Delecluse HJ, Kremmer E, Rouault JP et al. The expression of Epstein-Barr latent proteins is related to the pathological features of post-transplant lymphoproliferative disorders. Am J Pathol, 1995; 146:1113–1120

82. Chadburn A, Cesarman E, Knowles DM. Molecular pathology of posttransplantation lymphoproliferative disorders. Semin Diagn Pathol, 1997; 14:15–26

83. Swerdlow SH. Post-transplant lymphoproliferative disorders: a working classification. Curr Diagn Pathol, 1997; 4:28–35

CNS involvement in other types of lymphoproliferative disorders

84. Gianaris PG, Leestma JE, Cerullo LJ et al. Castleman's disease manifesting in the central nervous system: case report with immunological studies. Neurosurgery, 1989; 24:608–613

85. Lacombe MJ, Poirier J, Caron JP. Intracranial lesion resembling giant lymph node hyperplasia. Am J Clin Pathol, 1983; 80:721–723

86. Severson GS, Harrington DS, Weisenburger DD. Castleman's disease of the leptomeninges: a report of three cases. J Neurosurg, 1988; 69:283–286

87. Ferry JA, Harris NL, Picker LJ. Intravascular lymphomatosis malignant angioendotheliomatosis. A B-cell neoplasm expressing surface homing receptors. Mod Pathol, 1988; 1:444–452

88. Au WY, Shek WH, Nicholls J et al. T-cell intravascular lymphomatosis angiotropic large cell lymphoma: association with Epstein-Barr viral infection. Histopathology, 1997; 31:563–567

89. Vieren M, Sciot R, Robberecht W. Intravascular lymphomatosis of the brain: a diagnostic problem. Clin Neurol Neurosurg, 1999; 101:33–36

90. Jalkanen S, Aho R, Kallojoki M. Lymphocyte homing receptors and adhesion molecules in intravascular malignant lymphomatosis. Int J Cancer, 1989; 44:777–782

91. Klein R, Mullges W, Bendszus M et al. Primary intracerebral Hodgkin's disease: report of a case with Epstein-Barr virus association and review of the literature. Am J Surg Pathol, 1999; 23:477–481

92. Deckert-Schluter M, Marek J, Setlik M. Primary manifestation of Hodgkin's disease in the central nervous system. Virchows Archiv, 1998; 432:477–481

93. Ashby MA, Barber PC, Holmes AE et al. Primary intracranial Hodgkin's disease. Am J Surg Pathol, 1988; 12:294–299

94. Higgins SA, Peschel RE. Hodgkin's disease with spinal cord compression. A case report and a review of the literature. Cancer, 1995; 75:94–98

95. Kleinschmidt-DeMasters BK, Filley CM, Bitter MA. Central nervous system angiocentric angiodestructive T-cell lymphoma (lymphomatoid granulomatosis) Surg Neurol, 1992; 37:130–137

96. Jaffe ES, Wilson WH. Lymphomatoid granulomatosis: pathogenesis, pathology and clinical implications. Cancer Surveys: Lymphoma, 1997; 30:233–248

97. Katzenstein AL, Carringtron CB, Liebow AA. Lymphomatoid granulomatosis. A clinicopathologic study of 152 cases. Cancer, 1979; 43:360–373

98. Schmidt BJ, Meagher-Villemure K, Del Carpio J. Lymphomatoid granulomatosis with isolated involvement of the brain. Ann Neurol, 1984; 15:478–481

99. Kokmen E, Billman JK Jr, Abell MR. Lymphomatoid granulomatosis clinically confined to the CNS. Arch Neurol, 1977; 34:782–784

100. Michaud J, Banerjee D, Kaufmann JCE. Lymphomatoid granulomatosis involving the central nervous system: complication of a renal transplant with terminal monoclonal B-cell proliferation. Acta Neuropathol, 1983; 61:141–147

101. Bodensteiner DC, Skikne B. Central nervous system involvement in mycosis fungoides: diagnosis, treatment and literature review. Cancer, 1982; 15:1181–1184

102. Tacconi L, Eccles S, Johnston FG et al. Mycosis fungoides with central nervous sytem involvement – a case report: T-cell lymphoma of the brain. Surg Neurol, 1995; 43:389–392

103. Lundberg WB, Cadman EC, Skeel RT. Leptomeningeal mycosis fungoides. Cancer, 1976; 38:2149–2153

104. Zonenshayn M, Sharma S, Hymes K et al. Mycosis fungoides metastasizing to the brain parenchyma: case report. Neurosurgery, 1998; 42:933–937

105. Bayliss KM, Kueck BD, Hanson CA et al. Richter's syndrome presenting as primary central nervous system lymphoma. Am J Clin Pathol, 1990; 93:117–123

106. Civit T, Coulbois S, Baylac F et al. Waldenstrom's macroglobulinemia and cerebral lymphoplasmocytic proliferation: Bing and Neel syndrome. Apropos of a new case. Neurochirurgie, 1997; 43:245–249

107. Schweechheimer K, Hashemian A, Ott G et al. Primary spinal epidural malifestation of malignant lymphoma. Histopathology 1996; 29:265–269

108. Grant JW, Kaech D, Jones DB. Spinal cord compression as the first presentation of lymphoma – review of 15 cases. Histopathology, 1986; 10:1191–1202

109. Epelbaum R, Haim N, Ben-Shahar M et al. Non-Hodgkin's lymphoma presenting with spinal epidural involvement. Cancer, 1986; 58:2120–2124

110. Haddad P, Thaell JF, Kiely JM et al. Lymphoma of the spinal extradural space. Cancer, 1976; 38:1862–1866

111. Lyons MK, O'Neill BP, Marsh WR et al. Primary spinal epidural non-Hodgkin's lymphoma. Report of eight patients and review of the literature. Neurosurgery, 1992; 30:675–680

112. Perry JR, Deodhare SS, Bilbao JM et al. The significance of spinal cord compression at the initial manifestation of lymphoma. Neurosurgery, 1993; 32:157–162

113. Salvati M, Cervoni L, Artico M et al. Primary spinal epidural non-Hodgkin's lymphomas: a clinical study. Surg Neurol, 1996; 46:339–343

114. Mascalchi M, Torselli P, Falaschi F et al. MRI of spinal epidural lymphoma. Neuroradiology, 1995; 37:303–307

115. Singer CRJ. Multiple myeloma and related conditions. Br Med J, 314:960–963

116. Benson WJ, Scarffe JH, Todd ID. Spinal cord compression in myeloma. Br Med J, 1979; 9:1541–1544

117. Gahrton G. Treatment of multiple myeloma. Lancet, 1999; 353:85–86

118. Truong LD, Kim HS, Estrada R. Meningeal myeloma. Am J Clin Pathol, 1982; 78:532–535

119. Slager UT, Taylor WF, Opfell RW et al. Leptomeningeal myeloma. Arch Pathol Lab Med, 1979; 103:680–682

120. Benli K, Inci S. Solitary dural plasmacytoma: case report. Neurosurgery, 1995; 36:1206–1209

121. Wiltshaw A. The natural history of extramedullary plasmacytoma and its relation to multiple myeloma. Medicine, 1976; 55:217–238

122. Wisniewski T, Sisti M, Inhirami G et al. Intracerebral solitary plasmacytoma. Neurosurgery, 1990; 27:826–829

123. Le Marc'hadour F, Fransen P, Labat-Moleur F et al. Intracranial plasma cell granuloma: a report of four cases. Surg Neurol, 1994; 42:481–488

124. Figarella-Branger D, Gambarelli D, Perez-Castillo M et al. Primary intracerebral plasma cell granuloma: a light, immunocytochemical, and ultrastructural study of one case. Neurosurgery, 1990; 27:142–147

125. Chamberlain MC. A review of leptomeningeal metastases in pediatrics. J Child Neurol, 1995; 10:191–199

126. Neglia JP, Meadows AT, Robison LL et al. Second neoplasms after acute lymphoblastic leukemia in childhood. N Engl J Med, 1991; 325:1330–1336

127. Blatt J, Oshan A, Gula MJ et al. Second malignancies in very long-term survivors of childhood cancer. Am J Med, 1992; 93:57–60

128. Bojsen-Moller M, Neison JL. CNS involvement in leukaemia. An autopsy study of 100 consecutive patients. Acta Pathol Microbiol Immunol Scand, 1983; 91:209–216

129. Arboix A, Besses C. Cerebrovascular disease as the initial clinical presentation of haematological disorders. Eur Neurol, 1997; 37:207–211

130. Cramer SC, Glaspy JA, Efird JT et al. Chronic lymphocytic leukemia and the central nervous system: a clinical and pathological study. Neurology, 1996; 46:19–25

131. Elliott MA, Letendre L, Li CY et al. Chronic lymphocytic leukaemia with symptomatic diffuse central nervous system infiltration responding to therapy with systemic fludarabine. Br J Haematol, 1999; 104:689–694

132. Yamamoto K, Hamaguchi H, Nagata K et al. Isolated recurrence of granulocytic sarcoma of the brain: successful treatment with surgical resection, intrathecal injection, irradiation and prophylactic systemic chemotherapy. Jpn J Clin Oncol, 1999; 29:214–218

133. Mostafavi H, Lennarson PJ, Traynelis VC. Granulocytic sarcoma of the spine. Neurosurgery, 2000; 46:78–83

Histiocytic disorders

134. Favara BE, Feller AC, Pauli M et al. Contemporary classification of histiocytic disorders. The WHO Committee on Histiocytic/Reticulum Cell Proliferations Reclassification Working Group of the Histiocyte Society. Med Pediatr Oncol, 1997; 29:157–166

135. Ladisch S. Langerhans' cell histiocytosis. Curr Opin Hematol, 1998; 5:54–58

136. Willis B, Ablin A, Weinberg V et al. Disease course and late sequelae of Langerhans' cell histiocytosis: 25 year experience at the University of California, San Francisco. J Clin Oncol, 1996; 14:2073–2082

137. Kilpatrick SE, Wenger DE, Gilchrist GS et al. Langerhans' cell histiocytosis histiocytosis X of bone. A clinicopathologic analysis of 263 pediatric and adult cases. Cancer, 1995; 76:2471–2484

138. Grois N, Tsunematsu Y, Barkovitch AJ et al. Central nervous system disease in Langerhans' cell histiocytosis. Br J Cancer, 1994; 23:24–28

139. Poe LB, Dubowy RL, Hochhauser L. Demyelinating and gliotic cerebellar lesions in Langerhans' cell histiocytosis. Am J Neuroradiol, 1994; 15:1921–1928

140. Kim EY, Choi JU, Kim TS et al. Huge Langerhans' cell histiocytosis granuloma of choroid plexus in a child with Hand-Schuller-Christian disease. Case report. J Neurosurg, 1995; 83:1080–1084

141. Willman CL, Busque L, Griffith BB. Langerhans' cell histiocytois histiocytosis X – a clonal proliferative disease. N Engl J Med, 1994; 331:154–160

142. Mader I, Stock KW, Radue EW et al. Langerhans' cell histiocytosis in monozygote twins: case reports. Neuroradiology, 1996; 38:163–165

143. Adle-Biassette H, Chetritt J, Bergemer-Fouquet AM et al. Pathology of the central nervous system in Chester–Erdheim disease: report of three cases. J Neuropathol Exp Neurol, 1997; 56:1207–1216

144. Wright RA, Hermann RC, Parisi JE. Neurological manifestations of Erdheim–Chester disease. J Neurol Neurosurg Psychiatry, 1999; 66:72–75

145. Veyssier-Belot C, Cacoub P, Caparros-Lefebvre D. Erdheim–Chester disease. Clinical and radiologic characteristics of 59 cases. Medicine (Baltimore), 1996; 75:157–169

146. Chetritt J, Paradis V, Dargeree D et al. Chester–Erdheim disease: a neoplastic disorder. Hum Pathol, 1999; 30:1093–1096

147. Kim M, Provias J, Bernstein M. Rosai-Dorfman disease mimicking multiple meningioma: case report. Neurosurgery, 1995; 36:1185–1187

148. Jones RV, Colegial CH, Andriko JW. Extranodal sinus histiocytosis with massive lymphadenopathy. Rosai-Dorfman disease of the central nervous system. J Neuropathol Exp Neurol, 1997; 56:613

149. Resnick DK, Johnson BL, Lovely TJ. Rosai-Dorfman disease presenting with multiple orbital and intracranial masses. Acta Neuropathol, 1996; 91:554–557

150. Haddad E, Sulis ML, Jabado N et al. Frequency and severity of central nervous system lesions in hemophagocytic lymphohistiocytosis. Blood, 1997; 89:794–800

151. Henter JI, Nennesmo I. Neuropathologic findings and neurologic symptoms in twenty-three children with hemophagocytic lymphohistiocytosis J Pediatr, 1997; 130:358–365

152. Kollias SS, Ball WSJ, Tzika AA et al. Familial erythrophagocytic lymphohistiocytosis: neuroradiologic evaluation with pathologic correlation. Radiology, 1994; 192:743–754

153. Imashuku S. Advances in the management of hemophagocytic lymphohistiocytosis. Int J Hematol, 2000; 71:1–11

154. Muenchau A, Laas R. Xanthogranuloma and xanthoma of the choroid plexus: evidence for different etiology and pathogenesis. Clin Neuropathol, 1997; 16:72–76

155. Hicks MJ, Albrecht S, Trask T et al. Symptomatic choroid plexus xanthogranuloma of the lateral ventricle. Case report and brief review of xanthogranulomatous lesions of the brain. Clin Neuropathol, 1993; 12:92–96

12 Metastatic tumours

Metastatic tumours represent the largest category of neoplasms involving the central nervous system (CNS).[1–4] Within this category, most tumours occur as intraparenchymal deposits within the brain,[5] but other sites may be involved including the spinal cord, cranial and spinal nerves, pineal gland and pituitary gland. Metastatic tumours may also primarily involve the subarachnoid space and thence spread into the brain, cranial nerves, spinal nerves or spinal cord.[6–10] Metastatic tumours can also produce damage to the CNS by mechanical compression, particularly when they occur in the spinal epidural space or the vertebral column. This chapter will consider metastatic tumours within the anatomical categories of intraparenchymal, leptomeningeal, epidural and bone metastases.

As a group, metastatic CNS tumours represent a major cause of morbidity and mortality in patients with primary tumours arising elsewhere in the body and not infrequently are the final cause of death in such patients, even when the primary tumour has been treated successfully.[1,3] The clinical and socioeconomic impact of these lesions is therefore in proportion to their frequency, and as survival times for patients with cancers outside the CNS increase, the incidence of metastases within the CNS may show a corresponding rise.

Incidence

Metastatic tumours are by far the commonest neoplasms in the CNS; the total number of metastatic tumours diagnosed on an annual basis outnumbers the total combined numbers for all other tumours arising in the CNS.[1–4] It is, however, difficult to calculate the precise incidence of metastatic tumours within the CNS, since many of these neoplasms occur in terminally ill patients with metastases elsewhere in the body and in whom no further investigation or treatment is possible. Estimates for the incidence of these tumours therefore come from both clinical data (based largely on neuroradiological findings) and from large autopsy series.[1–4] These have indicated that the age-related incidence of metastatic tumours is somewhat similar to those of primary tumours in the CNS, with a small peak occurring under the age of 10 in children with malignant embryonal neoplasms and leukaemia, and a second much larger peak in the sixth and seventh decades of life.[11,12] Brain metastases in patients with systemic malignancy have been reported in around 15–40% of cases, depending on case selection and whether or not a histological diagnosis has been made.[1,2,4,11,13] Since the accurate diagnosis of brain metastases depends upon multimodal investigation, it is difficult to extrapolate much of the information in historical series into contemporary clinical practice.

It has been suggested that younger patients with any given type of cancer are more susceptible to the develop-ment of metastatic neoplasms in the CNS than older patients with a corresponding tumour.[11] The underlying reasons behind this observation are uncertain, but it does not appear to be related to the length of patient survival and may therefore reflect a difference in tumour biology in relation to age, with certain tumours pursuing a more aggressive biological behaviour in younger patients, e.g. in breast carcinoma. Up to 15% of patients with a systemic malignancy will present with metastatic tumours involving the CNS before the primary tumour has declared itself clinically.[2,3,13,14] In many of these cases, the primary tumour becomes evident on a more detailed clinical and radiological assessment, but in a small percentage of cases autopsy will be required to establish the primary site of the tumour.

The relative frequency with which different primary tumours metastasise to the CNS is markedly variable, but several large studies have identified reproducible trends (Table 12.1). Carcinomas of the lung, breast and kidney and malignant melanoma are by far the commonest primary neoplasms which metastasise to the CNS. Lung cancer is the largest single category, but there is variability within this group of tumours; small cell anaplastic carcinoma and adenocarcinoma metastasise more frequently than squamous cell carcinoma. Conversely, certain tumours will metastasise only very infrequently to the CNS including most types of sarcoma, and carcinomas of the ovary, uterus, bladder and prostate.[15–26] Similar findings have been reported in surveys of leptomeningeal metastases, but in spinal epidural and bone metastases this general trend is not reproduced.

Intraparenchymal brain metastases account for 15–20% of all tumours investigated in neurosurgical departments (this is likely to represent an underestimate of total cases, for reason discussed above).[1,3,4] There is evidence from ongoing studies that the overall incidence of brain metastases is increasing; this has been attributed to improved therapy for the primary systemic and metastatic systemic disease.[2,4] Longer survival of such

Table 12.1 Metastatic brain tumours in relation to sex and age (commonest at top)[1,3,4,11,12,14]

Males	Females	Children
Lung carcinoma	Breast carcinoma	Acute leukaemia
Renal carcinoma	Lung carcinoma	Neuroblastoma
Malignant melanoma	Renal carcinoma	Embryonal rhabdomyosarcoma
Lymphoma	Malignant melanoma	Lymphoma
Colorectal carcinoma	Lymphoma	Nephroblastoma
Gastric carcinoma	Thyroid carcinoma	
Germ cell tumours	Uterine and germ cell tumours	

patients appears therefore to increase the likelihood of developing brain parenchymal metastases at a later date. This trend is reflected in historical data: analysis of autopsies shows that up to 37% of patients with disseminated malignancy have cerebral parenchymal metasses.[5,9]

There are clear-cut sex differences in the relative incidence of metastatic parenchymal brain tumours, with breast carcinoma being the commonest single type of tumour in women, whereas lung cancer is the commonest single type in males (Table 12.1).[1,2] As the incidence of lung cancers increase in females, this trend may eventually become reversed, with lung cancer representing the commonest primary tumour for metastatic parenchymal brain tumours in both sexes. For these reasons, it is difficult to obtain precise figures for the relative frequency of metastatic tumours for any tumour type, but it has been estimated that the distribution of primary sites of tumours in patients with intraparenchymal brain metastases includes 45% with lung tumours, 24% with breast carcinoma and 12% with malignant melanoma.[1–4,15,16,22,24] In contrast, there are other much rarer tumours which frequently spread to the CNS, although accounting for only a small percentage of the total number of metastatic tumours, the best example of which is choriocarcinoma.[27] Patients with germ cell tumours of the testis have been reported to develop cerebral parenchymal metastases in 15–25% of patients;[2–4,11,14] with increased cure rates for primary germ cell tumours at this site (particularly seminoma) it is anticipated that the number of patients with CNS metastases will therefore decline.

Aetiology

The spread of tumours from a primary site in the body to other organs is a complex process which is becoming increasingly understood (see Refs 2 and 28 for reviews). It is not possible to consider these complex biological issues in detail here, but it is appropriate to discuss the particular stages in metastasis which are relevant to the CNS. Although there is evidence for lymphocyte tracking through the brain which might be of relevance to the spread of lymphoid neoplasms, it is generally accepted that the overwhelming majority of tumours metastasise to the CNS by the bloodstream.[29,30] To invade the CNS, blood borne tumour cells must attach to capillary endothelial cells, disrupt and pass through the blood–brain barrier and adapt and respond to the CNS microenvironment.[29,30] Our understanding of the genetic determinants of invasion and metastasis is far from complete, but the differential expression of certain antigens on tumour cells appears to influence invasion and metastasis, e.g. in colonic carcinoma expression of CD44R1 appears to favour metastasis.

Neoplastic cells can be shed into the circulation either individually or in clusters, most of which will not result in the establishment of a metastatic deposit. However, it appears that the arterial circulation is the most important route for metastases to the brain, and it has been suggested that tumour cell 'emboli' can travel to the brain from either a primary or metastatic tumour in the lungs.[28] Alternative routes of spread include the venous route, involving Batson's venous plexus, resulting in vertebral column, epidural and possibly spinal cord metastases.[28]

Tumour cells can enter the CNS from blood vessels either in the parenchyma, the choroid plexus or in the subarachnoid and subpial spaces. There appears to be a relationship between the overall distribution of the metastases in the brain and the relative regional blood flow. Most intraparenchymal cerebral metastases occur at the temporal-parieto-occipital junction, in the vascular boundary zone where the terminal branches of the middle cerebral artery are located.[31] In the cerebellum, metastases tend to occur at the boundary zone between the superior and inferior cerebellar arteries. Metastases are usually located at the junction between the grey and white matter in the brain; the reason for this longstanding observation is still unclear, but may relate to local differences in blood flow or tissue oxygenation at these sites which favours the establishment and growth of metastases.[2,28,31] Metastatic lesions in the cerebellum and brain stem occur at a relatively high incidence in relation to the weight and volume ratio of these structures to the cerebral hemispheres.[28,31] This may relate in part to the spread of tumours to these sites via Batson's venous plexus, particularly with primary tumours arising in the gastrointestinal tract and kidney. Spinal intradural and intraparenchymal metastases are becoming increasingly diagnosed in clinical practice as a result of the widespread use of magnetic resonance imaging (MRI) techniques.[32]

The biological and genetic alterations which occur in metastatic tumours within the CNS are poorly understood. It has been observed that the proliferative potential of most brain metastases is high, and usually greater than in the primary tumour.[33] Although in individual tumour types there may be genetic alterations that favour invasion and metastasis,[34–39] few studies have investigated these abnormalities in a range of metastatic tumours in the brain. One recent study employed a comparative genomic hybridisation technique to investigate chromosomal abnormalities in 42 metastatic brain tumours.[40] The investigators found a common pattern of abnormalities, particularly involving chromosomal regions 1q23, 8q24, 17q24–25 and 20q13. Comparison with primary tumours suggested a clonal origin, with the possibility that specific genetic lesions are associated with tumour spread into the CNS.

Clinical features

Metastatic tumours in the CNS present with a wide range of clinical signs and symptoms. It has been estimated that neurological signs and symptoms occur in up to two-thirds of patients with brain metastases, but patients with widespread small metastatic deposits may have a relatively 'silent' clinical picture, which in the context of disseminated malignancy elsewhere in the body may go undiagnosed unless the appropriate neuroradiological investigations are performed. In patients with intra-parenchymal brain metastases, the clinical features depend on the location and number of the tumours; solitary metastatic deposits occur most frequently in the posterior fossa[13,14,41] where the presenting symptoms are confined to those of cerebellar dysfunction and raised intracranial pressure with hydrocephalus. Patients with multiple intraparenchymal brain metastases will present with a wide range of clinical signs and symptoms relating to the sites of involvement and the space occupying effects of these masses.[2,9,10] Haemorrhage is a particularly common occurrence in metastatic malignant melanoma and choriocarcinoma, but is by no means confined to metastatic deposits from these tumours alone. Other vascular complications of metastatic neoplasms include stroke, neoplastic aneurysms and subdural haemorrhage.[2,10,42]

Intraparenchymal metastatic deposits in the spinal cord occur much less frequently than in the brain and present with symptoms relevant to the site of the deposit. Cranial and spinal nerve root metastases are also uncommon as isolated phenomena[5,9] and present most often with isolated nerve palsies or radicular pain. Nerve root invasion is more likely to occur as a complication of malignant meningitis.[9]

Radiology

Metastatic tumours in the CNS are best detected on contrast enhanced MRI scans, which have been shown by numerous studies to be more sensitive and specific than other imaging techniques.[43,44] MRI studies have indicated that around 50% of brain metastases are solitary, with two lesions detectable in 20% of cases; the remainder comprise multiple lesions.[44] Marked vasogenic oedema and an accompanying mass effect are characteristic MRI features of intraparenchymal brain metastases. These appear as foci of increased signal intensity on T1-weighted images, with larger lesions occasionally exhibiting a non-enhancing core, representing central necrosis (Fig. 12.1).[45] Metastatic intraparenchymal deposits tend to be spherical in outline and peripherally located, usually at a grey–white matter junction. T2-weighted images show metastatic tumours to have decreased signal density relative to brain, but the surrounding vasogenic oedema exhibits increased intensity and is much better observed on T2-rather than T1-

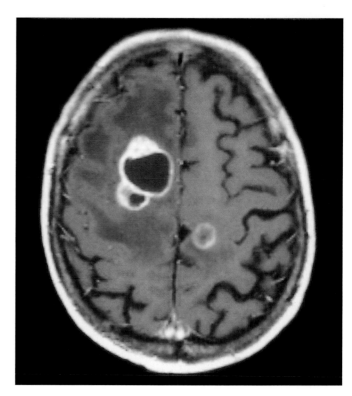

Fig. 12.1 Metastatic lung carcinoma. This scan shows multiple enhancing nodules with a cavitating necrotic centre deep in the cerebral hemispheres, characteristic of metastatic deposits. (Courtesy of D Collie, Edinburgh.)

weighted images.[44,45] Contrast enhanced MRI with gadolinium further enhances the neuroradiological detection of metastases both in the brain and in the sub-arachnoid space.[45–48] Metastatic deposits of melanoma, choriocarcinoma and teratoma are often accompanied by haemorrhage within the tumour deposits.[44] Subarachnoid deposits of carcinoma, lymphoma and leukaemia appear as multiple small focal (often nodular) contrast-enhancing lesions which are most easily identified in the posterior fossa or spinal meninges.[48–51] MRI and computerised tomography (CT) scans are also useful for the investigation of spinal epidural deposits and vertebral bone deposits; other investigations such as CT myelography are also helpful in defining the site and size of the lesions.[44]

Pathology

Macroscopic features

Metastatic tumours in the brain parenchyma form discrete deposits which are usually rounded and appear sharply demarcated from the adjacent brain (Fig. 12.2). The tumour deposits may be haemorrhagic or necrotic, particularly in the centre of larger lesions. Either solitary or multiple deposits may be present; solitary deposits are most often identified in the cerebellum or brain stem. The relative frequencies of metastatic tumour sites in the CNS are summarised in Table 12.2; tumours which tend to form solitary or multiple metaststic deposits are listed in Table 12.3. Intraparenchymal brain metastases are usually accompanied by marked vasogenic oedema, potentiating the mass effect and resulting in brain herniation in extreme cases (Fig. 12.3). This effect can be enhanced further if significant haemorrhage has occurred within the tumour deposits. Intraparenchymal metastases may also coexist with deposits in the leptomeningeal space, either focally attached to the dura mater, or with widespread infiltration of the subarachnoid space (carcinomatous meningitis). Under these circumstances the arachnoid appears thickened and opaque, either in a diffuse distribution, or around blood vessels or with multiple small nodules frequently measuring less than 2 mm in diameter (Fig. 12.4). Larger deposits attached to the dura mater may resemble meningiomas because of their well circumscribed and rounded outlines, but unlike meningiomas, these often invade the adjacent cerebral cortex. Metastatic deposits within the spinal cord parenchyma are less commonly identified (Fig. 12.5), but small nodules of tumour on the spinal nerve roots are not an uncommon finding in patients with carcinomatous meningitis (Fig. 12.6).

Intraoperative diagnosis

The cytological features of metastatic tumours in the CNS depend greatly on the primary tumour source; most tumours that are resected or biopsied are metastatic carcinomas in the cerebral hemispheres or cerebellum.

Table 12.2 Sites for metastatic tumours in the CNS[2,5–10,13–16]

Site	Frequency (%)	Tumour type
Cerebrum (frontotemporal)	70	Metastatic carcinomas
Cerebellum (hemisphere)	17	Renal carcinoma Colorectal carcinoma Uterine carcinoma
Basal ganglia	2	Metastatic carcinomas
Spinal cord (parenchymal)	1	Metastatic carcinoma
Spinal epidural space	10	Lymphoma Metastatic carcinoma myeloma
Dura mater	Rare	Breast carcinoma Prostatic carcinoma

Table 12.3 Metastatic brain deposits in relation to cell type (commonest at top)[2,5,10,14,15,41,45]

Solitary deposits	Renal carcinoma Gastrointestinal tract carcinoma Breast carcinoma Prostatic carcinoma Uterine carcinoma
Multiple deposits (> 2)	Pulmonary adenocarcinoma Pulmonary small cell carcinoma Malignant melanoma Choriocarcinoma

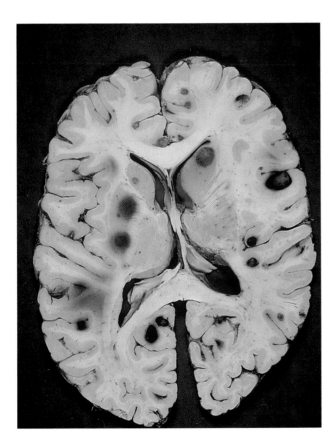

Fig. 12.2 **Metastatic melanoma.** Multiple pigmented deposits of malignant melanoma are characteristically located at grey/white matter junctions in the brain.

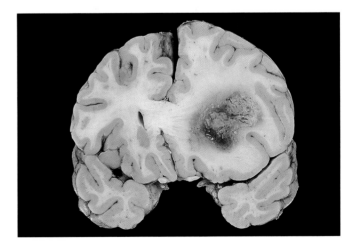

Fig. 12.3 **Metastatic melanoma.** A metastatic solitary deposit from a bronchial carcinoma. This is accompanied by extensive oedema, which potentiates the mass effect and contributes to intracranial herniation.

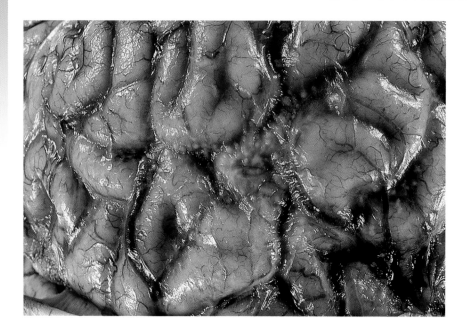

Fig. 12.4 **Metastatic breast carcinoma.** Multiple small nodular deposits of metastatic breast carcinoma in the subarachnoid space, closely related to blood vessels.

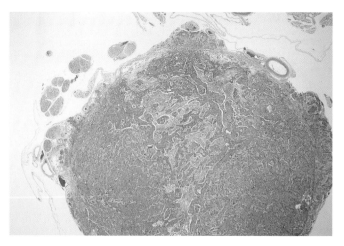

Fig. 12.5 **Metastatic lung carcinoma.** Intramedullary metastatic squamous carcinoma in the spinal cord. The carcinoma occupies most of the parenchyma. H & E.

Smear preparations from metastatic carcinomas show a population of pleomorphic tumour cells which exhibit considerable cohesion and are visible as irregular tumour cell clusters both adjacent to and spreading away from blood vessels (Fig. 12.7). Vascular endothelial hyperplasia is not a common feature and a gliofibrillary matrix is absent, but reactive astrocytes may be identified both within the tumour and particularly at the tumour margins. Cytological atypia and nuclear pleomorphism are usually pronounced, and mitotic figures and apoptotic nuclei are commonly identifiable in the tumour cell population. Metastatic carcinomas frequently contain multiple irregular nucleoli and exhibit cytological

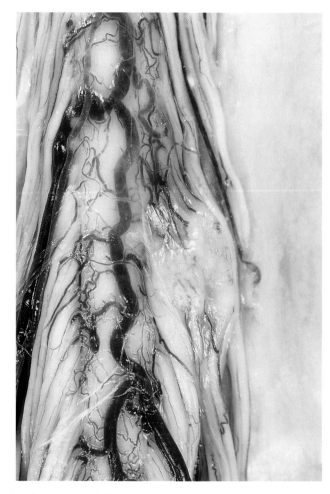

Fig. 12.6 **Metastatic lung carcinoma.** Metastatic lung carcinoma in the spinal canal, forming a large mass which tethers several nerve roots.

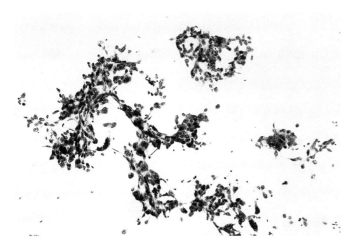

Fig. 12.7 **Metastatic lung carcinoma.** Smear preparation of a metastatic squamous cell carcinoma. This shows cohesive clusters of large cells with abundant cytoplasm and little endothelial proliferation. Toluidine blue.

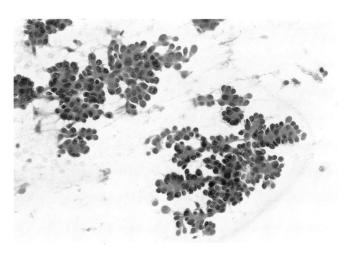

Fig. 12.8 **Metastatic thyroid carcinoma.** Smear preparation from a metastatic thyroid carcinoma. This shows cohesive clusters of cells with a well defined papillary pattern (see Figs 12.21 and 12.22 for the corresponding paraffin section). H & E.

features which vary according to the tumour differentiation (Figs 12.8 and 12.9). Squamous and glandular differentiation are usually clearly visible in smear preparations, while small cell carcinomas form irregular sheets of cohesive cells with relatively scanty cytoplasm which exhibit marked nuclear moulding. Haemorrhage and necrosis are frequently identifiable in smear preparations in all types of metastatic tumours.

Non-carcinomatous metastatic tumours may exhibit a wide range of morphologies; the most frequently encountered is metastatic melanoma in which the tumour cells characteristically have a large prominent nucleolus and a large quantity of cytoplasm which contains variable amounts of melanin pigment (Fig. 12.10). The tumour cells exhibit less cohesion in smear preparations than metastatic carcinoma, and tend to spread away from blood vessels in a monolayer. Certain tumours exhibit bizarre and spectacular cytological features, for example multinucleate giant cells in metastatic choriocarcinoma and strap cells in metastatic rhabdomyosarcoma (Fig. 12.11). Metastatic lymphomas contain a non-cohesive population of tumour cells whose nuclear features often indicate their lymphoid origin; most cases of metastatic CNS lymphoma are high grade B-cell non-Hodgkin's lymphomas with prominent populations of centroblasts and immunoblasts. A gliofibrillary matrix is also absent in these tumours, and unlike their intrinsic CNS counterparts, a marked perivascular orientation of the tumour cells is not common. The CNS is a common site for relapse of acute leukaemias in children, and although these are not always biopsied prior to treatment, it is essential to obtain adequate clinical information when interpreting the intraoperative cytological features, since many of these deposits are haemorrhagic and necrotic and can resemble intrinsic paediatric CNS

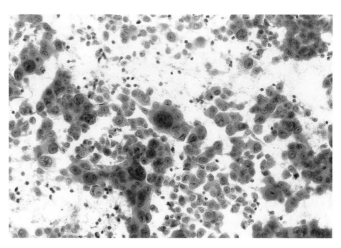

Fig. 12.9 **Metastatic lung carcinoma.** Smear preparation from a metastatic large cell anaplastic carcinoma of lung. This shows a population of pleomorphic tumour cells which contain prominent nucleoli in their enlarged nuclei. H & E.

tumours, including primary neuroectodermal tumours (PNET) in smear preparations.

Histological features

Cryostat sections Cryostat sections are a good way to investigate both the cytological appearances and architectural pattern in metastatic tumours at intraoperative diagnosis. Although lacking the fine nuclear detail visible in smear preparations, the overall growth pattern and relationship to adjacent brain tissue can be explored more fully in cryostat sections (Fig. 12.12). Although a wide range of cytological and histological features may be expected in metastatic tumours, they all share a characteristically well demarcated margin from the

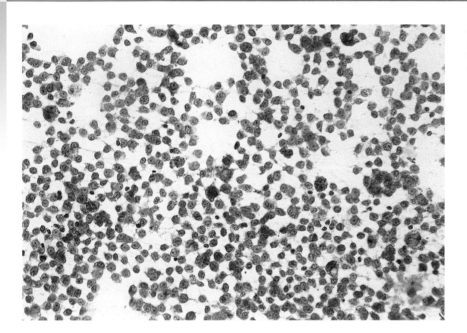

Fig. 12.10 **Metastatic melanoma.** Smear preparation from a metastatic malignant melanoma. A population of non-cohesive tumour cells of varying size is shown. Toluidine blue.

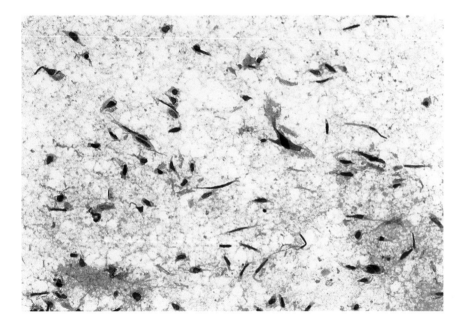

Fig. 12.11 **Metastatic sarcoma.** Smear preparation from a metastatic rhabdomyosarcoma in a 12-year-old male, which contains non-cohesive strap cells. H & E.

adjacent oedematous or gliotic brain, a high mitotic rate and multiple foci of necrosis in larger deposits (Fig. 12.13). Cryostat sections will allow the easy recognition of glandular and squamous differentiation in metastatic carcinomas, and the characteristic nuclear and cytoplasmic features of malignant melanoma are readily identifiable. Fine cytological detail in metastatic small cell carcinoma and lymphoma is, however, better appreciated in smear preparations. A pseudopapillary growth pattern is not uncommon in many types of metastatic carcinoma (usually as a result of accompanying necrosis) and is not confined to adenocarcinomas.

Microscopic features As mentioned above the general histological, cytological and immunocytochemical features of metastatic tumours within the parenchyma or in other regions of the CNS in general will reflect the primary tumours from which these arise. However, the degree of differentiation in the metastatic tumour may not be identical to that in the primary tumour and this has to be borne in mind when comparing the histological features of a metastatic deposit in a patient with a biopsy-proven primary tumour. In contrast to most intrinsic brain tumours, the metastatic deposits tend to have a well demarcated edge with surrounding oedema and gliosis, multiple areas of necrosis although nuclear pseudopalisading around necrotic foci is uncommon (Fig. 12.14). Vascular endothelial proliferation is not a consistent feature in metastatic tumours, but it may be identified at the margins of the lesion in the adjacent gliotic and oedematous brain. It can also occur in occasional tumours within the fibrovascular cores of tumour pseudopapillae; glomeruloid vascular tufts are an extreme example of this phenomenon. A perivascular lymphocytic infiltrate may also occur within and around metastatic tumours, presumably reflecting a host mediated immune response or a reaction to necrosis.

The interpretation of the histological features of the tumour cells should be informed by knowledge of the primary tumour diagnosis whenever possible. Morpho-logical assessment can usually identify major tumour categories, i.e. metastatic carcinoma, melanoma, lymphoma or others, and tinctorial stains, e.g. for glycogen, mucins, or melanin, can help clarify the initial morphological assessment (Figs 12.15–12.22).

Immunocytochemistry

Immunocytochemistry is invaluable for the assessment of cellular differentiation and can allow a precise categorisation of most metastatic CNS tumours.[41,52–55] This is of particular importance in patients who present with CNS metastases in whom the primary tumour is occult.[52,53] The approach to the investigation of a

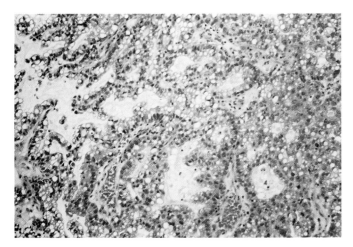

Fig. 12.12 **Metastatic lung carcinoma.** Cryostat section of a metastatic adenocarcinoma. A well defined papillary architecture is exhibited. H & E.

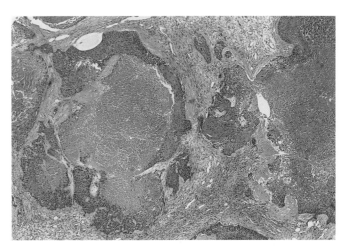

Fig. 12.14 **Metastatic squamous carcinoma.** Paraffin section carcinoma. Multiple irregular tumour deposits are shown with extensive necrosis in the centre of the larger lesions, which resembles a glioblastoma at low magnification. H & E.

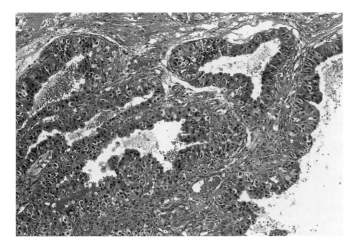

Fig. 12.13 **Metastatic ovarian carcinoma.** Cryostat section of a metastatic ovarian carcinoma. A composite glandular and solid architecture with foci of necrosis is shown. H & E.

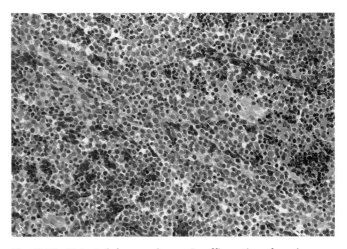

Fig. 12.15 **Metastatic lung carcinoma.** Paraffin section of a pulmonary small cell carcinoma. This demonstrates the nuclear moulding which is characteristic of these tumours, along with a variable quantity of pale staining cytoplasm around the nuclei. H & E.

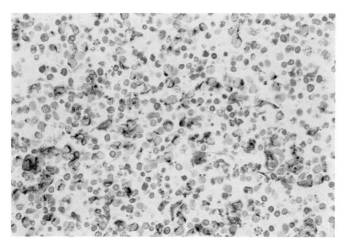

Fig. 12.16 **Metastatic lung carcinoma.** Immunocytochemistry for CAM5.2 in small cell pulmonary carcinoma. A characteristic dot-like positivity is shown in the paranuclear region of the cytoplasm.

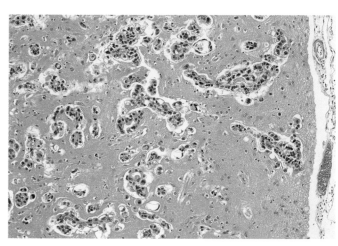

Fig. 12.19 **Metastatic breast carcinoma.** Infiltrating breast carcinoma in the cerebral cortex, composed of cords and clusters of tumour cells. H & E.

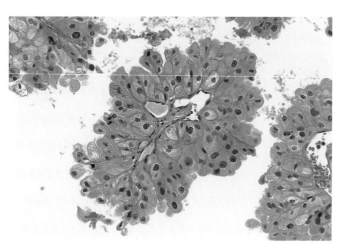

Fig. 12.17 **Metastatic renal carcinoma.** Paraffin sections of a metastatic renal carcinoma. A characteristic clear cell appearance is shown with a well defined cell wall and a pseudopapillary structure arranged around delicate fibrovascular stroma.

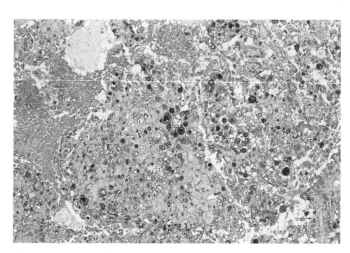

Fig. 12.20 **Metastatic breast carcinoma.** An Alcian blue/periodic acid–Schiff stain shows focal intense positivity in metastatic breast carcinoma.

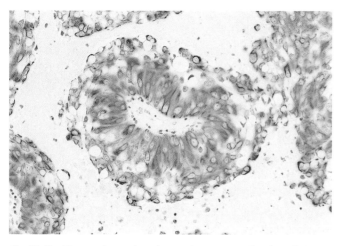

Fig. 12.18 **Metastatic renal carcinoma.** Immunocytochemistry for CAM5.2 shows variable positivity within the tumour cell population in the same case as Fig. 12.16.

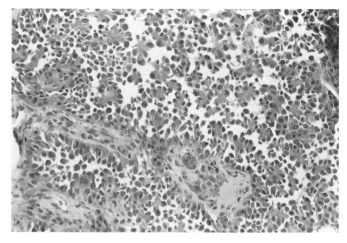

Fig. 12.21 **Metastatic papillary carcinoma of thyroid.** A similar architecture is shown to the smear preparation from the same case (Fig. 12.8). H & E.

metastatic tumour of unknown origin requires the use of an antibody panel, which is outlined in Table 12.4. After initial screening, further investigations including the use of 'cell-specific' antibodies, electron microscopy or molecular genetic techniques may be required for differential diagnosis and accurate classification (Figs 12.23–12.30).

Differential diagnosis

Differential diagnosis of metastatic tumours involving the CNS is a particular concern in patients in whom no primary tumour has been identified at the stage of clinical and radiological investigations. This is particularly likely to occur with carcinomas and malignant melanoma, since sarcomas and germ cell tumours, although capable of metastasis to the brain and spinal cord, usually spread through different sites in the body at a relatively late stage in disease progression when the primary tumour has declared itself. In contrast, patients with occult carcinomas in the lung, breast or kidney not infrequently present with metastatic deposits in the brain, liver or skeleton. Although the radiological appearances of metastatic carcinomas are usually

Table 12.4 Staining techniques useful in the diagnosis of metastatic neoplasms in the CNS[10,41,52–56]

Tinctorial stains
Glycogen and mucins
  Periodic acid–Shiff ± diastase,
  Alcian blue, mucicarmine

Melanin
  Masson Fontana / Singh

Antibodies
Initial panel
Epithelial membrane antigen, cytokeratins, glial fibrillary acidic protein

Cell-specific markers
Lung cancer: cytokeratin 7, surfactant
Breast cancer: cytokeratin 7, oestrogen and progesterone receptors
Gastrointestinal cancer: cytokeratin 20
Ovarian cancer: CA125
Neuroendocrine: chromogranins, peptides
Thyroid cancer: thyroglobulin
Prostate cancer: prostate specific antigen, prostatic acid phosphatase

Germ cell tumours
Placental alkaline phosphatase (see Chapter 10 for other germ-cell markers)

Sarcomas
Desmin, smooth-muscle actin, S-100

Malignant melanoma
S-100, HMB45, MART-1

Lymphoma
CD45, CD3, CD20 (see Ch. 11 for other lymphoma markers)

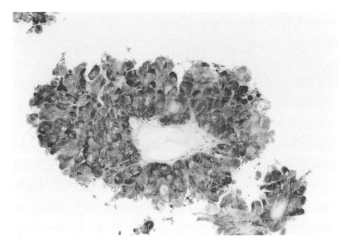

Fig. 12.22 **Metastatic thyroid carcinoma.** Immunocytochemistry for thyroglobulin in a metastatic papillary carcinoma of thyroid. This shows intense cytoplasmic positivity (same case as Figs 12.8 and 12.21).

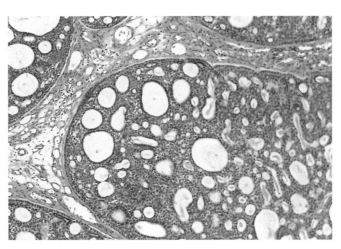

Fig. 12.23 **Metastatic adenoid cystic carcinoma.** A characteristic histological appearance with intense oedema and gliosis in the surrounding brain tissue is exhibited. H & E.

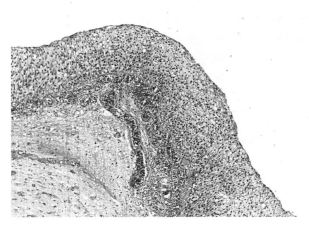

Fig. 12.24 **Metastatic bladder carcinoma.** Metastatic transitional cell carcinoma of the bladder forms the epithelial lining of a central cyst, with oedema, gliosis and haemorrhage in the adjacent brain. H & E.

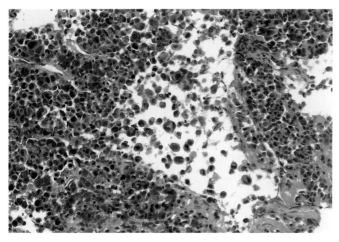

Fig. 12.25 **Metastatic melanoma.** Melanin pigmentation is variable. It often accumulates in macrophages within the tumour rather than the tumour cell population. H & E.

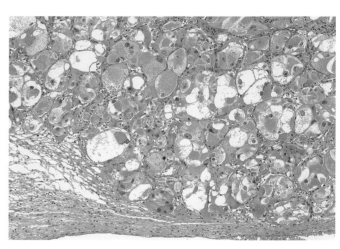

Fig. 12.28 **Metastatic alveolar soft part sarcoma.** This is characterised by a tumour population of large pleomorphic cells with bizarre nuclei and granular eosinophilic cytoplasm. H & E.

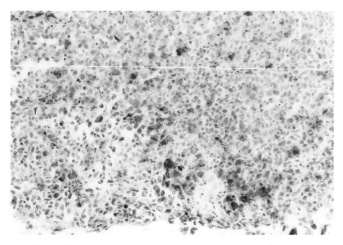

Fig. 12.26 **Metastatic melanoma.** HMB45 expression (red) is often focal commonly and it often appears most prominent in the larger tumour cells.

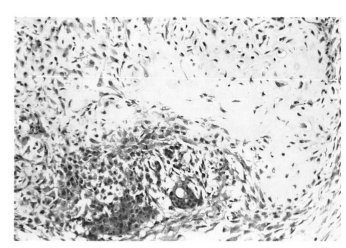

Fig. 12.29 **Metastatic teratoma.** An unusual combination of chondrosarcoma-like areas (top) and adenocarcinoma (bottom) are shown. H & E.

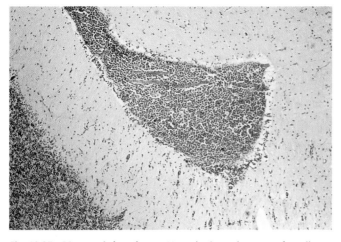

Fig. 12.27 **Metastatic lymphoma.** Note the irregular mass of small dark-staining cells in the subarachnoid space in the cerebellum (centre). The cells infiltrate the cortex and require distinction from the granular neurons (bottom left). H & E.

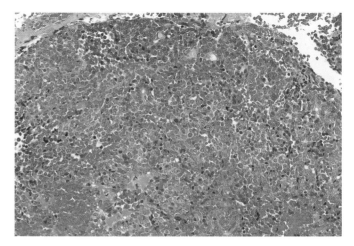

Fig. 12.30 **Metastatic neuroblastoma.** Primitive neuroblastic cells with evidence of rosette formation and widespread haemorrhage are present. H & E.

characteristic, confusion may arise with patients with rapidly growing *glioblastomas* accompanied by rapid progression of clinical signs and symptoms, and in whom neuroimaging studies can show an apparently multifocal lesion. In contrast, patients with solitary metastases within the brain parenchyma (particularly if no primary tumour is evident) may on neuroradiological grounds appear to have an intrinsic brain tumour (usually a *glioma*), or a *meningioma* if there is a dural attachment. Neurosurgical resections of metastatic lesions may also fail to distinguish between primary and metastatic lesions at the time of surgery since some gliomas (including *glioblastomas*) may appear to be relatively well circumscribed with an apparently clear plane of demarcation between the tumour and the adjacent brain. In contrast, some metastatic lesions, e.g. small cell carcinoma and melanoma, tend to infiltrate the adjacent brain parenchyma, resembling the growth pattern of an intrinsic glial tumour. Since central necrosis and haemorrhage may occur in both glioblastoma and metastatic carcinoma, these features cannot be relied upon to provide a distinction between the two entities. Primary intracerebral haemorrhage may also be confused clinically with metastatic carcinoma, particularly if multiple lesions are present, e.g. in the lobar haemorrhages characteristic of congophilic angiopathy.

Biopsy of metastatic tumours can usually result in an accurate diagnosis at the time of surgery. Differential diagnosis from intrinsic CNS tumours can often be resolved at this stage; cytological evidence of a glial origin for *glioblastomas* and other malignant gliomas is usually evident in smear preparations. Cryostat sections are particularly helpful in establishing the architectural pattern of a metastatic tumour and the characteristic areas of 'geographic' necrosis with nuclear pseudo-palisading can only be appreciated in cryostat sections from glioblastomas. Tumours which are extensively necrotic often cannot be diagnosed at the time of surgery, and careful examination of all the resected tissue at multiple levels through the paraffin block may be required in order to identify viable tissue on which a diagnosis can be made. This is a particular problem with glioblastomas, but necrosis can also occur in non-neoplastic inflammatory lesions (e.g. cerebral abscess and toxoplasmosis), and in cerebral infarction. The relatively uncommon *epithelioid glioblastoma* may resemble metastatic carcinoma in routinely stained preparations in terms of tumour cytology and architecture, but a careful search will usually reveal areas of typical glioblastoma and the characteristic widespread positivity for glial fibrillary acidic protein (GFAP) allows a distinction from metastatic carcinoma. It should be recalled that occasional metastatic neoplasms may exhibit focal (usually limited) positivity on immunocytochemistry for GFAP, possibly as a result of uptake of the protein from damaged parenchyma. The differential diagnosis of intraparenchymal metastatic deposits also includes *PNET*, particularly in adults. The cytological features of these tumours can be confused with those of metastatic small cell carcinoma in both smears and cryostat section preparations. Immunocytochemistry and electron microscopy can usually clarify the situation, since metastatic small cell carcinomas express cytokeratins and epithelial membrane antigen, whereas cerebral PNET usually do not express these antigens (EMA). Another tumour, the *rhabdoid/atypical teratoid tumour*, occurs mainly in children, and in routinely stained preparations which can resemble PNET, or metastatic neuroblastoma. Rhabdoid/atypical teratoid tumours express cytokeratins and EMA, but this usually occurs in the context of more widespread differentiation along muscle, neuroendocrine and mesenchymal lines, which allows it to be differentiated from other intrinsic and metastatic tumours.

A malignant papillary lesion in the brain is most likely to be a metastatic carcinoma, particularly metastatic adenocarcinoma, but in younger patients the possibility of a *choroid plexus tumour* should also be considered. Distinction between these entities is often difficult in young patients with solitary lesions at intraoperative diagnosis; since malignant choroid plexus tumours can also involve the cerebrospinal fluid (CSF) pathways; this creates further scope for diagnostic confusion with carcinomatous meningitis. Paraffin section histology is usually helpful in defining these two categories since choroid plexus tumours will express S-100 protein, carbonic anhydrase Type 2, cathepsin D and transthyretin (in addition to cytokeratin 7 (but not cytokeratin 20) and EMA);[54,55] electron microscopy may also be helpful in establishing the diagnosis (see Chapter 6).

The difficulty of examining the solitary posterior fossa metastasis in a patient with no known primary has already been discussed, but in the context of a patient with a family history of the von Hippel–Lindau syndrome this is particularly difficult, as renal carcinomas occur in this condition and may spread to the cerebellum. The cerebellum is also the commonest site for the *capillary haemangioblastomas* of the CNS, which are such a characteristic manifestation of this disorder. Both metastatic renal carcinoma and capillary haemangioblastoma are characterised by the presence of large irregular polygonal cells, often with a foamy appearance or clear cytoplasm. The differential diagnosis of haemangioblastomas is discussed in Chapter 14, but it should be noted here that these neoplasms do not express epithelial antigens such as cytokeratins or EMA.[56]

Metastatic malignant melanoma may be difficult to distinguish from a *primary melanoma* arising in the nervous system, although the latter are extremely uncommon and usually arise in the meninges, without the characteristic multifocal intraparenchymal location of metastatic deposits. Indeed, it is often wise to assume that any patient with a malignant melanoma involving the brain parenchyma has a metastasis until the possible primary sites have been excluded, since melanomas can arise at occult sites in the body including the upper respiratory tract, bladder and periungual regions.

Metastatic deposits occurring at particular sites within the cranial cavity have a wider range of differential diagnoses. Metastatic tumours occurring in the suprasellar region must be distinguished from *pituitary adenomas* or *craniopharyngiomas*. Neuroradiological studies are often invaluable in this respect, but it should be remembered that some 'locally infiltrative' pituitary tumours can appear markedly pleomorphic and exhibit mitotic activity, and the rare pituitary carcinoma can invade adjacent structures (Chapter 16). Craniopharyngiomas can usually be diagnosed on clinical and neuro-radiological grounds, but limited biopsy of part of the epithelium of the craniopharyngioma may result in diagnostic confusion with metastatic carcinoma, particularly squamous carcinoma. However, a distinction is often possible, even at intraoperative diagnosis, if adequate frozen section preparations are available to reveal the typical architecture of the common adamantinomatous type of craniopharyngioma. This distinction is more difficult in the less common *squamous papillary craniopharyngioma*, and diagnosis may be deferred until more detailed histological studies are performed on paraffin sections.

In the cerebellopontine angle, metastatic carcinoma can occur as a solitary lesion which requires distinction from *Schwannoma, choroid plexus papilloma or carcinoma*, or *meningioma*. In practical terms this should not present undue difficulties, since Schwannomas do not generally express epithelial markers such as cytokeratin or EMA (although focal positivity for both have been described in occasional cases). The distinction between metastatic carcinoma and choroid plexus tumours is discussed above. The distinction between *meningioma* and metastatic carcinoma is usually straightforward in the commoner histological subtypes of meningioma, but in the rarer types including the *clear cell, chordoid and papillary types* differential diagnosis is facilitated by immunocyto-chemistry and electron microscopy (see Chapter 13). Most meningiomas express EMA and vimentin, and focal expression of cytokeratins is not uncommon. Cytokeratin expression in metastatic carcinomas is more abundant and widespread, whereas vimentin positivity is less pronounced. The use of antibodies to specific epithelial products, for example thyroglobulin or prostate-specific antigen, can facilitate diagnosis in appropriate cases, but it should be recalled that many meningiomas express progesterone receptors, although immunoreactivity for oestrogen receptors is far less pronounced. The differential diagnosis of *atypical and malignant meningiomas* also includes metastatic sarcoma; the absence of reticulin expression in most meningiomas and appropriate immunocytochemistry (see Table 12.4) is particularly helpful. Electron microscopy is also most useful, since most meningiomas contain elongated and complex inter-digitations of the cell membranes, which are attached by hemisdesmosomes and other specialised cell junctions; this combination of features is unusual for both metastatic carcinoma and sarcoma.

It should also be recalled that metastatic carcinomas occasionally metastasise to other lesions in the CNS, most of which have been reported to occur in meningiomas (Figs 12.31 and 12.32).[57-59] Metastases to intrinsic tumours including gliomas have also been described, but these are much less common.[60,61] The tumours which metastasise to primary CNS neoplasms most frequently are carcinomas of the bronchus and breast.

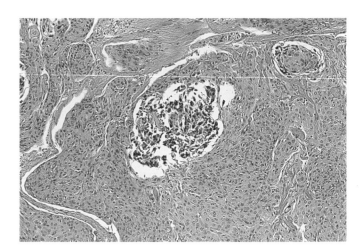

Fig. 12.31 **Metastatic carcinoma in meningioma.** This is clearly demarcated from the surrounding meningothelial meningioma cells. H & E.

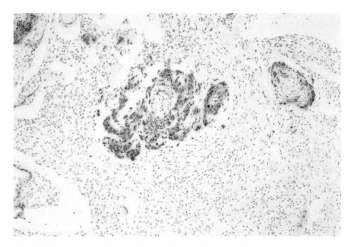

Fig. 12.32 **Metastatic carcinoma in meningioma.** Immunocyto-chemistry for CAM 5.2. Strong staining of the metastatic carcinoma is shown, but the meningioma is unstained (same case as Fig. 12.31).

In the pineal region, *pineoblastomas* may resemble small cell carcinomas of the lung in terms of their histology and architecture, but as mentioned above there are differences with respect to the expression of EMA and cytokeratins between these entities. Both *germinomas* and *teratomas* can be confused with metastatic carcinoma (particularly if a lymphocytic infiltrate is present – see Chapter 10), but these problems can usually be resolved easily by immunocytochemistry. With regard to primary pineal germ cell tumours, there is further scope for confusion with metastatic germ cell tumours, which are histologically indistinguishable. Relevant clinical information and neuroradiological data are clearly important in allowing this distinction to be made.

In addition to germ cell tumours, other non-epithelial tumours can metastasise to the CNS, particularly in children and young adults. These include a range of sarcomas (particularly osteogenic sarcoma, leiomyosarcoma, malignant fibrous histiocytoma and alveolar soft-part sarcoma) and paediatric tumours (Ewing's sarcoma, neuroblastoma and rhabdomyosarcoma). There is some evidence to suggest that the latter group is increasing in frequency as longer survival times are obtained with modern treatments, many of which do not cross the blood–brain barrier, leaving the CNS as a pharmacologically protected site. The same problem also arises in the management of acute leukaemias in childhood, when prophylactic irradiation and/or intrathecal cytotoxic dugs may be employed.

It may be difficult (if not impossible) to distinguish between primary and metastatic *cerebral lymphoma* in a patient with no apparent evidence of disease elsewhere in the body at the time of surgery. However, most primary CNS lymphomas have a characteristic cytological appearance, and are high grade malignant B-cell lymphomas (pleomorphic large cell type is commonest in the Revised European–American Classification of Lymphoid Neoplasms (REAL) classification). However, low grade primary CNS lymphomas have been reported, and ancillary investigations may be required, including thorough disease staging in the body. A close examination of the growth pattern of the tumour in the brain should be undertaken, since most primary brain lymphomas have a characteristic mode of growth involving expansion of the reticulin meshwork around the walls of blood vessels. This feature is uncommon in secondary lymphomas within the brain. Additional studies including the expression of Epstein–Barr virus related proteins and nucleic acids may be required for a more precise characterisation of the tumour. Primary brain lymphomas tend not to involve the CSF pathway at an early stage, but metastatic tumours can do this as a primary manifestation of disease, often accompanied by invasion of cranial or spinal nerve roots.

The ever increasing sophistication of diagnostic techniques for specific tumour types (including subgroups of carcinomas) have greatly facilitated accurate diagnosis of their corresponding metastatic deposits involving the CNS. The examples cited above are illustrative rather than comprehensive and further details of differential diagnosis are found in Table 12.4. As more patients with cancer survive for prolonged periods, as treatment for the primary tumour and its immediate complications improves, the enhanced survivals may well result in an increased frequency of metastatic deposits both within the CNS and in other parts of the body. Diagnostic vigilance is called for in patients with a past history of cancer, although it should be recalled that there is an association between certain types of intracranial tumours and carcinomas elsewhere in the body either as part of a recognised cancer syndrome (e.g. Li–Fraumeni syndrome) or by association, e.g. between breast carcinoma and meningiomas in female patients. The possible existence of several tumour types at once in the body will also inevitably lead to diagnostic confusion unless there is precise categorisation of these lesions. Finally, it is important to emphasise the need for adequate communication with clinical colleagues (neurologists, neurosurgeons and neuroradiologists) before reaching a diagnosis of metastatic carcinoma either at intraoperative diagnosis or when examining CSF specimens.

Therapy

Patients with brain metastases have for many years had very poor survival rates, with most patients dying within 1 year of diagnosis.[62–64] Most metastatic tumour deposits in the brain are relatively circumscribed (the commonest exceptions being metastatic melanoma and small cell lung carcinoma), although the extent of tumour involvement in histological terms usually exceeds the identifiable tumour margins seen on MRI scans and at surgery. This leads to difficulties in assessing the adequacy of surgical resection and this problem has led to attempts to remove all the contrast enhancing tissue, in some cases accompanied by the use of image guided frameless stereotaxis to remove multiple small deep-seated lesions.[64–66] This observation has also prompted the use of other focal treatments, including stereotactic radiosurgery and interstitial radiotherapy.[67–69]

Systemic disease is responsible for the death of at least 50% of patients with metastatic brain tumours and it is therefore essential to control the primary disease in order to improve survival figures.[63,64] It should be noted that brain metastases of unknown origin at the time of presentation are not at all uncommon and adequate neuropathological investigation and differential diagnosis is required in order to inform the search for the primary tumour.[64] The use of systemic chemotherapy may result in regression of brain metastases and a prolonged survival in patients with chemosensitive primary tumours including breast carcinoma, small cell lung carcinoma and germ cell tumours (including choriocarcinoma).[63] In the future, it is anticipated that a wider range of drugs will be available to treat chemosensitive brain metastases. Brain metastases are frequently accompanied by extensive vasogenic oedema, which contributes to the mass effect of the lesion. This is most often treated by a short course of corticosteroids.[62] Epileptiform seizures are not uncommon in patients with brain metastases and can be controlled by anticonvulsant drugs although these are not generally suited for prophylaxis.[64]

For patients with recurrent metastatic brain tumours, surgery can produce both symptomatic improvement and prolonged survival especially in patients with solitary metastases.[66,70] Neurosurgery is also indicated for life threatening mass effects and for larger lesions which require immediate decompression. Careful patient selection for surgery can also help; younger age and higher Karnofsky performance indicators at presentation are associated with better survival.[63,64] It has also been suggested that the number and location of metastatic tumours may also influence survival, but this has not been demonstrated universally, and it appears that the progression of the primary tumour and the sensitivity of the metastatic tumour to either focal or whole brain treatments are the predominant factors in determining patient outcome.

Metastatic tumours in the CSF pathway

As discussed above, metastases to the CNS can involve not only the brain parenchyma, but the pia and arachnoid mater and the dura mater; occasional metastases at these sites may exfoliate into the subarachnoid space, shedding malignant cells into the CSF at irregular intervals.[71-73] This process is not confined to metastatic carcinoma and may occur with other neoplasms, including lymphoma and leukaemia. The presence of extensive tumour deposits in the subarachnoid space can occasionally produce obstructive hydrocephalus,[71] but the widespread dissemination of tumour cells can produce a wide range of signs and symptoms including the non-specific features of headache, nausea and vomiting (usually attributable to hydrocephalus). This extensive involvement of the subarachnoid space can occur in the absence of solid intraparenchymal deposits, e.g. in diffuse invasion by a mucoid adenocarcinoma as a thin layer of cells. However, isolated cranial and spinal nerve palsies are a characteristic finding and may occur bilaterally in a non-symmetrical fashion. The optic nerves may also be involved, producing (often unilateral) visual disturbances, and both motor and sensory spinal nerves may

also be affected in an irregular distribution. Parenchymal invasion can occur at any site, with neoplastic cells infiltrating from the perivascular space.

The presence of metastases in the subarachnoid space is best identified by contrast enhanced MRI scans, which show small enhancing lesions in the arachnoid (best seen in the posterior fossa) (Fig. 12.33) and also on the cranial or spinal nerve roots, which may also appear irregularly thickened by tumour.[49,50]

Cytology

CSF cytology is required for confirmation of the diagnosis of carcinomatous meningitis, but initial examination of the lumbar CSF can a yield negative result and repeated examinations may be required in order to obtain a diagnostic sample.[74] Carcinomatous meningitis is frequently accompanied by a reduced level of CSF glucose relative to serum, but this finding is of supportive rather than diagnostic value. Metastatic tumours in the CSF pathway frequently cause a chronic inflammatory reaction in which the CSF contains increased numbers of lymphocytes and other mononuclear cells of monocyte/macrophage type.[74] This mononuclear reaction can be extreme in some cases, e.g. in the so-called

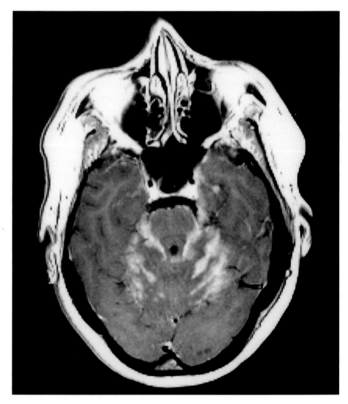

Fig. 12.33 **Carcinomatous meningitis.** Contrast-enhanced CT scan. This shows widespread enhancing leptomeningeal deposits around the cerebellar folia, upper pons and left trigeminal nerve. (Courtesy of D Collie, Edinburgh.)

'encephalitic' variant of malignant meningitis. It has been suggested that cisternal sampling of CSF may provide a higher diagnostic yield, but this method of sampling is much less convenient in general clinical practice.

The tumour types which are most likely to metastasise to the subarachnoid space (Table 12.5) are similar to those producing solid parenchymal metastases; it has been recorded that adenocarcinomas from the lung or lobular carcinoma of breast are particularly likely to disseminate to the CSF pathway.[72,74,75] Adenocarcinomas from other sites, including the lower gastrointestinal tract, pancreas, prostate and stomach have also been reported. The earlier literature has commented on the relatively high incidence of adenocarcinoma of stomach spreading to the CSF pathway,[71] but as the incidence of this tumour declines it has become relatively uncommon in current practice to see it involving the subarachnoid space. Malignant melanoma commonly involves the CSF pathway and in children the 'embryonal' tumours including neuroblastoma, embryonal rhabdomyosarcoma may involve the subarachnoid space; very occasionally, retinoblastoma can involve the subarachnoid space by direct invasion.

Most tumours involving the CSF pathway disseminate as single cells with occasional small clusters (Fig. 12.34); the larger clusters of malignant cells which typically occur in effusions into the pleural and peritoneal spaces are uncommon in the CSF. Most neoplastic cells are larger than the reactive mononuclear cells that usually accompany meningeal carcinomatosis (Fig. 12.35), but differential diagnosis on morphological terms alone is not always straightforward and reactive mononuclear cell populations can occasionally contain mitotic figures. The nucleus in carcinoma cells is usually large and irregular with multiple nucleoli and a coarse chromatin pattern. In adenocarcinomas, cytoplasmic vacuolation may be evident, and in malignant melanoma melanin pigmentation can occasionally be identified in tumour cells. Immunocytochemistry is of major value in confirming a diagnosis of meningeal carcinomatosis and a panel of antibodies can be employed to distinguish neoplastic cells from reactive mononuclear cells and glial cells (Figs 12.36 and 12.37). Further tumour cell subtyping using more specific antibodies e.g. HMB45 for malignant

melanoma, prostate-specific antigen, placental alkaline phosphatase (PLAP) for germ cell tumours, can also be employed (see Table 12.6 for a summary).

One major problem in diagnosing neoplastic involvement of the CSF pathway occurs in patients with systemic malignant lymphoma who present with neurological signs and symptoms. The differential diagnosis of a malignant lymphoma against a florid reactive mononuclear cell population is also difficult, and immunocytochemistry needs to be employed with care in order to identify the monoclonal population of neoplastic cells. Depending on the subtype of the primary lymphoma, a cytological distinction between neoplastic and reactive cells can be made on the basis of the cell size, nuclear morphology (particularly if large immunoblast-like cells are present), mitotic activity and immunophenotype. If a large quantity of CSF is available then flow cytometry

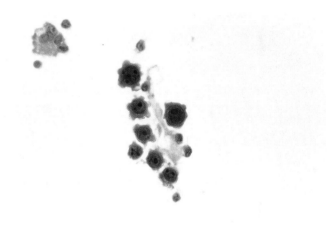

Fig. 12.34 **Carcinomatous meningitis.** CSF cytology in carcinomatous meningitis. A pleomorphic tumour cell population with large nuclei and prominent nucleoli is shown The primary tumour was a small cell anaplastic carcinoma in the lung. H & E.

Table 12.5 Tumours metastasising to the CSF pathway[8,9,12,47,48,72,74,75]

Adults	Children
Breast carcinoma	Acute leukaemia
Lymphoma	Lymphoma
Adenocarcinoma of lung	Neuroblastoma
Malignant melanoma	Retinoblastoma
Gastric carcinoma	
Small cell lung carcinoma	
Germ cell tumours	

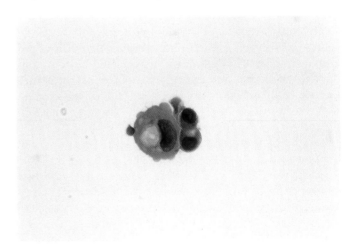

Fig. 12.35 **CSF metastases.** Metastatic adenocarcinoma in the CSF contains pleomorphic cells with intracytoplasmic vacuoles. H & E.

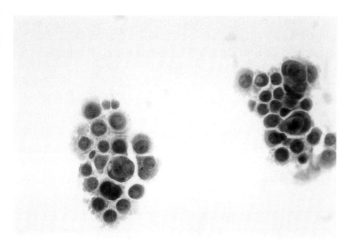

Fig. 12.36 **CSF metastases.** The CSF in metastatic breast carcinoma contains a mixture of lymphocytes, macrophages and large tumour cells. H & E.

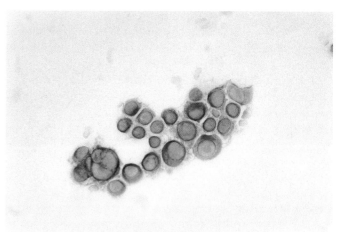

Fig. 12.37 **CSF metastases.** Immunocytochemistry for CAM 5.2. This shows strong cytoplasmic positivity in the tumour cells in a metastatic breast carcinoma in the CSF (same case as Fig. 12.36).

Table 12.6 Staining techniques for the investigation of malignant cells in the CSF[52–55,71,72,74]

Adults	Children
Initial screen EMA, cytokeratins, CD45, HMB45	*Initial screen* GFAP, synaptophysin, CD45
If epithelial cells present PAS / Alcian blue Epithelial cell specific markers, e.g. Oestrogen receptors, thyroglobulin, prostatic markers	*If blast cells present* CD screen for leukaemia / lymphoma (may require flow cytometry) *If no reaction obtained*
If lymphoid cells present CD3, CD20, CD68, CD79a	Desmin, n-myc and other markers for neuroblastoma and other embryonal tumours
If melanoma cells present Masson Fontana / Singh, S-100, HMB45	
If no reaction is obtained Placental alkaline phosphatase GFAP Sarcoma markers: desmin, actin, S-100	

EMA, epithelial membrane antigen; GFAP, glial fibrillary acidic protein; PAS, periodic acid–Schiff.

can reliably provide a detailed immunophenotype on the cellular infiltrates. Additional studies, including the demonstration of Epstein–Barr virus-related proteins and nucleic acids by immunocytochemistry or the polymerase chain reaction might be helpful in the characterisation of these tumours, but these are not in current diagnostic use on CSF specimens.

Details of the antibodies most useful in differential diagnosis of malignancy in the CSF are listed in Table 12.6. In paediatric practice this needs to be modified substantially to take into account the different range of tumours occurring in this age range, in particular to ensure that antibodies relevant the commoner tumours are employed, e.g. neuroblastoma and rhabdomyosarcoma.

The differential diagnosis of neoplastic cells in the CSF includes CSF involvement by primary CNS tumours;

neuroradiological findings are obviously of paramount importance in investigating this possibility and close attention to the cytological detail and immunophenotype of the tumour cells will also help resolve this problem. However, difficulties occasionally remain, for example in the distinction between cells from a *PNET* or metastatic small cell carcinoma in the CSF pathway.

In the differential diagnosis of metastatic tumour in the subarachnoid space, non-neoplastic processes must be considered, including infectious meningitis, particularly *tuberculous meningitis*, which can produce irregular thickening of the arachnoid with occasional small nodules which represent foci of granulomatous inflammation. Histological examination can usually distinguish between this and metastatic carcinoma; microbiological studies (including the polymerase chain reaction) for the relevant organisms will help resolve any diagnostic difficulties. The spinal nerves and cranial nerve roots may also be involved by metastatic carcinoma, producing ill-defined thickening either diffusely or in a more focal distribution which can be confused with the appearances of *chronic meningitis*. Earlier attempts to use specific forms of immunotherapy including radiolabelled monoclonal antibodies in a 'magic bullet' approach to patients with carcinomatous meningitis have not been adopted widely and it is accepted that patients with disseminated malignancy in the subarachnoid space have a poor outlook. However, this is not true for all tumours involving subarachnoid space, and in particular patients with malignant lymphoma in the CSF pathway may obtain a satisfactory response to the appropriate chemotherapy and radiotherapy.

Bone and epidural metastases

The vertebral bodies are common sites for metastatic tumours (see Table 12.7 for a summary). Metastases which occur initially within the bone of the vertebral column can spread into the spinal epidural space via the foramina around the intervertebral veins; occasional tumours can metastasise directly to the spinal epidural space.[76,77] These patterns of spread are somewhat modified for malignant lymphomas, which are more prone to involve the spinal epidural space by extension through the intervertebral foramen from adjacent paravertebral or retroperitoneal sites.

Patients with epidural metastases present with the signs and symptoms of spinal cord compression which is progressive and risks permanent cord damage unless treated.[76] The same applies for patients with osteolytic vertebral column metastases, as they will impinge upon the dura and may also result in collapse and pathological fracture of the vertebral body, thereby compressing the spinal cord and nerve roots and also potentially displacing in the intervertebral disc. Spinal cord infarction

has also been recorded under these circumstances as a consequence of vascular compression.[76] It is, however, extremely uncommon for the intervertebral disc to be involved by metastatic tumours within the adjacent vertebral body.[76,77] Spinal epidural metastases are usually solitary, with a rounded or lobulated outline and are characteristically associated with invasion of the vertebral column whilst sparing the intravertebral disc. Some retroperitoneal and pleural tumours (e.g. lymphoma, neuroblastoma, sarcoma and mesothelioma) can invade through the foramina of the spinal nerves, resulting in a dumb-bell-shaped mass which compresses the spinal cord and nerve roots.

Vertebral metastases are rounded lesions which result in extensive lysis in the adjacent bone accompanied by haemorrhage and collapse with resulting distortion of the vertebral column and spinal cord compression. These lesions are readily visualised in T1-weighted MRI scans as discrete, confluent or diffuse areas of low signal intensity.[32,45] The commonest neoplasms to involve the vertebral body are carcinomas of the lung, breast, kidney and prostate. For carcinomas of the breast (Figs 12.38 and 12.39) and lung, the thoracic spine is most commonly involved whereas prostatic carcinoma (Figs 12.40 and 12.41) usually involves the lumbar vertebral bodies initially. Prostatic carcinoma also differs from most others in that it produces an osteoblastic response which can occasionally be exuberant and compress adjacent sensory nerves, producing radicular pain. Most other carcinomas produce an osteolytic response which can result in vertebral collapse and pathological fracture. As mentioned above, intervertebral metastatic carcinoma can extend to involve the spinal epidural space, thereby potentiating spinal cord compression.[78]

Lymphoid neoplasms can also involve the epidural space and vertebral bodies (Figs 12.42–12.44). This can occur as a primary tumour, but secondary deposits are

Table 12.7 Differential diagnosis of tumours in the vertebral column and skull[44,45,76,77]

Tumours metastasising to bone
Lung cancer
Breast cancer
Prostatic cancer
Renal cancer
Multiple myeloma
Neuroblastoma (children)

Differential diagnosis
Primary bone tumours
Infection – tuberculosis and bacterial abscess
Metabolic bone disease, e.g. Paget's disease
Histiocytosis X
Meningioma infiltrating bone

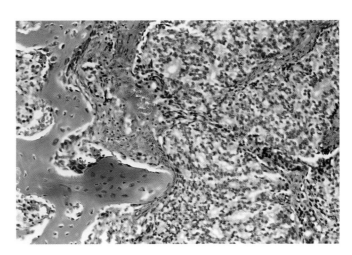

Fig. 12.38 **Bone metastases.** Extensive replacement of vertebral bone by metastatic breast carcinoma. H & E.

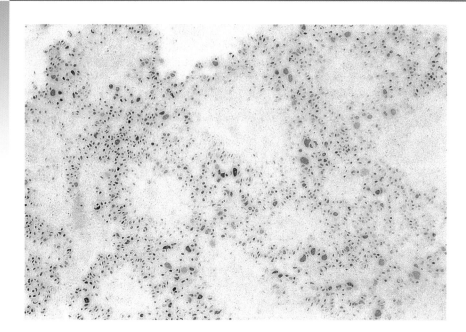

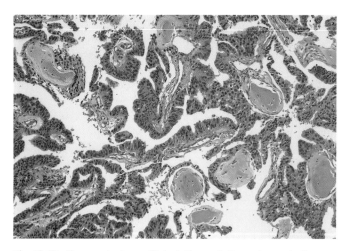

Fig. 12.40 **Bone metastases.** Metastatic prostatic carcinoma in the vertebral column. A prominent papillary pattern is shown. H & E.

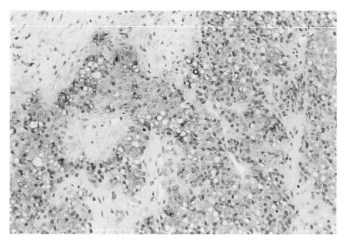

Fig. 12.41 **Bone metastases.** Metastatic prostatic carcinoma exhibits strong cytoplasmic positivity for prostatic acid phosphatase. (Same case as Fig. 12.40.)

more common, occurring most often in the midthoracic region. Most malignant lymphomas involving these sites are non-Hodgkin's lymphomas of high grade B-cell type; T-cell tumours rarely involve the spinal epidural space and Hodgkin's disease is extremely uncommon at this site. Multiple myeloma commonly involves the spinal epidural space and vertebral bodies and usually presents with bone pain in the back (see Chapter 11). Spinal cord compression can also occur in children as a result of epi- and intradural metastases from Ewing's sarcoma, neuroblastoma and Wilms' tumour. This has been reported in up to 5% of children in one recent series,[79] and was associated with a very short survival after diagnosis (median 2 months).

Differential diagnosis

The differential diagnosis for bony and epidural metastatic tumours is summarised in Tables 12.7 and 12.8. In the case of epidural metastases, the differential diagnosis for metastatic carcinoma is restricted, but for lymphoid tumours the distinction between a primary and secondary tumour is not always possible at initial diagnosis. Further clinical investigations and accurate disease staging are usually required for diagnosis before treatment can begin; this applies to both plasma cell tumours and non-Hodgkin's lymphomas. Distinction between a *meningioma* and a solitary dural deposit may be difficult in both clinical and radiological terms, unless

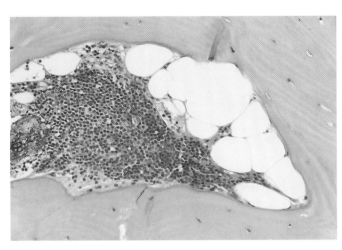

Fig. 12.42 **Bone metastases.** Metastatic lymphoma within the vertebral column often involves the marrow space. H & E.

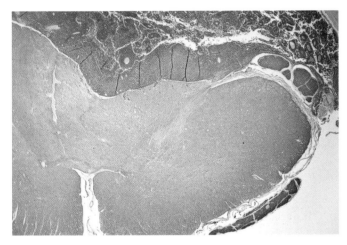

Fig. 12.43 **Epidural metastases.** Metastatic epidural lymphoma in the spinal subdural space, causing paraplegia as a result of spinal cord compression. H & E.

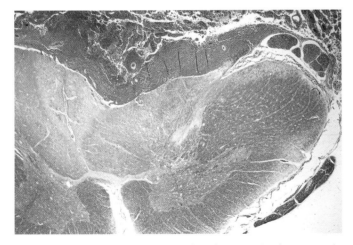

Fig. 12.44 **Epidural metastases.** Spinal cord compression by metastatic epidural lymphoma with marked pallor of myelin staining in the posterior columns (same case as Fig. 12.43). Luxol fast blue/Cresyl violet.

Table 12.8 Differential diagnosis of spinal epidural metastases[78–80]

Primary non-Hodgkin's lymphoma
Plasmacytoma/myeloma
Schwannoma or neurofibroma
Primary bone and cartilage tumours of vertebral column
Extraskeletal Ewing's tumour
Retroperitoneal and pleural tumours invading the epidural space
Tuberculoma
Paraspinal abscess
Herniated intervertebral disc

multiple lesions are present within the brain or spinal cord, or examination of CSF cytology has been positive. The distinction between non-neoplastic reactive processes, for example a *paraspinal abscess*, is usually straightforward. Some metastatic tumours, particularly breast carcinomas, produce an exuberant fibroblastic response and the identification of malignant cells is best achieved by immunocytochemistry. Occasionally, a *herniated intervertebral disc* is misdiagnosed as an epidural metastasis if herniation has occurred particularly in a central direction. This should not pose diagnostic difficulty on histological examination. The pathology of tumours arising in the epidural space and vertebral column are included in Chapter 18.

In the skull base region and in the vertebral column metastatic tumours need to be distinguished from *primary tumours of bone and cartilage, primary meningeal neoplasms* and *primary mesenchymal, non-meningothelial tumours*. The skull is involved by a similar range of metastatic tumours to the vertebral column; *metastatic carcinomas of the lung, breast, kidney and thyroid gland* are the commonest tumours. *Metastatic melanoma* and a range of *lymphoid neoplasms* may also involve the skull, particularly *multiple myeloma*, which usually exhibits a characteristic 'pepper-pot' appearance on plain X-ray films. The skull may be the presenting site of *Langerhans cell histiocytosis* (see Chapter 18) in the apparent absence of other lesions. The skull may also be involved by *primary tumours arising in adjacent structures including the paranasal sinuses and orbit*, which are considered more fully in Chapter 18. *Epidermoid and dermoid cysts* may involve the skull and a small biopsy of the lining squamous epithelium may produce confusion with metastatic squamous carcinoma, although careful review of the radiology and clinical details is usually helpful in clarifying this possibility. *Meningiomas* arising in the dura can occasionally infiltrate the skull and produce a marked hyperostosis (see Chapter 13). If the underlying meningioma has not been identified or diagnosed this may cause initial confusion with an infiltrating carcinoma, but the use of immunocytochemistry will help allow a distinction to be made (see above).

The prognosis for patients with spinal epidural deposits or vertebral bone deposits is somewhat better than those with intraparenchymal or subarachnoid CNS involvement, but the ultimate prognosis depends on the degree of tumour dissemination elsewhere in the body and the tumour type;[80] survival times for patients with solitary spinal epidural deposits of malignant lymphoma are better than those in patients with metastatic carcinoma or sarcoma.

REFERENCES

1. Johnson JD, Young B. Demographics of brain cancer. Neurosurg Clin N Am, 1996; 7:337–344
2. Henson RA, Urich H. Cancer and the nervous system. The neurological manifestations of systemic malignant disease. Oxford: Blackwell Scientific, 1982
3. Earle KM. Metastatic and primary intracranial tumors of the adult male. J Neuropathol Exp Neurol, 1954; 13:448–454
4. Counsell CE, Grant R. Incidence studies of primary and secondary intracranial tumors: a systematic review of their methodology and results. J Neurooncol, 1998; 37:241–250
5. Chason JL, Walker FB, Landers JW. Metastatic carcinoma in the central nervous system and dorsal root ganglia. Cancer, 1963; 16:781–787
6. Connolly ES Jr, Winfree CJ, McCormick PC et al. Intramedullary spinal cord metastasis: report of three cases and review of the literature. Surg Neurol, 1996; 46:329–337
7. Costigan DA, Windelman MD. Intramedullary spinal cord metastasis. A cliniopathological study of 13 cases. J Neurosurg, 1985; 62:227–233
8. Leonardi A, Dagnino N, Farinelli M et al. 'Pure' meningeal carcinomatosis as the autopsy-proven sole manifestation of an undetected cancer. Clin Neuropathol, 1992; 11:60–63
9. Lesse S, Netsky MG. Metastasis of neoplasms to the central nervous system and meninges. Arch Neurol Psych 1954; 72:133–153
10. Nussbaum ES, Djalilian HR, Cho KH et al. Brain metastases. Histology, multiplicity, surgery and survival. Cancer, 1996; 78:1781–1788
11. Aronson SM, Garcia JH, Aronson BE. Metastatic neoplasms of the brain: their frequency in relation to age. Cancer, 1964; 17:558–563
12. Bouffet E, Doumi N, Thiesse P et al. Brain metastases in children with solid tumors. Cancer, 1997; 79:403–410
13. Maesawa S, Kondziolka D, Thompson TP et al. Brain metastases in patients with no known primary tumor. Cancer, 2000; 89:1095–1101
14. Le Chevalier T, Smith FP, Caille P et al. Sites of primary malignancies in patients presenting with cerebral metastases. A review of 120 cases. Cancer, 1985; 56:880–882
15. Amer MH, Al-Sarraf M, Baker LH et al. Malignant melanoma and central nervous system metastases. Incidence, diagnosis, treatment and survival. Cancer, 1978; 42:660–668
16. Boogerd W, Vos VW, Hart AAM et al. Brain metastases in breast cancer, natural history, prognostic factors and outcome. J Neurooncol, 1993; 15:165–174
17. Burgess RE, Burgess VF, Dibella NJ. Brain metastases in small cell carcinoma of the lung. J Am Med Assoc, 1979; 242:2084–2088
18. Byrne TN, Cascino TL, Posner JB. Brain metastases from melanoma. J Neurooncol, 1983; 1:313–317
19. LeRoux PD, Berger MS, Elliott JP et al. Cerebral metastases from ovarian carcinomas. Cancer, 1991; 67:2194–2199
20. Lewis AJ. Sarcoma metastatic to the brain. Cancer, 1988; 61:593–601
21. Salvati M, Verconi L, Caruso R et al. Sarcoma metastatic to the brain: a series of 15 cases. Surg Neurol, 1998; 49:441–444
22. Srillet V, Catajar J-F, Croisile B et al. Cerebral metastases as first symptom of bronchogenic carcinoma. Cancer, 1991; 67:2935–2940
23. Yoshida S, Morii K, Watanabe M et al. Brain metastasis in patients with sarcoma: an analysis of histological subtypes. Surg Neurol, 2000; 54:160–164
24. Fernandez E, Maira G, Puca A et al. Multiple intracranial metastases of malignant melanoma with long-term survival. J Neurosurg, 1984; 60:621–624
25. Gay PC, Litchy WJ, Cascino TL. Brain metastases in hypernephroma. J Neurooncol, 1987; 5:51–56
26. Kaplan JG, DeSouza TG, Farkash A et al. Leptomeningeal metastases: comparison of clinical features and laboratory data of solid tumors, lymphomas and leukemias. J Neurooncol, 1990; 9:225–229
27. Ishizuka T, Tomoda Y, Kaseki S et al. Intracranial metastasis of choriocarcinoma. A clinicopathologic study. Cancer, 1983; 52:1896–1903
28. Willis RA. Pathology of tumours, 4th edn. London: Butterworth, 1967
29. Fidler IJ, Schackert G. Blood-brain barrier and pathogenesis of experimental brain metastasis. Cancer Bull, 1991; 43:33–40
30. Pauli BU, Lee C-L. Organ preference of metastasis. The role of organ-specifically modulated endothelial cells. Lab Invest, 1988; 58:379–387
31. Delattre JY, Krol G, Thaler HT et al. Distribution of brain metastases. Arch Neurol, 1988; 45:741–744
32. Edelson RN, Deck MDF, Posner JB. Intramedullary spinal cord metastases. Clinical and radiographic findings in 9 cases. Neurology, 1972; 22:1222–1231
33. Cho KG, Hoshino T, Pitts LH et al. Proliferative potential of brain metastases. Cancer, 1988; 62:512–515
34. Arnold SM, Young AB, Munn RK et al. Expression of p53, bcl-2, E-cadherin, matrix metalloproteinase-9, and tissue inhibitor of metalloproteinases-1 in paired primary tumors and brain metastasis. Clin Cancer Res, 1999; 5:4028–4033
35. Hamasaki H, Aoyagi M, Kasama T et al. GT1b in human metastatic brain tumors: GT1b as a brain metastasis-associated ganglioside. Biochim Biophys Acta, 1999; 1437:93–99
36. Hartsough MT, Steeg PS. Nm23-H1: genetic alterations and expression patterns in tumor metastasis. Am J Hum Genet, 1998; 63:6–10
37. Lloyd BH, Platt-Higgins A, Rudland PS et al. Human S100A4 (p9Ka) induces the metastatic phenotype upon benign tumour cells. Oncogene, 1998; 17:465–473
38. Ruan S, Fuller G, Levin V et al. Detection of p21WAF1/Cip1 in brain metastases. J Neurooncol, 1997; 37:461–474
39. Roetger A, Merschjann A, Dittmar T et al. Selection of potentially metastatic subpopulations expressing c-erbB-2 from breast cancer tissue by use of an extravasation model. Am J Pathol, 1998; 153:1797–1806
40. Petersen I, Hidalgo A, Petersen S et al. Chromosomal imbalances in brain metastases of solid tumors. Brain Pathol, 2000; 10:395–401
41. Deviri E, Schachner A, Halevy A et al. Carcinoma of lung with a solitary cerebral metastasis. Cancer, 1983; 52:1507–1509
42. Minette SE, Kimmel DW. Subdural hematoma in patients with systemic cancer. Mayo Clin Proc, 1989; 64:637–642
43. Bisese JH. MRI of cranial metastases. Semin Ultrasound CT, 1992; 13:473–483
44. Osborn AG. Diagnostic neuroradiology. St Louis: Mosby-Year Book, 1994
45. Ramsey RG. Neuroradiology, 3rd edn. Philadephia: WB Saunders, 1994
46. Peretti-Viton P, Margain D, Murayama N et al. Brain metastases. J Neuroradiol, 1991; 18:161–172
47. Yousem DM, Patrone PM, Grossman RI. Leptomeningeal metastases: MR evaluation. J Comp Assist Tomogr, 1990; 14:255–261
48. Watanabe M, Tanaka R, Takeda N. Correlation of MR and clinical features in meningeal carcinomatosis. Neuroradiology, 1993; 35:512–515
49. Sze G, Soletsky S, Bronen R et al. MR imaging of the cranial meninges with emphasis on contrast enhancement and meningeal carcinomatosis. Am J Roentgenol, 1989; 153:1039–1049
50. Gomori JM, Heching N, Siegal T. Leptomeningeal metastases: evaluation by gadolinium enhanced spinal magnetic resonance imaging. J Neurooncol, 1998; 36:55–60
51. Jackobs L, Kinkel WR, Vincent RG. Silent brain metastases from lung carcinoma determined by computerised tomography. Arch Neurol, 1997; 34:690–693
52. Ordóñez NG. Application of immunocytochemistry in the diagnosis of poorly differentiated neoplasms and tumors of unknown origin. Cancer Bull, 1989; 41:142–151
53. Williams GR. Unravelling the unknown primary. CPD Bull Cell Pathol, 1999; 1:140–143
54. Gyure KA, Molrrison AL. Cytokeratin 7 and 20 expression in choroid plexus tumors: utility in differentiating these neoplasms from metastatic carcinomas. Mod Pathol, 2000; 13:638–643
55. Perry A, Parisi JE, Kurtin PJ. Metastatic adenocarcinoma to the brain: an immunohistochemical approach. Hum Pathol, 1997; 28:938–943

56. Andrew SM, Gradwell E. Immunoperoxidase labelled antibody staining in differential diagnosis of central nervous system haemangioblastomas and central nervous system metastases of renal carcinomas. J Clin Pathol, 1986; 39:917–919

57. Bernstein RA, Grumet KA, Wetzel N. Metastasis of prostatic carcinoma to intracranial meningioma. J Neurosurg, 1983; 58:774–777

58. Chambers PW, Davis RL, Blanding JD Jr et al. Metastases to primary intracranial meningiomas and neurilemomas. Arch Pathol Lab Med, 1980; 104:350–354

59. Lodrini S, Savoiardo M. Metastases of carcinoma to intracranial meningioma: report of two cases and review of the literature. Cancer, 1981; 48:2668–2673

60. Tajika Y, Reifenberger G, Kiwit JC et al. Metastatic adenocarcinoma in cerebral astrocytoma: clinicopathological and immunohistochemical study with review of the literature. Acta Neurochir, 1990; 105:50–55

61. Le Blanc RA. Metastasis of bronchogenic carcinoma to acoustic neuroma. J Neurosurg, 1974; 41:614–617

62. Wright DC, Delaney TF, Buckner JC. Treatment of metastatic cancer to the brain. In: DeVita VT Jr, Hellman S, Rosenberg R, eds. Cancer: principles and practice of oncology, 4th edn. Philadelphia: Lippincott, 1993: pp 2170–2186

63. DeAngelis LM. Management of brain metastases. Cancer Invest, 1994; 12:156–165

64. Posner JB. Management of brain metastases. Rev Neurol, 1992; 48:477–487

65. Bindal RK, Sawaya R, Leavens ME et al. Surgical treatment of multiple brain metastases. J Neurosurg, 1993; 79:210–216

66. Patchell RA, Tibbs PA, Walsh JW et al. A randomised trial of surgery in the treatment of single metastases to the brain. New Eng J Med, 1990; 322:494–500

67. Sims E, Doughty D, Macaulay E et al. Stereotactically delivered cranial radiation therapy: a ten-year experience of linac-based radiosurgery in the UK. Clin Oncol, 1999; 11:303–320

68. Maor MH, Dubey P, Tucker SL et al. 'Stereotactic radiosurgery for brain metastases: results and prognostic factors. Int J Cancer, 2000; 90:157–162

69. Smalley SR, Laws ER Jr, O'Fallon JR et al. Resection for solitary brain metastasis. Role of adjuvant radiation and prognostic variables in 229 patients. J Neurosurg, 1992; 77:531–540

70. Sawaya R, Ligon BL, Bindal AK et al. Surgical treatment of metastatic brain tumors. J Neurooncol, 1996; 27:269–277

71. Grain GO, Karr JP. Diffuse leptomeningeal carcinomatosis. Clinical and pathologic characteristics. Neurology, 1955; 5:706–722

72. Iaconetta G, Lamaida E, Rossi A et al. Leptomeningeal carcinomatosis: review of the literature. Acta Neurol, 1994; 16:214–220

73. Kokkoris CP. Leptomeningeal carcinomatosis. How does cancer reach the pia-arachnoid? Cancer, 1983; 51:154–160

74. Bigner SH, Schold SC. The diagnosis of metastases to the central nervous system. Pathol Annu, 1984; 19:89–119

75. Lamovec J, Zidar A. Association of leptomeningeal carcinomatosis in carcinoma of the breast with infiltrating lobular carcinoma. Arch Pathol Lab Med, 1991; 115:507–510

76. Kakulas BA, Harper CG, Shibasaki K et al. Vertebral metastases and spinal cord compression. Clin Exp Neurol, 1978; 15:98–113

77. Barron KD, Hirano A, Araki S et al. Experiences with neoplasms involving the spinal cord. Neurology, 1958; 9:91–106

78. Byrne TN. Spinal cord compression from epidural metastases. New Eng J Med, 1992; 327:614–619

79. Bouffet E, Marec-Berard P, Thiesse P et al. Spinal cord compression by secondary epi- and intradural metastases in childhood. Childs Nerv Syst, 1997; 13:383–387

80. Nather A, Bose K. The results of decompression of cord or cauda equina compression from metastatic extradural tumors. Clin Orthop, 1982; 169:103–108

13 Meningiomas

The meninges, the tripartite coverings of the brain and spinal cord, are the site of a vast array of pathological lesions, many of which are commonly encountered by histopathologists. Although inflammatory lesions and secondary tumours do come within the pathologist's purview, primary tumours of the meninges are the most frequently observed lesions. Of these primary meningeal tumours, meningiomas are by far the most common, constituting a significant fraction of intracranial tumours at all neurosurgical centres. Other primary, non-meningothelial tumours of the meninges are discussed in Chapter 14.

Knowledge of select macroscopic and microscopic aspects of the meninges is helpful in understanding and evaluating meningeal tumours. The dura mater, the outermost membrane, is distinguished by its firm and thick appearance; hence the terms 'dura mater' ('tough mother') and 'pachymeninx' ('thick meninges'). The normal dura mater is a two-layered structure, the outer layer being closely affixed to the overlying skull and constituting part of the inner periosteum of the skull. In the setting of most meningeal tumours, the skull and dura mater thus constitute a outward barrier, encouraging neoplasms to grow inward to compress the underlying brain. However, this is a relative barrier, in that some tumours not only invade the dura mater but may transgress the skull itself to involve the soft tissues of the scalp. In the spinal region, the dura mater is not affixed to the surrounding spine, creating an actual epidural space; as a result, some spinal meningeal tumours may present in a primarily extradural location. Histologically, the dura mater is a paucicellular, densely collagenous structure containing scattered, large and patulous vascular channels. The cells have a rather non-descript fibroblastic appearance. The blood vessels consist of both venous conduits, including the large venous sinuses, as well as the branches of the meningeal arteries. Many meningiomas are attached to the overlying dura mater. In fact, frank invasion of the dura mater by meningioma is not unusual, and many tumours also invade into the dural venous sinuses. For these reasons, portions of dura mater are often removed along with meningeal tumours during neurosurgical procedures and thus come to histopathological attention.

Beneath the dura mater is the arachnoid mater, a 'spider-like' membrane that sends trabeculae to the surface of the brain and spinal cord. By definition, the arachnoid covers the subarachnoid space, through which courses the vital cerebrospinal fluid. The arachnoid is a membrane that is only a few cells thick, the outer cells being spindle shaped and resembling those seen in fibrous meningiomas, the inner cells being more polygonal in shape. Interspersed along the membrane are nests of meningothelial cells that are cytologically and architecturally identical to those found in meningothelial meningiomas, replete with whorls and psammoma bodies. Focally, these cells aggregate into grossly visible masses, the arachnoid or pacchionian granulations, which are conspicuous, vaguely papillary tufts of tissue that project into the dural venous sinuses. Cerebrospinal fluid from the subarachnoid space funnels into the dural sinuses, returning to the general circulation, via the arachnoid granulations. The arachnoid granulations are clustered in the meninges at locations where dural sinus drainage is most prominent, such as alongside the superior sagittal sinus and major sinuses at the skull base; interestingly, however, arachnoidal granulations are also present along the spinal arachnoid and along the optic nerves. This distribution closely mirrors that of meningiomas, providing, along with their histological appearance, another clue that meningiomas may be tumours derived from arachnoidal cells.

Arachnoidal cells are located in other places as well, accounting for the sometimes unexpected occurrence of those meningiomas unassociated with the dura mater. The best known of these are intraventricular meningiomas, arising from arachnoidal cells within the choroid plexus stroma. Such cells gain access to the inner reaches of the ventricular system during embryological development, when infolding of the choroid plexus brings meningothelial tissues inward along the tela choroidea. Other, perhaps abnormal embryological variations may account for rests of arachnoidal cells in other cranial sites, such as the skull and scalp, that could provide an explanation for primary meningiomas in these locations. Presumably the rare occurrences of meningiomas in other, systemic organs also reflects some similar embryological misadventures.

Closest to the brain is the final meningeal covering, the pia mater, an inconspicuous cell layer that constitutes the outer limit of the brain and spinal cord proper, with tight attachments to the underlying central nervous system tissue. The 'pious mother' devoutly follows all of the contours of the brain, diving down into the Virchow–Robin spaces as well. While there is no evidence for meningeal tumours arising from pial cells, disruption of the integrity of the pial–glial barrier is a potentially ominous histological sign in evaluating meningeal tumours. Thus, histopathological examination of the pial surface of any brain fragments removed during meningioma resection is an important responsibility when evaluating these lesions.

Meningiomas are a histologically diverse group of tumours composed of neoplastic meningothelial cells. While the vast majority of meningiomas are associated with the dura and arachnoid maters, the cell of origin of the meningioma remains open to debate. Most authors support the notion that arachnoid cap cells are the most likely oncogenic target. As mentioned above, many meningiomas closely resemble normal arachnoidal cells and meningiomas frequent those sites where arachnoidal granulations are most common. Furthermore, most meningioma cells have immunohistochemical profiles similar to arachnoidal cells. Nonetheless, on gross examination, on neuroradiological examination and at surgery, meningiomas most often have a broad *dural* attachment. This gross affinity for the dura mater, however, belies their distinctly arachnoidal histology.

Complete pathological descriptions of meningioma date back to Louis in 1774, who described the characteristic fungal-like growths of the dura mater.[1] Until the early part of the twentieth century, however, descriptions were sporadic and terminology highly variable, with the tumours reported as psammomas, endotheliomas, meningoexotheliomas and arachnoidal fibroblastomas, among other names. The modern era of diagnosing and classifying meningiomas was heralded in by Cushing, who coined the term 'meningioma' in 1922[2] and published a number of systematic studies of these tumours. The 1938 Cushing and Eisenhardt monograph on meningiomas was seminal in defining this histologically diverse group of tumours.[3] Their original classification was complex, with nine major types of meningioma and 22 subtypes, but drew attention to the similarities among these histologically disparate lesions. Over the years, some entities have been added to the cadre of meningioma variants, while others have been reassigned to other tumour types. For instance, haemangiopericytic lesions are no longer considered meningothelial in origin and are treated as primary pericytic tumours of the meninges. On the other hand, new entities such as secretory and rhabdoid meningioma are clinicopathologically important variants that have rightfully found their places alongside the classical subtypes. The 1993 World Health Organisation (WHO) struck a practical and reasonable compromise among the various classification systems, but still left leeway for further refinements and improvements. The 2000 revision of the WHO system clarified some of these issues and provided additional diagnostic guidelines. The present chapter largely follows the 2000 WHO system.[4]

Most meningiomas are biologically benign tumours and are correspondingly assigned a WHO grade of I of IV. Nearly all of the histological subtypes of meningioma, despite their astounding variety, share similar benignant tendencies. Certain meningiomas, however, have an increased tendency to recur or follow an aggressive clinical course and are designated as WHO grade II (e.g. atypical meningioma) and WHO grade III [e.g. anaplastic (malignant) meningioma]. Atypical meningiomas have a substantially increased incidence of recurrence; malignant meningiomas have an even higher incidence of recurrence and may be associated with brain invasion or systemic metastasis. In contrast to the common adult glial tumours, however, meningiomas do not invariably display malignant progression; often multiple recurrences over many years retain the histological characteristics of the original tumour. Indeed, it is often the inability to

resect tumours completely, such as those that occur at the base of skull, that leads to recurrence, rather than the emergence of a more malignant subclone. Nonetheless, some meningiomas may progress from benign to atypical to malignant over time.

From a diagnostic point of view, therefore, there may be relatively little importance in distinguishing among the many benign variants of meningioma, but considerable clinical importance in identifying grade II and grade III tumours. Unfortunately, as discussed below, the criteria to identify these potentially clinically aggressive variants remain somewhat ill-defined. Some aggressive subtypes are diagnosed on the basis of histological features of rapid growth, for instance, mitotic activity and hypercellularity; others are diagnosed on the presence of frankly malignant clinical features such as systemic metastasis; and yet others on the presence of specific histological patterns such as papillary architecture. Along with improving microneurosurgical techniques to facilitate complete resections of deeply situated tumours, finding more objective means of identifying those lesions more likely to recur remains a major goal in improving meningioma therapy.

Incidence

Meningiomas occur at an incidence of approximately 6 per 100 000 persons[5] and are estimated to constitute between 13 and 26% of primary intracranial tumours. Meningiomas may be more common in Africa, where they may constitute up to 38% of all intracranial tumours; however, such estimates may reflect reporting or diagnosing biases rather than true differences. Patients with certain inherited tumour syndromes, however, have a markedly increased incidence of meningiomas. Most notable among these syndromes is neurofibromatosis 2 (NF2),[6] in which patients develop multiple meningiomas, Schwannomas and ependymomas in addition to other characteristic central and peripheral nervous system lesions such as meningioangiomatosis (see below and Chapter 19). Many patients with NF2 develop meningiomas; indeed, most severely affected NF2 patients, having the so-called Wishart variant, have multiple meningiomas. Meningiomas occur with an increased frequency in other, non-NF2 families with a hereditary predisposition to meningioma; affected family members often develop multiple meningiomas yet lack other characteristic and diagnostic features of NF2.[6,7] Patients with other rare tumour syndromes, such as Gorlin or Cowden syndromes, have developed multiple meningiomas, suggesting a link with these other diseases, but such patients have been exceedingly rare and the associations between meningioma and these rare syndromes remain uncertain.[8–10]

Atypical meningiomas constitute between 4.7 and 7.2% of meningiomas, although such estimates are highly dependent on differing histological definitions for atypical meningioma (see below). Malignant meningiomas are uncommon, comprising between 1.0 and 2.8% of meningiomas,[11–13] with the variation also probably reflecting differing criteria for diagnosing malignant meningioma.

Meningiomas are most common in middle-aged and elderly patients, although they occur both in children and in the very old. For both men and women, the peak occurrence is in the sixth and seventh decades.[14] Children show may some bias for developing more aggressive forms of meningioma, but certainly not all childhood meningiomas behave in an aggressive manner.[15–17] Meningiomas occurring in hereditary tumour syndromes such as NF2 typically occur in younger patients, and a meningioma presenting early in life should prompt a careful family history and examination for stigmata of NF2. In these hereditary settings, the tumours also do not necessarily act in a more aggressive fashion; indeed, the tumours are typically histologically benign.

In middle-aged patients with meningioma, there is a marked female bias, with a female:male ratio approaching 2:1.[14] In particular, spinal meningiomas show a marked preference for women. Childhood meningiomas display a male predominance.[15–17] Meningiomas associated with hereditary tumour syndromes occur equally in men and women. Atypical and anaplastic (malignant) meningiomas, however, may show a conspicuous male predominance.[18]

Site

The vast majority of meningiomas arise within the intracranial and intravertebral cavities. Within the intracranial cavity, as many as 40% of tumours occur over the cerebral convexities, with many associated closely with the falx cerebri (Figs 13.1 and 13.2). Falcine tumours may be bilateral, with mirror-image lesions on either side. The predilection for the falx may also be seen in patients with multiple meningiomas, who may develop many, nearly confluent falcine lesions. Along the parasagittal region, the majority are found in the middle third, with the anterior third the next most common site.[22] Other common intracranial sites include the sphenoid ridges, olfactory grooves, parasellar regions, optic nerve (Fig. 13.3), petrous ridges, tentorium cerebelli and posterior fossa. In some of these locales, the tumours lie in close proximity to dural venous sinuses, and invasion of the dural sinuses occurs moderately frequently in meningiomas (Fig. 13.4). Meningiomas also occur within the ventricular system, most often in the lateral ventricles, reflecting the infolding of meningothelial tissue that accompanies formation of the choroid plexus during embryogenesis; curiously, the left ventricle is involved more frequently than the right. More confusing, however, are the rare meningiomas that appear entirely intracerebral, lacking either surface or ventricular involvement. Spinal meningiomas are most

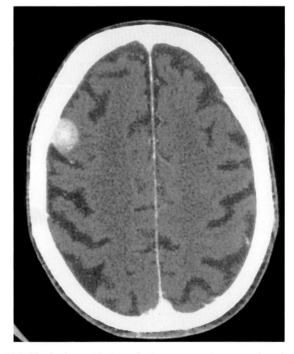

Fig. 13.1 **Meningioma.** Most meningiomas present on neuroimaging as discrete, dural-based, globular, enhancing masses, as noted in this contrast-enhanced, computerised tomography image of a convexity meningioma.

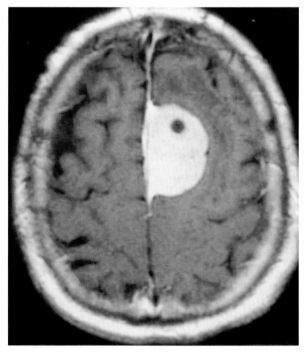

Fig. 13.2 **Meningioma.** A broad dural attachment and 'tail' is apparent on this T1-weighted, gadolinium-enhanced magnetic resonance image of a falcine meningioma. (Courtesy of Dr PW Schaefer, Boston, Massachusetts.)

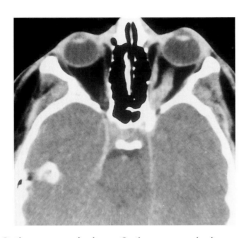

Fig. 13.3 **Optic nerve meningioma.** Optic nerve meningiomas enlarge the profile of the optic nerve as it passes through the orbit, as noted on computerised tomography scan.

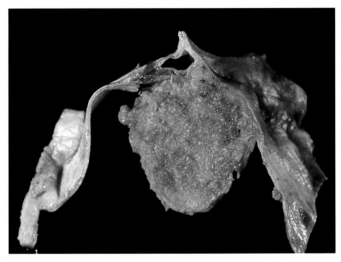

Fig. 13.4 **Parasagittal meningioma.** Parasagittal meningiomas often lie in close proximity to the superior sagittal sinus. Invasion of the sinus may occur and complicate total resection.

common in the thoracic region, where they tend to occupy more anterior and lateral positions than paraspinal Schwannomas (see Chapter 15).[19] Rarely, meningiomas of the spine may arise in an epidural location, most often in children and in males. Atypical and malignant meningiomas are more common on the falx and the lateral convexities than in other sites,[12] perhaps reflecting the general predisposition of meningiomas to occur in these sites. Finally, although rare, meningiomas have been reported as primary, usually benign tumours in many organs of the body, including the skull, nasal cavity, paranasal sinuses, oral cavity, parotid gland, ear, soft tissue of the neck, mediastinum, skin, peripheral nerve and lung.[23] For malignant meningiomas, metastatic deposits most often involve lung, liver, lymph nodes, bones and pleura, among other organs. Seeding of malignant meningioma via the subarachnoid space with drop metastases is exceedingly rare, but has been reported.[23]

Aetiology

The aetiology of most meningiomas remains unclear. To date, only radiation exposure and genetic factors have been clearly implicated, although hormonal alterations may play a role in meningioma development or growth and trauma has been suggested as a possible causative factor. Patients who have received radiation for a variety of therapeutic reasons have a predisposition to develop meningiomas in the field of radiation. Meningiomas have been induced by low, moderate and high dose radiation, with average time intervals to tumour appearance of 35, 26 and 19–24 years, respectively.[24] The vast majority of patients with radiation induced meningiomas have a history of low dose irradiation (800 cGy) to the scalp for tinea capitis; the second largest group of patients with radiation induced meningiomas received high-dose irradiation (greater than 2000 cGy) for primary brain tumours.[25] Given the relatively short survival of many patients radiated for primary brain tumours, it remains possible that the incidence of radiation induced tumours would be even higher if such patients survived longer. The literature suggests that radiation induced meningiomas are more commonly atypical or aggressive, with higher proliferation indices and multifocality, and occur in generally younger age groups.[25–27]

Genetic predisposition to meningiomas, as a result of alterations of a number of genes (see below), is certainly one aetiological factor. As mentioned above, meningiomas are a hallmark of NF2 (see Chapter 19).[6] The predisposition of NF2 patients to meningiomas implies that inactivating alterations of the *NF2* gene are important in the formation of meningiomas. This causal relationship is confirmed by the observation that sporadic meningiomas suffer mutations in the *NF2* gene as well (see below). Therefore, loss of function of the NF2 encoded protein, merlin, is a critical event in the genesis of at least some meningiomas. However, a number of families have an increased susceptibility to meningiomas, but do not have NF2.[6] At least some of these meningioma-only families do not show genetic linkage to the NF2 locus on chromosome 22q,[7] suggesting involvement of a second meningioma predisposition gene. The probability of such a second meningioma locus is strengthened by the finding that many sporadic meningiomas do not harbour either somatic *NF2* gene mutations or allelic loss of the long arm of chromosome 22q. The location of this second, early meningioma gene, however, has not been identified. Since some sporadic meningiomas that lack chromosome 22q loss have loss of the short arms of chromosomes 1 and 3,[28] chromosomes 1p and 3p may harbour another early meningioma gene and this possibility will need to be evaluated in non-NF2 meningioma families. Finally, the putative relationships of meningioma to Gorlin or Cowden syndrome[8–10] raises the possibility that alterations of the *PTCH* and *PTEN/MMAC1*, genes, respectively, could also be involved in meningioma tumorigenesis; indeed, occasional meningiomas harbour *PTCH* mutations.[29]

The role of sex hormones in the genesis of meningiomas is less clear. The over-representation of women among meningioma patients has suggested an aetiological role for sex hormones in these tumours. While estrogen receptor expression is very low or not detectable in the majority of meningiomas, approximately two-thirds of meningiomas express progesterone receptors,[30] with meningiomas from female meningioma patients more often expressing progesterone receptors than those from male patients. Whether the expression of these receptors is integral to meningioma formation and growth, however, remains to be determined. An association has also been reported between breast carcinoma and meningioma, again raising the possible role of sex hormones in meningioma formation. A number of patients have been reported with both breast carcinoma and meningioma, including patients with multiple meningiomas.[23] This association may be clinically important, as it should not be assumed that multiple dural masses in a patient with breast cancer are necessarily metastases. While the association between breast cancer and meningioma has been oft cited, this may simply represent the co-occurrence of two common tumours that affect older women rather than a significant biological association.[31] In this regard, it is interesting to note that alterations of the breast cancer-associated *BRCA1* and *BRCA2* genes do not occur in sporadic meningiomas.[32] Meningioma growth may also be accelerated during pregnancy and during the luteal phase of the menstrual cycle, again suggesting that hormonal factors may influence meningioma growth. In particular, meningiomas in the parasellar region have been noted to present or exacerbate during pregnancy, but this apparent preference for location may just reflect the greater likelihood of symptoms developing from tumours close to the optic pathways.[23] Thus a number of observations support the assertion that sex hormones and their receptors at least influence meningioma growth. Whether such alterations are in any way causative, however, remains unclear.

Other putative causative factors include trauma, as meningiomas have been noted at the sites of previous traumatic insults. Striking cases have included meningiomas developing around foreign bodies or at fracture lines from trauma.[23] However, such associations may be coincidental and proof of causation is lacking.

Clinical features

In general, the location of a meningioma dictates its clinical signs and symptoms, since meningiomas are usually slowly growing masses that elicit neurological signs and symptoms by compression of adjacent struc-

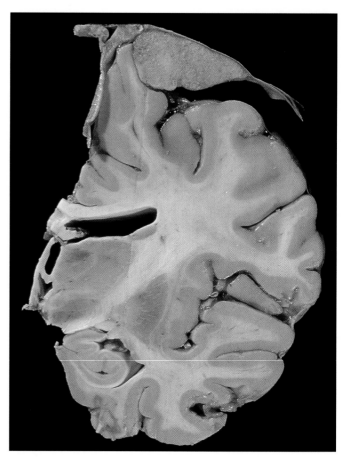

Fig. 13.5 **Meningioma.** Meningiomas tend to compress the adjacent brain and, in most cases, the tumour retracts easily from the brain.

tures (Fig. 13.5). Some tumours may grow to considerable size before causing clinical problems (Fig. 13.6), for instance olfactory groove tumours compressing one frontal lobe. Those lying alongside the upper falx may present primarily with lower extremity signs and symptoms, as they compress the regions of the motor and sensory cortices subserving leg functions. More laterally located convexity lesions may, on the other hand, primarily elicit hand and face signs and symptoms. Base of skull tumours may instead affect cranial nerve function directly as they entrap these structures, but often produce non-localising symptoms such as headache. In particular, sphenoid ridge tumours may present with painless unilateral exophthalmos, unilateral visual loss and/or ophthalmoplegia; olfactory groove lesions with central scotoma, ipsilateral optic atrophy, contralateral papilloedema and ipsilateral anosmia; tuberculum sellae masses with bitemporal haemianopsia and optic atrophy; cerebellopontine angle meningiomas with cerebellar signs and hearing loss; and foramen magnum tumours with spastic paresis and sensory findings in the upper extremities.[33] Other base of skull tumours present with extensive vascular involvement, wrapping around the carotid artery.

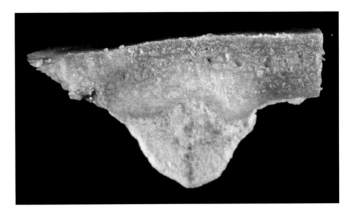

Fig. 13.7 **Osteoblastic meningioma.** Osteoblastic meningiomas may elicit hyperostosis of the overlying skull.

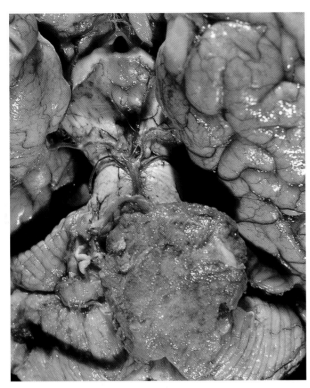

Fig. 13.6 **Meningioma.** Some meningiomas may attain considerable size without eliciting symptoms, as in this clival mass that was an incidental autopsy finding.

Meningiomas may also evoke underlying cerebral oedema which may itself cause neurological signs and symptoms. In some instances, peritumoral oedema may be marked and/or rapid in onset, simulating a more aggressive brain tumour at a clinical level. The presence of oedema may be related expression of various vascular permeability and angiogenic factors such as vascular endothelial growth factor/vascular permeability factor.[34] Headaches and seizures may also herald the presence of a meningioma, but are not as common as in other, more rapidly growing intracranial tumours. Uncommonly, meningiomas may present as skull or scalp nodules since some meningiomas invade the skull and overlying scalp; even less commonly, some meningiomas may induce overlying skull hyperostosis and present as a 'secondary' skull mass (Fig. 13.7).

Rarely, meningiomas may present with 'distant' findings. For instance, chordoid meningiomas may be associated with haematological abnormalities such as hypergammaglobulinaemia or anaemia,[35,36] while secretory meningiomas may present with elevated carcinoembryonic antigen (CEA) levels.[37] Rare erythropoietin producing meningiomas causing erythrocytosis have been reported.[38] Lastly, a considerable number of meningiomas may not elicit symptoms at all and are incidental findings on neuroradiological examination or at autopsy. These are often small tumours overlying 'non-eloquent' regions of the brain, but occasionally may be quite large. Certainly in patients with multiple meningiomas, many lesions are clinically silent.

Radiology

As many as 60% of meningiomas display some abnormalities on plain skull radiographs.[22] These changes include reactive hyperostosis and tumour calcification. Reactive hyperostosis occurs in up to one-quarter of cases and has been noted most often adjacent to convexity and parasellar masses. Calcification has been noted in about one-fifth of cases.[22] Less commonly on plain films, hypertrophied meningeal feeding vessels may highlight the vascular grooves on the inner table of the skull or unilaterally increase the size of the foramen spinosum. Rarely, meningiomas may be osteolytic. Computerised tomography scanning demonstrates meningiomas as isodense or slightly hyperdense masses which are sometimes calcified. Intense enhancement is noted following contrast administration (Fig. 13.1), but this may not be apparent in densely calcified masses. On T1-weighted magnetic resonance images, meningiomas are typically isointense to normal grey matter, but T2-weighted images variably show hypo- or hyperintensity.[22] Most hypointense lesions on T2-weighted images are fibrous or transitional, while meningothelial tumours are more often hyperintense on these images.[39] Secondary features such as cyst formation, oedema and calcification may also be discerned. After gadolinium administration, meningiomas uniformly display marked homogeneous enhancement (Fig. 13.2). A characteristic feature is the presence of a so-called 'dural tail' adjacent to the main mass, which can represent a triangular extension of tumour along the dura or a peritumoral collection of small blood vessels. Peritumoral vasogenic cerebral oedema is noted in approximately 50% of tumours[32] and is occasionally prominent, particularly in secretory variants[40] and in meningothelial tumours with so-called pericytosis.[41] Neuroimaging findings have not been consistently reliable in predicting tumour behaviour.

Pathology

Macroscopic features

The preferential locations of meningiomas have been reviewed in a previous section. While most of these locations are dural based, meningiomas may occur within the ventricles, rarely within the brain and in many extradural locations such as the skull, scalp, paraspinal soft tissues, and a variety of systemic organs (see above). With a few exceptions noted below, the location of the tumour does not correlate with particular macroscopic features. Nonetheless, meningiomas vary in their gross appearance to a remarkable degree. The classical appearance of a meningioma is a rubbery, well demarcated, rounded mass with a broad dural attachment (Fig. 13.8).[5,19–21] However, meningiomas vary from being soft and gelatinous to being firm and calcified. Some meningiomas are gritty on gross inspection, implying the presence of numerous psammoma bodies; such tumours are particularly common in the thoracic spinal cord of middle-aged women, but may be seen in other situations as well. Other meningiomas may be hard, secondary to bone formation within the lesion, or less commonly because of primary intraosseous growth of a meningioma with an osteoblastic reaction (Fig. 13.7). Most tumours have a smooth contour, but some lesions may be multilobular on sectioning (Fig. 13.9), and dumb-bell shaped masses may arise in locations where adjacent bony structures confine tumour growth. Occasionally, meningiomas may be grossly cystic, a finding that may be associated with microcystic changes as well. In certain

locations, meningiomas lack the typical rounded appearance. For instance, those growing along the sphenoid ridge may grow as a flat, infiltrative lesion of the dura, known as 'meningioma en plaque' (Fig. 13.10). Meningiomas of the optic nerve often grow as circumferential masses, encircling the optic nerve along its intraorbital path and sometimes infiltrating outside of the dural sheath (Fig. 13.11a,b). Most meningiomas are tan in colour (Fig. 13.8), varying from dark to light; highly vascular lesions may have a pink hue, while lipidised examples may be focally yellow.

Meningiomas usually compress the adjacent brain or spinal cord, but rarely display overt attachment or invasion of the brain (Fig. 13.5). In the event that a meningioma is

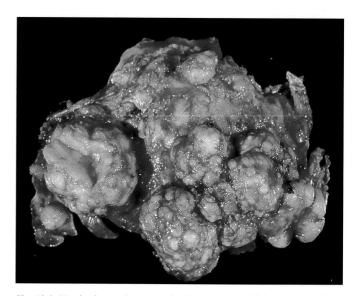

Fig. 13.9 **Meningioma.** Some meningiomas are multilobular, as in this large, recurrent tumour.

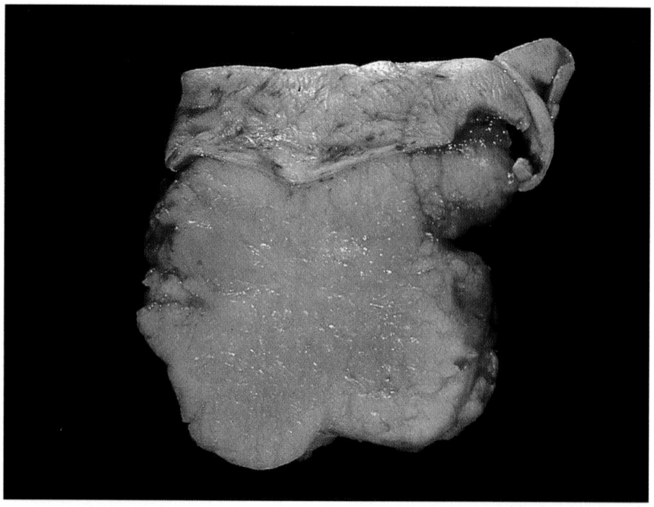

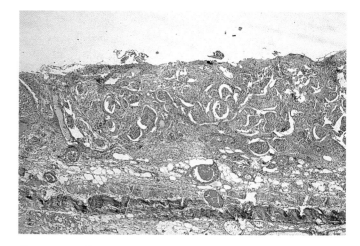

Fig. 13.10 **Meningioma 'en plaque'.** Some meningiomas, particularly those growing along the sphenoid ridge, grow as flat, 'en plaque' masses. These are often invasive of the dura, as demonstrated by this low power photomicrograph. H & E.

Fig. 13.8 **Meningioma.** Meningiomas often have a broad dural attachment. Their cut surfaces are usually light tan and homogeneous, sometimes with a nodular appearance.

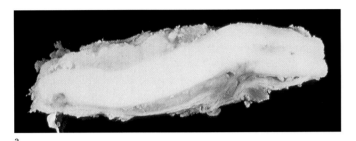

a

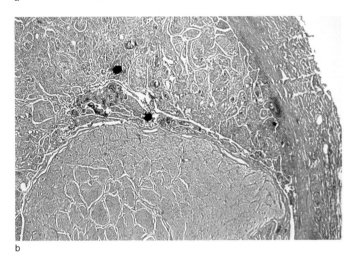

b

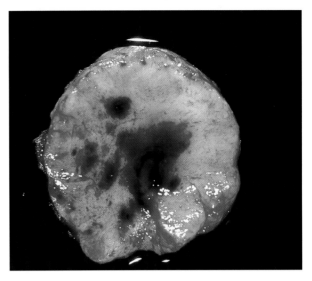

Fig. 13.12 **Atypical meningioma.** These more often show irregularities on their cut surfaces, as seen in this atypical meningioma with central haemorrhage. The tumours may also be darker tan in colour and softer than benign meningiomas.

Fig. 13.11 **Optic nerve meningioma.** Meningiomas of the optic nerve ensheath, but do not invade, the nerve. (a) Surgical resection specimen. (b) Low power photomicrograph demonstrating optic nerve, tumour and surrounding intact dura mater. H & E.

attached to the underlying brain, careful microscopic examination of the interface should be performed to determine whether brain invasion has taken place. Invasion of the dura and of nearby dural sinuses, on the other hand, is quite common; invasion of the dural sinuses does not necessarily indicate that the tumour will spread extracranially. Occasional meningiomas invade through dura to involve the skull, while other meningiomas incite an overlying hyperostosis of the skull (Fig. 13.7). Atypical and malignant meningiomas tend to be larger at operation than classical meningiomas,[12] tend to be less firm than most benign meningiomas, and may be more adherent to adjacent structures.

When assessing resected meningiomas, special attention should be paid to a number of issues. Any brain tissue affixed to the meningioma should be sampled to evaluate whether brain invasion has occurred, because of the potential importance of this histological finding in predicting tumour behaviour. Similarly, invasion of dural sinuses should be documented, as extensive dural involvement may provide an explanation for subsequent recurrence even in the setting of an ostensibly 'complete' resection. All meningiomas should be sectioned thinly and examined for grossly distinct regions that may imply histological diversity (Fig. 13.12). Comprehensive sampling

of such regions for histological examination is vital in ensuring that the lesion has been properly evaluated for features of atypical or malignant meningioma, since these diagnoses affect subsequent clinical follow-up and therapy. These issues are discussed in more detail below.

Histological features

Meningioma Meningiomas display a dazzling diversity of histopathological appearances.[5,19–21,23] From a diagnostic histopathological point of view, it is encouraging to know that relatively few of these distinct histological patterns have clinical importance. Most of the subtypes share a common clinical behaviour, with some exceptions noted below. It is, however, discouraging that the stunning histological diversity implies that meningiomas may microscopically mimic many other tumour types, including a number of malignant tumours, making their accurate diagnosis of great importance. Furthermore, histological features may be quite diverse within individual tumours. For this reason, large meningiomas should be sampled extensively, particularly in order to sample regions that may contain histological features that may suggest a greater likelihood of recurrence or aggressive clinical behaviour (see below).

Most meningiomas at least focally share certain basic histological features. Classical meningioma cells resemble those of the normal and reactive arachnoid. These cells are round-to-oval in shape with correspondingly round-to-oval nuclei. The nuclei are distinctive and are crucial for at first suggesting, and then confirming, the diagnosis of meningioma. Most nuclei are slightly oval with a delicate, euchromatic chromatin, without conspicuous nucleoli or chromatin clumping (Figs 13.13–13.16). Of particular help is the presence of intranuclear inclusions. These inclusions take on two forms. The first is a protrusion of usually eosinophilic cytoplasm into the nucleus, producing a sharply outlined pinkish pseudoinclusion that may be widespread in some lesions (Fig. 13.15). The second is a diffuse 'washing out' of the nuclei (Fig. 13.16) which, at the ultrastructural level, reflects extensive focal clearing of the chromatin. Again, this may be strikingly common in some tumours. The presence of these nuclear characteristics, while not pathognomonic, certainly should raise the likelihood of meningioma in the differential diagnosis. Careful searching will often reveal nuclei with such features even in fibrous meningiomas, in which the vast majority of nuclei have a rather featureless, fibroblastic

appearance. The cytoplasm of meningioma cells is eosinophilic and non-descript at the light microscopic level, being noteworthy primarily for the seeming absence of cytoplasmic borders that may create a so-called 'syncytial' appearance (Fig. 13.15). As discussed below, this reflects the intricate intercellular interdigitations that, although visible ultrastructurally, are beyond the resolution of the light microscope. Most meningiomas are moderately cellular tumours although, again, variety is the hallmark, with lesions ranging from low to focally high cellularity.

Two related histological features are also highly characteristic of meningiomas: cellular whorls and psammoma bodies. The presence of these structures should prompt careful consideration of meningioma in any differential diagnosis of an intracranial tumour.

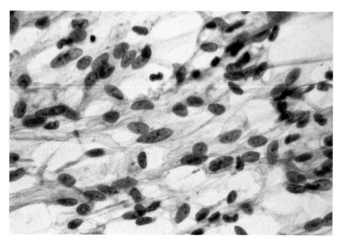

Fig. 13.13 **Meningioma.** Intraoperative smear preparations may be helpful in demonstrating the characteristic cytological features of meningioma. The features are oval nuclei with delicate euchromatin accompanied by light tapering cytoplasm. However, many meningiomas do not smear well as a result of their cohesiveness. H & E.

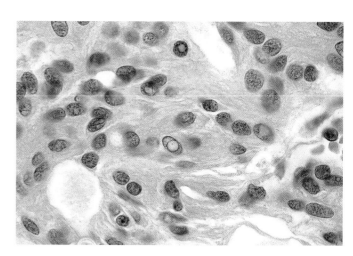

Fig. 13.15 **Meningioma.** The nuclei of meningiomas may have a characteristic appearance with oval nuclei having delicate euchromatin and 'Orphan Annie eye' inclusion. The cell borders are indistinguishable, giving a 'syncytial' impression. H & E.

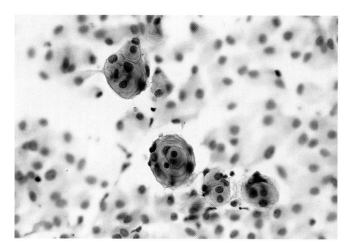

Fig. 13.14 **Meningioma.** Intraoperative touch preparations are often helpful in diagnosis, since intact cellular whorls have a propensity to 'pop out' onto the touch preps. H & E.

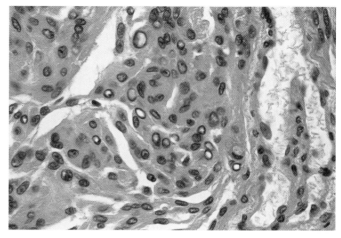

Fig. 13.16 **Meningioma.** Other nuclei in meningiomas have a 'washed out' look. H & E.

Cellular whorls are collections of cells arranged in a concentrically laminated fashion (Figs 13.14, 13.17 and 13.18). They are typically a few cell layers thick and range from being tightly to loosely wound. Cells in the centre of the whorls are polygonal, resembling typical meningothelial cells, sometimes harbouring intranuclear inclusions. Cells toward the outside of the whorls, however, are elongated as they stretch around the central cells, giving them a fibroblastic appearance more characteristic of the meningothelial cells seen in fibrous meningiomas. Tightly wound cellular whorls may be useful diagnostic findings on intraoperative touch preparations as these structures are readily transferred from the tumour to the touched glass slides (Fig. 13.14). Cellular whorls, however, while highly characteristic of meningioma, are not diagnostic; in particular, loose whorling can be seen in other tumours, including Schwannomas, sometimes raising difficult diagnostic questions in NF2 patients. A host of other tumours have also been shown to have whorl-like structures on occasion.[23]

Psammoma bodies are concentrically laminated calcifications that appear to arise initially within the centre of the cellular whorls (Figs 13.19 and 13.20). They vary from tiny, punctate mineral deposits no bigger than a single cell to large, lamellated structures that may almost be appreciated, at least on palpation, on macroscopic examination. As psammoma bodies enlarge, they typically obscure the underlying cellular whorl so that most psammoma bodies appear free within the lesions. Like cellular whorls, psammomas bodies are highly characteristic but not diagnostic of meningiomas, as they may also be seen in tumours such as Schwannomas and

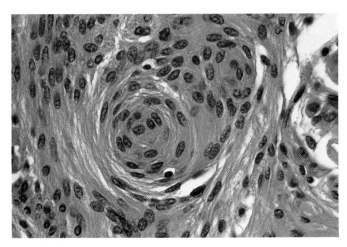

Fig. 13.17 **Meningioma.** Cellular whorls are characteristic of meningiomas, and may be found in most subtypes of meningioma. H & E.

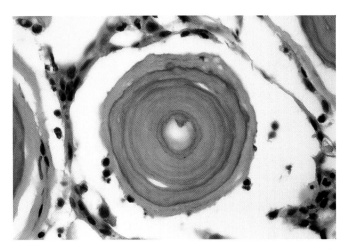

Fig. 13.19 **Meningioma.** Psammoma bodies are highly characteristic of meningiomas. Psammoma bodies are lamellated mineralisations that range in size from a few to hundreds of microns in size. H & E.

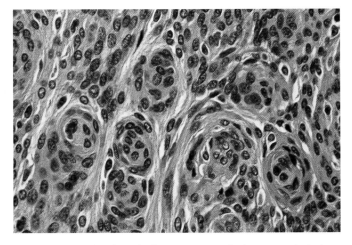

Fig. 13.18 **Transitional meningioma.** Some meningiomas, particularly transitional meningiomas, contain numerous whorls. When multiple, whorls tend to be more compact and tightly wound. H & E.

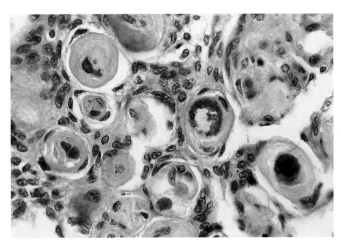

Fig. 13.20 **Meningioma.** Psammoma bodies have a range of appearances as they form in the centre of cellular whorls, from ill-defined concretions in intact whorls to larger lamellated mineralisations that replace whorls. H & E.

metastatic carcinomas that may enter the differential diagnosis, particularly paraspinal Schwannomas and rare metastatic tumours from the thyroid and ovary.

Despite the classic cytological characteristics, meningiomas nonetheless vary greatly in the degree to which these features are present and in their architectural patterns. This variability accounts for the wide range of meningioma subtypes. As mentioned above, over the years, different subtypes of meningioma have been included or removed as diagnostic entities from the various classification schemes. The present classification largely follows the 2000 WHO system,[4] with some additions and clarifications. The 2000 WHO classification is, in turn, a modification of the 1993 WHO system.[42] Of the various subtypes, meningothelial, fibrous and transitional meningiomas are by far the most common. Furthermore, many tumours show features intermediate between these common subtypes, again emphasising the relatively minor importance of subdividing the common variants.

Meningothelial meningioma In this classic and common variant, tumour cells generally form moderately cellular lobules (Fig. 13.21), surrounded by thin collagenous, vascular septae. Larger lobules should not be confused with 'sheeting' or loss of architectural pattern, seen in atypical meningiomas. Within the lobules, tumour cells appear to form a 'syncytium' as the delicate, intricately interwoven tumour cell processes cannot be discerned at the light microscopic level; this appearance has led to the alternative name 'syncytial' meningioma. The tumour cells closely resemble those of the normal arachnoid, and florid arachnoidal hyperplasia may simulate meningioma in small biopsy specimens (see below). Meningothelial tumour cells feature the classic cytological appearance for meningioma: oval nuclei and a delicate, even chromatin pattern. Nuclear inclusions in the form of cytoplasmic

pseudoinclusions and nuclear 'washing out' may be prominent in this subtype. Whorls and psammoma bodies are not as common in meningothelial meningioma as in other meningioma variants, but are found individually in many cases. When present, whorls tend to be less well formed and looser. Mutations of the *NF2* gene and allelic loss of chromosome 22q tend to be less common in this variant of meningioma, than in the other common subtypes, but the types of mutations are similar (see below). Most histologically described tumours in meningioma families that lack other features of NF2 have been of the meningothelial type.

Fibrous (fibroblastic) meningioma Fibrous meningioma is another classic and common variant. In fibrous meningioma, the tumour cells are predominantly spindle shaped, appearing somewhat fibroblastic (Fig. 13.22). However,

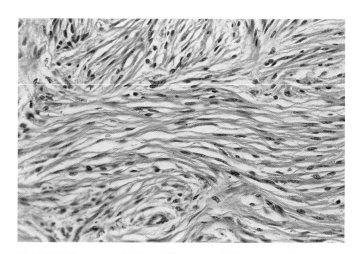

Fig. 13.22 **Fibrous meningioma.** Fibrous meningiomas contain elongated, fibroblast-like cells and intervening collagenous tissue. The cells are often arranged in fascicles. H & E.

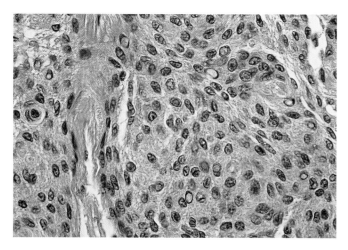

Fig. 13.21 **Meningothelial meningioma.** Meningothelial meningiomas often form lobules comprising cells with characteristic nuclear inclusions. Note the apparent 'syncytial' nature of these meningothelial cells. H & E.

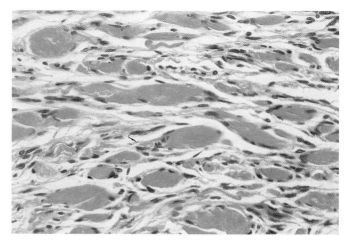

Fig. 13.23 **Fibrous meningioma.** Certain fibrous meningiomas feature extensive extracellular collagen deposition, as in this case in which broad eosinophilic collagen bands separate small groups of tumour cells. H & E.

cells with nuclear features characteristic of meningothelial meningioma are often found as well, which can be helpful in distinguishing fibrous meningiomas from other spindle cell tumours such as Schwannoma. In fibrous meningioma, the tumour cells form wide fascicles, with varying amounts of either interfascicular or intrafascicular, intercellular collagen and reticulin. In general, the fascicles of fibrous meningiomas are more organised than those of Schwannomas, which have a more haphazard fascicular pattern. In some cases, the amount of collagen may be striking (Fig. 13.23). Occasionally, the collagenous bands may be quite broad and may undergo dense calcification. Rare meningiomas have been reported with so-called 'amianthoid' collagen fibres, abnormally large, sometimes banded collagen fibres; these fibres may accumulate in a stellate pattern to form 'amianthoid' bodies.[43,44] Whorls and psammoma bodies are not as common in pure fibrous meningiomas as in other variants, but are nonetheless often present focally. Some authors have suggested that fibrous meningiomas are particularly common in patients with NF2.[1,45] In our experience and that of others, this has not been true, with NF2 patients developing all of the common subtypes of meningioma.[6,46] Some tumours reported to be fibrous meningiomas in NF2 patients may have been unusual Schwannomas, since distinguishing these two common tumours may be quite difficult in NF2 patients and may require immunohistochemistry. Nonetheless, somatic *NF2* gene mutations are particularly common in sporadic fibrous meningiomas, occurring in about 70% of cases, suggesting that somatic *NF2* gene alterations are related to the fibrous phenotype. To date, analysis of the types of *NF2* gene mutations in fibrous meningiomas has not provided insights into this relationship.

Transitional (mixed) meningioma These common tumours have features transitional between those of meningothelial and fibrous meningioma, hence the designation 'transitional' or 'mixed'. Lobular and fascicular arrangements are therefore present and regions of cytologically typical meningothelial cells are common (Fig. 13.24). Whorls are often conspicuous in this subtype, and may be tightly wound. Usually, meningothelial, fibrous and transitional regions mingle locally in these tumours, often within the same low-power microscopic field. Some tumours, however, have large, distinct areas of fibrous meningioma separated from regions of meningothelial meningioma; such tumours may also be designated as mixed or transitional, but do not have the same tendency to have numerous tight whorls. Psammoma bodies are frequent in transitional meningiomas, and it is the transitional meningioma with psammoma bodies that merges imperceptibly with the next histological subtype, psammomatous meningioma. Like fibrous meningiomas, transitional tumours commonly have *NF2* gene mutations. Again, however, the types of *NF2* mutations are similar to those observed in other subtypes.

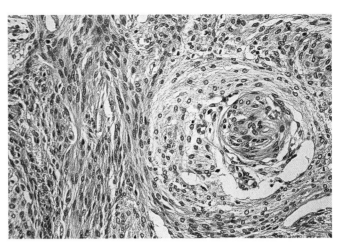

Fig. 13.24 **Transitional meningioma.** Transitional meningiomas display features of both meningothelial and fibroblastic meningiomas, often with numerous whorls. H & E.

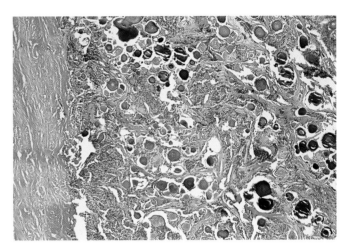

Fig. 13.25 **Psammomatous meningioma.** Meningiomas may be dubbed psammomatous when psammoma bodies become a dominant feature of the tumour, as seen in this spinal lesion. Note the portion of dura mater that is free of psammoma bodies. H & E.

Psammomatous meningioma This designation may be used for meningiomas with particularly abundant psammoma bodies (Fig. 13.25), although the degree of psammomatous change necessary for this diagnosis is not defined. Typically, the neoplastic cells in these tumours have a transitional appearance with whorls. Some tumours are almost replaced by psammoma bodies, requiring careful examination to identify intervening meningothelial cells. As psammoma bodies become particularly large, they may lose their circular appearance and assume less regular shapes. Psammomatous tumours characteristically occur in the thoracic spinal region, usually in middle-aged women, but may also have a predilection for the orbital region.

Angiomatous meningioma Angiomatous meningiomas have numerous, conspicuous blood vessels, at least in

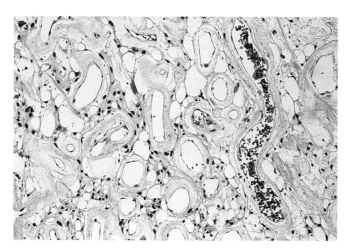

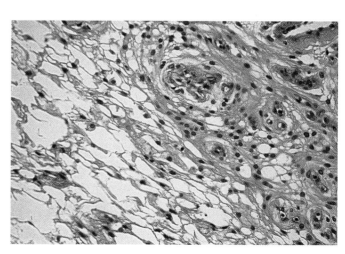

Fig. 13.26 **Angiomatous meningioma.** Angiomatous meningiomas have numerous small, hyalinised blood vessels. On occasion, relatively few meningothelial cells may remain, raising the differential diagnosis of a cavernous malformation. H & E.

Fig. 13.27 **Microcystic meningioma.** Microcystic meningiomas usually have regions of typical meningioma alternating with microcystic regions. H & E.

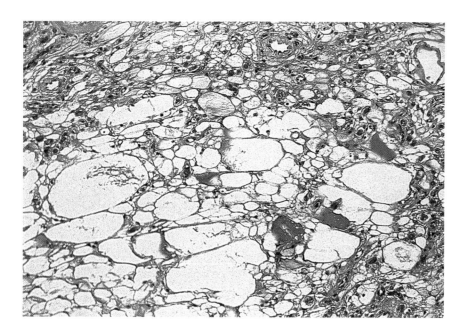

Fig. 13.28 **Microcystic meningioma.** Some microcystic meningiomas may show extensive microcyst formation, with larger, apparently coalescent cysts. H & E.

some parts of the tumour (Fig. 13.26). As a result, these tumours have also been termed 'highly vascular' meningiomas. Sometimes, the numerous blood vessels may obscure the background meningioma, but most tumours have clear regions of classical, usually meningothelial meningioma. In regions where the vascular channels overwhelm the meningothelial cells, the remaining meningioma cells may display considerable pleomorphism. The vascular channels may be small or medium sized and may be thin walled or have hyalinised, thickened walls. Most often the vessels are small with hyalinised walls. Differential diagnoses include vascular malformations and capillary haemangioblastoma, depending on the size of the meningiomatous vessels. This designation should not be equated with the obsolete term 'angioblastic

meningioma', as angiomatous meningiomas do not display aggressive clinical behaviour.

Microcystic meningioma This variant is characterised by focal regions of cells having elongated processes and a loose, mucinous background, giving the appearance of many small cysts among the cells (Figs 13.27 and 13.28). At the ultrastructural level, the small cystic structures are extracellular and may relate to focal detachment of desmosomes.[47] Some authors have suggested that the tumour cells bear more of a resemblance to arachnoidal trabecular cells, rather than to the arachnoidal cap cells, and that the microcystic spaces recapitulate small subarachnoid spaces. Most tumours have regions of classical, often meningothelial meningioma. As in the angiomatous meningioma, pleomorphic cells may also be numerous in this variant. And, again as in the angiomatous meningioma, the vessels of microcystic meningioma may show extensive hyalinisation. Occasionally, the histological appearance may mimic that of haemangioblastoma and some examples of the 'haemangioblastic variant of angioblastic meningioma' would now be classified as microcystic meningioma; the resemblance is heightened by the sometimes presence of foamy cells in this variant that may be histologically similar to the stromal cells of haemangioblastoma. The microcystic variant has also, for obvious reasons, been referred to as 'humid' meningioma (forme humide of Masson). No distinct clinicopathological associations have been made for microcystic meningioma, but these tumours may be associated with gross cystic changes.

Secretory meningioma The hallmark of secretory meningioma is the presence of pseudopsammoma bodies within an otherwise classical, usually meningothelial meningioma (Fig. 13.29). Pseudopsammoma bodies are small, round, eosinophilic, strongly periodic acid–Schiff (PAS) positive structures that often occur in clusters. On electron microscopic examination, these bodies are extracellular amorphous debris within well developed lumina that are replete with mature epithelial features such as tight junctions and villi. Thus, secretory meningioma has been considered the most epithelial of meningioma subtypes. The pseudopsammoma bodies stain immunohistochemically for CEA (Fig. 13.30) while the surrounding tumour cells are cytokeratin positive. Immunopositivity for human secretory component as well as immunoglobulin A (IgA) and IgM has also been noted, confirmed the truly secretory nature of these lesions.[48] The combined CEA and cytokeratin immunohistochemical staining pattern is unique among meningiomas, with other meningioma types only showing focal, light cytokeratin immuno-

positivity. Secretory meningiomas may be associated with elevated circulating CEA levels,[37] thus demonstrating a functionally secretory phenotype. Elevated CEA levels may be clinically significant in patients who also have breast carcinoma, since CEA levels are sometimes used as a marker of breast cancer recurrence. In addition, secretory meningiomas may present with prominent peritumoral cerebral oedema.[40,49] Secretory meningiomas have a marked female predominance and preferentially involve the frontal meninges and sphenoid ridge.[49]

Clear cell meningioma Clear cell meningiomas are uncommon subtypes that display prominent cytoplasmic vacuolation, often with clear, glycogen rich cytoplasm that stains for PAS. These tumours may be almost exclusively clear cell in nature (Fig. 13.31), with classic features of meningioma, such as whorls and nuclear pseudo-inclusions, being sparse in many cases. For this reason,

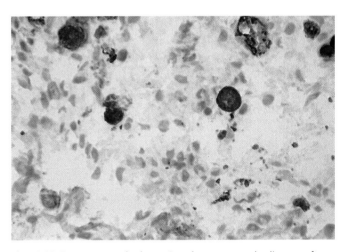

Fig. 13.30 **Secretory meningioma.** Pseudopsammoma bodies are often strongly immunopositive for CEA.

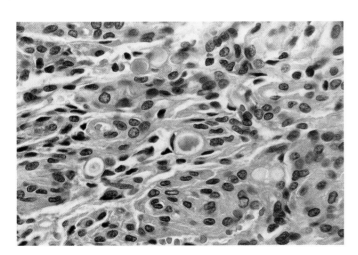

Fig. 13.29 **Secretory meningioma.** Secretory meningiomas have cytological features similar to meningothelial meningiomas, including the characteristic intranuclear inclusions. The diagnostic feature of secretory meningioma are the eosinophilic to lightly amphophilic globules known as pseudopsammoma bodies. H & E.

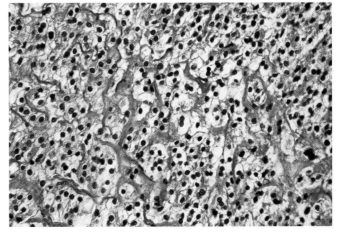

Fig. 13.31 **Clear cell meningioma.** As their name suggests, clear cell meningiomas have cleared out cytoplasm, histologically resembling tumours such as oligodendroglioma and neurocytoma. H & E.

Table 13.1 Histological variants of meningioma associated with recurrence and aggressive behaviour

Atypical meningioma	WHO grade II
Clear cell meningioma	WHO grade II
Chordoid meningioma	WHO grade II
Papillary meningioma	WHO grade III
Rhabdoid meningioma	WHO grade III
Malignant meningioma	WHO grade III
Meningiomas with brain invasion	
Meningiomas with high proliferative indices	

the diagnosis may rest on demonstrating epithelial membrane antigen (EMA) positivity or ultrastructural features of meningiomas, and excluding other clear cell tumours such as metastatic clear cell carcinomas, central neurocytomas or oligodendrogliomas (see below). There is a proclivity for the cerebellopontine angle and the cauda equina, but these tumours may occur supratentorially as well. Some reports have suggested that clear cell meningiomas, particularly intracranial lesions, may be associated with aggressive behaviour.[50] Thus, although these tumours are rare, their correct diagnosis is of great importance, both to exclude other unrelated tumours and to raise the possibility that the tumour may recur. As discussed in the section on atypical meningiomas, the clear cell phenotype is one of the few meningioma patterns that carry prognostic significance (Table 13.1) and warrants closer clinical attention. For this reason, clear cell meningioma is assigned a WHO grade of II of IV.

Chordoid meningioma Chordoid meningiomas contain nodules histologically similar to chordoma, with trabeculae of eosinophilic, vacuolated cells in a myxoid background (Figs 13.32 and 13.33). In most cases, the appearance is only vaguely chordoma-like, but some cases contain microscopic fields that appear nearly indistinguishable from classical chordoma. Fortunately, such chordoid areas are usually interspersed with typical regions of meningioma, facilitating the correct diagnosis. Chronic inflammatory cell infiltrates may be prominent in these tumours (Fig. 13.34), with conspicuous plasma cell infiltrates, and a few of these patients have haematological conditions consistent with Castleman's disease, dysgammaglobulinaemia[35] or hypochromic microcytic anaemia.[35,36] In some instances, the patient may present with the haematological condition. Also curious is the sometime spread of inflammatory infiltrates to involve the adjacent brain, creating an encephalitis-like histological appearance. Chordoid meningiomas have a greater tendency to recur after subtotal resections, and have therefore been designated WHO grade II of IV (Table 13.1).

Lymphoplasmacyte rich meningioma Some meningiomas feature copious chronic inflammatory infiltrates, often relegating the meningothelial component to the background (Fig. 13.35). The infiltrates are often rich in plasma cells, sometimes with numerous Russell bodies. Lymphoplasmacyte rich meningiomas may be more common in young patients. Care must be taken to avoid missing diagnoses of other meningeal-based haematologic conditions,[51] particularly since lymphoplasmacyte rich meningiomas may be associated with haematological abnormalities such as hypergammaglobulinaemia. Because primary meningeal haematologic conditions may elicit arachnoidal hyperplasia, the simple presence of a few meningothelial rests does not exclude a primary haematological proliferative or inflammatory process.

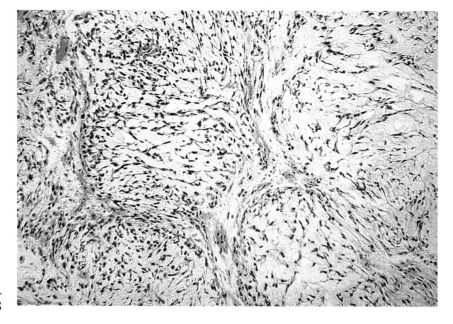

Fig. 13.32 **Chordoid meningioma**. These tumours have regions of typical meningioma along with lobules of less cellular, myxoid tissue resembling chordoma even on low power examination. H & E.

Metaplastic meningioma Mesenchymal differentiation is an uncommon but striking feature in some meningiomas. Meningothelial, fibrous or transitional tumours may display osseous (Figs 13.7 and 13.36), cartilagenous, lipomatous, myxoid or xanthomatous (Fig. 13.37) change. Osseous change may be extensive, creating a rock-like mass. Similarly, cartilagenous differentiation may be appreciated on macroscopic examination; when this rare feature is present, it is often associated with myxoid change. Focal xanthomatous change (Fig. 13.37), with typical meningothelial cells distorting by numerous intracytoplasmic lipid droplets, is common in otherwise typical meningiomas, but is usually not extensive enough to warrant a designation of xanthomatous meningioma.

Foamy histiocytes may also infiltrate meningiomas, creating xanthomatous foci. Such xanthomatous changes are histologically distinct from so-called lipomatous change, in which the cells are distorted by an apparently single large lipid droplet that creates an adipocyte-like appearance. The clinical significance of these changes is not clear, but histological distinctions can be made between these metaplastic variants and some of the above, more common subtypes.

Other histological variants At least three additional variants of meningioma exist: papillary, rhabdoid and oncocytic meningioma. Because papillary and rhabdoid meningiomas are usually associated with aggressive clinical courses, they are discussed below as subtypes of

Fig. 13.33 **Chordoid meningioma.** High power examination. This confirms the chordoid appearance, with trabeculae of more epithelioid cells in a myxoid matrix. H & E.

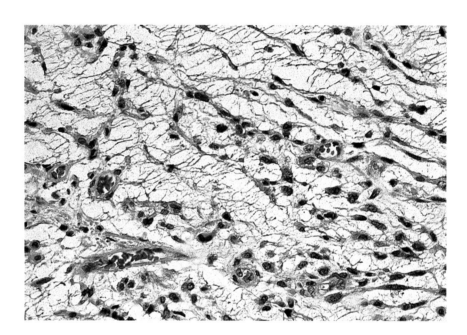

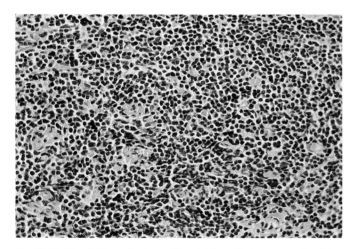

Fig. 13.34 **Chordoid meningioma.** Chordoid meningiomas may be rich in lymphoplasmacytic infiltrates. H & E.

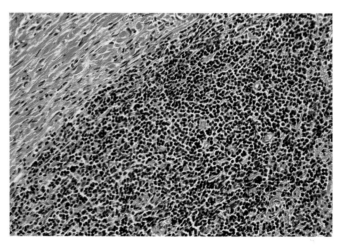

Fig. 13.35 **Lymphoplasmacyte rich meningioma.** Some meningiomas, which have been termed lymphoplasmacyte rich or inflammatory meningiomas, are notable for their dense inflammatory infiltrates. H & E.

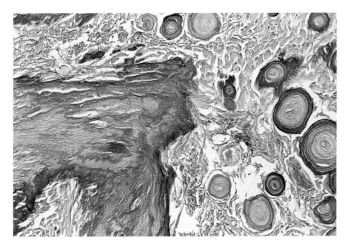

Fig. 13.36 **Osteoblastic meningioma.** Frank bone formation may occur in some meningiomas. This osteoblastic meningioma also has prominent, large psammoma bodies. H & E.

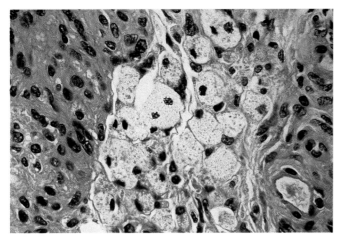

Fig. 13.37 **Meningioma.** Xanthomatous regions may be focal or diffuse within meningiomas. H & E.

atypical and malignant meningioma. Oncocytic meningioma is, as the name suggests, characterised by cells with finely granular cytoplasm that contains numerous mitochondria.[52] Although only one series of six cases has been reported, these tumours may be aggressive, with recurrences and brain invasion being common complications.[52] Further documentation of these rare tumours, however, is necessary before these tumours can be classified as definitely aggressive variants.

Atypical and malignant (anaplastic) meningioma Certain histological features are associated with an increased likelihood of meningioma recurrence and aggressive clinical behaviour. Meningiomas containing such features are designated as atypical meningioma or as malignant (anaplastic) meningioma, depending on the number and extent of the histological changes. From a clinico-pathological point of view, atypical meningiomas have an increased incidence of recurrence and are designated

WHO grade II of IV, while malignant meningiomas have a markedly increased chance of recurrence and may metastasise systemically; for this reason, they receive a WHO grade of III of IV. [Primary sarcomas of the meningiomas (see Chapter 14) are assigned a WHO grade of IV.]

Most authors agree that frequent mitoses, regions of hypercellularity, small cells with high nuclear cytoplasmic ratios and/or prominent nucleoli, patternless or sheet-like growth, necrosis, brain invasion and higher proliferation indices constitute worrisome histological features. Papillary architecture, 'rhabdoid' cytology and clear cell appearance (and perhaps oncocytic cytoplasm) are other histological features that may suggest an aggressive clinical course.

One relatively simple definition does not include brain invasion, considering brain invasion prima facie evidence of aggressive behaviour.[18] These authors define atypical meningioma as any histological variant of meningioma that displays at least one of the following:

1. Maximal mitotic rate greater than 4 per 10 high power fields.
2. Presence of at least three of four of the following morphologic features: sheeting architecture, hypercellularity, macronucleoli, small cell formation.[18]

In a study of malignant meningiomas, nuclear pleomorphism was present in 23 of 23 tumours, disorganised architecture in 22 of 22, necrosis in 20 of 23, prominent nucleoli in 17 of 23, and hypervascularity in 4 of 23, with 1 to 18 (mean 6.1) mitotic figures per 10 high power fields.[53] Another study emphasised lack of typical arrangement (i.e. patternless of sheet-like growth), a large number of mitoses, increased cellularity, focal necrosis, brain infiltration, pleomorphism and anaplasia for the diagnosis of anaplastic (malignant) meningioma.[54] One study regarded meningiomas as atypical or anaplastic (malignant) based on high cellularity, pleomorphism and the presence of mitotic figures; 6 of 34 cases showed only the above features and the remaining 28 also displayed one or more of the following 'ominous' variables: papillary formation, necrosis and invasion of the underlying brain.[55] The presence of atypical mitoses, together with poor cytological differentiation, has also been cited as an important prognostic criterion.[56]

The Helsinki group has proposed a simple and quantitative system for grading meningiomas that has proved predictive of tumour behaviour.[57] Six histological features are evaluated: loss of architecture, increased cellularity, nuclear pleomorphism, mitotic figures, focal necroses and brain infiltration. Except for brain infiltration, the features are each graded as 0 (absent) – 3; brain infiltration is either 0 (absent) or 3 (present). The grading points are simply added to yield benign, grade I tumours with 0–2 points; atypical, grade II tumours with 3–6 points: and anaplastic tumours with 7–11 points. This grading system correlates well with tumour doubling time, but has not gained widespread acceptance for routine grading.[18]

Thus, there are varying concepts as to which histological criteria are sufficient for diagnosing higher grade meningiomas and for accurately predicting recurrence. Furthermore, it has been difficult to quantify such features into a histological grading system that has acquired universal acceptance. Given that precise and universally accepted definitions are lacking, 'atypical meningioma' is usually diagnosed when several of the above features are present (see WHO definition below), whereas the diagnosis of 'anaplastic (malignant) meningioma' is restricted to tumours with frank anaplasia, very high mitotic activity and/or metastasis (see WHO definition below). Papillary architecture and rhabdoid cytological features necessitate diagnoses of papillary and rhabdoid meningioma, respectively, and these may be clinically aggressive as well. Because the evaluation of these histological features is of considerable importance in establishing the likelihood of recurrence and hence subsequent treatment, each meningioma requires considerable histological attention. We recommend submitting sufficient blocks for histological examination to provide representative sampling; for many laboratories, this results in approximately one block for every centimetre of tumour width. As mentioned below, special attention should be paid to submitting any attached cerebral parenchyma included in the resection specimen.

Atypical meningioma Atypical meningioma is a relatively recent diagnostic entity, which arose from the recognition that certain histological features, while not connoting overtly malignant behaviour in a meningioma, did indicate an increased incidence of local recurrence. For the patient with an atypical meningioma, this necessitates either closer postsurgical follow-up or adjuvant therapy, with the approach depending on the extent of resection and varying between clinical centres. As mentioned above, atypical meningiomas are not uncommon, constituting between 4.7 and 7.2% of meningiomas, depending on the criteria used for diagnosis.

Atypical meningioma was defined by the 1993 WHO as a meningioma 'in which several of the following features are evident: frequent mitoses, increased cellularity, small cells with high nuclear cytoplasmic ratios and/or prominent nucleoli, uninterrupted patternless or sheet-like growth and foci of "spontaneous" or geographic necrosis'. (Figs 13.38–13.42)[42] This description considers all relevant features but remains subjective.

Atypical meningiomas may occur in the background of almost any histological subtype of meningioma. By far, most of these tumours have a meningothelial appearance, although often with loss of the lobular and whorled architectural patterns. Certain variants, such as angiomatous meningioma, only rarely display any features of atypical meningioma, with the exception of nuclear pleomorphism. Other unique variants, such as secretory meningioma, can have atypical features. For this reason, every meningioma should be carefully scrutinised for features of atypical meningioma. Although not all clear cell and chordoid meningiomas act in an aggressive manner, a substantial fraction of these tumours recur. Similarly, papillary and rhabdoid meningiomas (see below) more often follow an aggressive clinical course. Therefore, these tumours, while not 'atypical meningiomas' by strict definition, may occupy a similar biological niche.

We consider atypical meningiomas as meningiomas that contain at least some of the following histological features: frequent mitoses (greater than 4 or 5 per 10 high

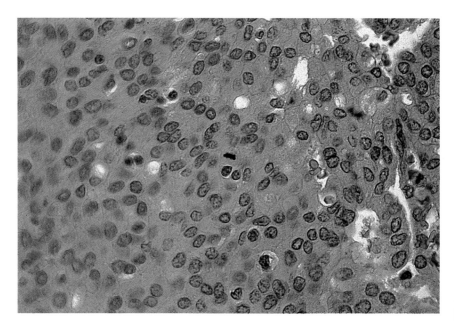

Fig. 13.38 **Atypical meningioma.** This tumour may look cytologically similar to benign meningiomas, but demonstrates loss of the normal architectural pattern ('sheeting') and mitotic activity. H & E.

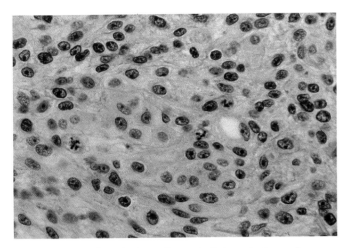

Fig. 13.39 **Atypical meningioma.** Some atypical meningiomas show brisk mitotic activity and prominent nucleoli. Well-demarcated cellular borders are also common in atypical meningiomas. H & E.

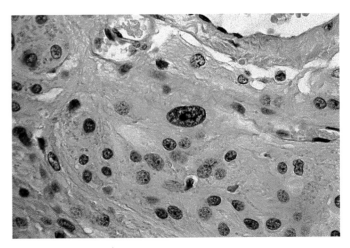

Fig. 13.40 **Atypical meningioma.** Nuclear pleomorphism may occur in atypical meningiomas, but may be noted in benign meningiomas as well. H & E.

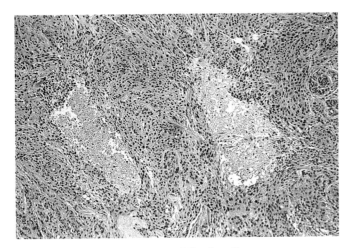

Fig. 13.41 **Atypical meningioma.** Multifocal small necroses are common in atypical meningiomas. H & E.

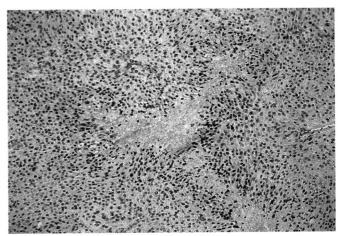

Fig. 13.42 **Atypical meningioma.** Necrotic regions in atypical meningiomas may appear similar to the perinecrotic pseudopalisading that is seen in glioblastomas. H & E.

power fields) (Fig. 13.39), regions of hypercellularity, small cells with high nuclear : cytoplasmic ratios, prominent nucleoli (Fig. 13.39), pleomorphic nuclei (Fig. 13.40), patternless or sheet-like growth (Fig. 13.38) and/or necrosis (Figs 13.41 and 13.42). With few exceptions, such as mitotic activity in excess of 4 or 5 mitoses per 10 high power fields, the presence of any one of these features is probably not sufficient for a diagnosis of atypical meningioma. For these reasons, the 2000 WHO definition of atypical meningioma is a meningioma having either:

1. 4 or greater mitoses per 10 high power fields; or
2. three or more of the following histological features: increased cellularity, small cells with high nucleus: cytoplasm ratios, prominent nucleoli, uninterrupted patternless or sheet-like growth, and foci of necrosis.[4]

Because of the importance attached to evaluating these histological features, they are discussed individually below.

Mitotic activity/proliferation indices Benign meningiomas may contain scattered mitotic figures, although not usually atypical mitotic figures. Such scattered mitotic activity, however, is not necessarily a worrisome histological feature. But when proliferative activity increases substantially, there is an increased likelihood of recurrence; in this instance, regardless of whether other features of atypical meningioma are present, a diagnosis of atypical meningioma may be rendered. Some definitions of atypical meningioma have in fact offered exact mitotic count criteria: for instance, atypical meningiomas as tumours with increased cellularity and at least four[18] or five[12] or six[58] mitotic figures in 10 high power fields. The major question is what number of mitoses is sufficient for the diagnosis of atypical meningioma. One reasonable estimate is a value of greater than 5 mitoses per 10 high power fields, i.e. that mitotic index of 5 or greater may be a critical criterion for predicting shorter disease-free interval.[12,18,58] Certainly, mitotic activity in this range should raise considerable concern of recurrence.

Because of the perceived vagaries of mitotic counts, there have been a number of attempts to correlate immunohistochemical proliferation indices with the likelihood of recurrence (see below). These have primarily involved using Ki-67/MIB-1 and anti-PCNA (proliferating cell nuclear antigen) antibodies. Since methodological differences prevent applying published values to other laboratories, the establishment of consistent cut-off values has failed to date. Nonetheless, elevated proliferation rates, perhaps those greater than approximately 5% in some laboratories, are generally associated with greater likelihood of recurrence. Such tumours could therefore be equated with atypical meningiomas, particularly for clinical purposes, although current definitions of atypical meningioma[4] do not take immunohistochemical proliferation indices into account.

Necrosis There are three general patterns of necrosis seen in meningiomas. Necrosis may occur in large, geographic regions, appearing ischaemic or infarctive in nature. Alternatively, necrosis may occur as multifocal, small regions of cell death, often with nuclear debris, in the centre of tumour lobules. Finally, single cell death may be noted in some meningiomas. In our opinion, while all three types of necrosis may be seen in atypical meningiomas, and are only occasionally noted in benign meningioma, only the multifocal, 'centrilobular' form of necrosis is highly characteristic of atypical meningioma. As opposed to the larger, infarctive necrosis, such centrilobular necrosis most likely reflects local outgrowth of tumour nutrient supply, that is, high tumour cell metabolic demand reflecting the presence of more active tumour cells. Indeed, tumours with necrosis have generally higher mitotic activity.[18] In some cases, these multifocal necroses may occur within hypercellular regions, creating a low power microscopic impression similar to the pseudopalisading of tumour cells around necrosis seen in glioblastomas. Such perinecrotic pseudopalisading may itself be predictive of recurrence.[18] In such situations, particular care must be taken on frozen section diagnosis to avoid misinterpretation of an atypical meningioma as a glioblastoma.

An important caveat in the assessment of necrosis in meningiomas is whether the tumour has been therapeutically embolised prior to resection.[59] Preoperative embolisation can obviously lead to tumour necrosis. Usually, this is of the large, geographic, infarctive type; nonetheless, we have seen cases in which otherwise benign-appearing meningiomas have characteristic 'centrilobular'-type necrosis following embolisation and we have interpreted this as secondary to embolisation. Postembolic necrosis may be associated with localised increases in labelling indices for proliferation markers.[60]

Lack of architectural pattern Most meningiomas have a conspicuous architectural pattern, whether it be lobular in meningothelial tumours, fascicular in fibrous tumours, and whorling in transitional and other forms. One of the most helpful features to prompt consideration of atypical meningioma is the 'lack' of such architectural patterns. Since most atypical meningiomas arise in the absence of a prior benign meningioma, and since there is no direct evidence that atypical meningiomas ever displayed any of these architectural features to begin with, such tumours probably 'lack' such features and have not actually 'lost' the architectural pattern.

The absence of these architectural patterns has been referred to as 'sheeting', since the tumour cells form large sheets of tumour cells, devoid of whorls or fascicles. One must be careful to avoid diagnosing large lobules in some meningothelial tumours as sheeting, since such lobules may achieve relatively large sizes. One helpful feature in assessing sheeting is evaluation of cytoplasmic borders. As mentioned above, meningothelial meningiomas have also been dubbed syncytial meningiomas because the extensive interdigitations of their cytoplasmic borders make the borders indistinguishable at light microscopic examination, creating the impression of a syncytium. Atypical meningiomas, perhaps because their cells are less 'differentiated', contain less extensive cellular interdigitations, resulting in distinctly visible cell borders on microscopic examination. The presence of such crisp borders suggests that such sheeting is real, and buttresses a diagnosis of atypical meningioma if other features are also present.

Regions of hypercellularity/high nuclear : cytoplasmic ratio Regions of hypercellularity and cells with high nuclear : cytoplasmic ratio often accompany one another in atypical meningiomas. Usually, one finds irregular, small islands of dense cellularity in which the cells have more hyperchromatic nuclei and relatively inconspicuous cytoplasm; some authors have termed this phenomenon 'small cell formation'.[18] Usually, such islands are not solitary in atypical meningiomas and are often punctuated by mitoses. While occasional hypercellular islands may be seen in benign meningiomas, these features usually indicate atypical meningioma. Similarly, the presence of many such hypercellular regions should prompt careful search for frankly anaplastic features.

Pleomorphism Nuclear pleomorphism is not, in and of itself, diagnostic of atypical meningioma. This is important since a considerable number of benign meningiomas display nuclear pleomorphism. Such nuclear variability ranges from minor differences in nuclear shape to marked changes in nuclear size and shape. In general, atypical meningiomas are accompanied by only modest nuclear pleomorphism, and large, bizarre cells are not characteristic. In certain variants, such as microcystic and angiomatous meningiomas, nuclear pleomorphism is a common histological feature, and in other benign meningiomas, large regions of pleomorphic cells may be noted, including bizarre, giant cells. Such features, while not necessarily indicative of atypical meningioma, should prompt further evaluation of the tumour for other features of atypical meningioma.

Prominent nucleoli Like pleomorphism, prominent nucleoli are not sufficient for a diagnosis of atypical meningioma. Usually, prominent nucleoli are accompanied by generalised nuclear pleomorphism. Nonetheless, the presence of prominent nucleoli should warrant a careful search for other features of atypical meningioma and many atypical meningiomas contain foci of cells with prominent nucleoli.

In some instances, in which some of these features are present, yet in insufficient quantities to warrant a diagnosis of atypical meningioma, we use the term 'meningioma with atypical features', describing the atypical features in a note. Such a descriptive diagnosis recognises the ill-defined border between benign and atypical meningioma, and conveys the need for somewhat closer postsurgical follow-up. Only long term follow-up of such cases will determine whether such intermediate cases conform to benign or to atypical meningioma, or occupy a true intermediate position.

Malignant (anaplastic) meningioma Malignant meningiomas are uncommon tumours, but important to distinguish from benign and atypical meningiomas because of their markedly more aggressive behaviour. While lower-grade meningiomas are often treated conservatively after complete surgical removal, sometimes with close follow-up alone, malignant meningiomas are usually treated with some form of ancillary therapy, commonly radiation therapy.

The criteria for the diagnosis of anaplastic (malignant) meningioma remained subjective until recently, with the 1993 WHO defining anaplastic meningioma as 'a meningioma exhibiting histological features of frank malignancy far in excess of the abnormalities noted in atypical meningioma. These include obviously malignant cytology, a high mitotic index and conspicuous necrosis'.[42] Furthermore, while some consider invasion of brain a hallmark of anaplastic meningioma,[61] the 1993 WHO did not necessarily endorse brain invasion as being diagnostic of malignancy,[42] and the 2000 WHO separates the issue of brain invasion from that of malignancy.[4]

The diagnosis of malignant meningioma hinges on three major criteria: frank histological anaplasia (Fig. 13.43), marked mitotic activity, and the presence of metastases (Fig. 13.44). Although brain invasion (Fig. 13.45) may be noted in malignant meningiomas, it is not required for diagnosis.

Since mitoses, lack of architectural pattern ('sheeting'), necrosis and nuclear atypia may accompany atypical meningiomas, the histological anaplasia of malignant

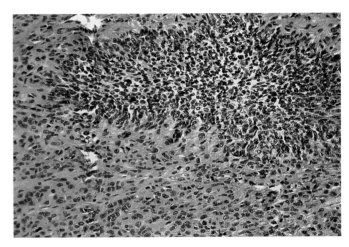

Fig. 13.43 **Malignant meningioma**. These tumours contain areas of frankly malignant neoplasia, as in this small cell anaplastic region in an otherwise classical meningioma. H & E.

meningioma must clearly exceed that of atypical meningioma. In most cases, this manifests as regions of mitotically-active spindle cells, with moderately large, hyperchromatic nuclei, in a coarsely fascicular pattern, an appearance similar to soft tissue spindle cell sarcomas seen in other parts of the body. In such a situation, while the malignant nature of the tumour is evident, its meningothelial histogenesis may be less evident. The focal presence of definite meningioma or, for recurrent tumours, the previous presence of a definite meningioma, is necessary to distinguish these tumours from primary sarcomas arising in the meninges (see Chapter 14). For most authors, the presence of such nigh-sarcomatous areas alongside more typical meningioma would be sufficient for a diagnosis of malignant meningioma. The 2000 WHO[4] defines malignant meningioma as having either:

1. 20 or greater mitoses per 10 high power fields; or
2. obviously malignant cytology (e.g. having an appearance similar to sarcoma, carcinoma or melanoma).

Metastasis and brain invasion in meningiomas

Metastasis The presence of metastatic systemic deposits from an intracranial meningioma is, in most cases, also sufficient for a diagnosis of malignant meningioma. Indeed, distant metastasis is the most feared complication of malignant meningioma. The most common sites for metastasis include the lung, pleura, liver, and bone, with multiple sites of metastasis common once spread has occurred. A number of caveats, however, must be raised in the assessment of meningioma metastasis.

One, rare reports have suggested that so-called 'benign metastasising meningioma' may exist as a distinct entity.[62] In this situation, a primary intracranial meningioma with benign histological features may be accompanied by isolated, histologically benign metastasis in the lung or

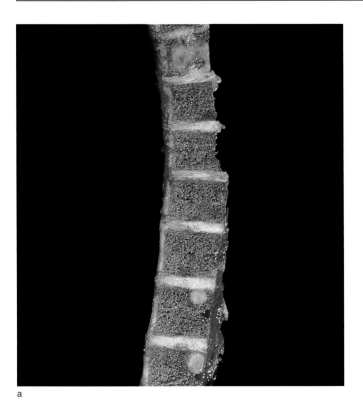

a

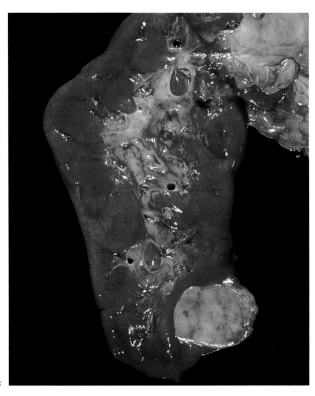

c

Fig. 13.44 **Metastatic meningioma.** Metastasis in malignant meningioma may affect organs such as the bone (a), liver (b) and kidney (c).

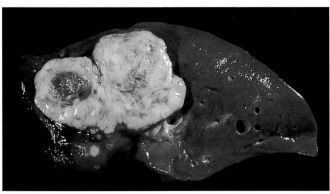

b

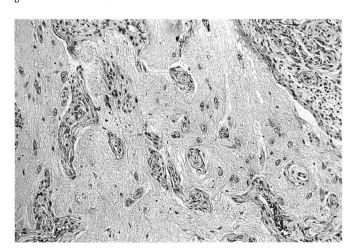

Fig. 13.45 **Meningioma: brain invasion.** Frank brain invasion often denotes a malignant meningioma, but may be observed in cytologically benign lesions as well. H & E.

liver; the removal of both may lead to a therapeutic cure, without further recurrences. Nonetheless, some tumours have subsequently pursued an aggressive course, either from the original tumour or the metastasis, and so the nosological position of this entity remains suspect.

Two, local sites do not qualify as sites of metastasis. For instance, extension of meningiomas into the overlying skull or through the skull to involve cranial soft tissues does not necessarily imply that the tumour will act in a malignant fashion. Indeed, resection of the overlying skull and soft tissue may effect a therapeutic cure. Similarly, invasion of the adjacent dural sinuses does not constitute evidence for malignancy or imply that the tumour will spread systemically. It is likely, however, that the more extensive the original tumour and the more infiltrative of adjacent vital structures, the more difficult a complete resection and the more likely subsequent local recurrences.

Three, meningiomas may occasionally arise primarily in extracranial sites and such rare instances should not be mistaken for metastatic disease. Favoured sites for extracranial primary meningiomas include the skin and the lung, but tumours have also been noted in the nasal cavity, paranasal sinuses, oral cavity, parotid gland, ear, soft tissue of the neck, mediastinum and peripheral nerves, in the absence of intracranial disease. These are typically meningothelial meningiomas with a benign appearance and can be cured by local excision.

Brain invasion Most meningiomas indent the brain and respect the pial barrier, allowing the neurosurgeon to dissect the tumour free of the underlying cerebral parenchyma. Nonetheless, some meningiomas adhere to the underlying brain and the neurosurgeon must remove superficial cerebral cortex along with the tumour. In all instances in which brain tissue is removed, a careful inspection of the attached brain is warranted. Approximately one-quarter of specimens that include brain parenchyma have brain invasion on microscopic examination.[18] On macroscopic examination of meningioma resection specimens, therefore, special attention should be paid to sampling any tissues that resemble cerebrum. And, on microscopic examination, close scrutiny should be applied to the interface between tumour and cerebrum.

Two general patterns of invasion may be encountered. The first is characterised by broad nodules of tumour superficially involving the Virchow–Robin spaces but with only mild gliosis of the adjacent parenchyma. Most authors do not consider this pattern of local involvement of Virchow–Robin spaces to be true invasion. The involvement is worth comment in histopathology reports, as it provides explanation for the tumour attachment to the brain as well as indication to the clinician that closer follow-up may be warranted if the excision was limited by the superficial brain involvement. Nonetheless, such localised Virchow–Robin space involvement does not necessarily imply that the tumour will act in a malignant fashion.

The second pattern is more worrisome and hence typical of aggressive, often malignant meningiomas. This pattern is characterised by invasion of the cortical parenchyma by single cells or small groups of tumour cells. Often such frank invasion is accompanied by marked gliosis of the parenchyma. In some resection specimens, the margin between the normal brain and tumour may not be oriented or well defined; in such samples, brain is seen as islands of gliotic neuropil entrapped among solid tumour. We interpret such a pattern as true parenchymal invasion, as it seems unlikely that such intimate admixture is a result of only superficial Virchow–Robin space involvement.

The role of true brain invasion still remains controversial. In the presence of a histologically anaplastic meningioma, true brain invasion simply confirms the diagnosis of malignant meningioma. In the presence of an atypical meningioma, the situation is less clear; some authors would favour a diagnosis of malignant meningioma in this situation, while others prefer 'atypical meningioma with brain invasion'. Certainly, such a situation necessitates further treatment, with most clinicians advocating adjuvant therapy for a tumor with both atypical features and brain invasion. When assessable, brain invasion is clearly a powerful predictor of recurrence.[18] In fact, when brain invasion is present, the presence of other adverse histological features does not appreciably affect recurrence-free survival times.[18]

Certain benign-appearing meningiomas may also invade the brain. Usually, such invasion is not true invasion, but occasionally true invasion may be present. True invasion does not necessarily imply a malignant course, but suggests that the tumour has a greater likelihood of recurrence (Table 13.1). Curiously, while histologically anaplastic meningiomas that invade the brain often display allelic loss of chromosome 10, a genetic feature of malignancy, invasive histologically benign tumours do not have this genetic feature, suggesting a basic biological difference between these entities.[63] From a clinical point of view, the presence of brain invasion in benign-appearing lesions should certainly warrant at least careful follow-up. Finally, the unusual lesion of meningioangiomatosis (see below) should not be confused with brain invasion.

A few histological variants of meningioma have been associated with more frequent recurrence and/or more aggressive behaviour. As discussed above, clear cell and chordoid meningiomas may have a high incidence of recurrence and may display aggressive behaviour. However, such behaviour does not consistently accompany clear cell cytology or chordoid patterns. Two histological variants, papillary and rhabdoid meningiomas, are associated with even greater likelihood of recurrence and aggressive behaviour. For these reasons, they are discussed as subtypes of malignant meningioma. Finally, the literature of the past few decades is strewn with reports of an aggressive variant of meningioma, known as 'angioblastic meningioma' and more specifically as the 'haemangiopercytic variant of angioblastic meningioma'. Because this entity is clinically, pathologically and genetically distinct from meningioma, it is now considered a primary haemangiopericytoma of the meninges.

Variants of malignant meningioma

Papillary meningioma Papillary meningioma is a meningioma defined by the presence of a perivascular papillary pattern in at least some part of the tumour (Fig. 13.46).[64] In most cases, the tumour has typical meningothelial features in some areas. The papillary configurations appear artefactual in many cases, as a result of tumour cells clinging to the blood vessels in an otherwise fractured specimen. The tumour cells may send broad processes down to the vessels walls, vaguely simulating perivascular pseudorosettes, and the vessels may be thick walled and hyalinised. In most cases, there are histological features such as mitotic activity that support the notion that such tumours may act in an aggressive manner. Local and brain invasion has been noted in 75%, recurrence in 55% and metastasis in 20% of papillary meningioma.[65] Because of their aggressive clinical behaviour, these tumours have been graded as WHO grade III. Papillary meningiomas tend to occur in

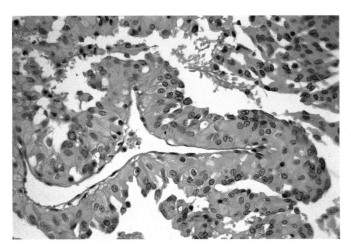

Fig. 13.46 **Papillary meningioma.** Papillary meningioma comprises at least focal accumulations of elongated tumour cells surrounding central vascular cores. H & E.

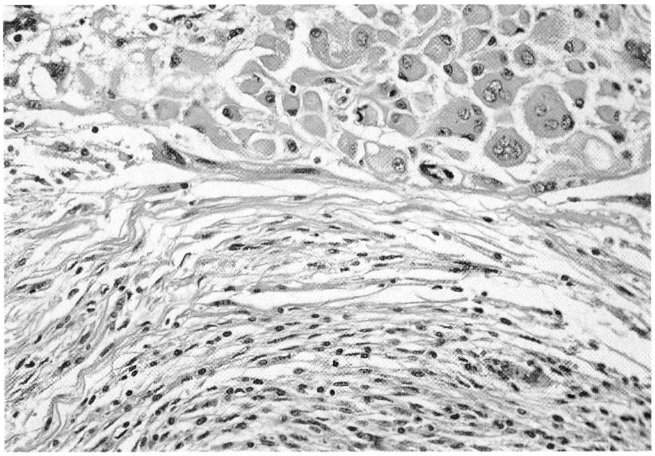

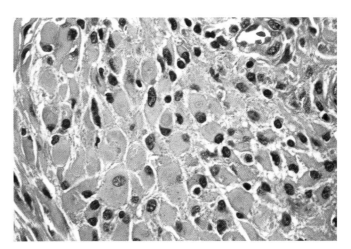

Fig. 13.47 **Rhabdoid meningioma.** Rhabdoid changes, as evidenced by the cluster of larger, epithelioid cells, may be focal within meningiomas. H & E.

children, with as many as 50% of such cases in children.[21] The curious histological appearance raises many other tumours in the differential diagnosis, including epithelial lesions such as metastatic carcinoma.

Rhabdoid meningioma Rhabdoid meningioma is a recently described variant of meningioma that is associated in most cases with aggressive clinical behaviour, in the form of numerous recurrences and sometimes metastasis.[66,67] Rhabdoid features may be focal (Fig. 13.47), with the background meningioma being otherwise typical, but rhabdoid regions may increase with subsequent recurrences; in some cases, rhabdoid features may only be apparent in recurrent tumours. Indeed, rhabdoid histology may be a hallmark of malignant progression in meningiomas.[67] Rhabdoid regions are characterised by loosely cohesive cells that have eccentric nuclei, sometimes with prominent nucleoli, and cytoplasm containing globular hyaline material (Figs 13.48 and 13.49). The eccentric hyaline inclusions consist of whorls of intermediate filaments and entrapped organelles on ultrastructural examination. Immunohistochemical features of these tumours include the standard EMA (Fig. 13.50) and vimentin (Fig. 13.49) positivity, but occasional focal cytokeratin, S-100 or actin immunoreactivity.[67] Once rhabdoid features are present, mitotic figures and high Ki-67/MIB-1 labelling are evident. Most of these tumours also have features of malignant meningioma, either overt anaplasia, brain invasion or systemic metastasis, and therefore receive a WHO grade of III. The behaviour of rhabdoid meningiomas without clear histological features of malignancy remains to be determined.[67]

'Haemangiopericytic variant of angioblastic meningioma' It is important to emphasise that those tumours historically known as the haemangiopericytic variant of angioblastic meningioma are no longer considered true meningiomas, but are classified as dural haemangio-

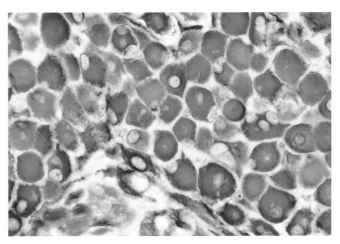

Fig. 13.48 **Rhabdoid meningioma.** Rhabdoid cells within meningiomas resemble rhabdoid cells in other human tumours, with eccentric nuclei, prominent nucleoli and globular eosinophilc cytoplasm. H & E.

Fig. 13.49 **Rhabdoid meningioma.** The rhabdoid appearance is emphasised by immunostaining for vimentin.

pericytomas. This reclassification, while wholly justified on clinical and biological grounds, does confuse review of the literature on aggressive meningiomas. These tumours are discussed in Chapter 14. Furthermore, rare tumours have reportedly shown features of both haemangiopericytoma and meningioma; the nosological position of these unusual lesions remains unclear.

Immunohistochemistry

The diagnosis of meningioma is usually readily made on standard light microscopic examination of haematoxylin and eosin-stained slides. Some meningiomas may not have classical light microscopic features, necessitating immunohistochemical assessment (Table 13.2). The most useful overall immunohistochemical marker of meningioma is EMA-positivity.[68] When present in a membranous pattern, the positivity is clear and helpful in establishing the diagnosis (Fig. 13.51). Diffuse or focal,

usually light cytoplasmic staining is less definitive for positivity, but is nonetheless common in meningiomas. Benign meningiomas usually stain for EMA, but EMA immunoreactivity is less consistent in atypical and malignant lesions. This is unfortunate, since the malignant lesions often pose the greatest differential diagnostic challenge. EMA staining is helpful in distinguishing meningioma from other brain tumours such as gliomas and Schwannomas, but not in the differential diagnosis with carcinoma, which, again, may be a major differential diagnostic entity in the assessment of dural-based malignant lesions. EMA staining is also helpful in distinguishing haemangiopericytoma from meningioma, since haemangiopericytomas are EMA-negative.

Vimentin positivity is found in all meningiomas, and is often strong (Fig. 13.49), but is of no great utility in terms of differential diagnosis. Immunopositivity for desmosome-related proteins, such as the desmoplakins, is also common in meningiomas, but is not often used in evaluating these

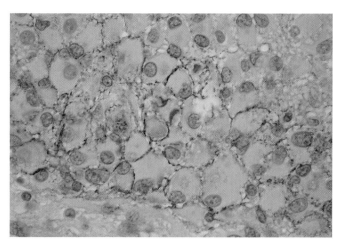

Fig. 13.50 **Rhabdoid meningioma.** Delicate membranous immunostaining for EMA. This may be present even in the rhabdoid cells of rhabdoid meningioma.

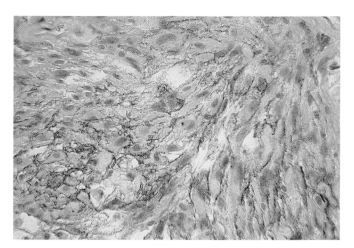

Fig. 13.51 **Meningioma.** EMA immunopositivity is typical of meningiomas. This may be helpful in establishing the diagnosis. EMA immunopositivity may follow the characteristic membranous appearance or have a more diffuse cytoplasmic quality.

Table 13.2 Immunohistochemistry in the differential diagnosis of meningiomas

Meningioma	EMA	CK	S-100	GFAP	CEA	CD34	Vimentin
All	+	–	+/–	–	–	–	+
Secretory	+	+	–	–	+	–	+
Metastasis							
Carcinoma	+	+	–	–	+/–	–	+
Sarcoma	specific lines of differentiation						+
Melanoma	–	–	+	–	–		+
Malignant glioma	–	–	+	+	–	–	+
Schwannoma	–	–	+	+/–	–	–	+
HPC	–	–	–	–	–	+/–	+
SFT	–	–	–	–	–	+	+

Abbreviations: CK = cytokeratin; HPC = haemangiopericytoma; SFT = solitary fibrous tumour; +/– = focal staining possible

tumours. Studies of S-100 protein have found varying positivity in meningiomas, but S-100 staining is not usually prominent. This may be useful in distinguishing meningioma from Schwannoma since Schwannomas are typically strongly positive for S-100 protein. Secretory meningiomas characteristically show strong positive staining for CEA in the pseudopsammoma bodies (Fig. 13.30) and for cytokeratins in the cells surrounding the pseudopsammoma bodies. None of the other meningioma subtypes, however, show conspicuous staining for these markers. Rare tumours with meningothelial features have been reported as staining for glial fibrillary acidic protein (GFAP),[69] but it has been unclear whether these represent true meningiomas or not.[70]

Immunohistochemistry has also been used to characterise some biological aspects of meningiomas. For instance, the extracellular matrix has been studied, showing the presence of type I, III, IV, V, VI, fibronectin and laminin.[71,72] Type I, III, IV and V collagens and laminin are found in the perilobular septae of meningothelial tumours, but among the tumour cells in fibrous lesions.[71] Various adhesion molecules are differentially expressed in meningiomas. Neural cell-adhesion molecule (NCAM) is widely expressed in meningiomas, most prominently in fibroblastic lesions.[73] CD44 and E-cadherin are also commonly expressed, both somewhat more in meningothelial and transitional tumours.[73,74] In malignant meningiomas, polysialylated NCAM expression occurs[73] and E-cadherin expression may be lost.[75] Integrin subunits are also commonly found in meningiomas, including various α subunits with 2 and alpha 6 expressed particularly in malignant meningiomas.[74]

Specific growth factors and their receptors are expressed in many meningiomas, including platelet derived growth factor (PDGF) ligands and receptors, epidermal growth factor and insulin-like growth factors.[76–78] Angiogenic factors and their receptors have also been demonstrated in meningiomas. For example, meningiomas that are densely vascular and those that elicit considerable peritumoral oedema produce both vascular endothelial growth factor/vascular permeability factor (VEGF/VPF) as well as VEGF/VPF receptors.[34,74] Endothelin-1 and endothelin receptors (ET-Ar and ET-Br) are also expressed in many meningiomas.[80]

Electron microscopy

Classical meningiomas have characteristic ultrastructural features that recall those of normal arachnoidal cap cells. Nuclear features largely recapitulate those seen at light microscopy, with euchromatin, cytoplasmic pseudo-inclusions and regions free of chromatin giving a 'washed-out' appearance. The cytoplasm is non-descript, with the exception of copious intermediate filaments, which correspond to the vimentin noted immunohistochemically.

These vimentin intermediate filaments end at desmosomal junctions, which may be numerous. Indeed, hemidesmosomes and desmosomes are highly characteristic of meningiomas, and their presence useful in the differential diagnosis with other central nervous system tumours. Also present are gap junctions. Most notable, however, particularly in meningothelial and transitional tumours, are the complex interdigitating cell processes. The interdigitations, not visible at the light microscopic level, producing the 'syncytial' appearance of many meningiomas.

At the ultrastructural level, cellular whorls consist of concentrically arranged cells surrounding calcified foci, collagen and reticulin fibres, and hydroxyapatite crystals. It is likely that centrally degenerating cells within whorls serve as nidi for mineralisation. Matrix vesicles produced by the adjacent meningothelial cells may provide a focus for calcification, with hydroxyapatite precipitating on collagen and reticulin.[81] Recent data suggest that expression of the calcium-binding phosphoprotein osteopontin may play a role in psammoma body development.[82]

Secretory meningiomas have ultrastructural features of extensive epithelial differentiation. These tumours form mature epithelial lumina, with tight junctions and villi, containing secreted, amorphous intraluminal products. On the other hand, fibrous meningiomas may display considerable amounts of extracellular type I collagen, including giant amianthoid collagen fibres.[43,44] Immunohistochemical studies have also shown collagen types III, IV and V, and laminin, with type IV collagen and laminin closely related to basement membrane material.[71] In microcystic meningiomas, the extracellular material is amorphous, presumably secreted by the tumours cells, which have many pinocytotic vesicles and complex Golgi apparatus. Cell processes in microcystic tumours are distorted by the extracellular material and are joined to one another by residual desmosomal junctions.

Because most meningiomas do not require ultrastructural examination for diagnosis, it is usually the less-differentiated tumours that come to electron microscopic evaluation. In these cases, the typical features are usually not overt. In general, it is the presence of desmosomes, hemidesmosomes and complex interdigitating cell processes that is most helpful in the ultrastructural confirmation of meningioma.

Proliferation indices

As expected, cellular proliferation increases with increasing degree of malignancy, from benign to atypical to malignant meningioma. This increase in proliferation is reflected in differences in mean doubling time, mitotic counts and immunohistochemical proliferation indices, as summarised below.

The mean doubling time for meningioma volume has been calculated as 415 days (range 138–1045) in benign, 178 days (34–551) in atypical, and 205 days (30–472) in anaplastic (malignant) meningioma, with the difference between benign and atypical/anaplastic being highly significant. Both mitotic index and the absence of calcification on computerised tomography scan correlate strongly with doubling time.[57] Tumour doubling times, estimated by serial computerised tomography scans, ranged in eight meningiomas from 8 to 440 days and showed a close inverse correlation with the 5-bromo-2′-deoxyuridine (BUdR) indices.[83]

Significant differences exist between tumour grades for mitotic indices (total counts per 10 high power fields) (0.08 ± 0.05 for benign, 4.75 ± 0.91 for atypical, and 19.00 ± 4.07 for malignant) and multivariate regression analysis has indicated that mitotic index greater than 6 may be a critical criterion for predicting shorter disease-free interval.[58]

BUdR indices are generally low in benign meningiomas. In one study of 178 meningiomas, 53 had BUdR indices greater than or equal to 1%; of these 53 tumours, 21 were diagnosed histopathologically as malignant meningioma. The mean BUdR index of recurrent tumours was significantly higher than that of the non-recurrent tumours (3.9% ± 2.6 versus 1.9% ± 1.0). Furthermore, the recurrence rate was 100% for tumours with labelling indices greater than or equal to 5%, 55.6% for those with labelling indices of 3–5%, and 30.6% for those with indices of 1–3%; the percentages of malignant meningiomas in these groups were 88%, 78%, and 19%, respectively.[84]

MIB-1/Ki-67 indices also show a highly significant increase from benign (mean 3.8% ± 3.09) to atypical (mean 7.17% ± 5.78) to anaplastic meningioma (mean 14.71% ± 9.76)[85] (Fig. 13.52). MIB-1 indices, however, may vary considerably among anaplastic meningiomas (from 1.3 to 24.2%; mean = 11.7%).[53] One study found that Ki-67 proliferation index was the most important criterion for distinguishing anaplastic meningioma (mean = 11%) from atypical meningioma (mean = 2.1%) and classical type (mean Ki-67 index: 0.7%).[86] One study has suggested that proliferation indices tend to be higher in meningiomas from male patients.[87] Another study has shown that proliferation indices are generally higher in meningiomas from NF2 patients.[46]

Flow cytometric studies have demonstrated approximately equal numbers of diploid and aneuploid meningiomas. Some reports have shown significant correlations between aneuploid tumours and features such as recurrence, pleomorphism, high cellular density, mitotic activity and brain and soft tissue infiltration.[88] From a practical point of view, however, flow cytometry has not to date had a major impact in the assessment of meningiomas.

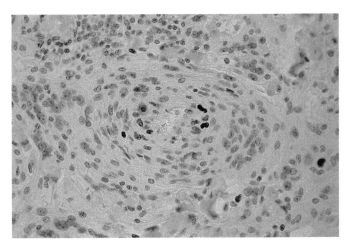

Fig. 13.52 **Meningioma.** Ki-67/MIB-1 labelling may vary within meningiomas. Some regions of this atypical meningioma demonstrate higher indices.

Table 13.3 Genetic alterations associated with meningioma

Benign
NF2 gene mutations and chromosome 22q loss
Chromosome 1p and 3p loss*
Chromosome Y loss (in males)
PTCH gene (chromosome 9q) mutations*

Atypical/malignant
Chromosome 1p loss
Chromosome 10 loss (morphologically malignant)
Chromosome 14q loss
TP53 mutations (rare) and chromosome 17p loss
CDKN2A/p16 gene (chromosome 9p) deletions (rare)
Chromosomes 6q, 9q and 18q loss*
Chromosome 17q23 amplification*
Chromosomes 1q, 9q, 12q, 15q, 17q and 20q gains*
(Loss of E-cadherin expression)

*Recent findings requiring confirmation

Molecular biology

Meningiomas were among the first solid tumours recognised to have cytogenetic alterations (Table 13.3).[89] Although a variety of cytogenetic changes have been noted in benign meningiomas, the most consistent change is deletion of chromosome 22.[90] Loss of chromosome 22 also occurs in recurrent and atypical meningiomas.[91] Molecular genetic findings have mirrored the above cytogenetic alterations, with polymorphic DNA markers demonstrating that approximately half of meningiomas exhibit allelic losses that involve band q12 on chromosome 22.[92–96] The NF2 gene, residing in this region on chromosome 22q (see Chapter 19), has now clearly been implicated as a tumour suppressor gene involved in sporadic and NF2-associated meningioma tumorigenesis.

Mutations in the NF2 gene are detected in up to 60% of the sporadic meningiomas.[97–100] The majority of the mutations are small insertions or deletions or nonsense mutations that affect splice sites, create stop codons or result in frameshifts. Mutations occur predominantly in the most 5′ two-thirds of the gene.[6] The predicted common effect of these mutations is a truncated, and presumably non-functional, merlin (Schwannomin) protein. The merlin protein is a member of the ERM (ezrin, radixin, moesin) family of proteins. These proteins form cellular links between the cell membrane and the actin cytoskeleton, participating in the production of cellular outpouchings and in signal transduction. How disruption of merlin function leads to tumorigenesis in arachnoidal cells, however, remains unclear.

Interestingly, the frequency of *NF2* gene mutations varies among the three most frequent meningioma variants. Both fibrous and transitional meningiomas carry *NF2* gene mutations in approximately 70 to 80% of the cases. In contrast, meningothelial meningiomas harbour *NF2* gene mutations in only 25% of the cases, suggesting that this variant has a genetic origin that is primarily independent of *NF2* gene alterations.[98] The observation of a close association of allelic loss of 22q with the fibrous meningiomas supports this hypothesis,[96] as does the observation that most non-NF2 meningioma families develop meningothelial tumours.[6] Furthermore, reduced merlin expression has been observed in different histopathological variants of meningioma variants, but is apparently rare in meningothelial tumours.[101] Interestingly, however, the types of *NF2* gene mutations do not differ significantly between tumour variants. In atypical and anaplastic (malignant) meningiomas, *NF2* gene mutations occur in approximately 70% of cases, matching the frequency of *NF2* mutations in benign fibroblastic and transitional meningiomas. These matching frequencies suggest that *NF2* gene mutations are not involved in progression to higher-grade meningiomas.

While it is likely that other genes beside *NF2* are involved in the formation of a substantial percentage of benign meningiomas, it is unclear whether these genes reside on the long arm of chromosome 22 or on other chromosomes. The close association of *NF2* mutations with allelic loss on chromosome 22 in meningiomas suggests that *NF2* is the major meningioma tumour suppressor gene on chromosome 22.[98] Nonetheless, some deletion studies of chromosome 22 have detected losses and translocations of genetic material outside of the *NF2* region, raising the possibility of a second chromosome 22 meningioma gene. One candidate gene is beta-adaptin, since it is located within a region homozygously deleted in a meningioma and shows reduced expression in some meningiomas; however, a partial mutational analysis of beta-adaptin did not reveal mutations.[102] Another chromosome 22q candidate gene is *MN1*, which is disrupted by a translocation in a meningioma.[103] However, convincing evidence that this gene plays a role in meningioma formation is also lacking. Recent comparative

genomic hybridisation studies have raised the possibility of candidate regions on chromosomes 1p and 3p involved in low grade meningioma formation specifically in cases that lack chromosome 22q aberrations.[23] A curious genetic change is the common loss of the Y chromosome noted in many meningiomas from male patients.[104]

Rare meningiomas also suffer *PTCH* mutations[24] and meningiomas have been reported in some patients with Gorlin syndrome,[9] suggesting that meningiomas may have alterations of the *PTCH* pathway. The protein encoded by *PTCH* participates in a signal transduction pathway, by acting as a receptor for the Sonic hedgehog protein; binding of Sonic hedgehog to the *PTCH* product prevents normal inhibition of the smoothened transmembrane protein. It remains to be shown whether meningiomas have other alterations of this pathway.

In atypical and malignant meningiomas, karyotypic abnormalities become more extensive.[105] Among the cytogenetic changes associated with meningioma, deletion of the short arm of chromosome 1[86] and loss of chromosome 14[106] have been most frequently observed. Correspondingly, at the molecular genetic level and by comparative genomic hybridisation, atypical and malignant meningiomas often exhibit allelic losses of chromosomal arms 1p, 6q, 9q, 10q, 14q, 17p and 18q, suggesting progression-associated genes at these loci.[63,95,107–109] Deletions of the short arm of chromosome 1 target the distal region, near the marker D1S496, at bands 1p34-1pter, a region which is often deleted in other human tumours.[110] Also of interest is the locus on chromosome 10 that is associated with malignant meningiomas, since allelic loss of this region is observed only in morphologically malignant lesions and not in cytologically benign meningiomas that invade the brain.[63] The *PTEN/MMAC1* gene on chromosome 10 does not appear to be the chromosome 10 tumour suppressor in malignant meningiomas.[111] Although allelic losses of chromosome 17p have been noted in higher-grade meningiomas, studies of the *TP53* gene on chromosome 17p have not shown significant gene alterations in meningiomas. Nonetheless, immunohistochemical positivity for p53 protein has been noted with some frequency in atypical meningiomas and rare anaplastic meningiomas suffer *TP53* gene mutations.[112] Mutations and deletions of the *p16/CDKN2* gene are also rare in meningiomas,[113] but have been noted in malignant meningiomas.[109] Loss of E-cadherin immunoreactivity is common in malignant meningiomas;[75] since E-cadherin may function as a tumour suppressor in epithelial tumours, loss of E-cadherin may play a role in the malignant progression of meningioma as well. Interestingly, E-cadherin is expressed in benign meningiomas invading dura, bone, brain, and muscle, but not in the majority of morphologically malignant meningiomas. In primary recurrent meningioma pairs, E-cadherin expression appears identical, except in cases with malignant progression, in which the malignant recurrence loses E-cadherin expression.[75] Most atypical and malignant meningiomas express telomerase, as do some benign meningiomas that have a tendency to recur, while ordinary benign meningiomas are only rarely telomerase- positive; this may suggest the emergence of immortal cell populations in higher-grade meningeal tumours.[114]

Amplification of known oncogenes is not a common feature of meningiomas. Comparative genomic hybridisation experiments have, however, recently demonstrated an amplification locus at 17q23 and a number of regions of chromosomal gain in higher-grade meningiomas, including chromosomes 1q, 9q, 12q, 15q, 17q and 20q.[109] The possible oncogenes residing at these chromosomal loci remain to be identified. A variety of growth factors are overexpressed in meningiomas and may therefore be implicated in meningioma formation. The B chain of the PDGF ligand and the beta chain of the PDGF receptor are cognately expressed in meningiomas, forming an autocrine stimulatory loop. Other growth factors such as basic fibroblast growth factor, epidermal growth factor and insulin-like growth factor I and II, are also expressed in some meningiomas at relatively high levels. It has been suggested that the relative level of insulin-like growth factor II to insulin-like growth factor binding protein 2 may be a marker for anaplasia in meningiomas, perhaps via stimulation of proliferation.[78] As mentioned earlier, expression of VEGF/VPF has been correlated with the presence of tumour-associated oedema.[34,79] Again, it remains to be shown how the expression of these growth factors actually effects tumorigenic changes in meningothelial cells.

Microsatellite instability is thought to result from mutations in DNA mismatch repair genes. One study reported microsatellite instability in 4 of 16 meningiomas.[115] A second study, however, showed no evidence for microsatellite instability in a series of 44 meningiomas.[108] In addition, patients with germline mismatch repair gene defects, such as occur in the Lynch syndromes, do not suffer from meningiomas, suggesting again that mismatch repair defects are not of primary importance in meningioma oncogenesis.

Clonality of meningiomas has also been an area of active investigation, with some interesting results emerging from such inquiries. Southern blot X chromosome inactivation studies in meningiomas have demonstrated that meningiomas are monoclonal tumours.[116] However, polymerase chain reaction (PCR)-based assays have hinted that a small fraction of meningiomas could be polyclonal.[117] Nonetheless, the Southern blot findings[116] and the observation that the overwhelming majority of meningiomas with *NF2* mutations only have a single mutation argues[98] for a clonal origin for these lesions. The clonality of multiple meningiomas has also been studied by X chromosome inactivation studies and by mutational analysis of the *NF2* gene in multiple tumours from single patients.[118–120] Strikingly, patients with three or more meningiomas have been shown to have either the same X chromosome inactivated or to carry the same *NF2* mutation in each of their lesions. These data provide strong evidence for a clonal origin of multiple meningiomas in patients with more than two lesions, with multiple lesions perhaps arising via spread. Patients with two meningiomas, however, have monoclonal tumours only in about half of the cases; the other half exhibit different *NF2* gene mutations in their respective tumours, indicating an independent origin for these lesions.[118] These results suggest that a significant number of multiple meningioma cases represent spread from a single, initial lesion.

Differential diagnosis

Most meningiomas present as slow growing, dural based lesions with characteristic neuroimaging features, so that the neurosurgeon has a high index of suspicion preoperatively that the tumour will be a meningioma. In addition, most meningiomas conform to one of the above-mentioned histological patterns. For these reasons, the majority of meningiomas do not pose diagnostic problems. Given the extraordinarily wide range of histological appearances seen in meningiomas, however, many tumour entities enter the differential diagnosis, particularly for tumours with unusual clinical or histological features (Table 13.4).

Cytological features may be of great importance in establishing the diagnosis, and touch and smear preparations are therefore recommended for intraoperative evaluations. Touch preparations will often yield cellular whorls and sometimes psammoma bodies in tumours that have these structures. Although smear preparations may not be optimal in highly collagenous, fibrous tumours, many meningiomas will smear well and will display characteristic cytological features. In particular, the euchromatic nuclei with pseudoinclusions are helpful in establishing the diagnosis. Frozen sections may be additionally helpful by demonstrating psammoma bodies as well as cellular whorls. Notably, however, cellular whorl-like structures have been noted in a variety of non-meningothelial human tumours, including metastatic carcinomas, metastatic melanoma and glioblastoma.[23]

Metastatic tumours

Metastatic tumours may mimic meningioma, particularly single metastatic lesions to the dura mater. This situation may be more common in the setting of breast or prostate carcinoma, which show a predilection for dural metastasis. In most cases, carcinomas are distinguished by their high mitotic rate and pleomorphism, but such features may be

Table 13.4 Differential diagnosis of meningiomas (after Scheithauer)[155]

Meningioma subtype	Differential diagnosis
Meningothelial (including atypical and malignant)	Metastatic carcinoma, melanoma, sarcoma Malignant glioma Arachnoidal hyperplasia Meningioangiomatosis
Fibrous	Schwannoma Astrocytoma, fibrillary and pilocytic Solitary fibrous tumour Other fibroblastic proliferations
Transitional	Same as above two categories
Psammomatous	Psammomatous Schwannoma Metastatic adenocarcinoma with psammoma bodies
Angiomatous	Vascular malformation Meningioangiomatosis
Microcystic	Haemangioblastoma Astrocytoma, fibrillary, protoplasmic and pilocytic
Secretory	Metastatic carcinoma
Clear cell	Oligodendroglioma Central neurocytoma Clear cell ependymoma Metastatic renal cell carcinoma
Chordoid	Chordoma
Lymphoplasmacyte-rich	Primary haematopoietic processes
Metaplastic	Primary mesenchymal lesions (e.g. osteoma)
Papillary	Metastatic papillary adenocarcinoma Metastatic melanoma Ependymoma Choroid plexus neoplasm
Rhabdoid	Metastatic rhabdoid tumour Metastatic carcinoma Malignant melanoma Malignant glioma Atypical teratoid/rhabdoid tumour Rhabdomyosarcoma
Oncocytic	Oncocytic tumours

combined in higher grade meningiomas as well. Typically, meningiomas lack the overtly epithelial characteristics of carcinomas, and the presence of glandular or squamous differentiation argues strongly against a diagnosis of meningioma. Nonetheless, some metastases may be poorly differentiated and impossible to distinguish at the light microscopic level from a malignant meningioma. Immunohistochemistry may be helpful in this situation, since even poorly-differentiated carcinomas often retain cytokeratin positivity, which is absent in most meningiomas (see Immunohistochemistry section, above). Although most diagnostic problems arise in the setting of a patient with no known primary, the presence of a known primary tumour, particularly breast carcinoma, does not argue against a coexistent meningioma, since the meningioma and breast carcinoma may be associated with one another. Finally, it is important to recall that metastatic carcinoma and meningioma may coexist, as meningiomas are the most common tumour to receive the albeit rare metastasis to an intracranial tumour. In this setting, the meningioma is often benign and the metastatic carcinomas stands out strongly. Metastatic sarcomas are vanishingly rare and usually present in the setting of a known primary sarcoma elsewhere. The rare primary sarcomas of the meninges are discussed elsewhere (Chapter 14); these are often anaplastic, spindle cell tumours that are distinguished from malignant meningiomas by the presence of specific avenues of mesenchymal differentiation and absence of meningothelial regions.

Malignant gliomas

Large irregular meningiomas that deeply indent or invade the brain may mimic malignant gliomas on neuroimaging. This confusion is confounded by the fact that malignant gliomas not uncommonly emerge from the brain parenchyma to involve the meninges. At surgery, the two tumour types may be difficult to distinguish on gross characteristics alone, particularly in the case of large, soft meningiomas. Fortunately, histological examination usually readily distinguishes gliomas from meningiomas, with gliomas demonstrating a fibrillary background, as well as endothelial proliferation and perinecrotic pseudopalisading in glioblastomas. As mentioned above, however, atypical and malignant meningiomas may show focal necroses, sometimes occurring within hypercellular foci that may resemble perinecrotic pseudopalisading. Most malignant gliomas will stain immunohistochemically for GFAP and S-100 protein, distinguishing them from meningiomas, which do not in general stain strongly for these markers. As mentioned above, rare meningiomas have been reported to be GFAP-positive but it remains unclear whether these are really meningiomas or unusual gliomas.[70]

Rare meningiomas may be associated with malignant gliomas in the setting of so-called sarcoglioma.[121] In this situation, usually malignant meningeal lesions may precede the development of an adjacent malignant glioma. Some of the reported meningeal lesions have been malignant meningiomas. Often the glial proliferation takes the form of entrapped islands of highly atypical astrocytic cells. While exceedingly rare, the possibility of such sarcogliomatous lesions may be entertained in a tumour with both meningothelial and glial appearances.

Schwannomas and NF2

Schwannomas may present a substantial differential diagnostic problem in meningioma diagnosis, particularly in posterior fossa tumours, in meningiomas with a fibroblastic appearance, and in patients with NF2. Often the neurosurgeon will reveal whether the tumour was dural-based or growing off a nerve, but in some regions this may not be entirely apparent. In the cerebellopontine angle, where this differential diagnosis may be most difficult, preoperative neuroimaging will usually demonstrate vestibular Schwannomas arising within the internal acoustic meatus and auditory canal, a location that is not consistent with a diagnosis of meningioma. In general, fibrous meningiomas present a more organised fascicular pattern than is seen in Schwannomas. Schwannomas often contain irregular, elongated pleomorphic nuclei and display distinct Antoni A and Antoni B areas along with Verocay bodies – although these features are unfortunately not common in cerebellopontine angle Schwannomas. The presence of strong S-100 staining also argues against a meningioma, and EMA-positivity is neither strong nor common in Schwannomas. On occasion, reticulin stains may be helpful in the differential diagnosis, since Schwannomas often contain copious basement membrane material around individual tumour cells; unfortunately, fibrous meningiomas may also contain reticulin-positive material and it is the fibrous meningioma that may be confused with Schwannoma.

NF2 patients present a special problem in the differential diagnosis of Schwannoma vs meningioma, since these patients are predisposed to the development of both of these tumour types. Indeed, finding a Schwannoma and meningioma in the same biopsy specimen is virtually pathognomonic of NF2.[122] Thus, the pathologist must be aware of the possibility of both Schwannoma and meningioma coexisting. More problematic in NF2 patients has been the occurrence of tumours with features hybrid between those of meningioma and Schwannoma. For instance, Schwannomas in these patients may show large, loose whorl-like patterns that may, at low power, have a meningioma-like appearance. Alternatively, meningiomas may have palisading regions that suggest Verocay bodies. In these difficult cases, we have found differential positivity for EMA and S-100 to be the best means for distinguishing between meningioma and Schwannoma.

Haemangioperictyoma

Haemangiopericytomas were previously classified as the haemangiopericytic variant of angioblastic meningioma, because of the general resemblance between haemangiopericytomas and meningiomas and because of the supposed presence of lesions with features of both haemangiopericytoma and meningioma. At low power microscopic examination, haemangiopericytomas are often remarkable for their 'staghorn' vascular pattern, in which thin walled blood vessels are distorted into thin, branching structures by the encroaching tumour cells. At high power examination, haemangiopericytomas are densely cellular, more so than most malignant meningiomas, and mitotic activity is sometimes brisk. The cells are arranged in a haphazard manner and have irregular, sometimes carrot shaped nuclei that are cytologically different from meningothelial cells. Haemangiopericytomas are EMA negative and vimentin positive on immunohistochemistry. Some studies have suggested that CD34 staining may be highly characteristic of haemangiopericytomas,[123] but others have found CD34 staining in meningiomas as well.[124] Reticulin staining may be useful, since haemangiopericytomas display extensive reticulin positivity surrounding individual tumour cells; in meningiomas, this is only seen in fibrous tumours, which do not histologically resemble haemangiopericytomas.

Solitary fibrous tumour

Solitary fibrous tumour of the meninges is a recently recognised tumour that resembles solitary fibrous tumours found in other sites in the body. It is a benign, paucicellular lesion in which spindle cells are found in a densely collagenous background. These tumours are characteristically strongly CD34 positive, separating them from fibrous meningiomas which typically only show faint CD34 positivity.[124]

Other differential diagnostic considerations

Specific subtypes of meningioma raise other specific entities in their differential diagnosis. Clear cell meningiomas naturally bring up other clear cell neoplasms as diagnostic possibilities. Oligodendrogliomas may be particularly problematic because oligodendrogliomas may show extensive meningeal involvement. However, the focal background fibrillarity, entrapped or neoplastic GFAP positive cells, single cell parenchymal infiltration and, if necessary, ultrastructural differences readily distinguish oligodendroglioma from clear cell meningioma. Furthermore, clear cell meningiomas are EMA positive and have ultrastructural characteristics of meningothelial cells. Central neurocytoma and clear cell ependymoma are separated on the basis of their typical intraventricular location and immunohistochemical positivity for neuronal (synaptophysin) and glial (GFAP, S-100) markers, respectively.

Microcystic meningiomas may be confused with primary haemangioblastomas of the meninges. Indeed, most tumours previously classified as the haemangioblastic variant of angioblastic meningioma are now considered microcystic meningioma. Primary meningeal haemangioblastomas are vanishingly rare and are essentially seen only in the setting of von Hippel–Lindau disease, in which meningiomas are not observed at increased frequencies. Chordoid meningiomas, in turn, raise the possibility of primary chordomas. Since most chordoid meningiomas contain regions of typical meningioma and do not occur in the midline regions frequented by chordoma, there is not usually diagnostic confusion between these entities. Furthermore, meningiomas do not display the strong cytokeratin and S-100 immunopositivity characteristic of chordomas. Finally, inflammation-rich meningiomas may mimic a variety of inflammatory meningeal lesions, such as plasma cell granuloma or Rosai–Dorfman disease,[51] and it is necessary to exclude specific haematological conditions in any lymphoplasmacyte-rich meningeal lesion.

Papillary meningiomas necessarily raise the possibility of other papillary, often epithelial tumours. This is especially significant since papillary meningiomas often contain histological features of malignancy, bringing a metastatic papillary carcinoma into the differential diagnosis. Again, strong cytokeratin positivity would favour a metastatic tumour, even in the absence of a known primary carcinoma. Other papillary tumours in the differential diagnosis may include ependymomas and choroid plexus tumours, although the intraventricular location of these tumours is unusual for meningioma. The presence of GFAP and/or cytokeratin positivity argue against a diagnosis of meningioma as the existence of GFAP-positive papillary meningiomas remains sub judice.

Rhabdoid meningiomas usually have fields of classical meningioma. Nonetheless, focally, these tumours may be confused with other tumours that have a rhabdoid cytology. Most classical rhabdoid tumours are lesions of childhood and therefore do not pose serious diagnostic challenges; such lesions include metastatic renal rhabdoid tumour, primary or metastatic rhabdomyosarcoma and atypical teratoid/rhabdoid tumour of the brain. None of these lesions shows features typical of meningioma, such as nuclear pseudoinclusions; in turn, rhabdoid meningiomas do not stain extensively for glial, neuronal or skeletal muscle immunohistochemical markers. Other tumours that affect adults, however, may have vaguely rhabdoid features and therefore enter the differential diagnosis. These include metastatic carcinomas with eccentric nuclei and hyalinised cytoplasm, malignant melanoma with prominent nucleoli, and gemistocytic astrocytomas with eccentric, eosinophilic cytoplasm. In certain cases, rhabdoid meningiomas have mimicked ependymomas when the cells had a pseudorosette-like appearance around hyalinised vessels.[67] In most cases, however, the presence of classical meningioma enables the diagnosis of rhabdoid meningioma; in others, immunohistochemistry for glial or melanoma markers will facilitate ruling out unusual astrocytomas or melanomas.

The rare oncocytic meningioma may raise the differential diagnosis of other intracranial granular cell lesions. These can usually be easily distinguished by the presence of light microscopic, immunohistochemical and ultrastructural meningothelial features in oncocytic meningiomas. The other major entities can be confirmed by immunohistochemical staining, with Schwann cell granular tumours staining for S-100, astrocytic granular cell lesions for GFAP and S-100, and carcinomas for cytokeratins.

Angiomatous meningiomas may raise the differential diagnosis of vascular malformations or of meningioangiomatosis (see below). Finally, for tumours of the cauda equina, paraganglioma must be considered, although the typical 'zellballen' are not readily confused with the whorls of meningioma and immunohistochemistry will easily separate these two entities.

Therapy and prognosis

The essential prognostic questions for meningiomas are prediction of recurrence and, for higher grade tumours, prediction of survival. The major clinical factor that impacts on whether meningiomas recur is the extent of surgical resection.[13] Subtotally resected tumours, even if histologically benign, have a substantial likelihood of recurrence.[18]

Surgery is therefore the mainstay of therapy for meningiomas.[33] At least for benign tumours, surgical extirpation holds the promise of a therapeutic cure. The extent of resection, however, is itself related to tumour site. Most convexity lesions can be removed surgically. Those involving major dural sinuses may be more difficult to resect in their entirety, although the utility of aggressive removal of all tumour from the sinuses has been debated.[33] Skull base meningiomas present a host of other problems related to their particular sites. Thus, the location of the tumour may affect the likelihood of recurrence, and if incompletely resected, even benign meningiomas may recur repeatedly. Furthermore, even after 'complete' resection, there is a substantial recurrence rate, with 7% recurring at 5 years, 20% at 10 years and 32% at 15 years.[125] Preoperative tumour embolisation may be utilised in order to reduce the tumoral vascular supply; at least theoretically, such an approach could reduce the incidence of recurrence if embolisation devascularised tumour foci that escaped surgical removal.[126]

Radiation therapy appears to reduce the risk of recurrence and increase the time to recurrence in subtotally resected meningiomas.[127,128] For instance, in one study, only 32% of irradiated, subtotally resected tumours recurred, compared with 60% of non-irradiated, subtotally resected lesions.[128] In addition, the median time to recurrence was 125 months for irradiated cases but only 66 months for non-irradiated patients. Some centres advocate the use of radiation therapy postoperatively, while others opt to delay radiation until recurrence has occurred, particularly in elderly patients.[33] The postsurgical treatment of atypical meningiomas varies, but patients with subtotally resected atypical meningiomas benefit similarly from the use radiation therapy.[129] For malignant meningiomas, tumours with a substantial chance of recurrence and of aggressive behaviour, radiation therapy is used regardless of the extent of resection. Furthermore, chemotherapy has been utilised in the therapy of malignant meningioma, primarily using sarcoma-type regimens.[33]

As noted above, certain histological variants, such as the papillary and rhabdoid meningioma, demonstrate a greater propensity for recurrence.[12] Overall, however, tumour grade (i.e. benign, atypical, malignant) provides the most useful histological predictor of the likelihood of recurrence. For instance, while histologically benign meningiomas have recurrence rates of about 7%, atypical meningiomas recur in 29–38% of cases and anaplastic (malignant) meningiomas have a recurrence rates of 50–78%.[12,13,86] Similarly, median times to recurrence correlate with grade, being 7.5, 2.4, and 3.5 years, in benign, atypical and malignant tumours, respectively.[13] Unfortunately, as discussed above, the assignment of these grades is somewhat subjective; thus, there have been numerous attempts to correlate specific histological features with recurrence. In one study, recurrent meningiomas showed significantly more hypercellularity and an increased mitotic rate, whereas nuclear pleomorphism, increased vascularity, and focal necroses were not more frequent in recurrent tumours.[130] Another study demonstrated seven histopathological features that correlated with recurrence: hypervascularity, haemosiderin deposition, growth of tumour cells in sheets, prominent nucleoli, mitotic figures, single-cell and small-group necrosis, nuclear pleomorphism, and overall atypical or malignant tumour grade; in addition, sheeting of tumour cells, prominent nucleoli, and the presence of less than 10% meningothelial pattern correlated with significantly abbreviated recurrence-free survival.[131] On the other hand, another report cited micronecrosis as the only histopathological feature associated with increased risk of meningioma recurrence: at 36 months, 32% of patients with micronecrosis were alive compared with 71% of patients without micronecrosis.[132] Interestingly, brain invasion was not associated with disease-free survival.[132] Furthermore, after recurrence, median survival was 7 months and did not correlate with any histopathological feature.[132]

Proliferation indices have been used for predicting recurrence and survival; these approaches are discussed in the 'Cellular proliferation' section above. Progesterone receptor status has also been correlated with recurrence. The absence of progesterone receptors, high mitotic index, and higher tumour grade were significant factors for shorter disease-free intervals in meningiomas; multivariate analysis showed that a three-factor inter-action model, with a progesterone receptor score of 0, mitotic index greater than 6, and malignant tumour grade, was a highly significant predictor for worse outcome.[133,134] Higher grade tumours more frequently lack progesterone receptors,[135] and progesterone receptor negative meningiomas tend to be larger than progesterone receptor positive tumours.[134]

Other meningothelial lesions

Meningioangiomatosis

Meningioangiomatosis is a curious and uncommon lesion that is histologically and histogenetically related to classical meningioma. As opposed to meningioma, however, meningioangiomatosis is not dural based; rather these lesions are usually intracortical, forming a firm, plaque-like widening of the cerebral cortex, although rare deep grey matter and brain stem lesions have been reported.[136]

Meningioangiomatosis occurs in two distinct clinical settings.[137] Sporadic cases of meningioangiomatosis usually present in children or young adults as seizures. In this setting, meningioangiomatosis is a single lesion and surgical removal often effects seizure control.[138–142] Patients with NF2 have a predisposition to develop meningioangiomatosis, with some patients developing mutliple intracranial lesions.[143–149] In the setting of NF2, however, the lesions are typically asymptomatic and are incidental discoveries at autopsy or on neuroradiological studies. From a genetic point of view, meningioangiomatosis is not a forme fruste of NF2, since sporadic cases of meningioangiomatosis do not suffer from constitutional *NF2* gene mutations.[137] More curiously, sporadic meningioangiomatosis cases do not demonstrate somatic mutations of the *NF2* gene, implying that *NF2* defects may have to be operative during development for this lesion to arise from an *NF2* defect.[137]

On gross examination, the external surface of the brain is covered by a firm whitish plaque, which obscures the usual translucent quality of the arachnoid. The cut surface typically demonstrates replacement or near-replacement of the cerebral cortex by white, firm tissue that stops abruptly at the grey–white matter junction (Figs 13.53 and 13.54). The intracortical lesion also has sharp boundaries, with abrupt transition to normal appearing cerebral cortex.

As the name suggests, meningioangiomatosis is a lesion comprised both meningothelial and vascular proliferation; some lesions demonstrate a preponderance of meningothelial cells and may rarely be associated with frank meningiomas;[150] other lesions feature conspicuous vascular channels lined by barely discernible arachnoidal cells (Figs 13.55 and 13.56). If, as in most cases, the meningothelial proliferation is more prominent, the low-power microscopic appearance is of multiple perivascular nodules within the cerebral cortex. On the other

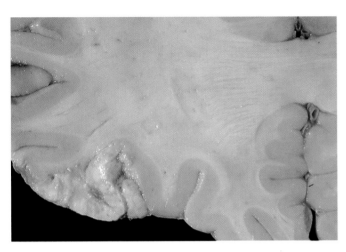

Fig. 13.53 **Meningioangiomatosis.** Meningioangiomatosis appears as a firm intracortical plaque, as noted in this inferior frontal example from a patient with NF2.

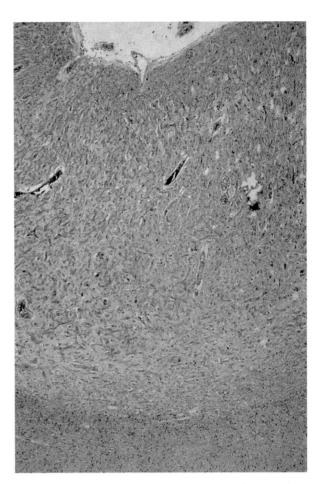

Fig. 13.54 **Meningioangiomatosis.** A trichrome stain illustrates the pervasive nature of meningioangiomatosis in the cerebral cortex, as well as its tendency not to involve the underlying white matter. Masson trichrome.

hand, cases with vascular prominence may display intense collagenous hyalinisation of the vascular walls. In general, the intervening cortex is gliotic, but the gliosis may be relatively inconspicuous. Neurofibrillary tangles have been described in the intervening neurons.[151] In sporadic cases of meningioangiomatosis, the intervening cortex is typically not dysplastic. In NF2 cases, the architecture of the intervening cortex may be distorted by the glial hamartomas that are pathognomonic of NF2.

Studies of proliferation markers have shown that these lesions have only rare proliferating cells and that the putative meningothelial cells are the dividing cells.[137,152] Immunohistochemical studies have not greatly clarified the nature of these lesions;[153,154] significantly, most are not EMA positive and therefore EMA immunonegativity should not dissuade one from a diagnosis of meningioangiomatosis.

Rare cases of meningioangiomatosis display mitotic activity and anaplastic nuclear features. In one case with these features seen by us, the lesion recurred multiple times over a series of years, a clinical course distinctly unusual for meningioangiomatosis. Therefore, it remains possible that anaplastic variants of meningioangiomatosis exist, but the entity remains sub judice until further cases are reported.

For the meningothelial predominant types of meningioangiomatosis, the differential diagnosis primarily includes invasive meningioma. As mentioned above, anaplastic features are rare in meningioangiomatosis and their presence should therefore make one carefully exclude the possibility of a malignant, invasive meningioma. Nonetheless, since some invasive meningiomas may have bland cytological features and primarily involve the Virchow–Robin spaces, the differential diagnosis with invasive meningioma may be difficult. The clinical, surgical and radiological features, however,

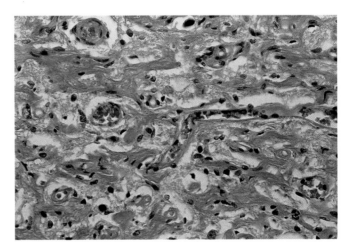

Fig. 13.55 **Meningioangiomatosis.** Some cases of meningioangiomatosis feature few meningothelial-type cells and moderate collagen deposition surrounding the cortical blood vessels, as noted on this trichrome stain.

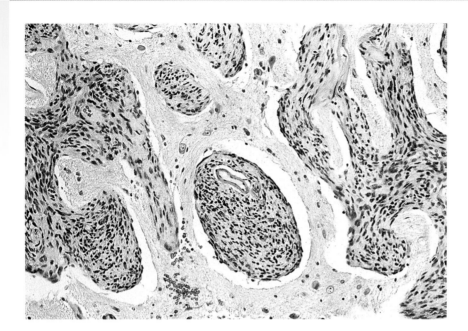

Fig. 13.56 **Meningioangiomatosis.** Other cases of meningioangiomatosis contain nodules of meningothelial cells, each associated with an intracortical blood vessel. H & E.

usually allow ready distinction between these possibilities, with a intracortical, plaque-like lesion in a young patient supporting a diagnosis of meningioangiomatosis over that of meningioma. Significantly, some reports have suggested that meningioangiomatosis is more likely to be accompanied by a frank meningioma in children, confusing the distinction between these entities in individual cases. Indeed, it remains possible that meningioangiomatosis is simply an intracortical meningioma, that the intracortical location predisposes to seizures and that the increased incidence of meningioangiomatosis in NF2 patients simply reflects the markedly increased incidence of meningiomas in these patients.

For the vascular predominant forms of meningioangiomatosis, the major differential diagnosis is with a primary vascular malformation. The plaque-like appearance, cortical location, lack of characteristic malformative blood vessels and typical lack of evidence of haemorrhage all argue against a diagnosis of a primary vascular malformation.

Arachnoidal hyperplasia

Hyperplasia of the arachnoid is an entity not often encountered in surgical neuropathology, but an entity of considerable diagnostic importance in a few instances. As discussed above, the normal arachnoid consists of nests of meningothelial cells that histologically and architecturally resemble minute meningothelial meningiomas. This resemblance extends to the presence of intranuclear inclusions, cellular whorls and psammoma bodies. These nests retain the ability to proliferate in response to adjacent pathological processes, including both neoplastic and inflammatory lesions. In such situations, the minute nests may become less inconspicuous nodules that are histologically indistinguishable from small meningothelial meningiomas. Clearly, biopsies of such nodules that miss the adjacent, inciting process may yield a false diagnosis of meningioma.

There are two sites which display a propensity for such arachnoidal hyperplasia and are therefore sites for which the pathologist must be particularly wary of jumping to a diagnosis of meningothelial meningioma. The most common is surrounding an optic nerve glioma. As opposed to optic nerve meningiomas, optic nerve gliomas do not transgress the sheath of dura mater surrounding the optic nerve. Nonetheless, their presence may incite significant arachnoidal hyperplasia so that a small biopsy will show changes consistent with meningothelial meningioma. Because of differences in both prognosis and treatment, the distinction between optic nerve meningioma and optic nerve glioma is of obvious importance. Therefore, the possible diagnosis, particularly at frozen section, of a meningothelial meningioma from the optic nerve region in a patient thought to have an optic nerve glioma on neuroimaging, should prompt a consultation between the neurosurgeon, neuroradiologist and neuropathologist to determine whether such a lesion is more likely to be arachnoidal hyperplasia overlying a glioma, or a true optic nerve meningioma. The clinical features of the case may also help, since optic nerve gliomas are typically tumours of children or young adults while optic nerve meningiomas more often affect middle-aged and elderly patients. A further distinction must be made in patients with NF; patients with NF1 often develop optic nerve gliomas, while patients with NF2 develop multiple meningiomas, including those of the optic nerve. Therefore, the diagnosis of optic nerve meningothelial meningioma should be held up to intense scrutiny in a young patient or a patient with NF1, and is more likely a misinterpretation of arachnoidal hyperplasia.

Although less well described, we have also noted arachnoidal hyperplasia adjacent to sellar region neoplasms, again creating the possibility that small biopsies that miss the adjacent tumour will be misinterpreted as meningothelial meningiomas. Therefore, the rendering of a diagnosis of meningothelial meningioma in a transsphenoidal tumour surgery in which the clinical and radiological features suggest a craniopharyngioma should raise the suspicion of arachnoidal hyperplasia and should prompt a search for further diagnostic tissue. We have also noted arachnoidal hyperplasia in association with inflammatory meningeal masses such as Rosai–Dorfman disease.

REFERENCES

1. Louis A. Mémoir sur les tumeurs fongueuses de la dure-mère. Mém Acad Roy Chir (Paris), 1774; 5:1–59
2. Cushing H. The meningiomas (dural endotheliomas). Their source and favoured seats of origin. Brain, 1922; 45:282–316
3. Cushing H, Eisenhardt L. Meningiomas: their classification, regional behavior, life history and surgical end results. Springfield IL,: Charles C. Thomas, 1938
4. Louis DN, Scheithauer BW, von Deimling A et al. Meningiomas. In: Kleihues P, Cavenee WK, eds. World Health Organization Classification of Tumours of the central nervous system. Lyon: IARC/WHO, 2000
5. Lantos PL, VandenBerg SR, Kleihues P. Tumours of the nervous system. In: Graham DI, Lantos PL, eds. Greenfield's neuropathology, vol. 2. London: Arnold, 1997
6. Louis DN, Ramesh V, Gusella JF. Neuropathology and molecular genetics of neurofibromatosis 2 and related tumors. Brain Pathol, 1995; 5:163–172
7. Pulst S-M, Rouleau GA, Marineau C et al. Familial meningioma is not allelic to neurofibromatosis 2. Neurology, 1993; 43:2096–2098
8. Louis DN, von Deimling A. Hereditary tumor syndromes of the nervous system: overview and rare syndromes. Brain Pathol, 1995; 5:145–151
9. Albrecht S, Goodman JC, Rajagopalan S et al. Malignant meningioma in Gorlin's syndrome: cytogenetic and p53 gene analysis. Case report. J Neurosurg, 1994; 81:466–471
10. Lyons CJ, Wilson CB, Horton JC. Association between meningioma and Cowden's disease. Neurology, 1993; 43:1436–1437
11. Mahmood A, Caccamo DV, Tomecek FJ et al. Atypical and malignant meningiomas: a clinicopathological review. Neurosurgery, 1993; 33:955–963
12. Maier H, Ofner D, Hittmair A et al. Classic, atypical, and anaplastic meningioma: three histopathological subtypes of clinical relevance. J Neurosurg, 1992; 77:616–623
13. Jaaskelainen J, Haltia M, Servo A. Atypical and anaplastic meningiomas: radiology, surgery, radiotherapy, and outcome. Surg Neurol, 1986; 25:233–242
14. Louis DN, Budka H, von Deimling A. Meningiomas. In: Kleihues P, Cavenee WK, eds. Pathology and genetics of tumours of the nervous system. Lyon: IARC, 1997
15. Sheikh BY, Siqueira E, Dayel F. Meningioma in children: a report of nine cases and a review of the literature. Surg Neurol, 1996; 45:328–335
16. Hope JK, Armstrong DA, Babyn PS et al. Primary meningeal tumors in children: correlation of clinical and CT findings with histologic type and prognosis. Am J Neuroradiol, 1992; 13:1353–1364
17. Erdincler P, Lena G, Sarioglu AC et al. Intracranial meningiomas in children: review of 29 cases. Surg Neurol, 1998; 49:136–140
18. Perry A, Salford SL, Scheithauer BW et al. Meningioma grading. An analysis of histologic parameters. Am J Surg Pathol, 1997; 21:1455–1465
19. Burger PC, Scheithauer BW. Tumors of the central nervous system. In: Rosai J, ed. Atlas of tumor pathology, 3rd series, Fascicle 10. Washington: Armed Forces Institute of Pathology, 1994
20. Burger PC, Scheithauer BW, Vogel FS. Surgical pathology of the nervous system and its coverings, 3rd edn. New York: Churchill Livingstone; 1991: pp 306–324
21. Russell DS, Rubinstein LJ. Pathology of tumours of the nervous system, 5th edn. Baltimore: Williams & Wilkins, 1989
22. Batnitzky S, Eckard DA. The radiology of brain tumors: supratentorial neoplasms. In: Morantz RA, Walsh JW, eds. Brain tumors: a comprehensive text. New York: Marcel Dekker, 1994
23. Kepes JJ. Meningiomas. New York: Masson, 1982
24. Kleinschmidt DeMasters BK, Lillehei KO. Radiation-induced meningioma with a 63-year latency period. J Neurosurg, 1995; 82:487–488
25. Harrison MJ, Wolfe DE, Lau TS et al. Radiation-induced meningiomas: experience at the Mount Sinai Hospital and review of the literature. J Neurosurg, 1991; 75:564–574
26. Musa BS, Pople IK, Cummins BH. Intracranial meningiomas following irradiation – a growing problem? Br J Neurosurg, 1995; 9:629–637
27. Mack EE, Wilson CB. Meningiomas induced by high-dose cranial irradiation. J Neurosurg, 1993; 79:28–31
28. Carlson KM, Bruder C, Nordenskjold M et al. 1p and 3p deletions in meningiomas without detectable aberrations of chromosome 22 identified by comparative genomic hybridization. Genes Chromosomes Cancer, 1997; 20:419–424
29. Xie J, Johnson RL, Zhang X et al. Mutations of the PATCHED gene in several types of sporadic extracutaneous tumors. Cancer Res, 1997; 57:2369–2372
30. Carroll RS, Glowacka D, Dashner K et al. Progesterone receptor expression in meningiomas. Cancer Res, 1993; 53:1312–1316
31. Jacobs DH, Holmes FF, McFarlane MJ. Meningiomas are not significantly associated with breast cancer. Arch Neurol, 1992; 49:753–756
32. Kirsch M, Zhu JJ, Black PM. Analysis of the BRCA1 and BRCA2 genes in sporadic meningiomas. Genes Chromosomes Cancer, 1997; 20:53–59
33. Levin VA, Leibel SA, Gutin PH. Neoplasms of the central nervous system. In: DeVita VT, Hellman S, Rosenberg SA, eds. Cancer: principles and practice of oncology. Philadephia: Lippincott-Raven, 1997
34. Goldman CK, Bharara S, Palmer CA et al. Brain edema in meningiomas is associated with increased vascular endothelial growth factor expression. Neurosurgery, 1997; 40:1269–1277
35. Kepes JJ, Chen WY-K, Connors MH et al. 'Chordoid' meningeal tumors in young individuals with peritumoral lymphoplasmacellular infiltrates causing systemic manifestations of the Castleman syndrome. Cancer, 1988; 62:391–406
36. Kobata H, Kondo A, Iwasaki K et al. Chordoid meningioma in a child. Case report. J Neurosurg, 1998; 88:319–323
37. Louis DN, Hamilton AJ, Sobel RA et al. Pseudopsammomatous meningioma with elevated serum carcino-embryonic antigen (CEA) – a true secretory meningioma. J Neurosurg, 1991; 74:129–132
38. Bruneval P, Sassy C, Mayeux P et al. Erythropoietin synthesis by tumor cells in a case of meningioma associated with erythrocytosis. Blood, 1993; 81:1593–1597
39. Elster AD, Challa VR, Gilbert TH et al. Meningiomas: MR and histopathologic features. Radiology, 1989; 170:857–862
40. Alguacil-Garcia A, Pettigrew NM, Sima AAF. Secretory meningioma. A distinct subtype of meningioma. Am J Surg Pathol, 1986; 10:102–111
41. Robinson JC, Challa VR, Jones DS et al. Pericytosis and edema generation: a unique clinicopathological variant of meningioma. Neurosurgery, 1996; 39:700–706
42. Kleihues P, Burger PC, Scheithauer BW. Histological typing of tumours of the central nervous system, 2nd edn. Berlin: Springer-Verlag, 1993
43. Harkin JC, Leonard GL. Abnormal amianthoid collagen fibers in meningioma. Acta Neuropathol, 1988; 76:638–639

44. Chuaqui R, Gonzalez S, Torrealba G. Meningothelial meningioma with 'amianthoid' fibers. Case report with ultrastructural study. Pathol Res Pract, 1992; 188:890–893

45. Schiffer D. Brain tumors, Berlin: Springer-Verlag, 1993

46. Antinheimo J, Haapasalo H, Haltia M et al. Proliferation potential and histological features in neurofibromatosis 2-associated and sporadic meningiomas. J Neurosurg, 1997; 87:610–614

47. Matsui S, Matsui T, Hirano A. Detachment of desmosomes in a microcystic meningioma. Noshuyo Byori, 1995; 12:85–89

48. Budka H. Hyaline inclusions (pseudopsammoma bodies) in meningiomas: immunocytochemical demonstration of epithel-like secretion of secretory component and immunoglobulins A and M. Acta Neuropathol, 1982; 56:294–298

49. Probst-Cousin S, Villagran-Lillo R, Lahl R et al. Secretory meningioma: clinical, histologic, and immunohistochemical findings in 31 cases. Cancer, 1997; 79:2003–2015

50. Zorludemir S, Scheithauer BW, Hirose T et al. Clear cell meningioma. A clinicopathologic study of a potentially aggressive variant of meningioma. Am J Surg Pathol, 1995; 19:493–505

51. Deodhare SS, Ang LC, Bilbao JM. Isolated intracranial involvement in Rosai–Dorfman disease: a report of two cases and review of the literature. Arch Pathol Lab Med, 1998; 2:161–165

52. Roncaroli F, Riccioni L, Cerati M et al. Oncocytic meningioma. Am J Surg Pathol, 1997; 21:375–382

53. Prayson RA. Malignant meningioma: a clinicopathologic study of 23 patients including MIB 1 and p53 immunohistochemistry. Am J Clin Pathol, 1996; 105:719–726

54. Inoue H, Tamura M, Koizumi H et al. Clinical pathology of malignant meningiomas. Acta Neurochir, 1984; 73:179–191

55. Chen WY, Liu HC. Atypical (anaplastic) meningioma: relationship between histologic features and recurrence – a clinicopathologic study. Clin Neuropathol, 1990; 9:74–81

56. Fabiani A, Trebini F, Favero M et al. The significance of atypical mitoses in malignant meningiomas. Acta Neuropathol, 1977; 38:229–231

57. Jaaskelainen J, Haltia M, Laasonen E et al. The growth rate of intracranial meningiomas and its relation to histology. An analysis of 43 patients. Surg Neurol, 1985; 24:165–172

58. Hsu DW, Pardo FS, Efird JT et al. Prognostic significance of proliferative indices in meningiomas. J Neuropathol Exp Neurol, 1994; 53:247–255

59. Ng HK, Poon WS, Goh K et al. Histopathology of post-embolized meningiomas. Am J Surg Pathol, 1996; 20:1224–1230

60. Paulus W, Meixensberger J, Hofmann E et al. Effect of embolization of meningioma on Ki-67 proliferation index. J Clin Pathol, 1993; 46:876–877

61. Alvarez F, Roda JM, Perez Romero M et al. Malignant and atypical meningiomas: a reappraisal of clinical, histological, and computed tomographic features. Neurosurgery, 1987; 20:688–694

62. Miller DC, Ojemann RG, Proppe KH et al. Benign metastasizing meningioma. J Neurosurg, 1985; 62:763–766

63. Rempel SA, Schwechheimer K, Davis RL et al. Loss of heterozygosity for loci on chromosome 10 is associated with morphologically malignant meningioma progression. Cancer Res, 1993; 53:2387–2392

64. Ludwin SK, Rubinstein LJ, Russell DS. Papillary meningioma: a malignant variant of meningioma. Cancer, 1975; 36:1363–1373

65. Pasquier B, Gasnier F, Pasquier D et al. Papillary meningioma: clinicopathologic study of seven cases and review of the literature. Cancer, 1986; 59:299–305

66. Kepes JJ, Moral LA, Wilkinson SB et al. Rhabdoid transformation of tumor cells in meningiomas: a histologic indication of increased proliferative activity: report of four cases. Am J Surg Pathol, 1998; 22:231–238

67. Perry A, Scheithauer BW, Stafford SL et al. 'Rhabdoid' meningioma: an aggressive variant. Am J Surg Pathol, 1998; 22:1482–1490

68. Schnitt SJ, Vogel H. Meningiomas. Diagnostic value of immunoperoxidase staining for epithelial membrane staining. Am J Surg Pathol, 1986; 10:640–649

69. Wanschitz J, Schmidbauer M, Maier H et al. Suprasellar meningioma with expression of glial fibrillary acidic protein: a peculiar variant. Acta Neuropathol, 1995; 90:539–544

70. Brat DJ, Scheithauer BW, Staugaitis SM et al. Third ventricular chordoid glioma: a distinct clinicopathological entity. J Neuropathol Exp Neurol, 1998; 57:283–290

71. Nitta H, Yamashima T, Yamashita J et al. An ultrastructural and immunohistochemical study of extracellular matrix in meningiomas. Histol Histopathol, 1990; 5:267–274

72. Ng HK, Wong AT. Expression of epithelial and extracellular matrix protein markers in meningiomas. Histopathology, 1993; 22:113–125

73. Figarella-Branger D, Pellissier JF, Bouillot P et al. Expression of neural cell-adhesion molecule isoforms and epithelial cadherin adhesion molecules in 47 human meningiomas: correlation with clinical and morphological data. Mod Pathol, 1994; 7:752–761

74. Figarella-Branger D, Roche PH, Daniel L et al. Cell-adhesion molecules in human meningiomas: correlation with clinical and morphological data. Neuropathol Appl Neurobiol, 1997; 23:113–122

75. Schwechheimer K, Zhou L, Birchmeier W. E-cadherin in human brain tumours: loss of immunoreactivity in malignant meningiomas. Virchows Arch, 1998; 432:163–167

76. Black P, Carroll R, Zhang J. The molecular biology of hormone and growth factor receptors in meningiomas. Acta Neurochir (Suppl), 1996; 65:50–53

77. Black PM, Carroll R, Glowacka D. Platelet-derived growth factor expression and stimulation in human meningiomas. J Neurosurg, 1994; 81:388–393

78. Nordqvist AC, Peyrard M, Pettersson H et al. A high ratio of insulin-like growth factor II/insulin-like growth factor binding protein 2 messenger RNA as a marker for anaplasia in meningiomas. Cancer Res, 1997; 57:2611–2614

79. Provias J, Claffey K, delAguila L et al. Meningiomas: role of vascular endothelial growth factor/vascular permeability factor in angiogenesis and peritumoral edema. Neurosurgery, 1997; 40:1016–1026

80. Pagotto U, Arzberger T, Hopfner U et al. Expression and localization of endothelin-1 and endothelin receptors in human meningiomas. Evidence for a role in tumoral growth. J Clin Invest, 1995; 96:2017–2025

81. Kubota T, Hirano A, Yamamoto S et al. The fine structure of psammoma bodies in meningocytic whorls. J Neuropathol Exp Neurol, 1984; 43:37–44

82. Hirota S, Nakajima Y, Yoshimine T et al. Expression of bone-related protein messenger RNA in human meningiomas: possible involvement of osteopontin in development of psammoma bodies. J Neuropathol Exp Neurol, 1995; 54:698–703

83. Cho KG, Hoshino T, Nagashima T et al. Prediction of tumor doubling time in recurrent meningiomas. Cell kinetics studies with bromodeoxyuridine labeling. J Neurosurg, 1986; 65:790–794

84. Shibuya M, Hoshino T, Ito S et al. Meningiomas: clinical implications of a high proliferative potential determined by bromodeoxyuridine labeling. Neurosurgery, 1992; 30:494–497

85. Maier H, Wanschitz J, Sedivy R et al. Proliferation and DNA fragmentation in meningioma subtypes. Neuropathol Appl Neurobiol, 1997; 23:496–506

86. Kolles H, Niedermayer I, Schmitt C et al. Triple approach for diagnosis and grading of meningiomas: histology, morphometry of Ki-67/Feulgen stainings, and cytogenetics. Acta Neurochir, 1995; 137:174–181

87. Matsuno A, Fujimaki T, Sasaki T et al. Clinical and histopathological analysis of proliferative potentials of recurrent and non-recurrent meningiomas. Acta Neuropathol, 1996; 91:504–510

88. Cruz Sanchez FF, Miquel R, Rossi ML et al. Clinico-pathological correlations in meningiomas: a DNA and immunohistochemical study. Histol Histopathol, 1993; 8:1–8

89. Zankl H, Zang KD. Cytological and cytogenetical studies on brain tumors. IV Identification of the missing G chromosome in human meningiomas as no. 22 by fluorescence technique. Humangenetik, 1972; 14:167–169

90. Zang KD. Cytological and cytogenetical studies on human meningiomas. Cancer Genet Cytogenet, 1982; 6:249–274

91. Arnoldus EP, Wolters LB, Voormolen JH et al. Interphase cytogenetics: a new tool for the study of genetic changes in brain tumors. J Neurosurg, 1992; 76:997–1003

92. Meese E, Blin N, Zang KD. Loss of heterozygosity and the origin of meningioma. Hum Genet, 1987; 77:349–351

93. Dumanski JP, Carlbom E, Collins P et al. Deletion mapping of a locus on human chromosome 22 involved in the oncogenesis of meningioma. Proc Natl Acad Sci U S A, 1987; 84:9275–9279

94. Dumanski JP, Rouleau GA, Nordeskjold M et al. Molecular genetic analysis of chromosome 22 in 81 cases of meningioma. Cancer Res, 1990; 50:5863–5867

95. Lindblom A, Ruttledge M, Collins VP et al. Chromosomal deletions in anaplastic meningiomas suggest multiple regions outside chromosome 22 as important in tumor progression. Int J Cancer, 1994; 56:354–357

96. Ruttledge MH, Xie YG, Han FY et al. Deletions on chromosome 22 in sporadic meningioma. Genes Chromosomes Cancer, 1994; 10:122–130

97. Trofatter JA, MacCollin MM, Rutter JL et al. A novel moesin-, ezrin-, radixin-like gene is a candidate for the neurofibromatosis 2 tumor suppressor. Cell, 1993; 72:791–800

98. Wellenreuther R, Kraus JA, Lenartz D et al. Analysis of the neurofibromatosis 2 gene reveals molecular variants of meningioma. Am J Pathol, 1995; 146:827–832

99. Papi L, De Vitis LR, Vitelli F et al. Somatic mutations in the neurofibromatosis type 2 gene in sporadic meningiomas. Hum Genet, 1995; 95:347–351

100. Lekanne Deprez RH, Bianchi AB, Groen NA et al. Frequent NF2 gene transcript mutations in sporadic meningiomas and vestibular schwannomas. Am J Hum Genet, 1994; 54:1022–1029

101. Lee JH, Sundaram V, Stein DJ et al. Reduced expression of schwannomin/merlin in human sporadic meningiomas. Neurosurgery, 1997; 40:578–587

102. Peyrard M, Fransson I, Xie YG et al. Characterization of a new member of the human beta-adaptin gene family from chromosome 22q12, a candidate meningioma gene. Hum Mol Genet, 1994; 3:1393–1399

103. Lekanne Deprez RH, Riegman PHJ, Groen NA et al. Cloning and characterization of MN1, a gene from chromosome 22q11, which is disrupted by a balanced translocation in a meningioma. Oncogene, 1995; 10:1521–1528

104. Logan JA, Seizinger BR, Atkins L et al. Loss of the Y chromosome in meningiomas. A molecular genetic approach. Cancer Genet Cytogenet, 1990; 45:41–47

105. Perry A, Jenkins RB, Dahl RJ et al. Cytogenetic analysis of aggressive meningiomas: possible diagnostic and prognostic implications. Cancer, 1996; 77:2567–2573

106. Schneider BF, Shashi V, von Kap herr C et al. Loss of chromosomes 22 and 14 in the malignant progression of meningiomas. A comparative study of fluorescence in situ hybridization (FISH) and standard cytogenetic analysis. Cancer Genet Cytogenet, 1995; 85:101–104

107. Simon M, von Deimling A, Larson J et al. Allelic losses on chromosomes 14, 10, and 22 in atypical and malignant meningiomas: A genetic model of meningioma progression. Cancer Res, 1995; 55:4696–4701

108. Simon M, Kokkino AJ, Warnick RE et al. Role of genomic instability in meningioma progression. Genes Chromosomes Cancer, 1996; 16:265–269

109. Weber RG, Bostrom J, Wolter M et al. Analysis of genomic alterations in benign, atypical, and anaplastic meningiomas: toward a genetic model of meningioma progression. Proc Natl Acad Sci U S A, 1997; 94:14719–14724

110. Bostrum J, Muhlbauer A, Reifenberger G. Deletion mapping of the short arm of chromosome 1 identifies a common region of deletion distal to D1S496 in human meningiomas. Acta Neuropathol, 1997; 94:479–485

111. Bostrom J, Cobbers JM, Wolter M et al. Mutation of the PTEN (MMAC1) tumor suppressor gene in a subset of glioblastomas but not in meningiomas with loss of chromosome arm 10q. Cancer Res, 1998; 58:29–33

112. Wang JL, Zhang ZJ, Hartman M et al. Detection of TP53 gene mutation in human meningiomas: a study using immunohistochemistry, polymerase chain reaction/single-strand conformation polymorphism and DNA sequencing techniques on paraffin-embedded samples. Int J Cancer, 1995; 64:223–228

113. Ono Y, Ueki K, Joseph JT et al. Homozygous deletions of the CDKN2/p16 gene in dural hemangiopericytomas. Acta Neuropathol, 1996; 91:221–225

114. Langford LA, Piatyszek MA, Xu R et al. Telomerase activity in ordinary meningiomas predicts poor outcome. Hum Pathol, 1997; 28:416–420

115. Pykett MJ, Murphy M, Harnish PR et al. Identification of a microsatellite instability phenotype in meningiomas. Cancer Res, 1994; 54:6340–6343

116. Jacoby LB, Pulaski K, Rouleau GA et al. Clonal analysis of human meningiomas and schwannomas. Cancer Res, 1990; 50(21):6783–6786

117. Zhu J, Frosch MP, Busque L et al. Analysis of meningiomas by methylation- and transcription-based clonality assays. Cancer Res, 1995; 55:3865–3872

118. Stangl AP, Wellenreuther R, Lenartz D et al. Clonality of multiple meningioma. J Neurosurg, 1997; 86:853–858

119. Larson JJ, Tew JM, Simon M et al. Evidence for clonal spread in the development of multiple meningiomas. J Neurosurg, 1995; 83:705–709

120. von Deimling A, Kraus JA, Stangl AP et al. Evidence for subarachnoid spread in the development of multiple meningiomas. Brain Pathol, 1995; 5:11–14

121. Lalitha VS, Rubinstein LJ. Reactive glioma in intracranial sarcoma: a form of mixed sarcoma and glioma ('sarcoglioma'): report of eight cases. Cancer, 1979; 43:246–257

122. Sobel RA. Vestibular (acoustic) schwannomas: histologic features in neurofibromatosis 2 and in unilateral cases. J Neuropathol Exp Neurol, 1993; 52:106–113

123. Renshaw AA, Paulus W, Joseph JT. CD34 and EMA distinguish dural hemangiopericytoma and meningioma. J Applied Histochem, 1995; 3:108–114

124. Perry A, Scheithauer BW, Nascimento AG. The immunophenotypic spectrum of meningeal hemangiopericytoma: a comparison with fibrous meningioma and solitary fibrous tumour of meninges. Am J Surg Pathol, 1997; 21:1354–1360

125. Mirimanoff RO, Dosoretz DE, Linggood RM et al. Meningioma: analysis of recurrence and progression following neurosurgical resection. J Neurosurg, 1985; 62:18–24

126. Nelson PK, Setton A, Choi IS et al. Current status of interventional neuroradiology in the management of meningiomas. Neurosurg Clin N Am, 1994; 5:235–259

127. Condra KS, Buatti JM, Mendenhall WM et al. Benign meningiomas: primary treatment selection affects survival. Int J Radiat Oncol Biol Phys, 1997; 39:427–436

128. Barbaro NM, Gutin PH, Wilson CB et al. Radiation therapy in the treatment of partially resected meningiomas. Neurosurgery, 1987; 20:525–528

129. Milosevic MF, Frost PJ, Laperriere NJ et al. Radiotherapy for atypical or malignant intracranial meningioma. Int J Radiat Oncol Biol Phys, 1996; 34:817–822

130. Jellinger K, Slowik F. Histological subtypes and prognostic problems in meningiomas. J Neurol, 1975; 208:279–298

131. de la Monte SM, Flickinger J, Linggood RM. Histopathologic features predicting recurrence of meningiomas following subtotal resection. Am J Surg Pathol, 1986; 10:836–843

132. McLean CA, Jolley D, Cukier E et al. Atypical and malignant meningiomas: importance of micronecrosis as a prognostic indicator. Histopathology, 1993; 23:349–353

133. Hsu DW, Efird JT, Hedley Whyte ET. Progesterone and estrogen receptors in meningiomas: prognostic considerations. J Neurosurg, 1997; 86:113–120

134. Brandis A, Mirzai S, Tatagiba M et al. Immunohistochemical detection of female sex hormone receptors in meningiomas: correlation with clinical and histological features. Neurosurgery, 1993; 33:212–217

135. Gabos S, Berkel J. Meta-analysis of progestin and estrogen receptors in human meningiomas. Neuroepidemiology, 1992; 11:255–260

136. Kollias SS, Crone KR, Ball WS et al. Meningioangiomatosis of the brain stem. J Neurosurg, 1994; 80:732–735

137. Stemmer-Rachamimov AO, Horgan M, Taratuto AL et al. Meningioangiomatosis is associated with neurofibromatosis 2 but not with somatic alterations of the NF2 gene. J Neuropathol Exp Neurol, 1997; 56:485–489

138. Sakaki S, Nakagawa K, Nakamura K et al. Meningioangiomatosis not associated with von Recklinghausen's disease. Neurosurgery, 1987; 20:797–801

139. Ogilvy CS, Chapman PH, Gray M et al. Meningioangiomatosis in a patient without von Recklinghausen's disease. J Neurosurg, 1989; 70:483–485

140. Harada K, Inagawa T, Nagasako R. A case of meningioangiomatosis without von Recklinghausen's disease. Report of a case and review of 13 cases. Childs Nerv Syst, 1994; 10:126–130

141. Kasantikul V, Brown WJ. Meningioangiomatosis in the absence of von Recklinghausen's disease. Surg Neurol, 1980; 15:71–75

142. Kunishio K, Yamamoto Y, Sunami N et al. Histopathologic investigation of a case of meningioangiomatosis not associated with von Recklinghausen's disease. Surg Neurol, 1987; 27:575–579

143. Bassoe P, Nuzum F. Report of a case of central and peripheral neurofibromatosis. J Nerv Ment Dis, 1915; 42:785–796

144. Feigin I. The nerve sheath tumor, solitary and in von Recklinghausen's disease; a unitary mesenchymal concept. Acta Neuropathol, 1971; 17:188–200

145. Foerster O, Gagel O. Ein fall von Recklinghausenscher krankheit mit funf nebeneinander bestehenden verschiedenartigen tumorbildungen. Z Ges Neurol Psychiatr 1932; 138:339–360

146. Hozay J. Une angioneuromatose meningo-encephalique diffuse. Rev Neurol, 1953; 89:222–236

147. Rodriguez HA, Berthrong M. Multiple primary intracranial tumors in von Recklinghausen's neurofibromatosis. Arch Neurol, 1966; 14:467–475

148. Rubinstein LJ. The malformative central nervous system lesions in the central and peripheral forms of neurofibromatosis. A neuropathological study of 22 cases. Ann NY Acad Sci, 1986; 486:14–29

149. Worster-Drought C, Carnegie Dickson WE, McMenemey WH. Multiple meningeal and perineural tumours with analogous changes in the glia and ependyma (neurofibroblastomatosis). Brain, 1937; 60:85–117

150. Blumenthal D, Berho M, Bloomfield S et al. Childhood meningioma associated with meningioangiomatosis. J Neurosurg, 1993; 78:287–289

151. Halper J, Scheithauer BW, Okazaki H et al. Meningio-angiomatosis: a report of six cases with special reference to the occurrence of neurofibrillary tangles. J Neuropath Exp Neurol, 1986; 45:426–446

152. Prayson RA. Meningioangiomatosis: a clinicopathologic study including MIB1 immunoreactivity. Arch Pathol Lab Med, 1995; 119:1061–1064

153. Goates JJ, Dickson DW, Horoupian DS. Meningioangiomatosis: an immunocytochemical study. Acta Neuropathol, 1991; 82:527–532

154. Paulus W, Peiffer J, Roggendorf W et al. Meningio-angiomatosis. Path Res Pract, 1989; 184:446–452

155. Scheithauer BW. Tumors of the meninges: proposed modifications of the World Health Organization classification. Acta Neuropathol, 1990; 80:343–354

14 Vascular, melanocytic and soft tissue tumours

Vascular tumours

Haemangioblastoma and haemangiopericytoma are the principal nervous system neoplasms associated with blood vessel elements, although neither is of entirely certain derivation. Endothelial lined vascular channels are a prominent component of both tumours, but in each case the vessels are of essentially normal architecture and it is only the stromal or intervascular cells which are definitely neoplastic. The majority of nervous system haemangiopericytomas and haemangioblastomas are topographically related to the leptomeninges, and they are listed in different subgroups of meningeal tumours in the current World Health Organisation (WHO) classification.[1] Haemangioblastomas are normally confined to the nervous system, but meningeal haemangiopericytomas are identical in most respects to their counterparts arising in systemic tissues. Rarely, the nervous system may be the primary site of other types of vascular neoplasm, including angiosarcomas and haemangioendotheliomas, and these are briefly discussed at the end of this account. Vascular malformations are described separately in Chapter 17 and hereditary angiomatous syndromes are included with other dysgenetic disorders in Chapter 19.

Haemangioblastoma

The term haemangioblastoma is attributed to Cushing and Bailey[2] and remains in current usage, despite the fact that 'haemangioblasts' are a purely hypothetical cell type, and the tumour is neither a primitive malignant lesion nor of certain angiogenic origin.[3,4] The older literature often refers to these tumours as angioblastic meningiomas, following the original classification of Cushing and Eisenhardt,[5] and until relatively recently the term haemangioblastic meningioma has been misleadingly applied to supratentorial tumours which are histologically identical to haemangioblastomas.[6,7] It is now clear, however, that a distinction can always be made between haemangioblastomas and true meningiomas, despite the fact that haemangioblastomas can sometimes be extraparenchymal in location and bear a superficial histological resemblance to angiomatous meningiomas.[8,9] In recognition that their cell of origin remains uncertain, haemangioblastomas appear under the heading 'meningeal tumours of uncertain histogenesis' in the current WHO classification.[1]

Incidence

Haemangioblastomas account for between 1 and 2% of all intracranial tumours in most reported series,[10,11] and about 7% of all posterior fossa neoplasms.[10,12] In the spinal cord the quoted incidence has varied from 1 to 6% of primary tumours, although the numbers have been small in some series and extramedullary tumours have not always been included.[13,14] Haemangioblastomas are more frequently encountered in Chinese populations than in Western ethnic groups.[15] They occur most often in young adults, where they may account for over 3% of all brain tumours.[12,16] The mean age of presentation is towards the end of the fourth decade of life[17,18] with a peak incidence between 30 and 50 years of age.[17,19] Cases presenting over the age of 60 are rare, although occasional patients over the age of 70 have been recorded.[17,18] The tumour is also rare under the age of 20 years[18,20] but exceptional cases have been reported in infants[21,22] and have even arisen congenitally.[23,24] When haemangioblastomas occur in the context of von Hippel–Lindau (VHL) disease, they typically present in a slightly younger age group compared to sporadic tumours, one study finding a mean age at presentation of 29 years compared to 42 years in cases lacking other evidence of the disease.[18] There is a pronounced bias towards males, with most studies reporting a sex ratio of about 2:1.[18,25]

Site

Haemangioblastomas are most frequently sited in the posterior fossa, which accounts for over 80% of all cases[18,26] (Fig. 14.1). Of these, some 80% are located in the cerebellar hemispheres and 13 to 14% in the vermis.[25,27] Although mostly intraparenchymal at these sites, the vast majority of the cerebellar tumours extend to the pial surface at one margin.[28] Less frequently, haemangioblastomas occur in the floor of the fourth ventricle, usually at its caudal end, in the region of the obex.[29,30] These intramedullary tumours may project out of the

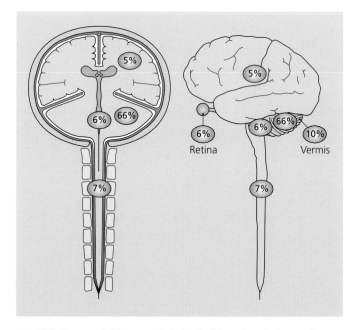

Fig. 14.1 **Haemangioblastoma**. Relative incidence in relation to site.

foramina of Lushka[31] and account for only about 7 or 8% of posterior fossa haemangioblastomas.[18,27] Supratentorial haemangioblastomas are also rare, although less than originally believed, owing to their earlier confusion with vascular meningiomas.[32] They probably represent about 5% of all cases[18] and occur in a variety of locations, including the pituitary stalk,[33] optic nerves[34] and third or lateral ventricles.[35,36] A proportion are hemispheric and superficial, and may show dural attachment[31] or lie entirely within the leptomeninges.[9] Both posterior fossa and supratentorial haemangioblastomas may be multiple at the time of presentation, especially in the context of VHL disease.[28,37] Spinal haemangioblastomas account for approximately 7% of all cases[18] and again may be multiple in cases of VHL disease.[38,39] They are usually posterior in location, involving the posterolateral sulcus or posterior spinal roots.[32,39] They are commonest in the cervical and thoracic regions,[40] but examples in the filum terminale have been reported.[41] About 60% of spinal tumours are entirely intramedullary, and approximately 30% are intradural but wholly or partly extramedullary.[40] These latter tumours are most likely to be attached to the posterior roots,[40,42] as are a further 10% or so of spinal haemangioblastomas which are distal enough to be entirely extradural and thus technically outside the central nervous system (CNS).[40,43] Finally, approximately 6% of all haemangioblastomas occur in the retina, and when in conjunction with similar tumours elsewhere in the neuraxis, these retinal tumours are always a manifestation of VHL disease.[12,18]

Genetics and the relationship with von Hippel–Lindau disease

VHL is an autosomal dominant familial tumour syndrome in which nervous system haemangioblastomas are associated with a variety of systemic tumours and cysts, including renal carcinomas (see Chapter 19 for a detailed description). The gene responsible for VHL acts as a tumour suppressor and occupies a single locus near the tip of the short arm of chromosome 3.[44,45] In individuals with the disease, inactivation of both copies of the gene is necessary for tumour genesis, and a 'second hit' somatic mutation occurs against the background of an inherited germline mutation.[45] The relationship between VHL and isolated, apparently sporadic cases of haemangioblastoma remains uncertain, and is complicated by the very wide spectrum of clinical manifestations seen in patients with the inherited gene defect.[46,47] Somatic mutations of the VHL gene have only been found in the cells of a proportion of isolated haemangioblastomas, suggesting a similar genetic aetiology in these cases but giving little information about the remaining ones.[48,49]

Assessing whether apparently isolated haemangioblastomas are part of VHL is of clear prognostic importance, but until germline genetic testing is widely available it will remain a difficult clinical problem. The haemangioblastomas occurring in association with the disease are histologically identical to those which are apparently isolated and sporadic lesions.[50] Moreover, a significant proportion of patients presenting with a single neuraxial haemangioblastoma have systemic lesions which are asymptomatic at the time of presentation, or harbour multiple haemangioblastomas which only become clinically manifest at a later date[26,50] The minimum diagnostic criteria for a definite clinical diagnosis of VHL[46] may be summarised as:

Either

1. At least two haemangioblastomas or typical visceral lesions in the absence of a positive family history;
or
2. a single haemangioblastoma or typical visceral lesion with an affected first degree relative.

However, the wide variation of manifestations and unpredictable temporal evolution of VHL has led many authorities to consider that all patients presenting with an isolated neuraxial haemangioblastoma should be investigated and followed up for manifestations of the disease, regardless of whether there is a family history or evidence of systemic lesions at the time of presentation.[50,51] In most clinical series, the proportion of patients with a solitary neuraxial haemangioblastoma in whom other evidence of VHL is detected either at presentation or during follow-up has been consistently quoted as about 23%,[26,50] although this figure would probably be higher if follow-up were longer and all cases were subjected to autopsy examination.[50,52] The condition is present in up to one-third of cases presenting with spinal as opposed to cerebellar haemangioblastomas,[40,43] and should be especially suspected if the spinal tumours are extramedullary lesions attached to nerve roots.[42,53]

Aetiology

The cellular derivation of haemangioblastomas remains controversial, particularly with regard to the true nature of the stromal cell component of the tumour.[31,54] The close topographical relationship of the leptomeninges in many cases has led to suggestions of an arachnoidal cell origin,[31] but there is not immunocytochemical or ultrastructural evidence to support this[55,56] and most authorities now consider that haemangioblastomas are quite distinct from true meningiomas of arachnoidal cell origin.[8,9]

The consistent finding of glial fibrillary acidic protein (GFAP) immunoreactivity in some haemangioblastomas raises the possibility of a glial origin for the tumour.[57,58] Many of the GFAP containing cells can be morphologically identified as incorporated reactive astrocytes,[59,60] but GFAP expression is also seen in some cells with stromal cell morphology,[55,61] although not in all cases.[62,63] When present, stromal cells expressing GFAP are mostly located near the margins of tumours that have an intense surrounding gliotic reaction, and they are not found in extramedullary haemangioblastomas or tumours in astrocyte free organ cultures.[31] Such observations have prompted suggestions that GFAP immunoreactivity in stromal cells may be due to passive uptake by non-glial tumour cells of extracellular protein derived from reactive astrocytes.[64,65] Some authors have emphasised the immunocytochemical heterogeneity of haemangioblastoma stromal cells[58,66] and suggested that only a proportion are true tumour cells, the remainder being reactive astrocytes which have undergone morphological transformation due to heavy lipidisation.[67,68] In either case, a true glial origin for haemangioblastomas currently seems unlikely, if not entirely excluded.

More recently, a neuroendocrine origin has been suggested, following reports of stromal cells showing immunocytochemical expression of various neuropeptides, including synaptophysin, somatostatin and substance P.[69,70] This has not been a consistent finding, however, and there is no other evidence to support a neuroendocrine lineage.[59]

Ultrastructural studies have tended to favour an angiogenic derivation of the tumour, despite initial suggestions that the capillary vessels were ultrastructurally normal and therefore not part of the tumour.[71] A number of studies have described endothelial cell features in some stromal cells[72,73] or even transitional forms between the two cell types,[74,75] suggesting that the stromal cells may either be vascular stem cells[75] or are perhaps derived directly from the capillary elements.[56] In support of this, endothelial transformation of stromal cells has been reported in vitro[76] and Weibel–Palade bodies have been described in stromal cells as well as in vascular endothelial cells of the tumour.[74,77] However, immunocytochemical studies have repeatedly shown the stromal cells to be antigenically distinct from endothelial cells, with no expression of factor VIII related antigen or *Ulex europaeus* agglutinin 1.[4,78] Those remaining in favour of an angiogenic origin have explained this by suggesting that the stromal cells are too undifferentiated or dedifferentiated to express endothelial antigens,[4,61] perhaps because they are mechanically excluded from forming vascular lumina by the presence of tumour basement membrane.[31]

Whatever their origin, there is now good evidence that the stromal cells are responsible for generating the rich neovascularisation seen in haemangioblastomas. They produce large amounts of both epidermal and vascular endothelial growth factors, which appear to interact with corresponding upregulated receptors on the tumour endothelial cells.[79,80]

Association with erythrocythaemia

Peripheral erythrocythaemia, often in excess of 180 g/l, is a recognised feature in patients with haemangioblastomas, and is present in about 40% of cases when the tumour is sited in the cerebellum.[3,27] It has also been reported in cases of supratentorial haemangioblastoma.[37,81] Erythrocythaemia is more common in cystic than solid tumours, although it may occur in either type.[27] Blood levels return to normal after excision of the tumour, unless this is incomplete or there are unsuspected multiple lesions.[27,82] In view of their common association with VHL disease, it should be noted that erythrocythaemia also occurs in up to 4% of renal carcinomas.[82] In haemangioblastomas, bioassay has shown greatly increased erythropoetic activity in the cyst fluid of up to 50% of cystic haemangioblastomas.[82,83] This increased activity is much less often found in cerebrospinal fluid (CSF) or serum[83,84] suggesting that the factor responsible is not always released from the tumour cyst.[83] Radioimmunoassay has confirmed that the factor produced by the tumour is erythropoietin, concentrated 1000-fold in the cyst fluid compared to serum.[85] However, the nature of the cells producing the erythropoietin is uncertain. Immunocytochemistry frequently demonstrates scattered cells in the tumours which react with antibodies to erythropoietin and renin substrate.[86] but at least some of these can be identified ultrastructurally as non-neoplastic mast cells.[87,88] In a smaller proportion of cases, positive staining cells which appear to be true tumour stromal cells have also been identified,[88] but it is not yet clear which cell type is responsible for the clinically active erythropoietin synthesis.

Clinical features

In the cerebellum, haemangioblastomas most frequently present with signs and symptoms of obstructive hydrocephalus and raised intracranial pressure.[12] There may also be clinical evidence of cerebellar dysfunction, such as nystagmus and cerebellar ataxia.[10] Cranial nerve palsies can occur, usually with involvement between the fifth and eighth cranial levels.[12,25] The duration of clinical history prior to presentation is typically between 6 months and 1 year, but in some cases symptoms may have been present for many years.[12,18] Where the tumour is sited in the medulla there is again usually evidence of raised intracranial pressure, but involvement of the floor of the fourth ventricle and the cervicomedullary junction may produce a variety of other signs and symptoms, including effortless vomiting, neurogenic hypertension, loss of involuntary respiratory drive and neck pain.[29]

In the spinal canal, extramedullary tumours are usually associated with early radicular pain because of spinal root involvement, whereas intramedullary lesions are more likely to present with increasing spastic paraparesis and a posterior column sensory deficit appropriate to the level of the tumour.[40] The associated syrinx cavities are often only manifest after radiological investigation or at autopsy examination.[38,40]

Supratentorial haemangioblastomas often resemble meningiomas in their clinical presentation.[12] Headache, epileptic seizures and alterations in mental state are all typical early manifestations, and depending on the precise site of the tumour there may also be localising deficits such as speech disturbance or hemiparesis.[37,89]

Rarely, either cerebellar or supratentorial haemangioblastomas may present acutely with intraparenchymal haemorrhage or bleeding into the subarachnoid space.[90,91] There are a number of anecdotal reports suggesting that pregnancy may precipitate the clinical presentation of haemangioblastomas,[18] possibly due to vascular engorgement of the tumour[92] or following a specific tumour growth response to raised progesterone levels.[93] In VHL disease, retinal haemangioblastomas may present with gradual deterioration of visual acuity or acute retinal detachment due to haemorrhage, and in some cases this can preceed the clinical manifestation of other neuraxis haemangioblastomas or systemic lesions[12,94] (see Chapter 19).

Radiology

Angiography has been the traditional radiological investigation of choice for intracranial haemangioblastoma, and remains an important diagnostic procedure despite the advent of computerised tomography (CT) and magnetic resonance imaging (MRI).[33,95] In addition to establishing the blood supply and vascular drainage of the tumour, angiography is a sensitive method of locating non-cystic examples[96] and allows detection of other, unsuspected tumours overlooked by localised scans.[12] For cystic tumours, CT allows precise definition of the cystic cavity and is often used in combination with angiography.[96,97] Solid tumours and mural tumour nodules are isodense with brain and not well seen in non-enhanced scans, but they show uniform, intense enhancement with intravenous contrast media.[12,97] MRI again allows good definition of tumour cysts, which are visible as well defined low signal areas, slightly hyperdense to CSF on T2-weighted images.[14,98] However, gadolinium administration is essential to identify the mural nodules of cystic lesions and to define the extent of solid tumours[14,99] (Fig. 14.2). MRI also allows visualisation of the larger abnormal vessels feeding and draining the tumour, which show as flow voids on T2-weighted images.[100] For spinal cord lesions, contrast enhanced CT allows good localisation[101] but the anatomical extent of the tumour and any associated syrinx cavity is more easily demonstrated using gadolinium enhanced MRI, which is now the investigation of choice for tumours at this site.[43,102]

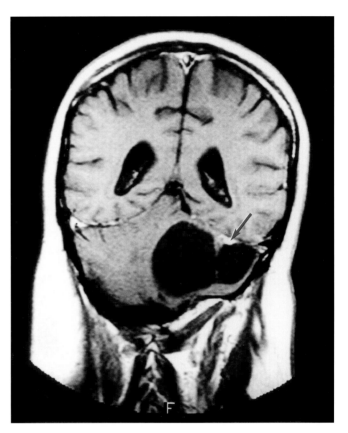

Fig. 14.2 **Haemangioblastoma**. Coronal T1-weighted MRI scan of a cystic posterior fossa example. A small mural nodule in the roof of the cyst is enhancing after administration of contrast material (arrow).

Pathology

Macroscopic features

Haemangioblastomas are well circumscribed red–brown tumours which may be totally intraparenchymal, partly extraparenchymal or entirely extra-axial (Fig. 14.3). The intraparenchymal tumours usually have a superficial margin at the pial surface, and this is often covered by ectatic and torturous superficial blood vessels. Supratentorial haemangioblastomas sometimes have a dural attachment and can grossly resemble meningiomas, especially when they are predominantly extraparenchymal. Intraventricular examples may appear macroscopically similar to ependymomas. In the spinal cord, extramedullary tumours are typically well defined masses growing out over the posterior surface of the cord, often with a foot-like extension into the cord parenchyma. They may also appear as discrete nodules attached to posterior nerve roots and can be multiple, especially in VHL disease. Something over two-thirds of haemangioblastomas at any site take the form of a large cystic cavity with a well defined, often quite small, mural nodule of haemorrhagic tumour embedded in the cyst wall.[18,40] The cyst usually contains yellow or rusty brown

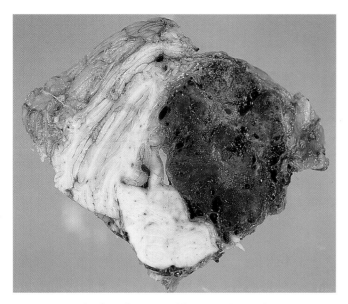

Fig. 14.3 **Posterior fossa haemangioblastoma**. This partly extraparenchymal, non-cystic tumour shows a typically variegated, red-brown cut surface and has well defined margins.

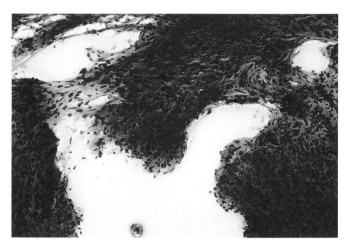

Fig. 14.4 **Haemangioblastoma**. Smear preparation. Swathes of tough and thickly smeared tumour tissue enclose irregular spaces. Foamy tumour cell cytoplasm is not usually apparent in smears, even at higher magnifications. Toluidine blue.

proteinaceus fluid which coagulates at room temperature. The cyst lining is smooth and opaque, and frequently shows haemorrhagic discolouration. In the spinal cord, the cysts are elongated syrinx cavities which may extend over several levels, both above and below the tumour. Both the solid tumours and mural nodules have a firm texture and very varied cut surface appearance (Fig. 14.3), with areas of old haemorrhage, numerous small cysts or blood filled cavernous spaces, and patchy yellow discolouration resulting from tumour lipidisation.

Intraoperative diagnosis

Haemangioblastomas are tough tumours and usually make rather unsatisfactory smear preparations. When smears are attempted, they are often quite thick and typically show elongated cells densely packed into broad trabeculae, which twist together to enclose irregular spaces (Fig. 14.4). The numerous blood vessels of the tumour are not very apparent. Individually smeared tumour cells with elongate, rather twisted nuclei may be visible in the spaces between the thickly smeared trabeculae, together with scattered haemosiderin laden macrophages. Occasional mast cells are also usually present, and contain brightly stained metachromatic granules if a toluidine blue stain us used. Foamy tumour cells are not usually identifiable. Smear preparations of haemangioblastomas can closely resemble those of meningeal haemangiopericytomas, and a definitive intra-operative diagnosis of haemangioblastoma is usually only possible using frozen sections, which reveal the vascular architecture and lipidised stromal cells typical of the tumour (Fig. 14.5).

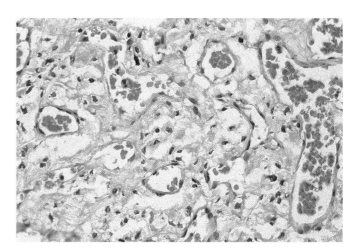

Fig. 14.5 **Haemangioblastoma**. Frozen sections are usually preferable to smears for intraoperative diagnosis, revealing the richly vascular architecture and intervascular stromal cells with small nuclei and abundant foamy or clear cytoplasm. H & E.

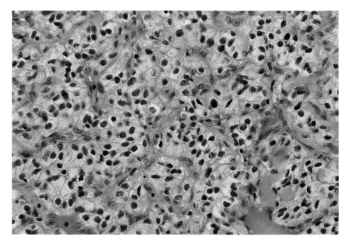

Fig. 14.6 **Haemangioblastoma**. Sheets of stromal cells with foamy cytoplasm are intersected by numerous capillary channels. H & E.

Fig. 14.7 **Haemangioblastoma**. The stromal cells in this tumour show marked pleomorphism, but there are no mitotic figures. H & E.

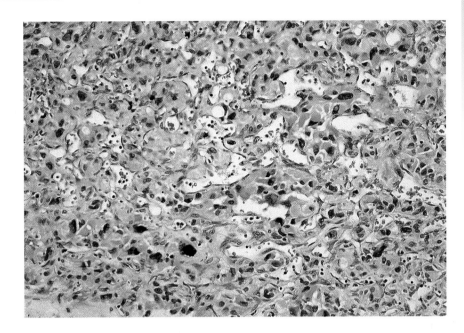

Fig. 14.8 **Haemangioblastoma**. Reticulin is forming a dense pericellular meshwork, in addition to outlining the vascular channels. Reticulin.

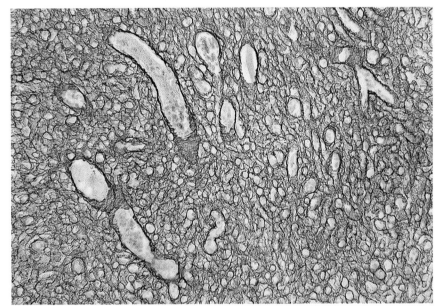

Histological features

Haemangioblastomas consist predominantly of an extensive meshwork of fine blood vessels and larger, sinusoidal, vascular spaces. They all have a capillary structure, with thin walls largely formed from plump endothelial cells. Between the vascular channels are variably abundant intervascular or stromal cells arranged in strands and packets (Fig. 14.6). These are large, rounded or polygonal cells with abundant cytoplasm and small, rounded, central or eccentrically placed nuclei. The cytoplasm may be pale and homogeneous, but is more often foamy in appearance and swollen by neutral lipid, which is sudanophil on frozen sections. There is some evidence that tumours without significant lipidisation of stromal cells tend to occur in a younger age group and are less often associated with erythrocythaemia.[27] The stromal cell nuclei may occasionally have a vacuolated appearance due to cytoplasmic invagination.[103] In some cases, pleomorphic, multinucleated or giant stromal cells may be found (Fig. 14.7), but mitotic figures are virtually never seen. Mast cells and phagocytes containing haemosiderin pigment are often intermingled with the stromal cells. Reticulin staining outlines the numerous capillaries and vascular channels, but usually there is also a dense pericellular reticulin meshwork surrounding individual stromal cells (Fig. 14.8). Occasionally, the tumours may show an architectural pattern more like that of para-

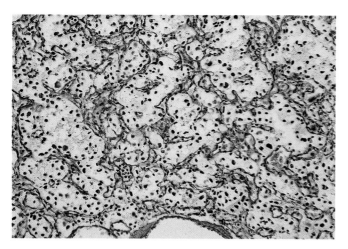

Fig. 14.9 **Haemangioblastoma**. In this example, reticulin is confined to blood vessel walls, creating a packeted appearance. Reticulin.

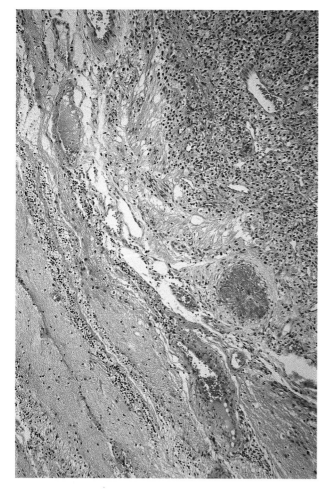

Fig. 14.10 **Haemangioblastoma**. The tumour is not encapsulated and merges with adjacent, gliotic cerebellar tissue towards the bottom left of the field. H & E.

gangliomas, with alveolar groups of stromal cells separated by flattened capillaries but not intersected by pericellular reticulin (Fig. 14.9).

Although grossly well demarcated, haemangioblastomas are not encapsulated and the tumour margins show infiltration of the adjacent leptomeninges and nervous tissue by proliferating capillary vessels (Fig. 14.10). In addition, there is usually quite florid reactive astrocytic proliferation and gliosis around the edges of the tumour, especially in cases with a long history, and entrapped islands of gliotic tissue may be identified quite deeply within the periphery of the tumour (see Immuno-cytochemistry, below). In some cases the astrocytic reaction may assume a neoplastic appearance in its own right, and it has been suggested this is the origin of some so-called 'angiogliomas'.[104] The cysts or spinal syrinx cavities are not formed from tumour tissue, but have a lining of densely matted gliotic tissue, often incorporating Rosenthal fibres and haemosiderin pigment (Fig. 14.11). They are thought to result from the accumulation of a tumour transudate, sometimes combined with the effects of recurrent haemorrhage.[18,40] Haemangioblastomas are low grade tumours and do not show intrinsic tumour necrosis or cytological evidence of malignancy, even in cases which are locally recurrent or in the rare examples which disseminate in the CSF pathways.[105]

Immunocytochemistry

Immunocytochemical staining for GFAP often shows reactive astrocytes trapped within the tumour, recognisable by their typical stellate morphology and irregular

Table 14.1   Haemangioblastoma: immunocytochemical staining

Epitope	Staining pattern
GFAP	Entrapped astrocytes (mostly marginal) Occasional stromal cells (faint)
S-100 protein	As for GFAP
Vimentin	Stromal cells
Neuron specific enolase	Stromal cells
Chromogranin	No staining
Polypeptide hormones	Variable
Cytokeratin	Usually no staining
Epithelial membrane antigen	No staining
Factor VIII related antigen	Vascular endothelial cells
Ulex europeus agglutinin 1	As for factor VIII

GFAP, glial fibrillary acidic protein

Fig. 14.11 **Haemangioblastoma**. In cystic tumours with a mural nodule, the cyst cavity is lined by densely matted, gliotic tissue. Numerous Rosenthal fibres are present. H & E.

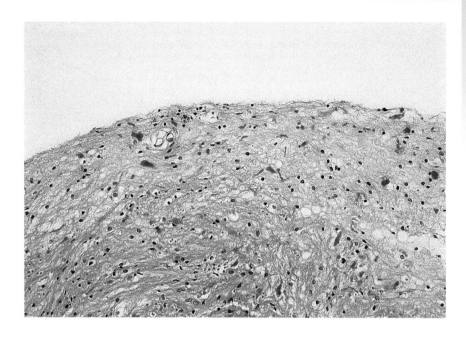

cell processes (Table 14.1).[60,78] They are mostly found near the tumour margins, adjacent to the surrounding gliotic nervous tissue, but may also be present deeper within the tumour.[54,61] In addition, a proportion of haemangioblastomas show scattered cells of stromal cell morphology which express both GFAP[43,62] and S-100 protein[55,58] (Fig. 14.12). These are again usually found near the gliotic margins of the tumour[65] and may be non-glial tumour cells which have absorbed extracellular protein leaked by adjacent reactive astrocytes,[64] or astrocytes which have been morphologically transformed by heavy lipidisation.[67,68] In either case it should be emphasised that these GFAP staining cells constitute only a small minority of the intervascular stromal cells in haemangioblastomas, and are only present in a proportion of cases, mostly those with a florid marginal gliotic reaction.[65] By contrast, the majority of stromal cells in most tumours react with antibodies to vimentin.[55,78] Stromal cells also consistently express neurone specific enolase (NSE) (Fig. 14.13),[106,107] although they do not stain for chromogranin.[54] There have been reports describing variable stromal cell immunoreactivity to a number of polypeptide hormones, including somatostatin and pancreatic polypeptide,[70] synaptophysin and substance P,[69,108] although this has not always been confirmed.[59]

In distinction from metastatic renal cell carcinoma, haemangioblastoma stromal cells are invariably unstained using antibodies to epithelial membrane antigen (EMA) and are not usually immunoreactive for cytokeratin,[54,107] although expression of the latter has occasionally been reported.[66] Antibodies to endothelial antigens such as *Ulex europeus* agglutinin 1 and factor VIII related antigen stain the endothelial cells lining the numerous vascular channels in the tumour, but not the stromal cells.[60,78] Antibodies to laminin show a different staining pattern to

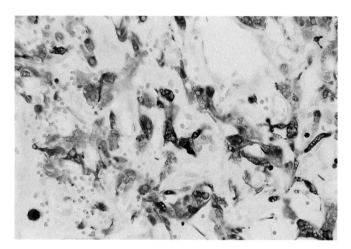

Fig. 14.12 **Haemangioblastoma**. This tumour contains cells with foamy cytoplasm and stromal cell morphology which stain strongly using immunocytochemistry for GFAP.

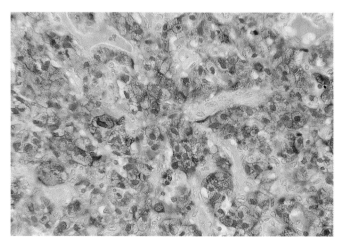

Fig. 14.13 **Haemangioblastoma**. The stromal cells stain consistently using immunocytochemistry for NSE.

that of reticulin impregnations, the reaction product being present only around the vascular channels and not in the intervascular spaces around stromal cells.[109] The wide spectrum of immunoreactivity of the stromal cells in haemangioblastomas has led to suggestions that they are a heterogeneous cell population,[58,66] and the results of immunocytochemistry need to be interpreted with care, particularly when using antibodies to GFAP and polypeptide hormones.

Electron microscopy

Numerous ultrastructural studies have established the presence of three main cell types in haemangioblastomas, with endothelial cells and pericytes forming the capillary channels and stromal cells arranged in between[76,110] (Fig. 14.14). The fine structure of the blood vessels is almost identical to that of normal capillaries. They are lined by a layer of endothelial cells, which are joined by elongated desmosome junctions and invested in a continuous outer basement membrane. Like normal capillary endothelial cells, their cytoplasm contains numerous pinocytotic vesicles and fine 7 nm filaments. The endothelial cells are surrounded by an incomplete layer of pericytes, which have a similar ultrastructural appearance but are not joined by desmosomes and are each enveloped by individual membranes. Although the relatively normal ultrastructure of the capillary channels has led some authors to conclude they are not an intrinsic element of the tumour,[71] the endothelial cells differ from those in non-neoplastic capillaries in showing membrane-bridged fenestrations.[71,111] Other reported abnormal features in the endothelial cell cytoplasm have included para-crystalline bodies,[112] giant pinocytotic vesicles[113] and embryonal type ciliary rootlets.[73]

The intervascular stromal cells have abundant electron lucent cytoplasm which contains a variable number of membrane bound lipid vascuoles separated by rather sparse organelles and glycogen granules. In some cases, there may also be prominent whorls of endoplasmic reticulum or annulate lamellae[71,75] (Fig. 14.14). The stromal cells generally lack endothelial features, but there are consistent reports of transitional forms showing isolated intercellular junctions, micropinocytotic vesicles and patchy basement membranes.[75,76] This suggests there may be a continuous morphological spectrum between the capillary lining cells and the intervascular stromal cells in haemangioblastomas.[56] In support of this, some studies have also described structures resembling endothelial cell Weibel–Palade bodies in the cytoplasm of some stromal cells.[74,77]

Proliferation indices

Analysis of cell replication in haemangioblastomas has confirmed the slow growth rate suggested by their

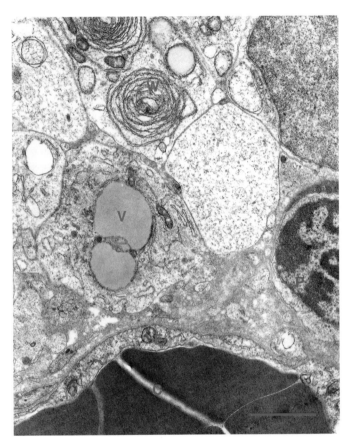

Fig. 14.14 **Haemangioblastoma**. The capillary channel (C) has a normal fine structure, with endothelial cells (E) surrounded by an incomplete layer of pericytes (P). The adjacent stromal cells contain lipid vacuoles (V) and whorls of endoplasmic reticulum (W). Electron micrograph. Bar = 2 μm.

benign histological features and relatively slow clinical evolution. Using the antibody Ki-67/MIB-1, which recognises cells in active phases of replication, less than 1% of haemangioblastoma cells are labelled, a rate which is similar to that found in benign meningiomas and Schwannomas.[114,115] A study of bromodeoxyuridine incorporation has reported a growth fraction slightly higher than that in Schwannomas, but still within the range seen in meningiomas and low grade glial tumours.[116]

Tissue culture

In tissue culture, haemangioblastomas produce strands or cords of proliferating endothelial cells growing out from the explant. These appear to represent rudimentary vascular buds, and have a branching pattern similar to that seen in the original tumour vessels.[117,118] Proliferating astrocytic and pial elements have also been described in the same cultures. One organ culture study has described the increasing development of basement membrane, micropinocytotic vesicles and intercellular junctions in association with cultured stromal cells, suggesting

Table 14.2 Haemangioblastoma: differential diagnosis

Meningeal haemangiopericytoma
Angiomatous meningioma
Metastatic renal cell carcinoma
Paraganglioma (cauda equina)
Angioglioma
Pilocytic astrocytoma (cyst wall)

progressive endothelial-like transformation and supporting the concept of a differentiating spectrum between the two cell types.[76]

Differential diagnosis

The main tumour types involved in the differential diagnosis of haemangioblastoma are listed in Table 14.2.

Meningeal haemangiopericytoma

Supratentorial haemangioblastomas may resemble meningeal haemangiopericytomas surgically and radiologically, especially if they are wholly or partly extraparenchymal and have a dural attachment. The intervascular cells of haemangiopericytomas differ from those in haemangioblastoma in showing a complete absence of lipidisation, and the vascular channels often have a distinctive staghorn pattern. Unlike haemangioblastomas, meningeal haemangiopericytomas usually show obvious high grade features, including a significant mitotic rate and foci of tumour necrosis. Immunocytochemical staining with antibodies to S-100 protein and GFAP may be confusing, especially near the reactive margins of either tumour, but expression of NSE may help to distinguish haemangioblastoma in many cases (Table 14.3).

Angiomatous meningioma

Many heavily vascularised meningiomas may undergo quite extensive xanthomatous change and thus show a superficial histological resemblance to haemangioblastomas. Unlike haemangioblastomas, however, they are always well encapsulated at their margins, and their vascular channels usually show prominent hyaline thickening. In addition, nests and whorls of typical meningothelial cells can nearly always be found in some areas of angiomatous meningiomas, even when they are heavily lipidised. Immunocytochemistry for NSE, GFAP and S-100 protein may all be useful in helping distinguish haemangioblastoma, especially since entrapped reactive glial elements are not usually found within the capsule of benign meningiomas (Table 14.3).

Metastatic renal cell carcinoma

Both renal cell carcinomas and haemangioblastomas occur in VHL disease, and a renal primary tumour may be clinically silent at the time of presentation of an intracranial metastasis. Particular care needs to be taken in patients presenting with a presumed recurrence from a previously treated tumour diagnosed as a haemangioblastoma. Mitoses and definite cytological evidence of malignancy may be hard to find in renal carcinoma metastases, and the vascular pattern is often similar to that of haemangioblastomas, although there is usually much less pericellular reticulin. Metastatic renal cell carcinoma is most easily distinguished by demonstrating immunocytochemical expression of epithelial antigens. EMA is not expressed by haemangioblastomas[119] and cytokeratin is confined to scattered stromal cells in a small proportion of cases.[66] An antibody to renal brush border antigen will also help to identify a renal metastasis where a positive result is obtained.

Paraganglioma

Solitary haemangioblastomas are well documented in the cauda equina region, but cannot be easily distinguished from paragangliomas arising at this site on clinical

Table 14.3 Distinguishing features of CNS vascular tumours

	Haemangiopericytoma	Haemangioblastoma	Angiomatous meningioma
Routine staining	Staghorn vascular pattern Mitoses Cytological atypia	Lipidisation of stromal cells Absence of malignant features	Hyalinised vessel walls Arachnoidal cells and whorls Absence of malignant features
Immunocytochemistry	NSE EMA ⎫ – no staining S-100 ⎬ GFAP ⎭	NSE – strains stromal cells EMA – no staining S-100 ⎫ – stain entrapped GFAP ⎬ glial elements and ⎭ some stromal cells	NSE – no staining EMA ⎫ – variable staining, S-100 ⎬ in some cases GFAP – no staining
Electron microscopy	Cytoplasmic filamentous densities Dense extracellular matrix No desmosomes	Cytoplasmic lipid vacuoles No desmosomes	Cytoplasmic interdigitations Desmosomes

EMA, epithelial membrane antigen; GFAP, glial fibrillary acidic protein; NSE, neuron specific enolase

grounds. The distinctive reticulin packeting of para-ganglioma cells is useful in most cases, but some haemangioblastomas can show a very similar pattern, with groups of stromal cells which lack pericellular reticulin and are enclosed by fine, flattened capillaries. Immunocytochemically, antibodies to NSE are unhelpful as both tumours show consistent positive staining of intervascular cells. Many of the neuroendocrine antigens found in paragangliomas have also been demonstrated in occasional stromal cells of some haemangioblastomas. Unlike paragangliomas, however, haemangioblastomas do not show immunoreactivity to chromogranin, and this should be the mainstay of the differential diagnosis between the two lesions.

Astrocytoma

Where a florid astrocytic reaction extends deeply in from the margins of a haemangioblastoma, the appearances can be difficult to distinguish from those of a heavily vascularised astrocytic tumour (angioglioma), especially if there is lipidisation of the astrocytic tumour cells.[104,120] However, angioglial tumours do not usually show the prominent pericellular reticulin meshwork seen in most haemangioblastomas and can also be distinguished by their lack of immunoreactivity to NSE. Immuno-cytochemical staining for GFAP and S-100 protein may be misleading, because the entrapped glial elements in some haemangioblastomas can be widespread and some stromal cells may express both these antigens.

A differential diagnosis of astrocytoma also needs to be considered when a cyst wall is biopsied in the absence of a radiologically or surgically identifiable mural tumour nodule. The tissue lining haemangioblastoma cysts may be difficult to distinguish from a low grade or pilocytic astrocytoma, although it is usually less cellular, more densely matted together and often contains more abundant haemosiderin pigment than expected in astrocytomas. Analysis of the cyst fluid may be useful in these circumstances, because haemangioblastoma cysts quite often contain detectable levels of erythro-poietin, even when there is no clinical evidence of erythrocythaemia.

Therapy

Surgical resection has been the traditional treatment of choice for solitary haemangioblastomas,[10,12] and modern microsurgical techniques have made this increasingly possible even in difficult sites such as the medulla and spinal cord.[29,121] For cystic tumours, the mural nodule must be identified and completely removed or the cyst will quickly recur,[10,12] but the cyst wall is not part of the tumour and does not need to be excised.[10,18] The removal of non-cystic tumours is more difficult, and in some cases the excision may have to be subtotal in order to safeguard

against increased surgical morbidity and mortality.[12,18] Preoperative radiotherapy[122] or embolisation[123] is some-times used to try and shrink the vascular supply of the tumour and aid the surgical resection. More recently, gamma knife radiosurgery has been shown to halt or reverse tumour growth in a high proportion of hae-mangioblastomas, and has been used successfully both as primary treatment and following subtotal surgical resection.[124,125] Where there are multiple haemangio-blastomas at presentation each case needs to be judged on its own merits, although one lesion is usually clinically dominant and excision of the others is likely to depend largely on surgical accessibility and their level of clinical symptomatology.[18] Radiosurgery is a particularly useful alternative to surgery in these circumstances, allowing treatment of multiple lesions in a single session with low morbidity.[124] In view of the frequency with which apparently solitary haemangioblastomas are associated with the subsequent development of multiple neuraxial lesions or renal carcinomas, all cases need to be thoroughly investigated for other systemic or nervous system manifestations at the time of initial presentation, and carefully followed up for a prolonged period.[50,52]

Prognosis

The long term prognosis is most favourable following successful, complete excision of the mural nodule from cystic cerebellar or supratentorial haemangioblastomas, where 5-year survival rates of up to 90% have been quoted.[12,18] There is now a negligible surgical mortality rate in such cases[61] and patients often die eventually from causes unrelated to the tumour.[12] The clinical relapse rate following apparently complete resection of an isolated haemangioblastoma is about 15%,[50,94] although this rises to over 25% of cases if there is evidence of multiple neuraxial lesions or VHL disease at the time of first presentation.[126] In some instances, clinical deterioration after total removal of a single tumour is due to a genuine local recurrence, and this may occur after many years.[127] In many cases, however, the subsequent clinical deterio-ration is due to the development of further primary tumours.[25,128] These may be multiple and at different sites from the original tumour, and again can take over a decade to become clinically manifest.[129] The development of multiple tumours is associated with a less favourable prognosis, largely due to the increased morbidity and mortality of repeated surgical interventions.[18]

Where excision of a solitary tumour has been incomplete, early recurrence of symptoms due to further tumour growth or cyst reaccumulation is to be expected in over half of the cases.[12,122] The overall mortality rate in this group of patients is also something over 50%, the majority of deaths being directly related to tumour recurrence or its treatment.[12,130] In occasional partially excised cases, however, there may be a long period of clinical remission, with 5 years or more before relapse due to local recurrence of tumour.[122]

Haemangioblastomas of the medulla have a rather poor prognosis compared to those at other sites, partly because they are usually solid and thus difficult to excise completely[18,131] and partly because of the risk of postoperative brain stem disturbances, especially the loss of involuntary respiratory drive.[132] Up to one-third of these cases may die due to early tumour recurrence or immediate postoperative complications.[30,133] Successful, total excision of brain stem haemangioblastomas has been reported, however, and those cases surviving the perioperative period can expect a good outcome in the longer term.[134] The prognosis in intramedullary spinal cord haemangioblastomas is also closely related to the success and completeness of surgical excision.[50] In many cases, total removal of the tumour is possible with the help of high resolution MR scanning and microsurgical techniques,[135] but preoperative clinical deficits persist in a proportion of cases because irreversible damage to the spinal cord parenchyma has already occurred by the time of surgery.[121]

Meningeal haemangiopericytoma

Meningeal haemangiopericytomas are closely related to haemangiopericytomas arising in systemic tissues and are now usually regarded as distinct from primary meningeal tumours of arachnoidal origin.[136,137] This separation is of more than just academic importance because of the aggressive biological behaviour and relatively poor prognosis of meningeal haemangiopericytomas compared to most meningiomas.[7,8] There has been much controversy in the past, however, and if the older literature is consulted it should be noted that these haemangiopericytomas were originally thought to be a variant of meningioma, and referred to variously as 'angioblastic' or 'haemangiopericytic' meningiomas.[5,7,138] The current WHO classification has entirely relinquished these terms, and groups cranial and spinal haemangiopericytomas with other malignant, non-meningothelial neoplasms which may arise in the leptomeninges.[1]

Incidence and site

Meningeal haemangiopericytomas account for 2–5% of all meningeal tumours.[139,140] They show a similar age distribution to that of haemangiopericytomas in extracranial sites, the majority of cases occurring in young adulthood and middle age.[140,141] There is a peak incidence between about 30 and 50 years of age[142] and the mean age at diagnosis has consistently been quoted as around 40 years.[136,143] Rarely, the tumour may present in infants[31,144]

and in some of these cases the history may suggest a congenital onset of tumour growth.[145,146] There is a consistent, but rather slight excess of male cases.[142,143]

Haemangiopericytomas may occur anywhere in the CNS, but they are usually related to the meninges and their distribution is similar to that of typical meningiomas.[143,147] The majority of cases are intracranial, where they most frequently arise in the parasagittal region near the vertex, over a cerebral convexity or at the skull base in the middle cranial fossa.[142] Tentorial and posterior fossa examples are rather less common.[142,148] The tumours are nearly all extraparenchymal and usually attached to the inner aspect of the dura,[147,148] although intraventricular examples have been reported, presumably arising in the choroid plexus.[149] Rare cranial sites include the pituitary fossa,[150] the pineal region[151] and the orbit, in relation to the optic nerve sheath.[152] About 7% of all cases are spinal in location[142] and these can be extramedullary, intradural lesions[153,154] or primarily extradural in origin.[155] Very rarely, intramedullary examples have also been described.[156] Although any spinal level may be involved, both intradural and extradural tumours are most frequent in the cervical and upper thoracic regions.[154,155]

Aetiology

Like their systemic counterparts, meningeal haemangiopericytomas are thought to take origin from differentiated vascular pericytes.[157] Electron microscopy of the meningeal tumours has demonstrated close ultrastructural similarities with the cells of systemic haemangiopericytomas.[158,159] Pericytes are closely related to smooth muscle cells and the ultrastructural evidence of leiomyoblastic differentiation found in both systemic and meningeal haemangiopericytomas is felt to be particularly suggestive of an origin from pericytes.[158,160] Immunocytochemistry again emphasises the similarity of meningeal haemangiopericytomas with their systemic counterparts, and most studies have failed to demonstrate EMA expression, as expected in meningiomas of arachnoidal cell origin.[55,159] Tissue culture has provided further evidence of both smooth muscle differentiation and a pericyte origin of the tumour.[161,162] The distinction from true meningiomas is underlined by cytogenetic studies, since both systemic and meningeal haemangiopericytomas lack the *NF2* gene alterations typical of meningiomas.[163] Furthermore, meningeal haemangiopericytomas have been found to show deletion of the *CDKN2A* gene, an alteration not found in meningiomas.[164] Claims of tumours showing a transition between haemangiopericytoma and typical meningioma[8,148] have not been substantiated in our clinical practice, although it remains theoretically possible that both arachnoidal cells and pericytes may arise from a common pluripotential mesenchymal stem cell.[31]

Clinical features

The clinical presentation of meningeal haemangio-pericytomas is similar to that of meningiomas at equivalent sites, although the history is often shorter and usually of only a few months duration.[7,12] In intracranial cases, the most common presenting complaint is headache.[12,136] Other clinical features often reflect the precise location of the tumour and may include focal seizures and paresis.[136] Spinal tumours typically present with increasing spastic paraparesis and sensory disturbance at an appropriate anatomical level.[154] In the cervical region there may also be upper limb deficits[154] and lumbosacral examples often cause low back pain with buttock or sciatic radiation.[165] Although they are very vascular tumours, CNS haemangiopericytomas have only very rarely been reported as presenting with acute haemorrhage.[166]

Radiology

Angiography remains an important part of preoperative assessment, if only to identify major feeding vessels.[167] Features which suggest a haemangiopericytoma rather than meningioma include rapid tumour filling, a dense, long lasting tumour blush and prominent, sinusoidal or corkscrew-like tumour vessels.[12,168] The appearances using CT are usually similar to those of meningiomas,[12] with strong enhancement after administration of contrast media and quite well defined tumour margins.[12,169] Irregularity of the margins, non-homogeneity of enhancement and the absence of calcification are all features more suggestive of haemangiopericytoma than meningioma, but are by no means specific for this diagnosis.[142,168] Using MRI, haemangiopericytomas again appear similar to meningiomas and enhance strongly after administration of gadolinium.[170]

Pathology

Macroscopic features

Haemangiopericytomas are firm, rounded and nodular tumours which have a very similar gross appearance to meningiomas. The majority are superficial lesions attached to the inner aspect of the dura, although their dural attachment is often broad compared to that of many typical meningiomas. They are mostly well circumscribed lesions, but there is not infrequently macroscopic evidence of infiltration into nervous system parenchyma. The external features are those of a highly vascular tumour, reddish in colour, and the texture is usually solid on cut section, without cysts, large vascular spaces or evidence of calcification.

Intraoperative diagnosis

Using smear preparations, haemangiopericytomas appear as highly cellular tumours, often with a loosely papillary

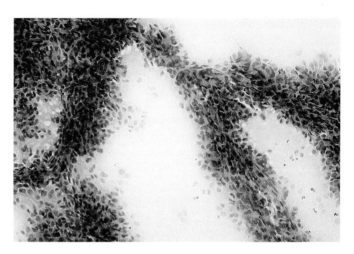

Fig. 14.15 Meningeal haemangiopericytoma. Smear preparation. The tumour is highly cellular and smears in a loose papillary pattern. The rich vasculature is less apparent than in paraffin sections. Toluidine blue.

pattern (Fig. 14.15). This is due to the tendency of tumour cells to cling to blood vessels, although it must be emphasised that the rich vasculature of the tumour is much less apparent in smears than in paraffin or frozen sections. The cells are densely aggregated and have ovoid or angulated, hyperchromatic nuclei. Mitotic figures are easily found in nearly all cases. The cell cytoplasm is scanty and ill defined, and individual cell boundaries are hard to identify, even where the tissue is more thinly smeared. Whorls are not present and the tumour is usually distinguishable from typical meningiomas on smear preparations. In cases of difficulty, H & E stained frozen sections will usually reveal the typical vascular architecture of the tumour, although it may also be helpful if a rapid reticulin preparation can be performed to outline the dense, pericellular reticulin pattern.

Histological features

The high cellularity of haemangiopericytomas is again apparent in paraffin sections. The tumour cells have an irregular, polygonal shape with ill-defined cytoplasmic margins and they are densely packed together in sheets (Fig. 14.16). There is no impression of a spindle cell or fascicular pattern and arachnoidal type cell whorls are absent. A looser, whorled arrangement of cells has been reported, but only in very occasional cases.[165] The tumour cell nuclei differ from those in most meningiomas in being flattened, angular and hyperchromatic. Mitoses are frequent in all cases (Fig. 14.17). The sheets of tumour cells are intersected by a rich meshwork of thin walled vascular channels lined by a single layer of flattened endothelial cells. Some of these channels are large and sinusoidal in pattern, often with a deeply indented, 'staghorn' profile[171] (Fig. 14.18). Many, however, are small, slit-like capillary structures, which are difficult to

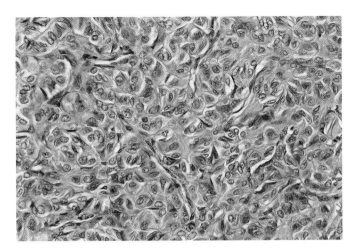

Fig. 14.16 **Meningeal haemangiopericytoma**. Sheets of irregular, polygonal cells are intersected by numerous, small, slit-like vascular channels. H & E.

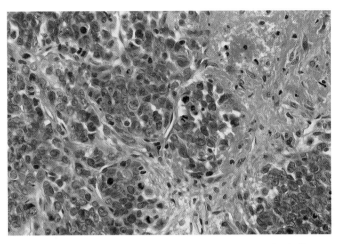

Fig. 14.17 **Meningeal haemangiopericytoma**. Numerous mitotic figures are visible and there is an area of tumour necrosis. H & E.

Fig. 14.18 **Meningeal haemangiopericytoma**. Larger vascular channels frequently have a deeply indented 'staghorn' profile, like those in the centre of this field. H & E.

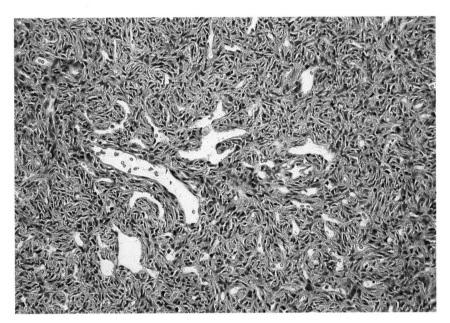

appreciate on routine stains but clearly outlined by reticulin impregnations. In most cases there is a dense meshwork of pericellular reticulin between the vascular channels, although this can vary in prominence in different areas of tumour (Fig. 14.19). Very occasionally, the tumours may show a prominent papillary architecture, with tumour cells arranged around fibrovascular stalks containing thick walled or hyalinised central blood vessels.[172] Meningeal haemangiopericytomas are encapsulated tumours which are initially separated from the underlying nervous parenchyma by a layer of collagenous tissue formed from altered leptomeninges. However, tumour tissue often extends into the dura in the area of macroscopic attachment, and in some cases there may also be extensive histological infiltration of the adjacent brain or spinal cord.

Immunocytochemistry

The immunocytochemical staining profile of CNS haemangiopericytomas is identical to that of their systemic counterparts.[55,159] The endothelial lectin *Ulex europeus* agglutinin 1 and factor VIII related antigen are both expressed by the endothelial cells lining the vascular channels, but not by the tumour cells in between[55,173] (Fig. 14.20). The tumour cells may express the endothelial antigen CD34, but only in about one-third of cases and in a weak and patchy fashion.[174] They react more consistently with antibodies to vimentin[55,174] (Fig. 14.21) but do not immunostain using antibodies to GFAP.[55,162] In contrast to haemangioblastomas, GFAP stained, entrapped astrocytic elements are not normally a feature of haemangiopericytomas, except at the margins of

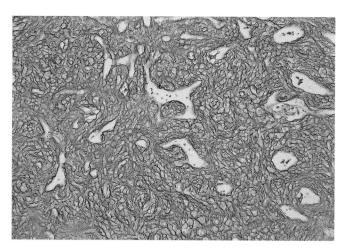

Fig. 14.19 **Meningeal haemangiopericytoma**. There is a dense meshwork of pericellular reticulin between the vascular channels. Reticulin.

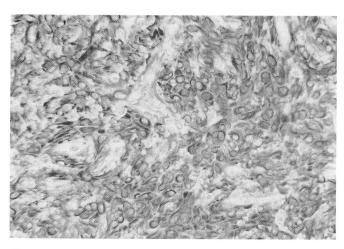

Fig. 14.21 **Meningeal haemangiopericytoma**. The tumour cells between the vascular channels stain consistently using immunocytochemistry for vimentin.

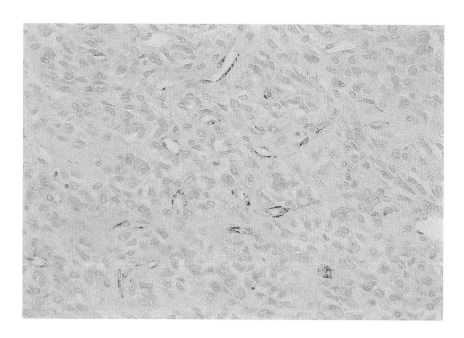

Fig. 14.20 **Meningeal haemangiopericytoma**. Immunocytochemistry for factor VIII related antigen stains the endothelial cells lining vascular channels but not the tumour cells in between.

those cases more extensively infiltrating nervous parenchyma. The tumour cells differ from those of most meningiomas in being uniformly unreactive with antibodies to S-100 protein[55,162] and EMA.[140,159] In most studies, there has been no immunocytochemical expression of cytokeratins,[15,159] but occasional positive staining cells have been described in a small proportion of reported cases.[174,175] Despite the ultrastructural evidence suggesting leiomyoblastic differentiation in these tumours, no tumour cell reactivity with antibodies to actin has been found[108] and expression of desmin is rare and focal.[174] Immunocytochemical expression of laminin is restricted to vascular basement membranes, and does not parallel the pericellular distribution of reticulin.[109,173]

Electron microscopy

Ultrastructurally, the appearances are again essentially similar to those of haemangiopericytomas arising in systemic tissues.[157] The tumour cells have polymorphic nuclei and electron lucent cytoplasm containing generally rather sparse organelles but prominent bundles of fine, 5–8 nm diameter microfilaments[158] (Fig. 14.22). In many cases these filaments are drawn into multiple, granular, electron dense condensations, both centrally and on the inner aspect of the cytoplasmic membranes.[162,176] Together with a tendency for juxtanuclear polarisation of organelles, these filamentous condensations have been interpreted as evidence of leiomyoblastic differentiation.[160,177] Pinocytotic vesicles have been observed in the tumour cells in some cases, but are not a consistent feature.[158] The tumour cells lack the desmosomes typical of meningiomas[177] and the only intercellular junctions present are occasional examples of the zonula adherentes type.[160] In most areas the cells are separated by patchy but often abundant, amorphous, electron dense extracellular matrix resembling basement membrane material.[160,162] This merges with distinct perivascular basement membranes, but between the tumour cells it takes the form of irregular masses and does not form a discrete membranous layer.[158] The numerous vascular channels have a largely normal ultrastructural appearance, although the endothelial cells show membrane bridged fenestrations.[56,178] Occasional pericytes are present outside the endothelial basement membranes of larger vessels, and these are separated from the tumour cells by their own intact basement membranes.[160]

Proliferation indices

Studies using the antibody Ki67 (MIB-1), which recognises actively replicating cells, have reported a proliferation

rate of anything between 9% and over 30% of cells in meningeal haemangiopericytomas.[179,180] This is similar to the rate found in high grade malignant gliomas, and contrasts with a figure of less than 1% of cells in typical meningiomas.[180] Silver staining of nucleolar organising regions (AgNors) in tumour cell nuclei has demonstrated a mean AgNor count per cell of over two, which is similar to that found in anaplastic meningiomas but significantly higher than in non-recurrent meningeal tumours.[181] Such studies support the clinical evidence that craniospinal haemangiopericytomas are biologically malignant tumours and further emphasises the need to recognise them as distinct from other types of meningeal tumour.[8,31]

Tissue culture

Cultured meningeal haemangiopericytomas have consistently shown a rapid and vigorous outgrowth from the explants, with a high mitotic rate.[148,162] In most studies the whorls typical of cultured meningiomas have not been seen,[161,162] although they were described in one early report.[138] Electron microscopy of the cultured cells has demonstrated pinocytotic vesicles and cytoplasmic filaments forming focal condensations[161,162] which have again been interpreted as evidence of smooth muscle differentiation.[162] In contrast to typical meningiomas, haemangiopericytic tumours do not form desmosomes in culture, intercellular junctions being represented only by occasional zonulae adherentes.[161] One study has described electron dense granular material in the extracellular space of in vitro specimens, similar to that seen in uncultured tumour tissue.[148] This material became more abundant with increasing time in culture until almost every cell was separately invested, suggesting that the tumour cells may be inherently capable of true basement membrane production.

Differential diagnosis

Haemangioblastoma

Supratentorial examples of haemangioblastoma may occasionally show a macroscopic resemblance to haemangiopericytomas, especially when they are non-cystic and attached to the dura. Histologically, haemangiopericytomas can be distinguished by their typical vascular pattern of slit-like capillaries and 'staghorn' sinusoids. They also lack the xanthomatous change frequently present in haemangioblastoma stromal cells. A high degree of mitotic activity is another important distinction and is never found in haemangioblastomas. Immunocytochemically, the most useful antibody is likely to be one recognising NSE, which is not found in haemangiopericytomas but is consistently expressed by haemangioblastoma stromal cells (Table 14.3, p. 393).

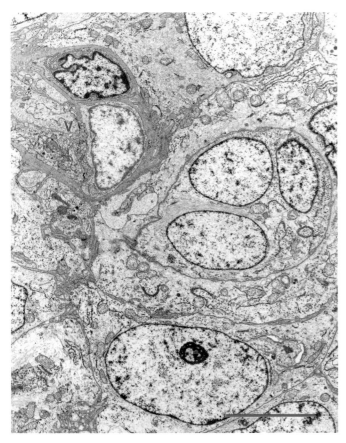

Fig. 14.22 **Meningeal haemangiopericytoma**. Ultrastructurally, the tumour cells have electron lucent cytoplasm containing sparse bundles of fine microfilaments. Electron dense intercellular matrix merges with the basal lamina material around a cross-cut vascular channel (V). Electron micrograph. Bar = 6 μm.

Angiomatous meningioma

These lesions are unlikely to be confused with haemangiopericytomas except perhaps on account of their prominent vascularity and meningeal location. They differ histologically from haemangiopericytomas in showing a low cellularity with no evidence of malignancy and a pronounced tendency to hyalinisation of vessel walls. In virtually all cases clumps of typical meningothelial cells can be found between the vascular channels, and in further distinction from haemangiopericytomas these intervascular cells may sometimes show immunocytochemical expression of S-100 protein or EMA.

Angiosarcoma

Although rare in the CNS, angiosarcomas may occur in a meningeal location and can be distinguished from haemangiopericytomas by the same criteria as in systemic sites. Most significantly, the vascular endothelial cells in haemangiopericytomas differ in having a normal, flattened morphology in paraffin sections, whereas the vascular lining cells inside the perivascular reticulin sheaths of angiosarcomas are neoplastic cells with atypical cytological features. In many cases these cells are not only rounded and pleomorphic, but are heaped up into solid papillary formations. Between the vessels, the stromal cells of haemangiopericytomas consistently form solid, epithelioid sheets, contrasting with the spindle celled, fascicular architecture typical of many angiosarcomas. Immunocytochemically, the two tumours can usually be distinguished using an antibody to factor VIII related antigen, which is expressed by intervascular cells in most angiosarcomas, and not just those surrounding vascular lumina.

Therapy

The primary treatment of choice for meningeal haemangiopericytomas is radical tumour resection at first operation.[12,142] A complete surgical removal of the tumour has a beneficial effect on survival[143,181] and is possible at favourable sites when a good surgical plane is present between the tumour capsule and the adjacent brain.[182] In a significant proportion of cases, however, total resection is not feasible because of widespread tumour infiltration of nervous parenchyma or extradural tissues.[136,183] Surgery may also be hindered by excessive intraoperative tumour haemorrhage, which can be difficult to control.[12] Both preoperative tumour embolisation[184,185] and prior irradiation[186] have been reported to be useful in reducing intraoperative bleeding and facilitating radical surgery. Postoperative radiotherapy has been shown to increase survival in several studies[143,147] and is advocated particularly where only partial resection has been possible.[185] In view of the high recurrence rate, some authorities recommend adjunct radiotherapy even after complete surgical excision.[142] Radiosurgery is claimed to produce dramatic, early shrinkage of small and medium sized intracranial haemangiopericytomas, and the gamma knife has been used successfully to control both new lesions and tumours which have recurred after surgery.[187]

Prognosis

Meningeal haemangiopericytomas are locally invasive tumours which can widely infiltrate adjacent nervous parenchyma, extradural connective tissue and bone.[183] They also have a marked tendency to recur locally after surgery, and the recurrence rate is much higher than that associated with either typical meningiomas[188] or haemangiopericytomas in systemic sites.[189] In some cases clinical relapse is associated with incomplete surgical excision, but recurrences may occur even when there has been an apparently complete removal of the lesion.[136] In either case, the development of clinical and radiological evidence of recurrence may be delayed for many years after first operation[190] and in one study the mean interval before relapse was 4 years.[142] Multiple, successive episodes of local tumour regrowth spanning a decade or more are by no means uncommon.[191,192] Reported series with long term follow-up have quoted a recurrence rate of between 65[143] and 80%[184] at 5 years after surgery, but this may rise to over 90% in patients surviving up to 15 years.[142] Metastatic spread to systemic sites is the other major complication of meningeal haemangiopericytomas, which show a similar metastatic potential to their systemic counterparts.[141] Common sites include lung, liver and bone,[143,147] including the spinal column,[190] pancreas[193] and kidneys.[194] As with local recurrences, distant metastases may develop after apparently complete removal of the primary tumour[136,190] and are increasingly likely to occur with more prolonged survival times.[142] Disease free intervals of up to 15 years have been reported before metastatic spread becomes clinically manifest,[190,193] and the mean interval from the time of first surgery to metastasis in large studies has consistently been more than 8 years.[136,142] In one series with longer follow-up, the incidence of postoperative metastatic spread rose to over 60% of cases after 15 years.[143]

In larger series, the overall mean survival from the time of diagnosis has been about 7 years.[136,143] Approximately three-quarters of deaths have been associated with local recurrences and one-quarter with systemic metastatic spread.[12] Although the initial survival rate of around two-thirds at 5 years is optimistic, this figure rapidly decreases with time and only about one-fifth of all cases can expect to survive for more than 15 years after the initial surgery.[142,143] Attempts have been made to predict the survival pattern on the basis of the histological appearance of the tumour,[147] but as with systemic haemangiopericytomas, there is no convincing evidence that the craniospinal lesions can be subclassified in this way.[189]

Miscellaneous vascular tumours

Angiosarcoma

Tissue with the histological features of angiosarcoma is most frequently encountered in the CNS as part of a gliosarcoma (see also Chapter 4). The sarcomatous part of these lesions often has a prominent and atypical vascular component, with secondary anaplastic changes in the vascular endothelial cells. In addition, the sarcomatous cells outside these vessels may express endothelial markers such as *Ulex europeus* agglutinin 1 and factor VIII related antigen.[195] The gliomatous and sarcomatous elements of gliosarcomas can be widely segregated in some cases, and a careful search for associated glial tumour is therefore necessary in any putative case of primary intracranial angiosarcoma.[31] Intracranial metastases from primary systemic angiosarcomas have also been reported,[196] and the possibility of a primary extracranial tumour must also be kept in mind in these circumstances.

Rarely, true angiosarcomas may arise de novo within the CNS, where they show a spectrum of histological and immunocytochemical features similar to those seen in their systemic counterparts.[197,198] Intracranial examples are often extraparenchymal lesions, apparently arising in the leptomeninges, but can also occur in deeper, predominantly intracerebral sites.[198] Those arising in the spine are again mostly extramedullary in location, although the spinal cord parenchyma may be secondarily infiltrated.[199,200] Reported cases have ranged in age from infancy to over 70 years.[198] Exposure to industrial solvents[201] and old surgical scarring[200] have both been anecdotally invoked as aetiological factors. The outcome following surgery has usually been poor for these tumours, with patients succumbing to local recurrence or systemic metastases,[198,202] but long term survival has been described in some cases following complete surgical excision.[198] Exceptionally, angiosarcomas may occur as primary tumours of peripheral nerves,[200,203] and focal angiomatous differentiation in more typical malignant peripheral nerve sheath tumours has also been described.[204] In either case, the development of angiosarcoma in the peripheral nervous system is most likely to occur in the context of von Recklinghausen's disease.[31,204]

Epithelioid haemangioendothelioma

This distinctive tumour was originally described in systemic sites in 1982.[205] Although found mostly in lung, liver or systemic soft tissues,[206,207] very rare examples have been reported in craniospinal locations.[208,209] Some of these have been extradural tumours, either cranially or in the spinal column,[209] but others have been intracerebral.[208,209] The histological appearances have been the same as for the systemic examples, with solid cords or nests of plump, epithelioid cells surrounded by reticulin sheaths and embedded in a myxoid background matrix.[208,209] The tumour cells typically show intracytoplasmic lumina, and larger, multicellular vascular channels are not a prominent feature. In some cases epithelioid haemangioendotheliomas may appear histologically similar to metastatic adenocarcinoma,[205] but they can be distinguished by an absence of cytokeratin expression and positive immunostaining of the tumour cells with antibodies to *Ulex europeus* agglutinin 1 and factor VIII related antigen.[209] The biological behaviour of these tumours is said to be intermediate between benign angiomas and angiosarcomas.[207]

Kaposi's sarcoma

This tumour is exceptionally uncommon in the CNS, and has only been described in patients suffering from AIDS.[210,211] The reported cases have almost invariably harboured similar systemic lesions, and the tumour should usually be regarded as metastatic when encountered in craniospinal locations in these patients.[210]

Melanocytic and soft tissue tumours

Melanocytic neoplasms

Melanocytes are present in small numbers within the pia mater around the base of the brain, particularly the ventral medulla and the upper cervical spinal cord. In caucasians, melanocytic pigmentation of the leptomeninges is seldom visible on macroscopic examination, but in normal dark skinned individuals faint pigmentation is occasionally visible to the naked eye in the leptomeninges over the ventral brain stem, upper cervical spinal cord and inferior frontotemporal lobes. Increased numbers of leptomeningeal melanocytes can occur in a variety of circumstances, accompanied by meningeal pigmentation on naked eye examination, for example during normal pregnancy and to a greater extent in neurocutaneous melanosis. In this disorder, neoplastic transformation of melanocytes in the meninges can result in diffuse melanocytosis, in which the neoplastic cells infiltrate throughout the subarachnoid space and can invade the underlying parenchyma.[212] More circumscribed melanocytic tumours, the melanocytoma and malignant melanoma, also rise in the meninges. Proliferations of CNS melanocytic cells may therefore occur in a variety of conditions and can result in benign or malignant melanocytic neoplasms which can be either diffuse or circumscribed; these will be considered under two major categories.

1. Diffuse melanocytic lesions – neurocutaneous melanosis

This unusual condition can present with a wide spectrum of clinical features, which have been encapsulated in diagnostic criteria initially proposed in 1972 and subsequently modified in 1991.[212] Neurocutaneous melanosis is described in Chapter 19.

2. Focal melanocytic lesions – meningeal melanocytoma

Incidence and clinical features

This is a circumscribed melanocytic tumour which is extremely uncommon, accounting for <0.1% of CNS tumours, but has probably been under-reported in the past; some of the earlier cases were described as a cellular blue naevus[213] and it is likely that confusion with melanotic Schwannomas and meningiomas has also occurred.[214] Melanocytomas occur across a wide age range in adults with a tendency to occur in the fifth decade, affecting females more often than males.[215–217] Two cases have been reported in association with ipsilateral oculodermal melanocytosis (congenital nevus of Ota).[218,219] Caucasians appear to be more likely to affected by melanocytomas than other races. These tumours present with signs and symptoms related to their site of origin and effects on adjacent structures, with myeloradiculopathy and cerebellar abnormalities most often recorded.[215–237] Supratentorial cases may present with seizures,[231] and one spinal melanocytoma presented with superficial siderosis of the CNS which resolved after the lesion was resected.[13] Neuroradiological studies show that melanocytomas appear isodense with grey matter of the brain on CT scans (Fig. 4.23), but show uniform enhancement after contast administration.[237] Melanocytomas are hyperintense on T1-weighted MRI scans and hypointense on T2-weighted MRI scans.[236]

Pathology

Melanocytomas usually occur as solid masses in the cranial or spinal compartments, particularly in the posterior fossa (in the region of the foramen magnum) and in the thoracic spinal canal, forming a dumb-bell shaped tumour situated in the region of the spinal nerve roots. Supratentorial lesions have been reported,[219,221,223,225,231] including a case in the region of the pineal gland.[220] Melanocytomas are predominantly dural based and grow as well circumscribed masses which may well be confused clinically with meningiomas.[217,222,226] The tumours are solitary and often encapsulated, with a striking degree of pigmentation which may vary from black to dark blue or a red–brown appearance depending on the

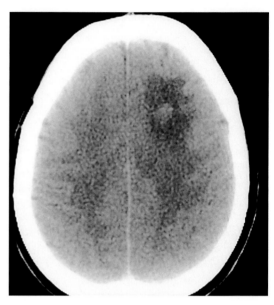

Fig. 14.23 **Melanocytoma.** Cranial CT scan after the administration of contrast. A uniformly enhancing well circumscribed melanocytoma with surrounding brain oedema is shown.

presence of haemorrhage.[217,224] Some lesions exhibit relatively scanty pigmentation (Figs 14.24 and 14.25).

Intraoperative diagnosis

Melanocytomas are not frequently encountered, so there are few decriptions of their appearances in smear preparations and cryostat sections. Smear preparations show a population of non-cohesive rounded or polygonal cells of varying size (Fig. 14.24). The nuclei are rounded, and usually contain a single prominent nucleolus. Melanin pigment may be present in large quantities within the tumour cells, or within macrophages within the tumour. A network of finely branching capillaries is usually present and may be accompanied by focal haemorrhage. There is no gliofibrillary background in the smears, and necrosis and mitotic activity are not detected. In cryostat sections, melanocytomas appear as solid tumours composed of pleomorphic rounded cells with varying melanocytic pigmentation. It is apparent that an unequivocal distinction from malignant melanoma cannot always be made at the time of intraoperative diagnosis, but distinction from a meningioma or nerve sheath tumour should be possible.

Histology

The histological features of meningeal melanocytomas are similar to those occurring in melanocytomas in the uvea and optic nerve head. CNS melanocytomas are generally composed of relatively monomorphic spindle, fusiform or epithelioid cells with round vesicular nuclei and prominent nucleoli.[215–217] The tumour cells are sometimes arranged in irregular aggregates, giving a 'packeted'

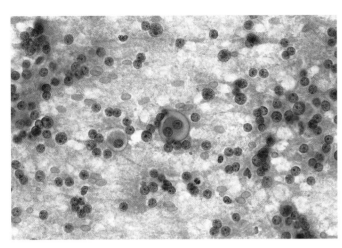

Fig. 14.24 **Melanocytoma.** Smear preparations show a population of non-cohesive tumour cells, including binucleate cells, with rounded nuclei and prominent nucleoli. Melanin pigmentation in this case is sparse. H & E.

appearance (Fig. 14.25). Abundant melanin is usually present in the cytoplasm and may also be detected in macrophages around blood vessels in the tumour. It may be necessary to bleach the melanin from histological sections in order to study the nuclear morphology, and before immunocytochemistry. Immunocytochemical studies have shown positivity for S-100 protein and vimentin in all cases, with positivity for HMB45 and NSE in a majority of cases, but a negative reaction for EMA, cytokeratin, 70 kDa neurofilament protein, Leu7 and GFAP.[213,215,217,222,225,232]

Differential diagnosis

As indicated above, the major differential diagnosis of melanocytomas includes *melanotic meningiomas and nerve*

sheath tumours (Table 14.4). Confusion with *meningiomas* has occurred in the past and, although it is accepted that classical meningiomas may occasionally contain melanin pigment, some previously reported cases of melanotic meningiomas are likely to represent meningeal melanocytomas. This difficulty can be resolved on immunocytochemistry, when melanocytomas will exhibit a negative reaction for EMA, and positive staining for NSE, S-100 protein and HMB45. Electron microscopy will also allow a distinction between these tumours, since melanocytomas lack the characteristic complex interdigitating cell processes and intercellular junctions which are characteristic of meningiomas.

Melanocytomas may also have been reported as *melanotic Schwannomas and neurofibromas* in the past. Melanocytomas have been reported to arise on spinal nerve roots and in the cerebellopontine angle, which can cause clinical confusion with a nerve sheath tumour. Immunocytochemistry should allow a distinction between nerve sheath tumours and melanocytomas, which can be reinforced on electron microscopy (Table 14.4), since melanocytomas lack the abundant pericellular basal lamina and long spacing collagen which are present in nerve sheath tumours.

A distinction from *primary* and *secondary malignant melanoma* in most cases is possible (Table 14.5), particularly when the clinical history, anatomical site of origin and neuroradiological features are taken into account. Melanocytomas exhibit a relatively homogeneous cytology and lack the nuclear pleomorphism, mitotic activity and necrosis that often occur in primary or secondary melanomas, and in our experience show a much lower cell proliferation index using Ki-67/MIB-1 antibodies. However, recurrent and locally invasive melanocytomas have been described,[216,217,223,228] and these can cause

Fig. 14.25 **Melanocytoma.** Supratentorial melanocytoma showing a prominent alveolar arrangement of the neoplastic epithelioid cells. Melanin pigmentation is variable both within tumour cells and in macrophages. Nuclear pleomorphism is not a conspicuous feature. H & E.

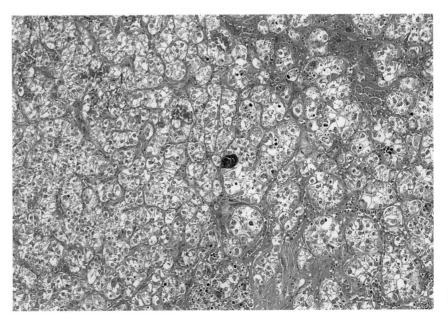

Table 14.4 Comparison between melanocytoma, meningioma and nerve sheath tumours (NST)

	Melanocytoma	NST	Meningioma
Age range	Adults, fifth decade	Adults, sixth decade	All ages
Sex incidence	F > M	F = M	F > M
Location	Spinal and cranial meninges	Sensory nerve roots	Cranial and spinal meninges
Immunocytochemistry	S-100, NSE, HMB45 positive; EMA negative	S-100 positive; HMB45, EMA negative	EMA, S-100 positive; HMB45 negative
Electron microscopy	Melanosomes, premelanosomes	Basal laminae, long spacing collagen	Interdigitating cell membranes, cell junctions

EMA, epithelial membrane antigen; NSE, neuron specific enolase

Table 14.5 Comparison between melanocytoma, primary and metastatic malignant melanoma

	Melanocytoma	Primary melanoma	Metastatic melanoma
Age (years)	Wide range	10–40	25–60
Site	Meningeal, focal	Meningeal, diffuse	Cerebral, multiple, expanding
Histology	Monomorphic spindle/epithelioid	Pleomorphic spindle/fusiform	Pleomorphic, necrotic
Mitosis	Usually absent	Widespread	Widespread
Haemorrhage	Usually absent	Common in large lesions	Common in all lesions

diagnostic difficulties which may not be easily resolved. A comparative flow cytometric study showed markedly different S-phase fractions and proliferative indices between melanocytomas and metastatic melanomas.[215]

Melanin deposition can also occur in *astrocytomas, ependymomas, primary neuroectodermal tumour (PNET), medulloblastomas* and in *teratomas*. However, the melanin deposition under these circumstances is usually not a major feature of the tumour and a histological distinction can normally be made without difficulty with reference to the predominant tumour cell type. The *melanotic PNET of infancy (melanotic progonoma)* can occur as a superficial cerebral tumour arising form the cranial bones or, more rarely, the brain;[237,238] the age of the patient and the primitive nature of the tumour cells in this extremely uncommon condition will allow a distinction from melanocytoma.

Therapy

Haemorrhage is a common feature, and often restricts the extent of surgical resection.[217,224] Necrosis is not a characteristic feature of melanocytomas and although mitotic activity is uncommon, it has been recorded.[217] Ploidy analysis by flow cytometry has shown that most melanocytomas are diploid, but aneuploidy has been detected and may be associated with a more aggressive clinical course.[215] Most melanocytomas are benign and cured by surgical resection. However, these tumours exhibit a spectrum of biological behaviour; tumour recurrence has been reported, occasionally accompanied by invasion of adjacent structures, including the dura, bone

and the spinal cord.[216,217,228] Tumour recurrence seems most likely when surgical resection has been incomplete. Because of this propensity for recurrence,[218] post-operative radiotherapy has been advocated, but its precise role is unclear at present.[217]

Malignant melanoma

Incidence and clinical features

Primary malignant melanomas of the meninges are extremely uncommon tumours which occur most often in the fourth decade of life, with a significant subset occurring in the first two decades, often in association with neurocutaneous melanosis.[240–259] Primary meningeal malignant melanoma is a common and well recognised complication in neurocutaneous melanosis (Chapter 19);[212] an association with the congenital naevus of Ota has been described on several occasions,[219,260–263] but there is not any convincing evidence of an association with the familial dysplastic naevus syndrome. The clinical features primary meningeal melanoma are non-specific and generally associated with the effects of raised intracranial pressure and the location of the tumour. However, patients may present with features suggestive of carcinomatous meningitis if the tumour has diffusely infiltrated the subarachnoid space.[241–243]

Neuroradiological studies show that meningeal malignant melanomas usually appear isodense with grey matter on CT scans, and exhibit marked diffuse enhancement after the administration of contrast.[244] The tumours appear hyperintense on T1-weighted MRI scans and hypointense on T2-weighted MRI scans, with dense enhancement after gadolinium administration.[241,244,247] The tumours are not all well circumscribed and diffuse intracranial meningeal enhancement in the region of the tumour is indicative of meningeal infiltration.[244] The presence of melanin in the tumour may be indicated by foci of T1 and T2 shortening in the brain parenchyma or meninges. Malignant melanomas are frequently accompanied by haemorrhage, which can substantially modify their appearances on MRI and CT scans.[249] Extensive haemorrhage or tumour infiltration of the subarachnoid space can result in obstructive hydrocephalus.[244]

Pathology

Most primary malignant melanomas arise in the leptomeninges; cases with a dural attachment can resemble a meningioma.[243] Diffuse meningeal spread is common, and in some cases CSF dissemination can be extensive, resulting in meningeal melanomatosis (Figs 14.26 and 14.27).[241,242,244,246,253] Under these circumstances, multiple tumour nodules can be present in a variety of sites in the subarachnoid space. Occasional cases present as a mass in the neural parenchyma including the spinal cord, but even these apparently intraparenchymal cases probably have an origin in the pial melanocytes.[247]

The high frequency of CSF involvement in malignant melanoma has allowed a diagnosis to be made on the basis of CSF cytology, where melanin containing tumour cells can be detected in cytospin preparations. Immunocytochemistry is useful in confirming the diagnosis,[242] using a panel of antibodies that should include S-100 protein, HMB45 and MART-1.

Intraoperative diagnosis of malignant melanoma is usually straightforward; in smear preparations, the tumour cells are non-cohesive and tend to spread in a monolayer away from the prominent blood vessels. Necrosis and haemorrhage may be detected in both smear preparations and cryostat sections. The tumour cells are markedly variable in size and shape and contain a variable quantity of melanin pigment (Fig. 14.28). The large rounded nuclei contain a single large nucleolus and mitotic figures may be present. It is, however, *not* possible to distinguish between a primary and metastatic malignant melanoma at intraoperative diagnosis based on the pathological features alone (see below under Differential diagnosis).

Histologically, CNS malignant melanomas exhibit considerable pleomorphism in terms of the nuclear morphology and cytological features, with a varying degree of pigmentation (Figs 14.29 and 14.30).[241] These tumours can closely resemble systemic melanomas, which adds substantially to the difficulty in establishing a diagnosis on presentation when the history is short and

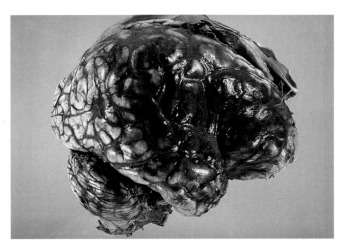

Fig. 14.26 **Malignant melanoma.** Leptomeningeal malignant melanoma with diffuse invasion over the right cerebral hemisphere.

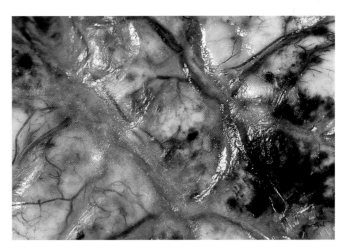

Fig. 14.27 **Malignant melanoma.** Multiple small tumour deposits are present in the leptomeninges in the contralateral hemisphere (same case as Fig. 14.26), indicating diffuse melanomatosis.

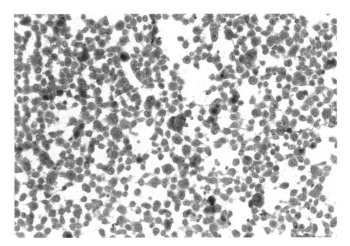

Fig. 14.28 **Malignant melanoma.** Smear preparations in a meningeal malignant melanoma. A dense population of non-cohesive pleomorphic cells are shown with rounded nuclei, prominent nucleoli and varying quantities of melanin pigment. H & E.

no other primary lesion can be identified. The cells within malignant melanomas can vary from small spindle shaped or fusiform cells to large epithelioid cells which can be bizarre and contain a multinucleate giant cell population. Some malignant melanomas may be amelanotic (Fig. 14.31), and a 'balloon cell' morphology has been described in a primary meningeal malignant melanoma.[254] Mitotic activity is generally widespread and necrosis and haemorrhage are frequent. The subarachnoid space can be extensively infiltrated by tumour cells. Invasion of the brain in spinal cord parenchyma is characteristic, but the presence of cells in the Vichow–Robin space must be distinguished from true parenchymal invasion. Immunocytochemical studies of primary meningeal melanomas shows similar features to melanocytomas and systemic malignant melanomas, with positivity for S-100 protein, NSE, HMB45 and MART-1.[243,244,264] The pattern of immunoreactivity in melanoma cells can vary within a tumour, particularly with HMB45 and MART-1 (Fig. 14.32). Malignant melanomas give a negative staining reaction with antibodies to EMA, cytokeratins and GFAP.

Differential diagnosis

The differential diagnosis of meningeal malignant melanoma is similar to that for melanocytoma. A distinction from *metastatic melanoma* is important (Table 14.5); this can be fraught with difficulty and calls for close liaison between the clinician, neuroradiologist and pathologist in investigating and excluding all other possible primary sites which can include the orbit, nail beds, gastrointestinal tract, urogenital tract and skin. *Melanocytoma* is also included in the differential diagnosis, but the greater extent of cellular atypia (particularly

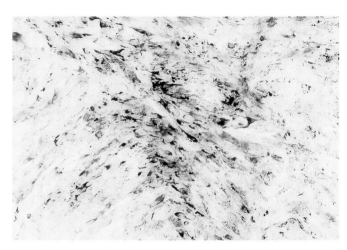

Fig. 14.30 **Malignant melanoma.** A Singh stain for melanin shows an irregular dispersion of melanin in both tumour cells and tumour associated macrophages in a meningeal malignant melanoma.

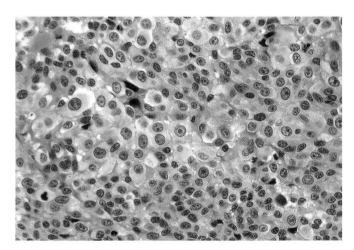

Fig. 14.31 **Malignant melanoma.** An amelanotic malignant melanoma with tumour cells containing a variable quantity of pale-staining cytoplasm. The tumour cell margins are well defined, and most of the cells contain a prominent large nucleolus. H & E.

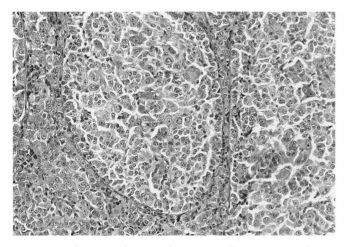

Fig. 14.29 **Malignant melanoma.** The tumour cells in a meningeal malignant melanoma tend to be arranged in large irregular groups, with markedly pleomorphic nuclei containing a prominent single nucleolus. This section has been bleached for melanin to display the nuclear details. H & E.

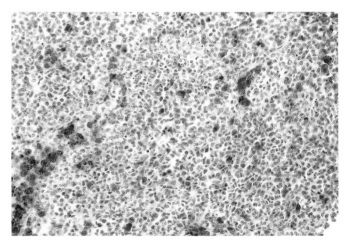

Fig. 14.32 **Malignant melanoma.** Immunoreactivity for HMB45 in a malignant melanoma is usually patchy, with positive staining (red) most evident in the larger tumour cells. Unbleached section.

the presence of giant tumour cells), nuclear pleomorphism, mitotic activity and necrosis usually allows a distinction to be made (Table 14.5). Melanocytomas do not spread in a diffuse manner in the leptomeninges, and CSF involvement has apparently never been reported in a melanocytoma. However, such a distinction can remain difficult and the diagnosis revised only in the light of further clinical follow-up information.[265]

The difficulties in making a diagnosis of malignant melanoma in relation to other primary pigmented tumours of the CNS mostly concerns *pigmented malignant peripheral nerve sheath tumours*. A distinction is usually possible according to the site of the tumour, its relation to nerve roots, the architectural pattern and cellular morphology. Immunocytochemical investigations may not completely resolve the differential diagnosis, since both groups of tumours will express S-100 protein, but HMB45 and MART-1 expression is usually confined to malignant melanomas and is not present in malignant peripheral nerve sheath tumours. Electron microscopy is frequently helpful in demonstrating the pericellular basal laminae and long spacing collagen which are characteristic of nerve sheath tumours, but are absent in melanomas.

Therapy

Most cases follow a rapidly progressive course, particularly in children and in young adults.[240,244] Primary meningeal malignant melanomas rarely metastasise to other organs;[251] occasional cases have disseminated following neurosurgical drainage for the relief of hydrocephalus.[252] The treatment of primary malignant melanoma in the CNS is difficult as the tumours are highly aggressive and relatively radioresistant. Craniospinal irradiation has been suggested because of the high frequency of CSF dissemination,[240,244] usually accompanied by combination chemotherapy. The response to chemotherapy (including interferon beta) is usually poor,[240,242,244] but one recent case has shown a good response to intrathecal recombinant interleukin-2.[248] Overall, the prognosis is extremely poor and most patients are dead within 1 year of diagnosis,[240] although longer survivals have been reported in children following craniospinal irradiation and combination chemotherapy.[244]

Soft tissue tumours

A wide range of both benign and malignant soft tissue (mesenchymal, non-meningothelial) tumours arise both in the CNS and in the meninges.[266–269] In the past, many of these have been confused with other tumours arising in these sites, particularly with meningiomas, and investigative data in these historical reports is inevitably limited. Advances in diagnostic techniques, particularly immunocytochemistry, have allowed a full appreciation of the wide range of differentiation that can occur in soft tissue tumours and an ever increasing number of distinct entities have been described.[266,267,270,271] Recent genetic analyses of soft tissue tumours have identified molecular markers which are linked to histopathologically defined tumour subtypes (see Refs 272 and 273 for reviews). These will allow further refinements in the classification of soft tissue tumours, and may also identify features which are of therapeutic and prognostic significance. Although these studies have been carried out on soft tissue tumours arising outside the CNS, preliminary data on their CNS counterparts suggest that the same molecular markers may be present. Further advances in this field are thus expected to aid the identification and classification of soft tissue tumours arising in the CNS.

In this section, soft tissue neoplasms are grouped according to their differentiation into tumours of adipose tissue, fibrous tissue, histiocytic tumours, smooth and striated muscle tumours and osteocartilaginous tumours (excluding those arising in the skull and vertebral column). Most of these tumours are extremely rare, many being described in a series of case reports.

Aetiological factors in primary intracranial sarcomas

Several examples of intracranial sarcoma, including fibrosarcoma, malignant fibrous histiocytoma, chondrosarcoma and osteogenic sarcoma, may occur several years after cranial irradiation, particularly for pituitary region tumours.[274–277] A meningeal sarcoma has recently been reported in a young child after 26 cycles of chemotherapy (alkylating agents plus etoposide) but without irradiation for an unrelated primary brain tumour.[278] However, in view of the occurrence of multiple primary brain brain tumours in families with the Li–Fraumeni syndrome and other familial genetic syndromes,[279] the possibility of an underlying genetic predisposition should always be investigated in such cases before an iatrogenic attribution is claimed.

Adipose tissue tumours

Lipomas are the commonest tumours of adipose tissue arising in the CNS and are thought to represent around 0.4% of all intracranial tumours and around 1% of all spinal tumours. Lipomas are described in Chapter 17.

Variants of lipoma which occur in the CNS include the angiolipoma, which has been reported to arise in the spinal and cranial meninges,[280,281] the hibernoma[282] and the osteolipoma.[283] These are all benign lesions which present clinically on account of their mass effect and compression of adjacent structures; the osteolipoma has been reported as an incidental finding at autopsy[283] and during surgery (Fig. 14.33). Surgical excision of these benign lesions is curative. Malignant lipomatous tumours are extremely

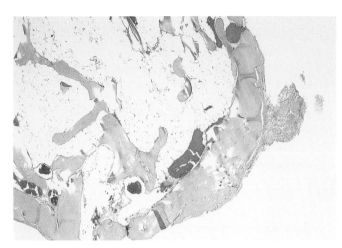

Fig. 14.33 **Osteolipoma.** Cerebral osteolipoma with a central component of mature adipose tissue surrounded by and partially invaginated by lamellar bone. This small lesion was an incidental finding at neurosurgery attached to the tentorium of the cerebellum.

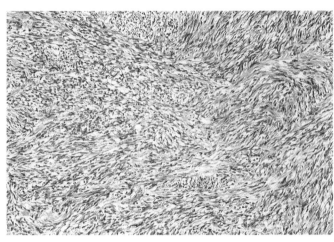

Fig. 14.34 **Solitary fibrous tumour.** Solitary fibrous tumour of the meninges. A population of bipolar tumour cells is arranged in dense interweaving fascicles. H & E.

uncommon in the CNS; liposarcomas have been reported as primary tumours in the meninges, with two cases occurring in association with a subdural haematoma.[284–286] The microscopic features of these cases included both well differentiated and pleomorphic histology.[284]

Fibrous tissue tumours

A wide range of fibrous tissue neoplasms occur within the CNS, most of which are extremely uncommon. As mentioned above, many of the historical reports of these entities can be questioned on the basis of the diagnostic techniques which were available at the time of publication. Benign fibromas occur extremely rarely and usually present in the first two decades of life as a meningeal mass which can be mistaken for a meningioma;[287] an intracerebral case has also been reported.[288]

Solitary fibrous tumour

Clinical and radiological features

A hitherto rare entity, the solitary fibrous tumour, has been reported with increasing frequency in recent years in the intracranial and spinal meninges.[289–304] These tumours are analogous to the solitary fibrous tumours occurring in the pleura. In the past, it is likely that these tumours were diagnosed as fibrous meningiomas or haemangiopericytomas;[303] to date over 20 cases have been reported, in patients with ages ranging from 11 to 73 years, with a tendency to occur most often around the fifth decade. Females appear to be affected slightly more often than males. One of the youngest patients with a solitary fibrous tumour was an 11-year-old male who

developed the lesion 29 months after surgery, irradiation and systemic chemotherapy for a pineal mixed germ cell tumour.[307]

The clinical manifestations of this lesion are similar to meningiomas; most patients present with signs and symptoms of a slowly enlarging lesion causing focal neurological dysfunction in adjacent structures and raised intracranial pressure. Neuroradiology shows solitary fibrous tumours to be isodense with grey matter and hypointense to white matter on unenhanced T1-weighted MRI scans, and hypodense to grey matter on T2-weighted scans.[291,296,298,304] The lesions usually exhibit uniform contrast enhancement, with peritumoral oedema contributing to the mass effect.

Pathology

Most lesions occur as an extra-axial mass attached to the dura mater; both intraspinal and intracranial cases have been reported, including lesions in the region of the tentorium and the cerebellopontine angle. Histologically, these lesions consist of irregularly elongated fusiform and spindle shaped tumour cells arranged in inter-connecting networks separated by dense collagenous connective tissue (Fig. 14.34). The tumour cells contain elongated nuclei with dispersed chromatin and without prominent nucleoli. Tumour vascularity is variable, but the blood vessels are usually surrounded by connective tissue and the lesions usually do not exhibit calcification or psammoma body formation (Fig. 14.35). Mitotic activity and necrosis are not usually a prominent feature in these tumours, but these have been reported in cases with an aggressive clinical course involving local recurrence and/or metastases[290,293,297] (see below). Immuno-cytochemistry allows a distinction from meningioma and

Fig. 14.35 **Solitary fibrous tumour**. The tumour cells contain elongated nuclei without prominent nucleoli. Fine bundles of collagen and small blood vessels are present in the background. H & E.

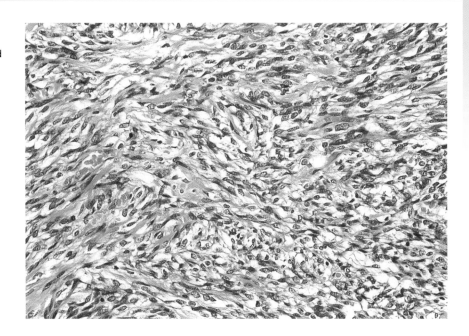

Table 14.6 Comparison of immunocytochemistry on solitary fibrous tumours, fibrous meningiomas and haemangiopericytomas[4,9,13,14,17]

Antibody	Solitary fibrous tumour	Fibrous meningioma	Haemangiopericytoma
EMA	–	++	–
Vimentin	++	++	++
CD34	++	–/+	–/+
PR	– –	+	–
S-100 protein	–	++	–
Factor XIIIa	+	++	–/+

EMA, epithelial membrane antigen; PR, progesterone receptor

(Table 14.6); since although vimentin is expressed in the tumour cells, solitary fibrous tumours stain positively for CD34 (Fig. 14.36), with a negative reaction for EMA and S-100 protein, unlike meningiomas. Electron microscopy shows neoplastic cells with the ultrastructural characteristics of fibroblasts rather than arachnoidal cells; interdigitating cell membranes and hemidesmosomes have not been reported.

Differential diagnosis

In histological terms the major differential diagnosis includes *fibrous meningioma* and *haemangiopericytoma*. Immunocytochemistry and electron microscopy is usually helpful in these entities for establishing a diagnosis (Table 14.6). A clearcut distinction from a *haemangiopericytoma* may be difficult to achieve, but solitary fibrous tumours usually lack the conspicuous vasculature of haemangiopericytomas, and the pericellular pattern of reticulin deposition is more variable. Other connective tissue lesions, particularly a *leiomyoma*, *Schwannomas* and

neurofibromas, should also be considered in the differential diagnosis, but this can easily be resolved by the use of immunocytochemistry and electron microscopy. Solitary fibrous tumours will give a negative reaction on immunocytochemistry for smooth muscle actin and S-100 protein, while most leiomyomas and nerve sheath tumours give a negative reaction with antibodies to CD34. Only a few studies of proliferation markers in solitary fibrous tumours have been reported; these usually show low proliferation rates, but in one report this varied from 1 to 18% (mean value 4%).[290,293,303] The cells within a solitary fibrous tumour do not contain the intracytoplasmic actin filaments present in leiomyomas, and the long spacing collagen and relationship to nerve structures characteristic of nerve sheath tumours are also absent.

Therapy

The prognosis for most cases is excellent following surgical resection; one of the previous reported cases

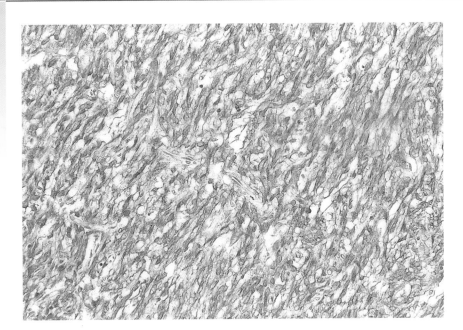

Fig. 14.36 **Solitary fibrous tumour.**
Immunocytochemistry for CD34 shows a positive
reaction in most of the cells within a solitary
fibrous tumour of the meninges (same case as
Fig. 14.35).

originally diagnosed as a low grade fibrosarcoma exhibited mitotic activity but did not recur at 10 years after initial surgery. Incompletely excised tumours may recur locally.[290] Malignant forms of solitary fibrous tumour with increased cellularity, nuclear atypia, necrosis and widespread mitotic activity have been described in the pleura, and one similar case has been described recently in the meninges, which recurred locally three times over a 10-year period and then metastasised to the lungs and soft tissues.[297] It is apparent that this tumour, which is being recognised increasingly as a primary meningeal lesion, can exhibit a spectrum of clinical and biological behaviour; careful histopathological assessment is therefore required in order to assess the possibility of aggressive growth and metastases, and to avoid confusion with other potentially aggressive tumours, particularly the haemangiopericytoma.

Other fibrous tissue tumours

Other fibrous tumours occurring in the CNS include the *fibromatoses*, which occur in the meninges as cytologically benign locally infiltrative lesions composed of elongated fibroblasts within collagen bundles.[305–307] These unusual conditions have a clear-cut malignant potential. *Pseudo-tumoral cranial fasciitis* can occur in childhood and is related to nodular fasciitis occurring at other sites in the body.[308] Rapid growth within the deep scalp can occur but usually there is no intradural component and the lesion has no malignant potential. These conditions can be confused histologically with *hypertrophic cranial pachymeningitis*, which is a reactive condition resulting in progressive dural thickening and fibrosis occurring in association with chronic inflammation and autoimmune diseases.[309]

Intracranial fibrosarcomas have been described in the literature,[310–317] although it is likely that many of the earlier reported examples may represent other types of connective tissue tumour which were not identified as specific entities until appropriate ultrastructural and immunocytochemical investigations were available. However, it is recognised that primary fibrosarcomas may occur in the cranial and spinal meninges as sporadic tumours; the cranial examples have been described in association with a subdural haematoma and intratumoral haemorrhage.[312,316] Familial cases,[317] cases described in association with neurofibromatosis,[314] or with an astocytoma arising in the lesion[315] would probably benefit from re-examination using current diagnostic methods. The occurrence of fibrosarcoma as a consequence of previous cranial irradiation[316] is also described above. A recent case has been reported in a child treated with combination chemotherapy (but not irradiation) for a glioblastoma.[318]

Histiocytic tumours

Benign fibrous histiocytomas have been reported very rarely as primary tumours in the meninges in children and young adults.[319] Histologically, these tumours comprise an admixture of fibroblasts and rounded histiocytic cells arranged in a prominent storiform pattern, with a basement membrane which can be demonstrated on stains for reticulin and containing foci of chronic inflammatory cells and occasional giant cells. Many of the initial reports of this lesion were subsequently found to be pleomorphic xantho-astrocytomas on review with immunocytochemistry for GFAP.[320]

Malignant fibrous histiocytomas are also uncommon, and have been described as primary tumours in the CNS across a wide age range.[321–330] Most arise in the meninges, but intracerebral examples have been reported.[322,327,328] One example occurred in association with a thoracolumbar meningomyelocele[324] and several reports of radiation induced malignant fibrous histiocytomas exist.[323,326] The tumours are malignant and invade the meninges, dura mater, bone and brain.[321–336] One case exhibited CSF dissemination.[321] The tumours are not associated with any specific neuroradiological or clinical features.

On histological examination, the tumour cells are markedly more pleomorphic than in their benign counterparts, although the storiform growth pattern is usually maintained and is associated with foci of necrosis and mitotic activity, with occasional examples having pronounced inflammatory cell components. A wide range of cell types may be present, including large multinucleate giant cells, histiocyte-like cells, macrophages, fibroblasts and myofibroblasts (Figs 14.37 and 14.38). The differential diagnosis includes other sarcomas, glioblastoma and gliosarcoma; immunocytochemistry for GFAP and S-100 protein is usually helpful in establishing a diagnosis. Some tumours, however, may express GFAP, particularly at the interface with neural tissue. This can cause problems in histological interpretation,[331] particularly with the differential diagnosis of gliosarcoma or glioblastoma. The tumour cells do not usually express a full macrophage/histiocyte phenotype and immunocytochemistry for macrophage markers, e.g. alpha-1 antichymotrypsin or CD68 may be negative.

Malignant fibrous histiocytomas are generally unresponsive to irradiation and chemotherapy, and most patients are dead within 1 year of diagnosis. One case with pulmonary metastases has been reported.[321]

Smooth and striated muscle tumours

Leiomyomas have been reported as primary intracranial tumours in young adults, although they are extremely uncommon.[332,333] They are usually attached to the dura, and present with non-specific features relating to their mass effect and compression of adjacent structures. Their predominant histological features are patterns of fascicles of eosinophilic spindle cells (Fig. 14.39), which may be confused with Schwannomas, particularly since nuclear palisading may also occur. Leiomyomas can also occur as diffuse leptomeningeal tumours which may be confused with meningiomas.[334] These difficulties can be resolved on immunocytochemistry, since leiomyomas express smooth muscle actin (Fig. 14.40), which is absent from the tumour cells in Schwannomas and meningiomas. A rare vascular variant, the angioleiomyoma, has also been described as a primary intracranial tumour.[335]

Dural leiomyomas and leiomyosarcomas have been reported in patients with AIDS;[336–339] interestingly, these lesions expressed Epstein–Barr virus related proteins in the nucleus of the tumour cells. Leiomyosarcomas have also been described in immunocompetent adults; most occur as dural based lesions (Fig. 14.41),[341–343] and a rare example has arisen within a teratoma in the pineal region.[344]

Histologically, leiomyosarcomas are composed of irregular fascicles of elongated cells with a variable quantity of eosinophilic cytoplasm. The cells may contain perinuclear vacuoles, and usually have a high mitotic rate (Fig. 14.42). Necrosis and haemorrhage may also

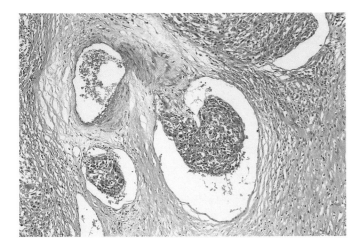

Fig. 14.37 **Malignant fibrous histiocytoma.** Invasion of blood vessels within the dura mater by malignant fibrous histiocytoma. H & E.

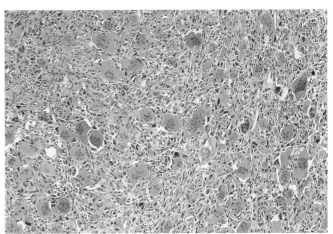

Fig. 14.38 **Malignant fibrous histiocytoma.** A large number of multinucleate giant cells are surrounded by a mixed population of mononuclear cells, including fibroblasts and macrophages (same case as Fig. 14.37). H & E.

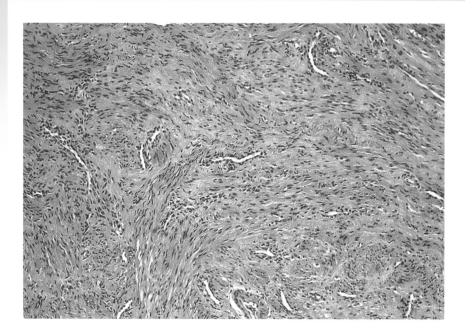

Fig. 14.39 **Leiomyoma.** Leiomyoma of the meninges with numerous prominent branching blood vessels embedded in dense smooth muscle tissue. H & E.

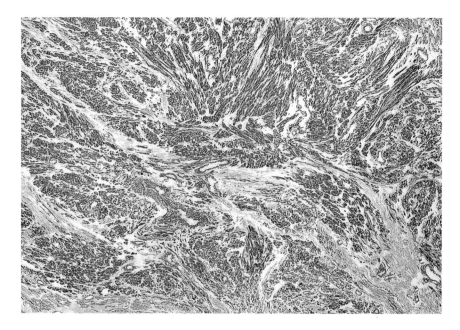

Fig. 14.40 **Leiomyoma.** Immunocytochemistry for smooth muscle actin. A strong positive reaction is shown within the tumour cells in the leiomyoma, and in the blood vessel walls.

occur in these malignant tumours. Their differential diagnosis includes rhabdomyosarcoma, malignant nerve sheath tumour, malignant teratoma and glioblastoma/gliosarcoma.

Immunocytochemistry shows leiomyosarcomas consistently to express smooth muscle actin, but not usually desmin, S-100 protein, placental alkaline phosphatase or GFAP. Leiomyosarcomas do not respond consistently to irradiation and chemotherapy; most patients are dead within 1–2 years of diagnosis.

A recent report has described two cases of primary meningeal sarcoma with both leiomyoblastic and meningothelial differentiation.[346] The tumour cells varied in shape from spindle cells to round/polygonal cells, which gave a positive reaction on immunocytochemistry for smooth muscle actin. The precise relationship of this apparently novel entity to other soft tissue or meningothelial tumours requires further investigation.

Rhabdomyomas are uncommon benign lesions of childhood and early adult life, consisting almost entirely of mature striated muscle, which tend to arise on the intracranial portion of cranial nerves.[347–349] The presence of mature adipose tissue[347] has led to the suggestion that these lesions should be considered as choristomas[348] rather than true neoplasms. Diagnostic confusion can arise with the uncommon skeletal muscle heterotopias, most of which occur in the meninges around the ventral pons.[350]

Their malignant counterpart, rhabdomyosarcoma, is one of the more commonly encountered forms of malignant mesenchymal tumour which arises in the CNS. Most rhabdomyosarcomas occur in midline structures including the region of the fourth ventricle and the brain stem, lumbar sacral cord and filum terminale across a wide age range, including infants.[351–359] One case occurred in association with hypomelanosis of Ito in a child,[359] and one case arose in a ventricle after resection of hyperplastic choroid plexus.[354] However other sites can be involved including the cerebral hemispheres, basal ganglia and leptomeninges. Rhabdomyosarcomas are invasive tumours with no specific neuroradiological or clinical features.

Most examples are embryonal rhabdomyosarcomas which consist of small malignant pleomorphic tumour cells containing eosinophilic cytoplasm. Other subtypes of rhabdomyosarcomas may contain strap cells, which can be identified at intraoperative diagnosis, particularly in smear preparations (Fig. 14.43) Strap cells and cross striations are often difficult to demonstrate in embryonal rhabdomyosarcomas and immunocytochemistry for myoglobin, actin and desmin help confirm the diagnosis (Figs 14.44 and 14.45).[355,357] Ultrastructural studies are also helpful in the identification of myosin and actin filaments.[355] It should also be recalled that rhabdomyosarcoma can occur as a component of other brain tumours such as *PNET/medullomyoblastoma, gliosarcoma* and *malignant teratoma*. The differential diagnosis also includes *leiomyosarcoma* and other tumours which may exhibit

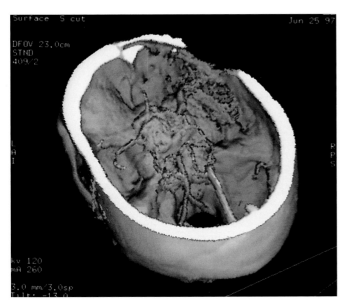

Fig. 14.41 **Leiomyosarcoma.** Three-dimensional reconstruction of a surface rendered contrast enhanced CT scan. A large leiomyosarcoma is shown which has arisen in the meninges and is invading the skull base.

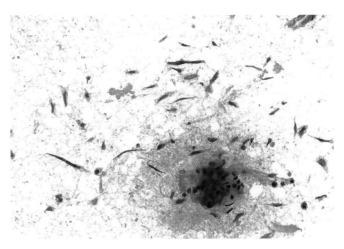

Fig. 14.43 **Rhabdomyosarcoma.** Smear preparation in primary rhabdomyosarcoma of the meninges containing several irregular elongated strap cells. H & E.

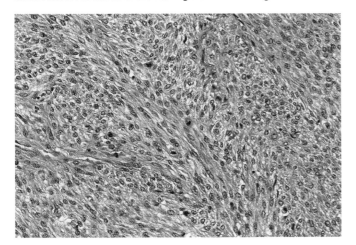

Fig. 14.42 **Leiomyosarcoma.** Leiomyosarcoma (same case as Fig. 14.41) showing dense fascicles of tumour cells. Widespread mitotic activity is shown but only a mild to moderate degree of nuclear pleomorphism. H & E.

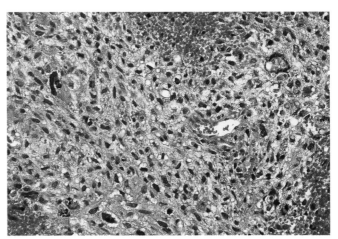

Fig. 14.44 **Rhabdomyosarcoma.** Primary rhabdomyosarcoma of the meninges containing very occasional strap cells, but composed predominantly of a population of pleomorphic polygonal cells with variable quantities of cytoplasm. H & E.

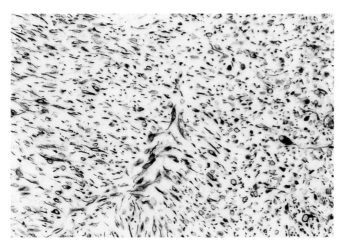

Fig. 14.45 **Rhabdomyosarcoma.** Immunocytochemistry for desmin. A strong positive reaction is shown in the tumour cells within a rhabdomyosarcoma, particularly in the large elongated cells.

rhabdoid features, including *meningiomas, glioblastomas* and *rhabdoid/atypical teratoid* tumours. A very rare tumour, the *malignant ectomesenchymoma* can occur in the CNS as a mixed tumour composed of ganglion cells and neuroblastic elements, with one or more mesenchymal elements including rhabdomyosarcoma.[360]

Osteocartilaginous tumours

Benign osteocartilaginous tumours occur very infrequently in CNS, mostly with a dural origin. Osteomas are particularly uncommon[361,362] and some of the reported cases may well represent reactive conditions, for example in patients with renal failure.[363] A differential diagnosis from similar tumours arising in the bone of the skull requires expert neuroradiological assessment and histological differentiation from dural calcification and ossification (e.g. as a result of trauma, or as a consequence of metabolic disease) is essential.

Chondromas have been reported more frequently, but they are still very uncommon lesions.[364–367] These lobulated and well circumscribed lesions occur over a wide age range, arising in the cranial dura. Some can reach a large size[365] or undergo cystic change.[364] Most of these lesions have been cured by surgery, but malignant progression of chondroma to chondrosarcoma has been reported.[370]

Primary osteosarcomas have only been described very occasionally in the CNS, arising in the brain[371–373] or in the dura mater,[374,375] usually in adolescents and young adults. One case has been reported to arise from an epidermoid cyst within the cerebellum,[376] and a further meningeal lesion arose in association with a glioblastoma,[377] apparently not representing a radiation induced tumour. These malignant tumours invade brain, dura mater and bone and usually respond poorly to irradiation and chemotherapy.

Chondrosarcomas occur infrequently as primary lesions in the CNS; by far the commonest of these is the mesenchymal chondrosarcoma (see below). Differentiated chondrosarcomas may arise in the cranial dura[378,379] and one example of a radiation induced tumour has been reported in the cerebellum.[380] These tumours are usually lobulated, with a poorly defined border with the meninges or brain (Fig. 14.46). Their histological features are similar to chondosarcomas occurring in the skull base or vertebral column; neoplastic chondrocytes are present in variable numbers in a cartilaginous stroma which may contain prominent blood vessels (Fig. 14.47). Mitotic figures are usually present, and larger lesions may exhibit necrosis, haemorrhage and cystic degenation. The main differential diagnosis is mesenchymal chondrosarcoma (see below) or chordoma. Chondrosarcomas express S-100 protein (Fig. 14.48), but not cytokeratins, which are expressed in chordomas. Most of these lesions exhibit low grade malignancy with recurrence and local invasion reported as characteristic features.[381] However, a more frankly malignant course with recurrence and systemic metastases has been reported.[381,382]

The CNS is the commonest site of extraosseous mesenchymal chondrosarcoma. These tumours usually occur in children and young adults with no gender preference, but occasional cases in the CNS have been reported in older adults.[381–391] They can be confused with cranial or spinal meningiomas in neuroradiological investigations and in their clinical presentation. Histological examination shows a characteristic mosaic pattern of pale staining chondroid tissue with more compact cellular aggregates of fusiform or poorly differentiated cells (Fig. 14.49), with a palisading architecture and prominent blood vessels. Chondroblastic features are present in the less cellular areas (Fig. 14.50) and occasional cases with osteoid formation have been described; diagnosis in the absence of these chondroid areas can be difficult as immunocytochemistry is not always helpful in characterising the small cell population. The small tumour cell population stains with antibodies to Leu7, vimentin and NSE, but not usually with antibodies to S-100 protein, EMA, cytokeratins, desmin, actin or synaptophysin.[389,390,392] The cartilaginous component expresses S-100 protein. Genetic alteration of TP53 appears to be a relatively uncommon event in mesenchymal chondrosarcoma;[393] recent studies have demonstrated expression of genes associated with both chondrogenesis and osteogenesis, with evidence of transdifferentiation of neoplastic chondrocytes to osteoblast-like cells.[394]

The differential diagnosis for mesenchymal chondrosarcomas is influenced by the predominant cell type; tumours without cartilaginous differentiation and with a major small cell component can be confused with a *haemangiopericytoma*, particularly if the vascular component

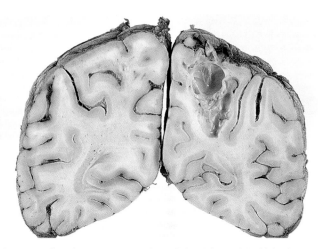

Fig. 14.46 **Chondrosarcoma.** Invasion of the right occipital lobe by a chondrosarcoma arising in the overlying dura mater.

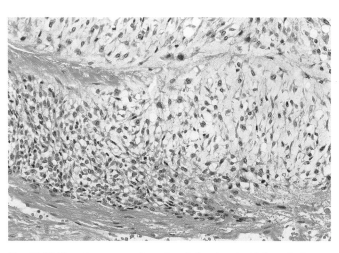

Fig. 14.47 **Chondrosarcoma.** Densely cellular chondroid tissue is shown with marked nuclear pleomorphism and prominent vascular channels (same case as Fig. 14.46). H & E.

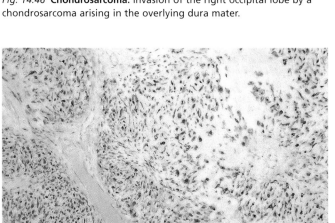

Fig. 14.48 **Chondrosarcoma.** Immunocytochemistry for S-100 protein. A positive reaction is shown in both the nuclei and cytoplasm of tumour cells within a chondrosarcoma (same case as Fig. 14.46).

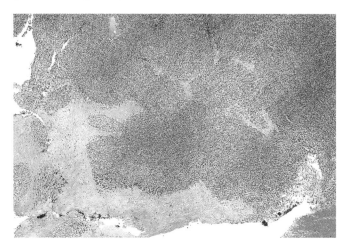

Fig. 14.49 **Mesenchymal chondrosarcoma.** Extensive dural invasion by a mesenchymal chondrosarcoma with a predominant population of small poorly differentiated tumour cells. H & E.

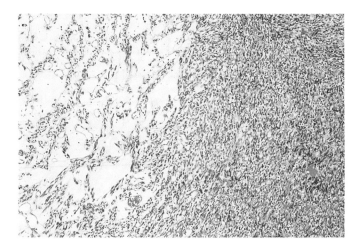

Fig. 14.50 **Mesenchymal chondrosarcoma.** Pale-staining areas within a mesenchymal chondrosarcoma contain chondroid tissue, surrounded by a large aggregate of small fusiform cells. H & E.

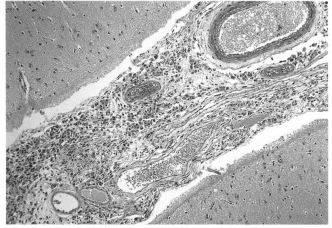

Fig. 14.51 **Meningeal sarcomatosis.** Meningeal sarcomatosis with extensive infiltration of the subarachnoid space by a population of non-cohesive tumour cells with a variable quantity of eosinophilic cytoptasm. The primary tumour was a rhabdomyosarcoma arising in the meninges. H & E.

is prominent. This difficulty can be resolved by a careful search for cartilaginous tissue, and by attention to the nuclear features, since haemangiopericytomas usually have larger and more elongated nuclei. Immunocytochemistry is not always helpful in this circumstance. Other differential diagnoses for small cell tumours include PNET (particularly if rosette-like structures are present) and othe 'round cell' neoplasms. Tumours with prominent osteocartilaginous differentiation need to be distinguished from a differentiated chondrosarcoma or osteogenic sarcoma by a careful search for the small cell component.[394]

Mesenchymal chondrosarcomas are locally aggressive tumours, and the prognosis is substantially affected by the completeness of surgical excision. Studies using cell proliferation markers and flow cytometry have suggested that tumours with high labelling indices and a high S-phase fraction may be associated with a poor outcome.[389,392] Tumour recurrence and systemic metastases have been reported in mesenchymal chondrosarcomas.[395]

Meningeal sarcomatosis

In the past, this lesion has been referred to as meningeal meningiomatosis and comprises extensive and diffuse involvement of the meninges by a malignant 'spindle cell' or mesenchymal tumour (Fig. 14.51),[396–406] often without an accompanying primary tumour mass. The clinical features can resemble those of meningoencephalitis and most cases occur in adults, although occasional examples have been recorded in childhood. Both the cranial and spinal meninges can be involved and the tumour growth is usually complicated by obstructive hydrocephalus. Review of earlier reported cases has revealed that these include examples of diffuse meningeal infiltration by other neoplasms, comprising carcinoma, lymphoma, glioblastoma or medulloblastoma.[399,403] Advances in immunocytochemistry should now allow the more precise use of this term, as non-mesenchymal tumours invading the subarachnoid space in the absence of an obvious primary lesion should be readily characterised and the use of the term 'meningeal meningiomatosis' for this condition should be avoided.[396]

REFERENCES

Vascular tumours

1. Kleihaus P, Burger PC, Scheithauer BW et al. Histological typing of tumours of the central nervous system, 2nd edn. Berlin: Springer, 1993
2. Cushing H, Bailey P. Tumours arising from the blood vessels of the brain. Springfield: Thomas, 1928
3. Silver ML, Hennigar G. Cerebellar haemangioma (haemangioblastoma): A clinicopathological review of forty cases. J Neurosurg, 1952; 9:484–492
4. McComb RD, Jones TR, Pizzo SV et al. Localisation of factor VIII/von Willebrand factor and glial fibrillary acidic protein in the haemangioblastoma; implications for stromal cell histogenesis. Acta Neuropathol (Berl), 1982; 56:207–213
5. Cushing H, Eisenhardt L. The meningiomas. The classification, regional behaviour, life history and surgical end results. Springfield: Thomas, 1938
6. Zulch KJ. Histological typing of tumours of the central nervous system. Geneva: World Health Organisation, 1979
7. Pitkethly DT, Hardman JM, Kempe LG et al. Angioblastic meningiomas. Clinicopathologic study of 81 cases. J Neurosurg, 1970; 32:539–544
8. Kepes JJ. Meningiomas. Biology, pathology and differential diagnosis. New York: Masson, 1982
9. Lee RK, Kishore PRS, Willfsberg E et al. Supratentorial leptomeningeal haemangioblastoma. Neurology, 1978; 28:727–730
10. Obrador S, Martin-Rodriquez JGT. Biological factors involved in the clinical features and surgical management of cerebellar haemangioblastomas. Surg Neurol, 1977; 7:79–85
11. Zimmerman HM. Introduction to tumours of the central nervous system. In: Minckler J, ed. Pathology of the nervous system, vol. 2. New York: McGraw-Hill, 1971: pp 147–151
12. Cobb CA, Youmans JR. Sarcomas and neoplasms of blood vessels. In: Youmans JR, ed. Neurological surgery, 3rd edn, vol. 5. Philadelphia: Saunders, 1990: pp 3152–3170
13. Fornari M, Pluchino F, Solero CL et al. Microsurgical treatment of intramedullary spinal cord tumours. Acta Neurochir Suppl (Wien), 1998; 43:3–8
14. Isu T, Abe H, Iwasaki Y et al. Diagnosis and surgical treatment of spinal haemangioblastoma. No Shinkei Geka, 1991; 19:149–155
15. Ng HK, Poon WS, South JR et al. Tumours of the central nervous system in Chinese in Hong Kong: A histological review. Aust N Z J Surg, 1988; 58:573–578
16. Bennett WA. Primary intracranial neoeplasms in military age group. World War 2 Mil Surg, 1946; 99:594–652
17. Resche F et al. Round table: Intratentorial hemangioblastoma. Neurochirurgie, 1985; 31:91–149
18. Jeffreys R. Clinical and surgical aspects of posterior fossa haemangioblastoma. J Neurol Neurosurg Psychiatry, 1975; 38:105–111
19. Zulch KJ. Brain tumours. Their biology and pathology, 3rd edn. Berlin: Springer-Verlag, 1986: pp 400–407
20. Craig W McK, Keith HM, Kernohan JW. Tumours of the brain occurring in childhood. Acta Psychiat (Kbh), 1949; 24:375–390
21. Mock A, Levi A, Drake JM. Spinal hemangioblastoma, syrinx and hydrocephalus in a two year old child. Neurosurgery, 1990; 27:799–802
22. Tomasello F, Albanese V, Iannotti F et al. Supratentorial hemangioblastoma in a child. J Neurosurg, 1980; 52:578–583
23. Janisch W, Schreiber D, Martin H et al. Primary intracranial tumors as cause of death in the fetus and infant. Zentralbl Allg Pathol, 1984; 129:75–89
24. Roig M, Ballesca M, Nevarro C et al. Congenital spinal cord haemangioblastoma: Another cause of spinal cord section syndrome in the newborn. J Neurol Neurosurg Psychiatry, 1988; 51:1091–1093
25. Olivecrona H. The cerebellar angioreticulomas. J Neurosurg, 1952; 9:317–330
26. Neumann HP, Eggert HR, Weigel K et al. Hemangioblastomas of the central nervous system. A 10-year study with special reference to von Hippel–Lindau syndrome. J Neurosurg, 1989; 70:24–30
27. Jeffreys R. Pathological and haematological aspects of posterior fossa haemangioblastoma. J Neurol Neurosurg Psychiatry, 1975; 38:112–119
28. Kawano T, Iwamoto K, Mori K et al. Multicentric hemangioblastomas in the cerebellum. Surg Neurol, 1985; 24:677–680
29. Sanford RA, Smith RA. Hemangioblastoma of the cervicomedullary junction. Report of three cases. J Neurosurg, 1986; 64:317–321
30. Tognetti F, Galassi E, Servadei F et al. Haemangioblastomas of the brain stem. Neurochirurgia (Stuttg), 1986; 29:230–234
31. Russell DS, Rubinstein LJ. Pathology of tumours of the nervous system, 5th edn. London: Edward Arnold, 1989: pp 639–663
32. Ferrante L, Acqui M, Mastronardi L et al. Supratentorial hemangioblastoma. Report of a case and review of the literature. Zentralbl Neurochir, 1988; 49:151–161
33. Grisoli F, Gambarelli D, Raybaud C et al. Suprasellar hemangioblastoma. Surg Neurol, 1984; 22:257–262

34. Nerad JA, Kersten RC, Anderson RL. Hemangioblastoma of the optic nerve. Report of a case and review of literature. Ophthalmology, 1988; 95:398–402

35. Katayama Y, Tsubokawa T, Miyagi A et al. Solitary hemangioblastoma within the third ventricle. Surg Neurol, 1987; 27:157–162

36. Ho Ys, Plets C, Goffin J et al. Hemangioblastoma of the lateral ventricle. Surg Neurol, 1990; 33:407–412

37. Ishwar S, Taniguchi RM, Vogel FS. Multiple supratentorial hemangioblastomas: Case study and ultrastructural characteristics. J Neurosurg, 1971; 35:396–405

38. Enomoto H, Shibata T, Ito A et al. Multiple hemangioblastomas accompanied by syringomyelia in the cerebellum and the spinal cord. Surg Neurol, 1984; 22:197–203

39. Fox JL, Bashir R, Jinkins JR et al. Syrinx of the conus medullaris and filum terminale in association with multiple hemangioblastomas. Surg Neurol, 1985; 24:265–271

40. Browne TR, Adams RD, Roberson GH. Haemangioblastoma of the spinal cord. Review and report of five cases. Arch Neurol, 1976; 33:435–441

41. Wolbers JG, Ponssen H, Kamphorst W. Hemangioblastoma of the cauda equina. Clin Neurol Neurosurg, 1985; 87:55–59

42. Hurth M. Les Hémangioblastomes intra-rachidiens. Neurochirurgie (Suppl.1) 1975; 21:1–136

43. Murota T, Symon L. Surgical management of hemangioblastoma of the spinal cord; A report of 18 cases. Neurosurgery, 1989; 25:699–708

44. Latif F, Tory K, Gnarra J et al. Identification of the Hippel–Lindau disease tumour suppressor gene. Science, 1993; 260:1317–1320

45. Neumann HP, Lips CJ, Hsia YE et al. von Hippel–Lindau syndrome. Brain Pathol, 1995; 5:181–193

46. Grossman M, Melmon KL. von Hippel–Lindau disease. In: Vinken PJ, Bruyn GW, eds. Handbook of clinical neurology, vol. 14. The phakomatoses. Amsterdam: North Holland, 1972: pp 241–259

47. Horten WA, Wong V, Eldridge R. von Hippel–Lindau disease. Clinical and pathological manifestations in nine families with 50 affected members. Arch Int Med, 1976; 136:769–777

48. Maher ER, Iselius L, Yates JR et al. von Hippel–Lindau disease: a genetic study. J Med Genet, 1991; 28:443–447

49. Kanno H, Kondo K, Ito S et al. Somatic mutations of the von Hippel–Lindau tumour suppressor gene in sporadic central nervous system haemangioblastomas. Cancer Res, 1994; 54:4845–4847

50. Boughey AM, Fletcher NA, Harding AE. Central nervous system haemangioblastoma; a clinical and genetic study of 52 cases. J Neurol Neurosurg Psychiatry 1990; 53:644–648

51. Michels VV. Investigative studies in von Hippel–Lindau disease. Neurofibromatosis, 1988; 1:1159–163

52. Huson SM, Harper PS, Hourihan MD et al. Cerebellar haemangioblastoma and von Hippel–Lindau disease. Brain, 1986; 109:1297–1310

53. Ismail SM, Cole G. von Hippel–Lindau syndrome with microscopic hemangioblastomas of the spinal nerve roots. J Neurosurg, 1984; 60:1279–1281

54. Frank TS, Trojanowski JQ, Roberts SA et al. A detailed immunohistochemical analysis of cerebellar hemangioblastomas: An undifferentiated mesenchymal tumor. Mod Pathol, 1989; 2:638–651

55. Moss TH. Immunohistochemical characteristics of haemangiopericytic meningiomas: Comparison with typical meningiomas, haemangioblastomas and haemangiopericytomas from extracranial sites. Neuropathol Appl Neurobiol, 1987; 13:467–480

56. Cervos-Navarro J. Electronermikroskopie der Hämangioblastome des ZNS und der angioblastischen meningiome. Acta Neuropathol (Berl), 1971; 19:184–207

57. Pasquier B, Lachard A, Pasquier D et al. Glial fibrillary acidic protein and central nervous system tumors. Immunohistochemical study of a series of 207 cases. 2: Medulloblastomas. Haemangioblastomas. Other tumors. Discussion. Ann Pathol, 1983; 3:203–211

58. Tanimura A, Nakamura Y, Hachisuka H et al. Hemangioblastoma of the central nervous system: Nature of the stromal cells as studied by the immunoperoxidase technique. Hum Pathol, 1984; 15:866–869

59. Grant JW, Gallagher PJ, Hedinger C. Haemangioblastoma. An immunohistochemical study of ten cases. Acta Neuropathol (Berl), 1988; 76:82–86

60. Holt SC, Bruner JM, Ordonez NG. Capillary hemangioblastoma. An immunohistochemical study. Am J Clin Pathol, 1986; 86:423–429

61. Hashimoto H, Tsunoda S, Tada T et al. Hemangioblastomas of the central nervous system: Immunohistochemical and ultrastructural study. Neurol Med Chir (Tokyo), 1990; 30:371–376

62. Gottschalk J, Szymas J. Significance of immunohistochemistry for neuro-oncology VI. Occurrence, localization and distribution of glial fibrillary acid protein(GFAP) in 820 tumors. Zentralbl Allg Pathol, 1987; 133:319–330

63. Alles JU, Bosslet K, Schachenmayr W. Haemangioblastoma of the cerebellum – an immunocytochemical study. Clin Neuropathol, 1986; 5:238–241

64. Mannoji H, Takieshita I, Fukui M et al. Immunohistochemical studies of hemangioblastoma with glial fibrillary acidic protein. No To Shinkei, 1983; 35:1207–1216

65. Deck JHN, Rubinstein LJ. Glial fibrillary acidic protein in stromal cells of some capillary haemangioblastomas: significance and possible implications of an immunoperoxidase study. Acta Neuropathol (Berl), 1981; 54:173–181

66. Hufnagel TJ, Kim JH, True LD et al. Immunohistochemistry of capillary hemangioblastoma. Immunoperoxidase-labelled antibody staining resolves the differential diagnosis with metastatic renal cell carcinoma, but does not explain the histogenesis of the capillary hemangioblastoma. Am J Surg Pathol, 1989; 13:207–216

67. Jurco S III, Nadji M, Harvey DS et al. Hemangioblastomas; histogenesis of the stromal cells studied by immunocytochemistry. Human Pathol, 1982; 13:13–18

68. Kepes JJ, Rengachary SS, Lee SH. Astrocytes in hemangioblastomas of the central nervous system and their relationship to stromal cells. Acta Neuropathol (Berl), 1979; 47:99–104

69. Becker I, Paulus W, Roggendorf W. Histogenesis of stromal cells in cerebellar hemangioblastomas. An immunohistochemical study. Am J Pathol, 1989; 134:271–275

70. Ismail SM, Jasani B, Cole G. Histogenesis of haemangioblastomas; an immunocytochemical and ultrastructural study in a case of von Hippel–Lindau syndrome. J Clin Pathol, 1985; 38:417–421

71. Castaigne P, David M, Pertuiset B et al. L'Ultrastructure des hémangioblastomes du systeme nerveux central. Rev Neurol, 1968; 118:5–26

72. Kamitani H, Masuzawa H, Sato J et al. Capillary haemangioblastoma: histogenesis of stromal cells. Acta Neuropathol (Berl), 1987; 73:370–378

73. Kawamura J, Garcia JH, Kamijo Y. Cerebellar hemangioblastoma: histogenesis of stroma cells. Cancer, 1973; 31:1528–1540

74. Wei YQ, Hang ZB. Ultrastructural study of 9 cases of cerebellar hemangioblastoma. Chung Hua Ping Li Hsueh Tsa Chih, 1989; 18:62–64

75. Chaudhry AP, Montes M, Cohn GA. Ultrastructure of cerebellar hemangioblastoma. Cancer, 1978; 42:1834–1850

76. Spence AM, Rubinstein LJ. Cerebellar capillary hemangioblastoma; its histogenesis studied by organ culture and electron microscopy. Cancer, 1975; 35:326–341

77. Ho KL. Ultrastructure of cerebellar capillary haemangioblastoma. 1. Weibel–Palade bodies and stromal cell histogenesis. J Neuropathol Exp Neurol, 1984; 43:592–608

78. Ironside JW, Stephenson TJ, Royds JA et al. Stromal cells in cerebellar haemangioblastomas; an immunocytochemical study. Histopathology, 1988; 12:29–40

79. Wizigmann-Voos S, Breier G, Risau W et al. Up-regulation of vascular endothelial growth factor and its receptors in von-hippel-Lindau disease-associated and sporadic hemangioblastomas. Cancer Res, 1995; 55:1358–1364

80. Bohling T, Hatva E, Kujala M et al. Expression of growth factors and growth factor receptors in capillary hemangioblastoma. J Neuropath Exp Neurol, 1996; 55:522–527

81. Perks WHY, Cross JN, Sivapragasam S et al. Supratentorial haemangioblastoma with polycythaemia. J Neurol Neurosurg Psychiatry, 1976; 39:218–220

82. Waldman TA, Levin EH, Baldwin M. The association of polycythaemia with a cerebellar haemangioblastoma. Am J Med, 1961; 31:318–324

83. Jeffreys RV, Napier JA, Reynolds SM. Erythropoetin levels in posterior fossa haemangioblastoma. J Neurol Neurosurg Psychiatry, 1982; 45:264–266

84. Jankjovic GM, Ristic MS, Pavlovic-Kentera V. Cerebellar hemangioblastoma with erythropoietin in cerebrospinal fluid. Scand J Haematol, 1986; 36:511–514

85. Horton JC, Harsh GR 4th, Fisher JW et al. von Hippel–Lindau disease and erythrocytosis; radioimmunoassay of erythropoietin in cyst fluid from a brainstem hemangioblastoma. Neurology, 1991; 41:753–754

86. Böhung T, Haltia M, Rosenlöf K et al. Erythropoetin in capillary haemangioblastoma. An immunohistochemical study. Acta Neuropathol (Berl), 1987; 74:324–328

87. Kamitani H, Masuzawa H, Sato J et al. Erythropoietin in haemangioblastoma: immunohistochemical and electron microscopy studies. Acta Neurochir (Wien), 1987; 85:56–62

88. Tachibana O, Yamashima T, Yamashita J. Immunohistochemical study of erythropoietin in cerebellar hemangioblastomas associated with secondary polycythemia. Neurosurgery, 1991; 28:24–26

89. Faiss J, Wild G, Schroth G et al. Multiple supratentorial haemangioblastomas following primary infratentorial manifestation. Clin Neuropathol, 1991; 10:21–25

90. Cerejo A, Vaz R, Feyo PB et al. Spinal cord hemangioblastoma with subarachnoid hemorrhage. Neurosurgery, 1990; 27:991–993

91. Wakai S, Inoh S, Ueda Y et al. Hemangioblastoma presenting with intraparenchymatous hemorrhage. J Neurosurg, 1984; 61:956–960

92. Kasarskis EJU, Tibbs PA, Lee C. Cerebellar hemangioblastoma symptomatic during pregnancy. Neurosurgery, 1988; 22:770–772

93. Martinez R, Marcos ML, Figueras A et al. Estrogen and progesterone receptors in intracranial tumors. Clin Neuropharmacol, 1984; 7:338–342

94. Palmer JJ. Haemangioblastomas: A review of eighty-one cases. Acta Neurochir (Wien), 1972; 27:125–148

95. Lee SR, Sanches J, Mark AS et al. Posterior fossa hemangioblastomas; MR imaging. Radiology, 1989; 17:463–468

96. Reynier Y, Baldini M, Hassoun H et al. Haemangioblastoma of the brain. Computed tomography and angiographic studies in 17 patients. Acta Neurochir (Wien), 1985; 74:12–17

97. Chen JK. CT scans in the diagnosis of cerebellar hemangioblastomas. Analysis of 21 cases. Chung Hua Shen Ching Ching Shen Ko Tsa Chih, 1990; 23:377–378

98. Weiss T, Mitsch E, Kazner E. Cystic changes of the posterior cranial fossa on the nuclear magnetic resonance tomogram. ROFO, 1986; 145:590–597

99. Anson JA, Glick RP, Cromwell RM. Use of gadolinium-enhanced magnetic resonance imaging in the diagnosis and management of posterior fossa hemangioblastomas. Surg Neurol, 1991; 35:300–304

100. Elster AD, Arthur DW. Intracranial hemangioblastomas: CT and MR findings. J Comput Assist Tomogr, 1988; 12:736–739

101. O'Keefe T, Ramirez H Jr, Huggins MJ et al. Computed tomography detection of cervical spinal cord hemangioblastoma; a case report. J Comput Assist Tomogr, 1985; 9:249–252

102. Silbergeld J, Cohen WA, Maravilla KR et al. Supratentorial and spinal cord hemangioblastomas; gadolinium enhanced MR appearance with pathologic correlation. J Comput Assist Tomogr, 1989; 13:1048–1051

103. Love JC, Harkin JC. Haemangioblastomas with cystic stromal cell nuclei. Acta Neuropathol (Berl), 1985; 67:160–162

104. Bonnin JM, Pena CE, Rubinstein LJ. Mixed capillary hemangioblastoma and glioma. A redefinition of the 'angioglioma'. J Neuropathol Exp Neurol, 1983; 504–516

105. Mohan J, Brownell B, Oppenheimer DR. Malignant spread of haemangioblastoma: report on two cases. J Neurol Neurosurg Psychiatry, 176; 39:515–525

106. Feldenzer JA, McKeever PE. Selective localisation of -enolase in stromal cells of cerebellar haemangioblastomas. Acta Neuropathol (Berl), 1987; 72:281–285

107. Gouldesbrough DR, Bell JE, Gordon A. Use of immunohistochemical methods in the differential diagnosis between primary cerebellar haemangioblastoma and metastatic renal carcinoma. J Clin Pathol, 1988; 41:861–865

108. Theunissen PH, Debets Te Baerts M, Blaauw G. Histogenesis of intracranial haemangiopericytoma and haemangioblastoma. An immunohistochemical study. Acta Neuropathol (Berl), 1990; 80:68–71

109. Giordana MT, Germano I, Giaccone G et al. The distribution of laminin in human brain tumours: An immunohistochemical study. Acta Neuropathol (Berl), 1985; 67:51–57

110. Moss TH. Tumours of the nervous system. An ultrastructural atlas. London: Springer-Verlag, 1986: pp 113–118

111. Fukushima M, Shibata S, Inoue M et al. Ultrastructure of capillary permeability in human brain tumors. 3: Mechanisms of contrast enhancement in non-glial tumors. No Shinkei Geka, 1986; 14:317–323

112. Ho KL. Ultrastructure of cerebellar capillary hemangioblastoma. III. Crystalloid bodies in endothelial cells. Acta Neuropathol (Berl), 1985; 66:117–126

113. Ho KL. Ultrastructure of cerebellar capillary hemangioblastoma. V. Large pinocytic vacuolar bodies (megalopinocytic vesicles) in endothelial cells. Acta Neuropathol (Berl), 1986; 70:117–126

114. Burger PC, Shibata T, Kleihues P. The use of the monoclonal antibody Ki-67 in the identification of proliferating cells; application to surgical neuropathology. Am J Surg Pathol, 1986; 10:611–617

115. Patsouris E, Stocker U, Kallmeyer V et al. Relationship between Ki-67 positive cells, growth rate and histological type of human intracranial tumors. Anticancer Res, 1988; 8:537–544

116. Yoshi Y, Maki Y, Tsuboi K et al. Estimation of growth fraction with bromodeoxyuridine in human central nervous system tumors. J Neurosurg, 1986; 65:659–663

117. Pomerat CM. Dynamic neuropathology. J Neuropathol Exp Neurol, 1955; 14:28–38

118. Unterharnscheidt FJ. Routine tissue culture of CNS tumours and animal implantation. Prog Exp Tumour Res, 1972; 17:111–150

119. Clelland CA, Treip CS. Histological differentiation of metastatic renal carcinoma in the cerebellum from cerebellar haemangioblastoma in von Hippel–Lindau's disease. J Neurol Neurosurg Psychiatry, 1989; 52:162–166

120. McComb RD, Eastman PJ, Hahn FJ et al. Cerebellar hemangioblastoma with prominent stromal astrocytosis: diagnostic and histogenetic considerations. Clin Neuropathol, 1987; 6:149–154

121. Seifert V, Trost HA, Stolke D. Microsurgery of spinal angioblastoma. Neurochirurgia (Stutt), 1990; 33:100–105

122. Smalley SR, Schomberg PJ, Earle JD et al. Radiotherapeutic considerations in the treatment of hemangioblastomas of the central nervous system. Int J Radiat Oncol Biol Phys, 1990; 18:1165–1171

123. Eskridge JM, McAuliffe W, Harris B et al. Preoperative endovascular embolisation of craniospinal hemangioblastomas. Am J Neuroradiol, 1996; 17:525–531

124. Patrice SJ, Sneed PK, Flickinger JC et al. Radiosurgery for hemangioblastoma: results of a multiinstitutional experience. Int J Rad Oncol Biol Phys, 1996; 35:493–499

125. Niemela M, Lim YJ, Soderman M et al. Gamma knife radiosurgery in 11 hemangioblastomas. J Neurosurg, 1996; 85:591–596

126. de la Monte SM, Horowitz, SA. Hemangioblastomas: clinical and histopathological factors correlated with recurrence. Neurosurgery, 1989; 25:695–698

127. Vinas FJ, Horrax G. Recurrence of cerebrellar hemangioblastoma after 22 years – operation and recovery. J Neurosurg, 1956; 13:641–646

128. Hoff JT, Ray BS. Cerebral haemangioblastoma occurring in a patient with von Hippel–Lindau disease. J Neurosurg, 1968; 28:365–368

129. Bataille B, Roualdes G, Babin P et al. Supratentorial hemangioblastoma. Neurochirurgie, 1988; 34:348–351

130. Young S, Richardson AE. Solid haemangioblastomas of the posterior fossa; radiological features and results of surgery. J Neurol Neurosurg Psychiatry, 1987; 50:155–158

131. Okawaza SH. Solid cerebellar hemangioblastoma. J Neurosurg, 1973; 39:514–518

132. Nakamura N, Sekino H, Taguchi Y et al. Successful total extirpation of hemangioblastoma originating in the medulla oblongata. Surg Neurol, 1985; 24:87–94

133. Singounas EG. Haemangioblastomas of the central nervous system. Acta Neurochir (Wien), 1978; 44:107–113

134. Djindjian M. Successful removal of a brainstem hemangioblastoma. Surg Neurol, 1986; 25:97–100

135. Xu QW, Bao WM, Mao RL et al. Magnetic resonance imaging and microsurgical treatment of intramedullary hemangioblastoma of the spinal cord. Neurosurgery, 1994; 35:671–675

136. Goelliner JR, Laws ER, Soule EH et al. Haemangiopericytoma of the meninges: Mayo Clinic experience. Am J Clin Pathol, 1978; 70:374–380

137. Zimmerman HM. Vascular tumours of the brain. In: Vinken PJ, Bruyn GW, eds. Handbook of clinical neurology, vol. 18. Amsterdam: North Holland, 1975: pp 269–298

138. Muller J, Mealey J. The use of tissue culture in differentiation between angioblastic meningioma and haemangiopericytoma. J Neurosurg, 1971; 34:341–348

139. Skullerud K, Loken AC. The prognosis in meningiomas. Acta Neuropathol (Berl), 1974; 29:337–344

140. Iwaki T, Fukui M, Takeshita I et al. Hemangiopericytoma of the meninges: a clinicopathologic and immunohistochemical study. Clin Neuropathol, 1988; 7:93–99

141. Schroder R, Firsching R, Kochanek S. Hemangiopericytoma of meningiomas. II. General and clinical data. Zentralbl Neurochir, 1986; 47:191–199

142. Guthrie BL, Ebersold MJ, Scheithauer BW. Neoplasms of the intracranial meninges In: Youmans JR, ed. Neurological surgery, 3rd edn, vol. 5. Philadelphia: Saunders, 1990: pp 3250–3315

143. Guthrie BL, Ebersold MJ, Scheithauer BW. Meningeal hemangiopericytoma: histological features, treatment, and long-term follow-up of 44 cases. Neurosurgery, 1989; 25:514–522

144. Sakaki S, Nakagawa K, Kimura H et al. Intracranial meningiomas in infancy. Surg Neurol, 1987; 28:51–57

145. Peace RJ. Congenital neoplasm of brain of new-born infant: report of case with necropsy. Am J Clin Pathol, 1954; 24:1272–1275

146. Blank W, Spring A, Giesen H et al. Intracranial hemangiopericytoma in a child. Klin Padiatr, 1988; 200:422–425

147. Mena H, Ribas JL, Pezeshkpour GH et al. Hemangiopericytoma of the central nervous system: a review of 94 cases. Hum Pathol, 1991; 22:84–91

148. Horten BC, Urich H, Rubinstein LJ et al. The angioblastic meningioma: A reappraisal of a nosological problem. Light-, electron-microscopic, tissue and organ culture observations. J Neurol Sci, 1979; 31:387–410

149. McDonald JV, Terry R. Haemangiopericytoma of the brain. Neurology, 1961; 11:497–502

150. Mangiardi JR, Flamm ES, Cravioto H et al. Hemangiopericytoma of the pituitary fossa: case report. Neurosurgery, 1983; 13:58–62

151. Lesoin F, Bouchez, B, Krivosic I et al. Hemangiopericytic meningioma of the pineal region. Case report. Eur Neurol, 1984; 23:274–277

152. Boniuk M, Messmer EP, Font RL. Hemangiopericytoma of the meninges of the optic nerve. A clinicopathologic report including electron microscopic observations. Ophthalmology, 1985; 92:1780–1787

153. Krugliask L, Barmeir E, Maroko I et al. Malignant spinal hemangiopericytoma, with benign radiological appearance. J Radiol, 1984; 65:485–487

154. Pitlyk PJ, Dockerty MB, Miller RH. Hemangiopericytoma of the spinal cord. Report of three cases. J Neurology, 1965; 15:649–653

155. Harris DJ, Fornasier WL, Livingstone KE. Hemangiopericytoma of the spinal canal. Report of three cases. J Neurosurg, 1978; 49:914–920

156. Ujiie H, Kubo O, Shimizu T et al. Intramedullary hemangiopericytoma of the spinal cord: case report and review of the literature. No Shinkei Geka, 1990; 18:273–277

157. Hahn MJ, Dawson R, Esterly JA et al. Haemangiopericytoma. An ultrastructural study. Cancer, 1973; 31:255–261

158. Popoff NA, Malinin TI, Rosomoff HL. Fine structure of intracranial hemangiopericytoma and angiomatous meningioma. Cancer, 1974; 34:1187–1197

159. D'Amore ES, Manivel JC, Sung JH. Soft-tissue and meningeal hemangiopericytomas: an immunohistochemical and ultrastructural study. Hum Pathol, 1990; 21:414–423

160. Pena CE. Intracranial haemangiopericytoma. Ultrastructural evidence of its leiomyoblastic differentiation. Acta Neuropathol (Berl), 1975; 33:279–284

161. Kawano H, Hayashi M, Kabuto M et al. An immunohistochemical and ultrastructural study of cultured intracranial hemangiopericytoma. Clin Neuropathol, 1988; 7:105–110

162. Nakamura M, Inoue HK, Ono N et al. Analysis of haemangiopericytic meningiomas by immunohistochemistry, electron microscopy and cell culture. J Neuropath Exp Neurol, 1987; 46:57–71

163. Joseph JT, Lisle DK, Jacoby LB et al. NF2 analysis distinguishes haemangiopericytoma from meningioma. Am J Pathol, 1995; 147:1450–1455

164. Ono Y, Ueki K, Joseph JT et al. Homozygous deletions of the CDKN2/p16 gene in dural hemangiopericytomas. Acta Neuropathol (Berl), 1996; 91:221–225

165. Bridges LR, Roche S, Nashef L et al. Haemangiopericytic meningioma of the sacral canal. A case report. J Neurol Neurosurg Psychiatry, 1988; 51:288–290

166. Leber GL, Fabinyi GC. Subarachnoid haemorrhage due to cauda equina haemangiopericytoma. Aust N Z J Surg, 1990; 60:69–70

167. Yagishita A, Hassoun J, Vincentelli F et al. Neuroradiological study of hemangiopericytomas. Neuroradiology, 1985; 27:420–425

168. Servo A, Jaaskelainen J, Wahlstrom T et al. Diagnosis of intracranial haemangiopericytomas with angiography and CT scanning. Neuroradiology, 1985; 27:38–43

169. Kolawole TM, Patel PJ, Boshra Y et al. Orbital and intracranial haemangiopericytoma. Case report with a short review. Eur J Radiol, 1988; 8:106–108

170. Parizel PM, Degryse HR, Gheuens J et al. Gadolinium-DOTA enhanced MR imaging of intracranial lesions. J Comput Assist Tomogr, 1989; 13:378–385

171. Von der Stein B, Schröder R. Three dimensional reconstruction of some vessel types in meningeal hemangiopericytoma. Clin Neuropathol, 1991; 10:279–284

172. Ludwin SK, Rubinstein LJ, Russell DS. Papillary meningioma: a malignant variant of meningioma. Cancer, 1975; 36:1363–1373

173. Böhling T, Paetau A, Ekblom P et al. Distribution of endothelial and basement membrane markers in angiogenic tumors of the nervous system. Acta Neuropathol (Berl), 1983; 62:67–72

174. Perry A, Scheithauer BW, Nascimento AG. The immunophenotypic spectrum of meningeal hemangiopericytoma: a comparison with fibrous meningioma and solitary fibrous tumour of meninges. Am J Surg Pathol, 1997; 21:1354–1360

175. Holden J, Dolman CL, Churg A. Immunohistochemistry of meningiomas including the angioblastic type. J Neuropathol Exp Neurol, 1987; 46:50–56

176. Itoh Y, Kowada M, Sakamoto T et al. Electron microscopic study of metastatic hemangiopericytic meningioma. No Shinkei Geka, 1984; 12:1187–1193

177. Pena CE. Meningioma and intracranial haemangiopericytoma. A comparative electron microscopic study. Acta Neuropathol (Berl), 1977; 39:69–74

178. Ramsey MJ. Fine structure of haemangiopericytoma and haemangioendothelioma. Cancer, 1966; 19:2005–2018

179. Boker DK, Stark HJ. The proliferation rate of intracranial tumors as defined by the monoclonal antibody KI 67. Application of the method to paraffin embedded specimens. Neurosurg Rev, 1988; 11:267–272

180. Roggendorf W, Schuster T, Peiffer J. Proliferative potential of meningiomas determined with monoclonal antibody Ki-67. Acta Neuropathol (Berl), 1987; 73:361–364

181. Jaaskelainen J, Servo A, Haltia M et al. Intracranial hemangiopericytoma: radiology, surgery, radiotherapy, and outcome in 21 patients. Surg Neurol, 1985; 23:227–236

182. Stone JL, Cybulski GR, Rhee HL et al. Excision of a large pineal region hemangiopericytoma (angioblastic meningioma, hemangiopericytoma type). Surg Neurol, 1983; 19:181–189

183. Berlit P, Pfiester P, Mattern I et al. Invasive meningioma of the anterior cranial fossa. Report of 2 cases. Nervenarzt, 1986; 57:649–653

184. Ciappetta P, Celli P, Palma L et al. Intraspinal hemangiopericytomas. Report of two cases and review of the literature. Spine, 1985; 10:27–31

185. Muller JP, Destee A, Verier A et al. Intraspinal hemangiopericytoma. 2 cases and review of the literature. Neurochirurgie, 1986; 32:140–146

186. Fulkum M, Kitamur K, Ohgama S et al. Radiosensitivity of meningioma – analysis of five cases of highly vascular meningioma treated by preoperative irradiation. Acta Neurochir (Wein), 1977; 36:47–60

187. Coffey RJ, Cascino TL, Shaw EG. Radiosurgical treatment of recurrent hemangiopericytomas of the meninges: preliminary results. J Neurosurg, 1993; 78:903–908

188. de la Monte SM, Flickinger J, Linggood RM. Histopathologic features predicting recurrence of meningiomas following subtotal resection. Am J Surg Pathol, 1986; 10:836–843

189. Backwinkel KD, Diddams JA. Haemangiopericytoma: Report of a case and comprehensive review of the literature. Cancer, 1970; 25:896–901

190. Russell T, Moss T. Metastasising meningioma. Neurosurgery, 1986; 19:1028–1030

191. Palkovic S. Multiple recurrence of an intracranial hemangiopericytoma. Neurosurg Rev, 1987; 10:233–236

192. Petito CK, Porro RS. Angioblastic meningioma with hepatic metastasis. J Neurol Neurosurg Psychiatry 1971; 34:541–545

193. Tanabe S, Soeda S, Mukai T et al. A case report of pancreatic metastasis of an intracranial angioblastic meningioma (hemangiopericytoma) and a review of metastatic tumor to the pancreas. J Surg Oncol, 1984; 26:63–68

194. Palacios E, Azar-Kia B. Malignant metastasising angioblastic meningiomas. J Neurosurg, 1975; 42:185–188
195. Slowik F, Jellinger K, Gaszo L et al. Gliosarcomas: histological, immunohistochemical, ultrastructural, and tissue culture studies. Acta Neuropathol (Berl), 1985; 67:201–110.
196. Kuratsu J, Beto H, Kochi M et al. Metastatic angiosarcoma of the brain. Surg Neurol, 1991; 35:305–309
197. Paulus W, Slowik F, Jellinger K. Primary intracranial sarcomas: histopathological features of 19 cases. Histopathology, 1991; 18:395–402
198. Mena H, Ribas JL, Enzinger FM. Primary angiosarcoma of the central nervous system. Study of eight cases and review of the literature. J Neurosurg, 1991; 75:73–76
199. Turner OA, Kernohan JW. Vascular malformations and vascular tumours involving the spinal cord. Arch Neurol Psychiatry 1941; 46:444–463
200. Kristoferitsch W, Jellinger K. Multifocal spinal angiosarcoma after chordotomy. Acta Neurochir (Wien), 1986; 79:145–153
201. Charman HP, Lowenstein DH, Cho KG et al. Primary cerebral angiosarcoma. Case report. J Neurosurg, 1988; 68:806–810
202. Abbott KH, Love JG. Metastasising intracranial tumours. Ann Surg, 1943; 118:343–352
203. Brickun AS, Rushton HW. Angiosarcoma of venous origin arising in the radial nerve. Cancer, 1977; 39:1556–1558
204. Ducatman BS, Scheithauer BW. Malignant peripheral nerve sheath tumors with divergent differentiation. Cancer, 1984; 15:1049–1057
205. Weiss SW, Enzinger FM. Epithelioid haemangioendothelioma. A vascular tumour often mistaken for carcinoma. Cancer, 1982; 50:970–987
206. Weiss SW, Ishak KG, Dail DH et al. Epithelioid hemangioendothelioma and related lesions. Semin Diagn Pathol, 1986; 3:259–287
207. Ellis GL, Kratochvil FJ. Epithelioid hemangioendothelioma of the head and neck: a clinicopathologic report of twelve cases. Oral Surg Oral Med Oral Pathol, 1986; 61:61–68
208. Taratuto AAL, Zurbriggen G, Sevlever G et al. Epithelioid hemangioendothelioma of the central nervous system. Immunohistochemical and ultrastructural observations of a pediatric case. Pediatr Neurosci, 1988; 14:11–14
209. Kepes JJ, Rubinstein LJ, Maw G et al. Epithelioid haemangiomas (hemangioendotheliomas) of the central nervous system and its coverings. A report of three cases. J Neuropathol Exp Neurol, 1986; 45:319
210. Gray F, Gherardi R, Scaravilli F. The neuropathology of the acquired immune deficiency syndrome (AIDS). Brain, 1988; 111:245–264
211. Staurou D, Mehraein P, Mellert W et al. Evaluation of intracerebral lesions in patients with acquired immunodeficiency syndrome. Neuropathological findings and experimental data. Neuropath Appl Neurobiol, 1989; 15:207–222

Melanocytic tumours

212. Kadonaga JN, Frieden IJ. Neurocutaneous melanosis: definition and review of the literature. J Am Acad Dermatol, 1991; 24:55
213. Lach B, Russell N, Benoit B et al. Cellular blue nevus ('melanocytoma') of the spinal meninges. Electron microscopic and immunohistochemical features. Neurosurgery, 1988; 22:773–780
214. Limas C, Tio FO. Meningeal melanocytoma ('melanotic meningioma'). Its melanocytic origin as revealed by electron microscopy. Cancer, 1972; 30:1286–1294
215. Glick R, Baker C, Husain S et al. Primary melanocytomas of the spinal cord: a report of seven cases. Clin Neuropathol, 1997; 16:127–132
216. Jellinger K, Bock F, Brenner H. Meningeal melanocytoma. Report of a case and review of the literature. Acta Neurochir, 1988; 94:78–87
217. Clarke DB, Leblanc R, Bertrand G et al. Meningeal melanocytoma. Report of a case and a historical comparison. J Neurosurg, 1998; 88:116–121
218. Botticelli AR, Villani M, Angiari P et al. Meningeal melanocytoma of Meckel's cave associated with ipsilateral Ota's nevus. Cancer, 1983; 21:2304–2310
219. Balmaceda CM, Fetell MR, Powers J et al. Nevus of Ota and leptomeningeal melanocytic lesions. Neurology, 1993; 43:381–386

220. Suzuki T, Yasumoto Y, Kumami K et al. Primary pineal melanocytic tumour. Case report. J Neurosurg, 2001; 94:523–527
221. Prabhu SS, Lynch PG, Keogh AJ et al. Intracranial meningeal melanocytoma: a report of two cases and review of the literature. Surg Neurol, 1993; 40:516–521
222. Litofsky NS, Zee C-S, Breeze RE et al. Meningeal melanocytoma: diagnostic criteria for a rare lesion. Neurosurgery, 1992; 31:945–948
223. Kawaguchi T, Kawano T, Kazekawa K et al. Meningeal melanocytoma in the left frontal region. Brain Tumor Pathol, 1998; 15:58–62
224. Matsumoto S, Kang Y, Sato S et al. Spinal meningeal melanocytoma presenting with superficial siderosis of the central nervous system. Case report and review of the literature. J Neurosurg, 1998; 88:890–894
225. Maiuri F, Iaconetta G, Benveniti D et al. Intracranial melanocytoma: case report. Surg Neurol, 1995; 44:556–561
226. Ruelle A, Tunesi G, Andrioli G. Spinal meningeal melanocytoma. Case report and analysis of diagnostic criteria. Neurosurg Rev, 1996; 19:39–42
227. Park SH, Park HR, Ko Y. Spinal meningeal melanocytoma. J Korean Med Sci, 1992; 7:364–368
228. Steinberg JM, Gillespie JJ, MacKay B et al. Meningeal melanocytoma with invasion of the thoracic spinal cord. Case report. J Neurosurg, 1978; 48:818–824
229. Gardiman M, Altavilla G, Marchioror L et al. Meningeal melanocytoma: a rare lesion of the central nervous system. Tumori, 1996; 82:494–496
230. Ibanez J, Weil B, Ayala A et al. Meningeal melanocytoma: case report and review of the literature. Histopathology, 1997; 30:576–581
231. Leonardi MA, Lumenta CB, Stolzle A et al. Unusual clinical presentation of a meningeal melanocytoma with seizures: case report and review of the literature. Acta Neurochir, 1998; 140:621–628
232. O'Brien TF, Moran M, Miller JH et al. melanocytoma. An uncommon diagnostic pitfall in surgical neuropathology. Arch Path Lab Med, 1995; 119:542–546
233. Hirose T, Horiguchi H, Kaneko F et al. Melanocytoma of the foramen magnum. Pathol Int 1997; 47:155–160
234. Uematsu Y, Yukawa S, Yokote H et al. Meningeal melanocytoma: magnetic resonance imaging characteristics and pathological features. Case report. J Neurosurg, 1992; 76:705–709
235. Winston KR, Sotrel A, Schmitt S. Meningeal melanocytoma. Case report and review of the clinical and histological features. J Neurosurg, 1987; 66:50–57
236. Czarnecki EJ, Silbergleit R, Gutierrez JA. MR of spinal meningeal melanocytoma. AJNR. Am J Neuroradiol, 1997; 18:180–182
237. Chen CJ, Hsu YI, Ho YS et al. Intracranial meningeal melanocytoma: CT and MRI. Neuroradiology, 1997; 39:811–814
238. Rege JD, Shet T, Sawant HV et al. Cytologic diagnosis of a melanotic neuroectodermal tumor of infancy occurring in the cranial bones. Diagn Cytopathol, 1999; 21:280–283
239. Rickert CH, Probst-Cousin S, Blasius S et al. Melanotic progonoma of the brain: a case report and review. Childs Nerv Syst, 1998; 14:389–393
240. Makin GW, Eden OB, Lashford LS et al. Leptomeningeal melanoma in childhood. Cancer, 1999; 86:878–886
241. Reyes-Mugica M, Chou P, Byrd S et al. Nevomelanocytic proliferations in the central nervous system of children. Cancer, 1993; 72:2277–2285
242. Koyama T, Ogawa M, Kurata S et al. Meningeal malignant melanoma in a child: immunological diagnosis. Acta Paediatr Jpn, 1992; 34:173–178
243. Barut S. Primary leptomeningeal melanoma simulating meningioma. Neurosurg Rev, 1995; 18:143–147
244. Allcutt D, Michowiz S, Weitzman S et al. Primary leptomeningeal melanoma: an unusually aggressive tumor in childhood. Neurosurgery, 1998; 32:721–729
245. Macfarlane R, Marks PV, Waters A. primary melanoma of the dura mater. Br J Neurosurg, 1989; 3:235–238
246. Thorton C, Brannan F, Hawkins SA et al. Primary malignant melanoma of the meninges. Clin Neuropathol, 1988; 7:244–248
247. Magni C, Yapo P, Mocaer J et al. Primary intramedullary melanoma. Apropos of a case. J Neuroradiol, 1996; 23:41–45
248. Fatallah-Shaykh HM, Zimmerman C, Morgan H et al. Response of primary leptomeningeal melanoma to intrathecal recombinant

interleukin-2. Case report. Cancer, 1996; 77:1544–1550

249. Kimura H, Itoyama Y, Fujioka S, Ushio Y. Neurocutaneous melanosis with intracranial malignant melanoma in an adult: a case report. No Shinkei Geka, 1997; 25:819–822

250. Lamas E, Diez Lobato R, Sotelo T et al. Neurocutaneous melanosis. Report of a case and review of the literature. Acta Neurochir, 1977; 36:93–105

251. Kaplan AM, Itabashi HH, Hanelin LG et al. Neurocutaneous melanosis with malignant leptomeningeal melanoma. A case with metastases outside the nervous system. Arch Neurol, 1975; 32:669–671

252. Gattuso P, Carson HJ, Attal H et al. Peritoneal implantation of meningeal melanosis via ventriculoperitoneal shunt: a case report and review of the literature. Diagn Cytopathol, 1995; 13:257–259

253. Bamborschke S, Ebhardt G, Szelies-Stock B et al. Review and case report. Primary melanoblastosis of the leptomeninges. Clin Neuropathol, 1985; 4:47–55

254. Adamek D, Kaluza J, Stachura K. Primary balloon cell malignant melanoma of the right temporo-parietal region arising from meningeal naevus. Clin Neuropathol, 1995; 14:29–32

255. Haddad FS, Jamali AF, Rebeiz JJ et al. Primary malignant melanoma of the gasserian ganglion associated with neurofibromatosis. Surg Neurol, 1991; 35:310–316

256. Jaenisch W, Schreiber D, Guthert H. Primare melanome der ZNS. Neuropathologie Tunoren des Nervensystems. Stuttgart: Gustav Fischer, 1988

257. Larson III TC, Houser OW, Onofrio BM et al. Primary spinal melanoma. J Neurosurg, 1987; 66:47–49

258. Ozden B, Barlas O, Hacihanefioglu U. Primary dural melanomas. Report of two cases and review of the literature. Neurosurgery, 1984; 15:104–107

259. Rodriguez, Gaetani P, Danova M et al. Primary solitary intracranial melanoma: case report and review of the literature. Surg Neurol, 1992; 38:26–37

260. Theunissen P, Spincemaille G, Pannebakker M et al. Meningeal melanoma associated with nevus of Ota: case report and review. Clin Neuropathol, 1993; 12:125–129

261. Hartmann LC, Oliver GF, Winkelmann RK et al. Blue nevus and nevus of Ota associated with dural melanoma. Cancer, 1989; 64:182–186

262. Sagar HJ, IIgren EB, Adams CB. Nevus of Ota associated with meningeal melanosis and intracranial melanoma. J Neurosurg, 1983; 58:280–283

263. Enriquez R, Egbert B, Boock J. Primary malignant melanoma of central nervous system. Pineal involvement in a patient with nevus of Ota and multiple pigmented skin nevi. Arch Pathol, 1973; 95:392–395

264. Jungbluth AA, Busam KJ, Gerald WL et al. An anti-melan-A monoclonal antibody for the detection of malignant melanoma in paraffin-embedded tissues. Am J Surg Pathol, 1998; 22:595–602

265. Marchiori G, Trincia G, Tonetto G, Baratto V, Cusumano S. Malignant meningeal melanoma. Ital J Neurol Sci, 1998; 19:37–40

Soft tissue tumours

266. Jellinger K, Paulus W. Mesenchymal, non-meningothelial tumors of the central nervous system. Brain Pathol, 1991; 1:79–87

267. Merimsky Ol, Lepechoux C, Terrier P et al. Primary sarcoma of the central nervous system. Oncology, 2000; 58:210–214

268. Paulus W, Slowik F, Jellinger K. Primary intracranial sarcomas: histopathological features of 19 cases. Histopathology, 1991; 18:395–402

269. Burger PC, Scheithauer BW. Tumors of the central nervous system. Fascicle 1 Atlas of tumor pathology. Washington DC: Armed Forces Institute of Pathology, 1994

270. Demirtas E, Ersahin Y, Yilmaz F et al. Intracranial meningeal tumours in childhood: a clinicopathologic study including MIB-1 immunohistochemistry. Pathol Res Pract, 2000; 196:151–158

271. Enzinger FM, Weiss SW. Soft tissue tumors, 3rd edn. St Louis: Moseby, 1995

272. Hibshoosh H, Lattes R. Immunohistochemical and molecular genetic approaches to soft tissue tumor diagnosis: a primer. Semin Oncol, 1997; 25:515–525

273. Ladanyi M, Bridge JA. Contribution of molecular genetic data to the classification of sarcomas. Hum Pathol, 2000; 31:532–538

274. Pieterse S, Dinning TA, Blumbergs PC. Postirradiation sarcomatous transformation of a pituitary adenoma: a combined pituitary tumor. Case report. J Neurosurg, 1982; 56:283–286

275. Nishio S, Morioka T, Inamura T et al. Radiation-induced brain tumours: potential late complications of radiation therapy for brain tumours. Acta Neurochir, 1998; 140:763–770

276. Waltz TA, Brownell B. Sarcoma: a possible late result of effective radiation therapy for pituitary adenoma. Report of two cases. J Neurosurg, 1966; 24:901–907

277. Schrantz JL, Araoz CA. Radiation induced meningeal fibrosarcoma. Arch Pathol, 1972; 93:26–31

278. Duffner PK, Krischer JP, Horowitz ME et al. Second malignancies in young children with primary brain tumors following treatment with prolonged postoperative chemotherapy and delayed irradiation: a Pediatric Oncology Group study. Ann Neurol, 1998; 44:313–316

279. Gainer JV, Chou SM, Chadduck WM. Familial cerebral sarcomas. Arch Neurol, 1975; 32:665–668

Adipose tissue tumours

280. Preul MC, Leblanc R, Tampieri D et al. Spinal angiolipomas. Report of three cases. J Neurosurg, 1993; 78:280–286

281. Pirotte B, Krischek B, Levivier M et al. Diagnostic and microsurgical presentation of intracranial angiolipomas. Case report and review of the literature. J Neurosurg, 1998; 88:129–132

282. Chitoku S, Kawai S, Watabe Y et al. Intradural spinal hibernoma: case report. Surg Neurol, 1998; 49:509–512

283. Sinson G, Gennarelli TA, Wells GB. Suprasellar osteolipoma: case report. Surg Neurol, 1998; 50:457–460

284. Sima A, Kindblom LG, Pelletieri L. Liposarcoma of the meninges. Acta Pathol Microbiol Scand, 1976; 8f4:306–310

285. Kothandaram P. Dural liposarcoma associated with subdural hematoma. Case report. J Neurosurg, 1970; 33:85–87

286. Cinalli G, Zerah M, Carteret M et al. Subdural sarcoma associated with chronic subdural hematoma. Report of two cases and review of the literature. J Neurosurg, 1997; 86:553–557

Fibrous tissue tumours

287. Reyes-Mugica M, Chou P, Gonzalez-Crussi F et al. Fibroma of the meninges in a child: immunohistological and ultrastructural study. Case report. J Neurosurg, 1992; 76:143–147

288. Palma L, Spagnoli LG, Yusuf MA. Intracerebral fibroma: light and electron microscopic study. Acta Neurochir, 1985; 77:152–156

289. Brunori A, Cerasoli S, Donati R et al. Solitary fibrous tumor of the meninges: two new cases and review of the literature. Surg Neurol, 1999; 51:636–640

290. Carneiro SS, Scheithauer BW, Nascimento AG et al. Solitary fibrous tumor of the meninges: a lesion distinct from fibrous meningioma. A clinicopathologic and immunohistochemical study. Am J Clin Pathol, 2000; 106:217–224

291. Challa VR, Kilpatrick SE, Ricci P et al. Solitary fibrous tumor of the meninges. Clin Neuropathol, 1998; 17:73–78

292. Gentil Perret A, Mosnier JF, Duthel R et al. Solitary fibrous tumor of the meninges. Ann Pathol, 1999; 19:532–535

293. Hasegawa T, Matsuno Y, Shimoda T et al. Extrathoracic solitary fibrous tumors: their histological variability and potentially aggressive behaviour. Hum Pathol, 1999; 30:1464–1473

294. Morimitsu Y, Nakajima M, Hisaoka M et al. Extrapleural solitary fibrous tumor: clinicopathologic study of 17 cases and molecular analysis of the p53 pathway. APMIS, 2000; 108:617–625

295. Mosnier JF, Perret AG, Scoazec JY et al. Expression of beta2 integrins and macrophage-associated antigens in meningeal tumours. Virchows Arch, 2000; 436:131–137

296. Nawashiro H, Nagakawa S, Osada H et al. Solitary fibrous tumor of the meninges in the posterior cranial fossa: magnetic resonance imaging and histological correlation – case report. Neurol Med Chir, 2000; 40:432–434

297. Ng HK, Choi PC, Wong CW et al. Metastatic solitary fibrous tumor of the meninges. Case report. J Neurosurg, 2000; 93:490–493

298. Nikas DC, De Girolami U, Folkerth RD et al. Parasagittal solitary fibrous tumor of the meninges. Case report and review of the literature. Acta Neurochir, 1999; 141:307–313

299. Perry A, Scheithauer BW, Nascimento AG. The immunophenotypic spectrum of meningeal hemangiopericytoma: a comparison with fibrous meningioma and solitary fibrous tumor of the meninges. Am J Surg Pathol, 1997; 21:1354–1360

300. Prayson RA, Estes ML, McMahon JT et al. Meningeal myofibroblastoma. Am J Surg Pathol, 1993; 17:931–936

301. Rodriguez LJ, Lopez J, Marin A et al. Solitary fibrous tumor of the meninges. Clin Neuropathol, 2000; 19:45–48

302. Slavik T, Bentley RC, Gray L et al. Solitary fibrous tumor of the meninges occurring after irradiation of a mixed germ cell tumor of the pineal gland. Clin Neuropathol, 1998; 17:55–60

303. Suzuki SO, Fukui M, Nishio S et al. Clinicopathological features of solitary fibrous tumor of the meninges: An immunohistochemical reappraisal of cases previously diagnosed to be fibrous meningioma or hemangiopericytoma. Pathol Int, 2000; 50:808–817

304. Yaghmai R, Karpinski NC, Wong WH et al. Dura based occipital mass in 41 year old female. Brain Pathol, 1998; 8:411–412

305. Kril M. Dural fibromatosis. J Neurosurg, 1992; 77:163–164

306. Quest DO, Salcman M. Fibromatosis presenting as a cranial mass lesion; case report. J Neurosurg, 1976; 44:237–240

307. Mitchell A, Scheithauer BW, Ebersold MJ et al. Intracranial fibromatosis. Neurosurgery, 1991; 29:123–126

308. Lauer DH, Enzinger FM. Cranial fasciitis of childhood. Cancer, 1980; 45:401–406

309. Tanaka M, Suda M, Ishikawa Y et al. Idiopathic hypertrophic cranial pachymeningitis associated with hydrocephalus and myocarditis: remarkable steroid-induced remission of hypertrophic dura mater. Neurology, 1996; 46:554–556

310. Malat J, Virapongse C, Palestro CJ et al. Primary intraspinal fibrosarcoma. Neurosurgery, 1986; 19:434–436

311. Gaspar LE, Mackenzie IR, Gilbert JJ et al. Primary cerebral fibrosarcomas. Clinicopathologic study and review of the literature. Cancer, 1993; 72:3277–3281

312. Cinalli G, Zerah M, Cartaret M et al. Subdural sarcoma associated with chronic subdural hematoma. Report of two cases and review of the literature. J Neurosurg, 1997; 86:553–557

313. Henry JM, Leestman JE. Astrocytoma arising in meningeal fibrosarcoma. Acta Neuropathol, 1973; 23:334–337

314. Savitz MH, Lestch SD, Goldstein HB et al. Fibrosarcoma of the spinal meninges in a case of neurofibromatosis. Mt Sinai J Med, 1982; 49:344–348

315. Schrantz JL, Araoz CA. Radiation induced meningeal fibrosarcoma. Arch Pathol, 1972; 93:26–31

316. McDonald P, Guha A, Provias J. Primary intracranial fibrosarcoma with intratumoral hemorrhage: neuropathological diagnosis with review of the literature. J Neurooncol, 1997; 35:133–139

317. Gainer JV, Chou SM, Chadduck WM. Familial cerebral sarcomas. Arch Neurol, 1975; 32:665–668

318. Kaminshi JM, Yang CC, Yagmai F et al. Intracranial fibrosarcoma arising after chemotherapy alone for glioblastoma multiforme in a child. Pediatr Neurosurg, 2000; 33:257–260

Histiocytic tumours

319. Lam RM, Colah SA. Atypical fibrous histiocytoma with myxoid stroma: a rare lesion arising from dura mater of the brain. Cancer, 1979; 43:237–245

320. Kepes JJ. 'Xanthomatous' lesions of the central nervous system: definition, classification and some recent observations. Prog Neuropathol, 1979; 4:179–213

321. Akimoto J, Takeda Y, Hasue M et al. Primary meningeal malignant fibrous histiocytoma with cerebrospinal dissemination and pulmonary metastasis. Acta Neurochir, 1998; 140:1191–1196

322. Biegel JA, Perilongo G, Rorke LB et al. Malignant fibrous histiocytoma of the brain in a six-year-old girl. Genes Chromosomes Cancer, 1992; 4:309–313

323. Gonzalez-Vitale JC, Slavin RE, McQueen JD. Radiation-induced intracranial malignant fibrous histiocytoma. Cancer, 1976; 37:2960–2963

324. Helle TL, Hanbey JW, Becker DH. Meningeal malignant fibrous histiocytoma arising from a thoracolumbar myelomeningocele. Case report. J Neurosurg, 1983; 58:593–597

325. Kalyanaraman UP, Taraska JJ, Fierer JA et al. Malignant fibrous histiocytoma of the meninges. Histological, ultrastructural, and immunocytochemical studies. J Neurosurg, 1981; 55:957–962

326. Leung GI, Yip P, Fan YW. Spontaneous epidural haematoma associated with radiation-induced malignant fibrous histiocytoma. J R Coll Surg Edinb, 1999; 44:404–406

327. Martinez-Salazar A, Supler M, Rojiani AM. Primary intracerebral malignant fibrous histiocytoma: immunohistochemical findings and etiopathogenetic considerations. Mod Pathol, 1997; 10:149–154

328. Roosen N, Cras P, Paquier P et al. Primary thalamic malignant fibrous histiocytoma of the dominant hemisphere causing severe neuropsychological symptoms. Clin Neuropathol, 1989; 8:16–21

329. Sima AA, Ross RT, Hoag G et al. Malignant intracranial fibrous histiocytomas. Histologic, ultrastructural and immunohistochemical studies of two cases. Can J Neurol Sci, 1986; 13:138–145

330. Swamy KS, Shankar SK, Asha T et al. Malignant fibrous histiocytoma arising from the meninges of the posterior fossa. Surg Neurol, 1986; 25:18–24

331. Paulus W, Peiffer J. Does the pleomorphic xanthoastrocytoma exist? Problems in the application of immunological techniques to the classification of brain tumors. Acta Neuropathol, 1988; 76:245–252

Smooth and striated muscle tumours

332. Kroe DJ, Hudgins WR, Simmons JC et al. Primary intrasellar leiomyoma. Case report. J Neurosurg, 1968; 29:189–191

333. Lin SL, Wang JS, Huang CS et al. Primary intracerebral leiomyoma: a case with eosinophilic inclusions of actin filaments. Histopathology, 1996; 28:365–369

334. Janisch W, Janda J, Link I. Primary diffuse leptomeningeal leiomyomatosis. Zentralbl Pathol, 1994; 140:195–200

335. Lach B, Duncan E, Rippstein P et al. Primary intracranial pleomorphic angioleiomyoma – a new morphologic variant. An immunohistochemical and electron microscopic study. Cancer, 1994; 74:1915–1920

336. Bargiela A, Rey JL, Diaz JL et al. Meningeal leiomyoma in an adult with AIDS: CT and MRI with pathological correlation. Neuroradiology, 1999; 41:696–698

337. Bejjani GK, Sdtopak B, Schwartz A et al. Primary dural leiomyosarcoma in a patient infected with human immunodeficiency virus: case report. Neurosurgery, 1999; 44:199–202

338. Brown HG, Burger PC, Olivi A et al. Intracranial leiomyosarcoma in a patient with AIDS. Neuroradiology, 1999; 41:35–39

339. Morgello S, Kotsianti A, Grumprecht JP et al. Epstein–Barr virus-associated dural leiomyosarcoma in a man infected with human immunodeficiency virus. Case report. J Neurosurg, 1997; 86:883–887

340. Steel TR, Pell MF, Turner JJ et al. Spinal epidural leiomyoma occurring in an HIV-infected man. Case report. J Neurosurg, 1993; 79:442–445

341. Karpinski NC, Yaghmai R, Barba D et al. A 26 year old HIV positive male with dura based masses. Brain Pathol, 1999; 9:609–610

342. Asai A, Yamada H, Murata S et al. Primary leiomyosarcoma of the dura mater. Case report. J Neurosurg, 1988; 68:308–311

343. Kidooka M, Okada T, Takayama S et al. Primary leiomyosarcoma of the spinal dura mater. Neuroradiology, 1991; 33:173–174

344. Louis DN, Richardson EPJ, Dickersin GR et al. Primary intracranial leiomyosarcoma. Case report. J Neurosurg, 1989; 71:279–282

345. Skullerud K, Stenwig AE, Brandtzaeg P et al. Intracranial primary leiomyosarcoma arising in a teratoma of the pineal area. Clin Neuropathol, 1995; 14:245–248

346. Sugita Y, Shigemori M, Harada H et al. Primary meningeal sarcomas with leiomyoblastic differentiation: a proposal for a new subtype of primary meningeal sarcomas. Am J Surg Pathol, 2000; 24:1273–1278

347. Vandewalle G, Brucher JM, Michotte A. Intracranial facial nerve rhabdomyoma. Case report. J Neurosurg, 1995; 83:919–922

348. Zwick DL, Livingston K, Clapp L et al. Intracranial trigeminal nerve rhabdomyoma/choristoma in a child: a case report and discussion of possible histogenesis. Hum Pathol, 1989; 20:390–392

349. Lee JI, Nam DH, Kim JS et al. Intracranial oculomotor nerve rhabdomyoma. J Neurosurg, 2000; 93:715

350. Fix SE, Nelson J, Schochet SS Jr. Focal leptomeningeal rhabdomyomatosis of the posterior fossa. Arch Pathol Lab Med, 1989; 113:872–873

351. Celli P, Cervoni L, Mraglino C. Primary rhabdomyosarcoma of the brain: observations on a case with clinical and radiological evidence of cure. J Neurooncol, 1998; 36:259–267

352. Dropcho EJ, Allen JC. Primary intracranial rhabdomyosarcoma: case report and review of the literature. J Neurooncol, 1987; 5:139–150

353. Ferracini R, Poggi S, Frank G et al. Meningeal sarcoma with rhabdomyoblastic differentiation: case report. Neurosurgery, 1992; 30:782–785

354. Herva R, Serlo W, Laitinen J et al. Intraventricular rhabdomyosarcoma after resection of hyperplastic choroid plexus. Acta Neuropathol (Berl), 1996; 92:213–216

355. Kobayashi S, Hirakawa E, Sasaki M et al. Meningeal rhabdomyosarcoma. Report of a case with cytologic, immunohistologic and ultrastructural studies. Acta Cytol, 1995; 39:428–434

356. Smith MT, Armbrustmacher VW, Violett TW. Diffuse meningeal rhabdomyosarcoma. Cancer, 1981; 47:2081–2086

357. Taratuto AL, Molina HA, Diez B et al. Primary rhabdomyosarcoma of brain and cerebellum. Report of four cases in infants: an immunohistochemical study. Acta Neuropathol, 1985; 66:98–104

358. Tomei G, Grimoldi N, Gappricci E et al. Primary intracranial rhabdomyosarcoma: report of two cases. Childs Nerv Syst, 1989; 5:246–249

359. Xu F, DeLas Casas LE, Dobbs LJ Jr. Primary meningeal rhabdomyosarcoma in a child with hypomelanosis of Ito. Arch Pathol Lab Med, 2000; 124:762–765

360. Paulus W, Slowik F, Jellinger K. Primary intracranial sarcomas: histopathological features of 19 cases. Histopathology, 1991; 18:395–402

Osteocartilaginous tumours

361. Aoki H, Nakase H, Sakaki T. Subdural osteoma. Acta Neurochir, 1998; 140:727–728

362. Choudhury AR, Haleem A, Tjan GT. Solitary intradural intracranial osteoma. Br J Neurosurg, 1995; 9:557–559

363. Fallon MD, Ellerbrake D, Teitelbaum SL. Meningeal osteomas and chronic renal failure. Hum Pathol, 1982; 13:449–453

364. Hadadian K, Abtahii H, Asil ZT et al. Cystic falcine chondroma: case report and review of the literature. Neurosurgery, 1991; 29:909–912

365. Kurt E, Beute GN, Sluzewski M et al. Giant chondroma of the falx. Case report and review of the literature. J Neurosurg, 1996; 85:1161–1164

366. Mapstone TB, Wongmongkolrit T, Roessman U et al. Intradural chondroma. A case report and review of the literature. Neurosurgery, 1983; 12:111–114

367. Nakazawa T, Inoue T, Suzuki F et al. Solitary intracranial chondroma of the convexity dura: case report. Surg Neurol, 1993; 40:495–498

368. Salazar C, Oommen KJ, Sobonya RE. Silent solitary right parietal chondroma resulting in secondary mania. Clin Neuropathol, 1993; 12:325–329

369. Takano M, Oka H, Kawano N et al. Dural chondroma with fat tissue. Acta Neurochir, 1997; 139:690–691

370. Miyamori T, Mizukoshi H, Yamano K et al. Intracranial chondrosarcoma – case report. Neurol Med Chir (Tokyo), 1990; 30:263–267

371. Bauman GS, Wara WM, Ciricillo SF et al. Primary intracerebral osteosarcoma: a case report. J Neurooncol, 1997; 32:209–213

372. Reznik M, Lenelle J. Primary intracerebral osteosarcoma. Cancer, 1991; 68:793–797

373. Sipos EP, Tamargo RJ, Epstein JI et al. Primary intracerebral small-cell osteosarcoma in an adolescent girl: report of a case. J Neurooncol, 1997; 32:169–174

374. Bar-Sela G, Tsuk-Shina T, Zaaroor et al. Primary osteogenic sarcoma arising from the dura mater: case report. Am J Clin Oncol, 2001; 24:418–420

375. Bonilla F, Provencio M, Salas C et al. Primary osteosarcoma of the meninges. Ann Oncol, 1994; 5:965–966

376. Cannon TC, Bane BL, Kistler D et al. Primary intracerebellar osteosarcoma arising within an epidermoid cyst. Arch Pathol Lab Med, 1998; 122:737–739

377. Couldwell WT, Scheithauer BW, Rice SG et al. Osteosarcoma of the meninges in association with glioblastoma. Acta Neurochir, 1997; 139:684–689

378. Lee YY, Van Tassel P, Raymond AK. Intracranial dural chondrosarcoma. Am J Neuroradiol, 1988; 9:1189–1193

379. Oruckaptan HH, Berker M, Soylemezoglu F, Ozcan E. Parafalcine chondrosarcoma: an unusual localization for a classical variant. Case report and review of the literature. Surg Neurol, 2001; 55:174–179

380. Bernstein M, Perrin RG, Platts ME et al. Radiation-induced cerebellar chondrosarcoma. Case report. J Neurosurg, 1984; 61:174–177

381. Forbes RB, Eljamel MS. Meningeal chondrosarcomas: a review of 31 patients. Br J Neurosurg, 1998; 12:461–464

382. el-Gindi S, Abd-el-Hafeez M, Salama M. Extracranial skeletal metastases from an intracranial meningeal chondrosarcoma. Case report. J Neurosurg, 1974; 40:651–653

383. Ranjan A, Chacko G, Joseph T et al. Intraspinal mesenchymal chondrosarcoma. Case report. J Neurosurg, 1994; 80:928–930

384. Rodda RA, Franklin CI. Intracranial meningeal chondrosarcoma – probable mesenchymal type. Aust N Z J Surg, 1984; 54:387–390

385. Parker JR, Zarabi MC, Parker JC. Intracerebral mesenchymal chondrosarcoma. Am J Clin Lab Sci, 1989; 19:401–407

386. Scheithauer BW, Rubinstein LJ. Meningeal mesenchymal chondrosarcoma: report of 8 cases with review of the literature. Cancer, 1978; 42:2744–2752

387. Cho BK, Chi JG, Wang KC et al. Intracranial mesenchymal chondrosarcoma: a case report and literature review. Childs Nerv Syst, 1993; 9:295–299

388. Huckabee RE. Meningeal mesenchymal chondrosarcoma of the spine; a case report. J Magn Reson Imaging, 1991; 1:93–95

389. Rushing EJ, Armonda RA, Ansari Q et al. Mesenchymal chondrosarcoma: a clinicopathologic and flow cytometric study of 13 cases presenting in the central nervous system. Cancer, 1996; 77:1884–1891

390. Swanson PE, Lillemoe TJ, Manivel JC et al. Mesenchymal chondrosarcoma. An immunohistochemical study. Arch Pathol Lab Med, 1990; 114:943–948

391. Sato K, Kubota T, Yoshida K et al. Intracranial extraskeletal myxoid chondrosarcoma with special reference to lamellar inclusions in the rough endoplasmic reticulum. Acta Neuropathol, 1993; 86:525–528

392. Demirtas E, Ersahin Y, Yilmaz F et al. Intracranial meningeal tumours in childhood: a clinicopathologic study including MIB-1 immunohistochemistry. Pathol Res Pract, 2000; 196:151–158

393. Park YK, Park HR, Chi SG et al. Overexpression of p53 and rare genetic mutation in mesenchymal chondrosarcoma. Oncol Rep, 2000; 7:1041–1047

394. Aigner T, Loos S, Muller S et al. Cell differentiation and matrix gene expression in mesenchymal chondrosarcomas. Am J Pathol, 2000; 156:1327–1335

395. Reif J, Graf N. Intraspinal mesenchymal chondrosarcoma in a three-year old boy. Neurosurg Rev, 1987; 10:311–314

Sarcomatosis

396. Budka H, Pilz P, Guseo A. Primary leptomeningeal sarcomatosis. Clinicopathological report of six cases. J Neurol, 1975; 211:77–93

397. Garbes AD. Cytologic presentation of primary leptomeningeal sarcomatosis. Acta Cytol, 1984; 28:709–712

398. Licandro AM, Girodano R, Morra M. Leptomeningeal sarcomatosis. Report of a clinical case. Acta Neurol, 1987; 9:297–301

399. Lukes SA, Wollmann R, Stefannson K. Meningeal sarcomatosis and multiple astocytomas. Arch Neurol, 1983; 40:179–182

400. Pfluger T, Weil S, Weis S et al. MRI of primary meningeal sarcomas in two children: differential diagnostic considerations. Neuroradiology, 1997; 39:225–228

401. Prabhu SR, Purandare SM. Primary diffuse sarcomatosis of leptomeninges (a case report). Indian J Cancer, 1972; 9:83–85

402. Reynier Y, Hassoun J, Vittini F et al. Meningeal fibrosarcomas. Neurochirurgie, 1984; 30:1–10

403. Slowinski J, Adamek D, Krygowska-Wajs A et al. Sarcomatosis of leptomeninges, brain and spinal cord coexisting with von Reckinghausen's neurofibromatosis. A case report and review of the literature. Folia Neuropathol, 1995; 33:135–140

404. Tachibana O. Meningeal sarcomatosis. Ryoikibetsu Shokogun Shirizu, 2000; 28:161–163

405. Thibodeau LL, Ariza A, Piepmeier JM. Primary leptomeningeal sarcomatosis. Case report. J Neurosurg, 1988; 68:802–805

406. Vieweg UI, Synowitz HJ, Minda R et al. Primary leptomeningeal sarcomatosis in a 26 year old patient. Neurochirugia, 1993; 36:213–215

15 Tumours of peripheral nerves

Classification

The World Health Organisation (WHO) classification of tumours of peripheral nerves recognises a wide variety of entities, listed in Table 15.1. Non-neurogenic tumours are also encountered (Table 15.2). In addition a variety of other lesions can be confused with tumours of peripheral nerve, including reactive, hyperplastic and hamartomatous lesions.[1,2]

Anatomy and histology of peripheral nervous system

The peripheral nervous system is composed of *nerves* and *ganglia*.

A *nerve* is a collection of axons, linked together by support tissue into an anatomically defined trunk. The axons may be either motor or sensory, myelinated or non-myelinated.

A *ganglion* is a peripheral collection of nerve cell bodies together with efferent and afferent axons, and support cells. Ganglia may be sensory (e.g. spinal sensory ganglia), or contain the cell bodies of autonomic nerves (i.e. sympathetic or parasympathetic ganglia).

A *peripheral nerve* is composed of: axons; Schwann cells, which may form myelin; perineural cells that ensheath fascicles; spindle shaped fibroblast support cells, which produce fibrocollagenous tissue; blood vessels and lymphatics; and variable numbers of adipocytes.

There are three compartments of support tissue in a nerve trunk, the endoneurium, perineurium and epineurium (Fig. 15.1).

Endoneurium is composed of longitudinally orientated collagen fibres, extracellular matrix material rich in glycosaminoglycans, and sparse fibroblasts. It surrounds the individual axons and their associated Schwann cells, as well as capillary blood vessels.

Perineurium surrounds groups of axons and endoneurium to form small bundles (fascicles). It is composed of a variable number (typically seven to eight) of concentric layers of epithelial-like flattened cells termed perineural cells separated by layers of collagen. The cells are joined by junctional complexes and each layer of cells is surrounded by an external lamina.

Epineurium is an outer sheath of loose fibrocollagenous tissue, which binds individual nerve fascicles into a nerve trunk. The epineurium may also include adipose tissue, as well as a main muscular artery supplying the nerve trunk.

Nerves vary in their relative composition of myelinated and non-myelinated fibres from one anatomical site to

Table 15.1 WHO classification of peripheral nerve tumours

Benign tumours of peripheral nerve
Schwannoma (neurilemoma, neurinoma)
   Conventional
   Cellular
   Plexiform
   Melanocytic

Neurofibroma
Plexiform neurofibroma

Perineurioma
Intraneural perineurioma
Soft tissue perineurioma

Granular cell tumour

Malignant tumours of peripheral nerve
Malignant peripheral nerve sheath tumour (MPNST)
Epithelioid MPNST
MPNST with divergent mesenchymal and or epithelial
   differentiation
Melanotic MPNST
Melanotic psammomatous MPNST
Malignant granular cell tumour

Table 15.2 Non-neurogenic tumours of peripheral nerve

Meningioma[1]
Paraganglioma[187–194]
Lipoma[195]
Angioma[196]
Haemangioblastoma[294]
Adrenal adenoma[197]
Lymphoma[198]
Amyloidoma[199]
Inflammatory pseudotumour[200]

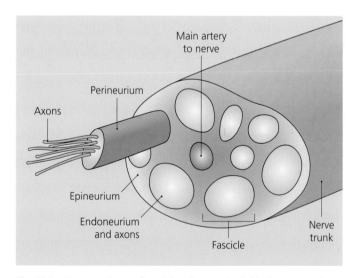

Fig. 15.1 **Support tissue of peripheral nerve.** Individual axons and their associated Schwann cells are surrounded by endoneurium, and bound into fascicles by the epithelial-like perineurium. The epineurium binds individual fascicles into a nerve trunk, and may contain the main muscular artery supplying the nerve trunk.

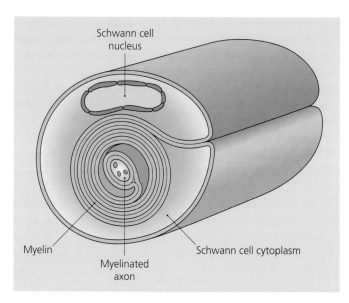

Fig. 15.2 **Myelinated axon.** The myelin sheath is formed from the fused cell Schwann cell membranes, which wrap concentrically around a central axon. Each myelinating Schwann cell will only associate with a single axon. Compare with the arrangement for unmyelinated axons shown in Figure 15.3.

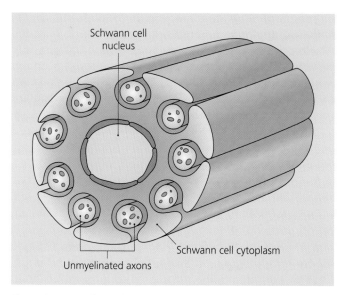

Fig. 15.3 **Unmyelinated axon.** Some Schwann cells support a number of unmyelinated axons, which bury themselves in the Schwann cell cytoplasm without invoking myelin sheath formation. Compare with the arrangement for myelinated axons shown in Figure 15.2.

another. Myelinated fibres in a typical peripheral nerve in the lower limb of an adult vary in diameter from 2 to 17 m (including myelin), there being a bimodal distribution with peaks around 5 m and 13 m.

Ganglia of the peripheral nervous system, which may be either sensory or autonomic, are composed of: neuron cell bodies; support cells termed satellite cells or capsular cells, regarded as specialised Schwann cells; axons; and fibroblastic cells producing loose fibrocollagenous support tissue. The *neuron cell bodies* are large; they have abundant cytoplasm containing Nissl substance and large nuclei with prominent nucleoli.

The *Schwann cells* support both myelinated and non-myelinated axons. In routine histological preparations of peripheral nerve Schwann cell cytoplasm is generally indistinct. In longitudinal sections nuclei are elongated and tapering, while in transverse section they have an oval or rounded profile.

Schwann cells show strong immunoreactivity for S-100 protein as well as CD56 (Leu7). Some Schwann cells may also express glial fibrillary acidic protein (GFAP). The external lamina associated with Schwann cells can be detected by immunostaining for type IV collagen or laminin.

Ultrastructurally, each Schwann cell has a well defined external lamina which separates the cell from the endoneurium. Myelin is formed from the fused cell membrane of Schwann cells which enwrap axons (Fig. 15.2). The membrane is modified by incorporation of specific lipids and proteins. In addition to producing myelin, Schwann cells

also support non-myelinated axons, which bury themselves into the Schwann cell cytoplasm (Fig. 15.3).

Benign tumours of peripheral nerve

Schwannoma

There are four types of Schwannoma, conventional, cellular, plexiform and melanocytic. Of these the conventional Schwannoma is by far the most common.

Cell biology and genetics

The majority of Schwannomas are solitary, sporadic tumours but there are syndromic associations:

- Neurofibromatosis type 2 (NF2) (Chapter 19) is associated with development of bilateral vestibular Schwannomas and multiple peripheral Schwannomas.
- Multiple peripheral Schwannomas may be seen in the condition of Schwannomatosis.[3–5]
- Carney's complex is associated with psammomatous melanotic Schwannomas.[6]
- Uncommon phenotypes of neurofibromatosis have been delineated including the syndrome of multiple naevi, multiple Schwannomas and multiple vaginal leiomyomas.[7]

The *NF2* gene has been implicated in the formation of both inherited (NF2) as well as sporadic Schwannomas. The *NF2* gene is a tumour suppressor gene producing the protein merlin (also called Schwannomin by some groups).[8] Absent merlin expression is seen by Western blotting in all Schwannomas. In patients with NF2, loss of both *NF2* alleles and merlin occur early in Schwann cell tumorigenesis, before the tumourlet stage.[9] In one study recurrent clonal chromosome aberrations seen in Schwannomas included loss of 22q material, loss of a sex chromosome, and trisomy 7.[10] Mice expressing a mutant merlin protein specifically in Schwann cells show a high prevalence of Schwann cell derived tumours and Schwann cell hyperplasia.[11] NF2 is discussed in more detail in Chapter 19.

Growth rates of Schwannomas have been mostly studied in relation to vestibular nerve tumours. The growth rate of Schwannomas has been measured on serial computerised tomography (CT) and magnetic resonance imaging (MRI) scans and is very variable. This is also supported by slow but variable cell proliferation rates in tumours. In one study, the mean tumour growth rate was 1.16 mm/year (range: 0.75–9.65 mm/year) with significant tumour growth seen in 36.4%, insignificant growth in 50%, and negative growth in 13.6% of lesions. The growth rate of cerebellopontine angle (CPA) tumours (1.4 mm/year) was significantly greater than that of internal auditary canal tumours (0.2 mm/year).[12]

Ki-67/MIB-1 immunostaining has been evaluated in vestibular Schwannomas showing a typically low labelling fraction.[13–15]

Conventional Schwannoma

Schwannomas are benign tumours of peripheral nerve derived from and composed of mature Schwann cells. They have also been termed neurilemomas or neurinomas in the past, although this usage is not now recommended.

Incidence and site

Schwannomas are very common tumours and occur at all ages with a peak incidence between the fourth and sixth decades. There is no sex diffence for peripheral Schwannomas, but there is a 2:1 female predominance for the small proportion of tumours that arise in the central nervous system.[16] In terms of aetiology there is an important association of Schwannomas with NF2, discussed in Chapter 19.

Schwannomas arise in a wide variety of anatomical sites[16], including:

- peripheral nerves in the extremities, head and neck;[17]
- spinal and cranial nerves[18] (particularly the vestibular nerve in the cerebellopontine angle (CPA);
- intracerebral;[19,20]
- intramedullary;[21]
- intraventricular;[22]
- sinonasal cavity or nasopharynx,[23] and
- visceral[24–29] sites.

Schwannomas mainly develop in relation to sensory nerves and are usually solitary tumours. Schwannomas that develop in association with NF2 may be multiple (Chapter 19). Schwannomas arising from the VIII cranial nerve are now termed vestibular Schwannomas, although they were usually referred to as 'acoustic neuromas' in the past.[30] Bilateral vestibular Schwannomas are diagnostic of NF2 (Chapter 19). Schwannomas arising from cranial nerves other than the VIII are more often than not associated with NF2. An incidence of 12 tumours per million population per year with a significant proportion of intracanalicular and small tumours has been estimated in Europe.[31]

Sporadic Schwannomas that arise from spinal nerve roots, either intradural or extradural, are most common in the lumbar region. Tumours may have both intradural as well as extradural components, so called 'dumb-bell' tumours. Schwannomas arising in the viscera are rare, generally sporadic, and are mainly seen in the gastro-intestinal tract.

Clinical features

Clinically Schwannomas present in a variety of ways reflecting a slow growing benign tumour with a slow pace of growth over a period of years. Most present as otherwise asymptomatic swellings, but some may present with local effects of growth and mass effect, including: nerve root compression, spinal cord compression, or the CPA syndrome.[12,18,30]

Radiological imaging of Schwannomas reveals them to be well circumscribed lesions that may have caused distortion or erosion of adjacent tissues through mass effect and local growth. CT scanning shows typically low attenuation lesions which are contrast enhancing. MRI shows high signal on T2-weighted scans with contrast enhancement.[32]

Pathology

Macroscopic features

The majority of Schwannomas are smooth, encapsulated lesions, which arise from an identifiable nerve in about half of cases seen pathologically. Tumours range in size from microscopic lesions to masses up to 12 cm in diameter. They are soft and rubbery in consistency with a cream or tan-coloured appearance on external and cut surfaces. On cut surface yellow areas can sometime be seen, believed to reflect areas of lipid accumulation. A thin capsule is evident in most tumours. Cystic change may be seen in some instances.[16,33]

Very small tumours may be intraneural, causing a fusiform swelling of a nerve. As the Schwannoma enlarges there is a tendency for the parent nerve to be displaced, such that it comes to lie in one part of the capsule. When a Schwannoma is excised with nerve attached the nerve fibres can generally either be traced as a broad bundle running around the eccentric tumour. Less commonly, the parent nerve becomes broadly stretched and incorporated into the tumour capsule.

Vestibular Schwannomas (acoustic neuromas) grow down into the vestibular nerve to involve the cochlear nerve by direct infiltration. Although often stated that they arise from the superior vestibular nerve, many probably originate in the inferior nerve.[30] Intralabyrinthine examples, originally only seen on labyrithectomy may now be detected with imaging.[34]

Small intracanalicular tumours are commonest in men and have an even range of incidence from 20 to 70 years. Lesions are very cellular and have few vessels.[35] Large lesions in the CPA are commonest in women. With increasing size tumours become heavily vascularised and collagenised. Vestibular tumours in children are also encountered, when they may be large and vascular lesions. Vestibular Schwannomas normally grow out into the CPA but transpetrous spread into the middle cranial fossa has been documented.

Intraoperative diagnosis

The diagnosis of a Schwannoma is usually clinically evident, based on location and imaging features. When faced with a sample from a CPA tumour suspected to be a Schwannoma it is important to be aware of other lesions that may arise in this locality. About 10% of CPA tumours turn out not to be vestibular Schwannommas: 3–4% meningiomas, 2–3% cholesteatomas, 1% facial nerve neuromas, 1% rarities including neuromas of other nerves, cysts, angiomas, gliomas, haemangioblastoma, metastatic carcinoma, lymphoma, lipoma, teratoma, rhabdomyosarcoma of middle ear, gliomangioma, and extension of bone tumours. Malignant peripheral nerve sheath tumours of the CPA are very rare.[32,33]

In smear preparations, tumours may not smear well owing to their tough consistency. When a smear is possible, the low power appearance is usually very suggestive, with the fascicles of cells in the Antoni A areas splaying out in an appearance that has been likened to twisted rope (Fig. 15.4). Higher magnification of the fascicles shows parallel streams of spindle cells with tapering nuclei (Fig. 15.5). In lesions with degenerative atypia, pleomorphic and hyperchromatic nuclei may be seen which should not be interpreted as indicating malignancy. Lymphoid cells and mast cells in the lesion may be prominent in smear preparations.

Frozen sections will generally show characteristic histological appearances to indicate a Schwannoma, as detailed below. In some lesions, focal necrosis and nuclear pleomorphism can lead the unwary to a mistaken

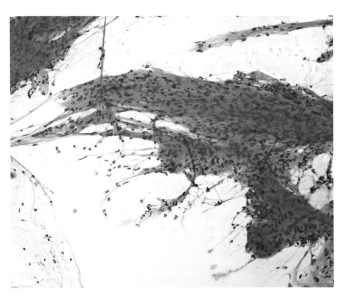

Fig. 15.4 **Schwannoma.** At low magnification fascicles of tumour composed of cohesive Antoni A tissue form intertwining cords of cells. H & E.

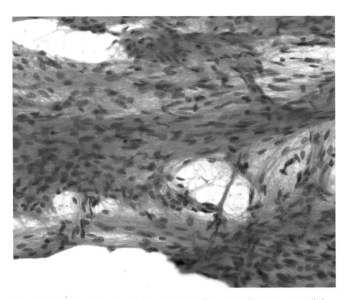

Fig. 15.5 **Schwannoma.** At higher magnification cells run in parallel bundles and have elongated nuclei with rounded ends. Cell bundles are thick and so it is necessary to focus through the section to appreciate the cellular detail. H & E.

opinion of a malignant tumour. Careful assessment for other features known to be associated with degeneration in a Schwannoma is the best safeguard to avoid this mistake.

Histological features

Schwannomas are composed of Schwann cells, seen as streams of elongated cells with tapering nuclei (Figs 15.6–15.10). Cells have small to moderate amounts of weakly eosinophilic cytoplasm with such indistinct borders that tumour appears as a pink-stained matrix containing tumour nuclei.

Two main patterns of cellular organisation are seen (Fig. 15.6):

1. compact areas where cells are arranged in streams and areas of palisading (Antoni A). In these areas nuclei are generally elongated and tapering;

2. loosely arranged cells often with areas of vacuolation and occasionally lipidisation (Antoni B). Schwann cells in these areas appear stellate and nuclei may not be elongated but have a rounder profile.

Verocay bodies are seen in a proportion of tumours in Antoni A regions. They are parallel arrays of tumour nuclei separated by the brightly eosinophilic compacted

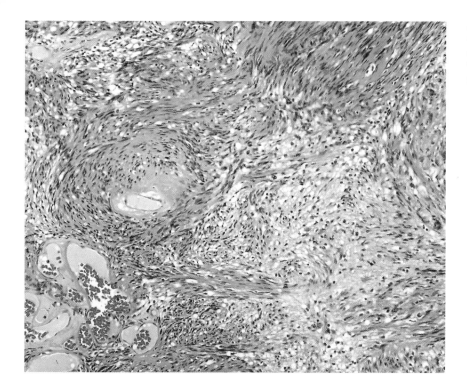

Fig. 15.6 **Conventional Schwannoma.** At low magnification Schwannomas are composed of swirls of compact Antoni A and loose Antoni B tissue with a generally prominent vascular pattern. H & E.

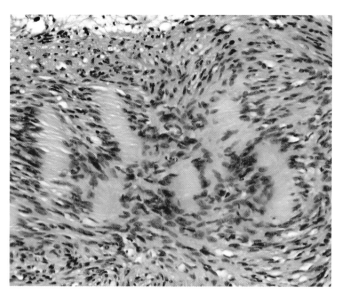

Fig. 15.7 **Conventional Schwannoma.** Verocay bodies can be identified in most Schwannomas as palisades of cells separated by pink-stained zones composed of cell processes. These areas stain with PAS. H & E.

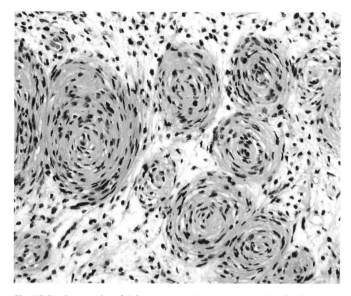

Fig. 15.8 **Conventional Schwannoma.** Concentric whorls of cells are prominent in some tumours which may cause confusion with some patterns of meningioma. H & E.

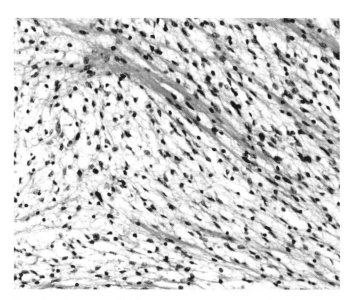

Fig. 15.9 **Conventional Schwannoma.** Loose Antoni B tissue is pale-staining and may appear myxoid. H & E.

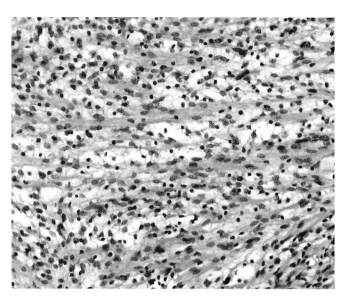

Fig. 15.10 **Conventional Schwannoma.** Lipidisation of cells and infiltration by lymphoid cells is a common finding in Antoni B areas. H & E.

cell membrane of Schwann cells (Fig. 15.7). These areas are periodic acid–Schiff (PAS) positive. Vessels are present in variable density within Schwannomas, the walls of which may show thickening and hyalinisation.

Schwannomas usually develop such that they peripherally displace the nerve from which they arise, hence axons are not generally seen within a Schwannoma. The prominent capsule around the tumour is derived from the attenuated perineurium and epineurium of the parent nerve.

Mitoses may be seen in conventional Schwannomas and do not imply malignancy. When a tumour has an Antoni A pattern with more than 4 mitoses per 10 high power fields, a diagnosis of cellular Schwannoma should be considered[36] (see later).

Secondary and degenerative changes are common in Schwannomas (Figs 15.11–15.16). Nuclei may become enlarged, hyperchromatic and pleomorphic (Figs 15.15, 15.16). This has been termed degenerative atypia and is a feature of benign lesions. It has been called 'ancient change' in a Schwannoma. Dense hyalinisation may be seen in some tumours, with much of the lesion replaced by poorly cellular dense hyaline collagenous material (Fig. 15.12). Cystic degeneration may be seen,[33] with cysts showing an almost epithelial lined appearance (Fig. 15.14). Such pseudoglandular spaces may dominate some Schwannomas. Immunohistochemistry shows no epithelial antigens expressed by the lining cells, which have the phenotype of Schwann cells.[37] Some tumours appear haemorrhagic, either focally or extensively. Bleeding into a tumour may have been the cause of a change in clinical features in some tumours.[38] Vascular proliferation may be a feature of some Schwannomas to the extent of simulating an

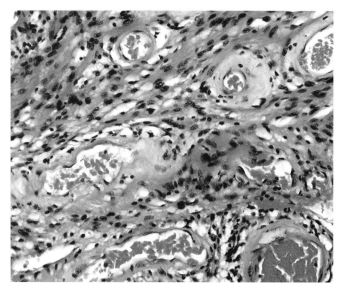

Fig. 15.11 **Conventional Schwannoma.** Hyalinisation of vessels and focal lymphocytic infiltration is common in most Schwannomas. H & E.

angioma. Phagocytic cells containing haemosiderin are common, representing resolution of previous intratumoral haemorrhage (Fig. 15.13). Lipidisation of cells is also a common feature together with focal infiltration with lymphocytes, plasma cells and mast cells (Fig. 15.10 and 15.11). Metaplastic formation of cartilage, bone and adipose tissue may be seen in some lesions.

Immunohistochemistry

Schwannomas are uniformly immunoreactive for S-100 protein, a useful and sensitive marker (Figs 15.17 and

15.18). CD56 (Leu7) positivity is also seen in a proportion of tumours, often in a focal pattern in Antoni A areas. GFAP may be detected in some tumours. Focal CD68 staining can also be seen in a proportion of cases. EMA immunoreactivity is confined to perineurial cells remaining around the tumour margins (Fig. 15.19).

Ultrastructural features

Schwann cells have long thin intertwined processes, many with adherens type junctions. Cells have a surrounding external basal lamina. In Antoni A areas and in Verocay bodies, the cellular background is composed of stacks of external lamina, thin cell processes and collagen fibres.

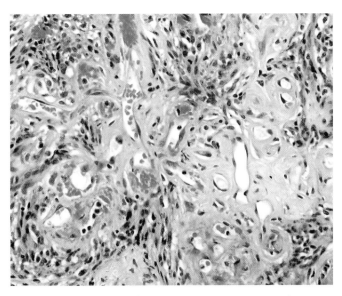

Fig. 15.12 **Conventional Schwannoma.** In some areas extensive hyalinisation is present. H & E.

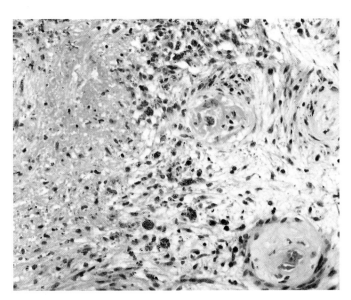

Fig. 15.13 **Conventional Schwannoma.** Areas of haemorrhage, necrosis and haemosiderin containing macrophages may be present. H & E.

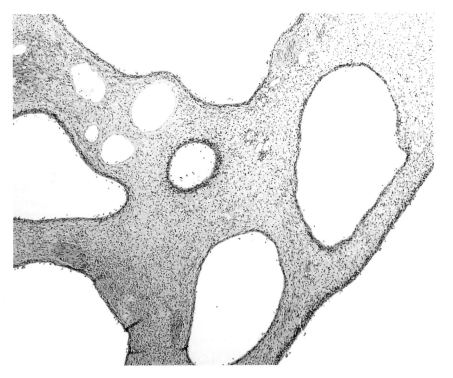

Fig. 15.14 **Conventional Schwannoma.** Pseudoglandular spaces are seen in a proportion of Schwannomas. These do not express epithelial antigens on immunohistochemistry. H & E.

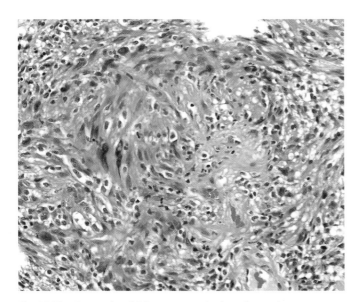

Fig. 15.15 **Conventional Schwannoma.** Ancient change is characterised by the presence of large, pleomorphic hyperchromatic nuclei. H & E.

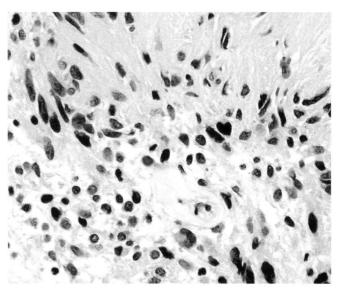

Fig. 15.16 **Conventional Schwannoma.** Nuclear hyperchromasia and pleomorphism are a reflection of degenerative atypia when seen in a Schwannoma. H & E.

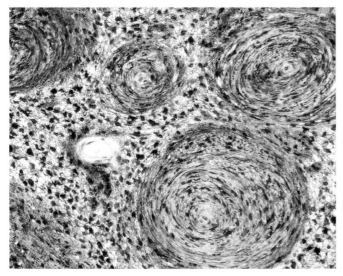

Fig. 15.17 **Conventional Schwannoma.** S-100 staining shows strong immunoreactivity in both Antoni A and B areas.

Ultrastructural examination does not have a routine place in the diagnosis of Schwannomas.[39]

Differential diagnosis

Several lesions may mimic the histological appearance of a conventional Schwannoma.

Cellular Schwannoma

If a lesion is cellular, composed of Antoni A pattern, with up to 4 mitoses per 10 high power fields a diagnosis of a cellular Schwannoma should be considered (see later).

Ancient naevus

Some melanocytic naevi may show ancient change and may resemble an ancient Schwannoma. Schwannomas may also be mistaken for a malignant melanoma on cytological grounds,[40] but this is more likely to be a problem with melanotic Schwannomas (see below).

Neurofibroma

When a Schwannoma is mainly composed of loose Antoni B tissue then it can look like a neurofibroma. The presence of a thick capsule (except in visceral or submucosal sites), areas of Antoni A patterning, lack of axons within the tumour, and a uniform pattern of S-100 protein immunoreactivity are all features that reinforce a diagnosis of Schwannoma. Some tumours appear to have features of both types of tumour.[41]

Leiomyoma

Diagnostic confusion mainly occurs in visceral, submucosal and soft tissue sites where leiomyomas may be common. The most important discriminant in modern pathological practice is immunohistochemical staining for smooth muscle, leiomyomas being S-100 negative but expressing desmin and smooth muscle actin (SMA).

Palisaded myofibroblastoma

This is a lesion that usually involves lymph nodes, characterised by a spindle cell and palisaded appearance which mimics Antoni A patterns of a Schwannoma with Verocay bodies. Like leiomyomas, these lesions are negative for S-100 protein but express SMA and desmin.

Other palisaded tumour types

Prominent cutaneous Schwannomas have been described, mainly seen in the head and neck region in adults. Such lesions may be confused with other tumour types showing a prominent palisading pattern. *Palisading leiomyoma* is immunoreactive for SMA and desmin. *Palisading cutaneous fibrous histiocytoma* and *myofibroblastic dermatofibroma* are variably positive for factor XIIIa, SMA and CD57. *Palisaded encapsulated neuromas* contain nerve fibres with myelin sheaths.[42]

Neuroblastoma

Benign Schwannomas have been described that mimic neuroblastoma (primitive neuroectodermal tumour). These lesions contain areas resembling neuroblastoma with rosette-like structures surrounded by small round cells. The cells are positive for S-100 protein, Leu7 and GFAP, but are negative for neurofilament protein, synaptophysin and MIC2. Ultrastructural examination confirms Schwannian features and does not show neuroendocrine granules.[43–45]

Therapy and prognosis

Conventional Schwannomas are benign tumours which do not recur when completely excised.[16] In surgery for Schwannomas of the vestibular nerve, conservation of the cochlear nerve is possible in some instances. In elderly patients with Schwannomas of the vestibular nerve, the risks of surgery sometimes have to be weighed against

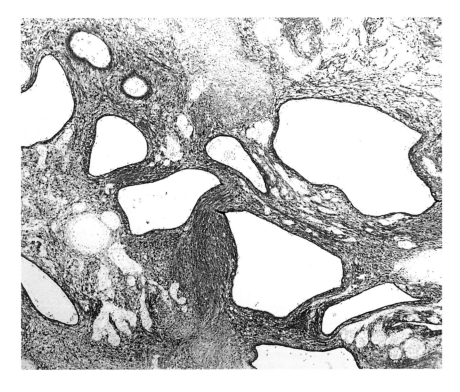

Fig. 15.18 **Conventional Schwannoma.** S-100 staining is intense in the lining of pseudoglandular spaces, confirming their Schwann cell origin.

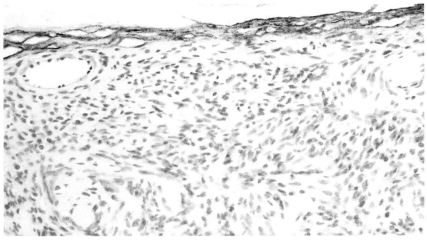

Fig. 15.19 **Conventional Schwannoma.** EMA immunoreactivity may be seen in perineurial cells remaining in the capsule of a Schwannoma.

the benefits of tumour removal. In some of these cases imaging has shown such a slow pace of growth that 'watchful waiting' has been advocated.[46,47] Stereotactic radiosurgery has been used to good effect in some cases. This causes coagulative necrosis of tumour.[48–50]

There is great surgical interest in whether it is possible to resect a vestibular nerve tumour to conserve hearing without recurrence. With interest in preservation of hearing function after tumour resection, aspects concerning resectability of tumours and risk of recurrence are evident.[51] Detailed pathological analysis of resected specimens has been performed and this reveals microscopic involvement of facial and cochlear nerves often not macroscopically evident at the time of surgery.[52,53] In another study, macroscopic adhesions to the cochlear nerve were seen in nine out of 12 cases, but not in the remaining three. Histology showed infiltration in all cases with no clear cleavage plane.[54] The fate of tumour rests has been studied in 14 patients using MRI with contrast. Persistent tumour was seen in 50% of patients, although none had new symptoms (mean 70 months) and the lesions were not visible on CT. Four out of seven cases showed enlargement of residual tumour.[55] Twenty-eight patients with surgery sparing cochlear and facial nerves were MRI scanned 5 years after surgery and showed no recurrence.[56]

Malignant change in a pre-existing Schwannoma is a very rare event but has been well documented[57–61] (see Chapter 19).

Cellular Schwannoma

This benign variant of a Schwannoma has a high cell density with a dominant Antoni A pattern and with absence of well-formed Verocay bodies.

Incidence and site

Cellular Schwannomas are generally solitary lesions and account for around 5% of all benign peripheral nerve sheath tumours. There is a female predominance and, while they occur in a wide age range including childhood, they are mainly seen in the fourth decade. Anatomically, cellular Schwannomas are mainly seen in the spinal, pelvic, mediastinal and retroperitoneal regions with fewer examples being encountered intracranially.[62–69] Unusual locations include nasopharynx,[23,67] female genital tract,[70] bronchus,[71] and colon.[72]

Clinical features

Clinical features associated with cellular Schwannomas are similar to those associated with conventional Schwannomas.[16]

Pathology

Macroscopic features

Macroscopically, cellular Schwannomas appear similar to conventional Schwannomas, as described above. The lesions are typically more uniform and have a firmer texture than a conventional Schwannoma.

Intraoperative diagnosis

Cellular Schwannomas generally produce smears that allow a diagnosis of a Schwann cell tumour. As with conventional Schwannoma, the low power appearance is the main clue to diagnosis, showing splaying out of bundles of spindle cells in a 'twisted rope' pattern (Fig. 15.4). Cell nuclei are tapering and may have a coarser chromatin pattern to that seen in conventional Schwannoma, with many lesions showing mitoses which should not be interpreted as indicating malignancy. Lymphoid cells and mast cells in the lesion are usually prominent in smear preparations from cellular Schwannomas.

Frozen sections will also show characteristic histological appearances to indicate a Schwannoma, as detailed below. Pronounced hyperchromasia of cells, epithelioid cells, mitoses in excess of 4 per ten high power fields, and large areas of geographic necrosis are features which should alert to the possibility of a malignant peripheral nerve sheath tumour (MPNST). In the setting of an intraoperative assessment it would be appropriate to advise the surgeon on the importance of achieving a complete local excision in such tumours, providing this is clinically feasible.

Histological features

Cellular Schwannomas show most of the histological features noted for conventional Schwannomas. They differ in having a high cellularity (Figs 15.20–15.22) with whorls and streaming fascicles of Schwann cells in an Antoni A pattern. In these areas nuclei are elongated and tapering and may show mild hyperchromasia. There is a degree of uniformity to the nuclei, with generally little pleomorphism seen (Fig. 15.21). Some nuclear palisading may be seen but this is generally not marked. Well formed Verocay bodies are not seen, representing a defining feature. Cellular whorls may be present in some tumours. Antoni B areas may be seen but in a minor proportion.

Mitotic figures are seen in the majority of these tumours, generally up to 4 per 10 high power fields (Fig. 15.20). Small numbers of cases have been observed with a typical clinical progression with higher mitotic activity.[36]

As with conventional Schwannomas degenerate changes may be seen:

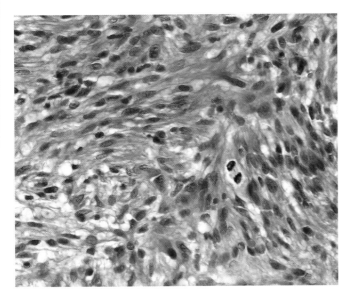

Fig. 15.20 **Cellular Schwannoma.** Cellular Schwannomas are composed of cohesive cells with frequent mitoses. Cellularity may be either uniform through the tumour or may be focal. H & E.

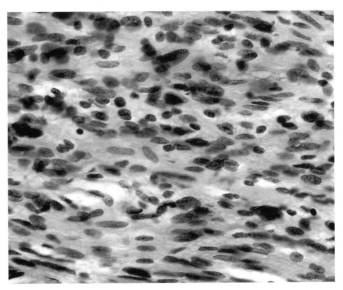

Fig. 15.22 **Cellular Schwannoma.** In a proportion of cellular Schwannomas degenerative nuclear atypia may be present. H & E.

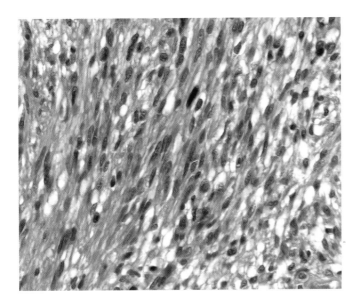

Fig. 15.21 **Cellular Schwannoma.** In most cellular Schwannomas nuclear pleomorphism is not marked but may be seen. H & E.

- vascular hyalinisation is common;
- aggregates of lymphoid cells are common;
- foam cells may be seen within tumour;
- haemosiderin laden cells may be seen but are generally not as frequent in this variant compared to conventional Schwannoma;
- microcystic change may be present, but large pseudoglandular cysts as seen in conventional Schwannoma are not typical;
- necrosis may be seen in small foci, typically in the absence of nuclear palisading;

- myxoid change can be seen focally in some lesions.
- some degenerative nuclear atypia may occur (Fig. 15.22)

Immunohistochemistry

S-100 immunoreactivity is seen in a strong uniform staining pattern and this is a useful feature in differential diagnosis. CD56 (Leu7) is seen in a small proportion of cases in a focal pattern. As with conventional Schwannoma, GFAP immunoreactivity may be present. Epithelial membrane antigen (EMA) immunoreactivity may be seen in residual perineurial cells. CD34 can be detected in dendritic cells (seen mainly in Antoni B areas) and beneath any residual perineurium.[73]

Assessment of cell proliferation using antibodies expressed by nuclei in the cell cycle shows values around 8%, with a wide variation.[36]

Ultrastructural appearance

Schwann cells in cellular Schwannomas show typical ultrastructural features with tapering cell processes invested by an external basal lamina. Adherens type junctions are seen as with conventional Schwannoma.[64]

Differential diagnosis

Malignant peripheral nerve sheath tumour (MPNST)

The histological features of a cellular Schwannoma must be distinguished from a well differentiated MPNST. Pronounced hyperchromasia of cells, epithelioid cells, mitoses in excess of 4 per 10 high power fields, and large areas of geographic necrosis are features which should alert to the possibility of a malignant peripheral nerve sheath tumour. This is supported by finding only patchy focal S-100 immunostaining. In contrast, the presence of Antoni A pattern tumour, foam cells, hyaline vessels, focal haemosiderin deposition and strong uniform S-100 protein expression support a diagnosis of a cellular Schwannoma.

Neurofibroma

Certain areas of cellular Schwannomas can have a loose pattern suggestive of a neurofibroma, raising the issue of whether the areas of high cellularity represent development of a MPNST in a neurofibroma. S-100 staining in cellular Schwannomas is generally strong and diffuse, in contrast to focal staining seen in neurofibromas.

Meningioma

Some cellular Schwannomas can be confused with meningiomas, especially those of fibroblastic pattern. In addition to their distinctive cellular and architectural features, meningiomas only show patchy focal immuno-staining with S-100 protein in contrast to the strong diffuse staining seen in cellular Schwannoma.

Leiomyosarcoma

The whorled pattern seen in some cellular Schwannomas may raise the possibility of a tumour of smooth muscle origin. This issue can best be resolved by application of a panel of immunochemical markers. S-100 immuno-reactivity will be lacking and muscle markers expressed in a tumour of smooth muscle origin.

Therapy and prognosis

Cellular Schwannomas are benign tumours but may undergo local recurrence if not completely excised. The mean time to recurrence in such lesions is around 7 years. No cases with metastatic spread have been reported.[64–66,68]

Plexiform Schwannoma

Incidence and site

This variant of Schwannoma is characterised by its plexiform, intraneural growth pattern. These are uncommon lesions which can occur at any age with no sex difference. The majority of tumours arise in subcutaneous tissues as solitary lesions although multicentric growth has been described.[5,74–78] Although the majority occur as sporadic tumours, some have been associated with NF2[79,80] (Chapter 19).

Pathology

Macroscopic features

When seen in surgical resections, plexiform Schwannomas appear as rubbery cream–yellow nodular lesions usually 1–3 cm in diameter, although uncommonly larger lesions have been described.

Histological features

The defining feature of this variety of Schwannoma is the presence of multiple nodules of tumour (Fig. 15.23). These are formed as a result of expansion of pre-existing nerve fascicles, as is the case with plexiform neurofibroma (see below). A capsule is usually apparent, if less well formed than in conventional Schwannoma. The tumour is generally of Antoni A pattern with little formation of Antoni B areas. The cytology and pattern of these Schwannomas are generally that of a conventional Schwannoma but plexiform cellular Schwannomas have been described. Such cellular lesions may be infiltrative and poorly defined.

Immunohistochemistry and electron microscopy

The immunohistochemical profile of this variant is the same as for conventional and cellular Schwannomas. Ultrastructural features are the same as for conventional Schwannoma.

Differential diagnosis

The multinodular pattern and predominant skin involvement for plexiform Schwannomas can lead to diagnostic confusion with four main entities.

Plexiform neurofibroma

Unlike the compact Antoni A pattern seen in most plexiform Schwannomas, neurofibromas are composed of cells

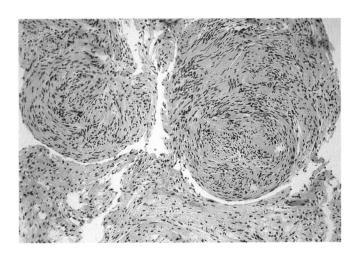

Fig. 15.23 **Plexiform Schwannoma.** Multiple nodules of tumour result from expansion of pre-existing nerve fascicles by Schwannoma. H & E.

with spindle cell nuclei separated by collagen bundles in a mucoid background stroma. Unlike Schwannomas, which show diffuse strong S-100 immunoreactivity, a neurofibroma only shows focal S-100 staining.

Palisaded encapsulated neuroma (solitary neuroma)

These are solitary, well circumscribed cutaneous hyperplastic lesions composed of Schwann cells formed into small fascicles and nodules. Axons are seen within lesions with special staining. Lesions are mainly encountered on the face.[81]

Traumatic neuroma

This is a reactive lesion caused by partial or complete transection of a nerve with local overgrowth. Lesions are generally ill-defined and composed of a haphazard proliferation of Schwann cells, perineurial cells and axons in a fibrocollagenous stroma.

Leiomyoma

Cutaneous leiomyomas may have a multinodular pattern, simulating a plexiform Schwannoma. The smooth muscle nature of the lesion is easily determined by lack of S-100 protein immunoreactivity and positive staining for desmin or smooth muscle actin.

Therapy and prognosis

This variant of Schwannoma is benign and complete excision is associated with cure.[76] Plexiform tumours which have a cellular Schwannoma pattern may be associated with local recurrence.

Melanotic Schwannoma

This variant of Schwannoma is very rare and is characterised by melanin pigmentation within tumour cells.

Clinical features

These lesions occur at any age between the second and ninth decade, mainly being seen in the fourth decade. Most tumours occur in relation to spinal nerves, with others involving autonomic nerves in the alimentary tract or other viscera. While the majority of lesions are solitary, multiple lesions are described in association with Carney's complex (lentiginous pigmentation; cardiac, skin or breast myxomas; pituitary endocrine abnormalities, and blue naevi).[6,82–84]

Pathology

Macroscopic appearances

Tumours vary in size, most being 4–5 cm in size at diagnosis. They are generally oval or sausage shaped,

circumscribed lesions but lack a capsule, differing in this respect from conventional Schwannomas. The colour of these lesions reflects their melanin content, varying from jet black through mottled black to dusky grey.

Histological features

There are two types of melanotic Schwannoma:

- *Conventional melanotic Schwannomas* These are mainly seen in spinal nerves although they have been described in other sites including the sympathetic chain, intramedullary spinal cord, cerebellum, orbit and soft tissues.[85–91] They are cellular and composed of plump spindle cell and epithelioid cells arranged in whorls and streaming fascicles, containing melanin pigment (Fig. 15.24). Nuclear palisading is not generally seen. Due to the often dense melanin deposition it is difficult to discern cytological details in these lesions unless melanin bleaching is performed. Nuclei are generally hyperchromatic and in some tumours degenerative atypia with mutinucleate cells is seen. Nuclear cytoplasmic pseudoinclusions may be seen.[92]
- *Psammomatous melanotic Schwannomas* These are mainly seen in autonomic/visceral locations. Approximately 50% of patients have Carney's complex. These lesions have the same Schwann cell arrangement as a melanotic Schwannoma with the additional feature of mineralised lamellar calcospherites. In many tumours, the cells develop large cytoplasmic vacuoles, to the extent that some areas of tumour resemble adipose tissue.[82]

Immunohistochemistry and electron microscopy

The Schwann cells in melanotic Schwannomas show strong diffuse immunoreactivity for S-100 protein and HMB45.

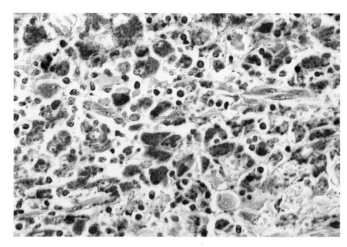

Fig. 15.24 **Melanotic Schwannoma.** Plump spindle celled and epithelioid Schwann cells are arranged in fascicles and contain melanin pigment. H & E.

Ultrastructural examination shows a Schwann cell morphology with interdigitating tapering processes associated with an external lamina and joined by adherens type junctions. Melanosomes are also visible in cells.[39,82,90,93,94]

Differential diagnosis

The main differential diagnostic problem lies in distinguishing a melanotic Schwannoma from other pigmented lesions.[16]

Pigmented neurofibroma

These lesions generally only show histological (as opposed to naked eye) evidence of pigmentation. The nuclei are like those of a neurofibroma, being elongated rather than the rounded nuclei seen in melanotic Schwannoma.[95]

Melanocytoma

These tumours characteristically arise in the meninges. While there are many overlapping features, melanocytomas lack external basal lamina around cells.[96]

Metastatic malignant melanoma

Cytologically, most metastatic malignant melanomas will show obvious nuclear atypia and other features of malignancy including obvious nuclear atypia, brisk mitotic activity and necrosis. Problems may be encountered when lesions are deeply pigmented and cytology is difficult to determine following melanin bleaching. Electron microscopy may be helpful in this differential diagnosis, by demonstrating conspicuous basal lamina in Schwann cell neoplasms.

Therapy and prognosis

While the majority of melanotic Schwannomas are benign lesions, approximately 10% may develop malignant change, with potential for metastatic spread. This generally develops after local recurrence following incomplete surgical excision. When lesions develop malignant change they are associated with mitotic figures, large nucleoli, nuclear pleomorphism and hyperchromatism.[92]

Neurofibroma

Neurofibromas are benign tumours of peripheral nerve composed of a mixture of three main cell types: Schwann cells, perineurial-like cells and fibroblasts.[16] Most tumours encountered are sporadic lesions, but some are associated with neurofibromatosis type 1 (NF1).[97] Neurofibromas are also associated with uncommon neurofibromatosis-variant syndromes including hereditary spinal neurofibromatosis, familial intestinal neurofibromatosis, autosomal dominant 'neurofibromas alone', Watson syndrome and Noonan/neurofibromatosis syndrome.[7]

Cell biology and genetics

Multiple neurofibromas are one of the characteristic features of NF1[98,99] (Chapter 19). There has been continued debate as to whether neurofibromas represent a neoplastic or hyperplastic phenomenon. Biological studies have shown that neurofibroma Schwann cells, in contrast to normal Schwann cells, can promote angiogenesis and invade basement membrane in an in vivo system.[100] In the same model, neurofibroma-derived fibroblasts neither promote angiogenesis nor show invasive capacity.[100] When grafted into nude mice, neurofibroma Schwann cells form progressive neurofibroma-like tumours.[101] Recent studies have shown that the *NF1* gene is involved in sporadic neurofibromas, as it is in NF1 related lesions.[102] The *NF1* gene product, neurofibromin, is thought to be a tumour suppressor and in patients with NF1, neurofibromas are believed to arise from NF1 inactivation in Schwann cells. One study has shown that fibroblasts isolated from neurofibromas have at least one normal *NF1* allele and express both NF1 mRNA and protein, but that S-100(+)cells, identified as Schwann cells, usually lack the NF1 transcript.[103] Most tumours are diploid, with about one-third being aneuploid.[104] The proliferative potential and growth rate of tumours has been investigated with Ki-67/MIB-1 immucytochemistry, the labelling index typically being around 5%.[105]

Clinical features

Clinically neurofibromas are very common tumours that can be seen at any age and with no sex specific preference.[16] Several clinical patterns of neurofibroma may be seen,[1,2,106] including localised cutaneous neurofibroma arising from peripheral cutaneous nerves; localised intraneural neurofibroma which may arise in any peripheral nerve from spinal nerve root to out to the periphery; plexiform neurofibromas, generally arising in large nerve trunks or plexuses; diffuse cutaneous neurofibroma, arising from peripheral cutaneous nerves; diffuse soft tissue neurofibroma, and, rarely, visceral neurofibromas.

Most tumours present as slow growing lesions with local swelling, often because of cosmetic concerns.

Pathology

Macroscopic features

Localised neurofibromas are typically soft, rounded, nodular lesions with a grey, glistening, sometimes gelatinous cut surface. Those arising in skin develop within the dermis with a loose covering of skin, often becoming polypoid.

Those arising in nerves produce a gelatinous fusiform swelling of the nerve. Most lesions range between 1 and 2 cm in size and are removed for cosmetic reasons. The vast majority of such lesions are seen as solitary tumours unassociated with NF1.[107]

Plexiform neurofibromas are uncommon and appear as tangled, gelatinous, thick tendrils involving the trunks of large nerves such as nerve plexuses. This pattern is often seen when neurofibromas affect visceral sites. In less common situations, this pattern may be seen expanding large fascicles in a major nerve such as the sciatic nerve. While sporadic plexiform neurofibromas have been described, there is a very strong clinical association of this type of neurofibroma with NF1, to the extent that diagnosing this type of tumour has been suggested a mandate to offer genetic counselling to an affected patient. This pattern of neurofibroma is also associated with a risk of subsequent neoplastic transformation.[106,108–111]

Diffuse neurofibromas are often ill-defined within soft tissues and composed of grey, soft glistening tissue. Those involving subcutaneous tissue are associated with loose, wrinkled overlying skin. This type of tumour has a stronger clinical association with NF1, often being encountered in children.[106] There is a low risk of malignant transformation in this pattern of tumour. Massive soft tissue neurofibromas are the least common pattern of diffuse tumour, seen only in patients with NF1, formerly termed elephantiasis neurofibromatosa.[106]

Intraoperative diagnosis

Requests for identification of a neurofibroma during surgery are not common in most clinical services. The most reliable way to do this is on a frozen section, rather than a smear.

A more demanding question that is sometimes asked of the pathologist is whether a lesion shows malignant change, usually in the context of a patient with known NF1. Given that such a decision may be problematic on conventional pathological examination of fixed embedded tissue, such a diagnosis must only be made with great caution using frozen section. While it is possible to tell a high grade malignant peripheral nerve sheath tumour from other pathologies, discriminating a low grade malignant lesion from a cellular neurofibroma or an atypical neurofibroma may not be possible.

Histological features

Neurofibromas are characterised by both cellular and stromal components. Both these components tend to develop within the existing structure of a nerve, such that in early lesions the tumour microarchitecture is aligned according to the original alignment and architecture of the nerve. In such early lesions a neurofibroma is typically well circumscribed from adjacent tissues and grows as a

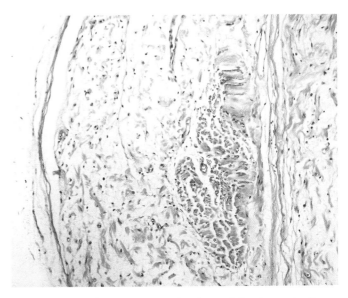

Fig. 15.25 **Neurofibroma.** A nerve showing early involvement with neurofibroma. A thin capsule lies over pale-staining hypocellular myxoid neurofibroma, with residual axons still preserved in the centre of the nerve. H & E.

fusiform enlargement of the parent nerve (Figs 15.25 and 15.26). With enlargement of a neurofibroma there is typically loss of orientation and the parent nerve becomes indistinguishable. Such later lesions typically become less well circumscribed and may show extension into adjacent tissues.

The cellular components of a neurofibroma can be divided into neoplastic, reactive and normal components. The neoplastic cells of a neurofibroma mainly have an elongated spindle cell morphology with smaller numbers of ovoid cells (Figs 15.27–15.31). In the majority of tumours cellularity in a neurofibroma is low. The cytoplasm of these cells is weakly eosinophilic and the cell margins are generally indistinct. Nuclei are elongated and have a wavy or curved morphology with generally uniform chromatin and small indistinct nucleoli (Fig. 15.27). In early lesions, such cells expand the endoneurial compartment of a nerve, sometimes being initially clustered circumferentially around existing myelinated axons in a pattern resembling that seen in a perineurioma or hypertrophic neuropathy (see below). In early lesions, neoplastic cells are aligned along the long axis of the nerve. In later lesions neoplastic cells develop a haphazard orientation. In most tumours nuclear pleomorphism and hyperchromasia of nuclei are not seen. Mitoses are rare in a benign neurofibroma and should occasion a careful search for other features of malignancy. The neoplastic spindle cells in a neurofibroma can be distinguished into Schwann cells, perineurial-like cells and fibroblasts using ultrastructural and immunohistochemical methods.

Variants of neurofibroma have been described based on variations of this cellular pattern:

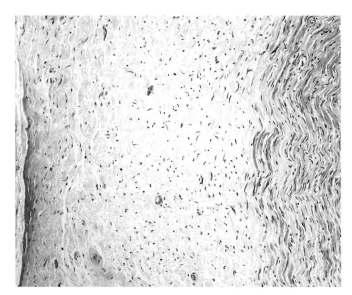

Fig. 15.26 **Neurofibroma.** This nerve shows a similar pattern of involvement with more marked deposition of pink-staining collagenous matrix material in the neurofibromatous areas. H & E.

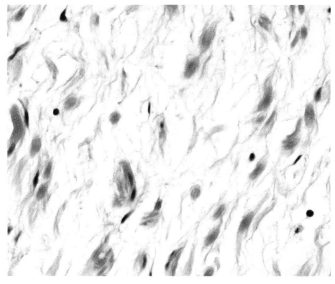

Fig. 15.27 **Neurofibroma.** Cytologically cells have wavy nuclei with tapering ends. In this example thin collagen bundles are widely separated by a myxoid stroma. H & E.

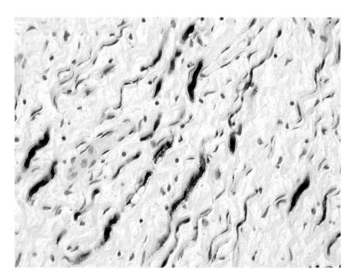

Fig. 15.28 **Neurofibroma.** Axons in affected nerve may be visible, separated by myxoid or collagenous stroma, and can be highlighted by specific immunochemical staining for neurofilament protein.

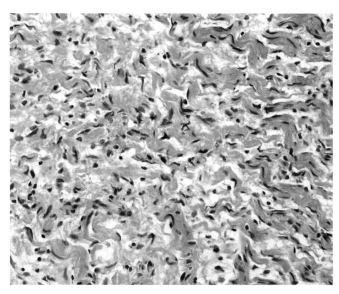

Fig. 15.29 **Neurofibroma.** In this example there is dense collagen deposition forming wavy bundles. Between these the spindle shaped neoplastic cells can be seen. H & E.

Atypical neurofibroma is defined when there is nuclear atypia (represented by nuclear hyperchromasia and pleomorphism) focally within an otherwise typical neurofibroma of low cellularity (Fig. 15.31). In the absence of mitoses and with a low cell proliferation index such changes have been interpreted as representing degenerative atypia, in a manner see more usually in Schwannomas.[1,104,112] Finding such changes in a cellular lesion or with evidence of cell proliferation would warrant consideration of MPNST.

Cellular neurofibroma has been defined where, in contrast to the usually low cellularity of a neurofibroma,

there is a dominant high cellularity, sometimes with small numbers of mitoses. This pattern must be distinguished from MPNST.[1,104,112] Cellular neurofibromas do not usually have the very high mitotic rate of malignant peripheral nerve sheath tumours, lack necrosis and have a relatively uniform background architecture without significant cytological atypia.

Pigmented neurofibromas have been described with spindle cells containing melanin.[95] In other tumours neuromelanin has been described.[113] Patterns resembling the tactile Meissnerian and Pacinian sensory structures can be seen in some neurofibromas, having given rise to

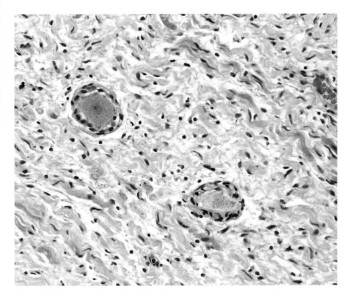

Fig. 15.30 **Neurofibroma.** This shows a dorsal root ganglion involved in neurofibroma. Such appearances can be confused with ganglioneuroma. H & E.

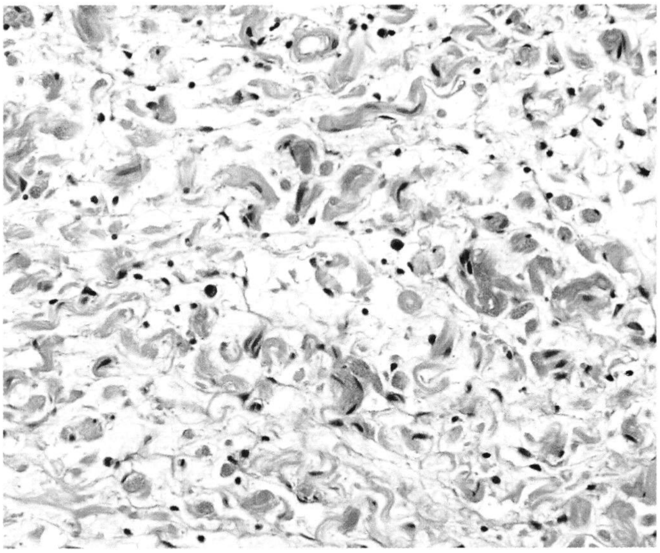

Fig. 15.31 **Atypical neurofibroma.** In some longstanding lesions focal degenerative atypia may be seen in nuclei. H & E.

the term *Pacinian neurofibroma* in the past.[114–120] These structures are S-100 positive and may have a rim of EMA immunoreactivity, and hence do not represent true differentiation into sensory tactile elements. Small cellular foci indistinguishable from Schwannoma can occur in some plexiform neurofibromas, raising issues of classification.[41]

Reactive cell populations are also present within neurofibromas. Some examples may be populated by large numbers of mast cells. Lymphoid cell and macrophage infiltration may be seen but this is generally minor, in contrast to that seen in a Schwannoma. The biological significance of these reactive cell populations is uncertain.[121]

Lastly, remnants of the normal nerve may be encountered within a neurofibroma, often only detected by special staining methods. These normal components include axons with associated Schwann cells, and intact perineurium.

The stromal components of a neurofibroma are a dominant component in most lesions. Collagen fibres surround cells and contribute to the wavy background fibrillarity dominant in most tumours (Fig. 15.29). In some tumours collagenisation is more marked, forming wide bundles running in haphazard directions. This pattern has been likened to the appearance of shredded, or grated, carrots. In some tumours collagen deposition can impart a palisaded pattern in a tumour, suggesting the possibility that the lesion is a Schwannoma.

Neurofibromas contain a mucopolysaccharide ground substance (extracellular matrix) which stains with Alcian blue. In some tumours this can be so pronounced as to impart a myxoid appearance. Blood vessels in neuro-

fibromas are typically thin walled and delicate; this is in contrast to those seen in Schwannomas, which are characteristically thick walled and hyalinised.

Neurofibromas often overrun local structures which become incorporated into a tumour. Ganglion cells may be seen in lesions involving a dorsal root (Fig. 15.30) or in visceral autonomic involvement, and such a pattern must be distinguished from a ganglioneuroma, best done by identifying intact satellite cells around the entrapped cells in a neurofibroma. In a similar way, skin appendages may be incorporated into cutaneous lesions, and must be distinguished from true epithelial elements in a peripheral nerve sheath tumour. As part of the pattern of tumour growth, a neurofibroma may show permeation of the connective tissue septa in adipose tissue or skeletal muscle.

Immunohistochemistry

S-100 is expressed in neurofibromas but in a focal and patchy pattern, in contrast with the diffuse and uniform staining seen in Schwannomas. EMA staining often shows an intact layer of perineurial cells around a neurofibroma, but EMA is not expressed within the lesion. This is in contrast to perineuriomas, and may assist in differential diagnosis where early neurofibromatous change in a nerve resembles this pattern of growth. Staining for neurofilament protein may reveal intact axons within a neurofibroma, usually in those tumours recognised anatomically to be involving a specific nerve. It is less often possible to demonstrate axons, or indeed intact perineurium, in diffuse forms of neurofibroma. Awareness of the pattern of CD34 expression by neurofibromas is important when considering the differential diagnosis with a dermatofibrosarcoma protruberans (DFSP). Neurofibromas have been shown to express CD34 but in a focal and consistent pattern. CD34 is detected in cells with a dendritic profile, being present in greatest numbers in myxoid areas, at the periphery of tumour lobules and in increased density adjacent to the perineurium.[73,122]

Ultrastructural features

Ultrastructural examination is generally not required in the diagnostic assessment of neurofibromas.[1,39,123] A mixture of cell types can be defined, comprising: Schwann cells, which form the largest proportion of cells and show characteristic ultrastructural features, with long tapering processes, few membrane associated vesicles, and an associated external basal lamina; perineurial-like cells, which are characterised by thin processes with abundant pinocytotic vesicles and an associated external basal lamina; and fibroblasts, which appear as process-bearing cells with abundant rough endoplasmic reticulum, reflecting their collagen synthesising role. Collagen fibres are intimately associated with the cellular components of the neurofibroma.

Differential diagnosis

The majority of neurofibromas pose little diagnostic problem on the basis of morphology and histology.

Schwannoma

In contrast to a Schwannoma, a neurofibroma typically lacks a capsule, has fine vessels, and shows few degenerative changes, including cysts (Fig. 15.31). The presence of Antoni A and B patterns and Verocay bodies is typical of a Schwannoma, not a neurofibroma.

Malignant peripheral nerve sheath tumour (MPNST)

Distinguishing a neurofibroma from a low grade MPNST is really only a problem when there is high cellularity or when there is significant nuclear atypia. If the lesion is of low cellularity and the only feature of concern is nuclear atypia then it is likely that the lesion represents an atypical neurofibroma.[1] In such circumstances a careful search confirming lack of mitotic activity backed up with a cell proliferation index, for example using Ki-67/MIB-1 immunostaining, can give reassurance in this diagnosis. Distinguishing between a cellular neurofibroma and a low grade malignant tumour is discussed below.

Dermatofibrosarcoma protruberans (DFSP)

Cutaneous neurofibromas may be confused with DFSP. Both lesions are composed of spindle cells with a frequent

wavy appearance to nuclei and collagenous stroma. Both diffuse cutaneous neurofibroma and DFSP infiltrate local tissues, especially dissecting into septa in subcutaneous fat. In addition to cytoarchitectural features of a prominent storiform pattern, immunostaining may be helpful. CD34 immunoreactivity is seen in a uniform strong pattern in DFSP, where it is seen only focally and in a non-uniform pattern in neurofibromas.[73] DFSP are not S-100 immunoreactive. Pigmented neurofibromas can be confused with a *pigmented DFSP* (Bednar tumour) which also contains melanin. However, a Bednar tumour shows a dominant storiform pattern, has strong immunoreactivity for CD34, and lacks the presence of scattered S-100 protein positive Schwann cells.[73,95]

Plexiform Schwannoma

Plexiform neurofibromas are generally easy to distinguish from plexiform Schwannomas on the basis of cytoarchitectural features and the pattern of S-100 protein staining. Another lesion that may resemble a plexiform neurofibroma is the *plexiform fibrohistiocytic tumour*, characterised by a myofibroblastic proliferation and including osteoclast-like giant cells.[124] These lesions lack S-100 protein immunoreactivity and have a pattern of immunoreactivity that goes with their fibrohistiocytic and myofibroblastic origin (CD68, SMA immunoreactive).

Ganglioneuroma

In visceral, autonomic and nerve root neurofibromas, entrapped ganglion cells may give the impression that the lesion is a ganglioneuroma. The best way to resolve this is to perform immunostaining for neurofilament protein, which will reveal if the ganglion cells lie within the remnants of an identifiable ganglion associated with axon bundles. Finding this microarchitectural feature is good reassurance that the lesion is not a ganglioneuroma. Additionally, the finding that the ganglion cells have intact, well formed satellite cells is a strong indication that these are entrapped structures. The satellite cells in a ganglioneuroma are typically poorly formed.

Therapy and prognosis

The clinical behaviour of neurofibromas is closely related to the clinicopathological subtype under consideration, especially whether the lesion is in a patient with NF1.[16] A dilemma in the management of neurofibromas involving large nerves is the need to sacrifice the parent nerve to achieve complete excision. Additionally, certain infiltrative soft tissue neurofibromas may be too extensive to allow local removal.

Sporadic solitary circumscribed neurofibromas, whether cutaneous or intraneural, have an excellent prognosis with a low chance of local recurrence if completely excised.

A further concern is the risk of development of malignant change in a neurofibroma that, for other reasons, cannot be surgically removed. This risk is highest in patients with NF1 and especially applies to plexiform neurofibromas. There is only a small risk for malignant change in localised intraneuronal and diffuse cutaneous neurofibromas.[16]

Perineurioma

These benign tumours have been identified relatively recently and their histogenesis related to true perineurial cells.[125] Three forms have been identified:

- intraneural perineurioma growing within nerves;
- soft tissue perineurioma with no obvious origin in a nerve, growing as a soft tissue mass;
- sclerosing perineurioma presenting as a cutaneous tumour.[126–128]

The resemblance of the intraneural perineurioma to several types of hypertrophic neuropathy led to the early belief that this lesion may have been a hyperplastic phenomenon, now refuted by recent insights.[129] The difficulty in identifying cells as perineurial cells in the context of a soft tissue tumour also led to the earlier term 'storiform perineurial fibroma' being applied to this entity.[130]

Cell biology and genetics

These tumours have been shown to be proliferations of perineural cells. They are not related to any recognised syndromes and have no identified aetiological factors. Monosomy of chromosome 22 has been identified in both intraneural and soft tissue types.[131,132] *NF2* mutations have also been detected in these tumours.[133] Cell proliferation studies using immunohistochemical staining for Ki-67/MIB-1 have shown labelling indices from 4 to 17%.[132]

Site and clinical features

Intraneural perineuriomas are typically seen in the first three decades with no sex difference. Lesions most often occur in the limbs and present with predominantly motor weakness in the distribution of the affected nerves. Imaging shows enlargement of the affected nerves. In contrast, *soft tissue perineurioma* has mainly been described in older adults with a female predominance, presenting with clinical features related to local mass effect. Most lesions occur in superficial soft tissues. *Sclerosing perineuriomas* usually present as painless lesions on the fingers or palm. A remarkable intracerebral perineurioma arising in the choroid plexus of the third ventricle has recently been reported.[134]

Pathology

Macroscopic features

Intraneural perineuriomas grow by diffuse expansion within the affected nerve, resulting in a uniform expansion of the diameter of the nerve trunk. An affected segment of nerve appears firm and grey over several centimetres. Some lesions have a plexiform pattern of growth.[135]

Soft tissue perineuriomas appear as circumscribed rounded lesions typically between 2 and 8 cm in diameter with larger examples being described. They have a grey coloured rubbery appearance on cut surface. These lesions are not generally associated with an identifiable nerve at surgical removal.

Sclerosing perineuriomas are generally well demarcated but non-encapsulated and have a firm consistency, ranged in size from 0.7 to 3.3 cm.[128]

Intraoperative diagnosis

It is uncommon for a surgeon to undertake a resection of an enlarged nerve where there is any preserved function without a clear diagnosis. A surgeon may request an intraoperative opinion to assist in planning the extent of surgery for an enlarged nerve where the diagnosis is unclear. The main question that is posed is whether a lesion represents a benign or malignant proliferation. In preoperative and intraoperative planning of a procedure, neurophysiology can be used to select a non-functional nerve or fascicle for biopsy. The pathologist will be presented with a fascicle of nerve, which should be orientated since attempting a diagnosis on small incisional biopsies is fraught with problems. Sections should be prepared in transverse orientation. The increased cellularity and nuclear size perceived in frozen section material can lead to confusion with other entities as discussed under differential diagnosis below. The most important aspect of obtaining a correct diagnosis is preparation of good quality transverse sections of the affected nerve, and identification of the typical onion-bulb pattern of growth. Making a diagnosis of an intraneural perineurioma is an indication for preservation of a nerve if there is function.

Another question posed during surgery concerns the extent of tumour and whether an excision margin is free of disease. This is usually in a case where an abnormal segment of nerve with no function is being removed with a view to nerve grafting. Assessment of excision margins is best achieved using transverse sections of the whole nerve, as focal involvement of fascicles has been documented in some cases.[130,134]

Histological features

In an *intraneural perineurioma*, the affected nerve shows cellular expansion corresponding to individual fascicles when seen at low magnification (Fig. 15.32). The typical appearance is that of concentric proliferation of spindle cells around nerve fibres in the endoneurium, producing an 'onion-bulb' appearance (Fig. 15.33). Larger concentric whorls may be present within fascicles, some encircling large bundles of original myelinated axons. Proliferation of similar cells may also be seen involving the perineurium, leading to cellular thickening and prominence of this structure. The cells have elongated, oval nuclei with stippled chromatin and inconspicuous nucleoli. There is minimal nuclear variation, an occasional larger cell being seen, and mitoses are rarely evident. As the lesion develops, growing along nerves, there is loss of myelin. In areas where there is minimal involvement, residual myelin may be seen in the centre of some of the 'onion-bulb' rings. While this appearance is best noted on transverse sections of nerve, longitudinal sections do not display this microanatomy, revealing a diffuse increase in spindle cells within the endoneurium.

Soft tissue perineuriomas have appearances that overlap with many soft tissue spindle cell tumours (Figs 15.34–15.37). Cells are arranged in layers and whorls with a focal storiform pattern. Cytologically, the cells have elongated tapering nuclei, often with a crimped or wavy profile, and indistinct cell borders. Cells may appear layered between sheets of collagen. When cells artefactually separate in histological preparations, many can be seen to have very long cell processes.

Fig. 15.32 **Perineurioma.** Intraneural perineurioma: low magnification showing diffuse nerve expansion. H & E.

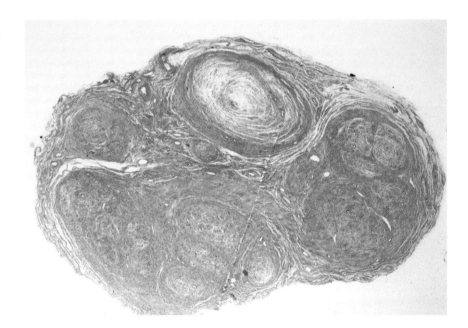

Fig. 15.33 **Intraneural perineurioma.** Onion-bulb appearance of perineurial cells wrapped around residual axons in the nerve.

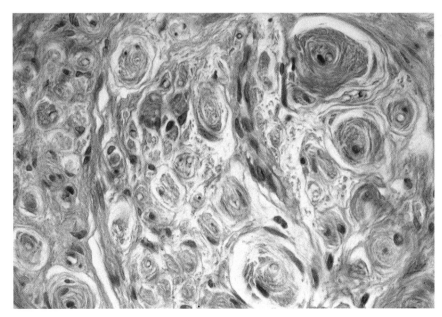

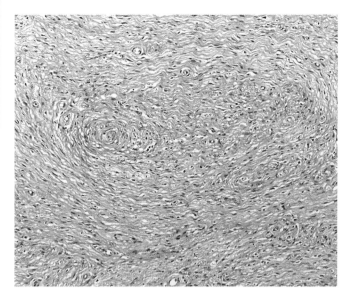

Fig. 15.34 **Soft tissue perineurioma.** At low magnification seen as a spindle cell tumour with ill-defined whorling pattern. H & E.

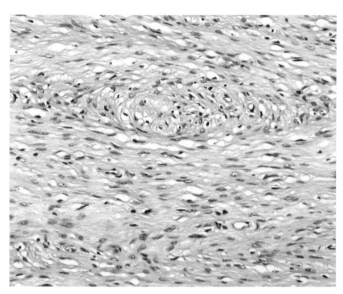

Fig. 15.35 **Soft tissue perineurioma.** Higher magnification highlights the ill-defined whorling pattern and details the nuclear cytology. H & E.

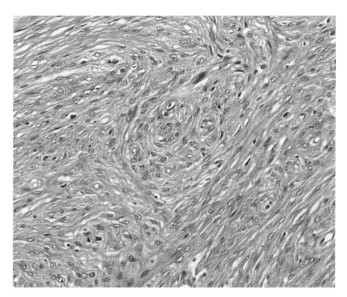

Fig. 15.36 **Soft tissue perineurioma.** Higher magnification highlights the ill-defined whorling pattern and details the nuclear cytology. H & E.

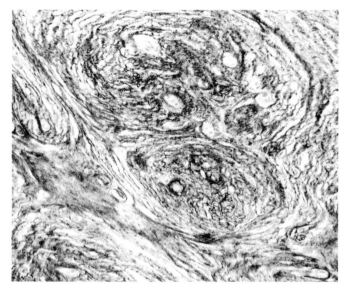

Fig. 15.37 **Soft tissue perineurioma.** EMA immunostaining shows whorled pattern and confirms perineurial cell phenotype.

Sclerosing perineuriomas show dense collagenisation, with variable numbers of small, epithelioid, and spindled cells showing trabecular and whorled (onion-bulb) growth patterns. Reticular perineuriomas are a recently described variant with a lace-like growth pattern and pale-staining fusiform cells.[136]

Immunohistochemistry

The key diagnostic finding is labelling of the proliferating cells for EMA, as seen in normal perineurial cells (Figs 15.37 and 15.38).[125,133,137,138] S-100 staining may label residual Schwann cells within the nerve, and may also stain remaining Schwann cells at the centre of some onion-bulb rings of proliferating cells (Fig. 15.39). If all of the circumferential cells label with S-100 then it is most likely that the lesion is a Schwann cell proliferation related to a localised or other form of hypertrophic neuropathy. Staining with neurofilament protein is a useful way of confirming that individual whorls of cells contain an original axon (Fig. 15.40).

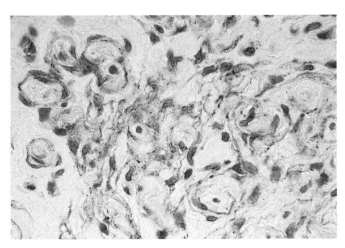

Fig. 15.38 **Intraneural perineurioma.** EMA immunostaining highlights perineurial cells in onion-bulb whorls.

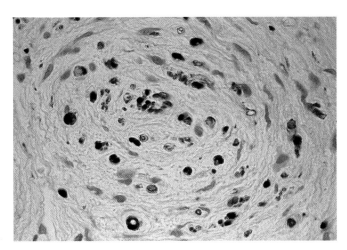

Fig. 15.39 **Intraneural perineurioma.** S-100 immunostaining shows residual Schwann cell myelin in the centre of some whorls but does not stain perineurial cells.

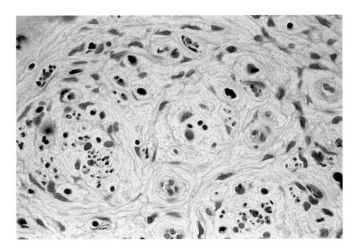

Fig. 15.40 **Intraneural perineurioma.** Neurofilament immunostaining identifies axons within whorls of perineurial cells.

Ultrastructural appearances

The perineurial cells that proliferate in an intraneural perineurioma have appearances of normal perineurial cells with intervening layers of collagen and associated external basal lamina. The characteristic whorls show axons with original Schwann cells surrounded by concentric layers of perineurial cells.[125,133,137]

Differential diagnosis

Localised hypertrophic neuropathy

This is a condition characterised by a reactive proliferation of Schwann cells forming 'onion-bulb' like structures within an expanded nerve. Such localised pathology must be distinguished from hereditary and autoimmune forms of demyelinating neuropathy. In contrast to perineuriomas, in which neoplastic cells label with EMA, the non-neoplastic Schwann cells in localised hypertrophic neuropathy label with S-100 and not with EMA. It is important to note that some authors have included localised hypertrophic neuropathy within the spectrum of perineurial cell proliferations.

Neurofibromas

In some patterns of neurofibroma, neoplastic cells can grow in a concentric pattern around the original axons within a nerve, simulating the pattern of growth in a perineurioma. Such cells in a neurofibroma are focally S-100 protein positive. Although some cells in neurofibromas are regarded as perineurial-like, based on ultrastructural characteristics, they do not show EMA immunoreactivity.

Malignant peripheral nerve sheath tumour

High cellularity in a nerve biopsy, especially if the sections being examined are of longitudinal orientation, can lead to a suspicion that a lesion is a low grade MPNST. Obtaining a transverse section of material is important to demonstrate the whorl-like arrangement of perineurioma. If not available, EMA staining will usually reveal the diagnosis of perineurioma.

Other spindle cell/collagenous proliferations

Soft tissue perineuriomas need to be distinguished from other spindle cell/collagenous proliferations. Modern diagnosis of soft tissue tumours now routinely incorporates immunohistochemical assessment, where the immunoreactivity of soft tissue perineuriomas for EMA is the mainstay of diagnosis. The sclerosing type of perineurioma needs to be distinguished from solitary fibrous tumour, which it can closely resemble, but which is CD34 immunoreactive.

Therapy and prognosis

Complete excision of soft tissue perineuriomas is associated with cure, with no reported cases of recurrence or metastasis. Such lesions are best regarded as low grade tumours with a capacity for local recurrence but not metastasis.

For intraneural perineuriomas, excision, when clinically indicated, is again associated with cure without recurrence or metastasis. The main issue in management of these lesions is establishing a diagnosis without compromising any residual function in the affected nerve.

Neurothekeoma

The neurothekeoma is a benign tumour composed of spindle cells and epithelioid cells that do not appear to have either Schwannian or perineurial cell origins.

Clinical features

Most tumours present as a solitary skin lesion. They are seen in the first three decades, with a slight female predominance. Lesions are commonest on the face, arms and upper back. Unusual sites include the tongue,[139] parasellar region,[140] cauda equina,[141] and intradural spine.[142] Clinically, the lesions are slow growing and appear as pale flesh coloured, smooth, domed lesions.

Pathology

Macroscopic features

When excised, neurothekeomas show a circumscribed pale tan firm appearance replacing the dermal and subcutaneous tissue affected.[143]

Histological features

Histologically, the tumour has a polylobated appearance with very many small pale-staining rounded nests separated by thin collagenous septa (Fig. 15.41). The nests are moderately cellular with a background pale mucoid matrix that can be stained with Alcian blue. The cells are plump and spindle shaped with some rounder epithelioid forms. These are focally cohesive and form small nests or whorls (Fig. 15.42). Nuclei are somewhat variable, with hyperchromatic forms and evident mitoses. Small numbers of multinucleate cells can be seen. A variant termed *cellular neurothekeoma* has been described in which low grade cytological atypia and mitotic activity are more common. Distinction from the more common myxomatous variants of neurothekeoma is based on the high cellularity in cell nests, inconspicuous myxomatous change, and a less defined lobular architecture with fewer collagenous septa. Such lesions can demonstrate a locally infiltrative pattern of growth.[144–146]

Immunohistochemistry

Immunohistochemistry generally shows absent S-100 or EMA staining. This is useful in the differential diagnosis of melanocytic lesions but S-100 staining has been seen in some myxoid lesions.[147,148] PGP9.5 is expressed by cells in neurothekeomas.[149]

Electron microscopy

Ultrastructural examination generally reveals absent Schwann cell differentiation[147] although cells with several patterns of differentiation have been described (including Schwann cell, smooth muscle cell, myofibroblast and fibroblast) with overlap with nerve sheath myxomas.[150]

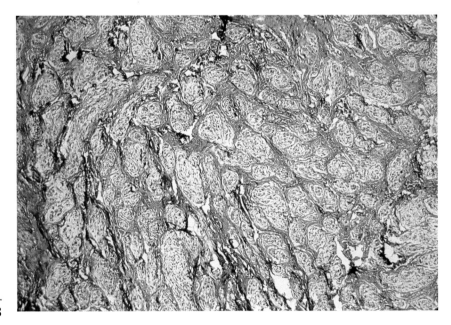

Fig. 15.41 **Neurothekeoma.** The tumour has a polylobated appearance with many small pale-staining rounded nests separated by thin collagenous septa. H & E.

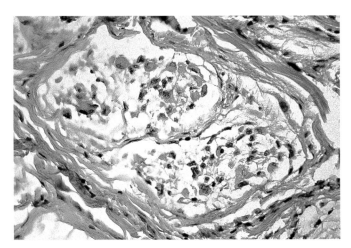

Fig. 15.42 **Neurothekeoma.** The nests contain cells in a background pale mucoid matrix. H & E.

Differential diagnosis

Nerve sheath myxoma

Nerve sheath myxoma generally has less cellular islands with a more dominant mucoid background (see below). Cells in this lesion stain with S-100, unlike neurothekeomas.

Melanocytic lesions

The spindle cells, epithelioid cells and nested pattern of neurothekomas often resemble a Spitz nevus. However in a neurothekeomas melanin is not seen and there is no epidermal involvement in the form of elements that might be interpreted as junctional nests. In a similar fashion some desmoplastic malignant melanomas can be confused with a neurothekeoma. Demonstration of melanin pigment and S-100 staining is usually helpful in this respect.[144] S-100 staining may be seen in myxoid neurothekeomas, but in such cases discrimination from melanocytic lesions is usually not a problem.

Malignant fibrohistiocytic lesions

Mitotic activity can be surprisingly high in a neurothekeoma and raise suspicion of a low grade myxoid malignant fibrous histiocytoma. This difficulty is best resolved on ultrastructural examination, but the rather restricted pattern of immunoreactivity in a neurothekeoma is also in contrast to a malignant fibrohistiocytic lesion (see Chapter 14).

Therapy and prognosis

Neurothekeomas and benign lesions and even those with mitotic activity usually do not recur after complete excision.[145] However recurrent lesions have been described.[151]

Nerve sheath myxoma

Nerve sheath myxomas are benign tumours composed of spindle cells with a Schwann cell phenotype set in a dominant mucoid matrix.

Clinical features

Nerve sheath myxoma is usually seen as a cutaneous tumour that presents as solitary skin lesion up to about 3 cm in size, most being seen when they reach just under 1 cm in size. They are detected in adults mainly between the ages of 30 and 60 years, with a female predominance. Lesions are commonest on the hands, face, neck and back. Clinically the lesions are slow growing and appear as pale flesh coloured smooth domed lesions.[152]

Pathology

Macroscopic features

Nerve sheath myxomas have a grey firm appearance, replacing the dermal and subcutaneous tissue affected.

Histological features

Histologically, these tumours have a polylobated appearance with pale-staining rounded nests separated by thin collagenous septa. Within the nests there is a dominant mucoid matrix, which stains strongly with Alcian blue and in which a mixture of multiprocessed and spindle cells are found. The mucoid matrix often contains pale 'bubbles' within a lightly basophilic background. The nuclei of the cells often run in small rows and streams. The nuclei are small and oval in shape with a stippled chromatin pattern. The cells have a small amount of eosinophilic cytoplasm and may show small vacuoles. Mitoses are not seen.

Immunohistochemistry

Immunohistochemistry shows S-100 reactivity in the cells within the mucoid matrix. Focal EMA immunoreactivity can be seen in some areas, possibly representing perineurial cells from a parent nerve.

Electron microscopy

Ultrastructural evidence points to a Schwann cell origin for these lesions, with cells surrounded by an external basal lamina.[150,153]

Differential diagnosis

In the differential diagnosis of these lesions several myxoid conditions of skin need to be considered including plexiform neurofibroma (p. 440), myxoid Schwannoma and neurothekeoma (p. 448).

Therapy and prognosis

These are benign lesions that usually do not recur if locally excised.

Benign granular cell tumour

These lesions are benign tumours that appear histogenetically related to Schwann cells. Other terms that have been used in the past to describe this lesion include granular cell myoblastoma and granular cell Schwannoma.

Clinical features

Clinically, benign granular cell tumours may be either single or multiple, most arising as subcutaneous or submucosal lesions on the tongue, and skin of the head, neck, breast, trunk and limbs. Examples have also been described from a wide variety of visceral sites.[154,174] They occur at all ages, with most being seen between the ages of 40 and 70 years. Tumours generally present because of local swelling. A characteristic, but not universal feature, is hyperplasia of overlying mucosal or epithelial tissues that may at times raise concerns of malignancy.

Pathology

Macroscopic features

The macroscopic appearances are variable and, although most tumours appear circumscribed, a proportion have ill-defined infiltrative margins. Because of their site, most lesions are encountered when small, about 1–2 cm in size although larger tumours have been described, for example in the breast. Lesions are firm and have a grey–yellow rubbery appearance on cut surface after fixation.

Histogical features

Granular cell tumours are composed of sheets and small lobules of cells separated by collagenous tissue which may be extensive in some cases.[175]

The neoplastic cells are large, having abundant bright eosinophilic granular cytoplasm, which stains intensely with PAS, and a rounded nucleus (Figs 15.43 and 15.44). Some cells have a more elongated appearance. Nuclei are generally monotonous and uniform, but in a small proportion of tumours clusters of pleomorphic or hyperchromatic nuclei can be seen. Mitoses are not generally seen. Tumour growth pattern is variable, with some growing as circumscribed nodules, while others have an infiltrative pattern extending into adipose tissue, muscle or involving small nerves. Lymphoid cell aggregates are a common finding within and around the tumour.

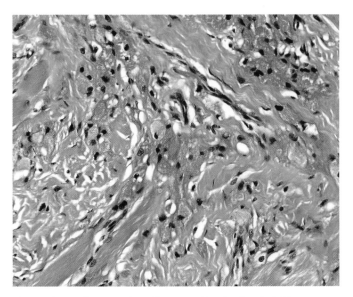

Fig. 15.43 **Benign granular cell tumour.** Neoplastic cells infiltrate between stroma and have abundant bright eosinophilic granular cytoplasm with a rounded nucleus. H & E.

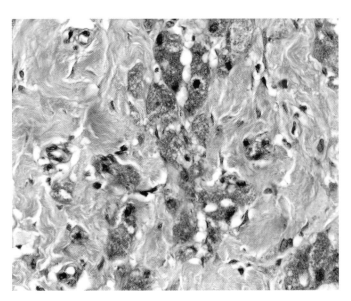

Fig. 15.44 **Benign granular cell tumour.** The neoplastic cells stain intensely with PAS.

Immunohistochemistry

Immunohistochemical staining is generally not necessary for establishing a diagnosis. Tumours show immunoreactivity for S-100 protein and neuron specific enolase. Some, but not all, tumours mark with Leu7. Markers of the lysosomal compartment are generally strongly expressed, such as CD68 and alpha-1 antichymotrypsin.[176,177] Some tumours express carcinoembryonic antigen-like immunoreactivity due to non-specific cross-reacting antigen.[178,181] Refuting previously suggested origins from muscle, granular cell tumours do not show immunoreactivity for muscle specific proteins.[177]

Electron microscopy

Granular cell tumours have a very distinctive appearance using electron microscopy. At low magnification the most obvious feature is the cell cytoplasm, which is packed with large, pleomorphic electron dense membrane bound bodies, representing large residual lysosomal bodies.[39,182,183] These are the correlates of the brightly eosinophilic cytoplasmic granules seen with light microscopy.

Differential diagnosis

Congenital granular cell tumour

Congenital granular cell tumour is a distinctive clinico-pathological entity, occurring in newborn children and situated on the alveolar ridge.[184] Although expressing CD68, these lesions are S-100 negative and lack the distinctive bodies seen within granules on ultrastructural examination.[176,177] These lesions are regarded as being histogenetically unrelated to granular cell tumours of Schwann cell derivation.

Granular smooth muscle tumour

Certain smooth muscle tumours may have a granular cytoplasm, an issue that is easily resolved by demonstrating expression of muscle specific proteins by immunohistochemistry.[130]

Astrocytic gliomas

Granular cell change may occur in astrocytic gliomas (Chapter 4). In addition to finding regions of more classical astrocytoma nearby, this diagnosis can be made by demonstrating GFAP immunoreactivity, since GFAP is not expressed in conventional granular cell tumours.[185,186]

Malignant granular cell tumour

The diagnosis of malignant granular cell tumour is problematic as most biologically malignant lesions have identical histology to the benign tumours. Features that would cause suspicion of a malignant granular cell tumour include anything more than focal nuclear atypia, clearly evident mitotic activity and the presence of necrosis (see section on malignant granular cell tumour on p. 457).

Therapy and prognosis

Granular cell tumours can be locally recurrent if incompletely excised. Complete local excision is recommended to minimise the risk of recurrence.

Benign non-neurogenic lesions, hamartomas and hyperplastic conditions

Peripheral nerve may be the site of origin of several non-neurogenic lesions, presenting as tumours, listed in Table 15.2 (also see p. 457).[1,187–200]

Several hyperplastic conditions may also arise from nerve:

- *Palisaded encapsulated neuroma*, also termed solitary circumscribed neuroma, is a cutaneous lesion composed of Schwann cells and axons. These are very common lesions that present commonly on the face[81] and also in oral mucosa.[201] They may be confused with Schwannomas, traumatic neuromas or leiomyomas.
- *Mucosal neuromas and mucosal neuromatosis* occur in multiple endocrine neoplasia type IIb. Lesions occur on the lips, eyelids and tongue as well as in the autonomic plexus of the gastrointestinal tract. Histologically, the lesions may be polypoid or diffuse and consist of greatly enlarged hypertrophied nerves.[202]
- *Localised hypertrophic neuropathy* is very rare and leads to enlargement of affected nerves.[1,203] The distinction of this condition from intraneuronal perineurioma has been discussed on p. 447.
- *Lipofibromatous hamartoma of nerve* is a rare benign condition characterised by overgrowth of the epineurial adipose tissue. This classically affects the hand and is associated with enlargement of the affected digit. Histologically there is diffuse interfascicular as well as perifascicular infiltration of nerve by mature adipose tissue. The intimate involvement of nerve trunks means that the fat cannot be dissected away from the fascicles.[195,204–214] These lesions must be distinguished from intraneural lipoma of nerve in which the lipoma is a discrete mass, pushing nerve fascicles around it rather than growing through them,[215] and lipoma of epineurium which compresses the nerve on one side. In both these lesions the lipoma can be shelled out from the involved nerve.
- *Neuromuscular choristomas* are rare lesions, termed benign Triton tumours by some authors in the past. They are composed of disordered skeletal muscle and proliferated nerve and are mainly seen in childhood, affecting large nerve trunks.[216,221]

Primary malignant tumours of peripheral nerve

MPNSTs

The lesions classified as primary malignant tumours of peripheral nerve are derived from specialised cells of the endoneurium and perineurium.[1,16,106] The term malignant peripheral nerve sheath tumour (MPNST) incorporates previously used terms such as neurofibrosarcoma and malignant Schwannoma. Tumours arising from the non-specialised connective tissue elements of the epineurium, even though they might arise from a nerve trunk, are conventionally regarded as extrinsic malignant soft tissue tumours.[16]

To define a tumour as being a MPNST a tumour must meet one of the following criteria.[1]

1. Arise from an identifiable peripheral nerve trunk and have histological features consistent with recognised types of MPNST.
2. Arise in a patient with known NF1 and show histological features conforming to a recognised type of MPNST (given that a patient has NF1 this allows inclusion of tumours without morphological demonstration of Schwann cell or perineurial cell differentiation).
3. Arise from an identifiable benign tumour of peripheral nerve, for example pre-existing Schwannoma, neurofibroma or ganglioneuroma.
4. Show histological features conforming to a recognised type of MPNST, with morphological evidence of Schwann cell or perineurial cell differentiation (this criterion excludes undifferentiated sarcomas arising in a patient without NF1).

The types of MPNST recognised in the WHO classification are shown in Table 15.1 (p. 426).

Cell biology and genetics

Although MPNSTs are not common neoplasms a sizeable percentage of these lesions arise in patients with NF1[98,99] (Chapter 19). NF1 is the most important risk factor for MPNST, accounting for as many as 50% at all MPNSTs. Patients with NF1 typically develop tumours earlier than those without NF1.[222,223] The risk of developing a MPNST in a patient with NF1 has been variably reported between 2 and 29%, different series being influenced by case ascertainment biases.[222] MPNSTs have also been described in segmental neurofibromatosis.[223] Previous irradiation is another risk factor for development of MPNST, with a typical long latent period between exposure and development of tumour.[225–228] Malignant change in a benign Schwannoma is a very rare event. MPNST may also rarely develop from a pre-existing ganglioneuroma or phaeochromocytoma.[59,62,63,229,230]

Mutation in the *NF1* gene is believed to be the most important predisposing molecular genetic event in the development of MPNST. Loss of both *NF1* alleles has been shown in MPNST in patients with NF1.[98,106] Loss of 17p in the majority of MPNST suggests that this region contains another tumour suppressor gene, the loss of

which is essential for malignant progression.[231] A strong candidate for this is *TP53*, supported by the finding of positive p53 staining in the majority of MPNSTs but absent staining in benign nerve sheath tumours.[105] The presence of *TP53* mutations has been documented in human MPNSTs,[232] and germline mutations of *TP53* have been used to model MPNSTs in mice,[233] thus implicating *TP53* in the formation of these malignancies. p53 staining has also been related to prognosis, suggesting that MPNSTs with absent staining have a better prognosis.[105,234] *TP53* is also implicated in formation of so-called malignant Triton tumour.[235]

Studies suggest that disruption of the pRB pathway is common in MPNST and in particular dose reduction of *CDKN2A* is particularly frequent, suggesting an important contribution to MPNST development. Deletion of the *CDKN2A* gene that encodes the p16 cell cycle regulatory protein has been implicated in tumour progression, being seen in about 50% of MPNSTs but not in neurofibromas.[236–238] On immunohistochemical analysis, while all neurofibromas express p16 protein, MPNSTs do not show p16 immunoreactivity suggesting that p16 immunohistochemistry may help in the distinction of neurofibromas from MPNST.[236] p27 nuclear expression has been demonstrated in most neurofibromas, but is absent in the majority of MPNSTs, which displayed only cytoplasmic staining. In this series cytoplasmic p27 expression was found to be a prognostic factor for poor survival in MPNSTs.[239] *Hras-I* point mutation has been demonstrated in 2/46 malignant peripheral nerve sheath tumours in one study.[240]

Cytogenetic studies have revealed a wide range of inconsistent changes.[10,241–244] Gains in chromosomes 7, 8q, 15q and 17q have been suggested as characteristic in malignant but not in benign peripheral nerve sheath tumours from patients with NF1.[245] The gain of both 7p15-p21 and 17q22-qter has been associated with a statistically significant poor overall survival rate in one series.[246] A tumour that demonstrated histology typical of a MPNST has been described with a variant form of the (X;18) translocation known to be associated with synovial sarcoma.[247] This has not been seen in other studies of small series of MPNST.[248]

Incidence and site

About 5% of all malignant soft tissue tumours are MPNSTs. They are mainly encountered between the third and sixth decades but may occur at any age, including a significant subset seen in childhood. MPNSTs typically develop in large nerve trunks, for example the sciatic nerve, brachial plexus and paraspinal nerves. Superficial soft tissue lesions are also commonly encountered and intraosseous lesions are also described. MPNSTs of cranial nerves are rare.

Clinical features

MPNSTs typically present with a rapidly growing mass or pain. In the setting of a patient with NF1, the development of increased growth, firmness or pain in a pre-existing neurofibroma should prompt consideration of whether malignant change has supervened.[222,228,249–258]

The imaging characteristics of MPNSTs are often indistinguishable from those seen in benign peripheral nerve tumours. In some lesions ill-defined margins suggesting local invasion may suggest malignancy.[259] The advent of novel imaging approaches, such as PET scanning, may provide a means for improved determination of tumour growth prior to biopsy.

Pathology

Macroscopic features

The gross appearance of MPNSTs is variable. In patients with NF1 there is often a pre-existing neurofibroma in which malignant change has supervened. Plexiform neurofibromas are especially at risk for developing malignant change.[108] In many instances surgical removal of a soft tissue mass will have been performed without macroscopic evidence of involvement of a nerve.

MPNSTs typically appear as firm, rubbery grey–yellow masses with necrotic areas commonly visible. The tumours may appear circumscribed by a collagenous pseudocapsule derived from adjacent tissues. MPNSTs, that arise in a pre-existing plexiform neurofibroma may maintain a lobulated plexiform pattern.[222]

Intraoperative diagnosis

Multidisciplinary management of malignancy depends on clinical imaging and pathological information prior to planning definitive treatment. Clinical and imaging features may not be able to predict the presence of a MPNST and so great reliance is placed on biopsy ascertainment. Given the potential for confusion between certain benign and malignant tumours of nerve, an intraoperative opinion based on frozen section is prone to errors of interpretation.

For low cellularity lesions, advise conservative surgery only and await full histological appraisal. For cellular lesions if the differential diagnosis lies between a MPNST and a cellular Schwannoma then conservative removal of the lesion is indicated, preserving functional nerve. This allows a formal diagnosis to be made on paraffin histology. If the lesion is a MPNST the relative merits of further surgery, with sacrifice of the parent nerve, can be discussed with the patient. Exceptionally, where sacrifice of the parent nerve is judged to be of no clinical consequence, a wide local excision might be appropriate in the face of a cellular lesion.

Histogical features

The diagnosis of MPNST must take into account the criteria listed above. Tumour heterogeneity is common and so histological sampling should include wide areas of tumour. Even when a surgeon has not been able to identify a parent nerve for a tumour, a careful macroscopic and histological search for nerve and benign peripheral nerve sheath tumour should be made by thorough and extensive tissue sampling of the tumour periphery. When nerve has been examined, separate blocking of the margins of excision is essential to assess completeness of excision.

MPNSTs are very cellular high grade spindle cell tumours with a background arrangement of sheets and fascicles of cells (Figs 15.45 and 15.46). In these high grade tumours, cell density may be variable, with stroma-rich cell-poor areas alternating with cell-rich stroma-poor regions. The background stroma may be collagenous or include myxoid areas. Vessels are thin walled and vascularity may be focally high. Cytologically, the cells typically have pleomorphic tapering nuclei with a coarse chromatin distribution and hyperchromatism. Mitoses are common, usually exceeding 4 per 10 high power fields.

A variety of histological patterns can be encountered in MPNSTs; these are worthy of note as they occur in other types of neoplasms and thus have the potential to cause diagnostic confusion. In particular, some tumours have a monomorphic appearance with a close fascicular 'herring bone' appearance, resembling a fibrosarcoma.[1,16] A distinction from fibrosarcoma can be made on the basis of immunocytochemistry (see below). MPNSTs frequently exhibit divergent differentiation. Approximately 15% of tumours show rhabdomyoblastic, glandular, squamous, osseous, cartilaginous or neuroendocrine elements (Figs 15.46–15.49 and 15.52). These derivatives all exhibit histological features of malignancy; two or more of these derivative elements may coexist. Glandular structures within MPNSTs may indicate either true glandular differentiation (when mucin secretion is demonstrable on a PAS or Alcian blue stain) or neuroendocrine differentiation, which can be confirmed on immunocytochemistry for chromogranin. The term malignant Triton tumour has been applied to MPNSTs with rhabdomyosarocomatous elements, within which strap cells maybe identified. However, strap cell differentiation is not evident in all cases, and a careful search for primitive rhabdomyoblasts (Fig. 15.48) is often aided by immunocytochemistry for desmin. MPNSTs with angiosarcomatous elements have also been described, but these appear to be exceptionally rare.[1,16,106,260–267]

Approximately 5% or MPNSTs exhibit epithelioid features, and in some cases this can represent the predominant (or exclusive) pattern. Irregular plump

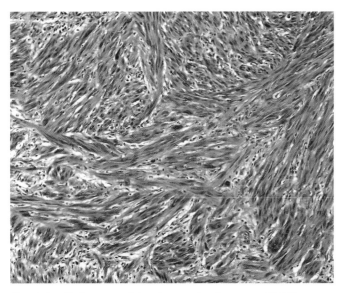

Fig. 15.45 **Malignant peripheral nerve sheath tumour.** MPNSTs are typically cellular high grade spindle cell tumours with a background arrangement of sheets and fascicles. H & E.

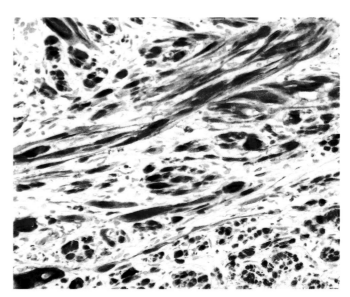

Fig. 15.46 **Malignant peripheral nerve sheath tumour.** S-100 immunostaining is positive in the majority of cases.

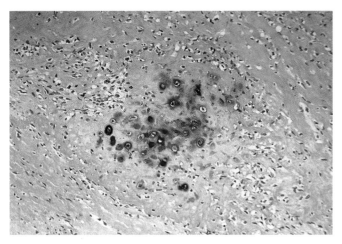

Fig. 15.47 **Malignant peripheral nerve sheath tumour.** Osseous differentiation. H & E.

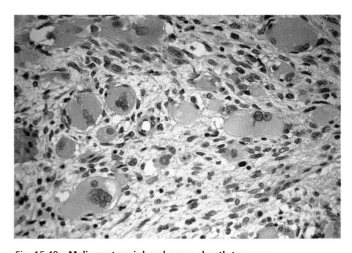

Fig. 15.48 **Malignant peripheral nerve sheath tumour.** Rhabdomyoblastic differentiation. H & E.

epithelial-like cells (Fig. 15.49) can often be confused with an epithelioid sarcoma (see below). Epithelioid MPNSTs appear to be softer and fleshier than conventional examples of this neoplasm, often with an ill-defined nodularity on cross-section. This form of MPNST appears to arise most often in the superficial soft tissues.[1,16,106,255,268–272] Many more MPNSTs have small focal areas of epithelial morphology, but this milder histological feature does not warrant a designation of epithelioid MPNST. In one series, 4% of MPNSTs exhibited perineural cell differentiation.[273] This unusual feature did not appear to be associated with neurofibromatosis type 1, and it was suggested that the prognosis for patients with MPNSTs showing perineural differentiation is more favourable than for those with conventional forms of the neoplasm.

Five cases of a primitive small round cell tumour have been described, located deep within the soft tissue of the trunks and limbs, apparently not in association with major nerves. These tumours do not exhibit the features of peripheral primitive neuroectodermal tumours, and it has been proposed that they may represent a small round cell type of MPNST.[274] However, this designation may be regarded as provisional until other examples are identified and more fully characterised by the use of extensive genetic investigations as well as histological, ultrastructural and immunocytochemical studies.

A small proportion of MPNSTs correspond to lower grade tumours and distinguishing these lesions from cellular or atypical neurofibromas may be problematic. It has been suggested that finding any mitotic activity in a plexiform neurofibroma or in a lesion that might be considered a cellular or atypical neurofibroma is indicative of malignant change. This view has been challenged and for diagnosis of a low grade MPNST it has been suggested that the following criteria should be met:[1]

1. Focal areas of high cell density in the lesion.
2. Nuclei in the lesion should be about three times larger than those seen in a typical neurofibroma.
3. Nuclei should be hyperchromatic.

Immunohistochemistry

Immunohistochemistry can play an important part in the diagnosis of MPNSTs. MPNSTs often show staining for S-100 protein, usually in a focal patchy distribution (Figs 15.46 and 15.51). Importantly some tumours are S-100 negative. Similarly, Leu7 immunostaining is also seen in a significant proportion of tumours, again in a focal patchy distribution.[261,275,276] Cytokeratin expression may be seen in some epithelioid MPNSTs. Most MPNSTs, including those that are EMA or AE1/AE3 positive, do not express cytokeratins 7 and 19 but glandular elements may express cytokeratin.[1,277] HMB45 is generally not expressed by MPNSTs, a useful finding when attempting to distinguish an epithelioid MPNST from metastatic malignant melanoma. However, some tumours have shown positive immunoreactivity[278] and not all malignant melanomas express this antigen.[65] If EMA staining is seen in significant numbers of spindle cells, perineurial differentiation in the MPNST should be considered.[279] EMA is also expressed in the glandular elements of MPNST with glandular differentiation. Neuroendocrine markers such as chromogranin-A and synaptophysin may identify glands in MPNST with glandular differentiation. Muscle specific actin and desmin immunostaining will reliably demonstrate areas of rhabdomyosarcomatous differentiation in tumours with divergent differentiation.

The main use of immunohistochemistry is in ascertaining the likely differentiation of a tumour. When taken with clinical and anatomical details, this may help identify a MPNST. For tumours that lack an association with a nerve in a patient without NF1, demonstration of S-100 and Leu7 immunoreactivity is particularly helpful in this regard.

Ultrastructural features

Most MPNSTs are poorly differentiated and so ultrastructural examination may not reveal specific evidence of Schwann cell or perineurial cell differentiation. Only a small proportion of MPNSTs show strong evidence of Schwann cell differentiation in the form of tapering cells, adherens type junctions and associated external lamina.

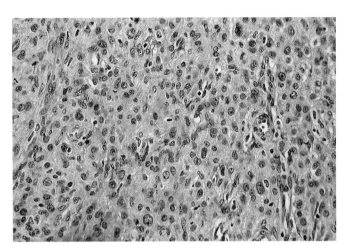

Fig. 15.49 **Epithelioid malignant peripheral nerve sheath tumour.** Epithelioid MPNST composed of plump cells with an ill-defined nested pattern. H & E.

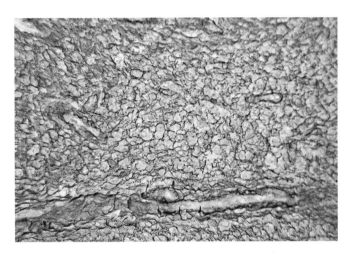

Fig. 15.50 **Epithelioid malignant peripheral nerve sheath tumour.** Reticulin staining highlights microscopic nested arrangement of cells.

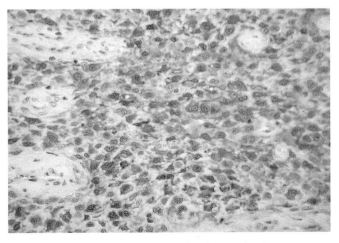

Fig. 15.51 **Epithelioid malignant peripheral nerve sheath tumour.** Strong S-100 immunoreactivity.

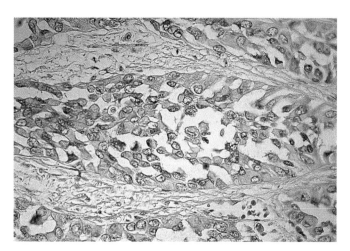

Fig. 15.52 **Epithelioid malignant peripheral nerve sheath tumour.** This tumour has a pseudo-glandular arrangement indicating marked epithelial differentiation. H & E.

A small number of tumours with perineurial cell maturation, including pinocytotic vesicles, have been described.[123,273,276,280,281]

Differential diagnosis

A panel of immunohistochemical studies is essential for the diagnosis of a MPNST and discrimination from other soft tissue sarcomas.

Cellular neurofibroma

The important distinction of low grade MPNSTs from cellular neurofibroma and atypical neurofibromas has been previously discussed (see p. 442). In particular, the absence of necrosis, the low mitotic rate and relatively uniform cytology of a cellular neurofibroma will aid the differential diagnosis.

Leiomyosarcoma

Leiomyosarcoma may resemble a MPNST but demonstration of wide expression of a muscle specific protein in the absence of S-100 protein expression is usually diagnostic.[16]

Fibrosarcomas

Fibrosarcomas lack Leu7 and S-100 protein immunoreactivity as well as showing ultrastructural features of fibroblastic maturation.[16]

Monophasic synovial sarcoma

Monophasic synovial sarcoma may be S-100 protein positive. It can be distinguished from MPNST by demonstrating cytokeratin or EMA in the spindle cells.[16,277,282,283] If EMA immunoreactivity is extensive, a diagnosis of MPNST with perineurial differentiation may be considered and

further evidence obtained by ultrastructural studies. The development of molecular assays for the diagnosis of synovial sarcoma also promises to clarify this differential diagnosis.[248]

Biphasic synovial sarcoma

Biphasic synovial sarcoma may be confused with a MPNST with glandular differentiation (Fig. 15.52). The glands in a MPNST may contain goblet cells, not seen in the glandular spaces in a synovial sarcoma. Immunostaining with synaptophysin or chromogranin-A will show reaction in the glands of a MPNST but not in synovial sarcoma.[16] Again, molecular assays for synovial sarcoma will clarify this differential diagnosis.[248]

Malignant melanoma and clear cell sarcoma

Epithelioid MPNST may be confused with malignant melanoma and clear cell sarcoma. In both instances absent HMB45 immunoreactivity in epithelioid MPNST helps with diagnosis.[16,284,285]

Epithelioid sarcoma

Epithelioid MPNST may also be confused with epithelioid sarcoma, a lesion that is usually S-100 negative and expresses cytokeratin.[16,286]

Neurotropic melanoma

Neurotropic melanoma may be confused with MPNST. Involved nerves show expansion of the perineurial space and occasionally the endoneurium by atypical melanocytic cells. While cranial nerves are uncommonly involved by MPNST, this is not the case for neurotropic melanoma. In contrast to the focal and patchy S-100 staining seen in most MPNST, cells of neurotropic melanoma are usually strongly and uniformly S-100 immunoreactive.[287,288]

Therapy and prognosis

MPNSTs are usually treated by wide primary excision. They frequently occur at sites that preclude radical or complete removal of the tumour and adjuvant radiotherapy is usually necessary. Even after wide local excision and with further adjuvant therapy MPNSTs have a poor prognosis. The 5-year survival is at most 40% with 10-year survival being significantly lower. Large tumours and those that have a paraspinal location are associated with an overall worse prognosis. Of less significant contribution to actuarial survival is the histological grade of the tumour. In general, the natural history of MPNSTs is that of local recurrence and metastatic spread, most commonly to the lungs.[106,222,228,249,250,252,256,257,289–291]

Malignant melanotic Schwannoma and malignant psammomatous melanotic Schwannoma

Melanotic Schwannomas may become malignant, usually in the setting of a local recurrence of a previously treated lesion. In such lesions nuclear atypia is generally present with abnormal mitoses. Necrosis is also a feature associated with malignancy. Unfortunately none of these histological features can be used in isolation to predict subsequent behaviour in these lesions. These findings are discussed with the benign counterparts earlier in this chapter.

Malignant granular cell tumour

These tumours are the malignant counterpart of benign granular cell tumours, described in detail on page 450. They tend to occur in adults and are most commonly reported in the thigh and upper limb. Despite the fact that oral locations are common for benign granular cell tumours, malignant examples are uncommon at this site.[16,292,293] The main problem with the histological assessement of malignant granular cell tumours in that metastatic spread has been documented in lesions where the primary tumour is histologically identical to proven benign lesions. The most reliable indicator that a granular cell tumour is malignant is demonstration of invasion of blood vessels or lymphatics. Local infiltration of adjacent nerve may be a feature of benign lesion and mitoses may also be present in benign lesions. Widespread nuclear atypia, with hyperchromatic and pleomorphic nuclei, is another feature suggesting malignancy (Fig. 15.53), but lesser degrees of nuclear atypia may be seen in benign lesions.

Six histological criteria have been proposed in the assessment of malignancy: Necrosis, spindling, vesicular nuclei with large nucleoli, mitotic activity (greater than 2 mitoses per 10 high power fields at 200 × magnification), high nuclear to cytoplasmic ratio, and widespread pleomorphism. Neoplasms that meet three or more of these criteria are classified as histologically malignant; those that meet one or two criteria are classified as atypical; and those that display only focal pleomorphism but fulfil none of the other criteria are classified as benign. In one study using these criteria, patients with benign multicentric and atypical granular cell tumours have had no metastases and no tumour deaths. Of cases with malignant granular cell tumour, 34% died of disease at a median interval of 3 years. There were local recurrences in 32% of malignant cases and metastases in 50% (median interval, 2 years). Adverse prognostic factors included local recurrence, metastasis, larger tumour size, older patient age, histological classification as malignant, presence of necrosis, increased mitotic activity, spindling of tumour cells, vesicular nuclei with large nucleoli, and Ki-67/MIB-1 labelling values greater than 10%.[292]

Non-neurogenic tumours of peripheral nerves

A wide range of non-neurogenic tumours of peripheral nerves and nerve roots have been reported (see Table 15.2, p. 426). The commonest of these is the paraganglioma, which most often arises in nerve roots in the region of the cauda equina.[187–194] Paragangliomas can readily be distinguished from neurogenic tumours by their characteristic histological, immunocytochemical and ultrastructural features (see Chapter 8). The other varieties of non-neurogenic tumours are all rare, and include haemangiomas of the spinal nerve root,[196] which can often be identified radiologically by their uniform enhancement with intravenous contrast. Both cavernous and capillary haemangiomas have been described, although the former are more common. Capillary haemangioblastomas have also been described in spinal nerve roots (in the cervical region and cauda equina). However, a rare example has been reported in the sciatic nerve.[294] Two cases have occurred in patients with von Hippel–Lindau disease; histological examination of these lesions showed features identical with cerebellar haemangioblastoma.

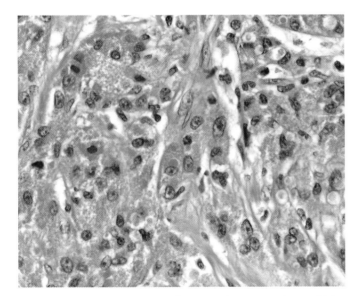

Fig. 15.53 **Malignant granular cell tumour.** The tumour shows a high nuclear cytoplasmic ration with prominent nucleoli. Nuclear atypia is pronounced when compared to a typical benign granular cell tumour. Vascular invasion was also present with other areas showing necrosis. H & E.

Lymphomas have occasionally been reported as a solitary tumour of peripheral nerves;[198] most are large B-cell high-grade non-Hodgkin's lymphomas. The tumours have a variable prognosis, which appears to be associated with expression of p16 (indicating *CDKN2A* gene deletion). Remarkably, adrenal adenomas have been reported on rare occasions in the intraspinal space, usually resulting in a extramedullary mass arising from a spinal nerve root. These tumours closely resemble similar lesions that occur rather more commonly at a variety of extraneural sites and can be identified readily by immunocytochemistry to demonstrate the presence of steroidogenic enzymes within the tumour cell cytoplasm.[197]

A variety of non-neoplastic tumour like masses have also been described in peripheral nerves, including fibrolipomas (lipofibromatous hamartoma), which have been reported mostly in the volar aspect of the upper limb, in association with the median nerve.[145] Inflammatory psuedo-tumours have also been described in peripheral nerves of both the upper and lower limbs. These rare lesions can be confused with lymphomas and malignant peripheral nerve sheath tumours, but a characteristic polymorphous reactive inflammatory infiltrate is demonstrable on immunocytochemistry.[200] Amyloidomas have very rarely been described in peripheral nerves.[199] The amyloid subtype involved is usually the amyloid light chain lambda type; deposits can occur in cranial and peripheral nerves and appear to be the product of a B-cell clone capable of terminal differentiation, with no evidence of disease progression into an aggressive or systemic neoplasm.

REFERENCES

Schwannoma

1. Scheithauer B, Woodruff J, Erlandson R. Tumors of the peripheral nervous system. Washington, DC : Armed Forces Institute of Pathology, 1999
2. Woodruff JM. Pathology of the major peripheral nerve sheath neoplasms. Monogr Pathol, 1996; 38:129–161
3. MacCollin M, Woodfin W, Kronn D et al. Schwannomatosis: a clinical and pathologic study. Neurology, 1996; 46:1072–1079
4. Evans DG, Mason S, Huson SM et al. Spinal and cutaneous schwannomatosis is a variant form of type 2 neurofibromatosis: a clinical and molecular study. Neurol Neurosurg Psychiatry, 1997; 62:361–366
5. Reith JD, Goldblum JR. Multiple cutaneous plexiform schwannomas. Report of a case and review of the literature with particular reference to the association with types 1 and 2 neurofibromatosis and schwannomatosis. Arch Pathol Lab Med, 1996; 120:399–401
6. Carney JA. The Carney complex (myxomas, spotty pigmentation, endocrine overactivity, and schwannomas). Dermatol Clin, 1995; 13:19–26
7. Ruggieri M. The different forms of neurofibromatosis. Childs Nerv Syst, 1999; 15:295–308
8. Gusella JF, Ramesh V, MacCollin M et al. Merlin: the neurofibromatosis 2 tumor suppressor. Biochim Biophys Acta, 1999; 1423:M29–36
9. Stemmer-Rachamimov AO, Ino Y, Lim ZY et al. Loss of the NF2 gene and merlin occur by the tumorlet stage of schwannoma development in neurofibromatosis 2. J Neuropathol Exp Neurol, 1998; 57:1164–1167
10. Mertens F, Dal Cin P, De Wever I et al. Cytogenetic characterization of peripheral nerve sheath tumours: a report of the CHAMP study group. J Pathol, 2000; 190:31–38
11. Giovannini M, Robanus-Maandag E, Niwa-Kawakita M et al. Schwann cell hyperplasia and tumors in transgenic mice expressing a naturally occurring mutant NF2 protein. Genes Dev, 1999; 13:978–986
12. Walsh RM, Bath AP, Bance ML et al. The natural history of untreated vestibular schwannomas. Is there a role for conservative management? Rev Laryngol Otol Rhinol, 2000; 121:21–26
13. Charabi S, Engel P, Charabi B et al. Growth of vestibular schwannomas: in situ model employing the monoclonal antibody Ki67 (MIB-1) and DNA flow cytometry [published erratum appears in Am J Otol 1996 Jul; 17(4):692]. Am J Otol, 1996; 17:301–306
14. Szeremeta W, Monsell EM, Rock JP et al. Proliferation indices of vestibular schwannomas by Ki67 (MIB-1) and proliferating cell nuclear antigen. Am J Otol, 1995; 16:616–619
15. Tsanaclis AM, Robert F, Michaud J et al. The cycling pool of cells within human brain tumors: in situ cytokinetics using the monoclonal antibody Ki67 (MIB-1). Can J Neurol Sci, 1991; 18:12–17
16. Weiss SW, Goldblum JR. Enzinger and Weiss's Soft Tissue Tumors, 4th ed. St Louis: CV Mosby, 2001.
17. Bruner JM. Peripheral nerve sheath tumors of the head and neck. Semin Diagn Pathol, 1987; 4:136–149
18. Osterhus DR, Van Loveren HR, Friedman RA. Trigeminal schwannoma. Am J Otol, 1999; 20:551–552
19. Sharma MC, Karak AK, Gaikwad SB et al. Intracranial intraparenchymal schwannomas: a series of eight cases. J Neurol Neurosurg Psychiatry, 1996; 60:200–203
20. Casadei GP, Komori T, Scheithauer BW et al. Intracranial parenchymal schwannoma. A clinicopathological and neuroimaging study of nine cases. J Neurosurg, 1993; 79:217–222
21. Binatli O, Ersahin Y, Korkmaz O et al. Intramedullary schwannoma of the spinal cord. A case report and review of the literature. J Neurosurg Sci, 1999; 43:163–167
22. Redekop G, Elisevich K, Gilbert J. Fourth ventricular schwannoma. Case report. J Neurosurg, 1990; 73:777–781
23. Hasegawa SL, Mentzel T, Fletcher CD. Schwannomas of the sinonasal tract and nasopharynx. Mod Pathol, 1997; 10:777–784
24. Prevot S, Bienvenu L, Vaillant JC et al. Benign schwannoma of the digestive tract: a clinicopathologic and immunohistochemical study of five cases, including a case of esophageal tumor. Am J Surg Pathol, 1999; 23:431–436
25. Nabeya Y, Watanabe Y, Tohnosu N et al. Diffuse schwannoma involving the entire large bowel with huge extramural development: report of a case. Surg Today, 1999; 29:637–641
26. Wada Y, Jimi A, Nakashima O et al. Schwannoma of the liver: report of two surgical cases. Pathol Int, 1998; 48:611–617
27. Daimaru Y, Kido H, Hashimoto H et al. Benign schwannoma of the gastrointestinal tract: a clinicopathologic and immunohistochemical study. [Review] [34 refs]. Hum Pathol, 1988; 19:257–264
28. Sarlomo-Rikala M, Miettinen M. Gastric schwannoma – a clinicopathological analysis of six cases. Histopathology, 1995; 27:355–360
29. Brown SZ, Owen DA, O'Connell JX et al. Schwannoma of the pancreas: a report of two cases and a review of the literature. Mod Pathol, 1998; 11:1178–1182
30. Consensus. The National Institutes of Health Consensus Development Conference on Acoustic Neuroma. In: Consensus Statement, 1991: pp 1–24
31. Tos M, Charabi S, Thomsen J. Increase of diagnosed vestibular schwannoma in Denmark. Acta Otolaryngol (suppl), 1997; 529:53–55
32. Suh JS, Abenoza P, Galloway HR et al. Peripheral (extracranial) nerve tumors: correlation of MR imaging and histologic findings. Radiology, 1992; 183:341–346
33. Charabi S, Mantoni M, Tos M et al. Cystic vestibular schwannomas: neuroimaging and growth rate. J Laryngol Otol, 1994; 108:375–379
34. Hermans R, Van der Goten A, De Foer B et al. MRI screening for acoustic neuroma without gadolinium: value of 3DFT-CISS sequence. Neuroradiology, 1997; 39:593–598
35. Neely JG, Hough J. Histologic findings in two very small intracanalicular solitary schwannomas of the eighth nerve. Ann Otol Rhinol Laryngol, 1986; 95:460–465
36. Casadei GP, Scheithauer BW, Hirose T et al. Cellular schwannoma. A clinicopathologic, DNA flow cytometric, and proliferation marker study of 70 patients. Cancer, 1995; 75:1109–1119

37. Ferry JA, Dickersin GR. Pseudoglandular schwannoma. Am J Clin Pathol, 1988; 89:546–552

38. Kim SH, Youm JY, Song SH et al. Vestibular schwannoma with repeated intratumoral hemorrhage. Clin Neurol Neurosurg, 1998; 100:68–74

39. Dickersin GR. The electron microscopic spectrum of nerve sheath tumors. Ultrastruct Pathol, 1987; 11:103–146

40. Kerl H, Soyer HP, Cerroni L et al. Ancient melanocytic nevus. Semin Diagn Pathol, 1998; 15:210–215

41. Feany MB, Anthony DC, Fletcher CD. Nerve sheath tumours with hybrid features of neurofibroma and schwannoma: a conceptual challenge. Histopathology, 1998; 32:405–410

42. Zelger BG, Steiner H, Kutzner H et al. Verocay body – prominent cutaneous schwannoma. Am J Dermatopathol, 1997; 19:242–249

43. Goldblum JR, Beals TF, Weiss SW. Neuroblastoma-like neurilemoma. Am J Surg Pathol, 1994; 18:266–273

44. Bhatnagar S, Banerjee SS, Mene AR et al. Schwannoma with features mimicking neuroblastoma: report of two cases with immunohistochemical and ultrastructural findings. J Clin Pathol, 1998; 51:842–845

45. Fisher C, Chappell ME, Weiss SW. Neuroblastoma-like epithelioid schwannoma. Histopathology, 1995; 26:193–194

46. Walsh RM, Bath AP, Bance ML et al. The role of conservative management of vestibular schwannomas. Clin Otolaryngol Allied Sci, 2000; 25:28–39

47. Walsh RM, Bath AP, Bance ML et al. Consequences to hearing during the conservative management of vestibular schwannomas. Laryngoscope, 2000; 110:250–255

48. Poen JC, Golby AJ, Forster KM et al. Fractionated stereotactic radiosurgery and preservation of hearing in patients with vestibular schwannoma: a preliminary report. Neurosurgery, 1999; 45:1299–1305

49. Noren G. Long-term complications following gamma knife radiosurgery of vestibular schwannomas. Stereotact Funct Neurosurg, 1998; 70:65–73

50. Pollock BE, Lunsford LD, Noren G. Vestibular schwannoma management in the next century: a radiosurgical perspective. Neurosurgery, 1998; 43:475–481

51. Post KD, Eisenberg MB, Catalano PJ. Hearing preservation in vestibular schwannoma surgery: what factors influence outcome? [see comments]. J Neurosurg, 1995; 83:191–196

52. Shea Jd, Hitselberger W, Benecke JJ et al. Recurrence rate of partially resected acoustic tumors. Am J Otol, 1985;107–109

53. Neely J. Hearing conservation surgery for acoustic tumors – a clinical-pathologic correlative study. Am J Otol, 1985; 143–146

54. Marquet J, Forton G, Offeciers F et al. The solitary schwannoma of the eighth cranial nerve. An immunohistochemical study of the cochlear nerve-tumor interface. Arch Otolaryngol Head & Neck Surg, 1990; 116:1023–1025

55. Lye R, Pace-Balzan A, Ramsden R et al. The fate of tumour rests following removal of acoustic neuromas: an MRI Gd-DTPA study. Br J Neurosurg, 1992; 6:195–201

56. Schessel D, Nedzelski J, Kassel E et al. Recurrence rates of acoustic neuroma in hearing preservation surgery. Am J Otol, 1992; 13:233–235

57. Robson DK, Ironside JW. Malignant peripheral nerve sheath tumour arising in a schwannoma. Histopathology, 1990; 16:295–297

58. Rasbridge SA, Browse NL, Tighe JR et al. Malignant nerve sheath tumour arising in a benign ancient schwannoma. Histopathology, 1989; 14:525–528

59. Nayler SJ, Leiman G, Omar T et al. Malignant transformation in a schwannoma. Histopathology, 1996; 29:189–192

60. Woodruff JM, Selig AM, Crowley K et al. Schwannoma (neurilemoma) with malignant transformation. A rare, distinctive peripheral nerve tumor. Am J Surg Pathol, 1994; 18:882–895

61. Mikami Y, Hidaka T, Akisada T et al. Malignant peripheral nerve sheath tumor arising in benign ancient schwannoma: a case report with an immunohistochemical study. Pathol Int, 2000; 50:156–161

62. Mariniello G, Horvat A, Popovic M, Dolenc VV. Cellular schwannoma of the hypoglossal nerve presenting without hypoglossal palsy. Clin Neurol Neurosurg, 2000; 102:40–42

63. Alberghini M, Zanella L, Bacchini P, Bertoni F. Cellular schwannoma: a benign neoplasm sometimes overdiagnosed as a sarcoma. Skeletal Radiol, 2001; 30:350–353

64. White W, Shiu MH, Rosenblum MK et al. Cellular schwannoma. A clinicopathologic study of 57 patients and 58 tumors. Cancer, 1990; 66:1266–1275

65. Lodding P, Kindblom LG, Angervall L et al. Cellular schwannoma. A clinicopathologic study of 29 cases. Virchows Arch Pathol Anat Histopathol, 1990; 416:237–248

66. Fletcher CD, Davies SE, McKee PH. Cellular schwannoma: a distinct pseudosarcomatous entity. Histopathology, 1987; 11:21–35

67. Henke AC, Salomao DR, Hughes JH. Cellular schwannoma mimics a sarcoma: an example of a potential pitfall in aspiration cytodiagnosis. Diagn Cytopathol, 1999; 20:312–316

68. Woodruff JM, Godwin TA, Erlandson RA et al. Cellular schwannoma: a variety of schwannoma sometimes mistaken for a malignant tumor. Am J Surg Pathol, 1981; 5:733–744

69. Deruaz JP, Janzer RC, Costa J. Cellular schwannomas of the intracranial and intraspinal compartment: morphological and immunological characteristics compared with classical benign schwannomas. J Neuropathol Exp Neurol, 1993; 52:114–118

70. Ellison DW, MacKenzie IZ, McGee JO. Cellular schwannoma of the vagina. Gynecol Oncol, 1992; 46:119–121

71. Nesbitt JC, Vega DM, Burke T et al. Cellular schwannoma of the bronchus. Ultrastruct Pathol, 1996; 20:349–354

72. Skopelitou AS, Mylonakis EP, Charchanti AV et al. Cellular neurilemoma (schwannoma) of the descending colon mimicking carcinoma: report of a case. Dis Colon Rectum, 1998; 41:1193–1196

73. Khalifa MA, Montgomery EA, Ismiil N et al. What are the CD34+ cells in benign peripheral nerve sheath tumors? Double immunostaining study of CD34 and S-100 protein. Am J Clin Pathol, 2000; 114:123–126

74. Megahed M. Plexiform schwannoma. Am J Dermatopathol, 1994; 16:288–293

75. Mannara GM, La Rosa FC, Marino F. Plexiform schwannoma of the cheek. J Laryngol Otol, 1999; 113:1034–1035

76. Fletcher CD, Davies SE. Benign plexiform (multinodular) schwannoma: a rare tumour unassociated with neurofibromatosis. Histopathology, 1986; 10:971–980

77. Hirose T, Scheithauer BW, Sano T. Giant plexiform schwannoma: a report of two cases with soft tissue and visceral involvement. Mod Pathol, 1997; 10:1075–1081

78. Woodruff JM, Marshall ML, Godwin TA et al. Plexiform (multinodular) schwannoma. A tumor simulating the plexiform neurofibroma. Am J Surg Pathol, 1983; 7:691–697

79. Val-Bernal JF, Figols J, Vazquez-Barquero A. Cutaneous plexiform schwannoma associated with neurofibromatosis type 2. Cancer, 1995; 76:1181–1186

80. Ishida T, Kuroda M, Motoi T et al. Phenotypic diversity of neurofibromatosis 2: association with plexiform schwannoma. Histopathology, 1998; 32:264–270

81. Dakin MC, Leppard B, Theaker JM. The palisaded, encapsulated neuroma (solitary circumscribed neuroma). Histopathology, 1992; 20:405–410

82. Carney JA. Psammomatous melanotic schwannoma. A distinctive, heritable tumor with special associations, including cardiac myxoma and the Cushing syndrome. Am J Surg Pathol, 1990; 14:206–222

83. Carney JA, Ferreiro JA. The epithelioid blue nevus. A multicentric familial tumor with important associations, including cardiac myxoma and psammomatous melanotic schwannoma. Am J Surg Pathol, 1996; 20:259–272

84. Carney JA, Stratakis CA. Epithelioid blue nevus and psammomatous melanotic schwannoma: the unusual pigmented skin tumors of the Carney complex. Semin Diagn Pathol, 1998; 15:216–224

85. Ranjan A, Chacko G, Chandi SM. Intracerebellar melanotic schwannoma: a case report. Br J Neurosurg, 1995; 9:687–689

86. Myers JL, Bernreuter W, Dunham W. Melanotic schwannoma. Clinicopathologic, immunohistochemical, and ultrastructural features of a rare primary bone tumor. Am J Clin Pathol, 1990; 93:424–429

87. Miller RT, Sarikaya H, Sos A. Melanotic schwannoma of the acoustic nerve. Arch Pathol Lab Med, 1986; 110:153–154

88. Kayano H, Katayama I. Melanotic schwannoma arising in the sympathetic ganglion. Hum Pathol, 1988; 19:1355–1358

89. Jensen OA, Bretlau P. Melanotic schwannoma of the orbit. Immunohistochemical and ultrastructural study of a case and survey of the literature. APMIS, 1990; 98:713–723

90. Font RL, Truong LD. Melanotic schwannoma of soft tissues. Electron-

microscopic observations and review of literature. Am J Surg Pathol, 1984; 8:129–138

91. Abbott AEJ, Hill RC, Flynn MA et al. Melanotic schwannoma of the sympathetic ganglia: pathological and clinical characteristics. Ann Thorac Surg, 1990; 49:1006–1008

92. Vallat-Decouvelaere AV, Wassef M, Lot G et al. Spinal melanotic schwannoma: a tumour with poor prognosis. Histopathology, 1999; 35:558–566

93. Erlandson RA. Melanotic schwannoma of spinal nerve origin. Ultrastruct Pathol, 1985; 9:123–129

94. Di Bella C, Declich P, Assi A et al. Melanotic schwannoma of the sympathetic ganglia: a histologic, immunohistochemical and ultrastructural study. J Neurooncol, 1997; 35:149–152

95. Fetsch JF, Michal M, Miettinen M. Pigmented (melanotic) neurofibroma: a clinicopathologic and immunohistochemical analysis of 19 lesions from 17 patients. Am J Surg Pathol, 2000; 24:331–343

96. Brat DJ, Giannini C, Scheithauer BW et al. Primary melanocytic neoplasms of the central nervous systems. Am J Surg Pathol, 1999; 23:745–754

Neurofibroma

97. Friedman JM. Epidemiology of neurofibromatosis type 1. Am J Med Genet, 1999; 89:1–6

98. Rasmussen SA, Friedman JM. NE1 gene and neurofibromatosis 1. Am J Epidemiol, 2000; 151:33–40

99. von Deimling A, Krone W, Menon AG. Neurofibromatosis type. 1: pathology, clinical features and molecular genetics. Brain Pathol, 1995; 5:153–162

100. Sheela S, Riccardi VM, Ratner N. Angiogenic and invasive properties of neurofibroma Schwann cells. J Cell Biol, 1990; 111:645–653

101. Muir D, Neubauer D, Lim IT et al. Tumorigenic properties of neurofibromin-deficient neurofibroma Schwann cells. Am J Pathol, 2001; 158:501–513.

102. Perry A, Roth KA, Banerjee R et al. NF1 deletions in S-100 protein-positive and negative cells of sporadic and neurofibromatosis 1 (NF1)-associated plexiform neurofibromas and malignant peripheral nerve sheath tumors. Am J Pathol, 2001; 159:57–61.

103. Rutkowski JL, Wu K, Gutmann DH et al. Genetic and cellular defects contributing to benign tumor formation in neurofibromatosis type 1. Hum Mol Genet, 2000; 9:1059–1066

104. Salmon I, Kiss R, Segers V et al. Characterization of nuclear size, ploidy, DNA histogram type and proliferation index in 79 nerve sheath tumors. Anticancer Res, 1992; 12:2277–2283

105. Liapis H, Marley EF, Lin Y et al. TP53 and Ki67 (MIB-1) proliferating cell nuclear antigen in benign and malignant peripheral nerve sheath tumors in children. Pediatr Dev Pathol, 1999; 2:377–384

106. Woodruff JM. Pathology of tumors of the peripheral nerve sheath in type 1 neurofibromatosis. Am J Med Genet, 1999; 89:23–30

107. Jelinek JE. Aspects of heredity, syndromic associations, and course of conditions in which cutaneous lesions occur solitarily or in multiplicity. J Am Acad Dermatol, 1982; 7:526–540

108. Waggoner DJ, Towbin J, Gottesman G et al. Clinic-based study of plexiform neurofibromas in neurofibromatosis l. Am J Med Genet, 2000; 92:132–135

109. Korf BR. Plexiform neurofibromas. Am J Med Genet, 1999; 89:31–37

110. Oliver DW, Wells FC, Lamberty BG et al. Massive plexiform neurofibroma of the sympathetic trunk. Eur J Cardiothorac Surg, 1999; 16:569–572

111. McCarron KF, Goldblum JR. Plexiform neurofibroma with and without associated malignant peripheral nerve sheath tumor: a clinicopathologic and immunohistochemical analysis of 54 cases. Mod Pathol, 1998; 11:612–617

112. Liapis H, Dehner LP, Gutmann DH. Neurofibroma and cellular neurofibroma with atypia: a report of 14 tumors. Am J Surg Pathol, 1999; 23:1156–1158

113. Fukuda T, Igarashi T, Hiraki H et al. Abnormal pigmentation of schwannoma attributed to excess production of neuromelanin-like pigment. Pathol Int, 2000; 50:230–237

114. Toth BB, Long WH, Pleasants JE. Central pacinian neurofibroma of the maxilla. Oral Surg Oral Med Oral Pathol, 1975; 39:630–634

115. Weiser G. An electron microscope study of Pacinian neurofibroma. Virchows Arch Pathol Anat Histol, 1975; 366:331–340

116. MacLennan SE, Melin-Aldana H, Yakuboff KP. Pacinian neurofibroma

117. King DT, Barr RJ. Bizarre cutaneous neurofibromas. J Cutan Pathol, 1980; 7:21–31

118. Levi L, Curri SB. Multiple Pacinian neurofibroma and relationship with the finger-tip arterio-venous anastomoses. Br J Dermatol, 1980; 102:345–349

119. MacDonald DM, Wilson-Jones E. Pacinian neurofibroma. Histopathology, 1977; 1:247–255

120. Bennin B, Barsky S, Salgia K. Pacinian neurofibroma. Arch Dermatol, 1976; 112:1558

121. Donhuijsen K, Sastry M, Volker B et al. Mast cell frequency in soft tissue tumors. Relation to type and grade of malignancy. Pathol Res Pract, 1992; 188:61–66

122. Weiss SW, Nickoloff BJ. CD-34 is expressed by a distinctive cell population in peripheral nerve, nerve sheath tumors, and related lesions. Am J Surg Pathol, 1993; 17:1039–1045

123. Erlandson RA, Woodruff JM. Peripheral nerve sheath tumors: an electron microscopic study of 43 cases. Cancer, 1982; 49:273–287

124. Zelger B, Weinlich G, Steiner H et al. Dermal and subcutaneous variants of plexiform fibrohistiocytic tumor. Am J Surg Pathol, 1997; 21:235–241

Perineurioma

125. Erlandson RA. The enigmatic perineurial cell and its participation in tumors and in tumorlike entities. Ultrastruct Pathol, 1991; 15:335–351

126. Smith K, Skelton H. Cutaneous fibrous perineurioma. J Cutan Pathol, 1998; 25:333–337

127. Sciot R, Cin PD, Hagemeijer A et al. Cutaneous selerosing perineurioma with cryptic NF2 gene deletion. Am J Surg Pathol, 1999; 23:849–853

128. Fetsch JF, Miettinen M. Sclerosing perineurioma: a clinicopathologic study of 19 cases of a distinctive soft tissue lesion with a predilection for the fingers and palms of young adults. Am J Surg Pathol, 1997; 21:1433–1442

129. Tsang WY, Chan JK, Chow LT et al. Perineurioma: an uncommon soft tissue neoplasm distinct from localized hypertrophic neuropathy and neurofibroma. Am J Surg Pathol, 1992; 16:756–763

130. Mentzel T, Dei Tos AP, Fletcher CD. Perineurioma (storiform perineurial fibroma): clinico-pathological analysis of four cases. Histopathology, 1994; 25:261–267

131. Giannini C, Scheithauer BW, Jenkins RB et al. Soft-tissue perineurioma. Evidence for an abnormality of chromosome 22, criteria for diagnosis, and review of the literature. Am J Surg Pathol, 1997; 21:164–173

132. Emory TS, Scheithauer BW, Hirose et al. Intraneural perineurioma. A clonal neoplasm associated with abnormalities of chromosome 22. Am J Clin Pathol, 1995; 103:696–704

133. Lasota J, Fetsch JF, Wozniak A et al. The neurofibromatosis type 2 gene is mutated in perineurial cell tumors: a molecular genetic study of 8 cases. Am J Pathol, 2001; 158:1223–1229

134. Giannini C, Scheithauer BW, Steinberg J, Cosgrave TJ. Intraventricular perineurioma: case report. Neurosurgery, 1998; 43:1478–1481

135. Zelger B, Weinlich G. Perineuroma. A frequently unrecognized entity with emphasis on a plexiform variant. Adv Clin Pathol, 2000; 4:25–33

136. Graadt van Rogen JF, McMenamin ME, Belchis DA et al. Reticular perineurioma: a distinctive variant of soft tissue perineurioma. Am J Surg Pathol, 2001; 25:485–493

137. Erlandson RA, Woodruff JM. Role of electron microscopy in the evaluation of soft tissue neoplasms, with emphasis on spindle cell and pleomorphic tumors. Hum Pathol, 1998; 29:1372–1381

138. Perentes E, Nakagawa Y, Ross GW et al. Expression of epithelial membrane antigen in perineurial cells and their derivatives. An immunohistochemical study with multiple markers. Acta Neuropathol, 1987; 75:160–165

Neurothekoma

139. Gallager RL, Helwig EB. Neurothekeoma–a benign cutaneous tumor of neural origin. Am J Clin Pathol, 1980; 74:759–764

140. Paulus W, Warmuth-Metz M, Sorensen N. Intracranial neurothekeoma (nerve sheath myxoma). Case report. J Neurosurg 1993; 79:280–282

141. Kaar GF, Bashir SH, N'Dow JM et al. Neurothekeoma of the cauda equina [letter]. J Neurol Neurosurg Psychiatry, 1996; 61:530–531

of the hand: a case report and literature review. J Hand Surg, 1999; 24:413–416

142. Paulus W, Jellinger K, Perneczky G. Intraspinal neurothekeoma (nerve sheath myxoma). A report of two cases. Am J Clin Pathol, 1991; 95:511–516

143. Breuer T, Koester M, Weidenbecher M et al. Neurothekeoma, a rare tumour of the tongue. ORL; J OtorhinoLaryngol Relat Spec, 1999; 61:161–164

144. Barnhill RL, Mihm MCJ. Cellular neurothekeoma. A distinctive variant of neurothekeoma mimicking nevomelanocytic tumors. Am J Surg Pathol, 1990; 14:113–120

145. Busam KJ, Mentzel T, Colpaert C et al. Atypical or worrisome features in cellular neurothekeoma: a study of 10 cases. Am J Surg Pathol, 1998; 22:1067–1072

146. Calonje E, Wilson-Jones E, Smith NP et al. Cellular 'neurothekeoma': an epithelioid variant of pilar leiomyoma? Morphological and immunohistochemical analysis of a series. Histopathology, 1992; 20:397–404

147. Barnhill RL, Dickersin GR, Nickeleit V et al. Studies on the cellular origin of neurothekeoma: clinical, light microscopic, immunohistochemical, and ultrastructural observations. J Am Acad Dermatol, 1991; 25:80–88

148. Husain S, Silvers DN, Halperin AJ et al. Histologic spectrum of neurothekeoma and the value of immunoperoxidase staining for S-100 protein in distinguishing it from melanoma. Am J Dermatopathol, 1994; 16:496–503

149. Wang AR, May D, Bourne P et al. PGP9.5: a marker for cellular neurothekeoma. Am J Surg Pathol, 1999; 23:1401–1407

150. Argenyi ZB, Kutzner H, Seaba MM. Ultrastructural spectrum of cutaneous nerve sheath myxoma/cellular neurothekeoma. J Cutan Pathol, 1995; 22:137–145

151. Allen PW. Myxoma is not a single entity: a review of the concept of myxoma. Ann Diagn Pathol, 2000; 4:99–123

Other benign nerve sheath lesions

152. Fletcher CD, Chan JK, McKee PH. Dermal nerve sheath myxoma: a study of three cases. Histopathology, 1986; 10:135–145

153. Angervall L, Kindblom LG, Haglid K. Dermal nerve sheath myxoma. A light and electron microscopic, histochemical and immunohistochemical study. Cancer, 1984; 53:1752–1759

154. Altaras M, Jaffe R, Bernheim J et al. Granular cell myoblastoma of the vulva. Gynecol Oncol, 1985; 22:352–355

155. Burton BJ, Kumar VG, Bradford R. Granular cell tumour of the spinal cord in a patient with Rubenstein-Taybi syndrome. Br J Neurosurg, 1997; 11:257–259

156. Conzen M, Schnabel R, Bruns B et al. Intracerebral granular cell tumor. Neurosurg Rev, 1987; 10:237–239

157. Critchley GR, Wallis NT, Cowie RA. Granular cell tumour of the spinal cord: case report. Br J Neurosurg, 1997; 11:452–454

158. Fletcher MS, Aker M, Hill JT et al. Granular cell myoblastoma of the bladder. Br J Urol, 1985; 57:109–110

159. Gal R, Dekel A, Ben-David M et al. Granular cell myoblastoma of the cervix. Case report. Br J Obstet Gynaecol, 1988; 95:720–722

160. Graziani N, Dufour H, Figarella-Branger D et al. Suprasellar granular-cell tumour, presenting with intraventricular haemorrhage. Br J Neurosurg, 1995; 9:97–102

161. Hori A, Altmannsberger M, Spoerri O et al. Granular cell tumour in the third ventricle. Case report with histological, electron-microscopic, immunohistochemical and necropsy findings. Acta Neurochir, 1985; 74:49–52

162. Kenefick C. Granular cell myoblastoma of the larynx. J Laryngol Otol, 1978; 92:521–523

163. Marchevsky AM. Mediastinal tumors of peripheral nervous system origin. Semin Diagn Pathol, 1999; 16:65–78

164. Matthews JB, Mason GI. Oral granular cell myoblastoma: an immunohistochemical study. J Oral Pathol, 1982; 11:343–352

165. Muthuswamy PP, Alrenga DP, Marks P et al. Granular cell myoblastoma: rare localization in the trachea. Report of a case and review of the literature. Am J Med, 1986; 80:714–718

166. Naraynsingh V, Raju GC, Jankey N et al. Granular cell myoblastoma of the breast. J R Coll Surg Edinb, 1985; 30:91–92

167. Orenstein HH, Brenner LH, Nay HR. Granular cell myoblastoma of the extrahepatic biliary system. Am J Surg, 1984; 147:827–831

168. Patel F. Granular cell tumour: an underdiagnosed cause of multifocal subcutaneous swellings. J R Soc Med, 1992; 85:578–579

169. Robertson AJ, McIntosh W, Lamont P et al. Malignant granular cell tumour (myoblastoma) of the-vulva: report of a case and review of the literature. Histopathology, 1981; 5:69–79

170. Rubesin S, Herlinger H, Sigal H. Granular cell tumors of the esophagus. Gastrointest Radiol, 1985; 10:11–15

171. Thomas de Montpreville V, Dulmet EM. Granular cell tumours of the lower respiratory tract. Histopathology, 1995; 27:257–262

172. Thunold S, Von Eyben FE, Maehle B. Malignant granular cell tumour of the neck: immunohistochemical and ultrastructural studies of a case. Histopathology, 1989; 14:655–657

173. Yanai-Inbar I, Odes HS, Krugliak P et al. Granular cell myoblastoma of the sigmoid colon. Dig Dis Sci, 1981; 26:852–854

174. Yasutomi T, Koike H, Nakatsuchi Y. Granular cell tumour of the ulnar nerve. J Hand Surg, 1999; 24:122–124

175. Ordonez NG. Granular cell tumor: a review and update. Adv Anat Pathol, 1999; 6:186–203

176. Junquera LM, de Vicente JC, Vega JA et al. Granular-cell tumours: an immunohistochemical study. Br J Oral Maxillofac Surg, 1997; 35:180–184

177. Filie AC, Lage JM, Azumi N. Immunoreactivity of S100 protein, alpha-1-antitrypsin, and CD68 in adult and congenital granular cell tumors. Mod Pathol, 1996; 9:888–892

178. Nielsen K, Paulsen SM, Johansen P. Carcinoembryonic antigen like antigen in granular cell myoblastomas. An immunohistochemical study. Virchows Arch Pathol Anat Histopathol, 1983; 401:159–162

179. Matthews JB, Mason GI. Granular cell myoblastoma: an immunoperoxidase study using a variety of antisera to human carcinoembryonic antigen. Histopathology, 1983; 7:77–82

180. Kaiserling E, Xiao JC, Ruck P et al. Aberrant expression of macrophage-associated antigens (CD68 and Ki-M1P) by Schwann cells in reactive and neoplastic neural tissue. Light- and electron-microscopic findings. Mod Pathol, 1993; 6:463–468

181. Kurtin PJ, Bonin DM. Immunohistochemical demonstration of the lysosome-associated glycoprotein CD68 (KP-1) in granular cell tumors and schwannomas. Hum Pathol, 1994; 25:1172–1178

182. Abenoza P, Sibley RK. Granular cell myoma and schwannoma: fine structural and immunohistochemical study. Ultrastruct Pathol, 1987; 11:19–28

183. Miettinen M, Lehtonen E, Lehtola H et al. Histogenesis of granular cell tumour – an immunohistochemical and ultrastructural study. J Pathol, 1984; 142:221–229

184. Tokar B, Boneval C, Mirapoglu S et al. Congenital granular-cell tumor of the gingiva. Pediatr Surg Int 1998; 13(:594–596

185. Geddes JF, Thom M, Robinson SF et al. Granular cell change in astrocytic tumors. Am J Surg Pathol, 1996; 20:55–63

186. Rickert CH, Kuchelmeister K, Gullotta F. Morphological and immunohistochemical characterization of granular cells in non-hypophyseal tumours of the central nervous system. Histopathology, 1997; 30:464–471

187. Aghakhani N, George B, Parker F. Paraganglioma of the cauda equina region – report of two cases and review of the literature. Acta Neurochir, 1999; 141:81–87

188. Moran CA, Rush W, Mena H. Primary spinal paragangliomas: a clinicopathological and immunohistochemical study of 30 cases. Histopathology, 1997; 31:167–173

189. Roche PH, Figarella-Branger D, Regis J et al. Cauda equina paraganglioma with subsequent intracranial and intraspinal metastases. Acta Neurochir, 1996; 138:475–479

190. Singh RV, Yeh JS, Broome JC. Paraganglioma of the cauda equina: a case report and review of the literature. Clin Neurol Neurosurg, 1993; 95:109–113

191. Orrell JM, Hales SA. Paragangliomas of the cauda equina have a distinctive cytokeratin immunophenotype. Histopathology, 1992; 21:479–481

192. Pigott TJ, Lowe JS, Morrell K et al. Paraganglioma of the cauda equina. Report of three cases. J Neurosurg, 1990; 73:455–458

193. Raftopoulos C, Flament-Durand J, Brucher JM et al. Paraganglioma of the cauda equina. Report of 2 cases and review of 59 cases from the iterature. Clin Neurol Neurosurg, 1990; 92:263–270

194. Ironside JW. Paraganglioma of the cauda equina [letter]. J Neurol Neurosurg Psychiatry, 1988; 51:740

195. Kameh DS, Perez-Berenguer JL, Pearl GS. Lipofibromatous hamartoma and related peripheral nerve lesions. South Med J, 2000; 93:800–802

196. Roncaroli F, Scheithauer BW, Krauss WE. Hemangioma of spinal nerve root. J Neurosurg, 1999; 91:175–180

197. Mitchell A, Scheithauer BW, Sasano H et al. Symptomatic intradural adrenal adenoma of the spinal nerve root: report of two cases. Neurosurgery, 1993; 32:658–661

198. Misdraji J, Ino Y, Louis DN et al. Primary lymphoma of peripheral nerve: report of four cases. Am J Surg Pathol, 2000; 24:1257–1265

199. Laeng RH, Altermatt HJ, Scheithauer BW et al. Amyloidomas of the nervous system: a monoclonal B-cell disorder with monotypic amyloid light chain lambda amyloid production. Cancer, 1998; 82:362–374

200. Weiland TL, Scheithauer BW, Rock MG et al. Inflammatory pseudotumor of nerve. Am J Surg Pathol, 1996; 20:1212–1218

201. Chauvin PJ, Wysocki GP, Daley TD et al. Palisaded encapsulated neuroma of oral mucosa. Oral Surg Oral Med Oral Pathol, 1992; 73:71–74

202. Morrison PJ, Nevin NC. Multiple endocrine neoplasia type 2B (mucosal neuroma syndrome, Wagenmann–Froboese syndrome). J Med Genet, 1996; 33:779–782

203. Suarez GA, Giannini C, Smith et al. Localized hypertrophic neuropathy. Mayo Clinic Proc, 1994; 69:747–748

204. Kameh DS, Perez-Berenguer JL, Pearl GS. Lipofibromatous hamartoma and related peripheral nerve lesions. South Med J, 2000; 93:800–802

205. Herrick RT, Godsil RDJ, Widener JH. Lipofibromatous hamartoma of the radial nerve: a case report. J Hand Surg, 1980; 5:211–213

206. Warhold LG, Urban MA, Bora FWJ et al. Lipofibromatous hamartomas of the median nerve. J Hand Surg, 1993; 18:1032–1037

207. Hauck RM, Banducci DR. The natural history of a lipofibromatous hamartoma of the palm: a case report. J Hand Surg 1993; 18:1029–1031

208. Steentoft J, Sollerman C. Lipofibromatous hamartoma of a digital nerve. A case report. Acta Orthopaed Scand, 1990; 61(2):181–182

209. Amadio PC, Reiman HM, Dobyns JH. Lipofibromatous hamartoma of nerve. J Hand Surg, 1988; 13:67–75

210. Gouldesbrough DR, Kinny SJ. Lipofibromatous hamartoma of the ulnar nerve at the elbow: brief report. J Bone Joint Surg, 1989; 71:331–332

211. Silverman TA, Enzinger FM. Fibrolipomatous hamartoma of nerve. A clinicopathologic analysis of 26 cases. Am J Surg Pathol, 1985; 9:7–14

212. Marom EM, Helms CA. Fibrolipomatous hamartoma: pathognomonic on MR imaging. Skeletal Radiol, 1999; 28:260–264

213. Canga A, Abascal F, Cerezal L Fibrolipomatous hamartoma of the median nerve. Case illustration. J Neurosurg, 1998; 89:683

214. Berti E, Roncaroli F. Fibrolipomatous hamartoma of a cranial nerve. Histopathology, 1994; 24:391–392

215. Houpt P, Storm van Leeuwen JB, van den Bergen HA. Intraneural lipofibroma of the median nerve. J Hand Surg 1989; 14:706–709

216. Tiffee JC, Barnes EL. Neuromuscular hamartomas of the head and neck. Arch Otolaryngol Head Neck Surg, 1998; 124:212–216

217. Bassett GS, Monforte-Munoz H, Mitchell WG et al. Cavus deformity of the foot secondary to a neuromuscular choristoma (hamartoma) of the sciatic nerve. A case report. J Bone Joint Surg, 1997; 79:1398–1401

218. Van Dorpe J, Sciot R, De Vos R et al. Neuromuscular choristoma (hamartoma) with smooth and striated muscle component: case report with immunohistochemical and ultrastructural analysis. Am J Surg Pathol, 1997; 21:1090–1095

219. Mitchell A, Scheithauer BW, Ostertag H et al. Neuromuscular choristoma. Am J Clin Pathol, 1995; 103:460–465

220. Awasthi D, Kline DG, Beckman EN. Neuromuscular hamartoma (benign triton tumor) of the brachial plexus. Case report. J Neurosurg, 1991; 75:795–797

221. Bonneau R, Brochu P. Neuromuscular choristoma. A cliniopathologic study of two cases. Am J Surg Pathol, 1983; 7:521–528

Malignant nerve sheath tumours

222. Hruban RH, Shiu MH, Senie RT et al. Malignant peripheral nerve sheath tumors of the buttock and lower extremity. A study of 43 cases. Cancer, 1990; 66:1253–1265

223. Ramanathan RC, Thomas JM. Malignant peripheral nerve sheath tumours associated with von Recklinghausen's neurofibromatosis. Eur J Surg Oncol, 1999; 25:190–193

224. Schwarz J, Belzberg AJ. Malignant peripheral nerve sheath tumors in the setting of segmental neurofibromatosis. Case report. J Neurosurg, 2000; 92:342–346

225. Foley KM, Woodruff JM, Ellis FT et al. Radiation-induced malignant and atypical peripheral nerve sheath tumors. Ann Neurol, 1980; 7:311–318

226. Navarro O, Nunez-Santos E, Daneman A et al. Malignant peripheral nerve-sheath tumor arising in a previously irradiated neuroblastoma: report of 2 cases and a review of the literature. Pediat Radiol, 2000; 30:176–180

227. Newbould MJ, Wilkinson N, Mene A. Post-radiation malignant peripheral nerve sheath tumour: a report of two cases. Histopathology, 1990; 17:263–265

228. Ducatman BS, Scheithauer BW, Piepgras DG et al. Malignant peripheral nerve sheath tumors. A clinicopathologic study of 120 cases. Cancer, 1986; 57:2006–2021

229. Ricci AJ, Parham DM, Woodruff JM et al. Malignant peripheral nerve sheath tumors arising from ganglioneuromas. Am J Surg Pathol, 1984; 8:19–29

230. Banks E, Yum M, Brodhecker C et al. A malignant peripheral nerve sheath tumor in associationwith a paratesticular ganglioneuroma. Cancer, 1989; 64:1738–1742

231. Rasmussen SA, Overman J, Thomson SA et al. Chromosome 17 loss-of-heterozygosity studies in benign and malignant tumors in neurofibromatosis type 1. Genes Chromosomes Cancer, 2000; 28:425–431

232. Menon AG, Anderson KM, Riccardi VM et al. Chromosome 17p deletions and TP53 mutations associated with the formation of malignant neurofibrosarcomas in Recklinghausen neurofibromatosis. Proc Nat Acad Sci U S A 1990; 87:5435–5439

233. Vogel KS, Klesse LJ, Veasco-Miguel S et al. Mouse tumor model for neurofibromatosis type 1. Science, 1999; 286:2176–2179

234. Halling KC, Scheithauer BW, Halling AC et al. TP53 expression in neurofibroma and malignant peripheral nerve sheath tumor. An immunohistochemical study of sporadic and NF1-associated tumors [see comments]. Am J Clin Pathol, 1996; 106:282–288

235. Strauss BL, Gutmann DH, Dehner LP et al. Molecular analysis of malignant triton tumors. Hum Pathol, 1999; 30:984–988

236. Nielsen GP, Stemmer-Rachamimov AO, Ino Y et al. Malignant transformation of neurofibromas in neurofibromatosis 1 is associated with CDKN2A/p16 inactivation. Am J Pathol, 1999; 155:1879–1884

237. Kourea HP, Orlow I, Scheithauer BW et al. Deletions of the INK4A gene occur in malignant peripheral nerve sheath tumors but not in neurofibromas. Am J Pathol, 1999; 155:1855–1860

238. Berner JM, Sorlie T, Mertens F et al. Chromosome band 9p21 is frequently altered in malignant peripheral nerve sheath tumors: studies of CDKN2A and other genes of the pRB pathway. Genes Chromosomes Cancer, 1999; 26:151–160

239. Kourea HP, Cordon-Cardo C, Dudas M et al. Expression of p27(kip) and other cell cycle regulators in malignant peripheral nerve sheath tumors and neurofibromas: the emerging role of p27(kip) in malignant transformation of neurofibromas. Am J Pathol, 1999; 155:1885–1891

240. Watanabe T, Sakamoto A, Tamiya S et al. H-ras-1 point mutation in malignant peripheral nerve sheath tumors: polymerase chain reaction restriction fragment length polymorphism analysis and direct sequencing from paraffin embedded tissues. Int J Mol Med, 2000; 5:605–608

241. Plaat BE, Molenaar WM, Mastik MF et al. Computer-assisted cytogenetic analysis of 51 malignant peripheral-nerve-sheath tumors: sporadic vs neurofibromatosis-type-1-associated malignant schwannomas. Int J Cancer, 1999; 83:171–178

242. Rao UN, Surti U, Hoffner L et al. Cytogenetic and histologic correlation of peripheral nerve sheath tumors of soft tissue. Cancer Genet Cytogenet 1996; 88:17–25

243. Mechtersheimer G, Otano-Joos M, Ohl S et al. Analysis of chromosomal imbalances in sporadic and NF1-associated peripheral nerve sheath tumors by comparative genomic hybridization. Genes Chromosomes Cancer, 1999; 25:362–369

244. Fletcher CD, Dal Cin P, de Wever I et al. Correlation between clinicopathological features and karyotype in spindle cell sarcomas. A report of 130 cases from the CHAMP study group. Am J Pathol, 1999; 154:1841–1847

245. Schmidt H, Taubert H, Meye A et al. Gains in chromosomes 7, 8q, 15q and 17q are characteristic changes in malignant but not in benign peripheral nerve sheath tumors from patients with Recklinghausen's disease. Cancer Letters, 2000; 155:181–190

246. Schmidt H, Wurl P, Taubert H et al. Genomic imbalances of 7p and 17q in malignant peripheral nerve sheath tumors are clinically relevant. Genes Chromosomes Cancer, 1999; 25:205–211

247. Vang R, Biddle DA, Harrison WR et al. Malignant peripheral nerve sheath tumor with a t(X;18). Arch Pathol Lab Med 2000; 124:864–867

248. van de Rijn M, Barr FG, Collins MH et al. Absence of SYT-SSX fusion products in soft tissue tumors other than synovial sarcoma. Am J Clin Pathol, 1999; 112:43–49

249. Ducatman BS, Scheithauer BW, Piepgras DG et al. Malignant peripheral nerve sheath tumors in childhood. J Neurooncol, 1984; 2:241–248

250. Casanova M, Ferrari A, Spreafico F et al. Malignant peripheral nerve sheath tumors in children: a single-institution twenty-year experience. J Pediatr Hematol Oncol, 1999; 21:509–513

251. Coffin CM, Dehner LP. Peripheral neurogenic tumors of the soft tissues in children and adolescents: a clinicopathologic study of 139 cases. Pediatr Pathol, 1989; 9:387–407

252. deCou JM, Rao BN, Parham DM et al. Malignant peripheral nerve sheath tumors: the St. Jude Children's Research Hospital experience. Ann Surg Oncol, 1995; 2:524–529

253. Hujala K, Martikainen P, Minn H et al. Malignant nerve sheath tumors of the head and neck: four case studies and review of the literature. Eur Arch Otorhinolaryngol, 1993; 250:379–382

254. Khan RJ, Asgher J, Sohail MT et al. Primary intraosseous malignant peripheral nerve sheath tumor: a case report and review of the literature. Pathology, 1998; 30:237–241

255. Misago N, Ishii Y, Kohda H. Malignant peripheral nerve sheath tumor of the skin: a superficial form of this tumor. J Cutan Pathol, 1996; 23:182–188

256. Shearer P, Parham D, Kovnar E et al. Neurofibromatosis type I and malignancy: review of 32 pediatric cases treated at a single institution. Med Pediatr Oncol, 1994; 22:78–83

257. Wanebo JE, Malik JM, VandenBerg SR et al. Malignant peripheral nerve sheath tumors. A clinicopathologic study of 28 cases. Cancer, 1993; 71:1247–1253

258. Wesche WA, Khare V, Rao BN et al. Malignant peripheral nerve sheath tumor of bone in children and adolescents. Pediatr Dev Pathol, 1999; 2:159–167

259. Stull MA, Moser RPJ, Kransdorf MJ et al. Magnetic resonance appearance of peripheral nerve sheath tumors. Skeletal Radiol, 1991; 20:9–14

260. Nagasaka T, Lai R, Sone M et al. Glandular malignant peripheral nerve sheath tumor: an unusual case showing histologically malignant glands. Arch Pathol Lab Med, 2000; 124:1364–1368

261. Daimaru Y, Hashimoto H, Enjoji M. Malignant peripheral nerve-sheath tumors (malignant schwannomas). An immunohistochemical study of 29 cases. Am J Surg Pathol, 1985; 9:434–444

262. Wong SY, Teh M, Tan YO et al. Malignant glandular triton tumor. Cancer, 1991; 67:1076–1083

263. Mentzel T, Katenkamp D. Intraneural angiosarcoma and angiosarcoma arising in benign and malignant peripheral nerve sheath tumours: clinicopathological and immunohistochemical analysis of four cases. Histopathology, 1999; 35:114–120

264. Sangueza OP, Requena L. Neoplasms with neural differentiation: a review. Part II: Malignant neoplasms. Am J Dermatopathol, 1998; 20:89–102

265. Morphopoulos GD, Banerjee SS, Ali HH et al. Malignant peripheral nerve sheath tumour with vascular differentiation: a report of four cases. Histopathology, 1996; 28:401–410

266. Rose DS, Wilkins MJ, Birch R et al. Malignant peripheral nerve sheath tumour with rhabdomyoblastic and glandular differentiation: immunohistochemical features. Histopathology, 1992; 21:287–290

267. Woodruff JM, Christensen WN. Glandular peripheral nerve sheath tumors. Cancer, 1993; 72:3618–3628

268. Eltoum IA, Moore RJr, Cook W et al. Epithelioid variant of malignant peripheral nerve sheath tumor (malignant schwannoma) of the urinary bladder. Ann Diagn Pathol, 1999; 3:304–308

269. Laskin WB, Weiss SW, Bratthauer GL. Epithelioid variant of malignant peripheral nerve sheath tumor (malignant epithelioid schwannoma). Am J Surg Pathol, 1991; 15:1136–1145

270. DiCarlo EF, Woodruff JM, Bansal M et al. The purely epithelioid malignant peripheral nerve sheath tumor. Am J Surg Pathol, 1986; 10:478–490

271. Woodruff JM, Chernik NL, Smith MC et al. Peripheral nerve tumors with rhabdomyosarcomatous differentiation (malignant Triton tumors). Cancer, 1973; 32:426–439

272. Woodruff JM. Peripheral nerve tumors showing glandular differentiation (glandular schwannomas). Cancer, 1976; :2399–2413

273. Hirose T, Scheithauer BW, Sano T. Perineurial malignant peripheral nerve sheath tumor (MPNST): a clinicopathologic, immunohistochemical, and ultrastructural study of seven cases. Am J Surg Pathol, 1998; 22:1368–1378

274. Abe S, Imamura T, Park P et al. Small round-cell type of malignant peripheral nerve sheath tumor. Mod Pathol, 1998; 11:747–753

275. Wick MR, Swanson PE, Scheithauer BW et al. Malignant peripheral nerve sheath tumor. An immunohistochemical study of 62 cases. Am J Clin Pathol, 1987; 87:425–433

276. Hirose T, Hasegawa T, Kudo E et al. Malignant peripheral nerve sheath tumors: an immunohistochemical study in relation to ultrastructural features. Hum Pathol, 1992; 23:865–870

277. Smith TA, Machen SK, Fisher C et al. Usefulness of cytokeratin subsets for distinguishing monophasic synovial sarcoma from malignant peripheral nerve sheath tumor. Am J Clin Pathol, 1999; 112:641–648

278. Shimizu S, Teraki Y, Ishiko A et al. Malignant epithelioid schwannoma of the skin showing partial HMB-45 positivity. Am J Dermatopathol, 1993; 15:378–384

279. Ariza A, Bilbao JM, Rosai J. Immunohistochemical detection of epithelial membrane antigen in normal perineurial cells and perineurioma. Am J Surg Pathol, 1988; 12:678–683

280. Fisher C. The value of electronmicroscopy and immunohistochemistry in the diagnosis of soft tissue sarcomas: a study of 200 cases. Histopathology, 1990; 16:441–454

281. Hirose T, Sumitomo M, Kudo E et al. Malignant peripheral nerve sheath tumor (MPNST) showing perineurial cell differentiation. Am J Surg Pathol, 1989; 13:613–620

282. Folpe AL, Schmidt RA, Chapman D et al. Poorly differentiated synovial sarcoma: immunohistochemical distinction from primitive neuroectodermal tumors and high-grade malignant peripheral nerve sheath tumors. Am J Surg Pathol, 1998; 22:673–682

283. Krane JF, Bertoni F, Fletcher CD. Myxoid synovial sarcoma: an underappreciated morphologic subset. Mod Pathol, 1999; 12:456–462

284. King R, Busam K, Rosai J. Metastatic malignant melanoma resembling malignant peripheral nerve sheath tumor report of 16 cases. Am J Surg Pathol, 1999; 23:1499–1505

285. Shah IA, Gani OS, Wheler L. Comparative immunoreactivity of CD-68 and HMB-45 in malignant melanoma, neural tumors and nevi. Pathol Res Pract, 1997; 193:497–502

286. Guillou L, Wadden C, Coindre JM et al. Proximal-type epithelioid sarcoma, a distinctive aggressive neoplasm showing rhabdoid features. Clinicopathologic, immunohistochemical, and ultrastructural study of a series. Am J Surg Pathol, 1997; 21:130–146

287. Mack EE, Gomez EC. Neurotropic melanoma. A case report and review of the literature. J Neurooncol, 1992; 13:165–171

288. Carlson JA, Dickersin GR, Sober AJ et al. Desmoplastic neurotropic melanoma. A clinicopathologic analysis of 28 cases. Cancer, 1995; 75:478–494

289. Vauthey JN, Woodruff JM, Brennan MF. Extremity malignant peripheral nerve sheath tumors (neurogenic sarcomas): a 10-year experience. Ann Surg Oncol, 1995; 2:126–131

290. Loree TR, North JHJ, Werness BA et al. Malignant peripheral nerve sheath tumors of the head and neck: analysis of prognostic factors. Otolaryngol Head Neck Surg, 2000; 122:667–672

291. Wong WW, Hirose T, Scheithauer BW et al. Malignant peripheral nerve sheath tumor: analysis of treatment outcome. Int J Radiat Oncol Biol Phys, 1998; 42:351–360

292. Fanburg-Smith JC, Meis-Kindblom JM, Fante R et al. Malignant granular cell tumor of soft tissue: diagnostic criteria and clinicopathologic correlation. Am J Surg Pathol, 1998; 22:779–794

293. Simsir A, Osborne BM, Greenebaum E. Malignant granular cell tumor: a case report and review of the recent literature. Hum Pathol, 1996; 27:853–858

Non-neurigenic tumours

294. Giannini C, Scheithauer BW, Hellbusch LC et al. Peripheral nerve hemangioblastoma. Mod Pathol, 1998; 11:999–1004

16 Pituitary fossa tumours

Pituitary adenomas: general features

Detailed classifications of pituitary adenomas correlate the differing ultrastructural and immunocytochemical properties of each tumour with their secretory capacity in vitro and in vivo.[1,2] It should be noted, however, that such subdivisions are not part of the current World Health Organisation (WHO) classification, which lists pituitary adenomas only as a single entity.[3] The scheme used here is based on that suggested by Kovacs and Horvath[2] and is shown in Table 16.1, together with the basic cytological and endocrinological properties of the different secretory subtypes. A full description of each of these, including summary tables, is given in the separate sections which follow this general account. Pituitary carcinomas, listed separately in the WHO classification, are rather controversial in significance and definition[2,4] and are discussed here under malignancy and invasion in pituitary adenomas.

Incidence

The incidence of pituitary adenomas presenting symptomatically during life is usually quoted as between 6 and 10% of all intracranial tumours.[1,5] Those without evidence of endocrine function tend to present in a slightly older age group, usually after the fifth decade of life, whereas most actively secreting adenomas manifest between 30 and 50 years of age.[1,2] Pituitary adenomas are uncommon in children, representing just 0.6% of all intracranial tumours in children under 12 years.[6] The majority of childhood adenomas are functioning and small, with an endocrinological presentation most often associated with prolactin secretion, or slightly less commonly as acromegaly or pituitary dependent Cushing's disease.[2,7]

Asymptomatic pituitary adenomas have been reported as an incidental finding in anything from 10 to 20% of cases in different autopsy series[8,9] and have a peak incidence in the seventh and eighth decades of life.[10] They are mostly prolactin containing or non-functioning tumours,[11] and are nearly always microadenomas less than 10 mm in diameter.[12]

Site

The overwhelming majority of pituitary adenomas arise in the anterior hypophysis and are initially intrasellar in location. It must be remembered, however, that these tumours have a marked tendency to grow beyond the bony confines of the pituitary fossa and occupy suprasellar or parasellar sites.[4,13] In addition, there are rare examples of true ectopic pituitary adenomas, arising out-

Table 16.1 Classification of pituitary adenomas

Tumour type	Tinctorial characteristics	Hormones produced	Cell population
1 *Growth hormone cell adenoma*			
Sparsely granulated	Chromophobe	Growth hormone	Monomorphic
Densely granulated	Acidophil	Growth hormone	Monomorphic
2 *Prolactin cell adenoma*			
Sparsely granulated	Chromophobe	Prolactin	Monomorphic
Densely granulated	Acidophil	Prolactin	Monomorphic
3 *Mixed growth hormone cell and prolactin cell adenoma*	Variable mixture of chromophobe and acidophil cells	Growth hormone and prolactin	Bimorphic
4 *Acidophil stem cell adenoma*	Chromophobe	Growth hormone and prolactin	Monomorphic
5 *Mammosomatotroph cell adenoma*	Acidophil	Growth hormone and prolactin	Monomorphic
6 *Corticotroph cell adenoma*			
Functioning			
Densely granulated	Basophilic	ACTH	Monomorphic
Sparsely granulated	Chromophobe	ACTH	
Non-functioning	Basophilic or chromophobe	ACTH	Three tumour subtypes
7 *Thyrotroph cell adenoma*	Chromophobe	TSH	Monomorphic
8 *Gonadotroph cell adenoma*	Chromophobe	FSH, LH, alpha subunit in varied combinations	Monomorphic Sex linked dichotomy
9 *Non-functioning adenoma*			
Non-oncocytic	Chromophobe	Scanty FSH, LH, alpha subunit or no hormones detected	Monomorphic
Oncocytic	Chromphobe or acidophil		
10 *Plurihormonal adenomas*	Variable	Two or three hormones in variable combinations	Monomorphic, biomorphic or trimorphic

ACTH, adrenocorticotropic hormone; FSH, follicle stimulating hormone; LH, luteinising hormone; TSH, thyroid stimulating hormone

side an entirely normal fossa. These have been described in the sphenoid air sinus[14,15] and in suprasellar locations, either attached to the upper part of the pituitary stalk[16] or within the inferior part of the third ventricle.[17,18] They are presumed to arise in ectopic nests of adenohypophyseal tissue, which are a not uncommon finding around the upper part of the pituitary stalk.[18]

Aetiology

At first sight, it seems likely that well differentiated adenomas producing a single hormone have arisen from the corresponding type of mature, secretory pituicyte in the anterior gland. Many types of adenoma, however, secrete two or more hormones and the cellular origins of these are less clear. In some cases, such tumours may consist of separate neoplastic cell populations, each corresponding to one of the different hormones produced. Examples include the relatively familiar mixed growth hormone cell and prolactin cell adenomal,[19] combinations such as adrenocorticotropic hormone (ACTH) and prolactin[20] and several rarer plurihormonal adenomas.[21] In other cases, plurihormonal tumours may be entirely monomorphic, consisting either of primitive cells presumed to be stem cells, as in the case of acidophil stem cell adenomas,[22] or well-differentiated cells able to produce more than one anterior gland hormone, like those in mammosomatotroph adenomas.[23] In some monomorphic plurihormonal adenomas, immuno-electronmicroscopic studies have demonstrated more than one hormone not only in the same cells, but in the same secretory granules.[24] It thus seems possible that all types of adenoma arise from a common pluripotential stem cell, and that the endocrine properties of each tumour depend on the degree and direction of differentiation following neoplastic transformation.[25] This view is given support by the finding that even plurihormonal pituitary adenomas are monoclonal when subjected to X-chromosome analysis, suggesting that neoplasia follows somatic mutation in a single progenitor cell.[26] A causative somatic mutation has been demonstrated in approximately 40% of growth hormone cell adenomas, which show acquired defects in the *GSPT1* oncogene.[27] The normal protein product (Gs) of this gene interacts with growth hormone releasing hormone (GHrh), allowing tight control of its trophic activity. Activating point mutations result in continuous GHrh-like stimulation, permitting autonomous proliferation and growth hormone secretion.[27] Mutations of the Gs protein have also been found in a small minority of both non-secretory and ACTH cell adenomas, indicating that this mechanism of tumorigenesis is not confined to growth hormone cell adenomas.[28,29] Activating mutations involving a second oncogene, H-*ras*, have only been found in a tiny minority of pituitary tumours, but significantly these have nearly

all involved metastasising carcinomas, suggesting a rare but late event in the progression of malignancy.[30] Further cytogenetic information comes from patients with multiple endocrine neoplasia type 1 (MEN-1), over half of whom develop pituitary adenomas in addition to other types of endocrine tumour.[31] The gene for MEN-1 lies on chromosome 11q13 and, unlike the *GSPT1* and H-*ras* genes, it functions as a typical tumour suppressor.[32] In patients inheriting the syndrome, one allele of the gene is inactivated by a germline mutation and tumorigenesis occurs only when a spontaneous somatic mutation affects the other allele. However, deletions of the *MEN-1* gene have also been found in varied types of pituitary adenoma from patients who have not inherited the syndrome, suggesting a causative role in some sporadic tumours as well the *MEN-1* related ones.[33] Finally, evidence is emerging that a novel tumour suppressor gene very close to the retinoblastoma locus *RB1* on 13q14 may be important in the genesis of a small minority of pituitary tumours with invasive or frankly malignant features.[34]

For some pituitary adenomas, the trigger for neoplasia may be physiological rather than genetic, with loss of negative feedback on the hypothalamus resulting in chronic stimulation of the relevant anterior gland cell type.[2] Rare examples of gonadotrophic cell and thyrotrophic cell adenomas have been described in patients with longstanding hypogonadism[35] or primary hypothyroidism[36] respectively, and ACTH secreting adenomas have occasionally arisen against a background of Addison's disease.[37] In rats[38] and exceptionally in humans,[39] pharmacological doses of oestrogen can lead to the development of prolactinomas, presumably also via hypothalamic mediation, although epidemiological studies have not shown any increased incidence of these tumours in large cohorts of women taking oestrogen-containing oral contraceptives.[40] Both ACTH and prolactin cell adenomas can sometimes occur in conjunction with hyperplasia of the same cell type, again suggesting that chronic hypothalamic stimulation may have preceded development of neoplasia in these cases.[41,42] However, hyperplasia has never been demonstrated in glands harbouring growth hormone secreting adenomas,[43] despite the evidence from the *GSPT1* gene that prolonged GHrh-like stimulation can lead to neoplastic transformation.[27]

Clinical features

Functioning pituitary adenomas may present with clinical evidence of abnormal hormone secretion, as described below in the sections covering individual adenoma subtypes. Larger adenomas, either functioning or endocrinologically silent, usually produce signs and symptoms relating to their mass effect, particularly if there is suprasellar extension or parasellar invasion.

Suprasellar extension commonly causes visual field defects due to pressure on the optic chiasm, which can be demonstrated clinically in a large proportion of adenoma patients on formal testing.[44,45] Superior bitemporal hemianopia is the earliest and commonest field disturbance, and is due to involvement of the chiasmatic decussating fibres.[44,46] Headaches are a frequent clinical feature of large pituitary adenomas and are the presenting complaint in about 20% of all cases.[47] Cranial nerve palsies occur in about 15% of cases and vary from an isolated third nerve palsy through to combined involvement of the fourth, fifth and sixth cranial nerves in tumours invading the cavernous sinus.[46,47] Direct pressure from tumours with large suprasellar extensions may also cause hypothalamic disturbances,[47] and even when there is no extrasellar extension, pressure on the adjacent normal gland may lead to generalised hypopituitism in some cases.[46,47] In addition, a moderate rise in serum prolactin levels may be caused by any pituitary adenoma exerting sufficient pressure on the pituitary stalk to interfere with the delivery of prolactin inhibiting factor from the hypothalamus to the anterior gland.[48] This phenomenon may also occur with non-pituitary-derived mass lesions in the sellar or suprasellar region[48] and should be considered as a cause for prolactinaemia if the serum levels are not raised above 150 ng/ml.[46] Pituitary apoplexy is the presenting syndrome in about 5% of all adenomas,[49] and is due to tumour swelling following massive haemorrhage or infarction. It typically manifests as an acute onset of severe headache together with sudden visual loss, meningism and ophthalmoplegia.[46,50]

Radiology

Plain skull X-rays have been largely superseded by magnetic resonance imaging (MRI) and computerised tomography (CT) scans in the investigation of pituitary tumours, but they remain a sensitive method of demonstrating ballooning or erosion of the fossa if the tumours are large.[47] Tumour calcifications are only very rarely detected.[51] The results with CT are dependent on tumour size, and an abnormality may not be apparent in a significant proportion of microadenomas less than 10 mm across.[46,52] For small intrasellar tumours, suspicious CT changes include increased gland size, low density areas, stalk shift, elevation of the diaphragma and erosion of the fossa floor.[46] MRI is particularly good for visualising the extrasellar extent of large adenomas[53] (Fig. 16.1) and is probably more sensitive than CT in detecting the presence of cavernous sinus invasion by smaller tumours.[46] Some intrasellar microadenomas may also be visualised, but, as with CT, a significant proportion of the smallest tumours may remain undetected even after administration of contrast media.[54,55] Using

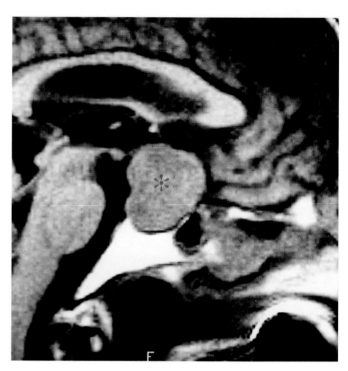

Fig. 16.1 **Invasive pituitary adenoma.** Sagittal T1-weighted magnetic resonance scan of an invasive pituitary adenoma (asterisk). The tumour is expanding the fossa and has a large suprasellar extension.

non-enhanced scans, larger adenomas show a variable intensity relative to normal gland on T1-weighted images but are usually hyperintense with T2 weighting.[46,53]

Pathology

Macroscopic features

Microadenomas are usually defined as being less than 10 mm in diameter. They are not associated with bony changes and are entirely contained within a fossa of normal dimensions. In post-mortem specimens, a coronal section through the decalcified bony pituitary fossa block usually reveals a circumscribed, often haemorrhagic nodule surrounded by a crescentic rim of compressed anterior gland. Asymptomatic microadenomas are multiple in about 0.9% of cases, and some autopsied pituitary glands may contain as many as three separate tumours.[8] *Macroadenomas* may be classified as enclosed, i.e. enlarging the fossa but still confined by it, or frankly invasive.[56] As the tumours enlarge, they completely fill the enlarged fossa, the anterior gland becoming thinned beyond naked eye recognition (Fig. 16.2). The dura of the diaphragma is pushed intracranially in a dome-like fashion, easily visible after removal of the brain at autopsy. In adenomas with more extensive suprasellar growth, the optic chiasm either becomes stretched over the bulging diaphragma, sometimes forming a band-like constriction across the tumour, or it may be displaced

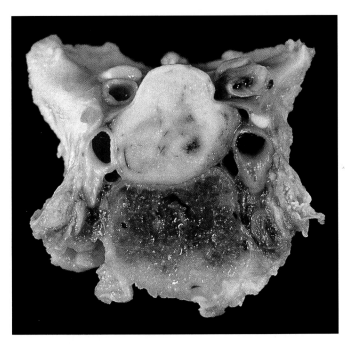

Fig. 16.2 **Enclosed pituitary adenoma.** Coronal section through an autopsy specimen of skull base. The tumour fills the expanded fossa and is pushing the diaphragma upwards in a dome-like fashion.

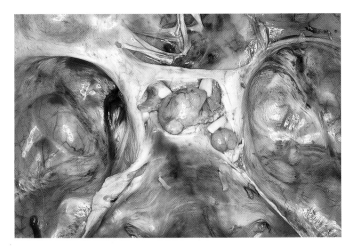

Fig. 16.3 **Invasive pituitary adenoma.** After removal of the brain at autopsy, the tumour can be seen to have ruptured up through the diaphragma and extends intracranially as a lobulated mass. A separate nodule emerges from the cavernous sinus on the right.

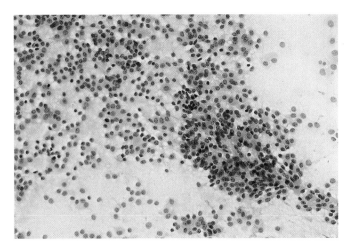

Fig. 16.4 **Pituitary adenoma.** Smear preparation. The cells have a uniform cytological appearance and smear easily away from the thin walled blood vessels. H & E.

cut section, the tumour tissue is grey and friable and often very haemorrhagic, especially after surgical intervention. Cystic spaces filled with proteinaceous or xanthochromic fluid are common, but macroscopic evidence of calcification is only rarely encountered.

Intraoperative diagnosis

Intraoperative diagnostic advice may be required where there is uncertainty over the nature of tumour tissue in the suprasellar or cavernous sinus regions, or alternatively when a surgeon is trying to determine whether intrasellar tissue is anterior gland or adenoma. Using smear preparations, pituitary adenomas spread very easily into an even, thin monolayer, although there may also be some papillary formations with cells clinging to the numerous thin-walled blood vessels (Fig. 16.4). The cytological appearances are usually remarkably uniform, with rounded cell nuclei, prominent nucleoli, and well-circumscribed perinuclear cytoplasm. There is little tendency for the cells to mould or adhere to each other in clumps, like those seen in smears of metastatic carcinoma. Tissue from the normal anterior gland shows a much greater variation in cytological appearance, due to the different populations of cells present in the gland (Fig. 16.5). When both gland tissue and adenoma are present in the same preparation, this is usually obvious, but otherwise distinguishing between the two can be difficult. The presence of mitoses or significant nuclear pleomorphism will obviously exclude normal gland tissue, although such features are uncommon in smears of adenomas. In some cases, a haematoxylin and eosin stain may help highlight the variations in cytoplasmic eosinophilia and cell size seen in normal gland tissue. Frozen sections may also be useful in this context, and have the added advantage that a reticulin preparation or

anteriorly. The largest tumours can rupture through the diaphragmatic dura, invaginating up into the base of the brain as a lobulated mass, incompletely covered by a thin membrane of altered leptomeninges (Fig. 16.3). Invasive adenomas may also extend laterally into the cavernous sinuses, wrapping around the internal carotid arteries, or erode through the floor of the fossa and protrude into the air sinuses as irregular, nodular masses. Such lateral and downward invasion need not necessarily be accompanied by significant suprasellar growth in all cases. On

rapid trichrome stain can be used to help in the distinction of tumour from gland tissue.

Histological features

The different cell types of the *normal anterior gland* are grouped in varying combinations into small or medium sized nests and cords, each enclosed by a prominent recticulin meshwork to create a prominent alveolar pattern (Figs 16.6 and 16.7a). The cell groups are separated by a rich meshwork of anastamosing, thin-walled, sinusoidal vascular channels. Growth hormone secreting cells make up about 50% of the anterior gland and are mostly concentrated in the lateral lobes. Their cytoplasm is strongly acidophilic using trichrome stains. Prolactin secreting cells have acidophil or chromophobe staining characteristics and are more randomly distributed in the gland, although with some tendency to condensation along the posterior margin. They constitute anything from 15 to 25% of the cell population. Corticotrophs constitute between 15 and 20% of the cells and are largely concentrated in the posterior median region. Their cytoplasm is strongly basophilic and periodic acid–Schiff (PAS)-positive on trichrome staining. Thyrotrophs are mostly situated in the anterior median region and account for only about 5% of the gland cells.

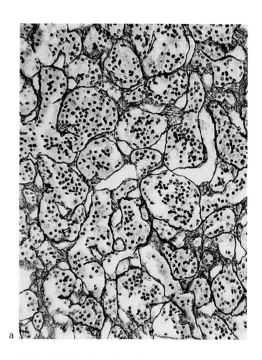

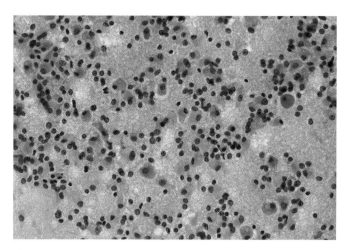

Fig. 16.5 **Anterior pituitary.** Smear preparation. There is a much more varied cytological appearance than in adenomas, reflecting the different types of cell normally present in the gland. H & E.

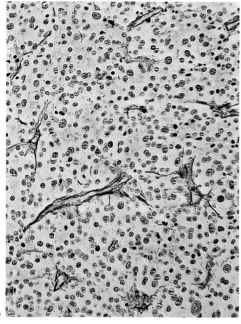

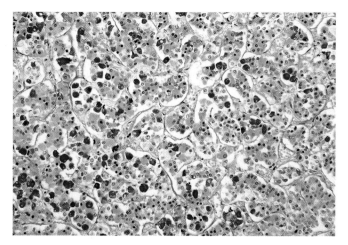

Fig. 16.6 **Anterior pituitary.** The cells have differing tinctorial properties using trichrome stains and are grouped in varying combinations into nests and cords. Orange-fuschin-green.

Fig. 16.7 **(a) Anterior pituitary gland.** Reticulin fibres enclose distinct packets of cells. **(b) Pituitary adenoma.** The reticulin architecture of the normal gland is effaced. Reticulin stain.

Their cytoplasm is weakly basophilic and PAS-positive. Gonadotrophs have similar tinctorial properties and are a randomly distributed, heterogeneous cell population comprising approximately 10% of the total.

In *pituitary adenomas*, the alveolar pattern and reticulin architecture of the normal gland is largely effaced in most cases (Fig. 16.7b). Depending on the secretory subtype, the commonest histological patterns are diffuse sheets of cells (Fig. 16.8) or a pseudopapillary pattern with palisades or rosettes of tumour cells arranged around vascular cores (Fig. 16.9). This latter pattern is often more apparent at the edges of tissue fragments where the vascular structures are less cohesive. There may also be a sinusoidal pattern similar to that of the normal gland, but without alveolar grouping of the cells. Using trichrome stains, the tinctorial properties of the tumour cell cytoplasm are again linked to the secretory subtype, as described in the sections that follow below. In some bimorphous or polymorphous adenomas, more than one population of cells may be apparent tinctorially, as for example with the mixture of chromophobe and acidophil cells seen in some mixed growth hormone cell-prolactin cell adenomas. It should be noted, however, that the results of trichrome staining vary widely with differences in tissue preservation, fixation or processing, and can be very misleading. Although these stains are useful in distinguishing gland tissue from tumour, the hormone typing of adenomas must depend on immunocytochemistry or electron microscopy, and cannot be attempted on the results of tinctorial stains alone.

Routine biopsies of pituitary adenomas frequently show acute interstitial haemorrhage, which is usually a

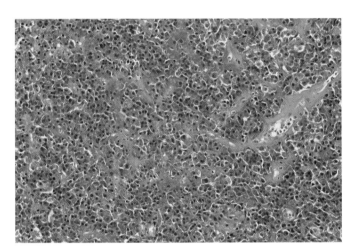

Fig. 16.8 **Pituitary adenoma.** In this densely granulated growth hormone cell tumour, the cells form diffuse sheets intersected by vascular channels. H & E.

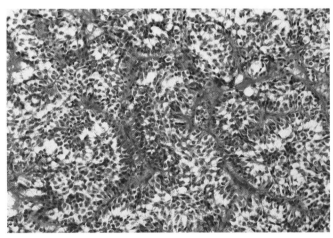

Fig. 16.9 **FSH-producing gonadotropin cell pituitary adenoma.** In this tumour, there is a pseudopapillary pattern, with palisades of cells arranged around vascular cores. H & E.

Fig. 16.10 **Pituitary adenoma.** A cholesterol granuloma is present, suggesting a previous episode of haemorrhage or infarction within the tumour. H & E.

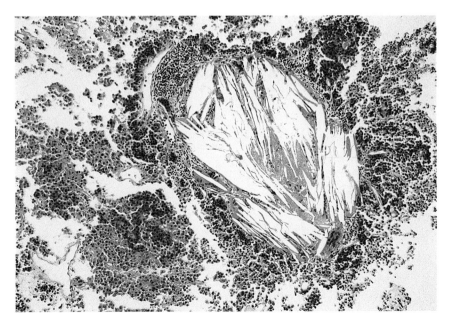

reaction to surgical manipulation of the tissue. In cases of pituitary apoplexy, the majority of the tissue can be effaced by recent haemorrhage, sometimes in conjunction with acute tumour necrosis. Evidence of old haemorrhage, including haemosiderin pigment, focal scarring and cholesterol granuloma formation, is found in a significant proportion of adenomas, even where there is no history of an acute clinical episode[57] (Fig. 16.10). Calcification is rather infrequent in pituitary adenomas and is most often encountered in non-functioning tumours or those secreting prolactin or growth hormone.[51,58]

Amyloid of endocrine origin, analogous to that found in medullary carcinoma of the thyroid gland, is present in up to about three-quarters of prolactin and growth hormone secreting adenomas.[59] Traces of amyloid have also been reported in some non-functioning and corticotrophic adenomas.[59] It is usually apparent on Congo or sirius red staining as faint deposits in the interstitium, especially around blood vessels, and is often sparse enough to be easily overlooked (Fig. 16.11). Very occasionally, the amyloid may take the form of massive, spherical crystals with a lamellated architecture.[60,61] The amyloid in pituitary adenomas is thought to be derived from constituents of the hormone secretory products of the tumour, and occasionally may immunostain with the appropriate hormone antibody.[60]

At the interface with anterior gland, most adenomas show a moderately well circumscribed margin abutting the compressed gland tissue (Fig. 16.12). There is no capsule, however, and entrapped, non-neoplastic anterior gland pituicytes are often present within the more peripheral part of the tumour. These entrapped cells are most readily visualised on immunocytochemical stains for the different anterior gland hormones. They may be of any or all hormone types, and are usually individually dispersed by the tumour tissue. In distinction from the appearances seen in plurihormonal adenomas, entrapped pituicytes are almost entirely confined to the peripheral part of the tumour, constitute less than 1% of the total tumour cell population and often have a stellate contour which contrasts with the rounded or polygonal adenoma cells.[62]

Immunocytochemistry

In addition to their individual reactions with antibodies to anterior gland hormones, all types of adenoma exhibit strong positive staining with antibodies to neurone specific enolase.[63] Positive immunostaining for chromogranin is found in adenomas secreting the glycoprotein hormones follicle stimulating hormone (FSH), luteinising hormone (LH), thyroid stimulating hormone (TSH) or alpha subunit, and in a proportion of apparently non-functioning tumours[64] (Fig. 16.13). Growth hormone secreting tumours may also show some focal positive staining for chromogranin, but prolactinomas and corticotroph tumours are likely to be unreactive.[64,65] All adenomas

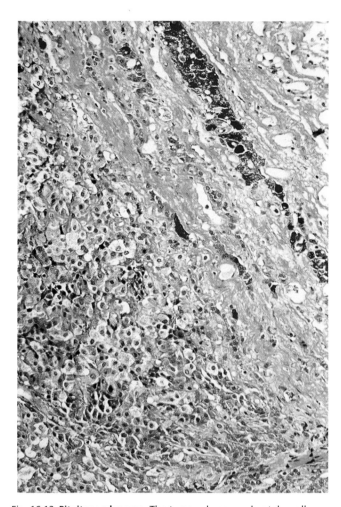

Fig. 16.12 **Pituitary adenoma.** The tumour has a moderately well defined margin and abuts directly onto adjacent, compressed anterior gland tissue (upper right). Orange-fuschin-green.

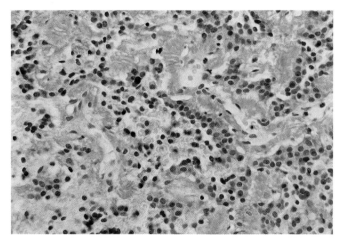

Fig. 16.11 **Prolactin cell pituitary adenoma.** Amyloid is present in the interstitium, especially around blood vessels. Sirius red.

producing growth hormone, prolactin or ACTH express low molecular weight cytokeratins, but in non-functioning tumours and those secreting the glycoprotein hormones, cytokeratin immunoreactivity can be weak or absent.[66,67] Adenoma cells do not express vimentin, glial fibrillary acidic protein or S-100 protein.[66,68] This is in contrast to folliculostellate cells, which are found in many pituitary adenomas, especially those secreting growth hormone or prolactin[69] (Fig. 16.14). Folliculostellate cells, are also present in the normal gland and are thought to be derived from secretory pituicytes which respond to a degenerating neighbour by encircling it and dedifferentiating.[70] They immunostain strongly with antibodies to S-100 protein and sometimes vimentin or glial fibrillary acidic protein (GFAP) but do not express cytokeratin or neuron specific enolase.[71]

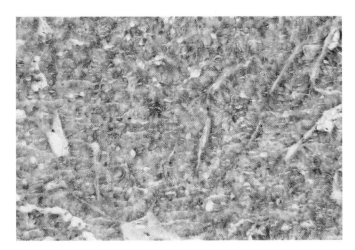

Fig. 16.13 **Pituitary adenoma.** In this example producing FSH and LH, there is widespread reactivity using immunocytochemistry for chromogranin.

Hyperplasia

Physiological hyperplasia of anterior pituitary gland cells is a reversible, non-autonomous process resulting from an alteration in endocrine homeostasis. The most obvious example is the hyperplasia of prolactin secreting cells which occurs during pregnancy.[2] *Pathological hyperplasia*, by contrast, is irreversible and autonomous, i.e. not dependent on the normal mechanisms of hypothalamic function. It most often affects corticotrophs in glands harbouring ACTH-cell adenomas, where it may be a cause of treatment failure following selective trans-phenoidal microadenectomy.[41,43] It may also rarely involve anterior gland prolactin cells adjacent to some prolactinomas,[2] but it has never been found in association with growth hormone producing adenomas.[43] Symptomatic and histologically verified pathological hyperplasia in the absence of an adenoma is exceedingly rare and has only been reported in cases of Cushing's disease.[72] Since a coexisting microadenoma can easily be missed during surgery, primary corticotroph hyperplasia should not be diagnosed purely on the results of a biopsy sample, but only after the entire gland has been removed and sectioned histologically.[73] The hyperplastic gland tissue shows widespread, nodular proliferation of corticotroph cells within expanded alveolar clusters. The reticulin structure of the gland is distorted but preserved and there is typically a transition from normal gland architecture at the margins of hyperplastic areas. Immunocytochemistry shows a clear excess of ACTH-staining cells within the expanded alveolar clusters, interspersed with only occasional cells of other hormonal types (Fig. 16.15).

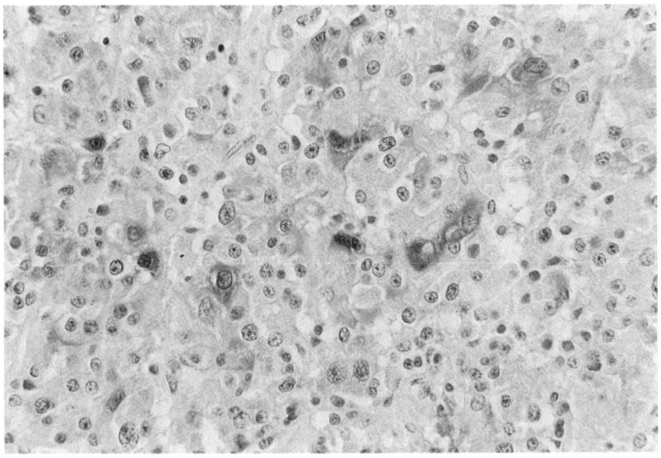

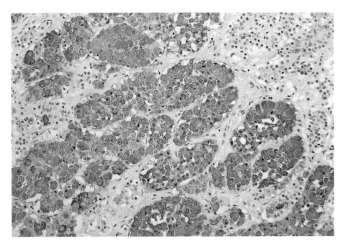

Fig. 16.14 **Growth hormone cell pituitary adenoma.** S-100 protein is expressed by folliculostellate cells present in the tumour, but not by the surrounding adenoma cells. Immunocytochemistry for S-100 protein.

Fig. 16.15 **Corticotroph hyperplasia.** The gland shows nodular proliferation of corticotroph cells within expanded alveolar clusters. ACTH immunocytochemistry.

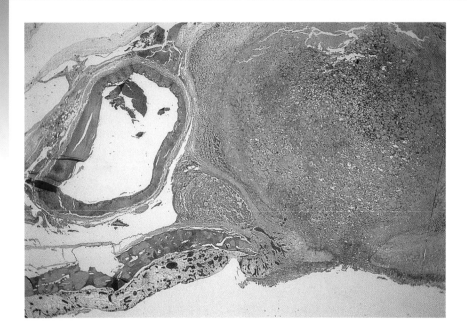

Fig. 16.16 **Invasive pituitary adenoma.** The tumour fills an enlarged fossa (upper right). A separate nodule (lower centre) has invaded laterally into the cavernous sinus and lies adjacent to the carotid artery. Much of the intrasellar part of the tumour has been surgically removed via a trans-sphenoidal approach (defect bottom right) and is replaced by blood and haemostatic material. H & E.

Malignancy and invasion

Pituitary adenomas show a marked natural tendency to infiltrate bone and local structures around the fossa. Some hormone subtypes, including Nelson syndrome adenomas, acidophil stem cell adenomas and thyrotroph cell adenomas, appear to have a greater invasive potential than others, but no adenoma is exempt from this behaviour.[74] Macroscopic invasion of the fossa walls occurs in about 35 to 40% of tumours,[75] and 10% of all cases show more extensive tumour spread into the cranial cavity, cavernous sinuses, orbits or air sinuses[76] (Fig. 16.16). Histological evidence of dural infiltration has been found in up to 98% of adenomas with a significant suprasellar extension.[75] By contrast, cytological features normally associated with malignancy, including mitoses, pleomorphism and giant cells, only occur in a small minority of pituitary adenomas (Fig. 16.17), and there is generally a very poor correlation between such cytological atypia and invasive behaviour.[2] Histologically uniform tumours may widely invade or even metastasise, whilst some with gross pleomorphism and atypical cytology may remain entirely intrasellar.[47] As a result, many authorities have rejected the concept of a 'malignant adenoma' and prefer to class pituitary adenomas simply as invasive or non-invasive on the basis of their observed behaviour.[2,4] The term 'pituitary carcinoma' can then be reserved specifically for those lesions which metastasise and are therefore unquestionably malignant.[2,4]

Metastatic spread may involve the cerebrospinal fluid (CSF) pathways or systemic sites, but in either case it is extremely rare.

1. *CSF dissemination* has been reported in Nelson syndrome[77,78] and tumours secreting growth hormone[79] or prolactin.[80,81] It usually follows surgery, typically after an interval of several years.[82] Most of the primary tumours show invasion and extrasellar extension at initial presentation, and they are often recurrent or incompletely excised lesions.[79,83] Some may have atypical histological features, although not always when initially biopsied.[78,83]

2. Of those tumours metastasising to *systemic sites*, about half have been non-functioning and the remainder have secreted growth hormone,[84] prolactin[85] or ACTH.[86] The primary tumours are again mostly invasive or recurrent lesions which have

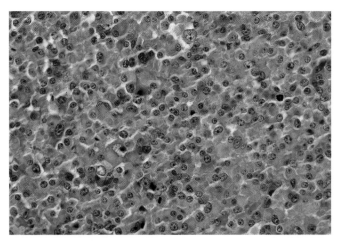

Fig. 16.17 **Non-functioning pituitary adenoma.** There is considerable cytological pleomorphism and several mitoses are visible. Despite this, there was no evidence of extrasellar invasion at surgery. H & E.

previously undergone incomplete surgical resection.[85,87] Some may have quite a uniform cytological appearance, although there is often a significant mitotic rate.[87]

Where the primary pituitary tumours are hormonally functional, the origin of both CSF and systemic tumour deposits can often be confirmed immunocytochemically by demonstrating the appropriate hormone in the metastatic tumour cells.[80,86]

Genetics and cell proliferation indices

An aneuploid DNA pattern is found in a high proportion of functioning adenomas, especially somatotroph and prolactin tumours, and is associated with both large size and a higher S-phase fraction than diploid adenomas.[88] Loss of heterozygosity involving several different chromosomes has been linked to invasive behaviour, and deletion of the *MEN-1* allele appears to be particularly significant in this context.[89] Proliferative activity assessed by nucleolar organiser region counts has been reported to be higher in macroadenomas than microadenomas[90] but no relationship has been found between the bromodeoxyuridine labelling index and either tumour size[91] or clinical evidence of malignancy.[92] By contrast, immunocytochemical staining for c-myc protein, which regulates gene expression of cell proliferation, has shown a good correlation between the percentage of positively labelled cells and subsequent malignant behaviour in pituitary adenomas.[92] Overtly malignant pituitary carcinomas which have metastasised show increased Ki67 (MIB-1) and TP53 labelling indices in the metastatic deposits compared to the primary tumours.[93] In apparently benign adenomas, a raised Ki-67/MIB-1 (S-phase) index is positively correlated with histological evidence of dural invasion[94] but there is little evidence of a consistent relationship between cell proliferation in adenomas and their hormonal subtype.[94] In one study assessing the proliferation index by bromodeoxyuridine incorporation, Nelson syndrome adenomas were found to have a significantly higher S-phase fraction, but amongst other tumours there was no correlation with secretory type.[91]

Differential diagnosis

Pituitary adenomas presenting a problem in differential diagnosis are likely to be endocrinologically silent tumours, but pituitary hormone immunocytochemistry may still permit a conclusive identification in many cases, since a proportion of clinically non-functioning adenomas are immunoreactive with antibodies to various anterior gland hormones, especially FSH, LH, TSH and alpha subunit. In addition, functioning prolactinomas in males or postmenopausal women and a small proportion of corticotroph adenomas may also present as endocrinologically silent mass lesions. Even when there is no expression of anterior gland hormones, pituitary adenomas can be distinguished from many other tumour types by ultrastructural demonstration of secretory granules. It must be remembered, however, that these are also an ultrastructural feature of neuronal tumours such as gangliocytoma or olfactory neuroblastoma. Other features which may be helpful in differential diagnoses are set out below and in Table 16.2, taking into account the location of the tumours surgically and radiologically. A more exhaustive list of lesions which may involve the sellar region is given in the last section of this chapter.

Intrasellar tumours

Metastatic carcinoma In contrast to many metastases, obvious cytological evidence of malignancy is rare in pituitary adenomas and mucin production does not occur. Care should be taken over the interpretation of isolated follicular structures, because epithelial remnants of Rathke's pouch can become entrapped in pituitary adenomas. In some cases, immunocytochemical staining for chromogranin may help to identify positively non-functioning adenomas which do not react with pituitary hormone antibodies. Unless the metastasis is of oat cell type, immunoreactivity for neuron specific enolase will also help to distinguish adenoma from metastasis.

Meningioma These may be entirely intrasellar or breach the diaphragma from above, producing a similar gross appearance to adenomas with a suprasellar extension. If typical arachnoidal features are not apparent histologically, immunocytochemistry can be used to look for evidence of anterior gland hormone production. Failing this, absence of neurone specific enolase but consistent expression of vimentin are the most reliable distinguishing features of meningiomas. Antibodies to chromogranin and cytokeratins may also be helpful, always remembering that scattered expression of cytokeratin to be expected in secretory meningiomas. The same principles apply in the distinction of adenomas from other soft tissue tumours which may arise in the pituitary fossa, including haemangiopericytomas and primary or metastatic sarcomas of various types.

Glial tumours Pilocytic astrocytomas of the posterior hypophysis should be clearly identifiable by their fibrillary glial morphology, expression of glial fibrillary acidic protein and absence of immunoreactivity for cytokeratin, neuron specific enolase and chromogranin. Rarely gangliogliomas or gangliocytomas may also occupy the pituitary fossa, and care should be taken not to misinterpret the results of immunocytochemistry for chromogranin and neuron specific enolase in these cases, especially where the glial elements are scanty or absent.

Table 16.2 Immunocytochemistry in the differential diagnosis of pituitary adenomas

Tumour type	Anterior gland hormones	Cytokeratin	Neuron specific enolase	Antibody epitope Chromogranin	S-100 protein	Vimentin	Placental alkaline phosphatase	GFAP	HCG
Pituitary adenomas	Variable +	Variable +	+	Variable +	–	–	–	–	Variable + if polyclonal
Metastatic carcinoma	–	+	–	–	–	–	–	–	–
Meningioma	–	+ if secretory	–	–	Variable +	+	–	–	–
Glioma/ganglioglioma	–	–	+ if ganglionic	–	+	Variable +	–	+	–
Germinoma	–	Focal +	–	–	–	–	+	–	Variable +
Granule cell tumour	–	–	Variable +	–	–	–	–	Variable +	–
Craniopharyngioma	–	+	–	–	–	–	–	–	–
Paraganglioma	–	+	+	+	–	–	–	–	–
Olfactory neuroblastoma	–	+	+	+	+	–	–	–	–

GFAP, glial fibrillary acidic protein; HCG human chorionic gonadotropin

Germinoma Ectopic, intrasellar pineal germinomas can usually be readily distinguished from pituitary adenomas by their typical appearance using routine histological stains. Where there is difficulty, expression of placental alkaline phosphatase is quite a reliable immunocyto-chemical feature. Germinomas may also express human chorionic gonadotrophin, but specific monoclonal anti-bodies to the beta part of the molecule must be used, because the alpha subunit is identical to that in the anterior pituitary glycoprotein hormones TSH, FSH and LH. Cytokeratins are focally expressed in some germinomas and are unlikely to be helpful in distinguishing them from pituitary adenomas.

Granular cell tumour Like germinomas, these are usually easily recognised by their typical cytological appearance, with eccentric nuclei and swollen cytoplasm filled with PAS-stained granular material. In the rare cases which are large, symptomatic and not obviously arising in the posterior hypophysis, distinction from PAS-positive corticotroph adenomas can be made using immuno-cytochemical staining for ACTH.

Lymphocytic hypophysitis This can sometimes present as an expanding sellar and suprasellar mass lesion, clinically indistinguishable from a pituitary adenoma. If there is hyperprolactinaemia due to stalk compression syndrome, a preoperative diagnosis of prolactinoma is often entertained. The patients are nearly always young women in the late stages of pregnancy or immediately post partum and no discreet tumour is found at surgery. The true diagnosis is readily apparent in biopsies, which show inflamed anterior gland tissue without any histo-logical evidence of adenoma.

Suprasellar tumours

In some cases, pituitary adenomas with large suprasellar extensions may produce little or no radiological evidence of sellar enlargement, and their initial differential diagnosis must take into consideration tumours arising primarily in a suprasellar location. These include metastases, germ cell tumours and meningiomas, which are all discussed above.

In addition, *craniopharyngiomas* may cause confusion with suprasellar extensions of pituitary adenomas if the typical cystic or adamantinous architecture is not apparent and there is no obvious squamous maturation or keratin production. If there is no anterior gland hormone immunoreactivity, the most useful way of dis-tinguishing a pituitary adenoma from craniopharyngioma is to demonstrate immunocytochemical expression of chromogranin or neuron specific enolase.

Parasellar tumours

In other cases, pituitary adenomas without gross sellar expansion or suprasellar extension may present primarily with invasion of the skull bone and air sinuses.

Nasopharyngeal carcinoma must be excluded in this context, particularly bearing in mind the non-keratinising form of this tumour. Pituitary adenomas without immuno-logical evidence of hormone production can usually be distinguished in the same way as from metastatic intrasellar carcinomas, by the demonstration of immunoreactivity for neuron specific enolase or chromogranin.

Olfactory neuroblastomas are usually readily identified by their typical fibrillar stroma, lobulated architecture and neuronal rosettes. Immunocytochemistry must be inter-preted with care, since olfactory neuroblastomas strongly express neuron specific enolase and some cells may also immunoreact with antibodies to cytokeratin and chromogranin. Unlike adenomas, however, they may sometimes also express neurofilament protein, and positive staining with antibodies to S-100 protein is typically found, especially around the margins of tumour cell lobules.

Paragangliomas may erode the skull base in the sellar region or even arise in an intrasellar location. They can closely resemble pituitary adenomas both histologically and immunocytochemically, and distinction between the two can be difficult. If there is no evidence of anterior gland hormone production, immunocytochemistry is unlikely to be of great help since both tumours can express cytokeratin, neuron specific enolase and chromogranin. The neurosecretory granules of either lesion can easily be confused ultrastructurally. A positive chromaffin reaction (if the fixative has contained chromate) or Gromelius stain may help identify paragangliomas if these rather fickle techniques can be made to work successfully. Otherwise reliance may have to be placed on the alveolar reticulin architecture typical of most paragangliomas.

Therapy and prognosis

Pituitary adenomas can be treated using surgery, radio-therapy, medical treatment or a combination of these. The types of drugs used in medical management and their effectiveness vary with different secretory subtypes of adenoma, and drug therapy is discussed in the individual sections which follow this account.

For most types of adenoma, surgery is now considered the primary treatment of choice,[95,96] with total excision as the aim wherever possible.[97] The development of trans-sphenoidal microsurgical techniques for selective adenectomy has advanced the treatment of micro-adenomas in particular, and in many cases offers the prospect of an immediate, permanent endocrine cure with preserved normal pituitary function.[45] For larger tumours, trans-sphenoidal surgery may still be indicated if the lesion is predominantly invading bone or air sinuses, but if there is a large suprasellar extension a transcranial approach is often necessary.[46] Total excision of invasive adenomas is often not possible using either technique, and many authorities favour limited surgery to relieve pressure symptoms in such cases, followed by radiotherapy.[98] Radiosurgery has been successfully used for surgically inaccessible tumours extending into the cavernous sinus and for small Cushing's disease adenomas,[99] but there is a high visual complication rate if it is used to treat to larger adenomas extending close to the chiasm.[100] In pituitary apoplexy, the acute threat to vision and even to life is such that emergency decompressive surgery, usually via a trans-sphenoidal route, is normally considered mandatory.[50]

A return of clinical signs and symptoms following surgery sometimes heralds a rapidly growing or frankly malignant adenoma, but it is more often the result of incomplete primary excision.[47] For microadenomas undergoing selective trans-sphenoidal surgery, the long-term recurrence rate for all types of adenoma taken together is usually quoted as between 5 and 7% of cases,[101,102] but recurrences virtually never occur in those instances where the tumour is positively identified at surgery and entirely removed.[97] The recurrence rate is rather higher for larger intrasellar adenomas approached trans-sphenoidally, especially when the tumour is tough or exceeds 2 cm in diameter.[103] Where only partial excision has been possible because of local invasion or significant suprasellar extension, local recurrences may be expected in up to 40% of cases in the longer term.[104] For such large and incompletely excised adenomas the recurrence rate is significantly reduced if postoperative radiation treatment is given.[105] An important long term complication in the treatment of pituitary adenomas is the development of endocrine deficiencies due to impairment of normal pituitary function. Long term pituitary deficiencies occur in less than one-fifth of cases undergoing trans-sphenoidal surgery without prior evidence of hypopituitism,[106] but where tumours are large enough to cause preoperative endocrine deficiencies, pituitary function deteriorates further after surgery in up to one-third of cases.[106] Radiotherapy, in distinction from radiosurgery, is also a particularly potent cause of delayed hypopituitism, and endocrine deficiencies have been reported in over half of irradiated cases in some long term follow-up studies.[107,108]

Pituitary adenomas: secretory subtypes

Growth hormone cell adenomas

Growth hormone secreting adenomas account for between 15 and 20% of all pituitary adenomas.[2,109] The relative sex incidence has either been reported as approximately equal or showing a slight predominance of males.[2,109] Although clinically regarded as a single tumour group, growth hormone secreting adenomas can be subdivided pathologically into sparsely granulated and densely granulated tumours (Table 16.3). In some series these have been almost equally common[2] while in others there has been a clear predominance of densely granulated lesions.[110] Occasionally both sparsely and densely granulated cells are found in the same tumour, suggesting cellular variation in the degree of hormone synthesis, secretion and storage, rather than origin from different precursor cells.[111] Immunoelectron microscopy has revealed alpha subunit in the same secretory granules as growth hormone in a significant proportion of otherwise typical growth hormone secreting tumours.[112,113] This finding has been supported by reports of raised serum alpha subunit levels in up to one-fifth of acromegalic patients[112] and indicates that many apparently dedicated growth hormone secreting adenomas may be more accurately classified as plurihormonal tumours. Approximately 40% of growth hormone cell adenomas have been shown to harbour activating mutations in the *GSPT1* oncogene, thought to produce autonomous proliferation due to unrestrained GHrh-like activity (see p. 467).[27]

Table 16.3 Growth hormone cell adenomas

	Sparsely granulated	Densely granulated
Clinical syndrome	Acromegaly or gigantism Tumour mass effects common	
Serology	Elevated growth hormone levels	
Tinctorial staining	Chromophobe	Acidophil
Immunocytochemistry	GH-positive, some cells Focal, paranuclear stain	GH-positive, most cells Uniform cytoplasmic stain
Electron microscopy	Pleomorphic nuclei Dispersed profiles RER Prominent Golgi body Sparse granules 100–300 nm diameter Paranuclear fibrous bodies	Uniform rounded nuclei Parallel stacks RER Prominent Golgi body Abundant granules 300–600 nm diameter

GH, growth hormone; RER, rough endoplasmic reticulum

Clinical features

The majority of growth hormone secreting adenomas present in the 30–50-year age group[2] and patients invariably display clinical evidence of acromegaly.[46] Men may also complain of impotence or loss of libido and a majority of premenopausal women will experience menstrual irregularity or amenorrhoea.[2] In the small proportion of cases presenting in adolescence, before closure of the epiphyseal plates, the clinical features are those of gigantism.[114] Over half of growth hormone secreting adenomas show suprasellar extension or local invasion by the time of presentation, and signs and symptoms of mass effect, including visual field defects, are a common finding.[56] Serum levels of growth hormone are invariably raised and are not correlated with the densely and sparsely granulated tumour types.[111]

Pathology

Histological features

Densely granulated growth hormone secreting tumours are typical acidophil adenomas, a majority of cells having strongly eosinophilic cytoplasm which is acidophilic using trichrome stains such as PAS-orange-green (Fig. 16.18). They mostly show a diffuse architectural pattern but can also be sinusoidal or trabecular in appearance. Nuclear pleomorphism is uncommon.

Sparsely granulated adenomas nearly always have a diffuse pattern and are more likely to show significant nuclear pleomorphism, including multinucleate cells. They are predominantly chromophobe tumours although very sparse acidophilic granules may be visible using trichrome stains. These stains may also show hyalinised, green cytoplasmic bodies indenting the cell nuclei, which are equivalent to the fibrous bodies visible ultrastructurally in these tumours.[2,115] Amyloid is present in a high proportion of growth hormone secreting tumours, either as sparse interstitial deposits or occasionally as large crystalline bodies.

Immunocytochemistry

In the densely granulated adenomas, most cells present show intense, pancytoplasmic immunocytochemical staining with antibodies to growth hormone[111] (Fig. 16.19). In sparsely granulated tumours, staining is usually evident in a smaller proportion of cells and is confined to a focal paranuclear area which is the site of the Golgi body[2,111] (Fig. 16.20). A significant proportion of otherwise typical growth hormone secreting adenomas also show immunocytochemical expression of alpha subunit, especially in cases where there are raised levels in the serum.[116]

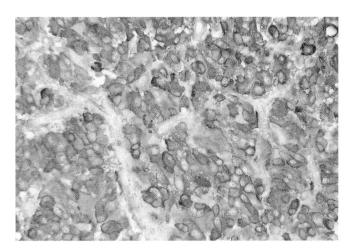

Fig. 16.19 **Densely granulated growth hormone cell adenoma.** There is dense, pancytoplasmic staining using immunocytochemistry for growth hormone.

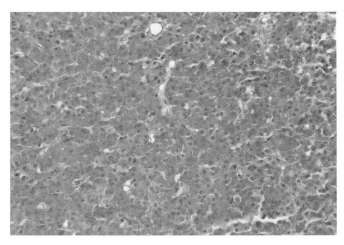

Fig. 16.18 **Densely granulated growth hormone cell ademona.** There is a diffuse architectural pattern and the cells are strongly acidophil. PAS-orange-green.

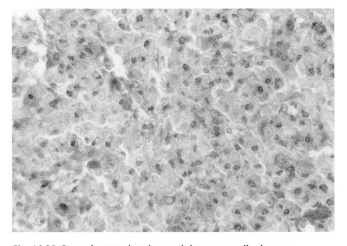

Fig. 16.20 **Sparsely granulated growth hormone cell adenoma.** Immunocytochemical staining for growth hormone is confined to focal, paranuclear areas of cell cytoplasm.

Electron microscopy

Densely granulated adenomas These consist of cells which are morphologically similar to normal anterior gland somatotrophs.[117,118] They have quite uniform features, with relatively abundant cytoplasm containing rough endoplasmic reticulum in well developed parallel stacks and a prominent Golgi body. The abundant secretory granules vary widely from less than 300 to over 600 nm in diameter, are electron dense and usually spherical in shape.

Sparsely granulated adenomas Compared to the densely granulated tumours, the cells in these adenomas have more pleomorphic nuclei and less abundant cytoplasm, with a greater tendency for the rough endoplasmic reticulum to be dispersed in short profiles.[118,119] The Golgi body is still well developed but is often indented or displaced by a globose, paranuclear accumulation of whorled microfilaments[117] (Fig. 16.21). These fibrous bodies are a characteristic hallmark of sparsely granulated growth hormone secreting adenomas and are found ultrastructurally in a high proportion of cells in most cases. They consist immunocytochemically of

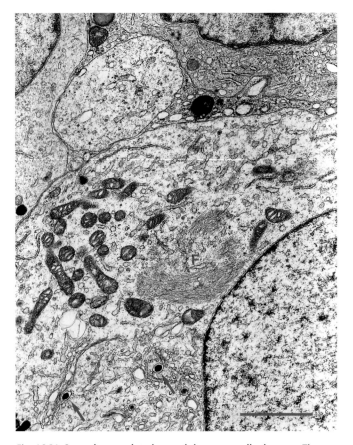

Fig. 16.21 Sparsely granulated growth hormone cell adenoma. The few secretory granules present are up to about 300 nm in diameter (arrows). This cell also contains a typical paranuclear bundle of microfilaments (F). Electron micrograph. Bar = 2 µm.

cytokeratin filaments.[120] The sparse, electron-dense, secretory granules are much smaller than in the densely granulated adenomas, usually measuring between 100 and 300 nm, and may be marginated.[118,119]

Therapy and prognosis

Surgical resection is the primary treatment of choice for most cases of growth hormone secreting adenoma, regardless of tumour size.[100,121] In large tumours where total resection is not possible, most authorities recommend postoperative radiotherapy.[98,122] Normalisation of serum growth hormone levels has been reported postoperatively in 65 to 80% of all intrasellar growth hormone secreting adenomas treated by trans-sphenoidal surgery,[121,123] and following selective microadenectomy a surgical cure may be expected in up to 90% of cases.[56] When tumour size or invasion precludes complete resection, normal serum growth hormone levels can still be achieved with radiotherapy in about 70% of cases.[121] In general, a better prognosis is associated with lower preoperative serum growth hormone levels and a densely granulated pattern of tumour.[122] Sparsely granulated growth hormone adenomas carry a poorer prognosis, since they are usually faster growing tumours which are more often large or invasive and have a higher tendency to recur postoperatively.[110] Trials of medical therapy with the dopamine agonists bromocriptine and pergolide have shown that only a small proportion of growth hormone secreting adenomas are endocrinologically responsive,[100,124] and radiological evidence of tumour shrinkage is exceptional even when a potent long-lasting agonist like cabergoline is used.[124,125] However, somatostatin analogues (e.g. octreotide) are much more effective at reducing serum growth hormone levels and may sometimes ameliorate the mass effects of larger tumours.[126] They have been used in presurgical preparatory therapy and also as an alternative to radiotherapy after surgery.[127]

Prolactin cell adenomas

Pituitary adenomas producing prolactin alone make up 30–40% of all adenomas.[2,128] Like growth hormone secreting adenomas, they can be subdivided pathologically into sparsely and densely granulated tumours, depending on the cellular dynamics of hormone production and secretion (Table 16.4). Densely granulated prolactinomas are rare and over 98% of cases have a sparsely granulated pattern.[2] Some cases of symptomatic prolactinoma are associated with prolactin cell hyperplasia in the adjacent anterior gland[42] but there is no evidence that this precedes neoplastic transformation or is the result of a primary hypothalamic or endocrine disturbance. Prolactinomas have been reported to develop in the presence of high circulating oestrogen levels in

Table 16.4 Prolactin cell adenomas

	Sparsely granulated	Densely granulated
Clinical syndrome	Premenopausal women: menstrual disturbance, galactorrhoea Postmenopausal women: mass effects only Men: infertility, loss of libido or mass effects only	
Serology	Prolactin levels raised, usually in excess of 150 ng/ml	
Tinctorial staining	Chromophobe	Acidophil
Immunocytochemistry	PRL-positive, some cells Focal, paranuclear stain	PRL-positive, most cells Uniform, dense staining
Electron microscopy	Uniform morphology Abundant stacks of RER Large Golgi body Numerous mitochondria Sparse granules 150–300 nm diameter Misplaced exocytosis	Pleomorphic nuclei Lamellar stacks RER Prominent Golgi body Abundant granules 200–1000 nm diameter, often pleomorphic

PRL, prolactin; RER, rough endoplasmic reticulum

animals[38] and vary rarely in man,[39] although long term use of the oral contraceptive pill does not appear to confer a greater risk of developing the tumour.[40]

Clinical features

Prolactinomas occur most commonly in young women, particularly in the 20–35-year age group.[118] The usual presenting features are primary or secondary amenorrhoea and infertility.[46,118] Spontaneous or expressible galactorrhoea is present in over two-thirds of such cases and weight gain is a common symptom.[129] In over half of these patients the tumours are microadenomas and there is no evidence of visual disturbance or other mass effect.[109] In postmenopausal women, however, the adenomas are mostly large and endocrinologically silent, presenting with the effects of local compression.[130] In adult males, the tumours are again usually macroadenomas[109] with a clinical presentation dominated by symptoms of mass effect.[131] In adolescent males, the presentation is typically that of delayed puberty and primary hypogonadism.[2] In either sex, serum prolactin levels are invariably raised and usually in excess of 150 ng/ml. Below that level, and especially below 100 ng/ml, the results need interpreting with care, since a similar rise can be produced non-specifically by any sellar or suprasellar mass lesion which compresses the pituitary stalk and interferes with delivery of prolactin inhibiting factor to the anterior gland.[46]

Pathology

Histological features

The sparsely granulated tumours have a diffuse or papillary pattern of cells and chromophobe properties on trichrome stains. Cystic change and calcospherites are commonly present and many cases show broad septa of hyalinised collagen (Fig. 16.22). Using Congo or sirius red stains, interstitial amyloid can be detected in a proportion of cases, and as in growth hormone adenomas it may occasionally take the form of large crystalline bodies.[132] The rare densely granulated prolactinomas are strongly acidophilic on trichrome staining.

Immunocytochemistry

In sparsely granulated prolactinomas, immunocytochemical staining with antibodies to prolactin is localised to a focal area near the nucleus which corresponds to the Golgi body[33] (Fig. 16.23). In densely granulated tumours, most cells present show heavy, pancytoplasmic staining.[133] Occasionally, tumours may be encountered with cells sharing both these staining patterns, supporting the concept that the differences between them are due to differing dynamics of hormone secretion and storage.[124] As with growth hormone secreting adenomas, a significant proportion of otherwise typical prolactinomas have been found to express alpha subunit, sometimes in association with raised serum levels[116] and these tumours should perhaps be more accurately classified as plurihormonal adenomas. The sparsely granulated prolactinomas are histologically, immunohistochemically and often endocrinologically indistinguishable from acidophil stem cell adenomas and electron microscopy is needed to exclude this diagnosis.

Electron microscopy

Sparsely granulated prolactinomas The cells are large, closely apposed and of fairly uniform morphology.[133,134] There is abundant rough endoplasmic reticulum, mostly in the form of parallel stacks or concentric whorls

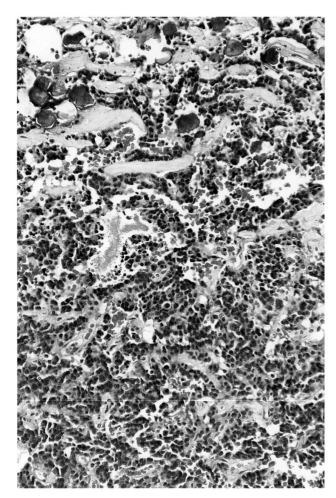

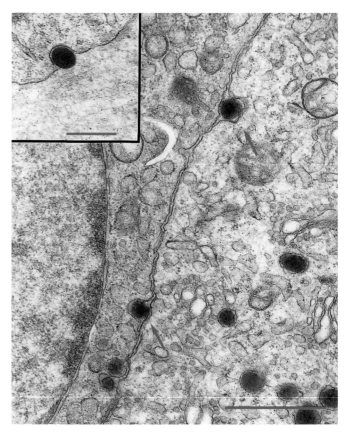

Fig. 16.24 Sparsely granulated prolactin cell adenoma. In misplaced exocytosis, secretory granules are extruded through the lateral aspects of cell membranes and become lodged between the closely apposed cell bodies (arrows). Electron Micrograph. Bar = 1 μm. Inset: In normal exocytosis, secretory granules are extruded apically into free extracellular space. Bar = 0.5 μm.

Fig. 16.22 Sparsely granulated prolactin cell adenoma. Sheets of cells are interspersed by septa of hyalinised collagen. Calcospherites are visible towards the top of the field. H & E.

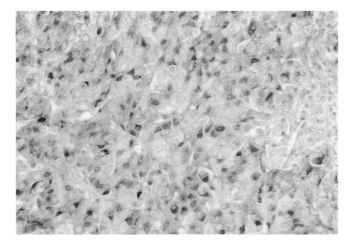

Fig. 16.23 Sparsely granulated prolactin cell adenoma. Immunocytochemical staining for prolactin is confined to focal, paranuclear areas of cell cytoplasm, corresponding to the sites of Golgi bodies.

(Nebenkern). The Golgi body is well developed and may occupy a considerable area of cytoplasm. Mitochondria are often numerous and oncocytic change may be seen in some cases.[135] The sparse secretory granules are electron dense, spherical or pleomorphic and mostly between 150 and 300 nm in diameter. The ultrastructural hallmark of sparsely granulated prolactinoma cells is misplaced exocytosis,[136] in which granules are extruded through the lateral rather than the apical aspects of the cell membranes and become lodged between adjacent cells (Fig. 16.24). Amyloid is visible ultrastructurally as compact bundles of typical 10–13 nm diameter fibrils, either within tumour cell cytoplasm or in the extracellular space[137] (Fig. 16.25).

Densely granulated prolactinomas The cells in these tumours are ultrastructurally similar to the prolactin secreting cells in the normal anterior gland.[118,133] Their nuclei are pleomorphic in outline and the abundant cytoplasm contains prominent lamellar stacks of rough endoplasmic reticulum. The Golgi body is well developed and there are numerous electron-dense, rather pleomorphic secretory granules. These vary greatly in size and can be anything from 200 to over 1000 nm in diameter.

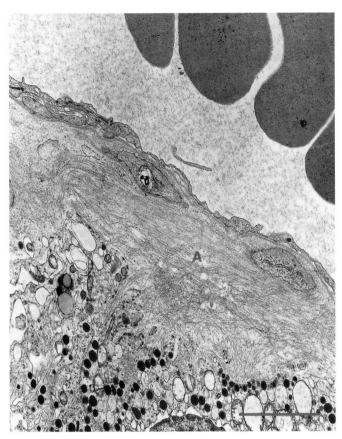

Fig. 16.25 **Sparsely granulated prolactin cell adenoma.** Amyloid is visible as bundles of 10–13 nm diameter fibrils (A) in the extracellular space around a capillary vessel. Electron micrograph. Bar = 3 μm.

Pathological effects of dopamine agonist therapy

The microscopic changes in prolactinomas after treatment with dopamine agonists such as bromocriptine are of interest because of the radiological evidence of tumour shrinkage which occurs in these tumours. After short term therapy, the pathological changes appear to represent a reversible involution of tumour cells, and include decreased intensity of cell staining with antibodies to prolactin and a decrease in the measured areas of cell cytoplasm, nucleus and nucleolus.[138,139] Electron microscopy shows a diminution in the amount of rough endoplasmic reticulum and Golgi profiles relative to cytoplasmic volume, but an increase in the number of secretory granules.[139] After longer periods of therapy, there is an increase in stromal fibrous tissue, which is initially perivascular in distribution.[140] Eventually more severe degenerative changes supervene, with islands of tumour cells enclosed by larger areas of hyalinised collagen and individual tumour cell necrosis[141] (Fig. 16.26). Such changes are clearly not reversible and have not been found to any significant degree in non-functioning or growth hormone secreting tumours undergoing similar treatment.[140,142]

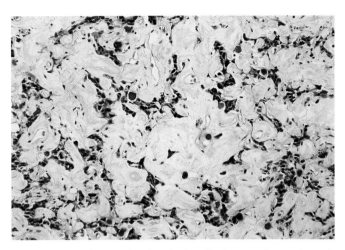

Fig. 16.26 **Sparsely granulated prolactin cell adenoma after prolonged bromocriptine therapy.** There is a marked increase in hyalanised stromal collagen, which encloses islands of residual tumour cells (compare Fig. 16.22). H & E.

Therapy and prognosis

Dopamine agonists such as cabergoline and bromocriptine are very effective in normalising serum prolactin levels and relieving endocrinological symptoms in a majority of prolactinomas.[125,143] There is significant shrinkage of the tumour mass in most macroadenomas and complete resolution of radiological abnormality in over two-thirds of microprolactinomas, often persisting some time after drug withdrawal.[125] In the longer term, however, the beneficial effects of these agents are dependent on continued treatment in all but a small proportion of patients. Even after treating for several years, stopping drug therapy is eventually associated with a renewed rise in prolactin levels and return of symptoms in a majority of cases.[144,145] As a result, surgery is still favoured as the definitive treatment for most prolactinomas, and particularly for microadenomas amenable to selective transsphenoidal adenectomy.[95] For larger tumours producing symptoms of mass effect, surgery can often be facilitated by using preoperative dopamine agonist therapy to reduce the tumour size.[46]

Following apparently total removal of smaller, intrasellar prolactinomas, an initial clinical cure has been reported in up to 80% of cases,[146,147] but for larger, extrasellar tumours the reported cure rate has usually been 50% or less.[148,149] Where there is invasive behaviour, a surgical cure can only be expected in a small minority of patients.[149] Long term follow-up studies have shown that even in cases apparently cured by successful surgical resection, one-sixth to one-third may be expected to show endocrinological and sometimes radiological evidence of tumour recurrence between 1 and 5 years postoperatively.[95,150] There is some evidence that postoperative radiotherapy may improve the long term prognosis,[151]

Table 16.5 Mixed prolactin cell and growth hormone cell adenomas

Clinical syndrome	Acromegaly or gigantism in all cases May be menstrual disturbance or diminished libido
Serology	Raised growth hormone and prolactin levels
Tinctorial staining	Variable mixture of acidophil and chromophobe cells
Immunocytochemistry	Variable mixture of GH-positive and PRL-positive cells Either may be diffuse or focal-paranuclear in staining pattern
Electron microscopy	Any combination of sparsely or densely granulated prolactin or growth hormone cells. The cell populations are morphologically distinct

GH, growth hormone; PRL, prolactin

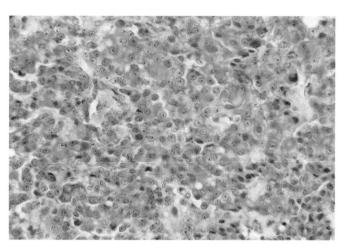

Fig. 16.27 Mixed sparsely granulated prolactin cell and densely granulated growth hormone cell adenoma. Trichrome staining shows a mixed population of chromophobe and acidophil cells. PAS-orange-green.

although radiation treatment is associated with a high incidence of delayed pituitary insufficiency.[152] Apart from tumour size, factors which have been linked with a better surgical outcome include lower preoperative serum prolactin levels, age below the mid-20s and a shorter duration of symptoms.[153] Prolactinomas show a wide variation in natural growth rate, however, and there are no pathological features which will predict the biological behaviour of the tumour.

Mixed prolactin cell and growth hormone cell adenomas

These are bimorphous tumours secreting growth hormone and prolactin from two separate populations of cells, either of which may be of sparsely or densely granulated type (Table 16.5). Although there are now arguments for including these tumours in the rapidly expanding group of plurihormonal tumours (see below) they are a relatively common and well circumscribed entity compared to other plurihormonal adenomas, and are usually classified separately. In most series, these lesions account for between 4 and 5% of all adenomas[2,128] and they are distributed approximately evenly between the sexes.[2]

Clinical features

All adult cases of combined growth hormone and prolactin secreting tumours have clinical changes of acromegaly, whilst those with onset of symptoms before the end of puberty usually show gigantism.[154,155] Serum levels of both growth hormone and prolactin are invariably raised[154,155] but the clinical effects of hyperprolactinaemia are not always evident.[154]

Pathology

Histological features

The tumour architecture is usually of diffuse pattern, although there may also be a sinusoidal arrangement. Trichrome stains most often show an obvious mixture of chromophobe and acidophilic cells (Fig. 16.27), but in some cases the vast majority of cells present can be of one or other tinctorial type. On clinical and histological grounds alone it is not possible to exclude a pure growth hormone secreting adenoma producing hyperprolactinaemia secondary to stalk compression, and immunocytochemistry is needed to make this distinction.

Immunocytochemistry

Immuncytochemistry shows a mixture of growth hormone and prolactin immunoreactive cells in variable proportions[154,155] (Fig. 16.28). In either case the staining may be heavy and pancytoplasmic (densely granulated), or focal and paranuclear in location (sparsely granulated).[2] Unless double labelling studies are undertaken, however, it can be difficult to be sure that the two hormones are expressed by separate populations of cells, and electron microscopy may be needed to exclude monomorphic types of growth hormone and prolactin producing tumours, i.e. acidophil stem adenoma and mammosomatotroph adenoma.

Electron microscopy

The two main populations of cells are ultrastructurally identical to the sparsely and densely granulated cells found in prolactinomas and growth hormone secreting adenomas[154,155] (Fig. 16.29). Any combination is possible, although a mixture of densely granulated growth hor-

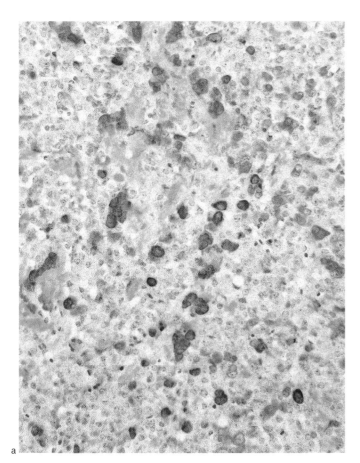

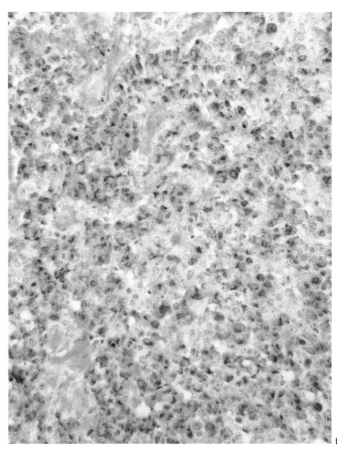

a   b

Fig. 16.28 **Mixed prolactin cell and growth hormone cell adenoma.** Adjacent sections of the same area of tumour show **(a)** Densely granulated growth hormone cells using immunocytochemistry for growth hormone and **(b)** Sparsely granulated prolactin cells using immunocytochemistry for prolactin.

mone cells and densely granulated prolactin cells has been least often reported.[118] Where one or both of the sparsely granulated cell types are present, these can be identified by the fibrous bodies typical of sparsely granulated growth hormone cells and/or the presence of misplaced exocytosis indicating sparsely granulated prolactin cells.[117] In contrast to acidophil stem cell adenomas and mammosomatotroph adenomas, the cell populations are always ultrastructurally distinct, and cells with combined features of growth hormone and prolactin production are not found.[154]

Therapy and prognosis

Surgery is usually the primary treatment of choice, with selective trans-sphenoidal adenectomy of small tumours and partial removal followed by radiotherapy where the lesions are very large or invasive. Dopamine agonists are very effective for short term control of endocrine symptoms and preoperative tumour shrinkage to facilitate surgery.[2] They are also more efficient at reducing serum growth hormone levels than is the case with pure growth hormone secreting tumours.[2,156] Prognostically, there is

nothing to suggest that these mixed adenomas have any particular tendency to be either slower growing or more aggressive than pure prolactinomas or pure growth hormone secreting tumours.

Acidophil stem cell adenomas

Acidophil stem cell adenomas are immature and rapidly growing monomorphic tumours capable of both growth hormone and prolactin production[22,157] (Table 16.6). Electron microscopy shows features suggesting synthesis of both hormones within the same cells,[157] and they are thought to be derived from a committed but shared precursor of anterior gland prolactin cells and somatotrophs.[22] Acidophil stem cell adenomas are quite rare tumours, constituting something between 2.5 and 4.5% of all pituitary adenomas.[2,157] They occur most frequently in younger adults and are uncommon over the age of 50 years.[22,157] Distribution between the sexes is about equal, but the average age of presentation in females is significantly younger than for males, with quoted means of mid-fourth decade for women and late fifth decade for men.[157]

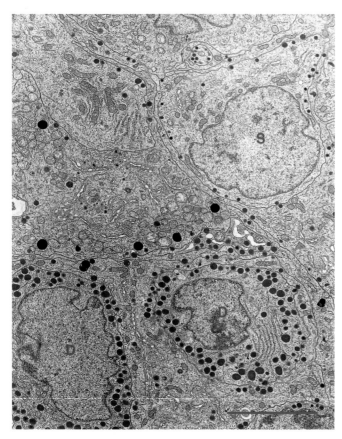

Fig. 16.29 **Mixed prolactin cell and growth hormone cell adenoma.** The tumour consists of ultrastructurally distinct populations of densely granulated growth hormone cells (D) and sparsely granulated prolactin cells (S). Electron micrograph. Bar = 5 μm.

Table 16.6 Acidophil stem cell adenomas

Clinical syndrome	Usually clinical manifestations of hyperprolactinaemia Acromegaly rarely Tumour mass effects common
Serology	Moderate elevation of prolactin levels Growth hormone raised only in a minority
Tinctorial staining	Chromophobe or faintly acidophil
Immunocytochemistry	PRL-positive. Diffuse or focal, paranuclear stain Variable GH-positive cells some cases only
Electron microscopy	Monomorphic, irregular cells Dispersed RER. Free ribosomes Small Golgi body Variable oncocytic change, maybe giant or ballooned mitochondria Sparse secretory granules 50–300 nm diameter Fibrous bodies and misplaced exocytosis, can occur in the same cells

GH, growth hormone; PRL, prolactin; RER, rough endoplasmic reticulum

Clinical features

A majority of cases present with clinical evidence of hyperprolactinaemia, and changes of acromegaly are rare.[22,157] Visual field defects and other results of local tumour compression are often present, since the lesions are usually large by the time of presentation.[22] Most show suprasellar extension or bony erosion of the fossa floor when first investigated, with involvement of the nasopharynx or sphenoid sinus in approximately 50% of cases.[157] Serum prolactin levels are usually raised, but less markedly so than with prolactinomas.[22,157] Elevation of growth hormone levels is only detected in a minority of cases.[22,157]

Pathology

Histological features

Histologically, the tumours consist of diffuse sheets of cells lacking any particular architectural features. Using trichrome stains the cell cytoplasm usually has chromophobe characteristics, although at high magnification very sparse acidophilic granules may be visible in some cases. In a proportion of cases, some of the cells show prominent, large cytoplasmic vacuoles (Fig. 16.30), which are thought to be derived from swollen giant mitochondria.[157]

Immunocytochemistry

Immunoreactivity with antibodies to prolactin is present in every case, though not in all cells present (Fig. 16.31a). The staining pattern may be pancytoplasmic or confined to a focal paranuclear area, as in sparsely granulated prolactinomas.[22] Staining with antibodies to growth hormone is very variable and may be entirely absent in

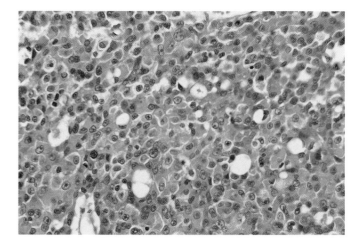

Fig. 16.30 **Acidophil stem cell adenoma.** The tumour cells have rounded vesicular nuclei and are arranged in diffuse sheets. Some of the cells present are distorted by large cytoplasmic vacuoles, thought to be derived from ballooned mitochondria. H & E.

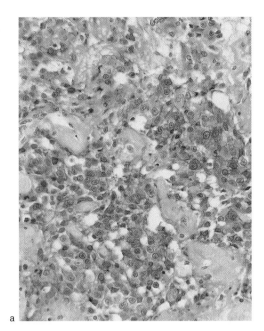
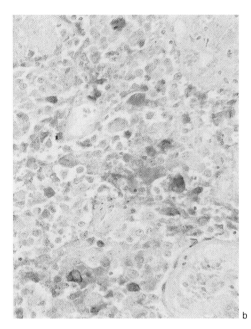

a
b

Fig. 16.31 **Acidophil stem cell adenoma. (a)** Many cells show diffuse cytoplasmic staining using immunocytochemistry for prolactin. **(b)** An adjacent section of the same area of tumour shows fewer, more faintly stained cells using immunocytochemistry for growth hormone.

some cases.[157] Where growth hormone reactivity is present, fewer cells are usually stained than with prolactin antibodies and with a less dense precipitate[22] (Fig. 16.31b). Where no growth hormone immunoreactivity is found, these tumours cannot be reliably distinguished from prolactinomas without electron microscopy, and even where growth hormone is detected, ultrastructural study is necessary to exclude mixed growth hormone cell and prolactin cell adenomas.

Electron microscopy

The tumour cells are monomorphic but immature in appearance with numerous free ribosomes.[22,157] There is commonly a degree of oncocytic change, with accumulation of deformed mitochondria. These often show loss of cristae and may contain tubular structures similar to distorted centrioles.[22] In some cases, massively ballooned mitochondria may be present, recognisable only by the double leaflets of their limiting membranes.[157] Secretory granules are sparse, mostly marginated and small, mostly measuring between 50 and 300 nm in diameter (Fig. 16.32). Fibrous cytoplasmic bodies, like those seen in sparsely granulated growth hormone adenoma cells, and misplaced exocytosis, typical of prolactin secretion, are both invariably present. These two features often occur together in the same cells, a phenomenon which is considered pathognomonic of acidophil stem cell adenomas.

Therapy and prognosis

Complete surgical resection is often not possible because acidophil stem cell adenomas are usually large and

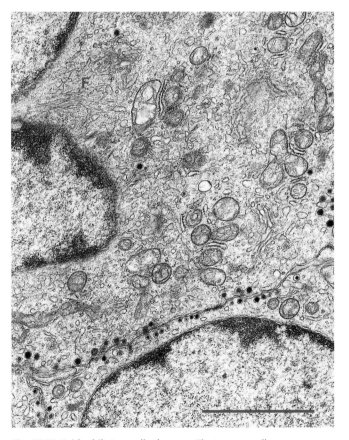

Fig. 16.32 **Acidophil stem cell adenoma.** The tumour cells are monomorphic and contain numerous, pleomorphic mitochondria. Sparse, small secretory granules are mostly marginated and examples of misplaced exocytosis can be found at high magnification. Fibrous cytoplasmic bodies are also a constant feature (F). Electron micrograph. Bar = 2 μm.

Table 16.7 Mammosomatotroph cell adenomas

Clinical syndrome	Acromegaly or gigantism
Serology	Elevated growth hormone levels PRL normal or mildly elevated
Tinctorial staining	Acidophilic
Immunocytochemistry	Variable degree of GH-positivity and PRL-positivity often within the same cells

Electron microscopy	Monomorphic. Large cells, uniform
	  nuclei
	Well developed stacks of RER
	Large Golgi body
	Abundant granules 100 → > 1000 nm
	  diameter, may appear as two
	  populations
	Whorled fibrous bodies in some cases
	Polymorphous exocytosis, with persisting,
	  discrete extracellular deposits

GH, growth hormone; PRL, prolactin; RER, rough endoplasmic reticulum

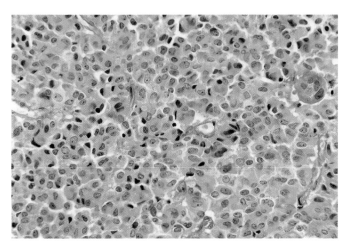

Fig. 16.33 **Mammosomatotroph adenoma.** There is a diffuse architectural pattern and the tumour cells have acidophilic cytoplasm. Orange-fuschin-green.

invasive tumours by the time of first presentation,[2] and postoperative radiotherapy is advisable in view of their aggressive biological behaviour. There is little information on long term prognosis, but the outlook must be guarded because of the rapid growth rate and likelihood of residual tumour.[157]

Mammosomatotroph cell adenomas

These are monomorphous tumours composed of cells which synthesise both prolactin and growth hormone[23,158] (Table 16.7). In contrast to acidophil stem cell adenomas they are well differentiated, slow growing tumours in which production of growth hormone predominates both clinically and immunocytochemically. Non-neoplastic mammosomatotroph cells are known to occur in the normal human anterior pituitary gland and are presumed to give rise to this type of adenoma.[2] Mammosomatotroph cell adenomas are very rare tumours and account for only about 1.5% of all pituitary adenomas.[2,158] They nearly always affect males, with a mean age of presentation in the mid-fifth decade.[158]

Clinical features

The clinical presentation is almost invariably one of acromegaly, often without visual impairment or other evidence of mass effect.[158,159] Gigantism has been described in one case with a clinical history dating back to excessive growth in childhood.[160] Serum growth hormone levels are always significantly raised, but prolactin levels are often within the normal range or only slightly elevated and there is usually no symptomatic evidence of hyperprolactinaemia.[158]

Pathology

Histological features

The histological appearance is very similar to that of densely granulated growth hormone cell adenomas, with acidophilic tumour cell cytoplasm and a diffuse architectural pattern[158] (Fig. 16.33). Immunocytochemistry is necessary to make the distinction between these two adenoma types.

Immunocytochemistry

There is strong immunoreactivity with antibodies to both prolactin and growth hormone (Fig. 16.34), and double labelling studies show that a majority of tumour cells contain both hormones.[23,158] In contrast to acidophil stem cell adenomas, staining with growth hormone antibodies is often more prominent than with prolactin antibodies. Unless electron microscopy or double labelling studies are undertaken, however, mammosomatotroph adenomas may be difficult to distinguish from other types of mixed growth hormone and prolactin secreting adenoma.

Electron microscopy

Mammosomatotroph cell adenomas are ultrastructurally monomorphous tumours which show some similarities with densely granulated growth hormone cell adenomas.[158,160] The cells are large and uniform, with electron lucent cytoplasm containing well developed stacks of rough endoplasmic reticulum, a large Golgi body and abundant secretory granules of widely varying size. It has been suggested that the latter fall into two populations: spherical, electron-dense, growth hormone-like granules mostly between 100 and 400 nm in diameter, and larger, more pleomorphic, prolactin-type

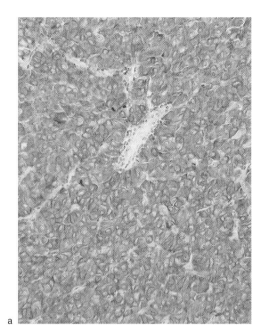
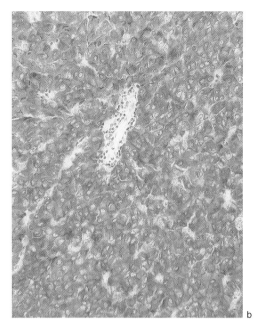

a   b

Fig. 16.34 **Mammosomatotroph adenoma.** Adjacent sections from the same area of tumour show an identical staining pattern using immunocytochemistry for **(a)** prolactin and **(b)** growth hormone.

granules with an irregular core and diameters which may be over 1000 nm.[158] Double labelling immunoelectron-microscopy techniques, however, have suggested that at least some granules contain both hormones.[159,160] Whorled, paranuclear fibrous bodies similar to those seen in sparsely granulated growth hormone cell adenomas are present in some cases.[158] Granule exocytosis is also a prominent feature of mammosomatotroph cell adenomas and may be misplaced between closely apposed cells.[160] In contrast to other prolactin synthesising adenomas, however, the extruded granules retain their density and compactness, even when in unrestricted extracellular space.[158] This has been considered a specific ultrastructural hallmark of mammosomatotroph adenomas.[2,158]

Therapy and prognosis

Total and selective trans-sphenoidal excision is the ideal and definitive treatment. At present, there is no information on the susceptibility of these adenomas to medical agents such as dopamine agonists. Mammosomatotroph adenomas are slow growing, well differentiated tumours which may be expected to have a good longer term outlook, especially if completely excised.[158]

Corticotroph cell adenomas

Functioning corticotroph adenomas

These are pituitary adenomas secreting ACTH either in the context of Nelson syndrome or as a cause of Cushing's disease (Table 16.8). Together, they have been estimated as comprising anything from 8 to 17% of all pituitary adenomas, the differences presumably reflecting referral practice.[2,109] Cushing's disease adenomas present most commonly in young adult life, with a mean age in the mid-fourth decade, and are very much more common in women than men.[109] Corticotroph adenomas are only rarely reported in patients with Addison's disease[37] and it seems unlikely that they are simply the direct result of prolonged hypocorticism. Nevertheless, corticotroph hyperplasia has been found in the anterior gland adjacent to some functioning corticotroph adenomas,[41,42] and occasional cases of Cushing's disease may be due to primary hyperplasia without adenoma formation.[72] The relationship between adenoma, hyperplasia and hypothalamic function remains rather unclear, but there is some in vitro evidence that even true adenoma cells may not be entirely autonomous of hypothalamic regulatory changes.[161] In Nelson syndrome, a pre-existing ACTH-secreting micro-adenoma is assumed to have been the cause of Cushing syndrome treated by bilateral adrenalectomy. The abrupt fall in circulating cortisol levels leads to failure of inhibitory feedback mechanisms and rapid growth of the adenoma.[2]

Clinical features

Pituitary dependent Cushing syndrome (i.e. Cushing's disease) is clinically similar to the syndromes resulting from primary adrenal gland hypersecretion or ectopic ACTH production.[2] The majority of Cushing's disease adenomas are microadenomas, and signs or symptoms relating to extrasellar extension are uncommon.[109,162] Pituitary dependence of the raised serum cortisol levels

Table 16.8 Functioning corticotroph cell adenomas

	Sparsely granulated	Densely granulated
Clinical syndrome	Cushing's disease	Cushing's disease
		Nelson syndrome
Serology	Cushing's: Raised cortisol, raised ACTH	
	Nelson: Raised ACTH, raised MSH	
Tinctorial staining	Chromophobe	Basophilic
Immunocytochemistry	Faintly ACTH-positive, some cells only	Strongly ACTH-positive
		May be endorphin, MSH or lipotrophin-positive
Electron microscopy	Less well differentiated cells, fewer organelles	Large cells, rounded nuclei
	Sparse, small granules	Parallel stacks RER
	Inconspicuous filaments	Prominent Golgi body
		Abundant granules, variable shape and density, 200–500 nm diameter
		Bundles of intermediate filaments

ACTH, adrenocorticotropic hormone; MSH, melanocyte stimulating hormone; RER, rough endoplasmic reticulum.

can be confirmed by the dexamethasone suppression test or raised serum levels of metyrapone. Raised serum ACTH levels will exclude primary adrenal disease but not the presence of an unsuspected ectopic ACTH secreting tumour.[46] In Nelson syndrome, bilateral adrenalectomy for Cushing syndrome is followed by hyperpigmentation, without return of Cushingoid features. In addition, there are usually visual disturbances or other mass effects of a rapidly enlarging pituitary tumour.[46] ACTH levels are abnormally raised but cortisol levels are dependent on therapeutic replacement.

Pathology

Histological features

The vast majority of functioning corticotroph adenomas are well differentiated, densely granulated tumours, which usually show a sinusoidal architectural pattern and are strongly basophilic when stained with trichrome combinations containing PAS or fuschin (Fig. 16.35). In Nelson syndrome, the adenoma cells tend to be even more densely granulated and basophilic than those in Cushing's disease. A very small minority of Cushing's disease adenomas are sparsely granulated, chromophobe tumours, usually showing a diffuse rather than a sinusoidal pattern. Crooke's hyaline change is a degenerative change of anterior gland corticotroph cells which occurs either in the presence of a functioning corticotroph adenoma or as a result of persistently raised serum cortisol levels of other aetiology.[163] Using trichrome stains it is visible as progressive cytoplasmic degranulation together with the development of a large paranuclear vacuole (Fig. 16.36). End-stage cells show only a thin marginal rim or perinuclear cluster of basophilic granules, the majority of the cytoplasm being replaced by green-

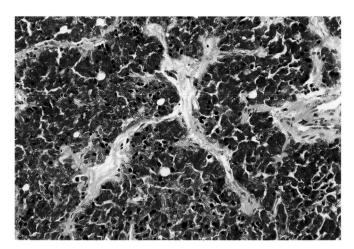

Fig. 16.35 **Densely granulated functioning corticotroph adenoma.** There is a prominent sinusoidal pattern and the tumour cells are strongly basophilic on trichrome staining. Orange-fuschin-green.

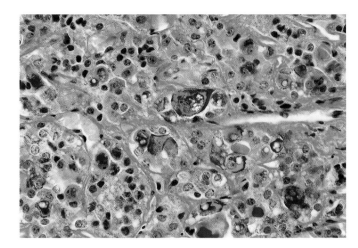

Fig. 16.36 **Crooke's hyaline change.** Anterior gland. Basophil cells (centre) show degranulation, vacuolation and green-staining, hyalinised cytoplasm. Orange-fuschin-green.

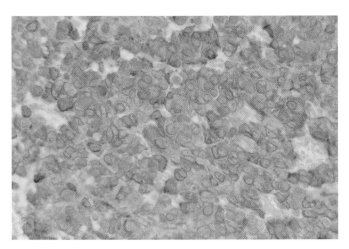

Fig. 16.37 **Densely granulated, functioning corticotroph adenoma.** The majority of tumour cells show strong uniform cytoplasmic staining using immunocytochemistry for ACTH.

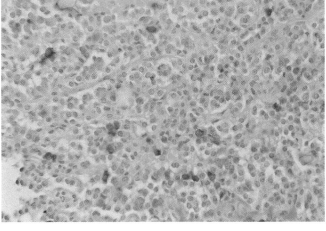

Fig. 16.38 **Sparsely granulated, functioning corticotroph adenoma.** There is faint staining in only a few cells using immunocytochemistry for ACTH (compare Fig. 16.37).

staining hyaline material. Exceptionally, a similar change has been observed in the tumour cells of functioning corticotroph adenomas.[164]

Immunocytochemistry

In Nelson syndrome tumours and densely granulated Cushing's disease adenomas, a majority of cells show strong, uniform cytoplasmic staining with antibodies to ACTH (Fig. 16.37), especially when using reagents active towards the C-terminal portion of the molecule.[2] In many of these tumours, positive-staining cells may also be found using antibodies to related neuropeptides, including beta-endorphin, beta-lipotropin and alpha or beta melano-cyte stimulating humone (MSH).[165,166] The sparsely granulated variant of functioning corticotroph adenomas shows rather faint staining with ACTH antibodies in only a small proportion of cells present[2] (Fig. 16.38). Immuno-cytochemistry has shown that the cytoplasmic hyaline material of Crooke's hyaline change is an accumulation of cytokeratin filaments.[167]

Electron microscopy

The cells of densely granulated Cushing's disease adenomas are well differentiated and ultrastructurally similar to normal anterior gland corticotrophs.[116,119] The numerous secretory granules are of variable shape and electron density, and may be anything between 200 and over 500 nm in diameter. Granule extrusion or exocytosis is not seen.[168] A characteristic ultrastructural feature of Cushing's adenomas is the presence of prominent, large bundles of 7–10 nm diameter cytoplasmic cytokeratin filaments. In anterior gland corticotroph cells affected by Crooke's hyaline change, similar filaments are massively accumulated together with lipofuscin bodies, and may fill the entire cytoplasm[169] (Fig. 16.39). In Nelson syndrome

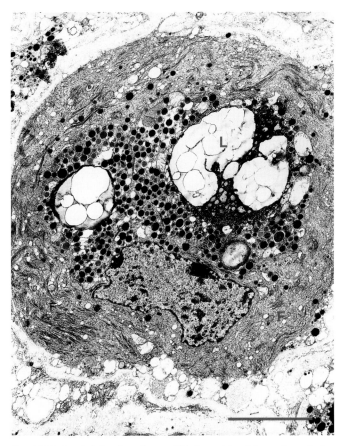

Fig. 16.39 **Crooke's hyaline change.** This basophil cell from the anterior gland adjacent to a corticotroph adenoma shows typical cytoplasmic accumulation of filamentous material (F) and vacuolated lipofuscin bodies (L). Electron micrograph. Bar = 4 µm.

tumours, the ultrastructural features are usually similar to those of Cushing's disease, but the cells tend to be more evenly and densely granulated, and bundles of cytokeratin filaments are sparse or absent.[119] Sparsely granulated

Cushing's adenomas have relatively poorly differentiated cells, with few organelles, sparse small secretory granules and inconspicuous cytoplasmic filaments.[2]

Therapy and prognosis

Selective trans-sphenoidal adenectomy is usually the treatment of choice for typical Cushing's micro-adenomas.[98,170] Where no tumour is found at surgery, or microadenectomy fails to produce an endocrinological cure, anterior gland corticotroph cell hyperplasia must be suspected, and either exenteration or irradiation of the fossa may be needed.[41,72] For larger corticotroph adenomas, especially the invasive lesions associated with Nelson syndrome, total removal may not be possible and postoperative radiotherapy has again been recommended.[98,171] Dopamine agonists, serotonin antagonists[172] and sodium valproate[173] have all been shown to reduce serum ACTH levels in Cushing's disease, but the need for indefinite treatment makes them unsuitable except as temporary, symptomatic measures.[172]

An initially successful outcome from surgery may be expected in up to 90% of patients with typical Cushing's microadenomas but in only about half that number of larger tumours with extrasellar extension.[109,170] Sparsely granulated Cushing's adenomas and Nelson syndrome tumours are usually more rapidly growing, invasive lesions and thus carry a correspondingly poorer prognosis.[2,171] Delayed tumour recurrence months or years after an initial surgical cure is a well documented phenomenon in Cushing's disease treated by trans-sphenoidal adenectomy.[174] It has been reported to occur in about 10% of all cases within 5 years of surgery[175] and is much more likely when the original tumours were large or invasive in nature.[170]

Non-functioning corticotroph adenomas

Very rarely, adenomas with immunocytochemical evidence of ACTH or endorphin synthesis can present as mass lesions without clinical evidence of Cushing's disease.[176,177] Reported cases account for about 6% of all pituitary adenomas and have occurred in a wide age range of patients but predominantly in women.[2,177] They appear to be a pathologically heterogeneous group of adenomas and have been divided into three subtypes on the bases of their immunocytochemical and electron microscopic features[2,177] (Table 16.9). Synthesis of abnormal forms of ACTH or defective granule release may account for the lack of clinical endocrinological response to the tumour.[176,178] However, some examples appear to have a latent capacity to convert to functioning tumours, with signs and symptoms of Cushing's disease developing later in the clinical course.[179,180]

Table 16.9 Non-functioning corticotroph cell adenomas

Clinical syndrome	Tumour mass effect only
Serology	No elevation of cortisol or ACTH levels
Tinctorial staining	Basophilic or chromophobe
Immunocytochemistry	ACTH positivity may be strong, variable or absent
Electron microscopy	May be (i) Identical to densely granulated functioning ACTH adenomas (ii) Less well differentiated with scanty organelles, irregular granules and no cytoplasmic filaments (iii) Large, pleomorphic cells with abundant organelles and filaments, but sparse, small granules

ACTH, adrenocorticotropic hormone.

Clinical features

Patients are eucorticoid and usually present with headaches, visual field disturbances or other mass effects of large, non-functioning adenoma.[176,179] Some cases may also have a history of loss of libido or other symptoms of raised serum prolactin due to stalk compression syndrome.[3] Serum levels of ACTH and cortisol are not elevated. An unusually high rate of acute tumour infarction and pituitary apoplexy has been reported in these tumours.[177]

Pathology

Histology and immunocytochemistry

Subtype 1 adenomas are strongly basophilic tumours of sinusoidal pattern which are heavily stained with antibodies to ACTH and are indistinguishable from Cushing's disease adenomas by light microscopy.[176,177] The remaining tumours are mostly of diffuse pattern and have chromophobe tinctorial characteristics using trichrome stains.[177] Those of subtype 2 show variable immunoreactivity for ACTH, whilst a third group shows weak or absent staining but may react with antibodies to alpha- or beta-endorphin.[2]

Electron microscopy

The basophilic adenomas are ultrastructurally similar to functioning densely granulated corticotroph adenomas, but may show prominent autophagic changes and accumulation of lysosomes.[176,177] The chromophobe but ACTH-expressing tumours differ in having less well developed cytoplasmic organelles, absent microfilaments, and secretory granules which are irregular or tear-drop in shape.[2] The third group of tumours consist

Table 16.10 Thyrotroph cell adenomas

Clinical syndrome	Usually hyperthyroidism and tumour mass effect
	May be tumour mass effect only, in longstanding primary hypothyroidism
Serology	Elevated serum TSH
	Raised T3 and T4 if clinically hyperthyroid
Tinctorial staining	Chromophobe
Immunocytochemistry	Beta TSH-positive, often focal staining
Electron microscopy	Small cells with cytoplasmic processes
	Well developed RER and Golgi body. Microtubules
	Sparse granules, often in processes, 100–200 nm diameter
	May also be poorly differentiated cells with sparse organelles

RER, rough endoplasmic reticulum; TSH, thyroid stimulating hormone.

Fig. 16.40 **Thyrotroph cell adenoma.** The results of immunostaining are frequently patchy and inconsistent, even when specific monoclonal reagents are used. Immunocytochemistry for beta-TSH.

of cells which are pleomorphic and mostly well differentiated but contain only sparse, small secretory granules less than 200 nm in diameter.[2]

Therapy and prognosis

Most cases present with visual disturbance due to large suprasellar extensions and require craniotomy for decompressive surgery. In many instances emergency surgical intervention is needed because of pituitary apoplexy.[177] In general, these tumours appear to have a rather poor prognosis because of their relatively large size at presentation and a tendency to rapid growth and recurrence.[177,178]

Thyrotroph cell adenomas

Thyrotroph cell adenomas are the rarest of all pituitary adenomas, making up barely 1% of the total[181,182] (Table 16.10). Most become symptomatic in middle life and there appears to be an approximately even distribution between the sexes.[182] A minority of patients have a history of longstanding hypothyroidism, and loss of negative feedback on the hypothalamus appears to play an important role in adenoma formation in these cases.[36,183]

Clinical features

The typical presentation is one of primary hyperthyroidism, usually with a diffuse thyroid goitre.[184,185] The pituitary tumours are often large in these patients, causing visual field disturbance or other evidence of mass effect.[183] Less often, the clinical presentation may be that of a non-functioning mass lesion, associated either with a euthyroid or a chronic hypothyroid state.[181,183] Serum levels of TSH are raised in all cases, and in

clinically hyperthyroid patients the levels of T3 and T4 are also usually elevated.[184,186] In addition, the serum often shows disproportionately high levels of the alpha subunit common to TSH, FSH and LH hormones.[186]

Pathology

Histology and immunocytochemistry

Thyrotroph cell adenomas usually have a sinusoidal architecture, often with prominent pseudorosettes around blood vessels. The tumour cell cytoplasm is chromophobic when trichrome stains are used. Most cases show at least some cells which react with antibodies to beta TSH, but the tumours are often difficult to immunostain and the results can be faint or very focal[181,183] (Fig. 16.40). If polyclonal reagents are used, cross-reactivity with FSH and LH should be expected, because of their common alpha subunit.[187] Very occasionally, immunoreactivity with antibodies to prolactin or growth hormone is also encountered[181] and such tumours might be better classified with the plurihormonal adenomas.

Electron microscopy

In some cases, the cells appear well differentiated and are ultrastructurally similar to the thyrotroph cells of the normal anterior pituitary gland.[182,188] Secretory granules are of uniform rounded shape and distributed either along cell body margins or in prominent cytoplasmic processes. In other tumours, the predominating cells are smaller with very sparse organelles and resemble non-functioning pituitary adenoma cells.[2,182] In either case, the secretory granules are scanty and small, usually between 100 and 200 nm in diameter, and granule exocytosis is not observed.[181]

Therapy and prognosis

Cases presenting with primary hyperthyroidism and/or visual defects due to suprasellar extension normally require urgent surgical treatment,[2,186] although there are anecdotal accounts of a dramatic primary response to continuous infusion of somatostatin analogues.[189] The majority of these thyrotroph cell adenomas have a relatively poor prognosis because of their large size by the time of presentation and marked tendency for rapid growth and local invasion.[184,185] Where only partial excision of the tumour has been possible, persistent, symptomatic elevation of TSH levels is likely even after radiotherapy,[186] and there is a very high mortality rate in these patients.[185,186] Tumours presenting in the context of longstanding hypothyroidism may respond well to simple thyroid hormone replacement therapy and are possibly not autonomous neoplasms.[2]

Gonadotroph cell adenomas

Gonadotroph cell adenomas are said to comprise between 2.5 and 6.0% of all adenomas,[2,190] but most figures quoted are likely to be an underestimate because of the high proportion of endocrinologically silent lesions, only identifiable by immunocytochemical or in vitro evidence of gonadotropin subunit production.[191,192] There is an approximately even distribution between the sexes and most of the tumours present in middle life, with a mean age in the fifth decade.[2,193] Occasional cases occur in the context of longstanding primary hypogonadism,[35] but in the majority of tumours there is no evidence that hypothalamic dysregulation plays a part in pathogenesis.[194] Gonadotroph cell adenomas may produce intact FSH or LH, their beta subunits or their common alpha subunit either individually or in almost any combination[191] (Table 16.11).

Clinical features

Most gonadotroph cell adenomas are large tumours with suprasellar extensions, and usually present purely as mass lesions, without any endocrinological signs or symptoms.[191,193] In a proportion of men, however, there may also be a history of impotence or secondary hypogonadism,[191,193] and some premenopausal women may suffer menstrual disturbances or even galactorrhoea.[193,194] The commonest serological abnormality in both sexes is elevation of FSH levels.[191] LH or its specific beta subunit may also be elevated in some cases,[193] although rarely in isolation,[190] and abnormal levels of free alpha subunit frequently accompany the other serum changes.[32,191] Rather uncommonly, raised alpha subunit levels may be the only serological abnormality associated with a pituitary adenoma, and a proportion of these tumours also appear to be gonadotropinomas, since they have been shown capable of FSH production in vitro.[191,195] Finally, some gonadotroph adenomas show no detectable serum abnormalities at all, and their distinction from non-functioning adenomas rests entirely on the results of immunocytochemistry or electron microscopy.[187,190]

Pathology

Histology and immunocytochemistry

Gonadotroph cell adenomas typically have a sinusoidal architectural pattern and are composed of elongate cells, often polarised into pseudorosettes around blood vessels (Fig. 16.41). Some cases may show oncocytic change but the cell cytoplasm is chromophobic with trichrome stains. Immunocytochemistry usually reveals some

Table 16.11 Gonadotroph cell adenomas

Clinical syndrome	Usually present with tumour mass effects
	May be impotence, menstrual disturbance or evidence of secondary hypogonadism
Serology	May be elevated FSH or FSH and LH, often with raised free alpha subunit
	No serum abnormalities in some cases
Tinctorial staining	Chromophobe
Immunocytochemistry	Patchy staining for FSH, LH, alpha subunit in any combination
Electron microscopy	Sex-linked dichotomy
	Females Well differentiated cells Cytoplasmic processes Vesicular (honeycomb) Golgi body
	Males More often smaller cells with less developed organelles

FSH, follicle stimulating hormone; LH, luteinising hormone.

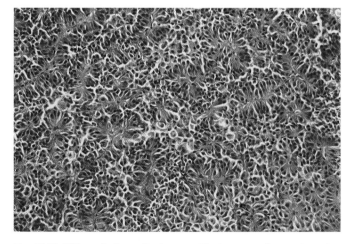

Fig. 16.41 **FSH-producing cell adenoma.** The tumour cells are elongate and polarised into pseudorosettes around vessels. H & E.

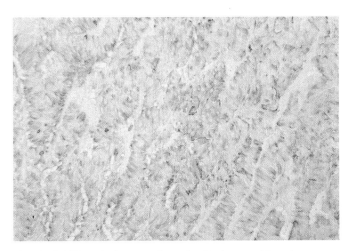

Fig. 16.42 **FSH-producing gonadotroph cell adenoma.** There is a prominent sinusoidal architecture. The tumour cells show patchy staining using immunocytochemistry for beta-FSH.

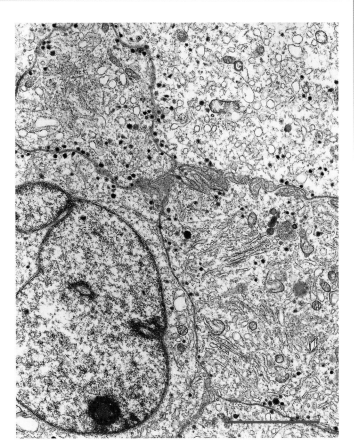

Fig. 16.43 **FSH-producing gonadotroph cell adenoma from a female patient.** Although the secretory granules are sparse and small, the cells are well differentiated and contain prominent Golgi bodies with dilated cisternae (G). Electron micrograph. Bar = 3 μm.

evidence of gonadotropin or alpha subunit production, even in those cases with no detectable serological abnormalities.[196] Like thyrotroph cell adenomas, however, these tumours are often difficult to immunostain, and the results are often very patchy and focal.[2] A majority of the tumours are immunoreactive with antibodies to beta-FSH or the whole FSH molecule[193,196] (Fig. 16.42) and a significant proportion also stain with antibodis to beta-LH.[187,196] Specific immunostaining for LH in the absence of FSH is rare.[117] If polyclonal antibodies are used, considerable cross-reactivity can be expected between the two hormones because of their common alpha subunit. Free alpha subunit can be detected immunocytochemically in most cases[2] and sometimes may be the only positive finding.[190,197]

Electron microscopy

Ultrastructurally, gonadotroph cell adenomas demonstrate a sex-related dichotomy.[198] In females, the cells are mostly well differentiated, with long cytoplasmic processes containing numerous microtubules. The Golgi bodies are usually large and may have a honeycomb appearance due to prominent vesicular dilation of their cisternae[196,198] (Fig. 16.43). This feature is lacking in male tumours, which are typically composed of smaller, less well differentiated cells with poorly developed cytoplasmic organelles.[196,198] In tumours of either sex, the secretory granules are sparse and small, usually less than 250 nm in diameter.[193,196] They are often in the cytoplasmic processes or at the perikaryal margins, but granule extrusion is not found.[168]

Therapy and prognosis

As with non-functioning adenomas, most gonadotroph cell adenomas are treated by surgical resection to relieve the mass effects of the tumour and safeguard against

further visual deterioration.[191] Where complete resection is not possible, or if hormone levels remain elevated postoperatively, then radiotherapy is usually advocated.[191] Dopamine agonists may be effective in reducing serum FSH levels in some cases[199] and luteinising releasing hormone agonists have also been reported to produce both serological and radiological improvement.[200] The long term prognosis must be guarded because of the large size and extrasellar extent of most cases at presentation.[187,191]

Non-functioning adenomas

Non-functioning tumours probably account for approximately one-quarter of all adenomas,[2,201] although in some series the proportion quoted has been as high as 50%.[202] The diagnosis is essentially one of exclusion using serology, electron microscopy and immunocytochemistry, and the incidence quoted will depend on the range and sensitivity of techniques used. Non-functioning adenomas are most likely to be a heterogeneous group of tumours which are too poorly differentiated to be associated with specific anterior gland cell lines.[130] In a significant proportion of cases, there is in vitro evidence that the cells are capable of producing one or more subunits of the glycoprotein hormones FSH, LH or TSH, and it seems likely that at least some so-called non-functioning adenomas represent incompletely differentiated gonadotropin cell adenomas.[201,203]

Clinical features

Non-functioning adenomas usually arise in an older age group than other types of adenoma and are rarely manifest before the fourth decade of life.[2,118] There is a marked bias towards the male sex.[2,118] The tumours are almost always large with extrasellar extension and present clinically with evidence of local compression and mass effect[201,204] (Table 16.12). In some patients there may be clinical or serological evidence of hyperprolactinaemia due to stalk compression syndrome[2] but in the majority of cases there is either no serological abnormality or simply evidence of generalised hypopituitism.[204]

Pathology

Histological features

Non-functioning adenomas typically show a diffuse architectural pattern, with small, rounded or polyhedral cells arranged in monotonous sheets (Fig. 16.44). In some cases, the cells are more elongate and form prominent pseudorosettes around blood vessels. In non-oncocytic tumours the cytoplasm is scanty and has chromophobe characteristics with trichrome stains. Where significant oncocytic change is present, the cells have more swollen and eosinophilic cytoplasm, which may be diffusely acidophilic on trichrome staining.

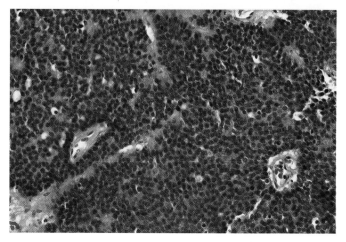

Fig. 16.44 Non-functioning adenoma. Uniform, small tumour cells with scanty cytoplasm are closely packed in diffuse sheets. H & E.

Immunocytochemistry

Using antibodies to anterior pituitary hormones, half or more of these adenomas can be expected to show isolated cells reacting positively with antibodies to FSH, LH, TSH or isolated alpha subunit.[205,206] Where such cells are at all numerous, however, a diagnosis of a specific functioning adenoma needs to be considered, and careful review of the results of serology and electron microscopy is advisable. In males or postmenopausal females, prolactin immunocytochemistry is particularly important for the distinction of a prolactin secreting adenoma from a non-functioning adenoma with stalk compression syndrome.

Electron microscopy

Non-oncocytic tumours consist of tightly apposed polyhedral cells with scanty, electron-lucent cytoplasm and poorly developed organelles.[117,119] The secretory granules are very sparse and small, usually measuring between 100 and 250 nm in diameter. They have wide, prominent, lucent halos between outer membrane and core, and are typically arranged in a single row immediately adjacent to the cell membrane (Fig. 16.45). Exocytosis is not seen.[168] There is often a variable degree of mitochondrial accumulation,[206] but in tumours with marked oncocytic transformation, the majority of cells have cytoplasm which is distended by tightly packed mitochondria.[207] The mitochondria in these cases are often enlarged or swollen and show a range of structural anomalies including tubular or concentric cristae and electron dense inclusions.[208]

Therapy and prognosis

Symptomatic non-functioning adenomas are normally treated surgically for relief of pressure effects, especially those due to chiasmatic compression.[96] Visual field

Table 16.12 Non-functioning adenomas

Clinical syndrome	Tumour mass effect. Older age group May be evidence of secondary hypoprolactinaemia
Serology	May be no abnormality, raised alpha subunit levels or secondary elevation of prolactin
Tinctorial staining	Usually chromophobe Oncocytic tumours may be diffusely acidophil
Immunocytochemistry	Some are entirely unreactive Others show scattered cells staining for FSH, LH, TSH or alpha subunit
Electron microscopy	Small polyhedral cells. Irregular nuclei Poorly developed RER and Golgi body Microtubules Sparse, marginated granules 100–250 nm diameter Oncocytic change common, may affect most cells

FSH, follicle stimulating hormone; LH, luteinising hormone; RER, rough endoplasmic reticulum; TSH, thyroid stimulating hormone.

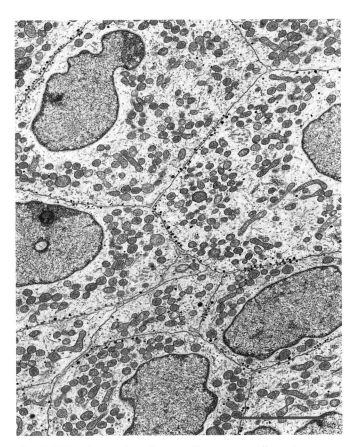

Fig. 16.45 **Non-functioning adenoma.** The sparse, small secretory granules are visible as black dots lined up along the inner aspects of the tumour cell membranes. There is a moderate degree of mitochondrial accumulation. Electron micrograph. Bar = 4 μm.

improvement has been reported in over 80% of cases following surgical decompression, even in patients with large tumours and significant preoperative deficits.[96,204] Dopamine agonist therapy has been claimed to improve visual field defects prior to surgery in some patients,[209] but there is no evidence that it is effective in reducing tumour size in the majority of cases.[210] Where excision has been incomplete, postoperative radiotherapy is usually recommended.[201,204] Even after an apparent surgical cure, delayed recurrence of tumour is less likely in patients receiving postoperative irradiation compared to those treated by surgery alone, where recurrences can be expected to occur in over 10% of cases.[204,211] The overall 10-year survival rate is between 80 and 90% when all cases are considered together,[129,212] but again the figures have been much less favourable for patients not receiving postoperative radiotherapy.[212]

Plurihormonal adenomas

These are a heterogeneous and increasingly reported group of adenomas which are capable of synthesising the hormones normally associated with two or more differ-

Table 16.13 Plurihormonal adenomas

Clinical syndrome	Most often acromegaly May be one or more of any endocrine syndromes Tumour mass effect common
Serology	Anterior gland hormones elevated in varied combinations
Tinctorial staining	Any staining result possible
Immunocytochemistry	Varied combinations of staining for two or more hormones Combined staining for GH, PRL and glycoprotein hormone subunits is commonest
Electron microscopy	May be monomorphic or separate cell populations typical of individual hormones present

GH, growth hormone; PRL, prolactin.

ent anterior gland cell lines[2,213] (Table 16.13). They are far more common than originally realised, and may account for as many as 10–15% of all pituitary adenomas.[213]

Aetiology

The derivation of plurihormonal adenomas is uncertain, but X-linked chromosome studies have suggested that they are of monoclonal origin, like other pituitary adenomas.[26] It is possible they are the result of dedifferentiation in a single mature cell line, which thereby acquires the ability to produce more than one hormone.[214] It is perhaps more likely, however, that they arise from a common precursor cell of the anterior gland, with their final morphological and functional properties depending on the degree and direction of subsequent differentiation.[25] There is also a suggestion that the *MEN-1* gene on chromosome 11 plays a particularly important role in the pathogenesis of plurihormonal adenomas, since cases of type 1 multiple endocrine neoplasia show an unusually large proportion of plurihormonal tumours compared with other types of adenoma.[31,213]

Clinical features

Approximately 80% of plurihormonal adenomas are macroadenomas, and they commonly produce signs and symptoms of mass effect.[213] Some cases present with clinical evidence of plurihormonal activity, as for example in patients with hyperthyroidism combined either with acromegaly[215] or features of hyperprolactinaemia.[216] More often, however, only one endocrine abnormality is apparent clinically. This is most often acromegaly,[213] although cases have also been described with clinically typical Cushing's disease,[24] hyperthyroidism[21] and prolactinaemia.[25]

Pathology

Immunocytochemical staining shows that the commonest variant of plurihormonal adenoma produces a combination of growth hormone, prolactin and one or more components of the glycoprotein hormones FSH, LH and TSH.[213] The latter are most often represented by TSH, but free alpha subunit or a mixture of beta subunits may also be present.[217] Other variants produce hormones associated with only two different cell lines, including alpha subunit and ACTH,[24] TSH and prolactin[21] and TSH with growth hormone.[215] In some cases, immunocytochemistry and electron microscopy demonstrate a monomorphic tumour, with the different hormones present in the same cells or even in the same secretory granules.[24,213] Other tumours consist of two or more distinct cell populations, each morphologically typical for the hormones they are producing.[21,27]

Tumours of the posterior hypophysis

The stromal cells of the posterior pituitary gland and stalk are modified glial cells known as pituicytes.[218] They are capable of a gliotic reaction similar to that seen elsewhere in the brain, and have both in vitro and immunocytochemical features similar to typical astrocytes, including expression of glial fibrillary acidic protein.[219] Ultrastructurally, several morphological variants of pituicyte are apparent, including astrocytic and granular-cell forms, which are felt to represent differing functional states of a single cell type.[220] Tumours purported to be derived from posterior gland pituicytes are very uncommon and have been the subject of varied and confusing nomenclature. They are not separately identified in the WHO classification, but the preferred terms in this text are neurohypophyseal astrocytoma and neurohypophyseal granular cell tumour.

Neurohypophyseal granular cell tumours

Incidence

Granular cell tumours of the neurohypophysis which are large enough to present symptomatically are extremely rare, with only a handful of reported cases.[221,222] Small nests of granular cells, however, are a relatively common incidental finding at autopsy and have been observed in anything from 5 to 17% of unselected post-mortem pituitary glands.[223,224] They are found with increasing frequency in old age and can be multiple.[224] They vary in size from clusters of only a few cells to nodules of about 1 mm in diameter and are usually too small to be visible to the naked eye.[225] The neoplastic potential and natural history of such tiny incidental lesions is uncertain, but it seems likely that the larger symptomatic tumours are derived from the same cells since their cytological features are identical.[226]

Aetiology

Granular cell tumours are a heterogeneous group of neoplasms which derive from different cells at different sites in the body.[227,228] In the neurohypophyseal lesions, tumour cells showing transitional features with the granular variant of normal pituicytes have been described[229] and it is most likely that these particular tumours are of pituicyte origin.[225,230] A majority of cases appear to lack the glial fibrillary acidic protein seen in pituicytes, but this may perhaps be explained by the excessive accumulation of granular material in the tumour cell cytoplasm.

Clinical features

The larger symptomatic tumours typically arise in middle life, usually presenting between the ages of 30 and 60 years.[221,222] Females are affected more frequently than males.[221] Nearly all patients have a history of headache and visual impairment due to suprasellar extension and pressure of the tumour on the optic chiasm or nerves.[226,231] Endocrine disturbances are less frequent, but some cases may have symptoms of secondary hyperprolactinaemia due to stalk compression,[221] and others have presented with diabetes insipidus or hypogonadism.[221,229] Involvement of the cavernous sinus is rare and cranial nerve palsies are not usually present.[225] Using CT scanning, the tumours typically appear as high density, sharply demarcated, suprasellar lesions with dense enhancement after administration of contrast media.[222]

Pathology

Macroscopic features

Symptomatic tumours arising in the posterior gland or lower stalk fill the pituitary fossa and extend upwards through the diaphragma to a varying degree. Those arising in the upper part of the stalk are essentially suprasellar lesions, which usually cause downward displacement of the diaphragma and compression of the sellar contents. At surgery, granular cell tumours appear as lobulated, well circumscribed and richly vascular lesions which displace or compress surrounding structures rather than infiltrate them. They are usually of whitish-pink colour and have a solid, homogeneous, appearance on cut section without cystic spaces.

Histological features

The cytological features of the small, incidental granule cell nests and the larger symptomatic tumours are

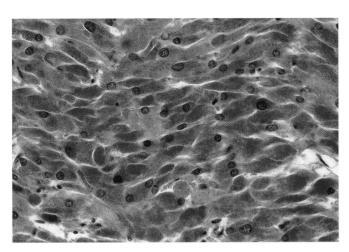

Fig. 16.46 Neurohypophyseal granular cell tumour. The cells have abundant, finely granular cytoplasm which is invariably PAS-positive and diastase resistant. PAS/diastase.

identical. They usually consist of sheets of large, ovoid or polyhedral cells with eccentric nuclei and abundant finely granular cytoplasm. In some cases, however, the cells are elongate or bipolar in shape and may be arranged in fascicles or loose whorls. Significant nuclear pleomorphism may be encountered in occasional cases, but mitotic figures are not found. The granular cytoplasm invariably shows diastase-resistant PAS staining, and this should be considered a prerequisite for making the diagnosis (Fig. 16.46). In some cases, the cytoplasmic granules may also stain positively with phosphotungstic acid haematoxylin. There is usually a dense meshwork of thin-walled capillary blood vessels, but connective tissue stroma is sparse.

Immunocytochemistry

The tumour cells do not immunostain with antibodies to neuron specific enolase or S-100 protein[228,232] and expression of glial fibrillary acidic protein is only found in a small proportion of cases.[218]

Electron microscopy

The tumour cell cytoplasm is swollen with a varied mixture of membrane-bound dense bodies, multivesicular bodies, lamellated membranous structures and vacuoles of differing size and shape.[233,234] These structures are all thought to represent autophagic lysosomal vacuoles.[233] In some cases cytoplasmic intermediate filaments and intercellular desmosome-like structures have also been described.[233] Basement membrane is present only where tumour cells abut onto areas of extracellular collagen.[233,234]

Differential diagnosis

The abundant, PAS-positive, granular cytoplasm makes granule cell tumours easy to distinguish from most other sella region neoplasms. Negative immunocytochemical staining for neuron specific enolase and anterior pituitary hormones will help avoid confusion with *pituitary adenomas*, especially the PAS-positive corticotroph adenomas. The PAS staining alone is usually sufficient to distinguish granule cell tumours from intrasellar or suprasellar *meningiomas* and the lack of cytokeratin expression will help exclude *metastatic carcinoma* or *craniopharyngioma*. *Gliomas* at this site are most often pilocytic and easily distinguished on basic histological criteria, but again the presence of strong, diastase resistant PAS staining makes a glial neoplasm unlikely. In *germinomas*, the PAS staining is diastase sensitive and the tumour cells usually express placental alkaline phosphatase and cytokeratin. *Paragangliomas* can be excluded by the lack of immunocytochemical staining for neurone specific enolase or chromogranin.

Therapy and prognosis

Symptomatic neurohypophyseal granular cell tumours are relatively benign neoplasms which should be surgically excised whenever possible.[222] Where there is very extensive suprasellar spread, surgery is probably best limited to biopsy of the lesion for tissue diagnosis and decompression of suprasellar structures.[221,222] Repeat excision is usually recommended if symptoms recur following initial surgery[222] and there is no evidence that postoperative radiotherapy is of value in such circumstances.[221,222] Most patients surviving surgery have remained alive and well after follow-up periods of 5 years and more,[235,236] and symptom free survivals of up to 12 years have been reported even where tumour excision has been incomplete.[221,222]

Neurohypophyseal astrocytoma

These rare tumours are presumed to arise from the pituicytes of the posterior gland or stalk because of their site and topographical extent. In most cases the histological appearances are identical to those of juvenile astrocytomas of the third ventricle region, and where there is extensive suprasellar spread of tumour the value of attempting to distinguish the two lesions is questionable. In a very small number of cases, however, the lesions are entirely intrasellar or even confined to the posterior lobe, and therefore more likely to be of pituicyte origin.[237–239] Such cases have usually presented clinically as pituitary adenomas, producing a variety of endocrine dyscrasias secondary to pressure on the stalk or anterior gland.[237,239] In some instances the tumours have been too small for reliable radiological detection[239] while other cases have been large enough to cause obvious elevation of the diaphragma.[237,238] Histologically, neurohypophyseal astrocytomas are well defined, typical pilocytic tumours, which compress rather than infiltrate the surrounding posterior gland.[237,238] The usual treatment is surgical excision via a trans-sphenoidal approach.[239] In one reported case, an entirely intrasellar astrocytoma recurred several years postoperatively with a large suprasellar extension,[237] but prognostic information is otherwise lacking.

Miscellaneous neoplasms and tumour-like conditions of the sellar region

Ganglioneuroma

These rare lesions may occur either alone or in association with a functioning pituitary adenoma. When present, the accompanying adenomas are most often growth hormone cell tumours presenting as acromegaly[240,241] although occasionally they may be Cushing's disease adenomas or symptomatic prolactinomas.[242] The presence of an associated ganglion cell lesion is not usually suspected until the adenoma is excised and examined histologically. The ganglionic element typically consists of randomly orientated, bizarre, multipolar neuronal cells embedded in an argyrophilic meshwork of neuritic processes.[242,243] The ganglion cells are sometimes bi- or trinucleate and Nissl substance can be demonstrated on cresyl violet staining. The relationship of the ganglionic tissue to the pituitary adenoma in these cases varies widely. In some instances, the ganglioneuroma may take the form of a discrete tumour, separate from the adjacent anterior gland adenoma.[242] In other tumours there are only small islands of ganglion cells, dispersed within an otherwise unremarkable functioning adenoma.[240,244] Occasionally, no discrete adenoma is found, but the ganglioneuromatous tissue contains isolated nests of functioning adenoma cells, identifiable only by immunocytochemical staining for the appropriate hormone.[245,246] In a minority of cases there are no associated elements of pituitary adenoma at all, and these tumours are often large enough to cause visual impairment due to suprasellar extension.[247,248] The histological appearance is that of an entirely typical ganglioneuroma, similar to those occurring elsewhere in the nervous system.[247,248] Such 'pure' lesions may originate in either the anterior or posterior lobes of the pituitary gland.

The neuronal cells of intrasellar ganglioneuromas are morphologically similar to the neurosecretory magnocellular neurones of the hypothalamus,[243,244] and it has been suggested that they may arise from aberrantly migrated hypothalamic elements.[245] This theory is supported by immunocytochemical studies demonstrating anterior gland hormone releasing factors in the ganglio-neuroma cells.[249,250] Where an associated pituitary adenoma is present, these hormone releasing factors have been appropriate to the adenoma cell type, and it seems likely that the adenomas may develop because of a trophic effect of the ganglion cells on the anterior gland tissue.[241,245] Where a functioning pituitary adenoma contains only microscopic islands of ganglionic cells, it is tempting to speculate that these are simply functioning ectopia and not part of a neoplastic process.[245,251] There seems little doubt, however, that at least some intrasellar ganglionic lesions are genuine neoplasms, since cases without associated adenomas can grow to a large size[247,248] and may even recur after excision.[248]

Post-irradiation sarcoma

These are malignant soft tissue tumours which develop in the pituitary fossa of patients who have undergone previous radiation treatment for pituitary adenomas.[252–254] They arise in the path of the therapeutic beam, and are caused by the effects of radiation on the local soft tissue elements.[252,255] The latent interval following radiotherapy varies from 2 to 20 years[254] and the reported cases have all received large, often multiple doses of radiation with a total in excess of 4000 cGy.[254,255] The tumours are usually large, rapidly growing lesions which aggressively infiltrate supra- and parasellar tissues including brain, but tend not to metastasise.[252,256] Histologically, they are highly malignant, pleomorphic spindle cell neoplasms with a high mitotic rate. Some appear totally undifferentiated whilst others show features of a fibrosarcoma.[254,255] The prognosis is extremely poor in these patients and most die from the effects of local tumour spread within 6 months of presentation, regardless of surgical intervention.[253,254]

Pituitary abscess

Pituitary abscesses most often present in a similar fashion to non-functioning pituitary adenomas, with headache, visual impairment, cranial nerve palsies and clinical evidence of hypopituitism.[257,258] There is usually no evidence of disseminated intracranial or systemic infection.[259] In a small proportion of cases, the intrasellar pus is associated with the presence of a pituitary adenoma or craniopharyngioma, but in the remainder there is no demonstrable tumour.[257] The pus from some intrasellar abscesses is sterile on culture[258] and even where no residual tumour tissue is found it has been suggested that these lesions may be the end result of massive infarction in a pituitary adenoma rather than a primary infective process.[260] In other cases, however, the pus is clearly generated by local infection, presumably blood-borne, and culture yields a variety of organisms including pneumococcus and *Staphylococcus aureus*.[257,261]

In some patients, rupture of infected pus into the subarachnoid space results in a potentially fatal meningitis,[257,258] but otherwise the prognosis is usually very favourable following trans-sphenoidal drainage and appropriate antibiotic therapy.[259]

Lymphocytic hypophysitis

Lymphocytic hypophysitis is an idiopathic inflammation of the anterior pituitary gland, usually affecting young women in the later stages of pregnancy or post partum.[262,263] Men are only rarely affected.[264] The condition typically manifests with multiple endocrine deficiencies or clinical evidence of prolactinaemia due to stalk compression syndrome.[262,265] Isolated endocrine deficiencies may also occur.[266] In some cases the presentation is that of an expanding sellar and suprasellar mass with visual field disturbance.[267,268] A clinical diagnosis of prolactinoma is often made under these circumstances, but no discreet tumour is found at surgery. Biopsies reveal anterior gland tissue with a dense infiltrate of B- and T-lymphocytes, plasma cells and occasional eosinophils. Lymphoid follicles may be present and the residual gland tissue is often fibrotic. The differential diagnosis for the pathologist includes fungal or tuberculous infection and sarcoid. In distinction, there are no granulomas in lymphocytic hypophysitis and organisms cannot be demonstrated, either histologically or in culture.[268] There is no association with systemic autoimmune disorders and the aetiology of the condition is unknown. Treatment consists of subtotal resection and decompression of the chiasm if there is evidence of mass effect, together with long-term pituitary supplements.[268]

Other lesions

Intrasellar origin

A number of neoplasms which are more typically found at other intracranial or spinal sites may occasionally arise within the pituitary fossa, including meningiomas,[269] haemangiopericytomas,[270] Schwannomas[271] and primitive neuroectodermal tumours[272] (Table 16.14). Cavernous haemangiomas can also occur within the sella.[273] Rathke's cleft cysts are discussed in Chapter 17. Germinomas and some teratoid neoplasms are sometimes intrasellar rather than suprasellar in location,[274,275] as are rare examples of craniopharyngioma.[276] Intrasellar metastases are usually a late feature of metastatic disease, but can also present symptomatically in the absence of a known primary tumour.[277,278]

Suprasellar origin

Tumours which may encroach on the pituitary fossa from a suprasellar origin include meningiomas, gangliogliomas

Table 16.14 Tumours and space occupying lesions of the sellar region

1. Intrasellar origin	Pituitary adenoma
	Granular cell tumour
	Pilocytic astrocytoma
	Gangliocytoma
	Metastasis
	Sarcoma
	Meningioma
	Haemangiopericytoma
	Schwannoma
	Germ cell tumours
	Haemangioma
	Rathke's cleft cyst
	Lymphocytic hypophysitis
2. Suprasellar origin	Meningioma
	Pilocytic astrocytoma
	Ganglioglioma
	Optic nerve glioma
	Germ cell tumour
	Craniopharyngioma
	Hypothalamic hamartoma
	Lipoma
	Dermoid and epidermoid cysts
	Sarcoid, tuberculosis
	Histiocytosis X
3. Skull base and air sinus origin	Chordoma
	Olfactory neuroblastoma
	Nasopharyngeal carcinoma
	Paraganglioma
	Plasmacytoma
	Mucocele (sphenoid)
	Primary bone and cartilage tumours
	Wegener granulomatosis

of the third ventricle region, optic nerve gliomas, germ cell tumours and craniopharyngiomas. Non-neoplastic space occupying lesions which typically involve the suprasellar region are discussed in Chapter 17 and include hypothalamic hamartomas, lipomas, dermoid and epidermoid cysts. Intracranial histiocytosis X has a particular predilection for the hypothalamic region and has been described in the older literature under the eponyms Gagel granuloma or Ayala disease.[279,280]

Skull base origin

A wide variety of tumours may also invade the pituitary fossa from the skull base or air sinuses, including chordomas, olfactory neuroblastomas, nasopharyngeal carcinomas, rhabdomyosarcomas[281] and primary neoplasms of bone and cartilage. Paragangliomas may invade upwards from jugulotympanic or carotid body sites, and can occasionally arise within the sella itself.[282] Solitary plasmacytomas may rarely involve the skull base and present as masses expanding the pituitary fossa.[283] Mucoceles of the sphenoid sinus often erode upwards into the fossa and can present both radiologically and clinically as pituitary tumours.[284] In addition to expanding the fossa and causing endocrine disturbances they can extend into the suprasellar region and cause visual disturbances due to chiasmatic compression.

REFERENCES

Pituitary adenomas: general references

1. Zülch KJ Brain tumours. Their biology and pathology, 3rd edn. Berlin: Springer-Verlag, 1986: pp 461–473
2. Kovacs K, Horvath E. Tumors of the pituitary gland. Atlas of tumour pathology, 2nd series, Fascicle 21. Washington: Armed Forces Institute of Pathology, 1986
3. Kleihaus P, Burger PC, Scheithauer BW et al. Histological typing of tumours of the central nervous system, 2nd edn. Berlin: Springer, 1993
4. Martins AN, Hayes GJ, Kempe LG. Invasive pituitary adenomas. J Neurosurg, 1965; 22:268–276
5. Schelin U. Chromophobe and acidophil adenomas of the human pituitary gland. A light and electron microscopic study. Acta Pathol Microbiol Scand (Suppl), 1962; 158:1–80
6. Ingraham FD, Matson DD. Neurosurgery of infancy and childhood. Springfield: Thomas, 1954
7. Richmond IL, Wilson CB. Pituitary adenomas in childhood and adolescence. J Neurosurg, 1978; 49:163–168
8. Kontogeorgos G, Kovacs K, Horvath E et al. Multiple adenomas of the human pituitary: A retrospective autopsy study with clinical implications. J Neurosurg, 1991; 74:243–247
9. Costello RT. Subclinical adenoma of the pituitary gland. Am J Pathol, 1936; 12:205–216
10. Siqueira MG, Guembarovski AL. Subclinical pituitary microadenomas. Surg Neurol, 1984; 22:134–140
11. Coulon G, Fellmann D, Arbez-Gindre F et al. Latent pituitary adenoma. Autopsy study. Sem Hop Paris, 1983; 59:2747–2750
12. Parent AD, Bebin J, Smith RR. Incidental pituitary adeneomas. J Neurosurg, 1981; 54:228–231
13. Hardy J, Vezina JL. Transphenoidal neurosurgery of intracranial neoplasm. Adv Neurol, 1976; 15:261–274
14. Lloyd RV, Chandler WF, Kovacs K et al. Ectopic pituitary adenomas with normal anterior pituitary glands. Am J Surg Pathol, 1986; 10:546–552
15. Tovi F, Hirsch M, Sacks M et al. Ectopic pituitary adenoma of the sphenoid sinus: report of a case and review of the literature. Head Neck, 1990; 12:264–268
16. Matsumura A, Meguro K, Doi M et al. Suprasellar ectopic pituitary adenoma: case report and review of the literature. Neurosurgery, 1990; 26:681–685
17. Kleinschmidt-DeMasters BK, Winston KR, Rubinstein D et al. Ectopic pituitary adenoma of the third ventricle. Case report. J Neurosurg, 1990; 72:139–142
18. Rothman LM, Sher J, Quencer RM et al. Intracranial ectopic pituitary adenoma. J Neurosurg, 1976; 44:96–99
19. Zimmerman EA, Defendi R, Frantz AG. Prolactin and growth hormone in patients with pituitary adeneomas: a correlative study of hormone in tumor and plasma by immunoperoxidase technique and radioimmunoassay. J Clin Endocrinol Metab, 1974; 38:577–585
20. Sherry SH, Guay AT, Lee AK et al. Concurrent production of adenocorticotropic and prolactin from two distinct cell lines in a single pituitary adenoma: a detailed immunohistochemical analysis. J Clin Endocrinol Metab, 1982; 55:947–955
21. Duello TM, Halami NS. Pituitary adenoma producing thyrotropin and prolactin. Virchows Arch (A), 1979; 376:255–265
22. Horvath E, Kovacs K, Singer W et al. Acidophil stem cell adeneoma of the human pituitary. Arch Pathol Lab Med, 1977; 101:594–599
23. Halmi NS. Occurrence of both growth hormone- and prolactin-immunoreactive material in the cells of human somatotropic pituitary adenomas containing mammotropic elements. Virchows Arch (A), 1982; 398:19–31
24. Berg KK, Scheithauer BW, Felix I et al. Pituitary adenomas that produce adrenocorticotropic hormone and alpha-subunit; clinicopathological, immunohistochemical, ultrastructural, and immunoelectron microscopic studies in nine cases. Neurosurgery, 1990; 26:397–403
25. Horvath E, Scheithauer BW, Kovacs K et al. Pituitary adenomas producing growth hormone, prolactin and one or more glycoprotein hormones; a histologic, immunohistochemical and ultrastructural study of four surgically removed tumors. Ultrastruct Pathol, 1983; 5:171–183
26. Herman V, Fagin J, Gonsky R et al. Clonal origin of pituitary adenomas. J Clin Endocrinol Metab, 1990; 71:1427–1433
27. Leon SP, Jiguang Z, Black P McL. Genetic aberrations in human brain tumours. Neurosurgery, 1994; 34:708–722
28. Tordjman K, Stern N, Ouaknine G et al. Activating mutations of the Gs alpha gene in non-functioning pituitary tumours. J Clin Endocrinol Metab, 1993; 77:765–769
29. Williamson EA, Ince PG, Harrison D et al. G-protein mutations in human pituitary adrenocorticotrophic hormone-secreting adenomas. Eur J Clin Invest, 1995; 25:128–131
30. Pei L, Melmed S, Scheithauer BW et al. H-ras mutations in human pituitary carcinoma metastases. J Clin Endocrinol Metab, 1994; 78:842–846
31. Scheithauer BW, Laws ER Jr, Kovacs K et al. Pituitary adenomas of the multiple endocrine neoplasia type I syndrome. Semin Diagn Pathol, 1987; 4:205–211
32. Larsson C, Nordenskold M. Multiple endocrine neoplasia. Cancer Surv, 1990; 9:703–723
33. Zhuang Z, Ezzat SZ, Vortmeyer AO et al. Mutations of the MEN 1 tumour suppressor gene in pituitary tumours. Cancer Res, 1997; 57:5446–5451
34. Pei L, Melmed S, Scheithauer BW et al. Frequent loss of heterozygosity at the retinoblastoma susceptibility gene (RB) locus in aggressive pituitary tumours: evidence for a chromosome 13 tumour suppressor gene other than RB. Cancer Res, 1995; 55:1613–1616
35. Nicolis G, Shimshi M, Allen C et al. Gonadotropin producing pituitary adenoma in a man with longstanding primary hypogonadism. J Clin Endocrinol Metab, 1988; 66:237–241
36. Fatourechi V, Charib H, Scheithauer BW et al. Pituitary thyrotropic adenoma associated with congenital hypothyroidism. Report of two cases. Am J Med, 1984; 76:725–728
37. Yanase T, Sekiya K, Ando M et al. Probable ACTH-secreting pituitary tumour in association with Addison's disease. Acta Endocrinol Copenh, 1985; 110:36–41
38. Furth J, Ueda G, Clifton KH. The pathophysiology of pituitaries and their tumours: methodological advances. In: Busch H, ed. Methods in cancer research, vol X. New York: Academic Press, 1973: pp 201–277
39. Gooren LJ, Assies J, Asscheman H et al. Estrogen-induced prolactinoma in a man. J Clin Endocrinol Metab, 1988; 66:444–446
40. Gordis L, Gold EB, Libauer C et al. Pituitary adenomas and oral contraceptives: a multicenter case-control study. Fertil Steril, 1983; 39:753–760
41. Lamberts SWJ, Stefanko SZ, de Lange SA et al. Failure of clinical remission after transsphenoidal removal of a microadenoma in a patient with Cushing's disease; multiple hyperplastic and edematous cell nests in surrounding pituitary tissue. J Clin Endocrinol Metab, 1980; 50:793–795
42. Saeger W. Die. Morphologie der paraadenomatösen Adenohypophyse. Virchows Arch (A), 1977; 372:299–314
43. Ludecke D, Kautzky R, Saeger W et al. Selective removal of hypersecreting pituitary adenomas. An analysis of endocrine function, operative and microscopical findings in 101 cases. Acta Neurochir, 1976; 35:27–42
44. Halle AA, Drewry RD, Robertson JT. Ocular manifestations of pituitary adenomas. South Med J, 1983; 76:732–735
45. Wilson CB, Dempsey LC. Transsphenoidal microsurgical removal of 250 pituitary adenomas. J Neurosurg, 1978; 48:13–22
46. Tindall GT, Barrow DL. Tumours of the sellar and parasellar area in adults. In: Youmans JR, ed. Neurological surgery, 3rd edn, vol 5. Philadelphia: Saunders, 1990: pp 3447–3498
47. Martins AN Pituitary tumours and intrasellar cysts. In: Vinken PJ, Bruyn GW, eds. Handbook of clinical neurology, vol. 17. Amsterdam: Elsevier, 1974: pp 375–439
48. Balagura S, Frantz AG, Housepian EM et al. The specificity of serum prolactin as a diagnostic indicator of pituitary adenoma. J Neurosurg, 1979; 51:42–46

49. Bozadzhieva EK, Andreeva MKh, Karagiozov LK et al. Pituitary apoplexy. Probl Endokrinol Mosk, 1987; 33:36–39

50. Szeifert G, Pasztor E, Czirjak S et al. Surgical treatment of pituitary apoplexy. Orv Hetil, 1989; 130:119–123

51. Rilliet B, Mohr G, Robert F et al. Calcifications in pituitary adenomas. Surg Neurol, 1981; 15:249–255

52. Davis PC, Hoffman JC Jr, Tindall GT et al. Prolactin-secreting pituitary microadeneomas; inaccuracy of high-resolution CT imaging. Am J Roentgenol, 1985; 144:151–156

53. Kucharczyk W, Davis DO, Kelly WM et al. Pituitary adenomas; high-resolution MR imaging at 1.5 T. Radiology, 1986; 161:761–765

54. Pojunas KW, Daniels DL, Williams AL et al. MR imaging of prolactin-secreting microadeneomas. Am J Neuroradiol, 1986; 7:209–213

55. Steiner E, Imhof H, Knosp E. Gd-DTPA enhanced high resolutions MR imaging of pituitary adenomas. Radiographics, 1989; 9:587–598

56. Laws ERJ, Piepgras DG, Randall RV et al. Neurosurgical management of acromegaly. J Neurosurg, 1979; 50:454–461

57. Kaplan B, Day AL, Quisling R et al. Hemorrhage into pituitary adenomas. Surg Neurol, 1983; 20:280–287

58. Kurisaka M, Mori K, Tindall GT et al. Pituitary adenoma calcification. No To Shinkei, 1986; 38:1187–1195

59. Saitoh Y, Mori H, Matsumo K et al. Accumulation of amyloid in pituitary adenomas. Acta Neuropathol (Berl), 1985; 68:87–92

60. Mori H, Mori S, Saitoh Y et al. Growth hormone-producing pituitary adenoma with crystal-like amyloid immunohistochemically positive for growth hormone. Cancer, 1985; 55:96–102

61. Paetau A, Partanen S, Mustajoki P et al. Prolactinoma of the pituitary containing amyloid. Acta Endocrinol Copenh, 1985; 109:176–180

62. Holcn S, Klinken L. Entrapped, non-neoplastic adenohypophycytes in human pituitary adenomas. Clin Neuropathol, 1990; 9:251–253

63. Asa SL, Ryan N, Kovacs K et al. Immunohistochemical localization of neuron-specific enolase in the human hypophysis and pituitary adenomas. Arch Pathol Lab Med, 1984; 108:40–43

64. Lloyd RV, Wilson BS, Kovacs K et al. Immunohistochemical localization of chromogranin in human hypophyses and pituitary adenomas. Arch Pathol Lab Med, 1985; 109:515–517

65. DeStephano DB, Lloyd RV, Pike AM et al. Pituitary adenomas. An immunohistochemical study of hormone production and chromogranin localization. Am J Pathol, 1984; 116:464–472

66. Hofler H, Denk H, Walter GF. Immunohistochemical demonstration of cytokeratins in endocrine cells of the human pituitary gland and in pituitary adenomas. Virchows Arch (A), 1984; 404:359–368

67. Ironside JW, Royos JA, Jefferson AA et al. Immunolocalisation of cytokeratins in the normal and neoplastic human pituitary gland. J Neurol Neurosurg Psychiatry, 1987; 50:57–65

68. Hayashi K, Hoshida Y, Horie Y et al. Immunohistochemical study on the distribution of alpha and beta subunits of S-100 protein in brain tumours. Acta Neuropathol (Berl), 1991; 81:657–663

69. Lauriola L, Cocchia D, Stentinelli S et al. Immunohistochemical detection of folliculo-stellate cells in human pituitary adenomas. Virchows Arch (B), 1984; 47:189–197

70. Horvath E, Kovacs K, Penzs G et al. Origin, possible function and fate of 'follicular cells' in the anterior lobe of the human pituitary. Am J Pathol, 1974; 77:199–212

71. Höfler H, Walter GF, Denk H. Immunohistochemistry of folliculo-stellate cells in normal human adenohypophyses and in pituitary adenomas. Acta Neuropathol (Berl), 1984; 65:35–40

72. McKeever PE, Koppelman MCS, Metcalf D et al. Refractory Cushing's disease caused by multinodular ACTH-cell hyperplasia. J Neuropathol Exp Neurol, 1982; 41:490–499

73. Burke CW, Adams CB, Esiri MM et al. Transsphenoidal surgery for Cushing's disease: does what is removed determine the endocrine outcome? Clin Endocrinol (Oxf), 1990; 33:525–537

74. Scheithauer BW, Kovacs KT, Laws ER Jr et al. Pathology of invasive pituitary tumors with special reference to functional classification. J Neurosurg, 1986; 65:733–744

75. Selman WR, Laws ER Jr, Scheithauer BW et al. The occurrence of dural invasion in pituitary adenomas. J Neurosurg, 1986; 64:402–407

76. Ahmadi J, North CM, Segall HD et al. Cavernous sinus invasion by pituitary adenomas. Am J Roentgenol, 1986; 146:257–262

77. Gatti G, Limone P. ACTH-producing hypophyseal carcinoma monitored by computed tomography. Diagn Imaging Clin Med, 1984; 53:292–297

78. Papotti M, Limone P, Riva C et al. Malignant evolution of an ACTH-producing pituitary tumor treated with intrasellar implantation of 90Y. Case report and review of the literature. Appl Pathol, 1984; 2:10–21

79. Hashimoto N, Handa H, Nishi S. Intracranial and intraspinal dissemination from a growth hormone-secreting pituitary tumor. Case report. J Neurosurg, 1986; 64:140–144

80. Gasser RW, Finkenstedt G, Skrabal F et al. Multiple intracranial metastases from a prolactin secreting pituitary tumour. Clin Endocrinol (Oxf), 1985; 22:17–27

81. Plangger CA, Twerdy K, Grunert V et al. Subarachnoid metastases from a prolactinoma. Neurochirurgia (Stuttg), 1985; 28:235–237

82. Duskova J, Chlumska A, Vilikusova E et al. Carcinoma of the hypophysis with acromegaly. Cesk Patol, 1984; 20:170–176

83. U SH, Johnson C. Metastatic prolactin-secreting pituitary adenoma. Hum Pathol, 1984; 15:94–96

84. Mountcastle RB, Roof BS, Mayfield RK et al. Pituitary adenocarcinoma in an acromegalic patient: response to bromocriptine and pituitary testing: a review of the literature on 36 cases of pituitary carcinoma. Am J Med Sci, 1989; 298:109–118

85. Cohen DL, Diengdoh JV, Thomas DG et al. An intracranial metastasis from a PRL secreting pituitary tumour. Clin Endocrinol (Oxf), 1983; 18:259–264

86. Casson IF, Walker BA, Hipkin LJ et al. An intrasellar pituitary tumour producing metastases in liver, bone and lymph glands and demonstration of ACTH in the metastatic deposits. Acta Endocrinol Copenh, 1986; 111:300–304

87. Graf CJ, Blinderman EE, Terplan KL. Pituitary carcinoma in a child with distant metastases. J Neurosurg, 1962; 19:254–259

88. Kontogeorgos G, Kapranos N, Rologis D et al. DNA measurement in pituitary adenomas assessed on imprints by image analysis. Anal Quant Cytol Histol, 1996; 18:144–150

89. Bates, AS, Farrell WE, Bicknell EJ et al. Alleleic deletion in pituitary adenomas reflects aggressive biological activity and has potential value as a prognostic marker. J Clin Endocrinol Metab, 1997; 82:818–824

90. McNicol AM, Colgan J, McMeekin W et al. Nucleolar organiser regions in pituitary adenomas. Acta Neuropathol (Berl), 1989; 77:547–549

91. Nagahima T, Murovic JA, Hoskino T et al. The proliferative potential of human pituitary tumours in situ. J Neurosurg, 1986; 64:538–593

92. Ikeda H, Yoshimoto T. The relationship between c-myc protein expression, the bromodeoxyuridine labeling index and the biological behaviour of pituitary adenomas. Acta Neuropathol (Berl), 1992; 83:361–364

93. Pernicone PJ, Scheithauer BW, Sebo TJ et al. Pituitary carcinoma: a clinicopathological study of 15 cases. Cancer, 1997; 79:804–812

94. Knosp E, Kitz K, Perneczky A. Proliferation activity in pituitary adenomas: measurement by monoclonal antibody Ki-67. Neurosurgery, 1989; 25:927–930

95. Fahlbusch R, Buchfelder M. Present status of neurosurgery in the treatment of prolactinomas. Neurosurg Rev, 1985; 8:195–205

96. Harris PE, Afshar F, Coates P et al. The effects of transsphenoidal surgery on endocrine function and visual fields in patients with functionless pituitary tumours. Q J Med, 1989; 71:417–427

97. Stern WE, Batzdorf U. Intracranial removal of pituitary adenomas; an evaluation of varying degrees of excision from partial to total. J Neurosurg, 1970; 33:564–573

98. Sheline GE, Ward WM. Radiation therapy of pituitary tumors. In: Youmans JR, ed. Neurological Surgery, 3rd edn, vol. 5. Philadelphia: Saunders, 1990: pp 3499–3504

99. Motti ED, Losa M, Pieralli S et al. Stereotactic radiosurgery of pituitary adenomas. Metab Clin Exp, 1996; 45:111–114

100. Rocher FP, Sentenac I, Berger C et al. Stereotactic radiosurgery: the Lyon experience. Acta Neurochir (Suppl), 1995; 63:109–114

101. Marguth F, Oeckler R. Recurrent pituitary adenomas. Neurosurg Rev, 1985; 8:221–224

102. Auer LM, Clarici GT. The first 100 transsphenoidally operated pituitary adenomas in a non-specialised centre; surgical results and tumour-recurrence. Neurol Res, 1985; 7:153–160

103. Lloyd RV, Chandler WF, McKeever PE et al. The spectrum of ACTH-producing pituitary lesions. Am J Surg Pathol, 1986; 10:618–626

104. Valtonen S, Myllymaki K. Outcome of patients after transcranial

operation for pituitary adenoma. Ann Clin Res, 1986; 18 (suppl 47): 43–45

105. Vlahovitch B, Reynaud C, Rhiati J et al. Treatment and recurrences in 135 pituitary adenomas. Acta Neurochir Suppl (Wien) 1988; 42:120–123

106. Nelson AT Jr, Tucker HS Jr, Becker DP. Residual anterior pituitary function following transsphenoidal resection of pituitary macroadenomas. J Neurosurg, 1984; 61:577–580

107. Snyder PJ, Fowble BF, Schatz NJ et al. Hypopituitarism following radiation therapy of pituitary adenomas. Am J Med, 1986; 81:457–462

108. Feek CM, McLelland J, Seth J et al. How effective is external pituitary irradiation for growth hormone-secreting pituitary tumors? Clin Endocrinol (Oxf), 1984; 20:401–408

Growth hormone cell adenomas

109. Wilson CB. A decade of pituitary microsurgery. The Herbert Olivecrona Lecture. J Neurosurg, 1984; 61:814–833

110. Smallman LA, Dunn PJ, Curran RC et al. Pituitary adenomas producing growth hormone in acromegalic patients. J Clin Pathol, 1984; 37:382–389

111. Trouillas J, Girod C, L'Heritier M et al. Morphological and biochemical relationships in 31 human pituitary adenomas with acromegaly. Virchow Arch (A), 1980; 389:127–142

112. Beck-Peccoz P, Bassetti M, Spada A et al. Glycoprotein hormone alpha-subunit response to growth hormone (GH)-releasing hormone in patients with active acromegaly. Evidence for alpha-subunit and GH coexistence in the same tumoral cell. J Clin Endocrinol Metab, 1985; 61:541–546

113. Osamura RY. Immunoelectron microscopic studies of GH and alpha subunit in GH secreting pituitary adenomas. Pathol Res Pract, 1988; 183:569–571

114. Zampieri P, Scanarini M, Sicolo N et al. The agromegaly-gigantism syndrome. Report of four cases treated surgically. Surg Neurol, 1983; 20:498–503

115. Schochet SS Jr, McCormick WF, Halmi NS. Acidophil adenomas with intracytoplasmic filamentous aggregates. Arch Pathol, 1972; 94:16–22

116. Ishibashi M, Yamaji T, Takaku F et al. Secretion of glycoprotein hormone alpha-subunit by pituitary tumors. J Clin Endocrinol Metab, 1987; 64:1187–1193

117. Esiri MM, Adams CBT, Burke C et al. Pituitary adenomas: immunohistology and ultrastructural analysis of 118 tumours. Acta Neuropathol (Berl), 1983; 62:1–14

118. Martinez AJ, Lee A, Moossy J et al. Pituitary adenomas; clinicopathological and immunohistochemical study. Ann Neurol, 1980; 7: 24–36

119. Horvath E, Kovacs K. Ultrastructural classification of pituitary adenomas. Can J Neurol Sci, 1976; 3:9–21

120. Neumann PE, Goldman JE, Horoupian DS et al. Fibrous bodies in growth hormone-secreting adenomas contain cytokeratin filaments. Arch Pathol Lab Med, 1985; 109:505–508

121. del Pozo C, Webb SM, Oliver B et al. Treatment of acromegaly. Results in 56 patients. Med Clin (Barc), 1990; 94:85–87

122. Roelfsema F, van Dulken H, Frolich M. Long-term results of transsphenoidal pituitary microsurgery in 60 acromegalic patients. Clin Endocrin (Oxf), 1985; 23:555–565

123. Grisoli F, Leclercq T, Jaquet P et al. Transsphenoidal surgery for acromegaly: long-term results in 100 patients. Surg Neurol, 1985; 23:513–519

124. Oppizzi G, Liuzzi A, Chiodini P et al. Dopominergic treatment of acromegaly: different effects on hormone secretion and tumor size. J Clin Endocrinol Metab, 1984; 58:988–992

125. Muratori M, Arosio M, Gambino G et al. Use of cabergoline in the long term treatment of hyperprolactinaemic and acromegalic patients. J Endocrinol Invest, 1997; 20:537–546

126. Tolis G. The role of somatostatin analogs in the treatment of acromegaly. Metab Clin Exp, 1996; 45:109–110

127. Fahlbusch R, Hongger J, Buchfelder M. Acromegaly – the place of the neurosurgeon. Metab Clin Exp, 1996; 45:65–66

Prolactin cell adenomas

128. Mukai K. Pituitary adenomas. Immunocytochemical study of 150 tumours with clinicopathologic correlation. Cancer, 1983; 52:648–653

129. Duello TM, Halmi NS. Immunocytochemistry of prolactin-producing human pituitary adenomas. Am J Anat, 1980; 158:463–469

130. Horvath E, Kovacs K. Identification and classification of pituitary tumours. In Cavanagh JB, ed. Recent advances in neuropathology. London: Churchill Livingstone, 1986: pp 75–93

131. Hulting AL, Muhr C, Lundberg PO et al. Prolactinomas in men: clinical characteristics and the effect of bromocriptine treatment. Acta Med Scand, 1985; 217:101–109

132. Bilbao JM, Horvath E, Hudson AR et al. Pituitary adenomas producing amyloid-like substance. Arch Pathol, 1975; 99:411–415

133. Kameya T, Tsumuraya M, Adachi I et al. Ultrastructure, immunohistochemistry and hormone release of pituitary adenomas in relation to prolactin production. Virchow Arch (A), 1980; 387:31–46

134. Dingehans KP, Assies J, Jansen N et al. Sparsely granulated prolactin cell adenomas of the pituitary gland. Correlation of ultrastructure with plasma hormone level. Virchow Arch (A), 1982; 396:167–186

135. Horoupian DS. Large mitochondria in a pituitary adenoma with hyperprolactinaemia. Cancer, 1980; 46:537–542

136. Horvath E, Kovacs K. Misplaced exocytosis. Distinct ultrastructural features in some pituitary adenomas. Arch Pathol, 1974; 97:221–224

137. Kubota T, Kuroda E, Yamashima T et al. Amyloid formation in prolactinoma. Arch Pathol Lab Med, 1986; 110:72–75

138. Schottke H, Saeger W, Ludecke DK et al. Ultrastructural morphometry of prolactin secreting adenomas treated with dopamine agonists. Pathol Res Pract, 1986; 181:280–290

139. Tindall GT, Kovacs K, Horvath E et al. Human prolactin-producing adenomas and bromocriptine: a histologic, immunocytochemical, ultrastructural and morphometric study. J Clin Endocrinol Metab, 1982; 55:1178–1183

140. Esiri MM, Bevan JS, Burke CW et al. Effect of bromocriptine treatment on the fibrous tissue content of prolactin-secreting and non-functioning macroadenomas of the pituitary gland. J Clin Endocrinol Metab, 1986; 63:383–388

141. Gen M, Uozumi T, Ohta M et al. Necrotic changes in prolactinomas after long term administration of bromocriptine. J Clin Endocrinol Metab, 1984; 59:463–470

142. Mori H, Maeda T, Saitoh Y et al. Changes in prolactinomas and somatotropinomas in human treated with bromocriptine. Pathol Res Pract, 1988; 183:580–583

143. Molitch ME, Elton RL, Blackwell RE et al. Bromocriptine as primary therapy for prolactin-secreting macroadenomas: results of a prospective multicenter study. J Clin Endocrinol Metab, 1985; 60:698–705

144. Zarate A, Canales ES, Cano C et al. Follow-up of patients with prolactinomas after discontinuation of long-term therapy with bromocriptine. Acta Endocrinol Copenh, 1983; 104:139–142

145. Johnston DG, Hall K, Kendall-Taylor P et al. Effect of dopamine agonist withdrawal after long-term therapy in prolactinomas. Studies with high-definition computerised tomography. Lancet, 1984; ii:187–192

146. Charpentier G, de Plunkett T, Jedynak P et al. Surgical treatment of prolactinomas. Short- and long-term results, prognostic factors. Horm Res, 1985; 22:222–227

147. Thomson JA, Teasdeale GM, Gordon D et al. Treatment of presumed prolactinoma by transsphenoidal operation: early and late results. Br Med J Clin Res, 1985; 291:1550–1553

148. Ciric I, Mikhael M, Stafford T et al. Transsphenoidal microsurgery of pituitary macroadenomas with long-term follow-up results. J Neurosurg, 1983; 59:395–401

149. Saitoh Y, Mori S, Arita N et al. Treatment of prolactinoma based on the results of transsphenoidal operations. Surg Neurol, 1986; 26:338–344

150. Maira G, Anile C, De Marinis L et al. Prolactin secreting adenomas: surgical results. Can J Neurol Sci, 1990; 17:67–70

151. Grigsby PW, Simpson JR, Emami BN et al. Prognostic factors and results of surgery and postoperative irradiation in the management of pituitary adenomas. Int J Radiat Oncol Biol Phys, 1989; 16:1411–1417

152. Grossman A, Cohen BL, Charlesworth M et al. Treatment of prolactinomas with megavoltage radiotherapy. Br Med J Clin Res, 1984; 288:1105–1109

153. Nelson PB, Goodman M, Maroon JC et al. Factors in predicting outcome from operation in patients with prolactin-secreting pituitary adenomas. Neurosurgery, 1983; 13:634–641

Adenomas producing growth hormone and prolactin

154. Corenblum B, Sirek AMT, Horvath E et al. Human mixed somatotrophic and lactotrophic pituary adenomas. J Clin Endocrinol Metab, 1976; 42:857–863

155. Guyda H, Robert F, Colle E et al. Histological, ultrastructural and hormonal characterisation of a pituitary tumour secreting both hGH and prolactin. J Clin Endocrinol Metab, 1973; 36:531–547

156. Lamberts SWJ, Klijn JGM, Kwa GH et al. The dynamics of growth hormone and prolactin secretion in acromegalic patients with 'mixed' pituitary tumours. Acta Endocrinol, 1979; 90:198–210

157. Horvath E, Kovacs K, Singer W et al. Acidophil stem cell adenoma of the human pituitary: clinicopathological analysis of 15 cases. Cancer, 1981; 47:761–771

158. Horvath E, Kovacs K, Killinger DW et al. Mammosomatotroph cell adenoma of the human pituitary; a morphologic entity. Virchow Arch (A), 1983; 398:277–289

159. Cameron S, Alien I, Ozo C et al. Clinical, biochemical and immunoelectron microscopical evidence of dual hormone production in a mammosomatotroph cell adenoma. J Pathol, 1990; 161:239–244

160. Felix IA, Horvath E, Kovacs K et al. Mammosomatotroph adenoma of the pituitary associated with gigantism and hyperprolactinaemia. A morphological study including immunoelectron microscopy. Acta Neuropathol (Berl), 1986; 71:76–82

Corticotroph cell adenomas

161. Horvath SE, Asa SL, Kovacs K et al. Human pituitary corticotroph adenomas in vitro: morphologic and functional responses to corticotropin-releasing hormone and cortisol. Neuroendocrinology, 1990; 51:241–248

162. Robert F, Hardy J. Human corticotroph cell adenomas. Semin Diagn Pathol, 1986; 3:34–41

163. Crooke AC. A change in the basophil cells of the pituitary gland common to conditions which exhibit the syndrome attributed to basophil adenoma. J Pathol Bact, 1935; 41:339–349

164. Felix IA, Horvath E, Kovacs K. Massive Crooke's hyalinization in corticotroph cell adenomas of the human pituitary. Acta Neurochir, 1982; 58:235–243

165. Wowra B, Peiffer J. An immunoperoxidase study of a human pituitary adenoma associated with Cushing's syndrome. Pathol Res Pract, 1984; 178:349–354

166. Charpin C, Hassoun J, Oliver C et al. Immunohistochemical and immunoelectron-microscopic study of pituitary adenomas associated with Cushing's disease. Am J Pathol, 1982; 109:1–7

167. Neumann PE, Horoupian DS, Goldman JE et al. Cytoplasmic filaments of Crooke's hyaline change belong to the cytokeratin class. An immunocytochemical and ultrastructural study. Am J Pathol, 1984; 116:214–222

168. Ryder DR, Horvath E, Kovacs K. Fine structural features of secretion in adenomas of human pituitary gland. Arch Pathol Lab Med, 1980; 104:518–522

169. Decicco A, Deker A, Yunis EJ. Fine structure of Crooke's hyaline change in the human pituitary gland. Arch Pathol, 1972; 94:65–70

170. Boggan JE, Tyrell JB, Wilson CB. Transsphenoidal microsurgical management of Cushing's disease. Report of 100 cases. J Neurosurg, 1983; 59:195–200

171. Wislawski J, Kasperlik-Zaluska AA, Jeske W et al. Results of neurosurgical treatment by a transsphenoidal approach in 10 patients with Nelson's syndrome. J Neurosurg, 1985; 62:68–71

172. Hirata Y, Nakashima H, Uchihashi M et al. Effects of bromocriptine and cyproheptadine on basal and corticotropin-releasing factor (CRF)-induced ACTH release in a patient with Nelson's syndrome. Endocrinol Jpn, 1984; 31:619–626

173. Koppeschaar HP, Croughs RJ, van't Verlaat JW et al. Successful treatment with sodium valproate of a patient with Cushing's disease and gross enlargement of the pituitary. Acta Endocrinol Copenh, 1984; 107:471–475

174. Sample CG, Thomson JA, Teasdale GM. Trans-sphenoidal microsurgery for Cushing's disease. Clin Endocrinol (Oxf), 1984; 21:621–629

175. Devoe DJ, Miller WL, Conte FA et al. Long-term outcome in children and adolescents after transsphenoidal surgery for Cushing's disease. J Clin Endocrinol Metab, 1997; 82:3196–3202

176. Hovacs K, Horvath E, Bayley TA et al. Silent corticotroph cell adenoma with lysosomal accumulation and crinophagy: a distinct clinicopathologic entity. Am J Med, 1978; 64:492–499

177. Horvath E, Kovacs K, Killinger DW et al. Silent corticotropic adeneomas of the human pituitary gland. A histologic, immunocytologic and ultrastructural study. Am J Pathol, 1980; 98:617–638

178. Reincke M, Allolio B, Saeger W et al. A pituitary adenoma secreting high molecular weight adrenocorticotropin without evidence of Cushing's disease. J Clin Endocrinol Metab, 1987; 65:1296–1300

179. Gogel EL, Salber PR, Tyrrell JB et al. Cushing's disease in a patient with a 'nonfunctioning' pituitary tumor. Spontaneous development and remission. Arch Intern Med, 1983; 143:1040–1042

180. Vaughan NJ, Laroche CM, Goodman I et al. Pituitary Cushing's disease arising from a previously non-functional corticotrophic chromophobe adenoma. Clin Endocrinol (Oxf), 1985; 22:147–153

Thyrotroph cell adenomas

181. Girod C, Trouillas J, Claustrat B. The human thyrotropic adenoma: pathologic diagnosis in five cases and critical review of the literature. Semin Diagn Pathol, 1986; 3:58–68

182. Saeger W, Lüdecke DK. Pituitary adenomas with hyperfunction of TSH. Frequency, histological classification, immunocytochemistry and ultrastructure. Virchow Arch (A), 1982; 394:255–267

183. Samaan NA, Osborne BM, Mackay B et al. Endocrine and morphologic studies of pituitary adenomas secondary to primary hypothyroidism. J Clin Endocrinol Metab, 1979; 45:903–911

184. Grisoli F, Leclercq T, Winteler JP et al. Thyroid-stimulating hormone pituitary adenomas and hyperthyroidism. Surg Neurol, 1986; 25:361–368

185. McCutcheon IE, Weintraub BD, Oldfield EH. Surgical treatment of thyrotropin-secreting pituitary adenomas. J Neurosurg, 1990; 73:674–683

186. Gesundheit N, Petrick PA, Nissim M et al. Thyrotropin-secreting pituitary adenomas: clinical and biochemical heterogeneity. Case reports and follow-up of nine patients. Ann Intern Med, 1989; 111:827–835

187. Cravioto H, Fukaya T, Zimmerman EA et al. Immunohistochemical and electron-microscopic studies of functional and non-functional pituitary adeneomas including on TSH secreting tumour in a thyrotoxic patient. Acta Neuropathol (Berl) 1981; 53:281– 292

188. Waldhausl W, Bratusch-Marrain P, Nowotny P et al. Secondary hyperthyroidism due to thyrotropic hypersecretion: study of pituitary tumour morphology and thyrotropin chemistry and release. J Clin Endocrinol Metab, 1979; 49:879–887

189. Caron P, Gerbeau C, Pradayrol L et al. Successful pregnancy in an infertile woman with a thyrotropin-secreting macroadenoma treated with somatostatin analog (octreotide). J Clin Endocrinol Metab, 1996; 81:1164–1168

Gonadotroph cell adenomas

190. Trouillas J, Girod C, Sassolas G et al. The human gonadotropic adenoma: pathologic diagnosis and hormonal correlations in 26 tumors. Semin Diagn Pathol, 1986; 3:42–57

191. Snyder PJ. Gonadotroph cell adenomas of the pituitary. Endocr Rev, 1985; 6:552–563

192. Takeuchi J, Handa H, Suda K et al. In vitro secretion of follicle-stimulating hormone by pituitary chromaphobe adenomas. Surg Neurol,1980; 14:303–309

193. Trouillas J, Girod C, Sassolas G et al. Human pituitary gonadotropic adenoma; histological, immunocytochemical, ultrastructural and hormonal studies in eight cases. J Pathol, 1981; 135:315–336

194. Moses N, Goldberg V, Gutman R et al. Combined FSH and LH secreting pituitary adenoma in a young fertile woman without primary gonadal failure. Acta Endocrinol Copenh, 1986; 112:58–63

195. Snyder PJ, Bashey HM, Phillips JL et al. Comparison of hormonal secretory behavior of gonadotroph cell adenomas in vivo and in culture. J Clin Endocrinol Metab, 1985; 61:1061–1065

196. Horvath E, Kovacs K. Gonadotroph adenomas of the human pituitary: sex-relating fine structural dichotomy. A histologic, immunocytochemical and electron microscopic study of 30 tumors. Am J Pathol, 1984; 117:429–440

197. Klibanski A, Ridgway EC, Zervas NT. Pure alpha subunit-secreting pituitary tumours. J Neurosurg, 1983; 59:585–589

198. Kontogeorgos G, Horvath E, Kovacs K. Sex-linked ultrastructural dichotomy of gonadotroph adenomas of the human pituitary: an electron microscopic analysis of 145 tumours. Ultrastruct Pathol, 1990; 14:475–482

199. Leese G, Jeffreys R, Vora J. Effects of cabergoline in a pituitary adenoma secreting follicle-stimulating hormone. Postgrad Med J, 1997; 73:507–508

200. Zarate A, Fonseca ME, Mason M et al. Gonadotropin-secreting pituitary adenoma with concomitant hypersecretion of testosterone and elevated sperm count. Treatment with LRH agonist. Acta Endocrinol Copenh, 1986; 113:29–34

Nonfunctioning and plurihormonal adenomas

201. Klibanski A. Nonsecreting pituitary tumors. Endocrinol Metab Clin North Am, 1987; 16:793–804

202. Martinez AJ. The pathology of nonfunctional pituitary adenomas. Semin Diagn Pathol, 1986; 3:83–94

203. Asa SL, Gerrie BM, Singer W et al. Gonadotropin secretion in vitro by human pituitary null cell adenomas and oncocytomas. J Clin Endocrinol Metab, 1986; 62:1011–1019

204. van Lindert EJ, Grotenhuis JA, Meijer E. Results of follow-up after removal of non-functioning pituitary adenomas. Br J Neurosurg, 1991; 5:129–133

205. Landolt AM, Heitz PU, Zenklusen HR. Production of the alpha-subunit of glycoprotein hormones by pituitary adenomas. Pathol Res Pract, 1988; 183:610–612

206. Kovacs K, Horvath E, Ryan N et al. Null cell adenoma of the human pituitary Virchow Archiv (A), 1980; 387:165–174

207. Kovacs K, Horvath E. Pituitary 'chromophobe' adenoma composed of oncocytes. A light and electron microscopic study. Arch Pathol, 1973; 95:235–239

208. Goebel HH, Schluz F, Rama B. Ultrastructurally abnormal mitochondria in the pituitary oncocytoma. Acta Neurochir, 1980; 51:195–201

209. D'Emden MC, Harrison LC. Rapid improvement in visual field defects following bromocriptine treatment of patients with non-functioning pituitary adenomas. Clin Endocrinol (Oxf), 1986; 25:697–702

210. Barrow DL, Tindall GT, Kovacs K et al. Clinical and pathological effects of bromocriptine on prolactin-secreting and other pituitary tumors. J Neurosurg, 1984; 60:1–7

211. Ebersold MJ, Quast LM, Laws ER Jr et al. Long-term results in transsphenoidal removal of nonfunctioning pituitary adenomas. J Neurosurg, 1986; 64:713–719

212. Sheline G. Treatment of chromophobe adenomas of the pituitary gland. In: Kohler P, Ross GI, eds. Diagnosis and treatment of pituitary tumors. New York: Elsevier, 1973: pp 201–216

213. Scheithauer BW, Horvath E, Kovacs K et al. Plurihormonal pituitary adenomas. Semin Diagn Pathol, 1986; 3:69–82

214. Kovacs K, Horvath E, Ezrin C et al. Adenoma of the human pituitary producing growth hormone and thyrotropin. Virchow Arch (A), 1982; 395:59–68

215. Carlson HE, Linfoot JA, Braunstein GD et al. Hyperthyroidism and acromegaly due to a thyrotropin- and growth hormone-secreting pituitary tumour. Lack of hormonal response to bromocriptine. Am J Med, 1983; 74:915–923

216. Jaquet P, Hassoun J, Delori P et al. A human pituitary adenoma secreting thyrotropin and prolactin: immunohistochemical, biochemical, and cell culture studies. J Clin Endocrinol Metab, 1984; 59:817–824

217. Hofland LJ, Van Koetsveld PM, Verleun TM et al. Glycoprotein hormone alpha-subunit and prolactin release by cultured pituitary adenoma cells from acromegalic patients; correlation with GH release. Clin Endocrinol, 1989; 30:601–611

Posterior hypophyseal tumours

218. Russell DS, Rubinstein LJ. Tumours of the neurohypophysis. In: Pathology of tumours of the nervous system, 5th edn. London: Edward Arnold, 1989: pp 376–380

219. Suess U, Pliska V. Identification of the pituicytes as astroglial cells by indirect immunofluorescence-staining for the glial fibrillary acidic protein. Brain Res, 1981; 221:27–33

220. Takei Y, Seyama S, Pearl GS et al. Ultrastructural study of the human neurohypophysis. II. Cellular elements of the neural parenchyma, the pituicytes. Cell Tissue Res, 1980; 205:273–287

221. Houtteville JP, Lechevalier B, Lecoq PJ et al. Pituicytome à cellules granulaires (christome) de la tige pituitaire. Rev Neurol, 1976; 132:589–604

222. Becker DH, Wilson CB. Symptomatic parasellar granular cell tumors. Neurosurgery, 1981; 8:173–180

223. Doron Y, Behar A. Bellar AJ. Granular-cell 'myoblastoma' of the neurohypophysis. J Neurosurg, 1965; 22:95–99

224. Shankun WM. The origin, histology and senescence of tumorettes in the human neurohypophysis. Acta Anat, 1953; 18:1–20

225. Kovacs K, Horvath E. Tumours of the pituitary gland. Atlas of tumour pathology, second series, Fascicle 21. Washington DC: Armed Forces Institute of Pathology, 1986

226. Burston J, John R, Spencer H. 'Myoblastoma' of the neurohypophysis. J Pathol Bacteriol, 1962; 83:455–461

227. Markesbery WR, Duffy PE, Cowen D. Granular cell tumours of the central nervous system. J Neuropathol Exp Neurol, 1973; 32:92–109

228. Ulrich JU, Heitz Ph-U, Fischer T et al. Granular cell tumours: evidence for heterogeneous tumor cell differentiation. Virchow Arch (B), 1987; 53:52–57

229. Liss L, Kahn EA. Pituicytoma. Tumour of the sella tissue. A clinico-pathologic study. J Neurosurg, 1958; 15:481–488

230. Massie AP. A granular-cell pituicytoma of the neurohypophysis. J Pathol, 1979; 129:53–56

231. Glazer N, Hauser H, Slade H. Granular cell tumour of the neurohypophysis. Am J Roentgenol, 1956; 76:324–326

232. Asa SL, Ryan N, Kovacs K et al. Immunohistochemical localisation of neuron-specific enolase in the human hypophysis and pituitary adenomas. Arch Pathol Lab Med, 1984; 108:40–43

233. Landolt AM. Granular cell tumours of the neurohypophysis. In: Ultrastructure of human sella tumors. Correlation of clinical findings and morphology. Acta Neurochir, 1975; Suppl 22;120–128

234. Popovitch ER, Sutton CM, Becker NH et al. Fine structure and histochemical studies of choristomas of the neurohypophysis. J Neuropathol Exp Neurol, 1970; 29:155–156

235. Satyamurti S, Huntingdon HW. Granular cell myoblastoma of the pituitary. J Neurosurg, 1972; 37:483–486

236. Symon L, Ganz JC. Chir B et al. Granular cell myoblastoma of the neurohypophysis. J Neurosurg, 1971; 35:82–89

237. Rossi ML, Bevan JS, Esiri MM et al. Pituicytoma (pilocytic astrocytoma) Case report. J Neurosurg, 1987; 67:768–772

238. Scothorne CM. Glioma of the posterior lobe of the pituitary gland. J Pathol Bacteriol, 1955; 69:109–112

239. Zhou ZS. Infundibuloma: report of 6 cases. Chung Hua Chung Liu Tsa Chih, 1990; 12:150–151

Other lesions

240. Burchiel KJ, Shaw CM, Kelly WA. A mixed functional microadenoma and ganglioneuroma of the pituitary fossa. J Neurosurg, 1983; 58:416–420

241. Schiethauer BW, Kovacs K, Randall RV et al. Hypothalamic neuronal hamartoma and adenohypophyseal neuronal choristoma: their association with growth hormone adenoma of the pituitary gland. J Neuropathol Exp Neurol, 1983; 42:648–663

242. Fischer EG, Morris JH, Kettyle WM. Intrasellar gangliocytoma and syndromes of pituitary hypersecretion. J Neurosurg, 1983; 59:1071–1075

243. Asa SL, Kovacs K, Tindall GT et al. Cushing's disease associated with an intrasellar gangliocytoma producing corticotrophin-releasing factor. Ann Int Med, 1984; 101:789–793

244. Asa SL, Bilbao JM, Kovacs K et al. Hypothalamic neuronal hamartoma associated with pituitary growth hormone cell adenoma and acromegaly. Acta Neuropathol, 1980; 52:231–234

245. Rhodes RH, Dusseau JJ, Boyd AS Jr et al. Intrasellar neural-adenohypophyseal choristoma. A morphological and immunocytochemical study. J Neuropathol Exp Neurol, 1982; 41:267–280

246. Kamel OW, Horoupian DS, Silverberg GD. Mixed gangliocytoma-adenoma: a distinct neuroendocrine tumor of the pituitary fossa. Hum Pathol, 1989; 20:1198–1203

247. Robertson DM, Hetherington RF. A case of ganglioneuroma arising in the pituitary fossa. J Neurol Neurosurg Psychiatry, 1964; 27:268–272

248. Serebrin R, Robertson DM. Ganglioneuroma arising in the pituitary fossa: a twenty year follow-up. J Neurol Neurosurg Psychiatry, 1984; 47:97–98

249. Bevan JS, Asa SL, Rossi ML et al. Intrasellar gangliocytoma containing gastrin and growth hormone-releasing hormone associated with a growth hormone-secreting pituitary adenoma. Clin Endocrinol (Oxf), 1989; 30:213–224

250. Li JY, Racadot O, Kujas M et al. Immunocytochemistry of four mixed pituitary adenomas and intrasellar gangliocytomas associated with different clinical syndromes: acromegaly, amenorrhea-galactorrhea, Cushing's disease and isolated tumoral syndrome. Acta Neuropathol, 1989; 77:320–328

251. Slowik E, Fazekas I, Balint K et al. Intrasellar hamartoma associated with pituitary adenoma. Acta Neuropathol (Berl), 1990; 80:328–333

252. Powell HC, Marshall LF. Ignelzi RJ. Post-irradiation pituitary sarcoma. Acta Neuropathol, 1977; 39:165–167

253. Shi T, Farrell MA, Kaufmann JC. Fibrosarcoma complicating irradiated pituitary adenoma. Surg Neurol, 1984; 22:277–284

254. Waltz TA, Brownell B. Sarcoma: a possible late result of effective radiation therapy for pituitary adenoma. J Neurosurg, 1966; 24:901–907

255. Greenhouse AH. Pituitary sarcoma. J Am Med Assoc, 1964; 190:269–273

256. Kovacs K, Horvath E. Tumours of the pituitary gland. In: Atlas of tumour pathology, 2nd series, Fascicle 21. Washington DC: Armed Forces Institute of Pathology, 1986

257. Domingue, JN, Wilson CB. Pituitary abscesses: report of seven cases and review of the literature. J Neurosurg, 1977; 46:601–608

258. Lindholm J, Rasmussen P, Korsgaard, O. Intrasellar or pituitary abscess. J Neurosurg, 1973; 38:616–619

259. Martins AN. Pituitary tumours and intrasellar cysts. In: Vinken PJ, Bruyn GW, eds. Handbook of clinical neurology, vol. 17. Amsterdam: North Holland, 1974: pp 375–439

260. Bjerre P, Riishede J, Lindholm J. Pituitary abscess. Acta Neurochir (Wien), 1983; 68:187–193

261. Hammann H de V. Abscess formation in the pituitary fossa associated with a pituitary adenoma. J Neurosurg, 1956; 13:208–210

262. Asa SL, Bilbao JM, Kovacs K et al. Lymphocytic hypophysitis of pregnancy resulting in hypopituitarism: a distinct clinicopathologic entity. Ann Int Med, 1981; 95:166–171

263. Cosman F, Post KD, Holub DA et al. Lymphocytic hypophysitis: report of three new cases and review of the literature. Medicine, 1989; 68:240–256

264. Riedl M, Czech T, Slootweg J et al. Lymphocytic hypophysitis presenting as a pituitary tumour in a 63 year old man. Endocrinol Pathol, 1995; 6:159–166

265. Cebelin MS, Velasco ME, De Las Mulas JM et al. Galactorrhea associated with lymphocytic adenohypophysitis. Br J Obstet Gynaecol, 1981; 88:675–680

266. Jensen MD, Handwerger BS, Scheithauer BW et al. Lymphocytic hypophysitis with isolated corticotropin deficiency. Ann Int Med, 1986; 105:200–203

267. Mayfield RK, Levine JH, Gordon L et al. Lymphoid adenohypophysitis presenting as a pituitary tumour. Am J Med, 1980; 69:619–623

268. Baskin DS, Townsend JJ, Wilson CB. Lymphocytic adenohypophysitis of pregnancy simulating a pituitary adenoma; a distinct pathological entity. J Neurosurg, 1982; 56:148–153

269. Watanabe M, Toyama M, Watanabe M et al. A case of intrasellar meningioma with panhypopituitism and hyperprolactinemia. No Shinkei Geka, 1987; 15:869–874

270. Kumar PP, Good RR, Skultety EM et al. Spinal metastases from pituitary hemangiopericytic meningioma. Am J Clin Oncol, 1987; 10:422–428

271. Perone TP, Robinson B, Holmes SM. Intrasellar Schwanoma: case report. Neurosurgery, 1984; 14:71–73

272. Schwartz AM, Ghatak NR, Laine FJ. Intrasellar primitive neuroectodermal tumor (PNET) in familial retinoblastoma: a variant of 'trilateral retinoblastoma'. Clin Neuropathol, 1990; 9:55–59

273. Buonaguidi R, Canapicci R, Mimassi N et al. Intrasellar cavernous hemangioma. Neurosurgery, 1984; 14:732–734

274. Andrew J, Kendall BE, Brook CD. Germinoma of the pituitary gland, a report of two cases. J Neurol Neurosurg Psychiatry, 1985; 48:589–592

275. Yamagami T, Handa H, Takeuchi J et al. Choriocarcinoma arising from the pituitary fossa with extracranial metastasis: a review of the literature. Surg Neurol, 1983; 19:469–480

276. Hiramatsu K, Takahashi K, Ikeda A et al. A case of intrasellar craniopharyngioma Tokai J Exp Clin Med, 1987; 12:135–140

277. Teears RJ, Silverman EM. Clinicopathologic review of 88 cases of carcinoma metastatic to the pituitary gland. Cancer, 1975; 36:216–220

278. Branch CL Jr, Laws ER Jr. Metastatic tumors of the sella turcica masquerading as primary pituitary tumors. J Clin Endocrinol Metab, 1987; 65:469–474

279. Bernald JD, Aguilar MJ. Localised hypothalamic histiocytosis X. Report of a case. Arch Neurol, 1969; 20:368–373

280. Kepes JJ, Kepes M. Predominantly cerebral forms of histiocytosis X. A re-appraisal of 'Gagel's hypothalamic granuloma' 'Granuloma infiltrans of the hypothalamus' and 'Ayala's disease', with a report of four cases. Acta Neuropathol, 1969; 14:77–98

281. Jalalah S, Kovacs K, Horvath E et al. Rhabdomyosarcoma in the region of the sella turcica. Acta Neurochir (Wien), 1987; 88:142–146

282. Asa SL, Kovacs K, Horvath E et al. Sellar glomangioma. Ultrastruct Pathol, 1984; 7:49–54

283. Evans PJ, Jones MK, Hall R et al. Pituitary function with a solitary intrasellar plasmacytoma. Postgrad Med J, 1985; 61:513–514

284. Nugent GR, Sprinkle P, Bloor BM. Sphenoid sinus mucocoeles. J Neurosurg, 1970; 32:443–451

17 Cysts and tumour-like lesions

Craniopharyngioma

Craniopharyngiomas are often grouped topographically with pituitary adenomas and other sellar region tumours, disregarding the varied aetiology of lesions at this site.[1–3] However, the close relationship between cranio-pharyngiomas, Rathke's cleft cysts and suprasellar epidermoid cysts provides an argument for classifying craniopharyngiomas alongside cysts and other tumour-like lesions of maldevelopmental origin,[4,5] a scheme which is adopted here (Table 17.1). Craniopharyngiomas display a wide variation of architectural patterns, but the World Health Organisation (WHO) classification[3] distinguishes two particular histological variants: solid, adult type tumours of papillary pattern, and those with a predominantly 'adamantinous' or basaloid architecture.[6,7]

Incidence

Craniopharyngiomas account for between 4 and 6% of all intracranial tumours in most large series and about 30% of lesions arising in the sellar region.[8,9] They are most common in children, where they have been estimated to represent 17% of supratentorial tumours[4] and over half of all sellar region neoplasms.[10] The mean age at presentation is towards the end of the third decade,[11,12] with a peak incidence between the ages of 10 and 20 years.[13,14]

The tumour has been described in neonates[15,16] and developing fetuses[17,18] although such cases are rare compared to those of later childhood. Occasional patients presenting over the age of 80 have also been reported,[11,19] but the incidence drops off markedly after the end of the sixth decade.[20] In childhood, males are affected significantly more often than females[9,13] whilst in adults the incidence is equally divided between the sexes.[21,22]

Site

The vast majority of craniopharyngiomas arise intracranially in the suprasellar region, but a proportion of these tumours extend in a dumb-bell fashion down through the diaphragma into the pituitary fossa.[9,11] In some cases the tumour may be small and entirely intrasellar in its extent.[11,23] The suprasellar tumours may lie either beneath, in front of or behind the optic chiasm[9] and can be large enough to extend into any of the main cranial compartments, including the posterior fossa.[11,24] Upward extension into the third ventricle is not uncommon, especially in large childhood craniopharyngiomas, and rare examples may be entirely intraventricular in location.[25,26] Although they can involve the pituitary fossa, craniopharyngiomas very rarely infiltrate parasellar or base of skull regions, and invasion of the cavernous sinuses or nasopharyngeal air spaces is rare.[5] Very occasionally, however, examples

Table 17.1 Cystic lesions of the sellar region

	Histology	Immunocytochemistry
Craniopharyngioma	Keratinising stratified squamous epithelium	CK + EMA } Focal, variable CEA
Epidermoid cyst	Keratinising stratified squamous epithelium	CK + EMA +
Dermoid cyst	Stratified squamous epithelium with poor maturation. Dermal appendages	CK + EMA +
Differentiated cystic teratoma	Any epithelial type Differentiated mesodermal elements	CK EMA } Variable CEA
Rathke's cleft cyst	Columnar or cuboidal epithelium. May be – cilia and goblet cells – pseudostratification – squamous metaplasia	CK + EMA + GFAP } Focal, variable S-100
Cysts of pituitary gland/adenoma	No epithelium Anterior gland/adenoma tissue Evidence of old haemorrhage	CK + Anterior gland hormones +
Mucocele	Normal respiratory mucosa	CK + EMA +
Arachnoid cyst	No epithelium Arachnoid membrane	VIM +

CK, cytokeratin; EMA, epithelial membrane antigen; CEA, carcinoembryonic antigen; GFAP, glial fibrillary acidic protein; S-100, S-100 protein; VIM, vimentin

may present in an infrasellar location, mostly lying within the paranasal air sinuses or nasopharynx and seeming to arise outside the cranial cavity.[27,28]

Aetiology

The cellular origin of craniopharyngiomas is a controversial issue which has still to be satisfactorily resolved. They are often assumed to take origin from small nests of squamous cells found incidentally in normal pituitary glands, mostly around the anterior margins of the stalk and at its junction with the anterior gland.[29] These were initially interpreted as remnants of Rathke's stomatodeal-hypophyseal cleft,[9] thus suggesting an embryological origin for the tumour.[30,31] Unlike craniopharyngiomas, however, the squamous cell nests have most often been described in adulthood, especially with increasing age,[29] and there is evidence that they may actually result from metaplastic transformation of anterior pituicytes.[4,32] This has led to suggestions that craniopharyngiomas may originate from metaplastic rather than embryonic elements.[4] Similar nests of squamous cells have occasionally been found in neonatal pituitary glands,[33] but at this age they would seem unlikely to be metaplastic in nature, and fetal or congenital cases of craniopharyngioma argue in favour of an embryological origin of the tumour in infants and young children.[15,16] One proposal resolving this dichotomy is that adult craniopharyngiomas derive from pituitary gland cells undergoing squamous metaplasia whilst the childhood tumours arise in embryological remnants of Rathke's cleft.[34] It is also possible that the squamous cell nests visible in normal glands do not give rise to craniopharyngiomas at all, and that even in adults the origin is from other, as yet unidentified elements persisting from the fetal stomatodeal-hypophyseal cleft of Rathke.[1] In keeping with this view are occasional reports of adult lesions which apparently show a transition between craniopharyngiomas and Rathke's cleft cysts, occupying both intra- and suprasellar compartments and lined by a mixture of stratified squamous and ciliated columnar epithelium.[35,36] Further evidence is provided by the rare finding of rudimentary tooth formation in otherwise typical examples of the tumour.[37,38] This suggests that the histological similarity between some craniopharyngiomas and the adamantinomas or ameloblastomas of the jaw may be more than fanciful, and that craniopharyngiomas perhaps arise from embryological elements which are misplaced from the stomatodeal end of Rathke's cleft, where ectoderm is present during development.[38,39]

Clinical features

In children, larger tumours commonly present with raised intracranial pressure caused by obstruction of cerebrospinal fluid (CSF) flow through the third ventricle.[9,34]

Growth retardation due to pituitary growth hormone deficiency is another typical feature of childhood craniopharyngiomas, and may antedate the final presentation by several years.[13,40] In adults, hydrocephalus and evidence of raised intracranial pressure are less often apparent than in childhood[9,20] and clinical evidence of pituitary or hypothalamic failure most often takes the form of menstrual disturbances, loss of libido or impotence.[12,20] Dementia or lesser degrees of intellectual impairment may also occur in adults with craniopharyngiomas, especially if the tumours are large.[20,34] Objective evidence of visual field impairment is common in all age groups, but often passes unnoticed by the patient, especially in childhood.[22,34] Unlike pituitary adenomas, craniopharyngiomas very rarely invade the skull base or cavernous sinuses, and cranial nerve palsies are not usually present except where very extensive tumours have grown into the posterior fossa.[9,11]

Radiology

Plain skull X-rays may show tumour calcification or erosion of the pituitary fossa, but are only abnormal in about three-quarters of cases.[11,14] Computerised tomography (CT) is the usual radiological investigation of choice, the three most diagnostic features being calcification, cyst formation and enhancement with contrast media[14,34] (Fig. 17.1). In cystic tumours, the cyst contents

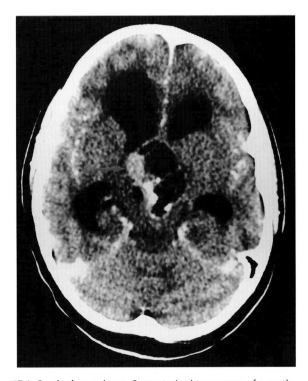

Fig. 17.1 **Craniopharyngioma.** Computerised tomogram of a partly cystic and partly solid tumour with dense flecks of calcification. The solid part of the tumour to one side of the cyst cavity is enhancing following administration of contrast medium (arrow).

are typically hypodense relative to CSF, and where it is present, contrast enhancement is confined to the cyst wall.[34,41] Magnetic resonance imaging (MRI) is very effective at defining the overall extent of the tumour, especially in the sagittal plane, but is less reliable than CT scanning for demonstration of calcification or cystic architecture.[42,43] Cystic areas have a very varied signal intensity in T1-weighted images,[43,44] although they more consistently show a high signal using T2-weighting.[42] Administration of gadolinium can help distinguish solid areas of tumour from cysts in some cases.[43]

Pathology

Macroscopic features

Craniopharyngiomas typically appear as lobulated tumours with a finely granular surface and a brown or greyish-pink colour. They vary greatly in size from less than 2 to over 15cm in maximum dimension, the larger lesions being more often found in children.[45] The smaller examples usually take the form of a dome-like mass sited over the diaphragma sellae, and may occasionally connect with the pituitary fossa via a dumbbell-like constriction at the level of the diaphragma. Larger tumours deeply invaginate the base of the brain in the interpeduncular region and produce considerable distortion of the optic chiasm, circle of Willis vessels and hypothalamic structures (Fig. 17.2). They may fill the third ventricle, extend anterolaterally into anterior or middle cranial fossa, or project caudally into the prepontine cistern and posterior fossa. The tumours have well defined, encapsulated, free surfaces, but they are nearly always

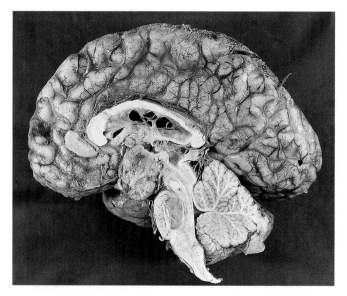

Fig. 17.2 **Craniopharyngioma.** This predominantly solid tumour is deeply invaginating the base of the brain and has a spongy cut surface flecked with calcification.

densely adherent to adjacent brain structures, from which they can be separated only with considerable difficulty. Cut section reveals very varied appearances depending on the architecture of the individual tumour. Well over half of craniopharyngiomas are entirely or predominantly cystic[11,14] and not uncommonly consist largely of a single, quite thin walled cystic cavity. Sometimes there are also areas of more solid tumour, which may appear spongy on cut section due to the presence of numerous smaller cystic spaces. Purely solid craniopharyngiomas are rather uncommon, and most likely to be encountered in adults with smaller tumours.[6,45] Craniopharyngioma cysts are typically filled by thick, brownish fluid which glistens due to the high cholesterol content and has been likened to engine lubricating oil. The cysts are either smooth walled or lined by numerous papillary projections of tumour tissue. Solid areas of tumour have a tough texture and are often flecked with yellow cholesterol deposits on cut section. They are also frequently gritty due to microcalcification and may sometimes contain larger areas of calcified material.

Intraoperative diagnosis

Where there is diagnostic doubt at the time of surgery, cyst fluid is not infrequently submitted for pathological analysis and can be most conveniently examined as a simple wet preparation using dark-ground optics. In most cases, fluid from a craniopharyngioma cyst examined in this way will be seen to contain cholesterol crystals with a typical notched, rhomboidal outline. Whilst not entirely specific, this finding is highly suggestive of craniopharyngioma, particularly if the site of the lesion and the oily macroscopic appearance of the fluid are taken into account. A similar examination can be carried out on cyst fluid obtained during drainage procedures performed prior to definitive surgery. Fine needle aspirate preparations can also be made from suitable pre- or intraoperative material[46] and may contain fragments of regular squamous epithelium in addition to macrophages and tissue debris. In the event of a more definitive tissue diagnosis being required at the time of surgery, frozen sections are likely to be needed, since the solid parts of craniopharyngioma are usually too tough to produce satisfactory smear preparations.

Histological features

The histological architecture of craniopharyngiomas varies widely, depending on the extent of cyst formation, the amount and configuration of stromal elements and the degree of degenerative change.

- *Solid areas of tumour* typically consist of broad anastamosing trabeculae or larger masses of epithelial tissue embedded in a collagenous matrix

(Fig. 17.3). The outermost layer of epithelial tissue abutting onto the connective tissue is formed from a basaloid palisade of columnar cells with central nuclei, often several cells in thickness. These are separated from the adjacent collagen by a continuous basement membrane. The arrangement is similar to that seen in the basal layer of the epidermis and has also been compared to that seen in odontogenic ameloblastoma. Towards the centre of larger epithelial masses, the cells are frequently arranged in looser sheets with a stellate outline and interconnecting cytoplasmic bridges like those in the prickle cell layer of normal epidermis (Fig. 17.4). There are often focal areas of squamous maturation, with compact whorls of keratinising cells and nodular masses of keratin. The tumour stroma consists of loose collagenous tissue in which there are

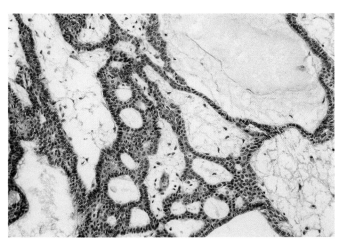

Fig. 17.3 **Craniopharyngioma.** The tumour consists of anastamosing cords of predominantly basaloid epithelial cells enclosing areas of loose collagenous matrix. H & E.

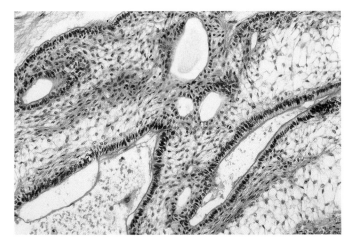

Fig. 17.4 **Craniopharyngioma.** The cells are forming basaloid palisades around small cystic spaces. Between these, there are looser sheets of stellate cells joined by tenuous cytoplasmic processes. H & E.

small blood vessels. Calcospherites are frequently present both in the epithelial and stromal areas, and there may be more extensive areas of calcification or even bone formation. Other common secondary changes include evidence of old and recent haemorrhage, collections of foamy macrophages and foreign-body giant cells, cholesterol clefts and patchy chronic inflammatory infiltrates.

• *Tumour cysts* are lined either by a simple layer of basaloid columnar cells or by stratified squamous epithelium of variable thickness. The cyst lining is again separated from the underlying collagenous tissue by a continuous basement membrane. The lining epithelium is often irregularly heaped up into solid masses of epithelial cells, sometimes incorporating buried foci of keratinisation or microcystic cavities (Fig. 17.5). The epithelium around larger cystic lumina may also show evidence of surface keratinisation, but there is no distinct granular cell layer like that seen in normal epidermis and epidermoid cysts, and intracytoplasmic keratohyaline granules are usually scarce. Not infrequently, the epithelial lining of cysts undergoes focal degeneration and is replaced by a granulomatous response consisting of foamy macrophages, giant cells, keratin masses and cholesterol clefts. The cyst lumina contain variable amounts of amorphous, eosinophilic, colloid-like material, often incorporating cholesterol clefts. There may also be separate masses of keratin, foamy macrophages and cell debris.

The WHO classification separately identifies cranio-pharyngiomas which show a predominantly papillary pattern, frequently with extensive squamous maturation, and those which have a mostly basaloid or 'adamantinous' arrangement.[3] The latter can be found in any age group, but a squamous-papillary pattern is most often encountered in adults.[6,7]

Where solid tumour or cyst walls abut onto brain, there is invariably a florid gliotic reaction with a broad surrounding zone of dense, fibrillar glial tissue and Rosenthal fibres. The histological margins of the tumour are not usually so well defined as they appear macroscopically, and there are often separate islands of tumour cells or masses of keratin embedded in the adjacent gliotic brain tissue (Fig. 17.6). Although this may give the appearance of tumour invasion, it should not be equated with true malignant change, which virtually never occurs in craniopharyngiomas. Mitoses are always very infrequent and despite peripheral budding of tumour into adjacent brain, most examples show no significant cytological pleomorphism. The few reports purporting to describe malignant transformation in craniopharyngioma have usually described locally recurrent or infiltrative behaviour without any specific cytological evidence of malignancy.[47,48] True carcinomatous change has occasionally been described in intracranial dermoid or epidermoid cysts, but these have only rarely been in a suprasellar location.[49] For practical purposes, it is therefore probably reasonable to regard craniopharyngiomas as lesions which are locally infiltrative but cytologically benign.[4]

Immunocytochemistry

The epithelial areas of craniopharyngiomas react variably and rather patchily with antibodies to cytokeratin,

depending on the molecular weight specificity of the reagents used. The staining reaction is strongest in focal areas of keratinous differentiation, and the outer basaloid cell layers of cysts and solid tumour lobules are unstained[50] (Fig. 17.7). In our hands, craniopharyngiomas also express epithelial membrane antigen and carcinoembryonic antigen, but the staining is more limited than with cytokeratin antibodies, and is usually confined to keratinous nests and the innermost surface of cyst walls. There is no immunocytochemical expression of the normal beta subunit of S-100 protein, but positive staining has been reported with an antibody to the alpha subunit.[51]

Fig. 17.5 **Cystic craniopharyngioma.** The cyst is lined by an irregular layer of partly stratified epithelium, incorporating smaller cystic spaces and nodular masses of keratin. H & E.

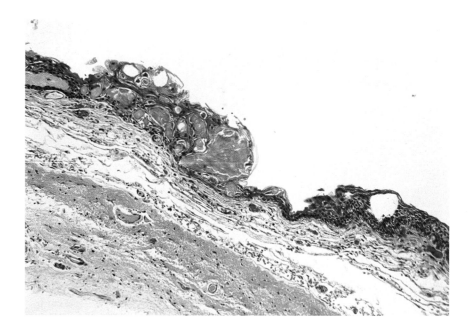

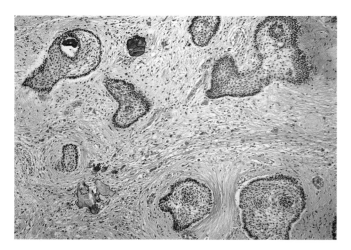

Fig. 17.6 **Craniopharyngioma.** Adjacent to the main tumour mass there are separate islands of tumour deeply embedded in gliotic brain tissue.

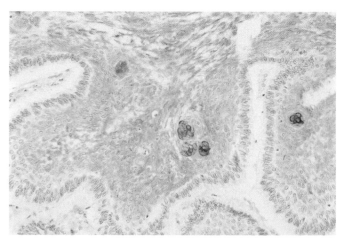

Fig. 17.7 **Craniopharyngioma.** Several small focal areas of squamous differentiation are strongly stained using immunocytochemistry for cytokeratin. Looser areas of tumour are only weakly reactive and the basaloid palisades are unstained. CAM5.2 antibody.

Electron microscopy

Ultrastructurally, the peripheral basaloid cells are separated from adjacent connective tissue elements by an intact basement membrane, and form a closely packed layer with little intervening intercellular space.[52,53] The cells are compact and polygonal in these marginal areas and there are abundant desmosome junctions. Towards the centre of the epithelial masses, the cells become stellate in outline and are joined to each other by long, tenuous cytoplasmic processes terminating in desmosome junctions (Fig. 17.8). These processes enclose large pockets of extracellular space and are covered by a broad, irregular layer of amorphous material which lacks the compact organisation of basement membrane.[53,54] In both areas, the cell cytoplasm is relatively electron dense and contains abundant 5 nm diameter tonofilaments. These are often arranged in well defined, separate bundles, which are the ultrastructural equivalent of keratohyaline granules[53,54] (Fig. 17.8). Keratinising foci are formed from disintegrating cells with an increased density of cytoplasmic tonofilaments.[52] Where mineralisation is taking place, the degenerating keratinised cells initially show hydroxyapatite crystal deposition within membrane bound vesicles.[55] These subsequently fuse with adjacent bundles of tonofilaments to form large, electron dense calcified masses. Small tumour cysts are lined by flattened epithelial cells which may bear microvilli on their luminal surfaces.[53,54] The cyst cavities typically contain cell debris and fibrillar material embedded in an electron dense matrix.

Tissue culture

Craniopharyngiomas show vigorous outgrowth in tissue and organ culture, producing epithelial sheets of well defined, polygonal cells joined by desmosomes.[56,57] The marginal layer of these cell sheets shows the same palisaded, basaloid arrangement as that seen in histological sections.[57,58] The cultured cells also retain the capacity to produce keratin nests and cystic cavities.[56,57] One study has described a more disorderly growth pattern in some craniopharyngiomas, with abundant microvilli and increased mitoses, and has correlated this with clinical evidence of a more aggressive growth pattern in the parent tumours.[58]

Differential diagnosis

Suprasellar epidermoid cyst

Many authors do not consider that there are sufficient grounds to justify distinction between cystic craniopharyngiomas and suprasellar epidermoid cysts[4,11] but there is controversy over this issue.[59] True epidermoid cysts are not generally considered to be neoplastic lesions, tend to occur in older age groups and show a slower natural progression than most craniopharyngiomas.[59] In pathological terms, however, there is considerable overlap between the two entities and there are no absolute distinguishing features. In general, epidermoid cysts are more likely to have solid, flaky keratinous contents rather than the oily fluid typical of craniopharyngiomas. Epidermoid cysts also tend to have a more uniform architecture with prominent squamous maturation than craniopharyngioma cysts and there is typically a distinct granular cell layer, like that in normal epidermis. It should nevertheless be acknowledged that there is a pathological spectrum between the two entities and it is probably unwise to attempt separate identification of a suprasellar epidermoid cyst in any but the most obvious cases.

Teratoma

Germ cell neoplasms of all types are common in the suprasellar region, especially in younger individuals, and well differentiated teratomas may be confused with craniopharyngiomas if they contain a prominent squamous

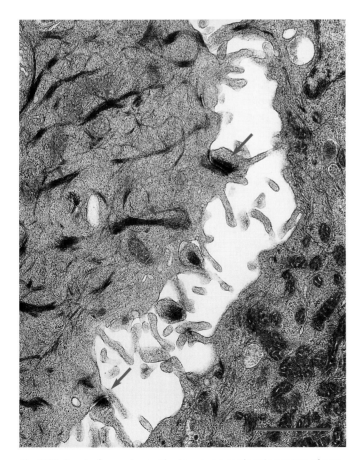

Fig. 17.8 **Craniopharyngioma.** The tenuous cytoplasmic process of two adjacent stellate tumour cells are joined to each other by desmosome junctions (arrows). Compact bundles of 5 nm cytoplasmic tonofilaments are present in one cell (arrow heads). Electron micrograph. Bar = 1 μm.

element. Craniopharyngiomas are purely squamous epithelial neoplasms, however, and the presence of recognisable tumour elements derived from mesodermal, endodermal or other ectodermal cell lines is in itself usually sufficient to distinguish a benign teratoma. The exception to this is the presence of tooth-like formations, since these may occur in otherwise typical craniopharyngiomas. In the case of less well differentiated teratoid neoplasms, distinction from craniopharyngioma may be helped by immunocytochemical staining with antibodies to human chorionic gonadotropin or alpha-fetoprotein.

Pituitary adenoma

This should be included as a differential diagnosis in tumours with an intrasellar component, especially if the lesion is solid and shows a predominantly basaloid or papillary architecture. Small nests of keratinising cells can be found in normal and neoplastic pituitary tissue, but the presence of more extensive squamous maturation and keratinisation is usually sufficient to identify craniopharyngiomas, even if they are entirely intrasellar in location. Immunocytochemical staining for cytokeratin may produce a positive result in either tumour, but expression of chromogranin or neuron specific enolase is only to be expected in pituitary adenomas. Antibodies to anterior gland hormones may also be helpful unless the pituitary tumour is entirely non-secretory.

Pilocytic astrocytoma

The broad zone of gliosis in brain tissue around craniopharyngiomas may have a histological appearance similar to that of juvenile pilocytic astrocytomas of the third ventricle region. Such gliotic tissue may comprise all or most of an attempted craniopharyngioma biopsy, especially if the tumour is predominantly cystic and the epithelial parts of the tumour have been destroyed by degenerative changes. The presence of cholesterol granulomas or keratin intermingled with the glial elements should arouse suspicion of a craniopharyngioma, and prompt a careful search through all the available biopsied tissue for epithelial elements. If cyst fluid is sampled, the oily liquid found in most craniopharyngiomas can usually be distinguished from the golden yellow proteinaceous contents of low grade astrocytoma cysts, which clots at room temperature and does not contain cholesterol crystals.

Metastatic carcinoma

Solitary metastases from unsuspected systemic malignancies are well documented in the sellar region and may be mistaken for a solid craniopharyngioma, especially if the primary tumour is a squamous carcinoma. Positive identification of such a metastasis will rely principally on the presence of histological and cytological features of malignancy, since these are virtually unknown in craniopharyngiomas.

Choroid plexus papilloma

Especially in younger age groups, these need to be considered in the differential diagnosis of those solid craniopharyngiomas which lie mostly or wholly within the third ventricle. The main histological distinguishing features of choroid plexus tumours are the orderly perivascular architecture of the papillary formations and the absence of stratified squamous differentiation or keratinisation. In difficult cases, immunocytochemical staining with antibodies to carbonic anhydrase C or transthyretin will help to identify positively a choroid plexus tumour.

Glioependymal cyst

Ependymal lined cysts of the third ventricle region can appear macroscopically similar to purely cystic craniopharyngiomas of suprasellar location, although the oily contents of craniopharyngiomas will contrast with the CSF-like fluid of glial cysts. Histologically, ependymal cysts can be readily distinguished by the paucity of surrounding connective tissue, the lack of stratified squamous elements and the presence of cilia on the luminal surface of the epithelium. Unlike craniopharyngiomas, the lining epithelium of ependymal cysts stains with antibodies to glial fibrillary acidic protein (GFAP) but not cytokeratin.

Therapy

Craniopharyngiomas are biologically benign lesions and therapy has traditionally been aimed at total surgical excision,[60,61] especially in children where radiotherapy may be less acceptable.[62,63] A trans-sphenoidal approach can be effective where tumour occupies the pituitary fossa, but is normally only undertaken in cases where there is sellar enlargement and only a small suprasellar component.[64,65] Larger suprasellar tumours are normally approached by a variety of transcranial routes, depending on their location and extent.[12,34] Attempts at total surgical removal of craniopharyngiomas have been greatly aided by modern microsurgical techniques,[66,67] but despite this complete excision is often not possible,[12,68] and where the tumours are large or awkwardly sited, an elective subtotal procedure may be better than risking damage to hypothalamic structures.[69] There is now little doubt that craniopharyngiomas are radiosensitive lesions[70,71] and most authorities recommend postoperative radiation therapy in cases where complete excision has not been possible or if the tumour recurs clinically.[71,72] The effectiveness of external radiotherapy has also led to suggestions that it should be given even where a radical removal of the tumour has been accomplished.[11,12]

For predominantly cystic craniopharyngiomas, simple drainage of the cyst contents may be effective in reducing pressure symptoms, both prior to surgery and in cases with cystic recurrence.[73,74] Cystic craniopharyngiomas have also been treated by instillation of a variety of radioisotopes directly into the cyst cavity, usually via a reservoir drainage system.[75,76] The clinical follow-up in these patients has been encouraging, with a high long term survival rate and radiological evidence of significant cyst shrinkage in a majority of cases.[77,78] It should be noted, however, that any solid areas of tumour are not affected by this form of treatment, and may enlarge sufficiently to necessitate subsequent surgery or external beam radiotherapy.[75,79]

Acute postoperative complications include diabetes insipidus,[12,80] Addisonian crisis[34,81] and a variety of hypothalamic disturbances.[34,82] In the longer term, the most common clinical problem in children is growth retardation and short stature, often necessitating long term growth hormone replacement therapy.[83,84] Adults also have an increased incidence of hypopituitary syndromes compared to their preoperative state,[9,85] and persistence of preoperative visual defects is common in both adults and children.[9]

Prognosis

The overall rate of tumour recurrence varies between 20% and 40% in different reported series,[60,86] but is dependent on the nature of the primary therapy. Clinical relapse due to further tumour growth is most likely after partial resection alone, and may be expected to occur in nearly all such cases within 10 years.[63,87] There is evidence that recurrence occurs less often in patients where the primary treatment has included radiotherapy, even if surgical intervention consists only of subtotal decompression.[87,88] Recurrences are said to be more likely in craniopharyngiomas with a largely basaloid or 'adamantinous' histological pattern compared to those adult tumours which show predominantly squamous epithelial differentiation.[6,89]

The best survival figures have been obtained in patients undergoing successful radical removal of tumour, with over 90% of cases surviving 5 years.[87,90] In some studies this figure has diminished after 5 years due to delayed tumour recurrences, but long term patient survival is clearly improved when postoperative radiotherapy is given. Patients receiving radiotherapy have shown 10-year survival rates of over 70% regardless of the extent of surgery, contrasting with figures of less than 50% for those undergoing surgery alone.[72,91] The site and size of craniopharyngiomas also affects their prognosis, and poorer results may be expected with lesions in a retrochiasmatic location,[9] or greater than 3 cm in maximum dimension.[11]

Nervous system cysts

The central nervous system is host to a wide variety of cysts of differing morphology and aetiology. Some are the result of a primary neoplastic process, as for example with the cysts typically associated with haemangioblastomas, craniopharyngiomas or astrocytomas, and these are discussed separately in the appropriate chapters concerned. Non-neoplastic cysts of the craniospinal axis can result from parasitic infections, notably cystercycosis and hydatid disease, or follow severe perinatal ischaemic insults. They may also form part of a complex malformation, such as a meningocele or the Dandy Walker syndrome. Such lesions are beyond the scope of this book. In addition, however, there is a group of non-neoplastic cysts which are mostly of congenital origin but can occur in the absence of other maldevelopmental abnormalities (Table 17.2). Cysts of this type may sometimes come to light incidentally during routine radiological investigation or at post-mortem examination, but they can also present clinically as space occupying lesions. Most of them are listed by the WHO under the heading 'Cysts and tumour-like lesions', although arachnoid, pineal, choroid plexus and perineurial cysts are not individually specified in that classification.[92]

Rathke's cleft cysts

Incidence and site

Small and asymptomatic cystic remnants of Rathke's cleft are a relatively common incidental finding in otherwise normal adult pituitary glands, and have been reported in up to one-quarter of glands sampled in some post-mortem series.[93,94] Larger, symptomatic cysts are very rare by comparison.[95,96] A review in 1991 found only 155 documented cases in the literature.[97] The age at presentation of these cysts has varied from the second to the eighth decade, with a mean in the fourth decade.[98,99] Females are more commonly affected than males.[97] The majority of symptomatic cysts are intrasellar lesions with a significant suprasellar extension, although some cases

---

Table 17.2 Primary non-neoplastic cysts of the nervous system
1. Rathke's cleft cyst
2. Epidermoid cyst
3. Dermoid cyst
4. Colloid cyst of the third ventricle
5. Enterogenous cyst
6. Neuroglial cyst
7. Congenital arachnoid cyst
8. Pineal cyst
9. Choroid plexus cyst
10. Perineurial cyst

remain confined by the sellar margins.[99,100] In a small proportion of cases, the cyst may also be entirely suprasellar in location, lying above a normal or compressed pituitary fossa.[98,101]

Aetiology

Rathke's cleft is a blind-ended evagination of the ectodermally- lined stomatodeum, which grows up to meet the primitive diencephalic vesicle during early embryogenesis, and subsequently differentiates into the elements of the anterior pituitary gland.[97,102] The original connection with the stomatodeum is lost, but fragments of the cleft persist in adults as microscopic cystic structures, mostly sited between the anterior and posterior lobes of the mature gland. These are lined by a similar epithelium to that of large Rathke's cleft cysts, and are considered by most authorities to be the origin of these larger, symptomatic cysts.[97,102] Cysts which are entirely suprasellar in location are similarly presumed to arise from remnants of Rathke's cleft which persist above the level of the diaphragma in the pituitary stalk.[97,98]

Some dissenting authors have proposed a neuro-epithelial origin for Rathke's cleft cysts, largely on the basis of histological similarities with colloid cysts and patchy immunocytochemical expression of GFAP,[103,104] but the frequent presence of squamous epithelial elements is generally quoted as a point of clear distinction from both colloid cysts and lesions of known neuroepithelial derivation.[105,106] Occasional examples of Rathke's cleft cyst exhibit a very prominent stratified squamous component, usually lying beneath the more typical lining epithelium, and this has been interpreted as evidence of a close aetiological relationship between cranio-pharyngiomas and Rathke's cleft cysts.[107,108] Even if both lesions share a common origin in embryological remnants of the fetal stomatodeal cleft, however, their subsequent differentiation is quite distinct, and in particular true neoplasia is not a feature of Rathke's cleft cysts.[108]

Clinical features

In adults, symptomatic Rathke's cleft cysts most commonly present with headache, pituitary dysfunction and visual field loss.[99,109] Larger lesions may also cause hypothalamic disturbances such as diabetes insipidus or lethargy.[95,110] Rarely, the clinical history may be that of recurrent episodes of aseptic meningitis due to cyst leakage into the subarachnoid space[111] and presentation as a bacterial abscess has also been reported.[102] Children most commonly present as pituitary dwarfs with failure of development of secondary sex characteristics.[99,110]

Radiology

Skull X-rays and CT show evidence of enlargement or erosion of the pituitary fossa in most cases of symptomatic Rathke's cleft cyst.[99,102] The lesions are typically hypo- or isodense to brain on CT scans and may be unenhanced following administration of contrast media or show only a thin ring of capsular enhancement.[99,112] Using MRI, different cysts have a very variable signal intensity using either T1- or T2-weighted images, and there may be considerable signal heterogeneity within individual lesions.[100,112]

Pathology

Macroscopic features

Small, asymptomatic cysts are mostly less than 5 mm in diameter and usually only become apparent if the pituitary gland is sectioned at autopsy.[93,94] About half such cases are less than 0.5 mm in size and may not be visible at all on naked eye examination.[94,113] Most symptomatic cysts are usually between 1 and 3 cm in maximum dimension.[100,114] On removing the brain at autopsy they typically appear as a smooth, glistening membrace bulging up through the diaphragma into the suprasellar region from the pituitary fossa. The intrasellar portion of smaller cysts is usually found embedded in the superior part of the gland, at the base of the infundibular stalk, but larger examples may appear to obliterate the pituitary gland entirely. The cyst wall is thin and translucent, and the contents may consist of opalescent mucous, clear colourless fluid, altered blood, or creamy purulent material.[102]

Histological features

The lining epithelium usually consists of columnar or cuboidal cells, which may be stratified in places and bear apical cilia or have a goblet cell appearance (Fig. 17.9). Beneath this is a sparse connective tissue layer in which

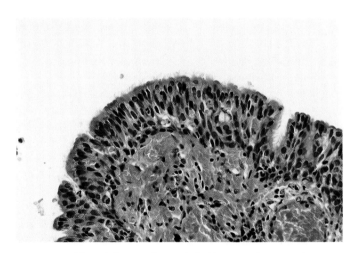

Fig. 17.9 **Rathke's cleft cyst.** The epithelial lining in this example consists of stratified columnar cells with apical cilia bordering the luminal surface. H & E.

simple gland-like structures may sometimes be embedded.[115] Using periodic acid–Schiff (PAS) and Alcian blue stains, mucin can be demonstrated both in the epithelial cell cytoplasm and over the apical surfaces of the cells. Particularly in larger examples, there may also be areas of stratified squamous epithelium with 'prickle cell' intercellular bridges. This is most often seen in the suprasellar part of a cyst and is often covered by a layer of ciliated columnar epithelium[115,116] (Fig. 17.10). Keratinisation is not seen. In some cases, the epithelial lining is extensively destroyed, leaving areas with only a thin connective tissue layer.

Immunocytochemistry

The typical cuboidal or columnar epithelial cells of Rathke's cleft cysts express both simple and complex type cytokeratins[117,118] and epithelial membrane antigen.[119] In many examples, and especially in smaller, asymptomatic cysts, there are occasional epithelial cells which coexpress GFAP and S-100 protein in addition to cytokeratin.[118,120]

Cells staining immunocytochemically with an antibody to carcinoembryonic antigen have also been reported.[119] The cells lining microscopic cystic remnants of Rathke's cleft often stain using antibodies to the anterior pituitary gland hormones, but this has not been found in the epithelium of larger symptomatic cysts.[116]

Electron microscopy

Ultrastructurally, the columnar epithelial cells either bear abundant apical cilia or have a goblet cell appearance, with luminal-surface microvilli and numerous membrane-bound secretory granules in the apical area of cytoplasm.[106,121] These cells are joined by lateral junctional complexes.[106] In addition, electron microscopy has confirmed the presence of true squamous cells, with cytoplasmic tonofilaments, desmosomes and intercellular bridges.[106,121] Small, wedge shaped basal cells abutting the epithelial basement membrane have also been described, and the overall ultrastructural appearance of the epithelium has been likened to that of sphenoid air sinus mucosa.[121]

Differential diagnosis

Craniopharyngioma

The distinction of Rathke's cleft cysts from purely cystic craniopharyngiomas or suprasellar epidermoid cysts is important in prognostic terms, and may necessitate frozen sections at the time of surgery. The main distinguishing features of Rathke's cleft cysts are the presence of ciliated or mucus-producing epithelium and the lack of keratinisation or horny pearl formation in stratified squamous areas.

Pituitary cysts

Significant and symptomatic cystic change in the anterior pituitary gland or its adenomas usually follows infarction or haemorrhage, and the cavities lack any epithelial lining.[122] Distinction from smaller Rathke's cleft cysts entirely embedded within the gland or an adenoma may also be helped by the presence of old blood pigment or cholesterol granuloma material.

Teratoma and dermoid cyst

The presence of a well differentiated cystic teratoma should be suspected if complex glandular formations or mesenchymal elements such as muscle or cartilage are present in the wall of the cyst. A dermoid cyst may similarly be distinguished by the presence of hairs or dermal adnexal structures beneath the epithelium, always bearing in mind that stratified squamous epithelium may be quite extensive in the suprasellar portion of some larger Rathke's cleft cysts.

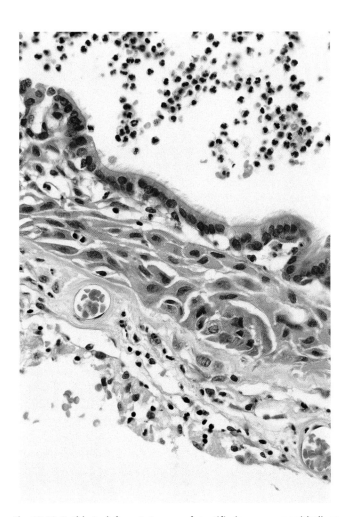

Fig. 17.10 **Rathke's cleft cyst.** A zone of stratified squamous epithelium lies beneath the luminal layer of ciliated columnar epithelium. H & E.

Arachnoid cyst

Arachnoid cysts may occur in a suprasellar location, sometimes with an intrasellar component as part of an 'empty sella syndrome'. Their walls consist of a membrane similar to normal arachnoid tissue and there is no epithelial lining comparable to that seen in Rathke's cleft cysts. It should be remembered, however, that the lining epithelium of Rathke's cysts can undergo extensive degeneration, leaving only a collagenous wall in some places.

Mucocele

Mucoceles of the sphenoid sinus may occasionally erode upwards into the sella or even suprasellar region, and both the macroscopic appearance of their contents and the histological features of the lining epithelium can be indistinguishable from those of Rathke's cleft cysts. Distinction between the two entities relies on radiographic or surgical evidence of their topographical extent, since Rathke's cleft cysts do not usually grow downwards through the sellar floor into adjacent air sinuses.

Therapy and prognosis

Rathke's cleft cysts are indolent, non-neoplastic lesions which enlarge very slowly with time. Once a craniopharyngioma has been excluded, conservative therapy is advocated by most authorities.[114,123] This consists of simple drainage of the cyst and biopsy or partial excision of the wall, usually via a trans-sphenoidal approach.[99,109] There is typically a rapid resolution of signs and symptoms following this procedure.[114,124] The prognosis for recovery of visual field defects is particularly encouraging, with significant improvement or a return to normal in a majority of cases.[123] Pituitary gland dysfunction may also resolve postoperatively, although in a rather smaller proportion of cases.[109] Even where there has been only simple biopsy of the cyst wall, clinical recurrences are very rare and may take over two decades to develop.[125,126] Where the cyst does reaccumulate sufficiently to cause symptoms, the patients respond well to a second drainage operation.[95,127] Aseptic meningitis due to contamination of CSF pathways by the cyst contents is a rare postoperative complication, and can usually be avoided if a trans-sphenoidal surgical approach is used.[96,128]

Epidermoid cysts

Incidence and site

Intracranial epidermoid cysts account for only 1% of all intracranial tumours if suprasellar examples are excluded.[105,129] Those occurring in the suprasellar region are generally regarded as a variant of craniopharyngioma,[130] although some authors advocate making a distinction between the two entities.[131] Aside from the sellar region, the cerebellopontine angles are by far the most common intracranial site for epidermoid cysts.[132] Less frequently, they may also occur in the cerebral hemispheres, the lateral ventricles, other major CSF cisterns at the base of the brain and in the orbits.[132,133] Unlike dermoid cysts, epidermoid cysts often occur laterally, without a particular preference for midline sites.[133]

In addition to those occurring within the cranial cavity, epidermoid cysts may also involve the bones of the middle ear region or the cranial vault.[134,135] The cranial vault examples are widely distributed and again not confined to the midline.[122] They most typically occur in the frontal bones either side of the sagittal suture and may be totally intraosseus, internal, external or dumb-bell in their extent.[135] All except the purely external examples may encroach on the cranial cavity.[136]

Epidermoid cysts are relatively rare in the spine and usually occur in thoracic or lumbar regions, with less of a predilection for the lumbosacral area than dermoid cysts (Table 17.3).[132,137] They may be intra- or extramedullary in location.[132]

Craniospinal epidermoid cysts present in a wide variety of age groups, but are most commonly diagnosed in young or middle aged adulthood.[132,138] Males are more commonly affected than females.[137,139]

Aetiology

Most craniospinal epidermoid cysts are presumed to arise from inclusion of embryonic ectodermal elements occurring during closure of the primitive neural groove or the more laterally placed secondary cerebral vesicles.[133,135] In distinction from dermoid cysts, this ectodermal sequestration is thought to occur at a relatively late point of embryogenesis, when the incorporated elements have already undergone a degree of epidermal differentiation.[137] Epidermoid cysts in the petrous bone, or so-called 'cholesteatomas', have traditionally been regarded as a separate entity, resulting from reactive inward growth of epithelial elements following chronic mastoid or middle ear infection.[133,140] In some cases, however, lesions at this site are deep seated without any evidence of previous suppurative disease, and a proportion may well be of similar congenital aetiology to those occurring elsewhere.[134,141] A history of previous penetrating trauma[142,143] or multiple lumbar punctures[144,145] has led to suggestions that some spinal epidermoid cysts may result from mechanical implantation of skin fragments into the spinal canal. Support for this theory comes from an animal study where epidermoid cysts were produced experimentally following implantation of skin into the neuraxis of rats.[146] Some authors have gone so far as to propose that spinal epidermoid cysts can be divided into two groups:

Table 17.3 Non-neoplastic cysts of the spine

	Preferred site	Histology	Other features
Epidermoid cyst	Thoracolumbar Posterior Intradural Intra/extramedullary	Keratinising stratified squamous epithelium	Rare compared with intracranial examples
Dermoid cyst	Lumbosacral Posterior Intradural Intra/extramedullary	Stratified squamous epithelium Poor maturation Dermal appendages	Commonly associated with posterior spina bifida
Enterogenous cyst	Cervical/upper thoracic Anterior or lateral Intradural Extramedullary	Cuboidal or columnar epithelium Mucin and goblet cells Rarely complex gastrointestinal mucosa	May be associated with anterior spinal defect or other vertebral anomaly
Neuroglial cyst	Any level Anterior or lateral Intradural Extramedullary	Cuboid or ciliated columnar ependymal epithelium	
Congenital arachnoid cyst	Thoracic Posterior Intra- or extradural Extramedullary	No epithelium Arachnoid membrane	Also acquired cysts due to adhesive arachnoiditis, usually lumbosacral
Perineurial cyst	Posterior sacral root At junction with dura	No epithelium Collagen and root tissue	Often an incidental finding

those where an associated malformation such as spina bifida indicates an embryonic origin of the cyst, and those where the history indicates that a traumatic or iatrogenic aetiology may be more likely.[142,147]

Associated lesions

A proportion of spinal epidermoid cysts, especially those in the lumbosacral region, occur in conjunction with spina bifida or other congenital abnormalities such as diastematomyelia.[142,147] Communication with the skin surface via a dermal sinus may also occur in some spinal and posterior fossa examples, although less consistently than with dermoid cysts.[142,148]

Clinical features

Patients with intracranial epidermoid cysts typically have a long history and gradual onset of symptoms, with headache and seizures as the most consistent complaints.[129,133] Suprasellar cysts usually present in a similar manner to craniopharyngiomas, with visual defects and pituitary or hypothalamic dysfunction, while cerebellopontine angle lesions may cause ataxia, nystagmus or palsies of the fifth to the eighth cranial nerves.[133,149] Less commonly, the presentation may involve recurrent episodes of aseptic meningitis due to leakage of cyst contents into the CSF pathways.[133,149] Epidermoid cysts in the petrous bone usually present as slowly progressive unilateral facial palsy, sometimes accompanied by deafness, and may

have no history of previous mastoid infection or otitis media.[141] Cysts in the cranial vault bones typically manifest as a painless, fluctuant scalp mass, but may be associated with headache or focal neurological signs if there is intracranial extension.[135,149]

Radiology

Using CT scans, intracranial and spinal epidermoid cysts are usually visible as non-homogeneous, hypodense lesions which do not enhance after administration of contrast media and have irregular, rather poorly defined margins.[139,150] The attenuation is often similar to that of CSF, and CT scans are generally rather poor at defining the precise margins of the lesion.[150] MRI is probably better at delineating the extent of the cysts, which have a signal intensity similar to fat on both T1- and T2-weighted images[139] (Fig. 17.11). Cranial vault cysts typically appear as rounded, well defined lytic defects with a sclerotic border on plain X-rays of the skull, and may be picked up as an incidental finding if they are small and mostly intraosseus.[135]

Pathology

Macroscopic features

Epidermoid cysts vary in size from a few millimetres to over 10 cm in diameter and have a characteristic macroscopic appearance, which often allows a diagnosis to be made on naked eye examination alone. They are rounded and slightly fluctuant masses with a smooth whitish capsule. This has a typical shining, silky appearance which has been compared to mother-of-pearl, and is often densely adherent to adjacent nervous tissue, dura or bone. It can be very thin in places and is easily torn in the most attenuated areas. The cysts are usually entirely filled by lamellated flakes of keratin which are pearly white with a friable, waxy texture (Fig. 17.12). They may be arranged in strikingly concentric layers, like an onion skin. The centre of larger cysts is sometimes degenerate, the keratin flakes being replaced by greasy brownish fluid.

Histological features

The cysts are lined by keratinising stratified squamous epithelium which forms well defined germinal, prickle cell, granular and corneal layers similar to those of normal skin. Lamellated keratin covers the innermost corneal layer and fills the cyst lumen. The epithelium rests on an outer layer of collagen, which is often very thin and does not contain glands or dermal appendages (Fig. 17.13). Calcification is uncommon. The collagen is usually closely applied to adjacent bone, meninges or brain. There is often a patchy chronic inflammatory infiltrate around the outer aspect of the capsule, and adjacent neural tissue almost always shows a zone of dense gliosis with Rosenthal fibres. In some larger cysts, there may be focal degeneration of the epithelial lining, and extruded keratin can extend deeply

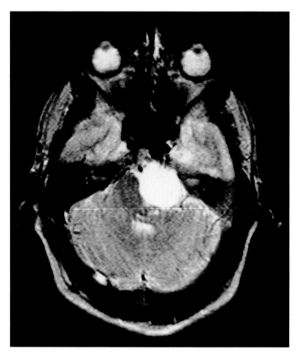

Fig. 17.11 **Epidermoid cyst in the cerebellopontine angle.** Horizontal T2-weighted magnetic resonance scan showing a well circumscribed lesion with high signal intensity, similar to that of fat.

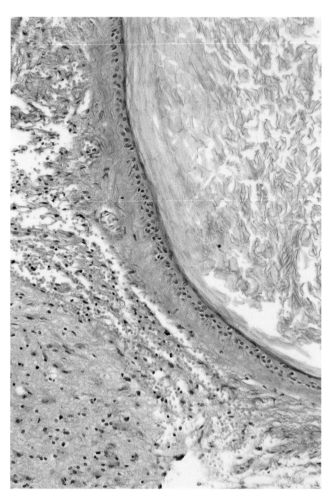

Fig. 17.13 **Epidermoid cyst in the cerebellopontine angle.** Lamellated collagen fills the cyst cavity (top right). The stratified squamous epithelial lining rests on a thin layer of collagen. Van Gieson.

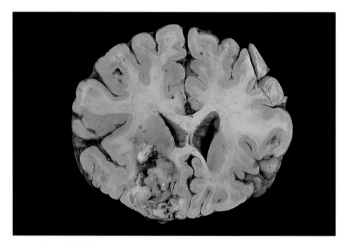

Fig. 17.12 **Epidermoid cyst.** This frontal lobe cyst contains nodular masses of pearly white keratin, which have ruptured out into the surrounding brain.

into adjacent brain or cord. A granulomatous reaction with foreign-body giant cells may be present in such areas, but in some cases isolated masses of leaked keratin may appear inertly embedded in gliotic brain without a significant inflammatory response. Where there has been significant cyst leakage into the CSF pathways, however, the leptomeninges nearly always show a widespread and florid inflammatory reaction including giant cells.

Immunocytochemistry

Most craniospinal epidermoid cysts show rather patchy and inconsistent staining reaction using antibodies to cytokeratins and epithelial membrane antigen (EMA). Where it is present, the expression of these antigens is usually restricted to the most superficial layer of the cyst epithelium. In contrast to cysts of neuroglial origin there is no immunoreactivity of the lining epithelium with antibodies to GFAP.

Malignant change

Malignant transformation of craniospinal epidermoid cysts is exceptionally rare, but there have been a number of reports of squamous carcinoma arising in histologically proven benign cysts. In some of these, a typical epidermoid cyst has been previously excised at the same site, often several years or even decades previously.[151,152] In other cases, often with a long clinical history, surgery at first presentation has revealed an epidermoid cyst containing focal areas of carcinoma.[153,154] In both instances, the patients have typically been middle aged males, and the lesions have been mostly sited in the cranial vault bones or the cerebellopontine angles.[151,155] In most cases, the squamous malignancies have been locally infiltrative and rapidly growing lesions, but distant metastases have not been reported.[152,154]

Differential diagnosis

Craniopharyngioma

The distinction of suprasellar epidermoid cysts from cystic craniopharyngiomas is often not considered justified, either on clinical or pathological grounds (see also p. 515).[105,130] Some authorities, however, maintain that epidermoid cysts at this site are slower growing lesions, more likely to occur in adults and to contain solid lamellated keratin than true craniopharyngiomas.[131] Histologically, there is considerable overlap between the two entities, but typical epidermoid cysts tend to have a more uniform epithelial architecture with a distinct granular cell layer and more orderly maturation/keratinisation.[131]

Teratoma and dermoid cyst

Epidermoid cysts are purely squamous epithelial lesions and a well differentiated teratoma should be suspected if there are any other tissues present in the cyst wall, such as glandular epithelium, cartilage or other mesenchymal elements. In the same way, a dermoid cyst can be distinguished by the presence of hairs or dermal appendages in the subepithelial connective tissue.

Metastatic carcinoma

Although malignant transformation may occur in craniospinal epidermoid cysts, it is exceptionally rare and for practical purposes the possibility of a metastatic squamous carcinoma must be considered if the lesion shows any evidence of cytological atypia or epithelial invasion of adjacent structures.

Enterogenous cyst

Spinal epidermoid cysts can usually be easily distinguished from enterogenous cysts by the exclusively stratified squamous nature of their lining epithelium. In some enterogenous cysts the glandular or ciliated lining can undergo squamous metaplasia, but this is usually focal and areas of more typical epithelium can nearly always be identified.

Colloid and neuroglial cysts

Neither colloid cysts or neuroglial cysts show evidence of squamous metaplasia and in most cases epidermoid cysts can again be easily identified by their squamous lining and keratinisation. If the epithelium is very attenuate, negative immunocytochemical staining for GFAP may help exclude a neuroglial cyst.

Therapy and prognosis

The ideal treatment for craniospinal epidermoid cysts is complete surgical removal,[139,156] but in many cases dense adherence of the capsule to adjacent brain, vessels, cord or nerve roots makes an attempt at radical resection of the cyst wall hazardous and unwise.[133,157] In such cases, surgery is probably best limited to removal of the keratinous contents, and partial stripping of the capsule where it is not stuck to vital structures.[133,156] Most cranial vault cysts, however, may be entirely resected quite safely unless there is significant intracranial extension.[135,136] Radiotherapy has no effect on residual cyst wall and symptomatic recurrences require further surgical debulking of the cyst contents.[135,156]

The most frequent postoperative complication following resection of intradural epidermoid cysts is a chemical meningitis due to leakage of keratin into the CSF pathways at the time of surgery.[139,158] In some cases this may produce long term meningeal scarring and hydrocephalus requiring CSF shunt insertion.[133] For patients surviving the postoperative period, the long term prognosis is generally good. Symptomatic recurrences are rare and usually delayed for many years, even when excision of the cyst wall has been incomplete.[139,149]

Dermoid cysts

Incidence and site

Dermoid cysts are less common in the cranial cavity than epidermoid cysts and have been estimated to comprise only about 0.3% of all intracranial tumours.[105,133] They are much more likely to occur at midline sites and are most frequent in the posterior fossa.[133,159] Like epidermoid cysts, they can also arise in the orbit, often with intracranial extension.[160,161] Dermoid cysts of the cranial vault are again usually in a midline location, and are encountered less often than intraosseus epidermoid cysts.[135] Subgaleal examples over the anterior fontanelle region typically present in childhood.[162,163] In the spine, dermoid cysts are more common than epidermoid ones and are nearly always sited in the lumbosacral region (Table 17.3).[137,164] In general, craniospinal dermoid cysts present at an earlier age than epidermoid cysts, the majority being diagnosed in children or young adults.[133,137]

Aetiology

Most dermoid cysts are presumed to have a similar aetiology to epidermoid cysts, arising from ectodermal elements which become sequestrated within the medullary folds or secondary cerebral vesicles of the developing neural tube as it closes during embryogensis.[105,137] It has been postulated that the entrapment of the ectodermal cells occurs at an earlier stage of embryogensis than those giving rise to epidermoid cysts, when they are still pluripotential cells capable of differentiating into both epidermal and dermal elements.[105] In rare cases, spinal dermoid cysts have manifested some years after surgical closure of myelomeningoceles in infants, leading to suggestions that some cases may be derived from iatrogenically implanted or inadequately excised dermal elements.[165,166] Dermoid cysts have also been produced by experimental neuraxial skin implantation in animals[146] but unlike epidermoid cysts, human cases have not been reported in association with previous lumbar punctures or spinal trauma.

Associated lesions

About half of all dermoid cysts are associated with other congenital malformations, most commonly spina bifida occulta and meningomyelocele.[133,166] The cysts usually occur at the same level as the spinal defect.[133] Dermal sinuses extending out through the bone to the skin surface are much more commonly associated with dermoid than epidermoid cysts and usually relate to those examples sited in the posterior fossa or spinal canal.[137,148]

Clinical features

Intracranial dermoid cysts tend to be associated with a more rapid onset of symptoms than epidermoid cysts, and raised intracranial pressure due to obstructive hydrocephalus is not uncommon as a presenting feature in posterior fossa examples.[133,159] Focal neurological deficits are varied and relate to the site of the lesion, but epileptic seizures are a particularly common feature.[149,167] In both posterior fossa and spinal cases there is quite frequently a skin dimple, hair tuft or discharging sinus visible in the midline skin at the level of the lesion.[137,159] Some cases may present with bacterial meningitis or abscess formation due to infection entering an associated dermal sinus.[148,159] As with epidermoid cysts, the clinical presentation may also rarely take the form of recurrent episodes of aseptic meningitis, due to leakage of cyst contents into the CSF pathways.[168,169]

Radiology

In CT scans, intracranial and spinal dermoid cysts typically appear as non-homogeneous lesions which do not enhance after administration of contrast media.[139] They are usually hypodense but have a wider range of attenuation values than seen in most epidermoid cysts.[139] Calcification is more often seen than in epidermoid cysts and CT scans may also help to demonstrate the presence of an associated dermal sinus track.[133] MRI shows a signal intensity similar to fat on both T1- and T2-weighted images, but the images tend to be more variegated than those of epidermoid cysts.[170,171]

Pathology

Macroscopic features

Dermoid cysts are well defined rounded masses with a firm outer capsule which varies greatly in thickness. It is often densely adherent to surrounding structures, including brain or spinal cord tissue. On cut section, the inner aspect of the capsule may be smooth or show small papillary projections. There are frequently plaques of calcified material. The cysts are filled by a thick, greasy, yellowish sebaceous material, typically with a variable number of matted, tangled hairs (Fig. 17.14). Very rarely, teeth may also be encountered.

Histological features

The cysts are lined by a stratified squamous epithelium which usually shows rather little in the way of maturation or keratin formation. In some places the epithelium is quite thin and flattened, but there may also be thicker areas where it becomes heaped up and more irregular. Deep to the epithelium is a zone of collagenous tissue

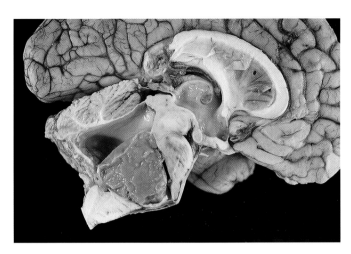

Fig. 17.14 **Posterior fossa dermoid cyst.** This thin walled cyst lies within the pons, adjacent to the fourth ventricle. It is entirely filled by greasy, yellow–green sebaceous material. No hairs are visible macroscopically.

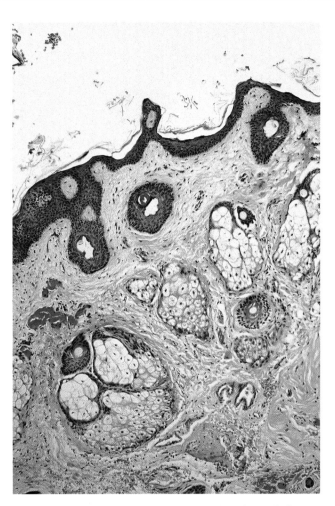

Fig. 17.15 **Dermoid cyst.** The thick collagenous layer beneath the stratified squamous epithelial lining contains numerous hair follicles and sebaceous glands. H & E.

which varies from a thin flattened layer to a broad zone which resembles dermis and contains skin appendages (Fig. 17.15). Hair follicles and sebaceous glands are the most commonly encountered appendages, but there may also be sweat glands. Rarely, foci of cartilage or bone are present. In addition, it is not uncommon to find focal areas of epithelial degeneration with a granulomatous inflammatory reaction, which can extend quite widely throughout the leptomeninges if there has been prior leakage or rupture of the cyst. Malignant change in dermoid cysts is even rarer than in epidermoid ones, with only a handful of reported cases.[153,172]

Differential diagnosis

The distinctive mixture of hairs and sebaceous material in dermoid cysts means they are often distinguishable from other cystic lesions on naked eye examination alone. Histologically, both the lack of keratinisation and the presence of hairs and dermal appendages will help differentiate from epidermoid cysts and craniopharyngiomas. Colloid and neuroglial cysts can easily be excluded by the presence of stratified squamous epithelium. Teeth, bone and cartilage may all occasionally occur in dermoid cysts, however, and the distinction from a well differentiated teratoma is rather more difficult. A careful search needs to be made for other tissue elements, particularly endodermal type glandular structures. It must be remembered that enterogenous cysts may undergo focal squamous metaplasia, but areas of typical ciliated and goblet cell epithelium can still usually be found and these do not occur in dermoid cysts. Solitary metastatic carcinomas are well documented in the cerebellopontine angle, and any cytological evidence of malignancy in the cyst epithelium should arouse suspicion of metastatic disease, especially in older age groups.

Treatment and prognosis

Treatment of craniospinal dermoid cysts consists of surgical excision, which should be as complete as possible.[133,139] In many cases, however, adherence of the cyst to surrounding structures precludes safe total removal of the capsule, especially in posterior fossa examples.[133,157] Cranial vault lesions and the ones occurring in the subgaleal anterior fontanelle region are an exception to this and can usually be totally excised.[135] In posterior fossa and spinal cases where there is an associated dermal sinus, it is important that this is identified preoperatively and excised with the cyst.[159] As with epidermoid cysts, aseptic meningitis is a recognised postoperative complication and follows leakage of the cyst contents into the subarachnoid space at the time of surgery.[105] The incidence of craniospinal dermoid cysts is too low for reliable prognostic comment, but even in partly excised cases recurrences have been infrequent, especially with the advent of modern microsurgical techniques.[149,157]

Colloid cysts of the third ventricle

Incidence and site

Colloid cysts of the third ventricle represent only 0.5 to 1% of all intracranial neoplasms,[173,174] although they account for 18% of tumours in the third ventricular region.[175] Up to 10% of cases have been reported as being an incidental autopsy finding[176] but a retrospective history of relevant symptoms can often be obtained in such circumstances, and the proportion of truly asymptomatic colloid cysts is almost certainly much smaller than this.[177] Of the cases diagnosed in life, a majority present in young and middle aged adults, and most published series give a mean age in the fourth or fifth decade.[178,179] Colloid cysts are rare in children, with only 2% of cases manifesting before the age of 10 years and just a handful of reports describing cases in infants less than 2 years old.[180] There is a variable but consistent bias towards the male sex.[177,178] By definition, colloid cysts are exclusively midline lesions of the third ventricle, the larger ones filling the ventricular cavity, the smaller ones usually sited anteriorly at the level of the foramen of Monro.[176] In some cases, small cysts may appear embedded in the base of the septum pellucidum between the fornices, whilst larger examples often show an attachment to the root of the choroid plexus on either side.[176,177] Cysts with the typical gelatinous contents of third ventricle colloid cysts are not found elsewhere in the nervous system, and the presence of this material is considered essential for the diagnosis.[105]

Aetiology

Colloid cysts are presumed to originate from persisting embryological remnants, but it is still not clear whether such sequestrated elements are of endodermal or neuroglial origin.[175] It was originally believed that the cysts derived from vestiges of the neural tube paraphysis vesicles, but these have an entirely glandular epithelium, and are now considered unlikely to be the embryonic structure responsible.[175,181] One hypothesis still supporting an origin from specialised neuroepithelial tissue is that the cysts derive from abnormal folding of the neural tube during early embryonic development of the choroid plexus, such that outward budding of the primitive tela choroidea results in an aberrant vesicle with the connective tissue layer on the outside.[175,182] More recently, however, there have also been suggestions that colloid cysts may be endodermally derived structures, analogous to enterogenous cysts of the spine.[183,184] Such suggestions have been largely based on electron microscopic study of the cysts, which have emphasised the similarity of the lining epithelium with that of the adult respiratory tract.[183,185] Using immunocytochemistry, the presence of epithelial antigens and lack of GFAP in colloid cyst epithelium has also been interpreted as indicating an endodermal origin.[184] A similar antigenic expression, however, might be expected in structures derived from choroid plexus and is probably unhelpful in distinguishing between a neuroglial and endodermal lineage.[105,186]

Clinical features

The most typical presenting feature of colloid cysts is intermittent headache, which is the initial symptom in over three-quarters of all cases.[133,178] The history of headaches may span a period of many years, but they may also present as a crescendo of increasingly severe episodes, necessitating emergency admission to hospital.[133,175] The pain is classically posture related and eased by changes of head position.[174,187] The mechanism behind the attacks of headache is uncertain, but hydrocephalus is present in a high proportion of cases and mobility of the cyst may allow intermittent obstruction of the foramina of Monro in a manner akin to a ball valve.[105,175] Other less common clinical presentations include transient attacks of paraparesis[175,188] and chronic, insidious dementia.[177,189] Although often quoted anecdotally, sudden unexpected death is a rare mode of presentation of colloid cysts, and in most fatal cases a relevant prior clinical history can usually be obtained, even if only retrospectively.[133,187]

Radiology

In a significant proportion of cases, the neurological examination is normal and radiology is vital in achieving the diagnosis.[177] Scans reveal obstructive hydrocephalus in the vast majority of symptomatic patients, and this is severe in about half of all cases at the time of presentation.[178] Using CT, the cysts themselves are most often hyperdense to brain, but they can also be isodense and are occasionally hypodense.[188,190] In the radiolucent cases the cysts may enhance after administration of contrast.[133] MRI provides good visualisation of the extent of the cysts and their relation to adjacent structures, but the colloid again produces differing appearances depending on its density and composition.[133,191] The signal may be hyper-, iso- or hypointense compared to brain on T1-weighted images and in some cases is heterogeneous.[191] T2-weighted images often show a central area of low signal and a rim which is of higher intensity.[181]

Pathology

Macroscopic features

Colloid cysts presenting symptomatically are usually much larger than those found incidentally at autopsy, and most measure between 1 and 3 cm in diameter.[176,177] They are unilocular, grape-like structures with a smooth, thin, membranous capsule. The colloid contents are visible through the capsule, and in the fresh state this typically gives the cysts an opalescent, greenish colour

(Fig. 17.16). They turn to a dull, opaque grey after fixation. On cut section, the colloid may be firm and hyaline in texture like soft cartilage, or of gelatinous, mucoid consistency. The texture and appearance of the colloid can vary considerably within a single cyst, and rather uncommonly areas of old or recent haemorrhage may be present. Sometimes the cysts are pendulous, freely mobile structures attached only by a pedicle to the tela choroidea in the anterior part of the third ventricle, but they can also be firmly adherent to the ventricle walls or to the pillars of the fornix.

Histological features

The lining of colloid cysts varies from a layer of flattened cuboidal or low columnar cells to well developed high columnar epithelium. The epithelial layer is usually only one cell thick, but some areas may show a degree of stratification with flattened basal cells that do not appear to reach the luminal surface. Ciliated areas are often present, especially when the cells are columnar in type (Fig. 17.17), and there may be interspersed goblet cells which stain positively with mucin stains. The epithelium can be focally destroyed in some cases, but a granulomatous reaction to the colloid is a rather infrequent finding.[192,193] The epithelial cells are bounded by a collagenous layer of variable thickness which may contain calcospherites and focal chronic inflammatory cell infiltrates. Very occasionally there are also subepithelial tubular spaces lined by similar epithelium to the main cyst lumen. The outer aspect of the connective tissue layer is often adherent to gliotic brain tissue or choroid plexus. The colloid within the cyst has a distinctive histological appearance and is essential in confirming the diagnosis. It is a homogeneous, amorphous material which encloses scattered exfoliated epithelial cells, macrophages, lymphocytes and polymorphs. It stains positively with both PAS and Alcian blue stains, and when these stains are combined, the Alcian blue positivity is often seen to be concentrated around the periphery. In some cases the colloid may also stain with mucicarmine.[194] Histochemical analysis has shown a heterogeneous mixture of complex lipids, fatty acids and cholesterol, consistent with a secretory product.[175]

Immunocytochemistry

The epithelial cells lining colloid cysts do not express GFAP but consistently react with antibodies to epithelial antigens, including cytokeratins and EMA.[186,195] The

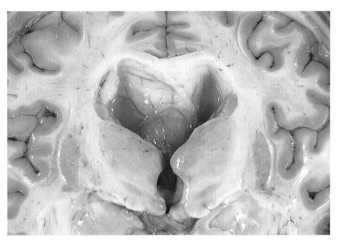

Fig. 17.16 **Colloid cyst.** The cyst has a smooth capsule and an opalescent, greenish colour in the unfixed state. This example was freely mobile and has been displaced upwards from its pedunculated attachment in the third ventricle.

Fig. 17.17 **Colloid cyst.** There is a lining of flattened cuboidal epithelium with focal areas of taller, ciliated columnar cells containing PAS-positive material. PAS/diastase.

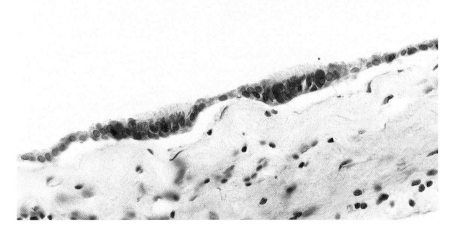

cytokeratins expressed include those normally associated with complex types of epithelium,[117] and where small basal cells are present beneath the outer epithelial layer, these are also stained.[184] EMA immunostaining is confined to the apical membranes of the epithelial lining cells.[184] Immunocytochemical staining with an antibody to carcinoembryonic antigen has also been described in one recent study.[195] In some cases the epithelium of colloid cysts may show focal staining using antibodies to S-100 protein,[119,195] but this has not been a consistent finding.[184]

Electron microscopy

The main epithelial cell types described in ultrastructural studies have been non-ciliated cells bearing only short apical microvillous processes, and tall columnar cells with cilia and longer microvilli projecting into the cyst lumen.[196,197] The non-ciliated cells show coating of their microvilli and apical membranes by a layer of finely granular, electron dense material.[185,196] They often have apical areas of cytoplasm packed with membrane bound granules, suggesting apocrine type secretory activity.[183,197] The ciliated columnar cells lack an apical surface coating, and in some cases their cilia show aberrant patterns of axial microtubules.[183] Both types of cells are joined by complex cytoplasmic interdigitations along their apposed lateral surfaces and junctional complexes near the apical margins.[183,198] Deep to the apical surface of the epithelium there are also occasional wedge shaped basal cells, squeezed between the other cell types and closely applied to the subepithelial basement membrane.[183,185] These show desmosome attachments to adjacent cells and contain cytoplasmic tonofilaments. Some reports have also described basal cells containing dense core vesicles, similar to the neurosecretory cells found in normal bronchial mucosa,[183] and the overall ultrastructural appearance of colloid cyst epithelium has been likened to that lining the mature respiratory tract.[183,185]

Differential diagnosis

The specialised site, macroscopic appearance and typical viscous contents of colloid cysts are usually sufficient to suggest the diagnosis at the time of surgery or autopsy, before histological sections are examined. Histologically, colloid cysts can be distinguished from dermoid, epidermoid or craniopharyngioma cysts by the presence of cilia and mucus production and the lack of squamous differentiation or keratinisation. It should be remembered, however, that the epithelial antigens expressed by squamous cysts are also present in colloid cyst epithelium. Both mucus production and cilia may also be present in the epithelium of Rathke's cleft cysts, but when suprasellar these often show areas of squamous metaplasia and their thin, watery contents contrast with the viscous, PAS stained material of colloid cysts. Both the epithelial lining and the viscous, mucous contents of mucoceles may appear similar to those of colloid cysts, but confusion between the two entities is unlikely since colloid cysts are always circumscribed, intraventricular lesions and lack the base of skull or air sinus component of mucoceles extending into the cranial cavity.

Therapy and prognosis

Colloid cysts are biologically benign lesions with the potential for complete cure, and although some reports have advocated simple CSF shunt insertion[199] or just careful follow-up,[178] most authorities favour complete surgical resection via a craniotomy.[159,179] Alternatively, the cysts can be aspirated, either stereotactically[188,190] or using a ventriculoscope if the ventricles are sufficiently dilated.[133] Although avoiding the risks of more major intracranial surgery, cyst aspiration may be unsuccessful if the lesion is too mobile to allow the capsule to be penetrated, or if the colloid content is too viscous.[133,188] There have been suggestions that the presence of high viscosity colloid which is unsuitable for aspiration may be predicted by the radiological appearances of the lesion, especially if the cyst is hyperdense on CT scans.[190]

Following complete excision the prognosis is excellent,[179] and symptomatic recurrences are very rare even when the cyst has been simply aspirated, leaving the capsule behind.[200] Malignant transformation of the cyst wall never occurs.[105] The most likely postoperative complications are epilepsy[177] or memory disturbance due to forniceal damage, particularly after transcallosal surgery.[112] Persistent hydrocephalus may also be a problem in some cases, and can require long term CSF diversion.[177,179]

Enterogenous cysts

Incidence and site

Enterogenous cysts, also referred to as neurenteric cysts, are rare congenital lesions occurring mainly in the spinal canal, where they account for about 0.4% of all spinal tumours.[201] They present clinically over a wide age range from birth to the fifth decade of life,[202,203] but a majority of cases are diagnosed in older children and young adults.[202,203] Males are affected more commonly than females.[202,204]

In the spine, enterogenous cysts are most commonly located in the cervical and upper thoracic regions (Table 17.3).[203,205] They are nearly always intradural extramedullary lesions,[204,206] although some may be partly buried within the spinal cord.[207,208] In contrast to teratomas, they are usually anterior or anterolateral to the cord, especially in the cervical region.[206,209] Very rarely, enterogenous cysts may also occur within the cranial cavity, most examples being sited in the vermis,[210] cisterna magna[211,212] or brain stem.[213,214] These posterior fossa cysts are again typically midline and extraparenchymal, lying within the subarachnoid space, although there are reports of cases which are intraparenchymal[215] or lateral in location.[216]

Aetiology

Spinal enterogenous cysts are generally believed to derive from an anomalous embryological connection between the primitive foregut and the developing neural tube, probably in association with splitting or reduplication of the intervening notochord.[203,206] This results in a spectrum of malformations of varying severity, depending on the degree to which the abnormal communication persists[202,203] (Fig. 17.18). The most extensive malformations consist of combined anterior and posterior spina bifida with complete posterior herniation of the gastrointestinal tract, and are only seen in aborted fetuses.[202,217] In less severely affected cases, the dysraphism is purely anterior and often compatible with life.[203,204] A proportion of intraspinal enterogenous cysts presenting in younger children show a persisting anterior connection with mediastinal cysts via defects in the vertebral bodies.[218,219] In later life, the vast majority of spinal enterogenous cysts

present as isolated anomalies without any evidence of anterior dysraphism, but these are nevertheless felt to have formed by the same basic embryological mechanism.[203,204] The initial splitting of the notochord may be a primary event, causing secondary adhesion and fistulation between the primitive gut and neural tube.[202,206] Alternatively, the notochord may fail to fuse because of abnormal persistence of the embryonic neurenteric canal, which connects it with the yolk sac during very early fetal development.[203,206] Intracranial enterogenous cysts have not been reported in association with skull base defects or persistent endodermal sinuses, but are thought to be the result of a similar sequence of embryological events to that postulated for the spinal examples.[212]

Associated abnormalities

Vertebral abnormalities are often found in association with spinal enterogenous cysts presenting in childhood and are said to be present in about 50% of cases when all age groups are taken together.[206] The associated anomalies are often relatively minor, and include vertebral fusion (Klippel–Feil syndrome), hemivertebrae, scoliosis, widened spinal canal, diastematomyelia and posterior spina bifida occulta.[203,207] Of more interest from an

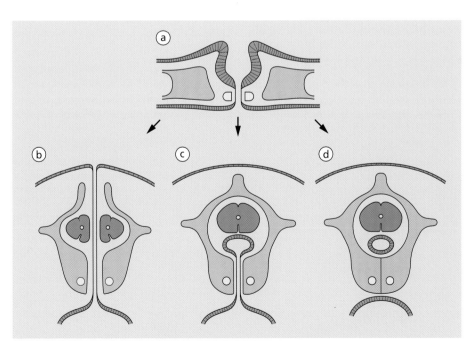

Fig. 17.18 Pathogenesis of spinal enterogenous cysts. (a) An anomalous connection is believed to form between the primitive foregut epithelium and the developing neural tube during early embryogenesis. This is thought to be associated with splitting of the notochord (yellow). Possible outcomes include **(b)** complete anterior and posterior spina bifida, **(c)** an enterogenous cyst in direct communication with a mediastinal cyst or the respiratory/ gastrointestinal tract via an anterior vertebral defect and **(d)** an isolated intraspinal cyst with a partly fused or entirely undetectable vertebral defect.

embryological viewpoint are the cases which are associated with similar enterogenous cysts in the mediastinal cavity, as outlined above. In some of these rare cases, there may be no vertebral anomaly or connection with the mediastinal cyst,[220] but in others the two cysts are joined by fibrous bands[221] or patent fistulae traversing a defect in the vertebral bodies.[222,223] Variants on this theme include cases of purely intraspinal enterogenous cysts in which an adjacent anterior vertebral defect is filled with cartilage,[217] and solitary mediastinal cysts which are joined to the anterior spinal dura by a blind ended, transvertebral fistula.[218,221]

Clinical features

Spinal enterogenous cysts usually present with focal spinal cord compression syndromes relating to the level of the lesion.[202,204] Pain is also a common symptom and often radiates in a nerve root distribution.[202] The clinical history is typically one of gradually progressive deterioration, often over several years, and the signs and symptoms have a characteristic tendency to fluctuate in severity.[202] Unusual presentations include recurrent meningitis due to a patent anterior spinal fistula[218,219] and respiratory distress caused by a coexisting mediastinal enterogenous cyst.[220,221] Enterogenous cysts in the posterior fossa may present with obstructive hydrocephalus, cerebellar symptoms or progressive brain stem dysfunction, depending on their location.[215,224] Headache in these cases is sometimes episodic or posture related.[211,212]

Radiology

Spinal enterogenous cysts have a rather non-specific appearance using computerised tomograms alone, but are better defined when CT myelography is used.[204,225] In rare cases where there is a patent anterior spinal fistula, this may also be outlined after myelography.[204] Plain X-rays are important to detect associated bony spinal abnormalities, including midline vertebral body defects.[204] With MRI, the lesions are usually uniformly hypointense to cord on T1-weighted images, and hyperintense on T2-weighted images, with a signal similar or slightly brighter than CSF.[225,226]

Pathology

Macroscopic features

The typical naked-eye appearance of spinal enterogenous cysts is that of a transparent, thin walled, smooth, rounded sac, either compressing the spinal cord or partly embedded within it. In cases with a more complex lining structure, the cyst wall may be focally thickened and opaque. The cysts usually contain clear, colourless fluid similar to CSF[202,227] but occasionally the contents are thicker and discoloured.[324]

Histological features

In the majority of enterogenous cysts, the lining consists of simple columnar epithelium resting on a thin outer layer of sparsely cellular collagen (Fig. 17.19). The cells may be of low or high columnar type and are frequently ciliated. Their cytoplasm stains positively with mucin stains, including PAS diastase, Alcian blue and mucicarmine. In addition, interspersed goblet cells are usually present. In some cases, the epithelium may show areas of stratification or pseudostratification, producing

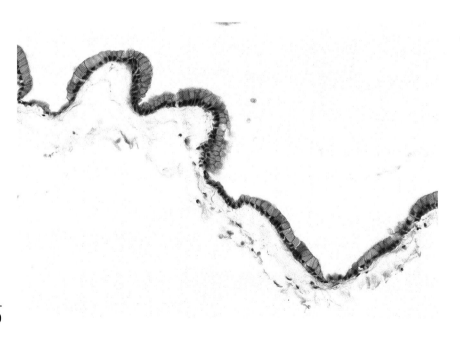

Fig. 17.19 **Spinal enterogenous cyst.** The wall of this cyst is lined by a single layer of columnar epithelium with mucus-filled goblet cells. There is a thin outer layer of collagen. H & E.

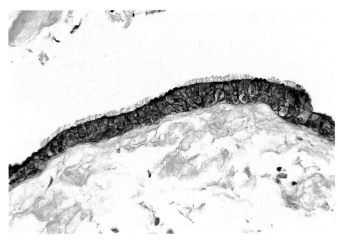

Fig. 17.20 **Spinal enterogenous cyst.** This example is lined by respiratory type epithelium with ciliated, pseudostratified columnar cells. The cells are strongly stained using immunocytochemistry for cytokeratin.

an appearance similar to adult respiratory tract epithelium (Fig. 17.20). Focal areas of non-keratinising squamous metaplasia may also be encountered.[214,228] Less commonly, the cyst wall may have a more complex structure resembling gastric[204,229] or oesophageal mucosa,[204,229] complete with appropriate submucosal glands and an underlying smooth muscle layer. The cysts with such complex linings tend to occur in a younger age group, and are more often associated with anterior fistulae, vertebral body defects and coexisting mediastinal cysts.[202,204]

Immunocytochemistry

The cells lining enterogenous cysts show positive immunocytochemical staining with antibodies to both EMA and cytokeratins[195,214] (Fig. 17.20). One study has indicated that the cytokeratins expressed are those normally associated with simple types of epithelium, contrasting with the complex-type cytokeratins of colloid and Rathke's cleft cysts.[117] The epithelial cells also have been found to express carcinoembryonic antigen in most studies where this has been looked for.[195,206] Focal positive staining of the lining epithelium with antibodies to S-100 protein has been described,[119,195] but the cells do not contain GFAP.[195,214]

Electron microscopy

Ultrastructurally, the epithelial cells either show abundant cilia protruding from their apical surfaces, or microvilli coated by a layer of electron dense material.[230,231] The apical portion of goblet-cell cytoplasm is filled with membrane bound secretory granules.[230] The lateral surfaces of the cells are joined by junctional complexes near the apical surface, and deep to this there are cytoplasmic interdigitations.[206,231] A continuous basement membrane separates the epithelial layer from the underlying collagen.[206,231] In areas with squamous metaplasia, the cells contain cytoplasmic tonofilaments and are joined by numerous desmosomes.[230] The ultrastructural features of enterogenous cysts have been likened to those of both colloid cysts and mature respiratory epithelium, supporting arguments for an endodermal derivation of colloid cysts.[231]

Differential diagnosis

Teratoma

Most enterogenous cysts are lined only by simple epithelium and can be distinguished from teratomas by the absence of other tissue elements in the cyst wall. Where the lining is more complex, however, as in cases with well developed gastric mucosa or focal squamous metaplasia, a well differentiated teratoma is more difficult to exclude. The presence of elements such as adipose tissue, cartilage or nervous tissue within the cyst wall suggests a teratoid origin, and suspicion of a teratoma should also be aroused by cysts which are posterior to the spinal cord, especially if they are in the lumbosacral region and associated with a meningocele or meningomyelocele.

Dermoid and epidermoid cysts

These can usually be clearly identified macroscopically by their characteristic caseous or pearly contents, which contrast with the thin fluid found in most enterogenous cysts. When squamous metaplasia occurs in enterogenous cysts, this is a focal, non-keratinising phenomenon, and remaining areas of ciliated, mucus producing epithelium can nearly always be identified to help exclude a dermoid or epidermoid cyst.

Neuroglial cysts

Like enterogenous cysts, these are usually thin-walled lesions which contain clear fluid and have a predominantly simple, ciliated epithelial lining. They may be distinguished using routine stains by the lack of squamous metaplasia or mucus production. Immunocytochemically, the epithelium expresses GFAP but not epithelial antigens such as the cytokeratins and carcinoembryonic antigen.

Arachnoid cysts

These are again thin walled lesions with CSF-like fluid contents, but can be distinguished from enterogenous cysts microscopically by the meningeal structure of their walls and the complete absence of an epithelial lining.

Therapy and prognosis

Enterogenous cysts are benign and potentially curable lesions which should be excised surgically as completely as possible.[202,204] A thoracotomy approach may be preferable for upper spinal examples and is mandatory for the repair of associated anterior spinal defects and fistulae.[204] As with many types of nervous system cyst, a safe total excision may be precluded by dense adherence of the membranous capsule to adjacent neural tissue or roots, particularly in cases which are wholly or partly intramedullary.[207] Treatment in such cases is best limited to drainage of the cyst contents and a limited removal of the more accessible parts of the cyst wall.[202,206]

The results of surgery are dependent on the severity of preoperative deficits and the presence of associated spinal malformations, but in most cases the prognosis is extremely favourable.[204,206] There is often a dramatic resolution of signs and symptoms following cyst excision, and complete neurological recovery can be expected in about 70% of all spinal cases.[202,203] Clinical recurrences are exceptionally rare even if the cyst wall has only been partly excised, and adhesive chemical meningitis is not normally encountered as a postoperative complication.[202]

Neuroglial cysts

Incidence and site

Neuroglial cysts are rare lesions which occur in a wide variety of sites throughout the neuraxis. They have an epithelial lining with the characteristics of ependymal or choroid plexus tissue. In the supratentorial compartment, neuroglial cysts most often take the form of large intrahemispheric cavities buried within cerebral white matter.[232,233] These are typically located in the frontal region, but any cerebral lobe may be affected.[234] Occasionally, they may be entirely extraparenchymal, usually lying over an indented cerebral convexity in the parasagittal region.[235,236] In the posterior fossa, neuroglial cysts may occur in the cerebellopontine angle region,[237,238] within the cavity of the fourth ventricle,[239,240] or entirely within the parenchyma of the brain stem or a cerebellar hemisphere.[241,242] In the spine, the cysts are typically intradural but extramedullary in location.[243] They may occur at any spinal level, but are usually anterior or anterolateral to the cord.[202,244] The intracranial cysts may manifest clinically at any age, although they most commonly present in adults.[230,234] Spinal examples are more often present in childhood.[202]

Aetiology

Intraparenchymal neuroglial cysts are generally believed to derive from neural tube lining elements which become sequestrated in the developing white matter during early embryogenesis.[233,241] Abnormal evagination of the neuroectoderm is thought to occur along the line of the choroidal fissure, at the junction of the differentiating ependyma and choroid plexus, thus explaining the mixed features of these two tissue elements in the cyst lining.[234,240] The extraparenchymal neuroglial cysts of the spine and cranial cavity are again felt to be of congenital origin, but in some cases may derive from ectopic glial elements in the leptomeninges, rather than primarily displaced neural tube lining elements.[235,237]

Clinical features

Supratentorial neuroglial cysts in adults usually present with a fairly short history and seizures are a common initial symptom.[234] There may also be a history of headaches, mental deterioration and varied focal neurological deficits, depending on the precise site of the cyst.[232,234] Posterior fossa examples typically present with cranial nerve palsies, focal brain stem dysfunction, or signs and symptoms of raised intracranial pressure due to hydrocephalus.[240,242] Spinal neuroglial cysts often have a longer clinical history, sometimes dating back to birth, and usually present with radicular pain or evidence of cord compression relating to the level of the lesion.[202,245] There have also been reports of cases presenting as recurrent episodes of chemical meningitis due to cyst leakage.[238]

Pathology

Macroscopic features

Intracerebral neuroglial cysts take the form of rounded, smooth-lined and uniloculate cavities buried within hemispheric white matter. They are typically large, and usually greater than 4 cm in diameter. They contain watery fluid which can be clear and CSF-like or turbid. There is no communication with the ventricular cavities, but some examples may have only a membranous roof bordering the pial surface. The extraparenchymal cysts have a thin, translucent wall and similar, watery contents. The cortical surface beneath extracerebral examples is usually markedly depressed and may show a pattern of rudimentary sulci or true polymicrogyria.[235] Spinal examples can extend over several anatomical segments and are either attached to nerve roots or to the surface of the cord by a small intramedullary component.

Histological features

The lining of neuroglial cysts varies from columnar, ependymal type epithelium to low cuboidal cells resembling those of choroid plexus tissue. The ependymal-like areas are frequently ciliated with blepharoplasts, and where the cysts are intraparenchymal the cells directly

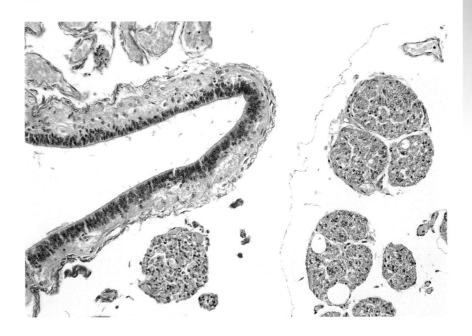

Fig. 17.21 **Extraparenchymal spinal neuroglial cyst.** There is an ependymal-like epithelial lining, which rests on a thin zone of central nervous tissue and is surrounded by a layer of collagen. Spinal roots lie alongside. Van Gieson.

abut onto adjacent white matter without intervening basement membrane or collagenous tissue. The areas of flattened or low cuboidal epithelium lack cilia and rest on a thin collagenous layer which can be easily overlooked unless connective tissue stains are performed. Cysts may show exclusively one or other type of epithelial lining or a mixture of the two. There are no goblet cells and stains for mucin are negative. Around intraparenchymal cysts, the neural tissue may appear entirely normal or mildly gliotic, but there is not usually evidence of previous haemorrhage or infarction. The unattached walls of extraparenchymal cysts sometimes show a thin layer of glial tissue between the epithelium and outer collagen, especially if the lining cells are of ependymal type[237,240] (Fig. 17.21). In some cases, rudimentary choroidal-like tufts of epithelium have been described projecting into the cyst lumen,[235] but in most examples the lining is flat and single layered.

Immunocytochemistry

The epithelial lining cells of neuroglial cysts show rather variable expression of GFAP, and may be negatively immunostained if they are of flattened, cuboidal type.[237,241] Absent expression of EMA, cytokeratin or carcino-embryonic antigen has been reported in one study of a cyst with a predominantly flattened epithelial layer.[237] Where an intermediate layer of glial tissue is present in extra-parenchymal cysts, this stains positively with antibodies to expected epitopes, including GFAP and S-100 protein.[237]

Electron microscopy

Ultrastructural studies have confirmed the mixture of ependymal and choroid plexus features in the cells lining neuroglial cysts.[234,246] Some cells contain glial-like arrays of cytoplasmic filaments and bear tall apical cilia, whilst others have only microvilli on their luminal surfaces. The cells are joined by lateral adherentes junctions and cytoplasmic interdigitations, and the basal aspects may rest on a basement membrane or abut directly onto neuroglial stroma.[237] The basal surfaces of some cells show evidence of pinocytotic vesicle formation, leading to suggestions that they may be capable of active transudation, as in choroid plexus epithelium.[234]

Differential diagnosis

Large intracerebral neuroglial cysts can be distinguished from porencephalic cysts by the presence of an epithelial lining, the lack of communication with the underlying ventricular cavity and the good preservation of adjacent brain tissue. Extraparenchymal neuroglial cysts, especially spinal ones, can be macroscopically indistinguishable from enterogenous cysts, but their lining epithelium lacks the mucin production and cytokeratin expression of the enterogenous lesions, and is usually simple rather than stratified or pseudostratified. Arachnoidal cysts may again appear similar on naked eye examination but they do not have the epithelial lining of neuroglial cysts. Dermoid and epidermoid cysts may be easily distinguished by their thick walls, typical solid contents and stratified squamous lining epithelium. In the third ventricle, most cysts are typical colloid cysts with characteristic, gelatinous, colloid contents, but some atypical examples lacking this material may be more accurately classified as neuroglial cysts. This is especially the case if the lining epithelium lacks evidence of mucin production or abuts neuroglial tissue without an intervening connective tissue layer.

Therapy and prognosis

Intraparenchymal neuroglial cysts, especially supratentorial examples, can be effectively treated by fenestration of the wall and establishing a drainage route to the ventricles or subarachnoid space.[232,234] Extraparenchymal cysts, including spinal examples, can sometimes be completely excised,[245] but removal may have to be subtotal in cases with an intramedullary extension.[202,247] The prognosis is excellent regardless of the site or extent of cyst wall excision, and in most cases there is rapid resolution of symptoms and neurological deficits.[202,232] Clinical recurrences are most unlikely, even in intracerebral cases where the treatment has been limited to simple fenestration and drainage.[234]

Congenital arachnoidal cysts

Incidence and site

These cysts are rare developmental lesions which occur in the absence of generalised leptomeningeal scarring. They are usually clearly distinguishable from the acquired cystic loculations of CSF seen in adhesive arachnoidopathy. Supratentorial examples account for over two-thirds of the congenital cysts in most series[248,249] and are most commonly sited in the Sylvian fissure region.[250] Other, much rarer supratentorial sites include the parasagittal convexity of a cerebral hemisphere, the interhemispheric fissure and the sellar or suprasellar region.[251,252] The majority of posterior fossa arachnoid cysts are sited either in the midline between the cerebellar hemispheres or in the cerebellopontine angle.[248,253] In the spine, congenital arachnoid cysts may be located either in the intradural or extradural compartments (Table 17.3).[254] The intradural cysts are commonest in young or middle aged adults[202,255] and are usually posterior to the spinal cord, in the low or midthoracic region.[255,256] Extradural spinal arachnoid cysts are typically posterolateral to the dural sheath and are again usually thoracic in location, although lumbar examples are also well documented.[257,258] They may occur in any age group, but most often present in the teenage years, more commonly in males than females.[257,258]

Aetiology

Intracranial congenital arachnoid cysts do not lie in the subarachnoid space per se, but within the thickness of a reduplicated arachnoid membrane, suggesting that they may result from focal splitting of the developing membrane during embryogenesis.[250,259] In the spine, the intradural cysts may result from localised abnormalities in the distribution of the arachnoid trabeculae[260] or from focal splitting of the septum posticum, a structure which normally divides the midline posterior subarachnoid space in cervical and thoracic regions.[254,255] Extradural spinal arachnoid cysts are thought to be caused by outward prolapse of arachnoidal tissue through points of weakness in the dura at its junction with the emerging spinal roots.[254,257] The majority of these spinal extradural cysts are thus effectively subarachnoid diverticulae with a patent transdural neck,[257,258] although in some cases this connection is assumed to have become obliterated subsequent to the formation of the cyst.[261] The spinal extradural arachnoid cysts are thought to enlarge because of pulsations in CSF pressure transmitted through their communication with the subarachnoid compartment.[257] For intradural arachnoid cysts, however, it is not clear whether enlargement is the result of a similar mechanism acting on a valve like flap in the cyst wall, or whether expansion occurs as a result of osmotic pressure gradients across an intact membrane.[259,262]

Clinical features

Large supratentorial arachnoid cysts frequently present in infants or young children with generalised head enlargement and widened sutures or a localised skull deformity.[263,264] In adults with cerebral convexity cysts, focal neurological deficits are more often a prominent feature, and most cases present with headache and other evidence of raised intracranial pressure.[248,256] Posterior fossa arachnoid cysts are most likely to cause an obstructive hydrocephalus, and in some cases the history may be episodic or posture related.[253,265] In infants, the presentation may again consist only of increasing head size and retarded development, but adult posterior fossa cysts often cause focal cerebellar or lower cranial nerve deficits appropriate to the site of the lesion.[249,254] In the spine, intradural arachnoid cysts typically present with a relatively long history of back pain, often without neurological deficit.[255] In the lumbosacral region the presentation may include radicular symptoms and simulate that of disc prolapse.[256,266] When the cysts are extradural, focal neurological deficits are said to be a more common clinical feature and there may also be associated minor bony abnormalities such as kyphoscoliosis.[254,257]

Radiology

Using both CT and MRI, arachnoid cysts appear as rounded, well defined, extra-axial, defects which have an attenuation identical to that of CSF and do not enhance following administration of contrast media.[249,252] Spinal cysts may be missed using myelography unless the patient is screened in prone and supine positions.[256,266] Most cases manifest as a simple block to the passage of dye, but in a proportion the cyst cavities may show delayed filling of the contrast medium.[266,267]

Pathology

Macroscopic features

Congenital arachnoid cysts are rounded, sac-like structures filled with clear fluid resembling CSF. The cyst walls are thin and transparent with smooth surfaces. Particularly in the supratentorial compartment, the cavities may be very large, often exceeding 10 cm in diameter, and can cause considerable indentation and displacement of adjacent neural structures (Fig. 17.22). In infants with cerebral convexity cysts there may also be prominent bulging and deformation of the overlying skull vault bones. In distinction from the acquired cystic spaces associated with adhesive arachnoidopathy, there is no generalised thickening or tethering of the surrounding leptomeninges, and congenital cysts are nearly always uniloculate structures which can be easily separated from the adjacent dural and pial surfaces. In the spine, both intradural and extradural cysts are typically elongate, sausage like structures extending over several anatomical levels. The intradural examples may be adherent to surrounding spinal nerve roots.

Histological features

The wall of congenital arachnoid cysts consists of a thin, vascularised collagenous membrane, either lined by a continuous layer of flattened arachnoidal cells or intermittent clusters of similar cells (Fig. 17.23). The appearances are usually histologically indistinguishable from the normal leptomeningeal membrane, although in some cases there can be focal hyperplasia of the arachnoid cells. Arachnoidal cell whorls and psammoma bodies

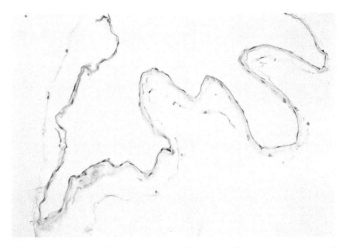

Fig. 17.23 **Congenital arachnoid cyst.** Histologically, the wall consists of a very thin collagenous membrane lined by flattened arachnoidal cells. H & E.

may also be present within the cyst wall. The cyst cavity is not traversed by trabeculae. In contrast to the meningeal adhesions in adhesive arachnoidopathy, congenital cyst walls do not contain inflammatory infiltrates or evidence of old haemorrhage. The underlying subpial cord or brain tissue usually appears normal or only mildly gliotic, and the outer cyst wall of intradural cases abuts directly onto the inner aspect of the dura. Electron microscopy has confirmed the arachnoidal nature of the cells in the cyst wall, which contain abundant intermediate type cytoplasmic filaments and are joined to each other by desmosomes.[250]

Differential diagnosis

Supratentorial arachnoid cysts can be distinguished from porencephalic defects by the presence of intact underlying cortical grey matter, without destructive changes or significant gliosis. Arachnoidal cyst walls differ from those of subdural hygromas in their absence of scarring, inflammatory infiltrates or old blood pigment. In the posterior fossa, midline interhemispheric cerebellar arachnoid cysts may grossly resemble those of the Dandy–Walker syndrome, but they are not associated with agenesis of the cerebellar vermis and the cyst wall lacks a neuroglial component. Other thin walled cysts with clear fluid contents which can macroscopically resemble arachnoid cysts include neuroglial cysts, Rathke's cleft cysts of the sellar region and enterogenous cysts in the intradural spinal compartment. Arachnoid cysts can be distinguished histologically from all these lesions by their typical leptomeningeal structure and by the absence of a true epithelial lining.

Therapy and prognosis

Congenital arachnoid cysts are usually treated by surgical excision of the cyst wall, since the contents

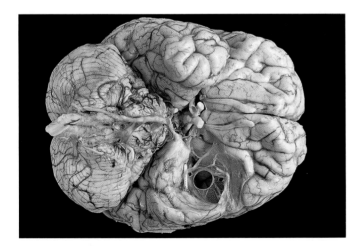

Fig. 17.22 **Congenital arachnoid cyst.** There is considerable indentation and distortion of the adjacent frontal and temporal lobes, transforming the left Sylvian fissure into a gaping, rounded cyst cavity lined by normal arachnoid. The outer part of the cyst wall consists only of translucent arachnoid membrane, which has ruptured and partly collapsed at the time of autopsy. A surgical drain lies in the collapsed cyst lumen.

reaccumulate after simple aspiration.[254,264] In some posterior fossa cases, a total removal of the cyst may be possible[253] but for large supratentorial cysts only the outer portion of the cyst wall can be safely resected.[248,268] Some authors advocate marsupialisation of these large cysts into the ventricular system or basal CSF cisterns.[251,268] Cystoperitoneal shunting has also been proposed, both as a primary procedure and as an adjunct to incomplete surgical excision of the cyst wall.[252,264] Marsupialisation and cyst cavity shunts have again been recommended for intradural spinal arachnoid cysts, especially when these are too adherent to spinal roots or the spinal cord to permit safe total removal of the cyst wall.[269,270] Spinal extradural cysts are nearly always amenable to safe total excision, but it is important to tie off any communication with the subarachnoid space and repair the dural defect.[257,259]

In the majority of cases, there is marked neurological improvement or complete cure following surgical excision,[248,258] although persistent deficits are likely in infants showing severe neurological disturbances from an early age.[268] Recurrences following adequate excision of the cyst wall are uncommon[248,253] and can normally be satisfactorily treated by further excision or shunting of the cyst cavity.[249,270]

CSF cysts in adhesive arachnoidopathy

Adhesive arachnoidopathy is a progressive scarring of the leptomeninges which may follow a variety of insults including trauma, meningitis, subarachnoid haemorrhage and chemical irritation by agents such as oily contrast media.[202] The thickening and tethering of the arachnoidal membrane is usually quite widespread and may result either in obliteration of the subarachnoid space or the formation of loculated CSF cavities bounded by adhesions.[105,271] Such cavities can occasionally increase in size, presumably due to hydrostatic pressure, and present symptomatically as space occupying lesions.[271] In some cases, the initial haemorrhage or infection may have occurred in infancy or in utero, and a positive clinical history may be lacking[105] (Fig. 17.24). The syndrome particularly affects the spinal canal, most often in a thoracolumbar distribution, where it may also result from spondylotic disease, disc prolapse, previous spinal surgery or back trauma.[272,273] Macroscopically, adhesive arachnoid cysts differ from congenital ones in being multiple or multiloculated. They are also surrounded by areas of generalised leptomeningeal thickening or tethering. Histologically, the acquired cyst walls are usually much thicker and more fibrous than those of congenital cysts, and often contain focal chronic inflammatory infiltrates or evidence of old haemorrhage. The natural history is typically one of insidiously progressive pain and neurological deficit, and the long term prognosis is generally rather poor despite attempts at surgical decompression.[202]

Pineal cysts

Small cysts in the pineal gland are found incidentally in about 1.5% of patients undergoing magnetic resonance scanning for other reasons, including the investigation of headache.[274,275] Rarely, pineal cysts may be 2 cm or more in diameter and present symptomatically with Parinaud syndrome of vertical gaze paralysis, or with raised intra-

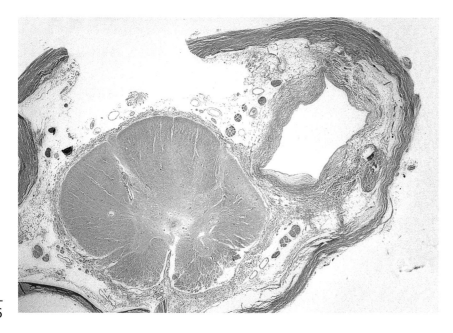

Fig. 17.24 **Spinal arachnoid cyst.** The cyst wall in this example was sclerotic and adherent to adjacent, thickened leptomeninges. The lesion was presumed to be acquired, although the cause of the scarring was not known. Van Gieson.

Fig. 17.25 **Symptomatic choroid plexus cyst of the fourth ventricle.** This cyst was lined by regular cuboidal epithelium and was in continuity with adjacent choroid plexus tissue. H & E.

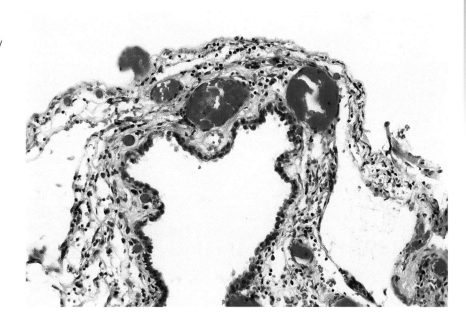

cranial pressure due to obstructive hydrocephalus.[274,276] Most of the symptomatic cysts occur in young adults and are estimated to account for only 4% of all pineal region tumours.[274,277] They have a signal density similar to CSF on CT and MRI scans, with rim-like enhancement of the capsule after administration of contrast media.[274,278] There is often surrounding calcification.[274] Macroscopically, the cysts have a smooth, yellowish-stained lining and usually contain brown or xanthochromic fluid. Histologically, they lack epithelium and are lined by a rim of compressed gliotic tissue, often including Rosenthal fibres and some admixed collagen. This lining abuts directly onto pineal gland parenchymal tissue. Where only small biopsy fragments of the cyst wall are available, a low grade cystic astrocytoma needs to be considered as a differential diagnosis. Small cysts found incidentally on MRI scanning can be managed conservatively with follow-up scans if appropriate,[274] while symptomatic cases are effectively cured by surgical excision of the cyst.[276,277] Some of the smaller examples may result from spontaneous degenerative changes within the pineal gland glial stroma[105,276] but the larger, symptomatic cysts are thought to be derived from persistent remnants of the fetal pineal diverticulum.[277,279]

Choroid plexus cysts

Small asymptomatic cysts of the choroid plexus are found incidentally in over a third of all autopsies.[280,281] They are usually less than 1 cm in diameter and are mostly lined by a thin layer of compressed connective tissue.[281] Such asymptomatic cysts are more often found in older age groups and are probably of degenerative aetiology.[281] Very uncommonly, larger cysts in the choroid plexus of the fourth or lateral ventricles can present with episodic headaches, probably due to intermittent obstruction of the ventricular system.[281,282] Some of these are lined by choroid plexus epithelium (Fig. 17.25) and even though they are intimately associated with normal plexus tissue, such lesions are probably best regarded as a form of developmental neuroglial cyst.[105,282] Large choroid plexus cysts are also found in around 3% of all second trimester fetuses screened by ultrasound examination.[283,284] Many of these are otherwise normal at birth, but about 6% have chromosome abnormalities, especially trisomy 18.[284,285] As a result, it has been suggested that such cases should undergo fetal karyotyping, particularly if ultrasound scans show any other anatomical abnormalities.[284,285]

Perineurial cysts

Perineurial cysts are fusiform, loculated cavities arising within spinal roots at their site of exit from the dura and their junction with the dorsal root ganglion (Table 17.3).[286,287] They mostly occur in posterior sacrococcygeal roots, although thoracic examples are documented.[288] The cysts vary from a few millimetres to 2 cm in diameter, and are either an incidental autopsy finding or present symptomatically with pain and sensory disturbance in a sciatic distribution.[287,288] They are often multiple, and can be detected radiologically using myelography or MRI.[286,288] Histologically, the cyst cavity is continuous with the perineurial space of the nerve root and lies inside the junction of arachnoid and perineurial membranes.[287] There is no epithelial lining and the cyst wall consists of

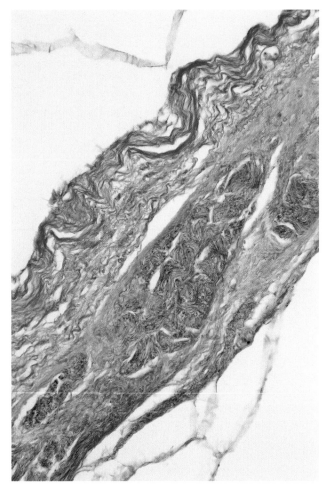

Fig. 17.26 **Sacral perineurial cyst.** The cyst cavity (top) is lined by dense collagenous tissue, but green-stained nerve root fibres are present within the wall. van Gieson/solochrome cyanine.

connective tissue intermingled with spinal root fibres and dorsal root ganglion cells (Fig. 17.26). The cysts are thought to result from degeneration within the nerve root sheath, possibly following localised inflammation or haemorrhage.[287,288] Symptomatic cases can be treated by surgical excision, although only the roof of the cyst can be removed if the nerve root is to be preserved.[288,289]

Nervous system lipoma

Incidence and site

Lipomas are rare at intracranial and intraspinal sites and account for less than 1% of nervous system tumours.[290] About 40% of *intracranial* lipomas are sited in the interhemispheric fissure over the corpus callosum[291,292] (Table 17.4), where they have been described as an incidental finding in 0.03% of cases in one large CT scan series.[293] Other typical intracranial sites are the quadrigeminal plate region[294,295] and the suprasellar cistern,

Table 17.4 Craniospinal lipoma – typical sites

Supratentorial	Interhemispheric (corpus callosum)
	Suprasellar (hypothalamic)
Infratentorial	Quadrigeminal plate
	Cerebellopontine angle
Spinal	Intradural: cervicothoracic, posterior
	Extradural: thoracic, posterior

where they are normally attached to the pituitary stalk or floor of the third ventricle.[292,296] Intracranial lipomas may also occupy a cerebellopontine angle,[297,298] but most are in midline sites.[299] *Intraspinal* lipomas are mostly intradural in location and account for between 1 and 2% of all primary spinal tumours.[300,301] They are typically posterior, midline lesions and occur most commonly in the thoracic region or at lower cervical levels.[301,302] High cervical lipomas extending above the foramen magnum are very uncommon.[303,304] Extradural spinal lipomas are again rare, accounting for only about 0.08% of primary spinal tumours.[301] They are also usually thoracic and posterior in location.[303,305] When symptomatic, both cranial and spinal lipomas usually present in children and young adults, with a fairly constant incidence throughout the first three decades of life.[301,302] Cases diagnosed symptomatically over the age of 60 years are very unusual and there is no sex bias.[301]

Aetiology

Intracranial and intradural spinal lipomas occur at sites where adipose tissue is not normally present, and are almost certainly maldevelopmental or hamartomatous lesions rather than true neoplasms.[301,306] They are usually intimately associated with meningeal tissue, and are felt most likely to be derived from aberrant differentiation of primitive mesenchymal elements persisting from an early stage of meningeal development.[294,306] In support of this concept, the sites of predilection of craniospinal lipomas are said to correspond to the temporal sequence in which the primitive meningeal matrix matures and disappears during normal embryogenesis.[202] In cases presenting in the second or third decade of life, it has been suggested that aberrant lipoid differentiation of the sequestered matrix elements may be stimulated by changes of hormonal environment associated with adolescence.[307] Embryonic inclusion of multipotential mesenchymal elements during closure of the neural tube has also been proposed as an aetiological mechanism for some nervous system lipomas, especially where there is an associated dysraphic abnormality.[301,306] In contrast to epidermoid cysts, however, lipomas thought to be the result of iatrogenic or traumatic implantation of subcutaneous fat have been exceptionally uncommon.[308]

Lumbosacral lipomas and lipomeningoceles

True intraspinal lipomas are normally held in distinction from the fatty masses which often form part of a lumbosacral spina bifida abnormality.[301,309] Such lesions always have a subcutaneous component which is in direct continuity with intraspinal fatty tissue via the posterior bony defect.[310,311] They also differ from purely intraspinal lipomas in having an exclusively lumbosacral location, a frequent association with spinal cord tethering, a typical presentation in very early life and a bias towards the female sex.[312] Where the dysraphic anomaly is severe, they are sometimes referred to as lipomeningoceles,[290,312] and they are probably best considered as being an integral part of a complex spinal malformation.

Associated lesions

Approximately 50% of intracranial lipomas are associated with various nervous system malformations,[292] including gliomeningeal heterotopia, micropolygyria and hemispheric hypoplasia.[313,314] Interhemispheric lipomas are particularly likely to be accompanied by partial or complete agenesis of the corpus callosum,[291,313] although it is not clear whether the lipoma prevents normal callosal development or simply develops at the site of a primary neural defect.[313] Dysraphic anomalies such as spina bifida and cleft palate have also been reported in association with intracranial lipomas.[294] Spina bifida occulta or other vertebral bony anomalies are found in association with about one-third of spinal intradural lipomas, but in contrast to lipomeningoceles, a low, tethered cord is uncommon.[301] Both cranial and spinal intradural lipomas may be multiple,[301,306] and spinal examples can occur in conjunction with quite separate subcutaneous lipomas at the same level.[301] Spinal extradural lipomas are not usually associated with neuraxial malformations, but patients quite often have other lipomas at systemic sites.[301] Adipose tissue is normally present in the spinal extradural space, and lipomas at this site probably have a closer aetiological relationship to their systemic counterparts than to intradural lipomas.[301]

Clinical features

About half of symptomatic intracranial lipomas present with seizures,[295,306] which are possibly caused by the effects of collagenous growth at the interface of adipose tissue and brain.[299] Some cases may also be associated with mental retardation or a history of non-localising headaches.[295] Larger lipomas in the quadrigeminal plate region may cause aqueduct compression and present acutely with raised intracranial pressure due to obstructive hydrocephalus.[315,316] Cerebellopontine angle lipomas are more likely to cause focal neurological deficits than lesions

at other intracranial sites, and can present with unilateral deafness, cerebellar disturbances or lower cranial nerve palsies.[295,317] Spinal lipomas may be a purely incidental finding or present with signs and symptoms of spinal cord compression appropriate to the level of the lesion.[301,302] The symptoms are typically of relatively short duration in cases of extradural spinal lipoma, but for intradural lesions the clinical history often dates back many years, with very gradually progressive clinical deterioration.[301,305]

Radiology

Craniospinal lipomas have the imaging characteristics of fat in both CT and MRI scans.[299,315] MRI scans show a homogeneous, high signal intensity on T1-weighted images and a very low attenuation with T2-weighting.[315,318] Using CT scans, lipomas appear as non-enhancing, very low density lesions with a signal intensity similar to that of dermoid cysts[295] (Fig. 17.27). Calcification can be present in larger corpus callosal lipomas, and this may be visible in CT scans and plain skull X-rays.[319,320]

Pathology

Macroscopic features

Craniospinal lipomas are lobulated masses of rubbery adipose tissue, which are invested in a well circum-

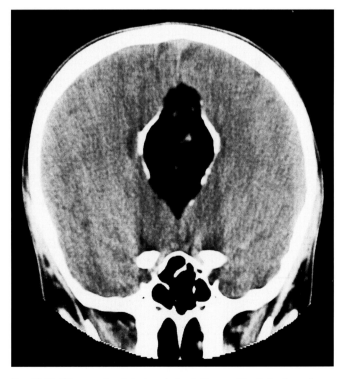

Fig. 17.27 **CT scan of an interhemispheric lipoma.** The fatty tissue has a very low signal intensity and lies between the cerebral hemispheres in the region of the corpus callosum. The lateral margins are outlined by high signal areas of calcification.

scribed, whitish fibrous capsule and covered by lepto-meninges. When viewed in cut section, their bright yellow colour contrasts with the dull greys of adjacent brain or spinal cord tissue, and irregular strands of whitish collagenous tissue can be seen to blend from their edges into the adjacent neural parenchyma. Interhemispheric lipomas are typically large, sausage shaped lesions which lie above an attenuate corpus callosum or occupy the defect caused by callosal agenesis (Fig. 17.28). Very large examples may project down into the lateral ventricles. The anterior cerebral arteries are usually deeply embedded in the lesion and may traverse its entire length. Lipomas in the suprasellar region are usually small, pea-sized nodules attached to the undersurface of the hypothalamus or pituitary stalk by a broad pedicle (Fig. 17.29). Spinal intradural lipomas tend to be elongate in shape, often extending over several segments. They are always firmly attached to the posterior cord surface and often have an extensive intramedullary component which may efface much of the cross-sectional area of the cord.

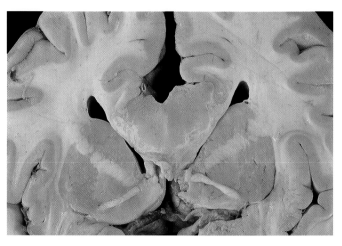

Fig. 17.28 **Interhemispheric lipoma.** The lesion bulges down into the lateral ventricles and displaces the cingulate arteries dorsally. Bright yellow fatty tissue contrasts with the grey colours of adjacent brain. White collagenous septae extend from the inferior margin of the lipoma into the attenuate corpus callosum beneath it.

Histological features

Microscopically, nervous system lipomas resemble those found elsewhere in the body and consist of lobules of mature adipose tissue intersected by variably dense collagenous septa. These collagenous bands often radiate deeply into adjacent brain or spinal cord, and may enclose separated islands of central nervous tissue at the periphery of the lesion. There is usually a marked reactive gliosis in the surrounding nervous parenchyma. Calcification is present in many larger lipomas and some may even be ossified.[306] As in systemic lipomas, the vascularity is very variable, but some examples show

quite prominent proliferation of small, thin walled vascular channels, and are often referred to as angiolipomas.[320] Angiomatous change is particularly common in spinal extradural lipomas.[321]

Differential diagnosis

The only serious diagnostic difficulty concerns the distinction of simple lipomas from well differentiated teratomas, which also tend to occupy similar sites in the neuraxis and may have a prominent adipose tissue component. The diagnosis may be made more difficult where otherwise apparently typical lipomas contain

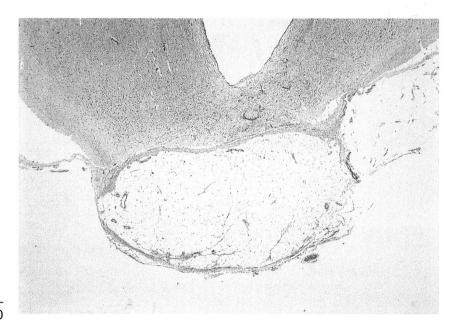

Fig. 17.29 **Suprasellar lipoma.** This example is small and well circumscribed but is densely adherent to the floor of the third ventricle. H & E.

ganglion cells or mature cartilage.[297,314] Where non-lipoid mesenchymal elements are present, teratoma should always be considered a possible diagnosis and the lesion extensively sampled for epithelial tissues or other more definite evidence of teratoid origin. In particular, it is clearly of prognostic importance to exclude the presence of poorly differentiated teratoid elements in areas not initially selected for histological examination.

Therapy and prognosis

The tenacious fibrous attachment of intradural lipomas to adjacent neural structures make radical excision dangerous or impossible in many cases, and most authorities advocate conservative management wherever possible.[297,306] This is particularly the case where epilepsy is the main clinical manifestation, since fits are rarely relieved by surgery.[299,320] Following attempted excision of callosal lipomas, a poor surgical outcome has usually been associated with damage to the anterior cerebral arteries or limbic pathways.[291,320] Brain stem dysfunction or multiple cranial nerve palsies may complicate excision of cerebellopontine angle lesions.[297,317] Where callosal or quadrigeminal plate lipomas are large enough to cause obstructive hydrocephalus, simple CSF shunting without attempted excision is normally advocated, and produces good long term results.[315,322] For spinal intradural lipomas causing cord compression, surgery is usually confined to a partial, intracapsular removal, and some cases may be best served by limiting the procedure to a simple decompressive laminectomy.[301,302] If the compressive symptoms recur, they normally respond to limited reoperation.[291] However, the situation is quite different for those spinal lipomas which are extradural. Here complete excision is normally possible, often with complete resolution of signs and symptoms.[301,305]

Hypothalamic neuronal hamartoma

Incidence, site and aetiology

Hypothalamic neuronal hamartomas are abnormal masses of brain tissue sited in the interpeduncular fossa adjacent to the floor of the third ventricle. They occupy the subarachnoid space between the mammillary bodies and the pituitary stalk, and are usually attached to the inferior aspect of the hypothalamus by a pedicle or narrow stalk of nervous parenchyma.[323,324] Occasionally there may be no neural connection with the underlying brain.[325] They are very rare lesions which occur more often in males than females[326] and are of presumed developmental aetiology.[323,326] Some cases occur in association with other congenital anomalies, including olfactory atresia and multiple systemic malformations.[324,327] Most of

these abnormalities can be dated to the period in early embryogenesis when the hypothalamus normally separates from the thalamus, and the hamartomas may be the result of a developmental insult interfering with this process.[324]

Clinical features

The most common clinical presentation is that of precocious puberty, usually manifesting in infancy or early childhood.[328,329] A degree of mental retardation is often present in these cases[328] and affected children may also display unusual laughing seizures, sometimes referred to as 'gelastic epilepsy'.[330,331] Less frequently, the hamartomas are found in adults presenting with acromegaly, usually in association with a functioning pituitary adenoma.[332,333] In rare instances, hypothalamic hamartomas are an incidental autopsy finding[325] or cause hydrocephalus due to third ventricular obstruction.[334]

Radiology

Hypothalamic hamartomas are visible on computerised tomograms as rounded, homogeneous masses in the interpeduncular cistern.[328,335] They are isodense with the adjacent brain and do not enhance after administration of contrast media.[335] MRI is probably better at delineating the extent of the lesion, because the abnormal tissue is strikingly hyperintense compared to brain when T2-weighted images are used.[336,337]

Endocrine function

A variety of tumours in the suprasellar region may cause precocious puberty as a result of non-specific mechanical interference with hypothalamic function,[338,339] but there is now good evidence that hypothalamic hamartomas produce their systemic endocrinological effects by specific hormonal modulation of the anterior pituitary gland.[333,340] In cases presenting with precocious puberty, immunocytochemical studies have demonstrated that the hamartomatous neurones are capable of synthesising gonadotropin releasing factors, which are thought to stimulate the anterior pituitary gland following direct secretion into the hypophyseal portal vascular system.[340,341] In acromegalic patients, the neurones in some hamartomas have shown immunocytochemical evidence of somatotrophin or growth hormone releasing factor production, which is presumed to provoke eventual pituitary adenoma formation by chronic overstimulation of the anterior gland somatotroph cells.[332,333] The situation here is analogous to that of the functioning pituitary adenomas associated with intrasellar gangliocytomas or ganglion cell nests (see Chapter 16).

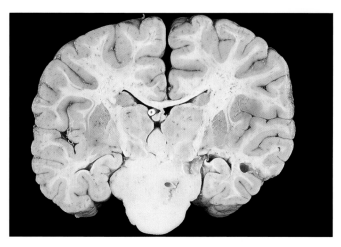

Fig. 17.30 **Hypothalamic neuronal hamartoma.** This quite large example has a broad base which merges with the floor of the third ventricle and extends into the ventricular cavity. The abnormal tissue is pale and featureless, enclosing a single large blood vessel.

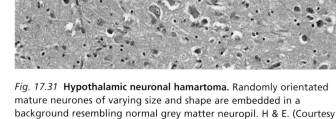

Fig. 17.31 **Hypothalamic neuronal hamartoma.** Randomly orientated mature neurones of varying size and shape are embedded in a background resembling normal grey matter neuropil. H & E. (Courtesy of Prof. M Esiri, Oxford, UK.)

Pathology

Macroscopic features

Hypothalamic hamartomas are smooth, lobulated masses which are covered by the leptomeninges of the inter-peduncular cistern. They vary in size from less than 1 cm to over 6 cm in diameter and the larger examples cause significant distortion of local structures, including the optic chiasm and pituitary stalk. In some cases the pituitary gland and stalk cannot be identified at post-mortem, possibly as a result of prolonged local compression.[324] The hamartomas are mostly well circum-scribed, pedunculated lesions, but some examples have a broad pedicle of tissue which merges with the underlying third ventricular floor. On cut section, the abnormal tissue has a homogeneous, greyish-white appearance, usually rather paler than cerebral grey matter (Fig. 17.30).

Microscopic features

The hamartomatous tissue consists of randomly arranged nests of mature neurones embedded in a fibrillary matrix resembling grey matter neuropil (Fig.17.31). The neurones vary widely in size and can be uni- or multipolar. Larger examples often have a chromatolytic appearance with eccentric nuclei and marginated Nissl substance, and these have been likened to the magnocellular neurones of the normal hypothalamus. Background neuritic processes usually lack an orderly structure, and glomeruloid nests of argyrophilic processes similar to senile plaques have been described.[325] Bundles of myelinated fibres may also be present.[342,343] There is often a significant degree of fibrillary gliosis, and the astrocytic cells present can be strikingly pleomorphic or multinucleated.[325] Mitotic figures and immature cellular elements are never seen,

but there may be a range of regressive changes, including hyalinisation, vascular thrombosis and mineralisation.[333] Electron microscopy has confirmed the neurosecretory nature of the larger neurones present, which contain well developed rough endoplasmic reticulum and Golgi bodies together with membrane bound neurosecretory granules.[333,340]

Differential diagnosis

The distinctive histological appearance of hypothalamic hamartomas means they are unlikely to be confused with suprasellar tumours such as lipomas, pituitary adenomas and craniopharyngiomas. They can be distinguished from teratomas by the lack of non-neural tissue elements and from pilocytic astrocytomas by their prominent neuronal component. Excluding a third ventricular ganglioglioma may be less straightforward, although most hamartomas differ from gangliogliomas in being obviously extracerebral, pedunculated lesions. Histo-logically, the typical grey matter neuropil and absence of ganglion cell atypia are helpful in the distinction of hamartomas from gangliomas. Pleomorphism of the glial elements needs to be interpreted with caution, as this can be a feature of either entity.

Therapy and prognosis

Hypothalamic hamartomas causing precocious puberty are usually treated by surgical excision of the abnormal tissue mass.[328,331] Where excision has been complete, abnormal sexual development has arrested or regressed in most cases, with resolution of disordered systemic gonadotropin levels.[329] Gelastic epilepsy has also been cured or improved by removal of the hamartoma.[331,344] There are no reports of neoplastic change or recurrence following surgery. In cases presenting with acromegaly due to an associated functioning pituitary adenoma, symptomatic relief may be obtained by transnasal resection of the adenoma.[333]

Neuroglial heterotopias

Meningeal glial heterotopia

Small islands of heterotopic central nervous tissue within the leptomeninges are a rather uncommon incidental autopsy finding in otherwise normal brains, but may be found in up to 25% of patients with other congenital abnormalities of the central nervous system.[345,346] Such asymptomatic heterotopia are not usually visible to naked eye examination, although some cases may show focally thickened, adherent meninges.[346] Very rarely, much larger extracerebral glial heterotopia may present clinically as mass lesions, either sited intradurally[347] or encapsulated within dural connective tissue.[348] The majority of meningeal glial heterotopia are sited over the anterior surface of the medulla or around the lumbosacral spinal cord, and they are relatively uncommon over the surfaces of the cerebral and cerebellar hemispheres.[346]

Pathology

Histologically, meningeal heterotopia consist of ovoid masses of glial tissue, with centrally grouped astrocytic nuclei and an outer, circumferential layer of glial fibres. They are usually entirely surrounded by a sheath of arachnoid tissue (Fig. 17.32). Ganglion cells are not usually present but over half of all cases contain ependymal cell nests or tubules. Mitotic figures and primitive elements are not seen. Although of no clinical significance in themselves, microscopic meningeal heterotopia are though to act as the source of both extracerebral astrocytomas[345,349] and diffuse leptomeningeal gliomatosis, especially where no intraparenchymal tumour is evident.[350,351]

Nasal glial heterotopia

Extracranial neuroglial heterotopia are most common in the region of the nose or nasopharynx and are developmental in aetiology, despite frequent use of the misleading term 'nasal glioma'. They are thought to result from entrapment of brain tissue as the anterior fontanelle closes during fetal development.[352,353] The mechanism is similar to that responsible for anterior encephaloceles, but in the case of nasal glial heterotopia the skull bones are presumed to fuse completely, leaving isolated or 'pinched off' extracranial nervous tissue without an intracranial connection.[354,355] The lesions are usually

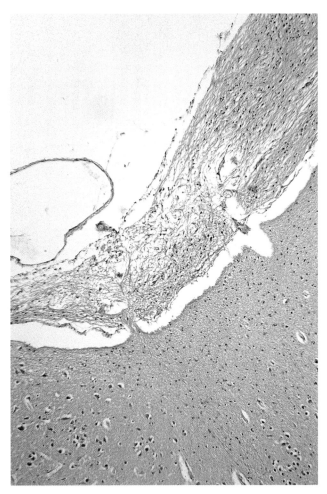

Fig. 17.32 **Meningeal glial heterotopia.** A mass of fibrillary glial tissue is lying over the cortical pial surface, ensheathed by a very thin layer of leptomeningeal collagen. Van Gieson.

diagnosed neonatally or in early infancy, and are more common in males than females.[356] Extranasal examples are sited over the bridge of the nose and present as a subcutaneous mass, typically with discolouration of the overlying skin.[352,354] The nose is often abnormally broad and there may also be hyperteliorism.[354] Slightly less commonly, the heterotopia take the form of an intranasal polyp, usually attached to the mucosa of the middle turbinate bone or high lateral wall of the nasal cavity.[354,357] These polyps can protrude visibly from one or other nostril, or may present with respiratory distress due to nasal obstruction.[357,355] Glial heterotopia can also occur within the cavity of the nasopharynx, usually with an attachment to the soft palate.[359,360] These again tend to present in early life with respiratory obstruction.[353]

Pathology

Nasal glial heterotopia are firm, irregular, rather elastic masses on gross examination and vary from pea size to several centimetres in diameter. Histologically, they consist of islands of mature central nervous tissue intersected by irregular collagenous septae. They are not encapsulated and may abut directly onto the overlying epidermis or respiratory mucosal epithelium (Fig. 17.33). The neural tissue consists mostly of astrocytic cells set in a fibrillary stroma of glial processes. Giant and multinucleated cells may be present but mitotic figures are virtually never seen. Mature ganglion cells and ependymal tubules are a rather infrequent finding, and are more likely to be encountered in nasopharyngeal examples.[353,359]

Differential diagnosis

Nasal glial heterotopia can easily be distinguished from olfactory neuroblastomas by the lack of immature or undifferentiated elements. The appearances are those of disorganised central nervous tissue rather than a glial neoplasm. Teratomas can be excluded by wide histo-logical sampling to confirm the absence of other tissue elements. The histological features in most cases are identical to those of anterior encephaloceles, and distinction between these two lesions relies on radiological exclusion of an anterior skull defect or intracranial connection.[361]

Therapy

Once a communicating encephalocele has been excluded, the heterotopia are usually treated by external resection, without the need for a craniotomy.[353,355] Recurrences are rare and are normally associated with incomplete primary resection.[353,358] Some recurrent examples appear to have enlarged due to autonomous growth, but these have not shown histological evidence of neoplastic transformation[354] and cure has normally been achieved by a repeated, more radical excision.[353] Local tissue invasion and metastatic spread have not been recorded, even in cases of clinical recurrence.[352]

Miscellaneous extracranial glial heterotopia

Extracranial central nervous tissue heterotopia are very uncommon outside the nasopharyngeal region, and nearly always occur in other areas of the head and neck. Reported sites include the orbit,[362] skull bones,[363] tongue,[364] middle ear,[365] lip[366] and scalp.[367] The lesions usually present in infancy as visible or palpable tissue masses, although some examples may be a purely incidental finding in later life.[363] The histological appearances are largely similar to those of nasal glial heterotopia, but in some cases neuronal, ependymal or choroid plexus elements may be a prominent feature,[364] and cerebellar differentiation has been described.[362] Exceptionally, heterotopic central nervous tissue has also been reported in the lungs of stillborn or otherwise healthy infants.[368] Such pulmonary glial heterotopia are sometimes found in association with anencephaly, and may result from fetal inhalation of brain fragments which become dispersed into the amniotic fluid during development.[369]

Vascular malformations

The characterisation of nervous system vascular malformations has been greatly influenced by angiographic studies, and their haemodynamic properties of are of considerable relevance to diagnosis, managment and prognosis.[370,371] In functional terms, the most important distinction is between arteriovenous malformations, or AVMs, which receive blood at arterial pressure directly from an arteriovenous fistula, and those malformations which involve only the capillary or venous systems.[371,372]

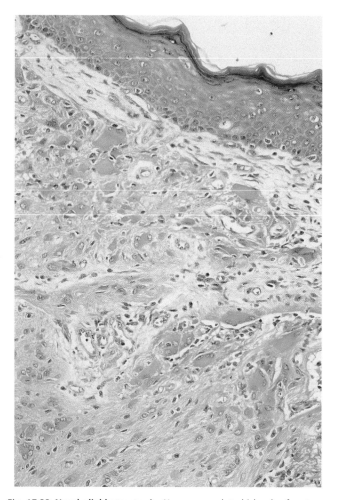

Fig. 17.33 Nasal glial heterotopia. Non-encapsulated islands of mature central nervous tissue are seen immediately deep to the nasal epidermis. The astrocytic cells show considerable pleomorphism but mitotic figures are not present. H & E.

Table 17.5 Classification of craniospinal vascular malformations

1. *Arterial fistula*
   Intracranial AVM   – Parenchymal
                                  – Vein of Galen
                                  – Transdural

   Spinal AVM   – Long dorsal (transdural fistula)
                                  – Glomus
                                  – Diffuse (juvenile)

2. *No arterial fistula*
   Capillary telangectasis
   Venous malformation   – Cavernous angioma
                                  – Venous angioma (varices)

The arterially fed AVMs are of greater clinical significance than purely capillary or venous malformations, and are associated with a considerably higher morbidity and mortality.[373,374] The subclassification of these two main groups of vascular malformation, however, is still rather controversial, particularly in regard to the various types of spinal AVM[372,375] and in the distinction of capillary from venous lesions.[376,377] Vascular malformations are not included in the WHO tumour classification[378] and the scheme suggested here takes into account the functional properties of each lesion as well as their pathological features (Table 17.5). Various types of vascular malformation also occur as part of complex hereditary disorders such as Sturge–Weber syndrome and hereditary haemorrhagic telangectasia, and these are dealt with in Chapter 19.

Arteriovenous malformations

(1) Intracranial parenchymal AVM

Incidence and site

AVMs account for between 1.5 and 4% of all brain tumours[379,380] and cases presenting with haemorrhage occur at about one-sixth the frequency of ruptured berry aneurysms.[381] Asymptomatic examples have been reported as an incidental post-mortem finding in 0.52% of cases in one large autopsy series.[382] There is no predilection for one or other sex.[381] Intracranial parenchymal AVMs are mostly supratentorial in location,[379] although posterior fossa examples may also occur.[383] The cerebral lesions are sited most commonly in the territory of middle cerebral artery supply, especially in the midparietal region[379] and are fed in descending order of frequency by branches of the middle, anterior and posterior cerebral arteries.[384] Draining veins are most commonly superficial convexity vessels, but some deep lesions drain into the vein of Galen, and these are described separately below. Rarer sites for cerebral AVMs include the choroid plexus[385] and

corpus callosum[386] and up to 4% of patients have lesions at multiple locations.[387] The optic pathways may also be affected, particularly in the Wyburn–Mason syndrome (see Chapter 19), where large malformations extend from the retina back into the brain via the optic nerve.[388]

Aetiology

In common with AVMs at other sites, the nidus of parenchymal brain AVMs acts as a true artery-to-vein shunt, without intervening capillary elements.[371,379] The abnormal vessels forming the fistula are presumed to be of congenital origin, and are thought to derive from focal persistence of embryological vascular channels which fail to differentiate normally into mature arterial, venous or capillary elements.[379] The arterial vessels feeding the lesion do not exhibit a normal autoregulatory response to changes in flow or pressure[371] and the surrounding brain tissue often becomes ischaemic due to cerebrovascular steal.[389,390] The progressive enlargement of cerebral AVMs is probably due to the sequential development of new collateral feeding arteries and draining veins, which form as a result of the continuous shunting of arterial blood into the venous system.[371]

Association with berry aneurysms

Between 6 and 9% of brain AVMs occur in conjunction with one or more berry aneurysms,[391,392] and about three-quarters of these cases present with a bleed from the aneurysm rather than the malformation.[393] The aneurysms are most commonly located proximal to the AVM on arterial branches acting as feeding vessels, but may also arise on vessels which appear to be unrelated to the fistula.[393] They are thought to form as a result of haemodynamic changes caused by the arteriovenous shunting through the AVM.[378]

Clinical features

Intracerebral AVMs most often become symptomatic in children or young adults, and are diagnosed increasingly rarely after the fourth decade of life.[379,384] The most common presentation is that of haemorrhage, which is especially associated with younger age groups and occurs in half to three-quarters of all cases.[381,394] The bleeding is more often intraparenchymal than subarachnoid or intraventricular, and is often less cataclysmic than that following berry aneurysm rupture, with a more subtle onset of headache and neurological deficit.[371] In some cases there may be a history of relatively mild, recurrent clinical episodes spanning a period of several years.[371] Over one-quarter of supratentorial AVMs present with epilepsy, often in older patients, and subsequent haemorrhage in these cases is unusual.[379,381] Sometimes there may also be progressive focal neurological deficits due to ischaemia of brain tissue adjacent to the lesion.[371,379]

Radiology

The radiological diagnosis is heavily dependent on angiography, which remains an essential investigation for the identification of arterial feeding vessels prior to surgery.[371,379] CT scans will identify the haematoma in lesions which have bled, and may also show the larger abnormal arteries and veins after contrast enhancement.[371] MRI usually provides better localisation of AVMs, even where there has not been haemorrhage. In customised sequences the abnormal vessels are clearly visible as low signal 'flow-voids', and in some circumstances magnetic resonance angiography is starting to supersede classical dye injection.

Pathology

Macroscopic features

The nidus of parenchymal AVMs consists of a tangled mass of irregular vascular channels which is bluish in colour in fixed specimens. The abnormal vessels vary in calibre but are often several millimetres in external diameter. In most cases, the lesions are quite superficial and have a pial component which is visible on external examination of the brain. The overlying leptomeninges are usually thickened and bloodstained, and the brain tissue adjacent to larger examples can be strikingly shrunken and atrophic. There is nearly always prominent hypertrophy of the leptomeningeal veins draining the lesion over a large area of the surface of the affected hemisphere. Unlike the draining veins, the hypertrophied feeding arteries tend to be buried deeper within brain substance, and are mostly concentrated in the Sylvian fissure when the lesions are fed by middle cerebral artery branches. In coronal section, superficially sited AVMs typically have a circumscribed, wedge shaped outline, with a broader base at the cortical surface tapering to an apex in deeper white matter. More centrally located examples may encroach on deep grey matter structures and partly occupy the ventricular cavities (Fig. 17.34).

Histological features

Microscopically, the lesions consist of a mass of vascular channels of widely varying calibre and configuration (Fig. 17.35). Some have the features of normal arteries or veins, but the majority are irregular cavernous spaces of very abnormal structure. Their walls vary greatly in thickness and individual examples may have both massively hypertrophied and very thin, attenuate areas in the same plane of section. Many of these abnormal vascular channels show proliferation of smooth muscle and elastic

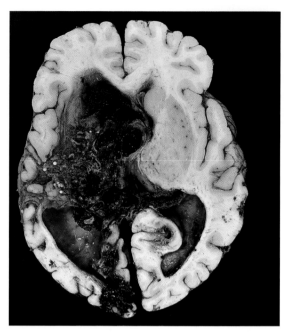

Fig. 17.34 **Intracerebral arteriovenous malformation.** This large, deep-seated example partly occupies the expanded left lateral ventricle and is associated with atrophy of the adjacent cerebral mantle. White intravascular embolisation spheres are visible towards the outer edge of the lesion.

tissue, giving the histological appearance of an irregularly arterialised vein. This constitutes an important distinction from the non-arterial types of vascular malformation, in which muscular hypertrophy and elastic tissue is lacking (Table 17.6). The abnormal vessels frequently show evidence of extensive thrombosis, organisation and recanalisation, and there may be calcification in thicker areas of vessel wall. The intervening and surrounding brain tissue is always markedly degenerate and gliotic, often with abundant deposition of old blood pigment and haemosiderin laden macrophages. Lesions examined after embolisation with cyanoacrylate derivatives show an intraluminal foreign-body giant cell reaction, sometimes with patchy mural necrosis, extravasated embolic material and chronic perivascular inflammatory infiltrates.[395,396]

Therapy and prognosis

If left untreated, approximately two-thirds of patients with AVMs in the brain will suffer a clinically significant haemorrhage[373,397] and this is associated with an immediate mortality rate of about 10%.[371,374] The prognosis following an initial bleed is less favourable when the lesion is sited in the posterior fossa.[373] Haemorrhage is more likely to occur in younger patients and those with smaller malformations[384,398] possibly as a result of the higher luminal pressures associated with such lesions.[371] The annual risk of haemorrhage has been estimated at 2–3%,

Fig. 17.35 Intracerebral arteriovenous malformation. The abnormal vascular channels have walls of a very variable thickness. Some show irregular proliferation of muscle and elastic tissue and resemble arterialised veins. Elastic/Van Gieson.

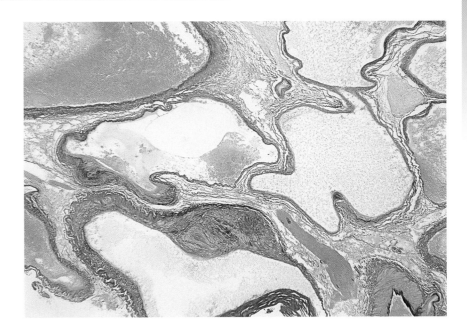

Table 17.6 Differential diagnosis of parenchymal vascular malformations

	Type of lesion	Most common sites	Appearances of abnormal vessels	Changes in adjacent nervous tissue
Parenchymal AVM	Arteriovenous fistula	Subpial cerebrum Thoracic cord	Irregular arterialised channels – hyaline sclerosis – muscular hypertrophy – elastic proliferation Thrombosis common	Gliosis and degeneration, usually marked Old blood pigment, macrophages May be ischaemic changes
Capillary telangectasis	Capillary anomaly	Brain stem	Dilated capillary channels Endothelium and basement membrane only Rarely calcified	Vessels widely separated by normal or mildly gliotic nervous tissue
Cavernous angioma	Venous anomaly	Temporal lobe Brain stem	Ectatic venous channels Variable hyaline thickening No muscular or elastic proliferation Thrombosis and calcification common	Little intervening nervous tissue in centre Gliosis and old haemorrhage around periphery
Venous angioma	Venous anomaly	Frontal and parietal white matter	Dilated veins in inappropriate location Normal histological structure or non-specific hyaline thickening	Vessels widely separated by normal or gliotic nervous tissue

with an overall mortality of 1% per year.[374,397] Following a first episode, the risk of rebleeding rises to about 6% in the ensuing year, but returns to the prehaemorrhage rate thereafter.[374,397]

The treatment of choice for smaller and surgically accessible AVMs is complete resection, combined with ligation or clipping of the main arterial feeding vessels.[379,399] In some suitable cases pre- or intraoperative embolisation is used to reduce the flow through the lesion prior to

excision.[400,401] The results of surgery depend on the size of the lesion and the eloquence of adjacent brain structures,[402] but in most series about 90% of cases have made a good recovery without subsequent haemorrhage.[398,403] Acute postoperative complications include bleeding and focal neurological deficits due to local ischaemia.[379,404] Epilepsy is another significant cause of postoperative morbidity, and is unlikely to resolve if it was the presenting clinical feature.[384] Angiographic embolisation with cyanoacrylate derivatives has also been used as the sole means of therapy in some larger or inaccessible lesions, particularly where the presentation has included progressive neurological deficit.[405,406] The results in such cases have been rather equivocal, but some studies have reported a decreased incidence in the rate of subsequent haemorrhage where lesions have not already bled.[406] Stereotactic radiosurgery (the so-called 'gamma knife') has also been used for inoperable cases,[407,408] and has been successful both in obliterating a significant proportion of smaller lesions[409,410] and in arresting progressive neurological deficits and seizures.[407] There have, however, been occasional reports of delayed cerebral radionecrosis following this procedure.[411]

(2) Arteriovenous fistulae involving the vein of Galen

These lesions, sometimes misleadingly referred to as 'aneurysms' of the vein of Galen, constitute a distinct subgroup of cerebral AVMs. The feeding vessels may be branches of the anterior or posterior cerebral arteries, choroidal arteries or anterior cerebellar vessels.[412,413] Drainage, however, is always directly into the vein of Galen, which is transformed into a huge, arterialised, fusiform sac, itself draining into the straight sinus[412] (Fig. 17.36). The massive arteriovenous shunting caused by these lesions typically presents in neonates as acute congestive heart failure,[413,414] and in some cases this may be complicated by associated congenital cardiac defects.[415] Haemodynamic steal may also result in massive neonatal cerebral infarction or periventricular leukomalacia.[416,417] Less commonly, the lesions manifest later in childhood or in early adult life, when the presentation is more often

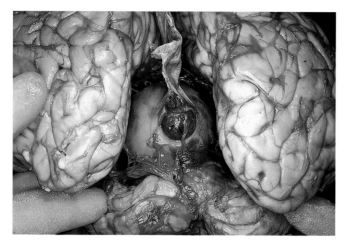

Fig. 17.36 **Vein of Galen arteriovenous fistula.** The vein of Galen is transformed into a large, aneurysmal sac, seen here between the occipital lobes.

one of hydrocephalus due to the local obstructive effect of the greatly enlarged vein of Galen.[413] Treatment in either case consists of ligation or clipping of the main feeding vessels, and removal of the venous sac itself is often not possible.[379,412]

(3) Intracranial transdural AVMs

These lesions consist of a small arteriovenous fistula within the thickness of the cranial dura which is fed by external branches of the carotid or vertebral arteries.[418,419] They represent between 10 and 15% of all intracranial AVMs.[418] In most cases the fistula is thought to be congenital in origin,[418,420] although a small proportion may develop as a result of major head trauma or sinus thrombosis.[419] In about three-quarters of all cases, the fistula is actually within the wall of the transverse or sigmoid sinuses, which act directly as draining vessels without involvement of intradural veins.[418,419] The presentation in such patients is usually that of tinnitus, head bruits, or headache and papilloedema due to increased intracranial venous pressure.[418] Occasionally a steal syndrome may cause neurological deficits due to cerebral ischaemia or focal infarction.[421] The remaining transdural AVMs drain into the cavernous sinus and present as a caroticocavernous fistula.[374] Unlike acquired fistulae, however, the shunt within the sinus wall is fed from extracavernous branches of the carotid artery.[419] These lesions may resolve spontaneously following thrombosis,[374] but the fistulae which drain into the transverse or sigmoid sinuses usually require embolisation or ligation of the feeding vessels, and preferably excision of the intradural shunt within the sinus wall.[418]

(4) Spinal AVMs

Selective spinal angiography has led to considerable advances in the categorisation of spinal AVMs, and from a previously rather confused and voluminous literature, the following classification has evolved:[375,422]

- *Long dorsal AVMs* These account for over 80% of all cases[423] and are the result of one or more transdural arteriovenous fistulae, usually sited where the radicular arteries enter the dural sleeve.[422] The fistulae lie within the thickness of the dura and are fed by branches of normal extradural segmental arteries.[424] Drainage is directly into the dorsal venous plexus of the cord, which is sinusoidal, arterialised and greatly hypertrophied.
- *Glomus AVMs* These are circumscribed AVMs similar to those found in the brain, and may be intra- or extramedullary in location.[375,422] They are often supplied by just a single intraparenchymal artery and again drain into the venous plexus of the cord.

- *Juvenile or diffuse AVMs* These are very large lesions fed by multiple intradural arterial feeding vessels, and they most commonly present in children. In most cases, the voluminous abnormal vascular channels fill the entire spinal canal and there is often extensive involvement of the cord parenchyma.[370,375] In contrast to the other two types, the abnormal intraspinal vasculature has a very high flow rate.

Incidence, site and aetiology

Most spinal AVMs are thought to be of congenital origin, although some examples of the long dorsal type may develop as the result of an acquired, post-traumatic transdural fistula.[424] Taken together, they have been estimated as accounting for anything between 3% and 11% of all spinal tumours.[375] With the exception of the juvenile type, they present most commonly in middle age, and are more common in males than females.[425,426] They most commonly affect thoracolumbar regions of the cord, although the abnormal vessels of the long dorsal and juvenile types often extend the entire length of the spinal canal.[426,427] In some patients, a cutaneous angioma may be present in the skin of the back overlying the affected levels of the spine.[370] Spinal AVMs, and particularly the long dorsal variety, are also associated with a chronic progressive form of myelomalacia, sometimes called Foix–Alajouanine disease,[427] which is thought to be due to the effects of chronic venous hypertension on the intraparenchymal vasculature of the cord.[423]

Clinical features

Spinal AVMs typically present with back pain, frequently radicular in nature, together with progressive cord dysfunction relevant to the site and extent of the lesion.[422,426] The neurological deficit is presumed to result from the accompanying myelomalacia, and frequently follows a step-like course, producing severe disability only a few years after the onset of symptoms.[422] An acute presentation due to haemorrhage is relatively uncommon and occurs only in about 10–15% of all cases.[422] The most relevant radiological investigation is selective spinal angiography, which is needed to identify the feeding vessel(s) prior to surgery. Myelography is rarely used now, but reveals the abnormal intradural vessels as serpiginous filling defects.[422,425] MRI is useful to assess the degree of spinal cord parenchymal damage, which is visible as areas of high signal with appropriate scan settings.[428]

Pathology

Macroscopic features

The long dorsal and diffuse types of spinal AVM lack a macroscopically obvious nidus but are associated with diffuse hypertrophy of vessels over the surface of the spinal cord. In the case of the long dorsal malformations, this is largely confined to the posterior aspect of the cord and typically has the appearance of an unusually prominent and convoluted posterior venous plexus (Fig. 17.37). Hypertrophy of the venous plexus is usually less prominent in glomus malformations, which have a similar naked eye appearance to AVMs of the brain. The spinal cord frequently appears shrunken and atrophic beneath the abnormal vasculature of diffuse and long dorsal lesions, and cut section may show extensive softening, discolouration and cavitation of medullary tissue.

Histological features

The histological features of glomus spinal AVMs are again similar to those of their cerebral counterparts, and the associated degenerative changes in the adjacent spinal cord parenchyma are usually quite localised.

In the juvenile type of malformation, the large and partly arterialised vascular channels do not form a discrete

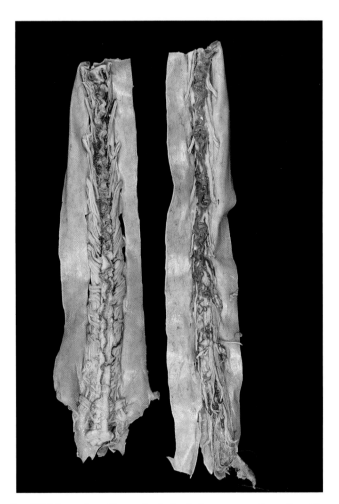

Fig. 17.37 **Long dorsal type of spinal arteriovenous malformation.** The posterior venous plexus of the spinal cord is abnormally tortuous and engorged.

focus, but fill the subarachnoid space, indenting the cord surface and extending widely into gliotic and degenerate underlying parenchyma.

In long dorsal malformations, the hypertrophied vessels are mostly confined to the posterior surface of the cord. They have the more regular microscopic features of previously normal veins which have become arterialised, showing uniform muscular hyperplasia and a diffuse proliferation of elastic tissue (Fig. 17.38). There may be evidence of thrombosis and recanalisation of these vessels, sometimes accompanied by a scanty perivascular lymphocytic infiltrate. In contrast to the juvenile lesions, there are no large arterialised vascular channels within the cord itself, but longer standing cases show the changes of diffuse myelomalacia or 'Foix–Alajouanine disease'. This usually takes the form of widespread, patchy demyelination and gliosis, often with areas of focal ischaemic degeneration and cystic cavitation. Small calibre parenchymal arteries and veins show a striking, hyaline sclerosis with progressive obliteration of the lumen, which is one of the most characteristic features of the condition. If the transdural shunt has been angiographically localised, it may be found by serially sectioning the specimen of surgically excised dura. As with intracranial transdural fistulae, the histological features of the shunt are those of a small, focal collection of irregular and partly arterialised vascular channels, embedded within the thickness of the dural membrane (Fig. 17.39).

Therapy and prognosis

The glomus type of spinal AVMs is most often treated by surgical excision, sometimes in association with pre-operative embolisation of the feeding vessels.[370,422] Embolisation alone often fails to ablate the lesion.[429] Embolisation also carries a significant risk of obstructing the normal blood supply to the cord, since collateral circulation is more limited than in most areas of the brain.[422] For the long dorsal type of lesion, it is now recognised that attempted surgical removal of the arterialised dorsal venous plexus is both unnecessary and often positively harmful.[370,423] Effective treatment depends on resection or ligation of the transdural fistula, which first needs to be accurately localised by selective spinal angiography.[422,423] Removal of the arteriovenous shunts usually halts further neurological deterioration and may produce dramatic clinical improvement,[423,430] but treatment needs to be given early, before irreversible degenerative changes have occurred in the cord.[430] The juvenile or diffuse form of spinal AVM carries a much less favourable prognosis than the other types and is not usually amenable to surgical resection.[370,422] Some cases may respond to ligation or embolisation of major feeding vessels[431] but these are very numerous and often cannot

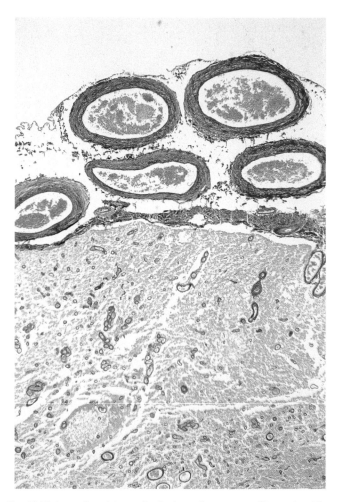

Fig. 17.38 **Long dorsal type of spinal arteriovenous malformation.** The hypertrophied vessels are confined to the surface of the spinal cord and have the regular architecture of veins which have become arterialised. Elastic/Van Gieson.

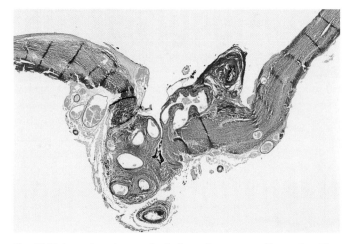

Fig. 17.39 **Long dorsal type of spinal arteriovenous malformation.** The transdural fistula consists of a focal collection of arterialised vascular channels embedded within the thickness of the dura. Elastic/Van Gieson.

be safely interrupted without risking ischaemic damage to the cord.[422]

Capillary telangiectases

Capillary telangiectases are an infrequent finding in the central nervous system, although the majority are small and asymptomatic and probably pass unnoticed.[432] They are most usually found in ventromedial areas of the brain stem, especially at the level of the pons[433] and may also occur in subcortical white matter of the cerebral hemispheres.[432,434] In some cases the lesions may be multiple,[376] especially in association with vascular dysgenetic syndromes such as ataxia telangiectasia[435] and hereditary haemorrhagic telangectasia[436] (see Chapter 19). The spinal cord is rarely affected.[376] Three-demensional study has shown irregular, multifocal dilatations of capillaries in the affected area, but no increase in capillary density as compared to the adjacent brain tissue.[434] The ectatic vessels drain into normal calibre venous channels.[434] Capillary telangiectases are most often an incidental autopsy finding[434] but some present symptomatically with acute haemorrhage,[433] and calcified examples in the temporal lobe may cause epilepsy.[437] In rare instances, large lesions in the brain stem have been associated with progressive neurological dysfunction without an episode of bleeding.[438]

Pathology

Macroscopically, telangectases are visible as rather poorly defined areas of reddish-grey discolouration with punctate foci resembling petechial haemorrhages. Cerebral subcortical examples tend to be wedge shaped, tapering into deeper white matter. Most are not much more than 1 cm in maximum dimension, but larger

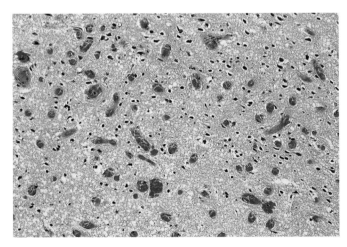

Fig. 17.40 **Frontal capillary telangiectasis.** There is a loose aggregation of dilated thin-walled capillary channels of varying calibre. The intervening nervous tissue is mildly gliotic with a few specks of haemosiderin pigment. H & E.

examples may occur.[438] Histologically, the appearances are those of a loose collection of irregularly dilated capillary channels varying widely in calibre (Fig. 17.40). The walls lack elastic or muscle tissue and usually consist only of a single endothelial layer supported by basement membrane. In distinction from cavernous angiomas, the vessel walls rarely show significant collagenous thickening and the intervening brain tissue is either normal or only very mildly gliotic. Even in rare cases where the capillary vessels are calcified, the lesions can usually be distinguished from calcified cavernous angiomas by the wide separation of individual vascular channels.[437] Where acute, fatal brain stem haemorrhage has occurred, the abnormal vessels of a telangectasis may be largely destroyed by bleeding, and can be difficult to demonstrate even after exhaustive histological sampling of autopsy tissue.

Venous malformations

(1) Cavernous angiomas

Incidence, site and aetiology

Cavernous angiomas of the nervous system present most commonly in children and young adults, and are more common in males than females.[439,440] A significant proportion of cases are familial[441] and some may be associated with similar angiomas in systemic sites.[432,442] Most authorities regard cavernous angiomas as quite distinct from capillary telangiectases, but both types of lesion may coexist in the same patient and examples with a transitional histological appearance have been described, suggesting a possible aetiological link between the two entities.[376,377] A majority of cavernous angiomas are supratentorial in location, most commonly involving the temporal lobe.[440,443] Other typical sites include the basal ganglia and the pons.[440] Rarely the optic pathways or spinal cord may also be involved.[440,444] Central nervous system cavernous angiomas are not infrequently multiple, and may present as part of a dominantly inherited syndrome with similar angiomas affecting skin and viscera (see Chapter 19)

Clinical features

Approximately one-third of symptomatic patients present with epilepsy, which is typically associated with heavily calcified lesions sited in or near the temporal lobe.[443,445] Acute haemorrhage occurs in a similar proportion of cases[439,445] and the annual risk of bleeding in untreated patients has been estimated as 0.7%.[446] About 10% of reported cases remain asymptomatic and are discovered incidentally at autopsy.[440] Like telangectases, cavernous angiomas do not have a direct arterial contribution and a significant proportion are angiographically occult.[445] The remainder typically appear as avascular areas with an early venous drainage phase.[371,440] Using CT most examples are hyperdense or heterogeneous lesions, which normally enhance with contrast media and often show prominent calcification.[440,445] The central areas of most cavernous angiomas also have a mixed signal intensity on magnetic resonance scans, but there is frequently a characteristic low density rim to the lesion.[371,440]

Pathology

Macroscopic features

Cavernous angiomas vary from pinhead to fist size, but most are in the region of 1–2 cm across. They are very well circumscribed, lobulated, dark red masses which are sometimes likened to a mulberry in external appearance. Cut section reveals a spongy network of blood-filled channels, often with extensive thrombosis and focal areas of calcification (Fig. 17.41). The adjacent brain tissue is usually shrunken and tough due to gliosis, and dis-

coloured by yellowish-brown blood pigment. Where the lesions are superficially sited, the overlying meninges are also discoloured by old haemorrhage, but in contrast to AVMs, there is no generalised hypertrophy of the surrounding meningeal veins.

Histological features

The dilated venous channels are of widely varying calibre and are lined by a single layer of flattened endothelium. Their walls are irregularly thickened by hyaline collagenous tissue (Fig. 17.42). There is no muscular hypertrophy or elastic lamina and elastic filaments are absent or extremely scanty. Many of the vessels show varying stages of thrombosis and recanalisation and there is often quite extensive intramural calcification. In the centre of the lesion the vessels are closely juxtaposed with little intervening brain tissue, but towards the margins they are separated by tongues of densely gliotic nervous parenchyma. This usually contains abundant old blood pigment and collections of macrophages, sometimes with cholesterol granulomata, giant cells and chronic inflammatory cells. Cavernous angiomas can be distinguished histologically from AVMs by the lack of muscular hypertrophy or elastic tissue in the vessel walls, and also by the absence of arteries in association with the lesion. The major differences from capillary telangectases are the close juxtaposition of the vascular channels, their thickened, hyaline walls and the degree of gliosis and degenerative change in adjacent brain tissue.

Therapy and prognosis

Symptomatic cavernous angiomas are normally treated by surgical resection,[440,447] the outcome depending on both the nature of initial presentation and the site of the lesion.[445] The best results are obtained with supratentorial angiomas presenting with epilepsy or mass effect, and there is much poorer prognosis in cases presenting with significant haemorrhage, especially those located in the brain stem.[445,448]

(2) Venous angiomas

Venous angiomas, also sometimes referred to simply as 'varices', consist of a group of small transcortical medullary veins which converge onto a large central draining vein within the brain parenchyma.[371,449] These large draining veins are often orientated radially to the pial surface and are presumed to represent a developmental anomaly, focally replacing the normal superficial draining system of the brain.[371] The angiomas may occur anywhere in the cerebrum or hindbrain, but are most common in the white matter of the frontal and parietal lobes and the cerebellum.[450,451]

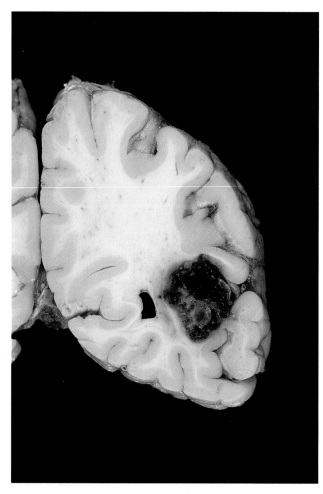

Fig. 17.41 **Occipital lobe cavernous angioma.** Cut section reveals a circumscribed mass of partly thrombosed vascular channels.

Fig. 17.42 **Cavernous angioma.** The dilated venous channels have irregularly thickened, hyalinised walls. They are closely apposed in the central area, but tongues of gliotic nervous tissue are visible around the margins of the field. H & E.

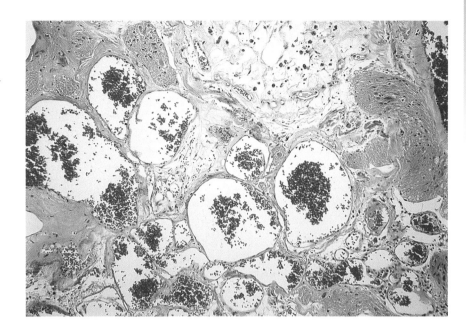

Clinical features

In the vast majority of cases, the lesions are asymptomatic and are discovered incidentally during radiological investigation for unrelated disorders.[372,450] A small number present clinically with headache, progressive neurological deficits or epilepsy.[449,450] Presentation with haemorrhage is rare and has been estimated to occur at a rate of only 0.15% per lesion-year.[451] The angiographic features are characteristic, and the lesions are often referred to as having a 'hydra' or 'caput medusa' appearance.[374,449] The large central draining veins are usually detectable as linear or serpiginous enhancing structures using CT, and may also be apparent as flow voids on magnetic resonance angiograms.[371,450]

Pathology

On gross examination of the brain, venous angiomas appear as small, rather ill-defined areas of discolouration in the subcortical white matter in which one or more dilated thin walled vessels may be visible (Fig. 17.43). Histologically, they consist of loose collections of dilated parenchymal veins of varying calibre (Fig. 17.44). The vessels lack a defined tunica media or elastic lamina and may either have an entirely normal histological structure or show non-specific hyaline thickening of their walls.[371,450] They differ from the vessels in cavernous angiomas in being widely separated by well preserved neural parenchyma.[450]

Therapy and prognosis

Death as a result of spontaneous haemorrhage from a venous malformation is exceptionally rare.[450] Some

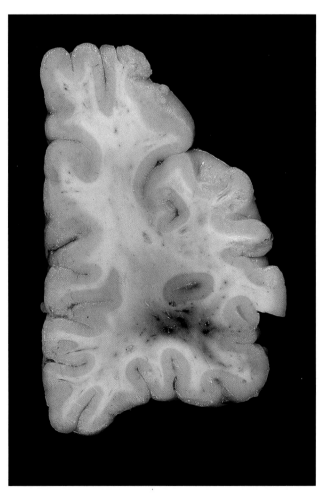

Fig. 17.43 **Venous angioma.** This lesion is visible macroscopically as a small focal collection of dilated venous channels within an area of discoloured white matter.

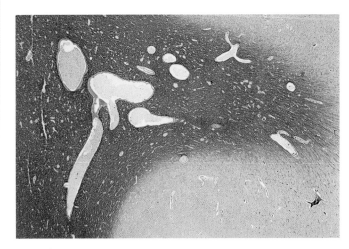

Fig. 17.44 **Venous angioma.** These malformations consist of loose collections of dilated parenchymal veins of variable calibre. The intervening white matter is well preserved histologically. Phosphotungstic acid haematoxylin.

patients presenting acutely due to bleeding recover without treatment and can be managed conservatively.[449,450] Where surgery is indicated, a favourable outcome may again be expected after drainage of the haematoma, with or without resection of the abnormal veins themselves.[450] In symptomatic cases without haemorrhage, a conservative approach is again usually advocated in view of the low incidence and risks of bleeding.[449,451] However, prophylactic surgery has been recommended for cerebellar examples, since these are said to be associated with an increased likeihood of life-threatening haemorrhage compared with those at other sites.[371]

REFERENCES

Craniopharyngioma

1. Burger PC, Vogel FS. Surgical pathology of the nervous system and its coverings. New York: Wiley, 1976: pp 425–437
2. Kovacs K, Horvath E. Tumours of the pituitary gland. Atlas of tumour pathology, second series, Fascicle 21. Washington DC: Armed Forces Institute of Pathology, 1986: pp 237–251
3. Kleihues P, Burger PC, Scheithauer BW et al. Histological typing of tumors of the central nervous system, 2nd edn. Berlin: Springer, 1993
4. Russell DS, Rubinstein LJ. Pathology of tumors of the nervous system, 5th edn. London: Arnold, 1989: pp 695–702
5. Zülch KJ. Brain tumours. Their biology and pathology, 3rd edn. Berlin: Springer, 1986: pp 426–432
6. Adamson TE, Wiestler OD, Kleihaus P et al. Correlation of clinical and pathological features in surgically treated craniopharyngiomas. J Neurosurg, 1990; 73:12–17
7. Sanford RA, Muhlbauer MS. Craniopharyngioma in children. Neurol Clin, 1991; 9:453–465
8. Lu DH, Xu QZ. Pathological analysis of 1458 cases of tumor in the sella turcica region. Chung Hua Chung Liu Tsa Chih, 1988; 10:205–208
9. Pertuiset B. Craniopharyngiomas. In: Vinken PJ, Bruyn GW, eds. Handbook of clinical neurology, vol. 18. Tumours of the brain and skull. Part III. Amsterdam: North Holland, 1975: pp 531–572
10. Koos WT, Miller MH. Intracranial tumors of infants and children. Stuttgart: Thieme, 1971: p 415
11. Petito CK, De Girolami U, Earle KM. Craniopharyngiomas. Cancer, 1976; 37:1944–1952
12. Baskin DS, Wilson CB. Surgical management of craniopharyngiomas: A review of 74 cases. J Neurosurg, 1986; 65:22–27
13. Banna M, Hoare RD, Stanley P et al. Craniopharyngioma in children. J Pediatr, 1973; 83:781–785
14. Banna M. Craniopharyngioma based on 160 cases. Br J Radiol, 1976; 49:206–223
15. Hurst RW, McIlhenny J, Park TS et al. Neonatal craniopharyngioma: CT and ultrasonographic features. J Comput Assist Tomogr, 1988; 12:858–861
16. Tabaddor K, Shulman K, Dal Canto MC. Neonatal craniopharyngioma. Am J Dis Child, 1974; 128:381–383
17. Bailey W, Freidenberg GR, James HE et al. Prenatal diagnosis of a craniopharyngioma using ultrasonography and magnetic resonance imaging. Prenat Diagn, 1990; 10:623–629
18. Janisch W, Flegel HG. Craniopharyngioma in a fetus. Zentralbl Allg Pathol, 1989; 135:65–69
19. Lederman GS, Recht A, Loeffler JS et al. Craniopharyngioma in an elderly patient. Cancer, 1987; 60:1077–1080
20. Russell RWR, Pennybacker JB. Craniopharyngioma in the elderly. J Neurol Neurosurg Psychiatry, 1961; 24:1–13
21. Banna M. Craniopharyngioma in adults. Surg Neurol, 1973; 1:202–204
22. Bartlett JR. Craniopharyngiomas. A summary of 85 cases. J Neurol Neurosurg Psychiatry, 1971; 34:37–41
23. Hiramatsu K, Takahashi K, Ikeda A et al. A case of intrasellar craniopharyngioma. Tokai J Exp Clin Med, 1987; 12:135–140
24. Shimada M, Tsugane R, Shibuya N et al. Craniopharyngioma with extension into the cerebellopontine angle. Case report. Tokai J Exp Clin Med, 1989; 14:113–116
25. Tkezaki K, Fujii K, Kishikawa T. Magnetic resonance imaging of an intraventricular craniopharyngioma. Neuroradiology, 1990; 32:247–249
26. Kunishio K, Yamamoto Y, Sunami N et al. Craniopharyngioma in the third ventricle: necropsy findings and histogenesis. J Neurol Neurosurg Psychiatry, 1987; 50:1053–1056
27. Hillman TH, Peyster RG, Hoover ED et al. Infrasellar craniopharyngioma: CT and MR studies. J Comput Assist Tomogr, 1988; 12:702–704
28. Byrne MN, Sessions DG. Nasopharyngeal craniopharyngioma. Case report and literature review. Ann Otol Rhinol Laryngol, 1990; 99:633–639
29. Luse SA, Kernohan JW. Squamous cell nests of pituitary gland. Cancer, 1955; 8:623–628
30. Erdheim J. Zur normalen und pathologischen Histologie der Glandula thyroidea, parathyroidea und hypophysis. Beitr Pathol Anat 1903; 33:158–236
31. Cushing H. Intracranial tumours. Springfield, Illinois: Thomas, 1932
32. Asa SL, Kovacs K, Bilbao JM. The pars tuberalis of the human pituitary. Virchows Archiv (A) 1983; 339:49–59
33. Goldberg GM, Eshbaugh DE. Squamous cell nests of the pituitary gland as related to the origin of craniopharyngiomas: a study of their presence in the newborn and infants up to age four. Arch Pathol Lab Med, 1960; 70:293–299
34. Carmel PW. Brain tumours of disordered embryogenesis. Craniopharyngioma. In: Youmans JR, ed. Neurological surgery, 3rd edn, vol. 5. Philadelphia: Saunders, 1990: pp 3223–3238
35. Goodrich JJ, Post MD, Duffy P. Ciliated craniopharyngioma. Surg Neurol, 1985; 24:105–111
36. Yoshida J, Kobayashi T, Kageyama N et al. Symptomatic Rathke's cleft cyst. Morphological study with light and electron microscopy and tissue culture. J Neurosurg, 1977; 47:451–458
37. Kalnins V, Rossi E. Odontogenic craniopharyngioma. A case report. Cancer, 1965; 18:899–906
38. Seemayer TA, Blundell JS, Wigglesworth FW. Pituitary craniopharyngioma with tooth formation. Cancer, 1972; 29:423–430
39. Bernstein ML, Buchino JJ. The histological similarity between craniopharyngioma and odontogenic lesions: a reappraisal. Oral Surg, 1983; 56:502–511
40. Sorva R Children with craniopharyngioma. Early growth failure and rapid postoperative weight gain. Acta Paediatr Scand, 1988; 77:587–592
41. Cabezudo JM, Vaquero J, Garcia de Sola R et al. Computer tomography with craniopharyngiomas: a review. Surg Neurol, 1981; 15:422–427
42. Freeman MP, Kessler RM, Allen JH et al. Craniopharyngiomas: CT

and MR imaging in nine cases. J Comput Assist Tomogr, 1987; 11:810–814

43. Pigeau I, Sigal R, Halimi P et al. MRI features of craniopharyngiomas at 1.5 Tesla. A series of 13 cases. J Neuroradiol, 1988; 15:276–287

44. Pusey E, Kortman KE, Flannigan BD et al. MR of craniopharyngiomas: tumour delineation and characterization. Am J Roentgenol, 1987; 149:383–388

45. Sorva R, Jaaskinen J, Heiskanen O. Craniopharyngioma in children and adults. Correlations between radiological and clinical manifestations. Acta Neurochir (Wien), 1987; 89:3–9

46. Mincione GP, Mincione F, Mennonna P. Cytological features of craniopharyngioma. Pathologica, 1991; 83:191–196

47. Nelson GLA, Bastian FO, Schlitt M et al. Malignant transformation in craniopharyngioma. Neurosurgery, 1988; B22:427–429

48. Grover WD, Rorke LB. Invasive craniopharyngioma. J Neurol Neurosurg Psychiatry, 1968; 31:580–582

49. Lewis AJ, Cooper PW, Kassel EE et al. Squamous cell carcinoma arising in a suprasellar epidermoid cyst. J Neurosurg, 1983; 59:538–541

50. Asa SL, Kovacs K, Bilbao JM et al. Immunohistochemical localisation of keratin in craniopharyngiomas and squamous cell nests of the human pituitary. Acta Neuropathol (Berl), 1981; 54:257–260

51. Hayashi K, Hoshida Y, Horie Y et al. Immunohistochemical study on the distribution of alpha and beta subunits of S-100 protein in brain tumours. Acta Neuropathol (Berl), 1991; 81:657–663

52. Landolt AM. Ultrastructure of human sella tumours. 7. Craniopharyngiomas. Acta Neurochir (Suppl), 1975; 22:104–119

53. Moss TH. Tumours of the nervous system. An ultrastuctural atlas. Berlin: Springer, 1986: pp 123–128

54. Ghatak NR, Hirano A, Zimmerman HM. Ultrastructure of a craniopharyngioma. Cancer, 1971; 27:1465–1475

55. Sato K, Kubota T, Yamamoto S et al. An ultrastructural study of mineralisation in craniopharyngiomas. J Neuropathol Exp Neurol, 1986; 45:463–470

56. Genth J, Gullotta F, Serra JP. Elektronenoptische und enzymhistochemische Vergleichsucheruchungen on Kraniopharyngiomen und ihren Gewebekulturen. Acta Neuropathol (Berl) 1974; 28:331–341

57. Unterharnscheidt FJ. Routine tissue culture of CNS tumours and animal implantation. Prog Exp Tumour Res, 1972; 17:111–150

58. Liszcak T, Richardson EP Jr, Phillips JP et al. Morphological, biochemical, ultrastructural tissue culture and clinical observations of typical and aggressive craniopharyngiomas. Acta Neuropathol (Berl), 1978; 43:191–203

59. Boggan JE, Davis RLO, Zorman G et al. Intrasellar epidermoid cyst. J Neurosurg, 1983; 58:411–415

60. Sorva R, Heiskanen O. Craniopharyngioma in Finland. A study of 123 cases. Acta Neurochir (Wien), 1986; 81:85–89

61. Pierre-Kahn A, Brauner R, Renier D et al. Treatment of craniopharyngiomas in children. Retrospective analysis of 50 cases. Arch Fr Pediatr, 1988; 45:163–167

62. Sorva R, Heiskanen O, Perheentupa J. Craniopharyngioma surgery in children: endocrine and visual outcome. Childs Nerv Syst, 1988; 4:97–99

63. Hoffman HJ, Kendrick EB, Humphreys RP et al. Management of craniopharyngioma in children. J Neurosurg, 1977; 47:218–227

64. Stolke D, Seifert V. Trans-sphenoid microsurgery of craniopharyngioma. Neurochirurgia (Stuttg) 1990; 33:106–109

65. Laws ER Jr. Trans-sphenoidal microsurgery in the management of craniopharyngioma. J Neurosurg, 1980; 52:661–666

66. Yasargil MG, Curcic M, Kis M et al. Total removal of craniopharyngiomas. Approaches and long-term results in 144 patients. J Neurosurg, 1990; 73:3–11

67. Al-Hefty O, Hassounah M, Weaver P et al. Microsurgery for giant craniopharyngiomas in children. Neurosurgery, 1985; 17:585–595

68. Hoffman HJ, De Silva M, Humphreys RP et al. Aggressive surgical management of craniopharyngiomas in children. J Neurosurg, 1992; 76:47–52

69. Amacher AL. Craniopharyngioma: the controversy regarding radiotherapy. Childs Brain, 1980; 6:57–64

70. Kramer SW, Southard M, Mansfields CM. Radiotherapy in the management of craniopharyngiomas. Am J Roentgenol, 1968; 103:44–52

71. Basaki M, Shitara N, Takakura K et al. Treatment of recurrent craniopharyngioma. No Shinkei Geka, 1988; 16:395–401

72. Manake S, Teramoto A, Takakura K. The efficacy of radiotherapy for craniopharyngioma. J Neurosurg, 1985; 62:648–656

73. Polz Tejera G, Sod L, Kotsilimbas D. Recurrent cystic craniopharyngioma management and course. Neurochirurgia (Stuttg), 1986; 29:48–49

74. Spaziante R, De Divigtiis E, Irace C et al. Management of primary or recurring grossly cystic craniopharyngiomas by means of draining systems. Topic review and 6 case reports. Acta Neurochir (Wien), 1989; 97:95–106

75. Backlund EO. Studies on craniopharyngiomas: III Stereotaxic treatment with intracystic yttrium-90. Acta Chir Scand, 1973; 139:237–247

76. Kobayashi T, Kageyama N, O'Hara K. Internal irradiation for cystic craniopharyngioma. J Neurosurg, 1981; 55:896–903

77. Saaf M, Thoren M, Bergstrand CG et al. Treatment of craniopharyngiomas: the stereotactic approach in a ten to twenty-three years' perspective. II Psychosocial situation and pituitary function. Acta Neurochir (Wien), 1989; 99:97–103

78. Munari C, Landre E, Musolino A et al. Long term results of stereotactic endocavitary beta irradiation of craniopharyngioma cysts. J Neurosurg Sci, 1989; 33:99–105

79. Rosenthal R, Gamroth A, Sturm V et al. Cystic craniopharyngiomas: computed tomography in the pretherapeutic evaluation and control of treatment results following intracystic contact irradiation. Strahlenther Onkol, 1987; 163:621–625

80. Bucci MN, Chin LS, Hoff JT. Perioperative morbidity associated with operative resection of craniopharyngioma: A review of ten years experience. Neurochirurgia (Stuttg), 1987; 30:135–138

81. Brauner R, Malandry F, Rappaport R et al. Craniopharyngioma in children. Endocrine evaluation and treatment. Apropos of 37 cases. Arch Fr Pediatr, 1987; 44:765–769

82. Griffiths AP, Henderson M, Penn ND et al. Haematological, neurological and psychiatric complications of chronic hypothermia following surgery for craniopharyngioma. Postgrad Med J, 1988; 64:617–620

83. Matson DD, Crigler JF. Management of craniopharyngioma in childhood. J Neurosurg, 1969; 30:377–390

84. Blethen SL, Weldon VV. Outcome in children with normal growth following removal of a craniopharyngioma. Am J Med Sci, 1986; 292:21–24

85. Sorva R, Heiskanen O, Perheentupa J. Craniopharyngioma in adults. Ann Clin Res, 1987; 19:339–343

86. Thomsett MJ, Conte FA, Kaplan SL et al. Endocrine and neurologic outcome in childhood craniopharyngioma. J Pediatr, 1980; 97:728–735

87. Carmel PW, Antunes JL, Chang CH. Craniopharyngiomas in children. Neurosurgery, 1982; 11:382–389

88. Fischer EG, Welch K, Shillito J Jr et al. Craniopharyngiomas in children. Long-term effects of conservative surgical procedures combined with radiation therapy. J Neurosurg, 1990; 73:534–540

89. Humphreys RP, Hoffman HJ, Hendrick EB. A long term postoperative follow-up in craniopharyngioma. Childs Brain, 1979; 5:530–539

90. Richmond IL, Wara WM, Wilson CB. Role of radiation therapy in management of craniopharyngiomas in children. Neurosurgery, 1980; 6:513–517

91. Tanaka T, Kobayashi T. The results of treatment of craniopharyngiomas in 33 children. No Shinkei Geka, 1988; 16:845–850

Cysts

92. Kleihaus P, Burger PC, Scheithauer BW et al. Histological typing of tumours of the central nervous system, 2nd edn. Berlin: Springer, 1993

93. Shanklin WM. On the presence of cysts in the human pituitary gland. Anat Rec, 1949; 104:379–407

94. Shanklin WM. Incidence and distribution of cilia in the human pituitary with a description of microfollicular cysts derived from Rathke's cleft. Acta Anat, 1951; 11:361–382

95. Eisenberg HM, Sarwar M, Schochet SS Jr. Symptomatic Rathke's cleft cyst. J Neurosurg, 1976; 45:585–588

96. Roux FX, Constans JP, Monsaingeon V et al. Symptomatic Rathke's cleft cysts; clinical and therapeutic data. Neurochirurgia (Stuttg), 1988; 31:18–20

97. Frazier CH, Alpers BJ. Tumours of Rathke's cleft. Arch Neurol Psychiat, 1934; 32:973–984

98. Barrow DL, Spector RH, Takei Y et al. Symptomatic Rathke's cleft cysts located entirely in the suprasellar region: review of diagnosis, management and pathogenesis. Neurosurgery, 1985; 16:766–772

99. Voelker JL, Campbell RL, Muller J. Clinical, radiographic, and pathological features of symptomatic Rathke's cleft cysts. J Neurosurg, 1991; 74:535–544

100. Kucharcyk W, Peck WW, Kelly WM et al. Rathke cleft cysts: CT, MR imaging, and pathologic features. Radiology, 1987; 165:491–495

101. Yuge T, Shigemori M, Tokutomi T et al. Entirely suprasellar symptomatic Rathke's cleft cyst. No Shinkei Geka, 1991; 19:273–278

102. Martins AN. Pituitary tumours and intrasellar cysts. In : Vinken PJ, Bruyn GW, eds. Handbook of clinical neurology, vol. 17. Tumours of the brain and skull. Amsterdam, North Holland, 1974: pp 375–439

103. Shuangshoti S, Netsky MG, Nashold BS Jr. Epithelial cysts related to sella turcica. Proposed origin from neuroepithelium. Arch Pathol, 1970; 90:444–450

104. Velasco MH, Roessmann U, Gambetti P. The presence of glial fibrillary acidic protein in the human pituitary gland. J Neuropathol Exp Neurol, 1982; 41:150–163

105. Russell DS, Rubinstein LJ. Pathology of tumours of the nervous system, 5th edn. London: Edward Arnold, 1989: pp 690–727

106. Diengdoh JV, Scott T. Electron-microscopical study of a Rathke's cleft cyst. Acta Neuropathol (Berl), 1983; 60:14–18

107. Goodrich JJ, Post KD, Duffy P. Ciliated craniopharyngioma. Surg Neurol, 1985; 24:105–111

108. Yoshida J, Kobayashi T, Kageyama N et al. Symptomatic Rathke's cleft cyst. Morphological study with light and electron microscopy and tissue culture. J Neurosurg, 1977; 47:451–458

109. Midha R, Jay V, Smyth HS. Transsphenoidal management of Rathke's cleft cysts. A clinicopathological review of 10 cases. Surg Neurol, 1991; B35:446–454

110. Rout D, Das L, Rao VRK et al. Symptomatic Rathke's cleft cysts. Surg Neurol, 1983; 19:42–45

111. Steinberg GK, Hoenig GH, Golden JB. Symptomatic Rathke's cleft cysts. J Neurosurg, 1982; 56:290–295

112. Nakasu Y, Isozumi T, Nakasu S et al. Rathke's cleft cyst: computed tomographic scan and magnetic resonance imaging. Acta Neurochir (Wien), 1990; 103:99–104

113. Keyaki A, Hirano A, Llena JF. Asymptomatic and symptomatic Rathke's cleft cysts. Histological study of 45 cases. Neurol Med Chir Tokyo, 1989; 29:88–93

114. Tindall GT, Barrow DL. Tumours of the sellar and parasellar area in adults. In : Youman JR, ed. Neurological surgery, 3rd edn. Philadelphia: Saunders, 1990: pp 3447–3498

115. Diengdoh JV, Griffiths D, Crockard HA. Rathke-cleft cyst. Clin Neuropathol, 1984; 3:72–75

116. Ikeda H, Yoshimoto T, Suzuki J. Immunohistochemical study of Rathke's cleft cyst. Acta Neuropathol (Berl), 1988; 77:33–38

117. Uematsu Y, Rojas Corona RR, Llena JF et al. Epithelial cysts in the central nervous system, characteristic expression of cytokeratins in an immunohistochemical study. Acta Neurochir (Wien), 1990; 107:93–101

118. Marin F, Boya J, Lopez Carbonell A et al. Immunohistochemical localization of intermediate filament and S-100 proteins in several non-endocrine cells of the human pituitary gland. Arch Histol Cytol, 1989; 52:241–148

119. Inoue T, Matsushima T, Fukui M et al. Immunohistochemical study of intracranial cysts. Neurosurgery, 1988; 23:576–581

120. Kasper M, Karsten U. Coexpression of cytokeratin and vimentin in Rathke's cysts of the human pituitary gland. Cell Tissue Res, 1988; 253:419–424

121. Matsushima T, Fukui M, Fujii K et al. Epithelial cells in symptomatic Rathke's cleft cysts. A light- and electron-microscopic study. Surg Neurol, 1988; 30:197–203

122. Rengachary SS, Kishore PRS, Watanabe I. Intradiploic epidermoid cyst of the occipital bone with torcular obstruction. J Neurosurg, 1978; 48:475–478

123. Fager CA, Carter H. Intrasellar epithelial cysts. J Neurosurg, 1966; 24:77–81

124. Baskin DS, Wilson CB. Trans-sphenoidal treatment of non-neoplastic intrasellar cysts. J Neurosurg, 1984; 60:8–13

125. Iraci G, Giordano R, Gerosa M et al. Ocular involvement in recurrent cyst of Rathke's cleft – case report. Ophthalmology, 1979; 11:94–98

126. Raskind R, Brown HA, Mathis J. Recurrent cyst of the pituitary: 26 year follow-up from first decompression. J Neurosurg, 1968; 28:595–599

127. Martinez LJ, Osterholm JL, Berry RG et al. Transsphenoidal removal of a Rathke's cleft cyst. Neurosurgery, 1979; 4:63–65

128. Verkijk A, Bots G Th AM. An intrasellar cyst with both Rathke's cleft and epidermoid characteristics. Acta Neurochir, 1986; 51:203–207

129. Ulrich J. Intracranial epidermoids. A study of their distribution and spread. J Neurosurg, 1964; 21:1051–1058

130. Petito CK, De Girolami U, Earle KM. Craniopharyngiomas. Cancer, 1976; 37:1944–1952

131. Boggan JE, Davis RL, Zorman G et al. Intrasellar epidermoid cyst. J Neurosurg, 1983; 58:411–415

132. MacCarty CS, Leavens ME, Love JG. Dermoid and epidermoid tumours in the central nervous system of adults. Surg Gynecol Obstet, 1959; 108:191–198

133. Carmel PW. Brain tumours of disordered embryogenesis. In: Youman JR, ed. Neurological surgery, 3rd edn. Philadelphia: Saunders, 1990: pp 3223–3249

134. Toglia JU, Netzky MG, Alexander E Jr. Epithelial (epidermoid) tumours of the cranium, their common nature and pathogenesis. J Neurosurg, 1965; 23:384–393

135. Gerlach J. Tumours of the cranial vault. In: Vinken PJ, Bruyn GW, eds. Handbook of clinical neurology, vol. 17. Tumours of the brain and skull. Part II. Amsterdam, North Holland, 1974: pp 104–135

136. Guridi J, Ollier J, Aguilera F. Giant intradiploic epidermoid tumor of the occipital bone: case report. Neurosurgery, 1990; 27:978–980

137. List CF. Intraspinal epidermoids, demoids and dermal sinuses. Surg Gynecol Obstet, 1941; 73:525–538

138. Love JG, Kernohan JW. Dermoid and epidermoid tumours (cholesteatomas) of central nervous system. J Am Med Assoc, 1936; 107:1876–1884

139. Yasargil MG, Abenathy CD, Sarioglu AL. Microneurosurgical treatment of intracranial dermoid and epidermoid tumours. Neurosurgery, 1989; 24:561–567

140. Pennybacker J Cholesteatoma of the petrous bone. Br J Surg, 1944; 32:75–78

141. Jefferson G, Smalley AA. Progressive facial palsy produced by intratemporal epidermoids. J Laryngol Otol, 1938; 53:417–443

142. Manno NJ, Uihlein A, Kernohan JW. Intraspinal epidermoids. J Neurosurg, 1962; 19:754–765

143. Smith CML, Timperley WR. Multiple intraspinal and intracranial epidermoids and lipomata following gunshot injury. Neuropathol Appl Neurobiol, 1984; 10:235–239

144. Batnitzky S, Keucher TR, Mealey J Jr et al. Iatrogenic intraspinal epidermoid tumours. J Am Med Assoc, 1977; 237:148–156

145. Blockey NJ, Schorstein J. Intraspinal epidermoid tumours in the lumbar region of children. J Bone Joint Surg, 1961; 43B:556–562

146. Van Gilder JC, Schwartz HG. Growth of dermoids from skin implants to the nervous system and surrounding spaces of the newborn rat. J Neurosurg, 1967; 26:14–20

147. Saunders RL. Intramedullary epidermoid cyst associated with a dermal sinus. J Neurosurg, 1969; 31:83–86

148. Schijman E, Monges J, Cragnaz R. Congenital dermal sinuses, dermoid and epidermoid cysts of the posterior fossa. Childs Nerv Syst, 1986; 2:83–89

149. Tytus JS, Pennybacker J. Pearly tumours in relation to the central nervous system. J Neurol Neurosurg Psychiatry, 1956; 19:241–259

150. Fein JM, Lipow K, Taate F et al. Epidermoid tumor of the cerebellopontine angle: Diagnostic value of computed tomographic metrizamide cysternography. Neurosurgery, 1981; 9:179–182

151. Yanai Y, Tsuji R, Ohmori S et al. Malignant change in an intradiploic epidermoid: report of a case and review of the literature. Neurosurgery, 1985; 16:252–256

152. Goldman SA, Gandy SE. Squamous cell carcinoma as a late complication of intracerebroventricular epidermoid cyst. Case report. J Neurosurg, 1987; 16:618–620

153. Lewis AJ, Cooper PW, Kassel EE et al. Squamous cell carcinoma arising in a suprasellar epidermoid cyst. J Neurosurg, 1983; 59:538–541

154. Nosaka Y, Nagao S, Tabuchi K et al. Primary intracranial epidermoid carcinoma. J Neurosurg, 1979; 50:830–832

155. Garcia CA, McGarry PA, Rodriguez F. Primary intracranial squamous cell carcinoma of the right cerebellopontine angle. J Neurosurg, 1981; 54:824–828

156. Keville FJ, Wise BL. Intracranial epidermoid and dermoid tumours. J Neurosurg, 1959; 16:564–569

157. Lunardi P, Missori P, Gagliardi FM et al. Long-term results of the surgical treatment of spinal dermoid and epidermoid tumors. Neurosurgery, 1989; 25:860–864

158. Peyton WT, Baker AB. Epidermoid, dermoid and teratomatous tumors of the central nervous system. Arch Neurol Psychiat, 1942; 47:890–917

159. Delong GR, Adams RD. Clinical aspects of tumours of the posterior fossa in childhood. In: Vinken PJ, Bruyn GW, eds. Handbook of clinical neurology, vol. 18. Tumours of the brain and skull. Part III. Amsterdam: North Holland, 1974: pp 387–411

160. Lane CM, Ehrlich WW, Wright JE. Orbital dermoid cyst. Eye, 1987; 1:504–511

161. Nugent RA, Lapointe JS, Rootman J et al. Orbital dermoids: features on CT. Radiology, 1987; 165:475–478

162. Martinez-Lage JF, Quinonez MA, Poza M et al. Congenital epidermoid cysts over the anterior fontanelle. Childs Nerv Syst, 1985; 1:319–323

163. Parizek J, Nemecek S, Nemeckova J et al. Congenital dermoid cysts over the anterior fontanel. Report on 13 cases in Czechoslovak children. Childs Nerv Syst, 1989; 5:234–237

164. de Baecque C, Snyder DH, Suzuki K. Congenital intramedullary spinal dermoid cyst associated with an Arnold–Chiari malformation. Acta Neuropathol (Berl), 1977; 38:239–242

165. Bryant H, Dayan AD. Spinal inclusion dermoid cyst in a patient with a treated myelocystocoele. J Neurol Neurosurg Psychiatry, 1967; 30:182–184

166. Scott RM, Wolpert SM, Bartoshesky LE et al. Dermoid tumours occurring at the site of previous myelomengocoele repair. J Neurosurg, 1986; 65:779–783

167. Fleming JFR, Botterell EM. Cranial dermoid and epidermoid tumours. Surg Gynecol Obstet, 1959; 109:403–411

168. Amendola MA, Garfinkle WB, Ostrum BJ et al. Preoperative diagnosis of a ruptured intracranial dermoid cyst by computerised tomography. J Neurosurg, 1978; 48:1035–1037

169. Boissonnot L, Drouineau J, Roualdes G et al. Spontaneous rupture of intracranial dermoid cyst. Clinical and radiological study. J Radiol, 1986; 67:917–919

170. Hudgins RJ, Rhyner PA, Edwards MSB. Magnetic resonance imaging and management of a pineal region dermoid. Surg Neurol, 1987; 27:558–562

171. Smith AS, Benson JE, Blaser SI et al. Diagnosis of ruptured intracranial dermoid cyst: value MR over CT. Am J Neuroradiol, 1991; 12:175–180

172. Gluszcz A. A cancer arising in a dermoid of the brain. J Neuropathol Exp Neurol, 1962; 21:383–387

173. Lobosky JM, Vangilder JC, Damasio AR. Behavoural manifestations of third ventricular colloid cysts. J Neurol Neurosurg Psychiatry, 1984; 47:1075–1080

174. Poppen JL, Reyes V, Horrax G. Colloid cysts of the third ventricle. J Neurosurg, 1953; 10:242–263

175. Pecker J, Guy G, Scarabin JM. Third ventricle tumours. In: Vinken PJ, Bruyn GW, eds. Handbook of clinical neurology, vol. 17. Tumours of the brain and skull, Part II. Amsterdam: North Holland, 1974: pp 446–450

176. Haymaker W, Yenermen MH. Pathological features of colloid cysts of the third ventricle. A consideration of 60 cases. Exc Med viii, Neurology, 1955; 8:788

177. Little JR, MacCarty CS. Colloid cysts of the third ventricle. J Neurosurg, 1974; 40:230–235

178. Camacho A, Abernathey CD, Kelly PJ et al. Colloid cysts: experience with the management of 84 cases since the introduction of computed tomography. Neurosurgery, 1989; 24:693–700

179. Fritsch H. Colloid cysts: a review including 19 own cases. Neurosurg Rev, 1988; 11:159–166

180. Buchsbaum HW, Colton RP. Anterior third ventricular cysts in infancy. J Neurosurg, 1967; 26:264–266

181. Kappers AJ. The development of the paraphysis cerebri in man with comments on its relationship to the intercolumnar tuberle and its significance for the origin of cystic tumours in the third ventricle. J Comp Neurol, 1955; 102:425–498

182. Shuangshoti S, Roberts MP, Netsky MG. Neuroepithelial (colloid) cysts. Pathogenesis and relation to choroid plexus and ependyma. Arch Pathol, 1965; 80:214–224

183. Ho KL, Garcia JM. Colloid cysts of the third ventricle: ultrastructural features are compatible with endodermal derivation. Acta Neuropathol (Berl), 1992; 83:605–612

184. Shibata T, Burger PC, Kleihues P. Origin of colloid cyst: immunoperoxidase study. No To Shinkei, 1987; 39:953–958

185. Ghatak NR, Kasoff I, Alexandre E Jr. Further observation on the fine structure of a colloid cyst of the third ventricle. Acta Neuropathol (Berl), 1977; 39:101–107

186. Meittinen M, Clarke R, Virtanen I. Intermediate filament proteins in choroid plexus and ependyma and their tumours. Am J Pathol, 1986; 123:231–240

187. Kelly R. Colloid cysts of the third ventricle. Analysis of twenty-nine cases. Brain, 1951; 74:23–65

188. Hall NA, Lunsford LD. Changing concepts in the treatment of colloid cysts. J Neurosurg, 1987; 66:186–191

189. Riddoch G. Progressive dementia, without headache or changes in the optic discs, due to tumours of the third ventricle. Brain, 1936; 59:225–233

190. Kondziolka D, Lunsford LD. Stereotactic management of colloid cysts: factors predicting success. J Neurosurg, 1991; 75:45–51

191. Wilms G, Marchal G, Van-Hecke P et al. Colloid cysts of the third ventricle: MR findings. J Comput Assist Tomogr, 1990; 14:527–531

192. Hadfield MG, Ghatak NR, Wanger GP. Xanthogranulomatous colloid cyst of the third ventricle. Acta Neuropathol (Berl), 1985; 66:343–346

193. Shuangshoti S, Phonprasert C, Suwanwela N et al. Combined neuroepithelial (colloid) cyst and xanthogranuloma (xanthoma) in the third ventricle. Neurology, 1975; 25:547–552

194. Mosberg WH Jr, Blackwood W. Mucus-secreting cells in colloid cysts of third ventricle. J Neuropathol Exp Neurol, 1954; 13:417–426

195. Mackenzie IR, Gilbert JJ. Cysts of the neuraxis of endodermal origin. J Neurol Neurosurg Psychiatry, 1991; 54:572–575

196. Hirano A, Ghatak NR. The fine structure of colloid cysts of the third ventricle. J Neuropathol Exp Neurol, 1974; 33:333–341

197. Landolt-Weber UM. Ultrastruktur einer Kolloidcyste des dritten ventrikels. Acta Neuropathol (Berl), 1973; 26:59–70

198. Coxe WS, Luse SA. Colloid cyst of third ventricle. An electron microscopic study. J Neuropathol Exp Neurol, 1964; 23:431–445

199. Hattab N, Freger P, Tadie M et al. Treatment of colloid cysts of the third ventricle by cerebrospinal fluid shunt. Neurochirurgie, 1990; 36:129–131

200. Bosch DA, Rahn T, Backlund EO. Treatment of colloid cysts of the third ventricle by stereotactic aspiration. Surg Neurol, 1978; 9:15–18

201. Fortuna A, Mercuri S. Intradural spinal cysts. Acta Neurochir, 1983; 68:289–314

202. Wilkins RH, Odom GL. Spinal intradural cysts. In: Vinken PJ, Bruyn GW, eds. Handbook of clinical neurology, vol. 20. Tumours of the spine and spinal cord. Part II. Amsterdam: North Holland, 1976: pp 55–102

203. Agnoli AL, Laun A, Schonmayr R. Enterogenous intraspinal cysts. J Neurosurg, 1984; 61:834–840

204. French BN. Midline, fusion defects and defects of formation. In: Youmans JR, ed. Neurological surgery, 3rd edn. Philadelphia: Saunders, 1990: pp 1201–1204

205. Kahn AP, Hirsch JF, daLage C et al. Les kystes enteriques intrarachidiens. A propos de trois observations. Neurochirurgie, 1971; 17:33–44

206. Whiting DM, Chou SM, Lanzieri CF et al. Cervical neurenteric cyst associated with Klippel–Feil syndrome: a case report and review of the literature. Clin Neuropathol, 1991; 10:285–290

207. Silvernal WI Jr, Brown RB. Intradmedullary enterogenous cyst. Case report. J Neurosurg, 1972; 36:235–238

208. Mizuno J, Fiandaca MS, Nishio S et al. Recurrent intramedullary enterogenous cyst of the cervical spinal cord. Childs Nerv Syst, 1988; 4:47–49

209. Rewcastle NB, Francoeur J. Teratomatous cysts of the spinal canal. With 'sex chromatin' studies. Arch Neurol Chic, 1964; 11:91–99

210. Challa VR, Markesbery WR. Infratentorial neuroepithelial cyst (colloid cyst). J Neurosurg, 1978; 49:457–459

211. Afshar F, Sholtz CL. Enterogenous cyst of the fourth ventricle. J Neurosurg, 1981; 54:836–838

212. Giombini S, Lodrini S, Migliavacca F. Intracranial enterogenous cyst. Surg Neurol, 1981; 16:271–273

213. Schelper RL, Kagan-Hallet KS, Huntingdon HW. Brainstem subarachnoid respiratory epithelial cysts: report of two cases and review of the literature. Hum Pathol, 1986; 17:417–422

214. Del Bigio MR, Jay V, Drake JM. Prepontine cyst lined by respiratory epithelium with squamous metaplasia: immunohistochemical and ultrastructural study. Acta Neuropathol (Berl), 1992; 83:564–568

215. Lach B, Russell N, Atack D et al. Intraparenchymal epithelial (enterogenous) cyst of the medulla oblongata. Can J Neurol Sci, 1989; 16:206–210

216. van der Wal AC, Troost D. Enterogenous cyst of the brainstem: a case report. Neuropediatrics, 1988; 19:216–217

217. Rhaney K, Barclay GPT. Enterogenous cysts and congenital diverticula of the alimentory canal with abnormalities of the vertebral column and spinal cord. J Pathol Bact, 1959; 77:457–471

218. Jackson FE. Neurenteric cysts. Report of a case of neurenteric cyst with associated chronic meningitis and hydrocephalus. J Neurosurg, 1961; 18:678–682

219. Millis RR, Holmes AE. Enterogenous cyst of the spinal cord with associated intestinal reduplication, vertebral anomalies and a dorsal dermal sinus. J Neurosurg, 1973; 38:73–77

220. Laha RK, Huestis WS. Intraspinal enterogenous cyst: Delayed appearance following mediastinal cyst resection. Surg Neurol, 1975; 3:67–70

221. Holcomb GW Jr, Matson DD. Thoracic neurenteric cyst. Surgery, 1954; 35:115–121

222. Dorsey JF, Tabrisky J. Intraspinal and mediastinal foregut cyst compressing the spinal cord. Report of a case. J Neurosurg, 1966; 24:562–567

223. Piramoon AM, Abbassioun K. Mediastinal enterogenous cyst with spinal cord compression. J Pediatr Surg, 1974; 9:543–545

224. Walls TJ, Purohit DP, Aji WS et al. Multiple intracranial enterogenous cysts. J Neurol Neurosurg Psychiatry, 1986; 49:438–441

225. Geremia GK, Russell EJ, Clasen RA. MR imaging characteristics of a neurenteric cyst. Am J Neuroradiol, 1988; 9:978–980

226. Esposito S, Nardi PV, Patricolo M et al. Enterogenous cyst of the spinal cord terminal cone. Clinical and radiological aspects (CT and MRI). J Neurosurg Sci, 1989; 33:287–289

227. Scoville WB, Manlapaz JS, Otis RD et al. Intraspinal enterogenous cyst. J Neurosurg, 1963; 20:704–706

228. Hoefnagel D, Benirscuke K, Duarte J. Teratomatous cysts within the vertebral canal. Observations on the occurrence of sex chromatin. J Neurol Neurosurg Psychiatry, 1962; 25:159–164

229. Knight G, Griffiths T, Williams I. Gastrocytoma of the spinal cord. Br J Surg, 1954–55; 42:635–638

230. Matsushima T, Fukim M, Egami H. Epithelial cells in a so-called intraspinal neurenteric cyst: a light and electron microscopic study. Surg Neurol, 1985; 24:656–660

231. Hirano A, Ghatak NR, Wisoff HS et al. An epithelial cyst of the spinal cord. An electron microscopic study. Acta Neuropathol (Berl), 1971; 18:214–223

232. Bouch DC, Mitchell I, Maloney AJF. Ependymal lined paraventricular cysts: a report of 3 cases. J Neurol Neurosurg Psychiatry, 1973; 36:611–617

233. Jakubiak P, Dunsmore RMK, Beckett RS. Supratentorial brain cysts. J Neurosurg, 1968; 28:129–136

234. Friede RL. Yasargil MG. Supratentorial intracerebral epithelial (ependymal) cysts: review, case reports and fine structure. J Neurol Neurosurg Psychiatry, 1977; 40:127–137

235. Palma L. Supratentorial neuroepithelial cysts. Report of two cases. J Neurosurg, 1975; 42:353–357

236. Shuangshoti S, Phisitbutr M, Kasantikul V et al. Multiple neuroepithelial (colloid) cysts: association with other congenital anomalies. Neurology, 1977; 27:561–566

237. Ho KL, Chason JL. A glioependymal cyst of the cerebellopontine angle: immunohistochemical and ulstructural studies. Acta Neuropathol (Berl), 1987; 74:382–388

238. Kuroda Y, Abe M, Nagumo F et al. Neuroepithelial cyst presenting as recurrent aseptic meningitis. Neurology, 1991; 41:1834–1835

239. Jan M, Ba Zeze CV, Velut S. Colloid cyst of the fourth ventricle: diagnostic problems and pathogenic considerations. Neurosurgery, 1989; 24:939–942

240. Sharpe JA, Deck JHN. Neuroepithelial cyst of the fourth ventricle. J Neurosurg, 1977; 46:820–824

241. Guerardi R, Lacombe MJ, Poirier J et al. Asymptomatic encephalic intraparenchymatous neuroepithelial cysts. Acta Neuropathol (Berl), 1984; 63:264–268

242. Mortara RH, Markesberg WR, Brooks WH. Pontine cyst presenting as trigeminal pain. Case report. J Neurosurg, 1974; 41:636–639

243. Morello G, Lombardi G. Choroido-ependymal cysts of the spinal roots: case report. J Neurosurg, 1964; 21:1103–1107

244. Moore MT, Book MH. Congenital cervical ependymal cyst. Report of a case with symptoms precipitated by injury. J Neurosurg, 1966; 24:558–561

245. Gainer JR Jr, Chou SM, Nugent GR et al. Ependymal cyst of the thoracic spinal cord. J Neurol Neurosurg Psychiatry, 1974; 37:974–977

246. Ghatak NR, Hirano A, Kasoff SS et al. Fine structure of an intracerebral epithelial cyst. J Neurosurg, 1974; 41:75–82

247. Wisoff MS, Ghatak NR. Ependymal cyst of the spinal cord. J Neurol Neurosurg Psychiatry, 1971; 34:546–550

248. Cilluffo JM, Onofrio BM, Miller RH. The diagnosis and surgical treatment of intracranial cysts. Acta Neurochir, 1983; 67:215–229

249. Galassi E, Tognetti F, Frank F et al. Infratentorial arachnoid cysts. J Neurosurg, 1985; 63:210–217

250. Rengachary SS, Watanabe I. Ultrastructure and pathogenesis of intracranial arachnoid cysts. J Neuropathol Exp Neurol, 1981; 40:61–83

251. Murali R, Epstein F. Diagnosis and treatment of suprasellar arachnoid cyst. J Neurosurg, 1979; 50:515–518

252. Lodrini S, Lasio G, Fornari M et al. Treatment of supratentorial primary arachnoid cysts. Neurochirurgie, 1985; 76:105–110

253. Little JR, Gomez Mr, MacCarthy CS. Infratentorial arachnoid cysts. J Neurosurg, 1973; 39:380–386

254. Di Rocco C. Arachnoid cysts. In: Youmans JR, ed. Neurological surgery, vol. 2, 3rd edn. Philadelphia: Saunders, 1990: pp 1299–1325

255. Kim JH, Shucart WA, Haimovici M. Symptomatic arachnoid diverticulae. Arch Neurol, 1974; 31L:35–37

256. Pau A, Viale Sehrbundt E, Turtas S. Spinal intradural arachnoid cysts. Neurochirurgia, 1982; 25:19–21

257. Cloward RB. Congenital spinal extradural cysts. Case report and review of literature. Ann Surg, 1968; 168:851–864

258. Davis CM Jr. Spinal extradural cyst. Case report and tabulation of previously reported cases. J Neurosurg, 1949; 6:251–254

259. Krawchenko J, Collins GH. Pathology of an arachnoid cyst. J Neurosurg, 1979; 50:224–228

260. Teng P, Papatheodrou C. Spinal arachnoid diverticula. Br J Radiol, 1966; 39:249–254

261. Lake PA, Minckler J, Scanlan RL. Spinal epidural cyst: theories of pathogenesis. Case report. J Neurosurg, 1974; 40:774–778

262. Kasdon DL, Douglas EZ, Brougham MF. Suprasellar arachnoid cyst diagnosed preoperatively by computerised tomographic scanning. Surg Neurol, 1977; 7:299–303

263. Aicardi J, Bauman F. Supratentorial extracerebral cysts in infants and children. J Neurol Neurosurg Psychiatry, 1975; 38:57–68

264. Anderson FM, Landing BH. Cerebral arachnoid cysts in infants. J Pediatr, 1966; 69:88–96

265. Mori K, Hayashi T, Handa K. Infratentorial retrocerebellar cysts. Surg Neurol, 1977; 7:135–142

266. Agnoli AL, Schonhayr R, Laun A. Intraspinal arachnoid cysts. Acta Neurochir, 1982; 61:291–302

267. Di Sclafani A, Canale DJ. Communicating spinal arachnoid cysts: diagnosis by delayed metrizamide computed tomography. Surg Neurol, 1985; 23:428–430

268. Galassi E, Piazza G, Gaist G et al. Arachnoid cysts of the middle cranial fossa: a clinical and radiological study of 25 cases treated surgically. Surg Neurol, 1980; 14:211–219

269. Palmer JJ. Spinal arachnoid cysts. Report of six cases. J Neurosurg, 1974; 41:728–735

270. Jensen FO, Knudsen V, Troesen S. Recurrent intraspinal arachnoid cyst treated with a shunt procedure. Acta Neurochir, 1977; 39:127–129

271. Starkman SP, Brown TC, Linell EA. Cerebral arachnoid cysts. J Neuropathol Exp Neurol, 1958; 17:484–500

272. Epstein JA, Epstein BS, Lavine LS et al. Obliterative arachnoiditis complicating lumbar spinal stenosis. J Neurosurg, 1978; 48:252–258

273. Stewart DH Jr, Red DE. Spinal arachnoid diverticula. J Neurosurg, 1971; 35:65–70

274. Fetell MR, Bruce JN, Burke AM et al. Non-neoplastic pineal cysts. Neurology, 1991; 41:1034–1040

275. Lum GB, Williams JP, Machen BC et al. Benign cystic pineal lesions by magnetic resonance imaging. J Comput Assist Tomogr, 1987; 11:228–235

276. Klein P, Rubinstein LJ. Benign symptomatic glial cysts of the pineal gland: a report of seven cases and review of the literature. J Neurol Neurosurg Psychiatry, 1989; 52:991–995

277. Vaquero J, Martinez R, Escandon J et al. Symptomatic cysts of the pineal gland. Surg Neurol, 1988; 30:468–470

278. Lee DH, Norman D, Newton TH. MR imaging of pineal cysts. J Comput Assist Tomogr, 1987; 1:586–590

279. Cooper E. The human pineal gland and pineal cysts. J Anat, 1932; 67:28–46

280. Shuangshoti S, Netsky MG. Neuroepithelial (colloid) cysts of the nervous system. Neurology, 1966; 16:887–903

281. Baker GS, Gottlieb CM. Cysts of the choroid plexus of the lateral ventricle causing disabling headache and unconsciousness. Proc Staff Meet Mayo Clin, 1956; 31:95–97

282. Inoue T, Kuromatsu C, Iwata Y et al. Symptomatic choroidal epithelial cysts in fourth ventricle. Surg Neurol, 1985; 24:57–62

283. Chinn DH, Miller EI, Worthy LM et al. Sonographically detected fetal choroid plexus cysts. Frequency and association with aneuploidy. J Ultrasound Med, 1991; 10:255–258

284. Gabrielli S, Reece EA, Pilu G et al. The clinical significance of prenatally diagnosed choroid plexus cysts. Am J Obstet Gynecol, 1989; 160:1207–1210

285. Platt LD, Carlson DE, Medearis AL et al. Fetal choroid plexus cysts in the second trimester of pregnancy: a cause for concern. Am J Obstet Gynecol, 1991; 164:1652–1656

286. French BN. Midline fusion defects and defects of formation. In: Youmans JR, ed. Neurological surgery, 3rd edn. Philadelphia: Saunders, 1990: pp 1210

287. Tarlov IM. Perineurial cysts of the spinal nerve roots. Arch Neurol Psychiat, 1938; 40:1067–1074

288. Tarlov IM. Spinal perineurial and meningeal cysts. J Neurol Neurosurg Psychiatry, 1970; 33:833–843

289. Tarlov IM. Cysts (perineurial) of the sacral roots. Another cause (removable) of sciatic pain. J Am Med Assoc, 1948; 138:740–744

Lipomas

290. Zülch KJ. Brain tumours. Their biology and pathology, 3rd edn. Berlin: Springer-Verlag, 1986: pp 441–445

291. List CE, Holt JF, Everett M. Lipoma of the corpus callosum. Am J Roentgenol, 1946; 55:125–134

292. Truwin CL, Barkovich AJ. Pathogenesis of intracranial lipoma: an MR study in 42 patients. Am J Roentgenol, 1990; 155:855–864

293. Gastaut M, Regis H, Gastaut JL et al. Lipomas of the corpus callosum and epilepsy. Neurology (NY), 1980; 30:132–138

294. Budka M. Intracranial lipomatous hamartomas (intracranial 'lipomas'). A study of 13 cases including combinations with medulloblastoma, colloid and epidermoid cysts, angiomatosis and other malformations. Acta Neuropathol (Berl), 1974; 28:205–222

295. Kazner E, Stockdorph O, Wende S et al. Intracranial lipoma. Diagnostic and therapeutic considerations. J Neurosurg, 1980; 52:234–245

296. Gaupp R, Jantz H. Zur Kasuistik der Balkenlipome Nervenarzt, 1942; 15:58–68

297. Christensen WN, Long DM, Epstein JI. Cerebellopontine angle lipoma. Hum Pathol, 1986; 17:739–743

298. Fukui M, Tanaka A, Kitamura K et al. Lipoma of the cerebellopontine angle. J Neurosurg, 1977; 46:544–547

299. Carmel PW. Brain tumours of disordered embryogenesis. In: Youmans JR, ed. Neurological surgery, vol. 5, 3rd edn. Philadelphia: Saunders, 1990: pp 3244–3246

300. Ehni G, Love JG. Intraspinal lipomas: report of cases. Review of the literature and clinical and pathological study. Arch Neurol Psychiat, 1945; 53:1–28

301. Giuffre R. Spinal lipomas. In: Vinken PJ, Bruyn GW, eds. Handbook of clinical neurology, vol. 20. Tumours of the spine and spinal cord, Part 2. Amsterdam: North Holland, 1976: pp 389–414

302. Caram PC, Scarcella G, Carton CA. Intradural lipomas of the spinal cord (with particular emphasis on the 'intramedullary' lipomas). J Neurosurg, 1957; 14:28–42

303. Fan CJ, Veerapen RJ, Tan CT. Subdural spinal lipoma with posterior fossa extension. Clin Radiol, 1989; 40:91–94

304. Kodama T, Numaguchi Y, Gellad FE et al. Magnetic resonance imaging of a high cervical intradural lipoma. Comput Med Imaging Graph, 1991; 15:93–95

305. Bender JL, Van Landingham JH, Manno NJ. Epidural lipoma producing spinal cord compression. J Neurosurg, 1974; 41:100–103

306. Zettner A, Netsky MG. Lipoma of the corpus callosum. J Neuropathol Exp Neurol, 1960; 19:305–319

307. Wilkins PR, Hoddinott C, Houriman MD et al. Intracranial angiolipoma. J Neurol Neurosurg Psychiatry, 1987; 50:1057–1059

308. Smith CML, Timperley WR. Multiple intraspinal and intracranial epidermoids and lipomata following gunshot injury. Neuropathol Appl Neurobiol, 1984; B10:235–239

309. Rogers HM, Long DM, Chou SN et al. Lipomas of the spinal cord and cauda equina. J Neurosurg, 1971; 34:349–354

310. Lassman LP, James CCM. Lumbosacral lipomas: critical survey of 26 cases submitted to laminectomy. J Neurol Neurosurg Psychiatry, 1967; 30:174–181

311. Pierre-Kahn A, Lacombe J, Pichon J et al. Intraspinal lipomas with spina bifida. Prognosis and treatment in 73 cases. J Neurosurg, 1986; 65:756–761

312. French BN. Midline fusion defects and defects of formation. In: Youman JR, ed. Neurological surgery, vol. 2, 3rd edn. Philadelphia: Saunders, 1990: pp 1185–1192

313. Kudoh H, Sakamoto K, Kobayashi N. Lipomas in the corpus callosum and the forehead associated with a frontal bone defect. Surg Neurol, 1984; 22:503–508

314. Schmid AK. A lipoma of the cerebellum. Acta Neuropathol (Berl), 1973; 26:75–80

315. Friedman RB, Segal R, Latchaw RE. Computerised tomographic and magnetic resonance imaging of intracranial lipoma. J Neurosurg, 1986; 65:407–410

316. Halmagyi GM, Evans WA. Lipoma of the quadrigeminal plate causing progressive obstructive hydrocephalus. J Neurosurg, 1978; 49:453–456

317. Pensak ML, Glasscook ME, Gulya AJ et al. Cerebellopontine angle lipomas. Arch Otolaryngol, 1988; 112:99–107

318. Uchina A, Maeoka N, Ohno M. Intracranial lipoma: MR imaging. Rinsho-Hoshasen 1989; 34:1591–1596

319. Cant WHP, Astey R. Lipoma of the corpus callosum. Arch Dis Child, 1952; 27:478–479

320. Gerber SS, Plotkin R. Lipoma of corpus callosum. J Neurosurg, 1982; 57:281–185

321. Takeuchi J, Handa H, Keyaki A et al. Intracranial angiolipoma. Surg Neurol, 1981; 15:110–113

322. Manganiello LOJ, Daniel EF, Hair LQ. Lipoma of the corpus callosum. J Neurosurg, 1966; 24:892–894

Hypothalamic neuronal hamartoma

323. Zülch KJ. Brain tumours. Their biology and pathology, 3rd edn. Berlin: Springer-Verlag, 1986: pp 447–450

324. Nurbhai MA, Tomlinson BE, Lorigan-Forsythe B. Infantile hypothalamic hamartoma with multiple congenital abnormalities. Neuropath Appl Neurobiol, 1985; 11:61–70

325. Bedwell SF, Lindenberg R. A hypothalamic hamartoma with dendritic proliferation and other neuronal changes associated with 'blastomastoid' reaction of astrocytes. J Neuropathol Exp Neurol, 1961; 20:219–236

326. Russell DS, Rubinstein LJ. Pathology of tumours of the nervous system, 5th edn. London: Edward Arnold, 1989: pp 710–721

327. Hennekam RC, Beemer FA, Van Merrienboer F et al. Congenital hypothalamic harmartoma associated with severe midline defect: a developmental field defect. Report of a case. Am J Med Genet Suppl, 1986; 2:45–52

328. Kyuma Y, Kuwabara T, Chiba Y et al. Controlling precocious puberty: surgical excision of hypothalamic hamartoma causing precocious puberty. No Shinkei Geka, 1986; 14:1095–1103

329. Northfield DWC, Russell DS. Pubertas praecox due to hypothalamic hamartoma: report of two cases surviving surgical removal of the tumor. J Neurol Neurosurg Psychiatry, 1967; 30:166–173

330. Berkovic SF, Andermann F, Melanson D et al. Hypothalamic hamartomas and ictal laughter: evolution of a characteristic epileptic syndrome and diagnostic value of magnetic resonance imaging. Ann Neurol, 1988; 23:429–439

331. Dammann O, Commentz JC, Valdueza JM et al. Gelastic epilepsy and precocious puberty in hamartoma of the hypothalamus. Klin Padiatr, 1991; 203:439–447

332. Asa SL, Scheithauer BW, Bilbao JM et al. A case for hypothalamic acromegaly: a clinicopathological study of six patients with hypothalamic gangliocytomas producing growth hormone releasing factor. J Clin Endocrinol Metab, 1984; 58:796–803

333. Schiethauer BW, Kovaks M, Randall RV et al. Hypothalamic neuronal hamartoma and adenohypophyseal neuronal charistoma: their association with growth hormone adenoma of the pituitary gland. J Neuropathol Exp Neurol, 1983; 42:648–663

334. Marcuse PM, Burger RA, Salmon GA. Hamartoma of the hypothalamus. Report of two cases with associated developmental defects. J Pediatr, 1953; 43:301–308

335. Nakagawa N, Takahashi M, Kohrogi Y et al. Neuroradiologic findings of hypothalamic hamartoma with emphasis on computed tomography. J Comput Assist Tomogr, 1986; 10:77–83

336. Kanazawa J, Uozumi T, Sakoda K et al. Magnetic resonance imaging of hypothalamic hamartoma. No Shinkei Geka, 1988; 16:585–588

337. Lona Soto A, Takahashi M, Yamashita Y et al. MRI findings of hypothalamic hamartoma: report of five cases and review of the literature. Comput Med Imaging Graph 1991; 15:415–421

338. Weinberger LM, Grant FC. Precocious puberty and tumors of the hypothalamus. Report of a case and review of the literature with a pathophysiologic explanation of the precocious sexual syndrome. Arch Int Med, 1941; 67:762–792

339. Poston H, Barber AH. External genital hypertrophy in infancy. Lancet, 1942; i:384–385

340. Judge DM, Kulin HE, Page R et al. Hypothalamic hamartoma. N Engl J Med, 1977; 296:7–10

341. Culler FL, James HE, Simon ML et al. Identification of gonadotropin-releasing hormone in neurones of a hypothalamic hamartoma in a boy with precocious puberty. Neurosurgery, 1985; 17:408–412

342. Richter RB. True hamartoma of the hypothalamus associated with pubertas praecox. J Neuropathol Exp Neurol, 1951; 10:368–383

343. Wolman L, Balmforth GV. Precocious puberty due to a hypothalamic hamartoma in a patient surviving to late middle age. J Neurol Neurosurg Psychiatry, 1963; 26:275–280

344. Machado HR, Hoffman HJ, Hwang PA. Gelastic seizures treated by resection of a hypothalamic hamartoma. Childs Nerv Syst, 1991; 7:462–465

Heterotopias

345. Abbott KH, Glass B. Intracranial extracerebral (leptomeningeal) glioma. Proc 2nd Int Cong Neuropath, Part 1. Amsterdam: Excerpta Medica, 1955: pp 165–168

346. Cooper IS, Kernohan JW. Heterotopic glial nests in the subarachnoid space: histopathologic characteristics, mode of origin and relation to meningeal gliomas. J Neuropathol Exp Neurol 1955; 10:16–29

347. Nishio S, Mizuno J, Barrow DL et al. Intracranial extracerebral glioneural heterotopia. Childs Nerv Syst, 1988; 4:244–248

348. Farhat SM, Hudson J-S. Extracerebral brain heterotopia. Case report. J Neurosurg, 1969; 30:190–194

349. Shuangshoti S, Kasantikui V, Suwanwela N et al. Solitary primary intracranial extracerebral glioma. J Neurosurg, 1984; 61:777–781

350. Ho K-L, Hoschner JA, Wolfe DE. Primary leptomeningeal gliomatosis. Symptoms suggestive of meningitis. Arch Neurol, 1981; 38:662–666

351. Kitahara M, Katahura R, Wada T et al. Diffuse form of primary leptomeningeal gliomatosis. J Neurosurg, 1985; 63:283–287

352. Davis EW. Gliomatous tumour in the nasal region. J Neuropathol Exp Neurol, 1942; 1:312–319

353. Hirsch LF, Stool SE, Langfitt TW et al. Nasal glioma. J Neurosurg, 1977; 46:85–91

354. Black BK, Smith DE. Nasal glioma. Two cases with recurrence. Arch Neurol Psychiat, 150; 64:614–630

355. Younus M, Coode PE. Nasal glioma and encephalocoele: two separate entities. Report of two cases. J Neurosurg, 1986; 64:516–519

356. Zülch KJ. Brain tumours. Their biology and pathology, 3rd edn.

Berlin: Springer-Verlag, 1986: pp 447–450

357. Deutsch HJ. Intranasal glioma. Am Otol Rhinol Laryngol, 1965; 74:637–644

358. Puppala B, Mangurten HH, McFadden J et al. Nasal glioma. Presenting as neonatal respiratory distress. Definition of the tumor mass by MRI. Clin Pediatr (Phila), 1990; 29:49–52

359. Bossen EH, Hudson WR. Oligodendroglioma rising in heterotopic brain tissue of the soft palate and nasopharynx. Am J Surg Pathol, 1987; 11:571–574

360. Low NL, Scheinberg L, Anderson DH. Brain tissue in the nose and throat. Pediatrics 1956; 18:254–259

361. Yeoh GP, Bale PM, de Silva M. Nasal cerebral heterotopia: the so-called nasal glioma of sequestered encephalocele and its variants. Pediatr Pathol, 1989; 9:531–549

362. Call NB, Bayliss MI. Cerebellar heterotopia in the orbit. Arch Ophthalmol, 1980; 98:717–719

363. Goldring S, Hodges FH III, Luse SA. Ectopic neural tissue of occipital bone. J Neurosurg, 1964; 21:479–484

364. Bychkov V, Gatti WM, Fresco R. Tumor of the tongue containing heterotopic brain tissue. Oral Surg Oral Med Oral Pathol, 1988; 66:71–73

365. Klein MV, Schwaighofer BW, Sobel DF et al. Heterotopic brain in the middle ear: CT findings. J Comput Assist Tomogr, 1989; 13:1058–1060

366. Pasyk KA, Argenta LC, Marks MW et al. Heterotopic brain presenting as a lip lesion. Cleft Palate J, 1988; 25:48–52

367. Musser AW, Campbell R. Nasal glioma. Report of an unusual case associated with multiple supragaleal nodules. Arch Otolaryngol, 1961; 73:732–736

368. Fuller C, Gibbs AR. Heterotopic brain tissue in the lung causing acute respiratory distress in an infant. Thorax, 1989; 44:1045–1046

369. Okeda R. Heterotopic brain tissue in the submandibular region and lung. Report of two cases and comments about pathogenesis. Acta Neuropathol (Berl), 1978; 43:217–220

Vascular malformations

370. Dichiro G, Werner L. Angiography of the spinal cord. J Neurosurg, 1973; 39:1–29

371. Stein BM, Solomon RA. Arteriovenous malformations of the brain. In: Youmans JR, ed. Neurological surgery, 3rd edn. Philadelphia: Saunders, 1990: pp 1831–1863

372. Jellinger K. Vascular malformations of the central nervous system: a morphological overview. Neurosurg Rev, 1986; 9:177–216

373. Fults D, Kelly DL. Natural history of arteriovenous malformations of the brain. A clinical study. Neurosurgery, 1984; 15:658–662

374. Wilkins RH. Natural history of intracranial vascular malformations. A review. Neurosurgery, 1985; 16:421–430

375. Ommaya AK, Dichiro G, Doppman J. Ligation of arterial supply in the treatment of spinal cord arteriovenous malformations. J Neurosurg, 1969; 30:679–692

376. Russell DS, Rubinstein LJ. Pathology of tumours of the nervous system, 5th edn. London: Edward Arnold, 1989: pp 727–746

377. Rigamonti D, Johnson PC, Spetzler RF et al. Cavernous malformations and capillary telangiectasia: a spectrum within a single pathological entity. Neurosurgery, 1991; 28:60–64

378. WHO Working Group. Histological typing of tumours of the central nervous system, 2nd meeting, Zurich. 1990

379. Pool JL. Arteriovenous malformations of the brain. In: Vinken PJ, Bruyn GW, eds. Handbook of clinical neurology, vol. 12. Vascular diseases of the nervous system, Part II. Amsterdam: North Holland, 1976: pp 227–266

380. Zülch KJ. Brain tumours. Their biology and pathology, 3rd edn. Berlin: Srpinger, 1986: pp 453–460

381. Perrett G, Nishioka H. Report on the cooperative study of intracranial aneurysms and subarachnoid hemorrhage. Section VI. Arteriovenous malformations. J Neurosurg, 1966; 25:467–490

382. McCormick WF. Pathology of vascular malformations of the brain. In: Wilson CB, Stein BM, eds. Intracranial arteriovenous malformations. Baltimore: Wiliams & Wilkins, 1984: pp 44–63

383. McCormick WF, Hardmann JM, Boulter TR. Vascular malformations (angiomas) of the brain with special reference to those occurring in the posterior fossa. J Neurosurg, 1968; 28:241–251

384. Parkinson D, Bachers G. Arteriovenous malformations. Summary of 100 consecutive supratentorial cases. J Neurosurg, 1980; 53:285–299

385. Britt RH, Silverberg GD, Ensmann DR et al. Third ventricular choroid plexus arteriovenous malformation simulating a colloid cyst. J Neurosurg, 1980; 52:246–250

386. Uchino A, Matsunaga M, Ohno M. Arteriovenous malformation of the corpus callosum associated with persistent primitive trigeminal artery: case report. Neurol Med Chir (Tokyo), 1989; 29:429–432

387. Willinsky RA, Lasjauniuas P, Terbrugge K et al. Multiple cerebral arteriovenous malformations (AVMs). Review of our experience from 203 patients with cerebral vascular lesions. Neuroradiology, 1990; 32:207–210

388. Fujita H, Nakano K, Kumon Y et al. A case of Wyburn–Mason syndrome. Rinsho Shinkeigaku, 1989; 29:1039–1044

389. Homan RW, Devous MD Sr, Stokely EM et al. Quantification of intracerebral steal in patients with arteriovenous malformation. Arch Neurol, 1986; 43:779–785

390. Tyler JL, Leblanc R, Meyer E et al. Hemodynamic and metabolic effects of cerebral arteriovenous malformations studied by positron emission tomography. Stroke, 1989; 20:890–898

391. Deruty R, Mottolese C, Soustiel JF et al. Association of cerebral arteriovenous malformation and cerebral aneurysm. Diagnosis and management. Acta Neurochir (Wien), 1990; 107:133–139

392. Havashi S, Arimoto T, Itakura T et al. The association of intracranial aneurysms and arteriovenous malformations of the brain. J Neurosurg, 1981; 55:971–975

393. Batjer H, Suss RA, Samson D. Intracranial arteriovenous malformations associated with aneurysms. Neurosurgery, 1986; 18:29–35

394. Thajeb F, Hsi MS. Cerebral arteriovenous malformation: report of 136 Chinese patients in Taiwan. Angiology, 1987; 38:851–858

395. Klara P, George E, McDonnell D et al. Morphological studies of human arteriovenous malformations. Effects of isobutyl 12-cyanoacrylate embolisation. J Neurosurg, 1985; 63:421–425

396. Vinters HV, Lundie MJ, Kaufman JCE. Long-term pathological follow-up of cerebral arteriovenous malformations treated by embolisation with bucrylate. New Eng J Med, 1986; 314:477–483

397. Graf CJ, Perrett GE, Torner JC. Bleeding from cerebral arteriovenous malformations as part of their natural history. J Neurosurg, 1983; 58:331–337

398. Guidetti B, DeLitala A. Intracranial arteriovenous malformations. Conservative and surgical treatment. J Neurosurg, 1980; 53:149–152

399. Yoshimoto T, Kayama T, Suzuki J. Treatment of cerebral arteriovenous malformation. Neurosurg Rev, 1986; 9:279–285

400. van Alphen HA. Intraoperative embolization of cerebral arteriovenous malformations. Neurosurg Rev, 1986; 9:77–86

401. Purdy PD, Samson D, Batjer HH et al. Preoperative embolization of cerebral arteriovenous malformations with polyvinyl alcohol particles: experience in 51 adults. Am J Neuroradiol, 1990; 11:501–510

402. Steinmeier R, Schramm J, Muller HG et al. Evaluation of prognostic factors in cerebral arteriovenous malformations. Neurosurgery, 1989; 24:193–200

403. Hernesniemi J, Keranen T. Microsurgical treatment of arteriovenous malformations of the brain in a defined population. Surg Neurol, 1990; 33:384–390

404. Miyasaka Y, Yada K, Ohwada T et al. Hemorrhagic venous infarction after excision of an arteriovenous malformation: case report. Neurosurgery, 1991; 29:265–268

405. Luessenhop AJ, Rosa L. Cerebral arteriovenous malformations. Indications for and results of surgery, and the role of intravascular techniques. J Neurosurg, 1984; 60:14–22

406. Luessenhop AJ, Presper JH. Surgical embolisation of cerebral arteriovenous malformations through internal carotid and vertebral arteries. Long term results. J Neurosurg, 1975; 42:443–451

407. Kjellberg RN, Hanamura T, Davis KR et al. Bragg–Peak proton beam therapy for arteriovenous malformations of the brain. N Engl J Med, 1983; 309:269–274

408. Phillips MH, Frankel KA, Lyman JT et al. Heavy charged-particle stereotactic radiosurgery: cerebral angiography and CT in the treatment of intracranial vascular malformations. Int J Radiat Oncol Biol Phys, 1989; 17:419–426

409. Loeffler JS, Rossitch E Jr, Siddon R et al. Role of stereotactic radiosurgery with a linear accelerator in the treatment of intracranial arteriovenous malformations and tumors in children. Pediatrics, 1990; 85:774–782

410. Souhami L, Olivier A, Podgorsak EB et al. Radiosurgery of cerebral arteriovenous malformations with the dynamic stereotactic irradiation. Int J Radiat Oncol Biol Phys, 1990; 19:775–782

411. Kaufman M, Swartz BE, Mandelkern M et al. Diagnosis of delayed cerebral radiation necrosis following proton beam therapy. Arch Neurol, 1990; 47:474–476

412. Gagnon J, Boileau G. Anatomical study of an arteriovenous malformation drained by the system of Galen. J Neurosurg, 1960; 17:75–80

413. Hoffman HJ, Chuang S, Hendrick EB et al. Aneurysms of the vein of Galen: experience at The Hospital for Sick Children, Toronto. J Neurosurg, 1982; 57:316–322

414. Pellegrino PA, Milanesi O, Saia OS et al. Congestive heart failure secondary to cerebral arterio-venous fistula. Childs Nerv Syst, 1987; 3:141–144

415. Crawford JM, Rossitch E Jr, Oakes WJ et al. Arteriovenous malformation of the great vein of Galen associated with patent ductus arteriosus. Report of three cases and review of the literature. Childs Nerv Syst, 1990; 6:18–22

416. Norman MG, Becker LE. Cerebral damage in neonates resulting from arteriovenous malformation of the vein of Galen. J Neurol Neurosurg Psychiatry, 1974; 37:252–258

417. Takashima S, Becker LE. Neuropathology of cerebral arteriovenous malformations in children. J Neurol Neurosurg Psychiatry, 1980; 43:380–385

418. Obrador S, Soto M, Silveba J. Clinical syndromes of arteriovenous malformations of the transverse-sigmoid sinus. J Neurol Neurosurg Psychiatry, 1975; 38:436–451

419. Malik GM, Pearce JE, Ausman JI et al. Dural arteriovenous malformations and intracranial haemorrhage. Neurosurgery, 1984; 15:332–339

420. Sakaki S, Furuta S, Fujita M et al. Dural arteriovenous malformation of the transverse and sigmoid sinus with special reference to its pathological features. Br J Neurosurg, 1991; 5:87–92

421. Tanaka K, Fujishima H, Motomura S et al. A case of dural arteriovenous malformation with bilateral thalamic infarction. No To Shinkei, 1986; 38:1005–1010

422. Stein BM, Solomon RA. Arteriovenous malformations of the spinal cord. In: Youmans JR, ed. Neurological surgery, 3rd edn. Philadelphia: Saunders 1990: pp 1918–1933

423. Oldfield EH, Dichiro G, Quindlen EA et al. Successful treatment of a group of spinal cord arteriovenous malformations by interruption of dural fistula. J Neurosurg, 1983; 59:1019–1030

424. Benhaiem N, Poirier J, Hurth M. Arteriovenous fistula of the meninges draining into the spinal veins. A histological study of 28 cases. Acta Neuropathol (Berl), 1983; 62:103–111

425. Yasargil MG. Intradural spinal arteriovenous malformations. In: Vinken PJ, Bruyn GW, eds. Handbook of clinical neurology, vol. 20. Tumours of the spine and spinal cord, Part II. Amsterdam: North Holland, 1976: pp 481–523

426. Aminoff MJ, Logue V. Clinical features of spinal vascular malformations. Brain, 1974; 97:197–210

427. Foix C, Alajouanine T. La myélite nécrotique subaiguë. Rev Neurol, 1926; 33:1–42

428. Isu T, Iwasaki Y, Akino M et al. Magnetic resonance imaging in cases of spinal dural arteriovenous malformation. Neurosurgery, 1989; 24:919–923

429. Miyamoto S, Kikuchi H, Nagata I et al. Problems in the embolization therapy of spinal arteriovenous malformation. No Shinkei Geka, 1988; 16:1067–1072

430. Logue V. Angiomas of the spinal cord: review of the pathogenesis, clinical features, and results of surgery. J Neurol Neurosurg Psychiatry, 1979; 42:1–11

431. Touho H, Karasawa J, Shishido H et al. Successful excision of a juvenile-type spinal arteriovenous malformation following intraoperative embolization. Case report. J Neurosurg 1991; 75:647–651

432. Zimmerman HM. Vascular tumours of the brain. In: Vinken PJ, Bruyn GW, eds. Handbook of clinical neurology, vol. 18. Tumours of the brain and skull, Part III. Amsterdam: North Holland, 1976: pp 270–284

433. Teilmann K. Hemangiomas of the pons. Arch Neurol Psychiat, 1953; 69:208–223

434. Blackwood W. Two cases of benign cerebral telangectasis. J Pathol Bacteriol, 1941; 52:209–212

435. Amromin GD, Boder E, Teplitz R. Ataxia-telangectasia with a 32 year survival. A clinicopathological report. J Neuropathol Exp Neurol, 1979; 38:621–643

436. Heffner RR Jr, Soutaire GB. Hereditory haemorrhagic telangectasia: neuropathological observations. J Neurol Neurosurg Psychiatry, 1969; 32:604–608

437. Vaquero J, Manrique M, Oya S et al. Calcified telangiectatic hamartomas of the brain. Surg Neurol, 1980; 13:453–457

438. Farrell DF, Forno LS. Symptomatic capillary telangectasis of the brainstem without haemorrhage. Report of an unusual case. Neurology, 1970; 20:341–346

439. Fortuna A, Ferrante L, Mastronardi L et al. Cerebral cavernous angioma in children. Childs Nerv Syst, 1989; 5:201–207

440. Requena I, Arias M, Lopez-Ibor L et al. Cavernomas of the central nervous system: clinical and neuroimaging manifestations in 47 patients. J Neurol Neurosurg Psychiatry, 1991; 54:590–594

441. Bicknell JM, Carlow TJ, Kornfeld M et al. Familial cavernous angiomas. Arch Neurol, 1978; 35:746–749

442. Wood MW, White RJ, Kernohan JW. Cavernous hemangiomatosis involving the brain, spinal cord, heart, skin and kidney. Clin Proc, 1957; 32:249–254

443. Kasantikiu V, Wirt TC, Allen VA et al. Identification of a brain stone as calcified hemangioma. J Neurosurg, 1980; 52:862–866

444. Manz HJ, Klein LH, Fermaglich J et al. Cavernous hemangioma of optic chiasm, optic nerves and right optic tract. Case report and review of literature. Virchow Arch (A), 1979; 383:225–231

445. Simard JM, Garcia-Bengochea F, Ballinger WE Jr et al. Cavernous angioma: a review of 126 collected and 12 new clinical cases. Neurosurgery, 1986; 18:162–172

446. Robinson JR, Awad IA, Little JR. Natural history of the cavernous angioma. J Neurosurg, 1991; 75:709–714

447. Ruel M, Keravel Y, Mignot B et al. Cerebral cavernoma: a rare vascular malformation. Presse Med, 1986; 15:1029–1032

448. Fahlbusch R, Strauss C. Surgical significance of cavernous hemangioma of the brain stem. Zentralbl Neurochir, 1991; 52:25–32

449. Numaguchi Y, Kitanura K, Fukui M et al. Intracranial venous angiomas. Surg Neurol, 1982; 18:193–202

450. Moritake K, Handa H, Mori K et al. Venous angiomas of the brain. Surg Neurol, 1980; 14:95–105

451. Neff NJ, Wemmer J, Heonig-Rigamanti K et al. A longitudinal study of patients with venous malformations. Documentation of a negligable haemorrage risk and benign natural history. Neurology, 1998; 50:1709–1714

18 Local extensions from adjacent tumours

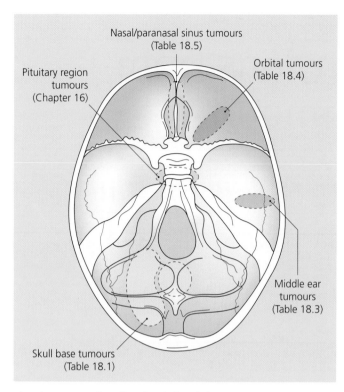

Fig. 18.1 **Tumours invading the skull and skull base.**

A wide range of tumours are routinely encountered in diagnostic surgical neuropathology which are not primary tumours of the nervous system. Many of these arise from adjacent structures (Fig. 18.1), particularly bone and soft tissues, and involve the nervous system by local extension.[1] These tumours may compress or invade the brain, spinal cord and nerve roots, and consequently patients are often referred to neurosurgeons for surgical management. This chapter will briefly present some of the diagnostic problems related to this group of tumours. Detailed discussions of primary bone tumours, soft tissue tumours, and lymphoid/haematological malignancies are beyond the scope of this book, and are covered in other learned texts.

Bone tumours and tumour-like conditions

The diagnosis of bone lesions can be complex; this is one area of diagnostic pathology where a multidisciplinary approach to diagnosis should always be made. A diagnosis should be the result of a careful review of clinical, imaging and histological information, particularly when small biopsy samples are being interpreted. The following account is a brief overview of the pathology of bone tumours and tumour-like lesions that may be encountered in neuropathological practice. In general, the amount of detail is proportionate to the frequency with which the

lesion is encountered in surgical neuropathology and the amount of information available in standard textbooks dealing with bone tumours.

Ecchordosis physaliphora

Notochordal remnants may form well defined solid and cystic structures termed ecchordosis physaliphora. These lesions are benign, but may become symptomatic through local pressure effects. Ecchordosis physaliphora has been mainly described as an incidental finding at post-mortem examination attached to the clivus or the basilar artery, often measuring only a few millimetres in diameter. Similar examples have also been described in the spine.[2,3]

Clinical features

Clinical signs and symptoms usually relate to compression of adjacent structures. There are only few clinical descriptions of symptomatic cases, prominent among which is a case where a large ecchordosis physaliphora caused a cerebrospinal fluid fistula, extending from the sphenoid sinus into the subarachnoid space of the prepontine cistern.[4] Haemorrhage is also well described in association with these lesions, which in a few rare instances may be fatal.[5,6] Magnetic resonance imaging (MRI) has shown ecchordoses as well defined, non-enhancing lesions of intermediate signal intensity on T1-weighted images and of low signal intensity on T2-weighted images.[3]

Pathology

These lesions appear as gelatinous, translucent masses. They may be approximately spherical or be flattened disk-like structures ranging in size from 4–5 mm up to examples 2–3 cm in diameter (Fig. 18.2). Ecchordosis physaliphora is composed of cords and ribbons of cells set in a matrix of connective tissue with a chondroid-like appearance. The histological appearances are identical to that seen in a chordoma, including immunohisto-chemical[7,8] and ultrastructural[9] aspects (see later). Necrosis and mitotic activity is exceptional in these lesions. The most important differential diagnosis is chordoma; despite the histological similarities, it is usually possible to use the site of origin to help distinguish between these lesions, since bony involvement is rare in ecchordosis, and extraskeletal chordomas arising adjacent to the basilar artery are extremely uncommon.

Therapy and prognosis

These lesions are believed to represent notochordal remnants (rather than neoplasms), a view supported by immunohistochemical and ultrastructural observations.

Fig. 18.2 **Ecchordosis physaliphora.** The lesion appears as a gelatinous, translucent, mass attached loosely to the basilar artery. This was an incidental post mortem finding.

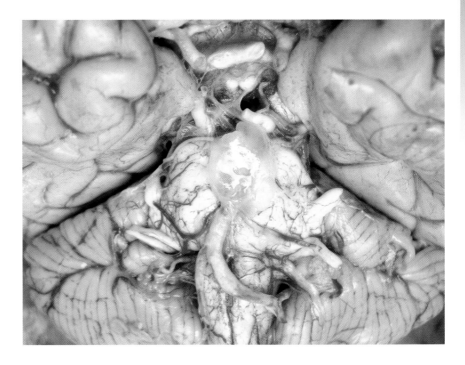

Since most intracranial examples are asymptomatic, there are very few cases reported in which treatment was required. Symptomatic intradural examples, by virtue of their location and lack of involvement of bone, are amenable to surgical resection and cure. However, there are so few descriptions of these lesions that experience of their biological behaviour and response to therapy is very limited.

Chordoma

Chordomas are infiltrative tumours of bone derived from notochord.[10] The nervous system is frequently involved by local extension of tumour; chordomas are one of the commonest bone tumours which present to neuro-pathologists for diagnosis. Chordomas arise along the craniospinal axis and are believed to derive from remnants of the fetal notochord. They account for about 8% of all primary malignancies of bone.[11] The commonest site is the sacrum, followed by the skull base (sphenoid and clivus), and then (less frequently) vertebral bodies. Examples arising from the pituitary fossa have also been described,[12] but are uncommon. Most chordomas occur in later adult life, but occasional cases in younger adults and even more rarely in children have been described.[13,14]

Clinical features and imaging

Clinical features relate to bone destruction (pain) and compressive effects of local growth on adjacent nerves.[15] Patients with chordomas usually suffer from headache;

cranial nerve palsies (particularly resulting in diplopia) are also common. Most patients with skull base chordomas develop a sixth nerve palsy followed by a visual field defect. Extension of the tumour around the brain stem may be accompanied by other cranial nerve palsies, e.g. VIII–XII nerves.

Chordomas are seen as osseodestructive, lobulated expansile lesions on imaging, typically appearing as well defined extradural tumours. Without contrast, the tumour appears isodense with brain, with focal calcification in a majority of cases. A lobulated, honeycomb appearance may be seen on MRI (Fig. 18.3) with gadolinium enhancement,[16,17] which can also demonstrate dural invasion. Surgical staging of spinal tumours can be performed,[18] but its prognostic significance is not fully established.

Pathology

Chordomas are lobulated grey, semitranslucent tumours of varying size; the sacral specimens can reach relatively large proportions. They are usually soft and gelatinous, sometimes with foci of calcification. A red–brown colour as a consequence of previous haemorrhage may also be present. The tumours are not encapsulated and may invade the dura to stretch cranial or spinal nerves, or displace blood vessels and the brain stem. Most are removed piecemeal during surgical procedures, giving rise to fragmented samples.

Intraoperative diagnosis

Chordomas generally produce satisfactory smear preparations in which cords and clusters of non-cohesive cells

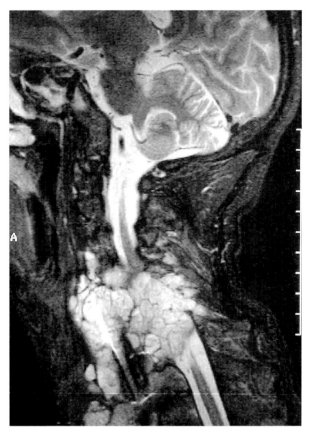

Fig. 18.3 **Chordoma.** MRI scan showing a lobulated chordoma involving the mid-cervical vertebrae, encroaching on and displacing the spinal canal.

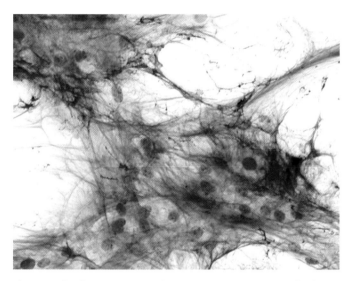

Fig. 18.4 **Chordoma.** Intraoperative smear preparations typically show discohesive tumour cells set in an abundant mucinous matrix. The matrix often stains metachromatically with toluidine blue. The tumour cells have uniform, rounded nuclei and abundant clear or vacuolated cytoplasm. Toluidine blue.

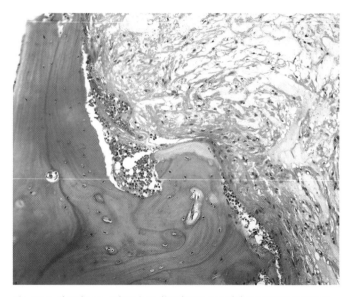

Fig. 18.5 **Chordoma.** When invading bone a nodular pattern may not be so evident and invasive tumour replaces marrow, destroying bone. H & E.

can be seen in a proteinaceous background (Fig. 18.4). Tumour cell vacuolation is generally evident in smears, allowing a diagnosis to be suggested. Frozen sections reflect the histological appearances discussed below, but ice crystal artefact can mask the typical appearances of physaliphorous cells. Occasional lymphocytes may also be present (see below).

Histological features

At low magnification, chordomas can be seen to be composed of nodules of cells within a mucoid matrix, separated by fibrocollagenous septa (Fig. 18.5). The cellular nodules appear as long cords and trabecular of epithelial cells set in a stroma composed of mucoid material. Conspicuous cytoplasmic vacuoles of varying size are generally present within tumour cells. The term physaliphorous cell is used to describe the large highly vacuolated cells seen in a chordoma (Figs 18.6–18.9). These cells have pink-staining cytoplasm and pleomorphic nuclei are generally rounded with a stippled chromatin pattern. Mitoses are generally few in number. The mucoid matrix stains strongly with Alcian blue, while the tumour cell cytoplasm is usually positive on a Periodic acid–Schiff

(PAS) stain. The fibrocollagenous septa frequently show a lymphocytic infiltrate (Fig. 18.10)

Some chordomas are characterised by a pleomorphic highly cellular spindle cell component showing mitotic activity (Figs 18.11 and 18.12). These have been being termed dedifferentiated chordomas and are associated with aggressive behaviour in relation to a standard cnordoma.[15,19–21] This histological appearance may occur as a de novo feature, or after therapy.[22]

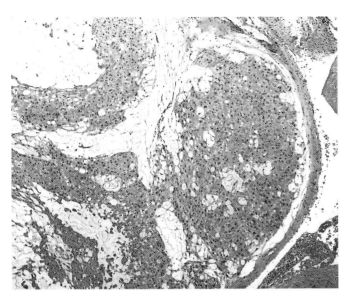

Fig. 18.6 **Chordoma.** Cellularity can vary in nodules from areas where cells form cohesive masses, as here, and mucoid stroma is focal, to tumours where mucoid stroma is dominant and cells are in low density. H & E.

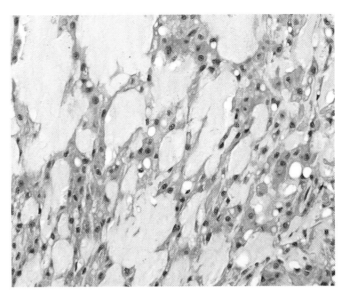

Fig. 18.7 **Chordoma.** In most tumours, cells appear as long cords and trabeculae of pink-staining epithelial cells set in a lightly basophilic mucoid stroma. Nuclear pleomorphism is generally not marked. H & E.

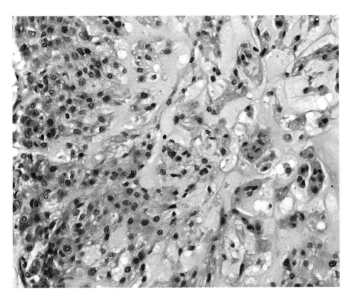

Fig. 18.8 **Chordoma.** Some tumours show focal high cellularity with nuclear pleomorphism and hyperchromatism. H & E.

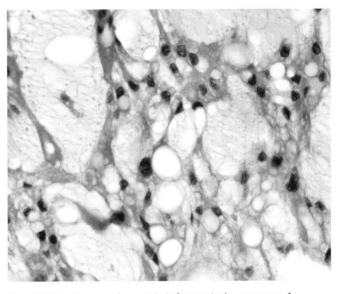

Fig. 18.9 **Chordoma.** A characteristic feature is the presence of conspicuous vacuoles in cells. The term physaliphorous cell is used to describe such highly vacuolated cells seen in a chordoma. H & E.

In some cases the background matrix of a chordoma appears cartilaginous (chondroid chordoma), raising the differential diagnosis of a chondroid neoplasm (chondrosarcoma). Immunocytochemical findings now suggest that the original suggestions that it was possible to distinguish a chondroid chordoma from a typical chordoma are incorrect. It has been proposed that chordomas (as defined by epithelial markers on immunocytochemistry) with a cartilage-like matrix be classified as hyalinised chordomas, rather than chondroid chordoma,[23–26] in order to avoid any further confusion.

Immunohistochemistry and ultrastructure

The epithelial cells in a chordoma stain with cytokeratin (Figs 18.13–18.16) and epithelial membrane antigen (EMA). Such epithelial markers stain about 93% of chordomas;[27,28] the tumour cells also exhibit S-100 immunoreactivity. Chondroid tumours do not stain for epithelial markers[23] but do express S-100. Chordomas express CK8/18, CK1/10, CK5 and CK19. CK20 is not expressed and CK7 is not usually detected, being seen in only one case in one series.[29–32] Electron microscopy

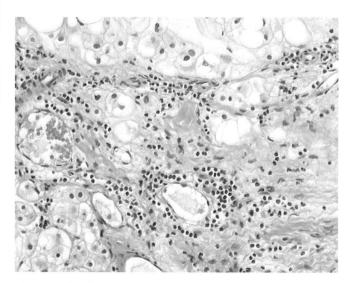

Fig. 18.10 **Chordoma.** A patchy lymphocytic infiltrate is often present in the fibrous septae which divide the tumour, and can be a prominent feature in some cases. H & E.

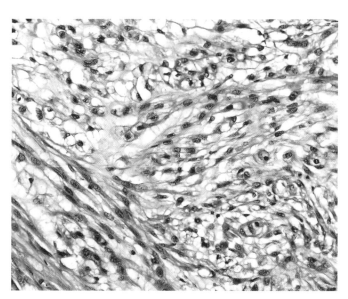

Fig. 18.11 **Dedifferentiated chordoma.** Dedifferentiation is seen as high cellularity and pleomorphism within chordoma. Vacuolation can still be evident. H & E.

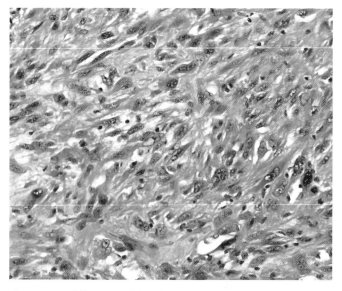

Fig. 18.12 **Dedifferentiated chordoma.** In some tumours dedifferentiation is seen as areas of undifferentiated malignant spindle cell tumour without special distinguishing morphological features. H & E.

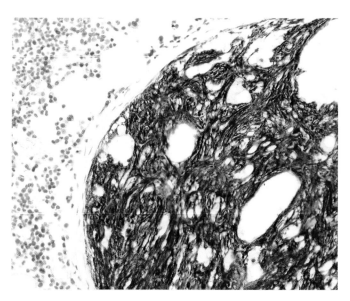

Fig. 18.13 **Chordoma immunohistochemistry.** Chordoma nodule in bone marrow stained for cytokeratin.

shows epithelial junctions between cells, confirming their epithelial phenotype. Mucin vacuolation and a prominent dilated endoplasmic reticulum around mitochondria are characteristic ultrastructural features for chordomas.

Proliferation indices and molecular biology

Chordomas are generally slow growing neoplasms, but tumours showing proliferation rates on Ki-67/MIB-1 immunocytochemistry in excess of 6% have been associated with faster growth.[33] Limited cytogenetic studies suggest possible recurring abnormalities, with chromosome 1p appearing to be involved frequently. Monosomies of 3, 4, 10 and 13 have been reported.[30] Involvement of band 21q22 in translocations has been found in two chordomas.[34] Familial cases have been described[35] and a tumour suppressor locus in familial and sporadic chordoma mapping to 1p36 has been identified.[36–40] Microsatellite instability has been detected in one study.[42]

A recent study of 16 chordomas by comparative genomic hybridisation and fluorescente in situ hybridisation suggested the involvement of tumour suppressor genes

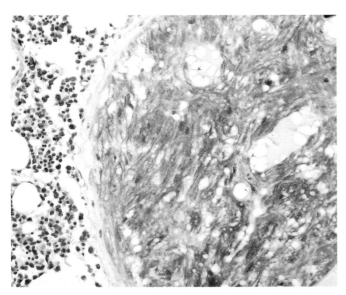

Fig. 18.14 **Chordoma immunohistochemistry.** Chordoma nodule in marrow stained for S-100.

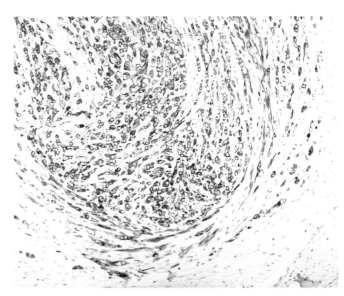

Fig. 18.15 **Chordoma immunohistochemistry.** Chordoma stained for cytokeratin highlighting a streaming pattern of cords of cells.

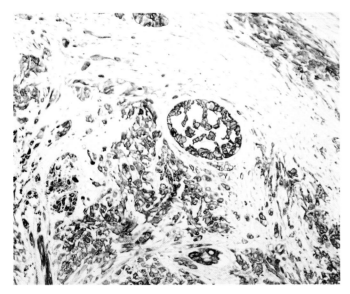

Fig. 18.16 **Chordoma immunohistochemistry.** Both spindle cell (dedifferentiated) and differentiated (glandular) patterns are immunoreactive for cytokeratin.

at 1p31 and 3p14, and an oncogene at 7q36 in the pathogenesis of chordomas.[41]

Differential diagnosis

The differential diagnosis of chordoma is wide, particularly for skull base lesions (see Table 18.1). Rarer bone tumours are summarised in Table 18.2.

Metastatic carcinoma

In smear or frozen section interpretation the presence of epithelial cells with vacuolation may suggest a metastatic

Table 18.1 Skull base tumours
Chordoma
Chondroma/chondrosarcoma
Meningioma
Schwannoma
Paraganglioma
Olfactory neuroblastoma
Salivary gland carcinoma
Nasopharyngeal carcinoma
Metastatic carcinoma

adenocarcinoma. In contrast to a metastasis, nuclei of a chordoma are generally regular and do not show the coarse chromatin pattern seen in most metastatic carcinomas. Immunohistochemical detection of carcinoembryonic antigen in some types of carcinomas has been suggested to be of diagnostic use.[43] Panels of cytokeratin antibodies can be useful in differential diagnosis.[29,31,32]

Chondrosarcoma

Examples of chordomas with a prominent cartilaginous matrix (the so-called chondroid chordoma) may resemble a low grade chondrosarcoma. Immunohistochemistry is the best way to resolve this diagnosis, as epithelial markers are not expressed in cartilaginous tumours.[28,44]

Chondromyxoid fibroma

These lesions have been described in relation to the clivus and mistaken for chordoma. These lesions, like chordoma, have a lobulated pattern of growth. The 'pale islands' of matrix contain spindle cells with heightened cellularity towards the periphery of the lobules, rather than epithelial looking cells as seen in chordoma. Immuno-cytochemistry for epithelial markers gives negative results, unlike in a chordoma.[45]

Chordoid glioma

This recently recognised glial tumour has histological features that resemble chordoma (see Chapter 4). These lesions usually occur within the third ventricle, but lesions have been described in the suprasellar region, a site recognised for chordoma.[46] Chordoid gliomas usually show glial fibrillary acidic protein expression, which is absent from a chordoma.

Chordoid meningioma

These tumours are composed of spindle or epithelioid cells arranged in clusters and cords in a myxoid matrix, resembling a chordoma (see Chapter 13). Such tumours also often have a lymphoid infiltrate, as do many chordomas.[47,48] A specific cytogenetic aberration has been described in these tumours, t(1;3).[49]

Parachordoma

In the periphery, outside the axial skeleton, an entity termed parachordoma has been described. This lesion tends to develop in muscle, adjacent to tendons, synovium and bone. These lesions have also been termed chordoid tumour, chordoid sarcoma and peripheral chordoma. These are very uncommon lesions which on light microscopy have morphological features identical to chordoma.[50] Immunohistochemistry shows positivity for cytokeratin and EMA[51] but the cytokeratin profile differs from that seen in chordoma. Where parachordoma express CK8/18, chordomas express CK8/18 and CK1/10.[30,52,53] Chordomas more frequently express cytokeratin (98% vs 66% in para-chordomas) and EMA (90% vs 20% in parachordomas).[54]

Therapy and prognosis

Chordomas require treatment with surgical resection and local radiotherapy to improve survival rates, reduce the incidence of local recurrence and improve the quality of the patient's life. Since these tumours are often sited close to vital structures, complete surgical resection is not usually possible. Since these vital structures are often also radiosensitive it is also often not possible to deliver a high dose of radiotherapy. Conventional postoperative radiotherapy is very useful in local palliation and is associated with an approximately 50% 5-year survival and 10-year survival of around 35%. Long term local control and cure are unfortunately rare.[55,56] Proton irradiation has been suggested to improve local tumour control.[55,57] Female sex, tumour necrosis in preradiation treatment biopsy, and tumour volume in excess of 70 ml have been suggested as independent predictors of

reduced survival after radiation therapy for skull base chordomas.[58] Metastasis is well documented and occurs in about a third of cases following initial therapy;[59–61] recurrence along the route of surgery has also been described.[62] The debate that has continued around the nosology of chordomas containing cartilaginous matrix probably has no pragmatic bearing on clinical outcome. There appear to be no significant survival differences between patients with cartilage containing tumours that are keratin immunopositive (hyalinised chordoma) or negative (chondrosarcoma).[63]

Fibrous dysplasia

Fibrous dysplasia of bone is a disorder of unknown aetiology which generally occurs in the first three decades of life and commonly affects the skull (particularly the frontal, facial sphenoid and ethmoid bones) and spine[64]. Lesions may be solitary or multiple and the disorder may be associated with disordered skeletal growth. An association is seen between polyostotic fibrous dysplasia and cutaneous lesions in Albright syndrome.[64]

Skull involvement produces structural abnormalities of the affected bones that cause compression of adjacent structures, especially manifest by cranial nerve defects. Orbital involvement commonly results in proptosis. Imaging studies show a variable appearance, which depends on the relative quantities of fibrous and osseous tissue in the lesion, but typical cases show a 'ground glass' lucency of bone with a surrounding sclerotic rim.[65]

Histology shows bone replaced by relatively loose sparsely cellular fibrovascular tissue from which haphazard

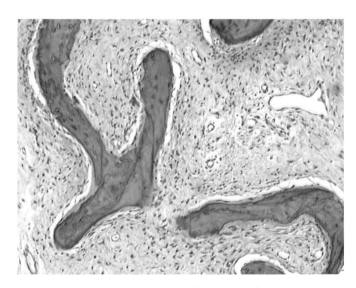

Fig. 18.17 **Fibrous dysplasia.** Towards the margins of the lesion, the fibrous stroma condenses to form numerous irregular bony spicules. These are formed of non-maturing woven bone, and osteoblastic activity is usually (although not always) absent. The bony spicules often have a characteristic 'fish hook' shape, as seen here. H & E.

trabeculae of woven bone 'condense out' to form islands and cords of mineralised bone (Fig. 18.17). Osteoblastic rimming of trabeculae is not usually present. Mature lesions contain a dense fibrous stroma with persistence of the woven bone trabeculae. Myxoid change, associated aneurysmal bone cyst change.[66] and the presence of islands of cartilage may lead to diagnostic uncertainty.[67] Some cases show areas resembling psammoma bodies and, in the context of a skull lesion, this may superficially resemble osseous meningioma.

The differential diagnosis of fibrous dysplasia is wide, particularly in terms of the radiological appearances. A distinction from an osteoma, an ossifying fibroma or the hyperostosis associated with a meningioma may be difficult in radiology, but a histological distinction is usually possible. However, the precise relationship between ossifying fibroma and fibrous dysplasia is uncertain.[67] Fibrous dysplasia is a benign condition which usually does not recur locally; polyostotic involvement is discussed above.

Aneurysmal bone cyst

This lesion are regarded as a locally aggressive but benign and reactive condition of unknown aetiology, resulting in cystic, expansile lytic lesions of bone, occasionally involving the skull[68–71] and vertebrae.[72,73] The lesion usually presents in the first three decades of life, and in the skull involves most often the occipital bone. Imaging shows a lytic lesion with expansion of the bone, typically

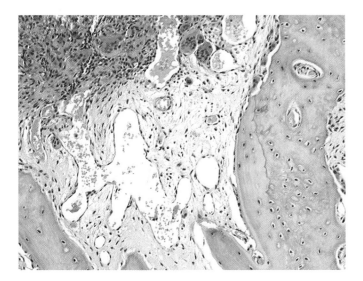

Fig. 18.18 **Aneurysmal bone cyst.** Immature lesions are dominated by a very cellular stroma containing numerous osteoclastic giant cells, as seen at the top left of this field. Later on, the stroma becomes much less cellular and bony trabeculae appear, with associated osteoblastic activity. Between these trabeculae there are numerous, thin-walled, ectatic vascular channels lined by flattened endothelium, as in the lower part of the figure. H & E.

preserving a thin shell of surrounding new bone. Histology is dominated by the presence of irregular blood containing cystic areas demarcated by prominent septa composed of plump fibroblasts in which giant cells are generally prominent and in which osteoid and bone are present (Fig. 18.18). Ectatic thin walled vascular channels may dominate in some areas and haemosiderin containing macrophages are also present in the majority of cases. Examples of solid aneurysmal bone cysts, composed of the spindle cell element are also described[74] (perhaps better termed giant cell reparative granulomas) but these are mainly described in peripheral sites. Areas resembling aneurysmal bone cyst can be seen in several types of primary bone tumour, especially fibrous dysplasia,[66] chondroblastoma[75] and giant cell tumours. They can also occur in relation to some types of osteosarcoma.[76] Caution therefore needs to be exercised in making the diagnosis in small or fragmented samples. Careful clinical and imaging correlation should be made before arriving at a diagnosis. Aneurysmal bone cysts are curable by complete resection, but may recur if resection is incomplete.

Paget's disease

Paget's disease is a bone disorder of unknown causation which typically involves many sites, including the femur, humerus, skull, vertebrae and ribs. The disease is characterised by exaggerated bone remodelling, in which abnormal osteoclastic bone resorption is accompanied by the formation of new bone.[77] It usually presents after the fourth decade of life, and affects males more often than females. Paget's disease is characterised by osseous thickening and distortion, which is evident on radiology. Early lesions can appear radiolucent and circumscribed, but as the disease progresses, bony resorption predominates and multiple trabeculae of new bone are formed, which appears radiodense.[78] In the final stages of the disease there is marked bony thickening, which in the skull can result in impingement on the foramen magnum and cranial nerve compression.[79] Histology shows excess activity of both osteoblasts and osteoclasts, resulting in disordered bony spicules with angular cement lines which are embedded in fibrous tisssue.

The differential diagnosis of Paget's disease is not usually the cause of major difficulty, but occasional cases have been confused with fibrous dysplasia, ossifying fibroma, osteoma or metabolic bone disease. Sarcomatous change is an uncommon but well recognised complication of Paget's disease;[80] osteogenic sarcoma is the commonest malignancy to occur under these circumstances (Fig. 18.19), but others have been described, including chondrosarcoma and giant cell tumour. The prognosis for patients with sarcomas in Paget's disease is particularly poor, with pulmonary metastases being present at an early stage in many cases.[80]

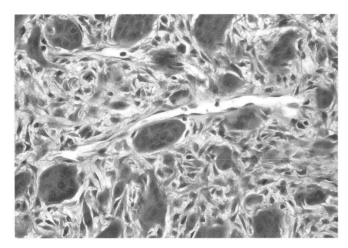

Fig. 18.19 **Osteogenic sarcoma in Paget's disease of the skull.** This is accompanied by large pleomorphic giant cell set within a matrix which contains irregular seams of osteoid. H & E.

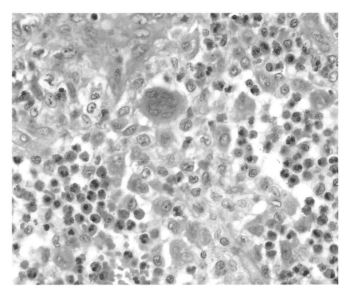

Fig. 18.21 **Langerhans cell histiocytosis.** Lesions are characterised by sheets of histiocytic cells intermixed with eosinophils and lymphocytes. Multinucleate giant cells are also seen but are generally in low frequency. H & E.

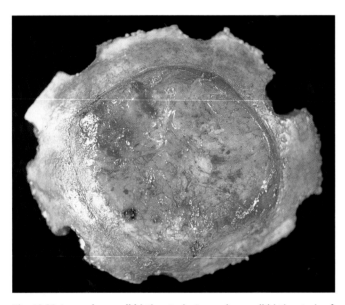

Fig. 18.20 **Langerhans cell histiocytosis.** Langerhans cell histiocytosis of the skull vault usually presents as a well demarcated exuberant lesion, which can be cured by complete resection.

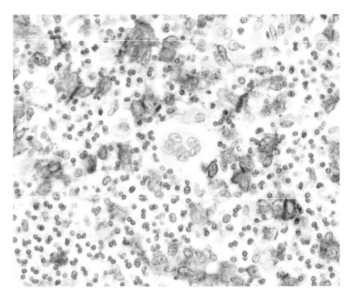

Fig. 18.22 **Langerhans cell histiocytosis.** Immunoreactivity for CD1a is seen in histiocytic cells.

Langerhans cell histiocytosis

These conditions are described in detail in Chapter 11 in relation to their intracranial pathology. The skull vault is a common site for development of eosinophilic granuloma, forming lytic lesions in bone with a sclerotic margin[81] (Fig. 18.20). Histology is characterised by sheets of histiocytic cells intermixed with and sometimes dominated by an accompanying admixture of eosinophils and lymphocytes, with small numbers of multinucleate cells (Fig. 18.21). The histiocytic cells are Langerhans cells and show immunoreactivity for S-100 and CD1a (Fig. 18.22). Ultrastructural examination will reveal characteristic Birbeck granules (see Chapter 11). Less commonly seen are examples of systemic Langerhans histiocytoses: Erdheim–Chester disease, a rare non-Langerhans cell histiocytosis, can also involve the orbit and skull,[82,83] and occasional cases can involve the brain (see Chapter 11).

Haemangioma of bone

Haemangiomas of bone[84] may affect the skull vault (particularly the parietal bone) as well as vertebrae. Most cases occur in middle age, with a female predominance,

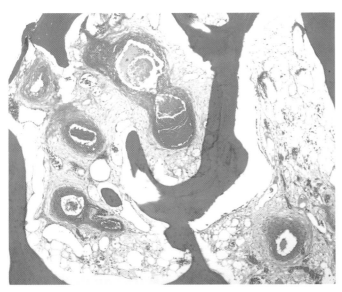

Fig. 18.23 **Haemangioma of bone.** Vascular channels with thick walls replacing marrow spaces. H & E.

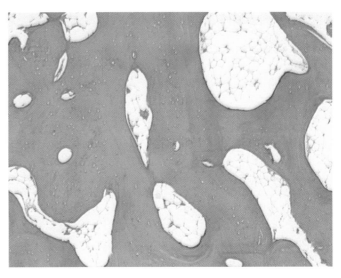

Fig. 18.24 **Osteoma.** Histologically, mature ivory osteomas constist of abnormally broad anastamosing trabeculae of dense lamellar bone enclosing small Haversian spaces. These spaces often contain adipose tissue rather than active marrow. H & E.

and present as a painful scalp mass. Imaging of bone frequently shows a 'honeycomb' pattern of radiating spicules, reflected by the histology which is characterised by vascular channels of varying size set between irregular trabeculae of lamellar bone (Fig. 18.23). These features allow a clear distinction in most cases from an aneurysmal bone cyst. This lesion is a cavernous angioma of bone and is cured by complete excision.

Osteoma

Osteomas are commonly seen in the skull affecting both inner or outer tables of the calvarium.[85] They usually occur as solitary lesions, most commonly involving the frontal bone or frontal sinus, but the other skull bones may be involved. The lesions usually present between the second and fourth decades of life, with a male predominance; facial asymmetry or cosmetic irregularity are the commonest presentations. Radiology shows a typically dense lesion with a well demarcated smooth outline of variable shape; an 'ivory button' is not uncommon. Macroscopically, osteomas are typically rock hard white dome shaped lesions, which frequently require prolonged decalcification prior to dissection. Histology shows broad interlinked trabeculae of lamellar bone with marrow spaces (Fig. 18.24). Osteoblasts are typically inconspicuous. Gardner syndrome includes a clinical triad of familial polyposis coli, osteomas and soft tissue tumours.[86] A classification for cranial osteomas has been proposed as follows:

1. intraparenchymal;
2. dural;
3. skull base; and
4. skull vault, the latter being subdivided into exostotic and enostotic variants.[87]

Osteomas are benign lesions which are cured by surgical resection.

Chondrosarcoma

Chondrosarcoma arising from bone (as opposed to chondrosarcoma arising from meninges – see Chapter 14) may occur in the skull base, where they are generally low grade lesions.[88,89] The main diagnostic problem in

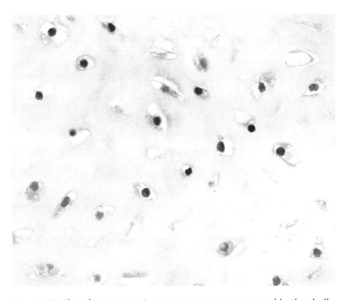

Fig. 18.25 **Chondrosarcoma.** In most tumours encountered in the skull base cellularity is low with minimal atypia. H & E.

arriving at a diagnosis in this site is in discriminating between a chondrosarcoma and a chordoma, discussed above. Histology shows a cartilaginous lesion with chondroid cells in lacunes within the chondroid matrix. In the majority of cases encountered in the skull there will be minimal nuclear atypia and rare mitoses (Figs 18.25–18.29), with occasional binucleate chondrocytes. Chondrosarcomas are graded on the basis of cellularity and nuclear cytology.[90] These lesions are locally aggressive and while they have a metastatic potential, this is typically low.[91] Histological examination of one large series showed that 51% of tumours were grade l, 11% grade II, 30% mesenchymal and 8% myxoid.[89] Another large series showed that 50.5% of tumours were grade 1, 28.5% had areas of grades 1 and 2, and 21% were pure grade 2 neoplasms.[90] Examples of high grade or dedifferentiated chondrosarcomas have been described in relation to the skull.[92,93] Some cases have been reported in association with Maffucci syndome.[94]

Plasmacytoma and myeloma

Involvement of the spine and skull is common in plasma cell neoplasia; these conditions are discussed in detail in Chapter 11.

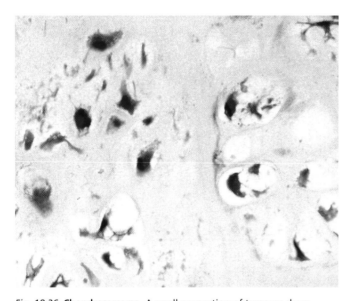

Fig. 18.26 **Chondrosarcoma.** A small proportion of tumours show significant cytological atypia. H & E.

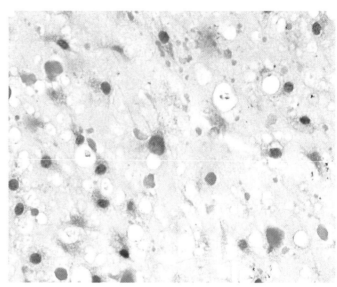

Fig. 18.27 **Chondrosarcoma.** In decalcified material nuclear staining may be difficult to assess. H & E.

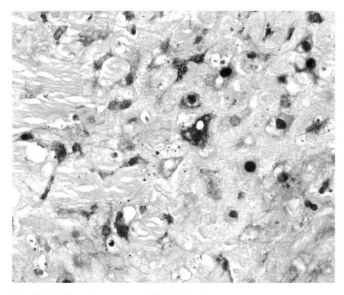

Fig. 18.28 **Chondrosarcoma.** Cells in chondrosarcoma are immunoreactive for S-100.

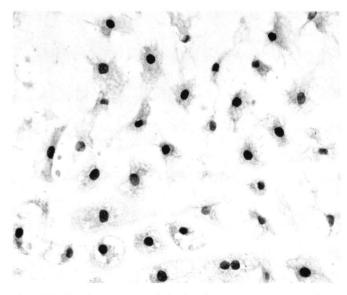

Fig. 18.29 **Chondrosarcoma.** Cells in chondrosarcoma are not reactive for cytokeratin, in contrast to chordoma. H & E.

Lymphoma and leukaemia

Lymphoma is commonly encountered in neuropathological practice as a result of extradural involvement and neurosurgical intervention to decompress the spinal cord. Secondary involvement of the nervous system by both lymphoma and leukaemia is also encountered; these conditions are discussed in more detail in Chapters 11 and 12. A problem is occasionally encountered in the recognition of primary B-cell lymphomas of bone. These lesions may have a deceptive spindle cell morphology and their true nature is only revealed on immunohisto-chemistry, when they express an expected pattern of lymphoid and B-cell markers.

Melanotic progonoma (melanotic neuroectodermal tumour of infancy)

This rare neoplasm occurs most often in children under 1 year of age, usually in the maxilla, but skull involvement has been reported and extremely rare cases appear to arise in the leptomeninges or brain.[95–99] Intracranial lesions usually involve the cerebellum and have occurred in an older group of patients (age range 3 months to 69 years).[97] The radiological features are non-specific, and most of the bone based tumours have a good prognosis if completely resected.[96] Histology shows a primitive neuro-ectodermal tumour with features of malignancy (mitotic activity, nuclear pleomorphism) that belie the benign behaviour in most cases. The tumour cells may be arranged in a variety of patterns, with solid, alveolar or tubular arrangements, often with a biphasic population of larger pigmented cells and smaller non-pigmented neuroblast like cells (Fig. 18.30).[99] As its name implies, melanin production in the tumour cell population is

usually a prominent feature (usually in large epithelioid cells), which facilitates diagnosis.

Malignant behaviour with local invasion and systemic metastases has been reported both in occasional bone tumours of this type, and rather more often in their central nervous system (CNS) counterparts.[97]

Uncommon bony lesions

Small series and individual case reports have documented involvement of the skull or spinal column in a wide variety of tumours for which most neuropathologists will have little practical experience (Table 18.2).[45,75,100–132] In modern clinical practice it would be unwise to attempt a diagnosis in an area outside one's day-to-day expertise. The diagnosis of bone tumours is a potential minefield, especially so with rare entities or common entities arising in an uncommon site. Close collaboration with a diagnostic service specialising in diagnosis of bone and soft tissue tumours is now an essential part of neuropathological practice.

Tumours of the ear and temporal bone

Tumours of the temporal bone or those arising in the ear may involve the nervous system and come to the attention of a surgical neuropathology service (Table 18.3).

> *Rhabdomyosarcomas* of the middle ear may extend to involve the cerebellopontine angle and this may be the main presenting feature of disease.[133–135]
> *Cholesteatomas* may also extend into the cerebellopontine angle.
> *Jugulotympanic paragangliomas* are been discussed in Chapter 8.

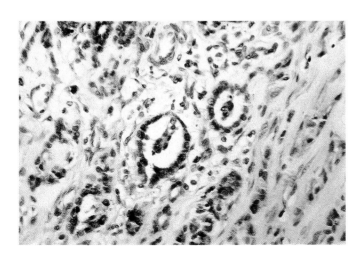

Fig. 18.30 **Melanotic progonoma.** This uncommon tumour is composed of a mixture of larger pigmented cells with a tubular arrangement and smaller non-pigmented primitive cells.

Table 18.2 Rare bone tumours and tumour-like lesions involving the skull[45,7–5,100–132]

Chondroma/osteochondroma
Osteoblastoma
Chondroblastoma
Chondromyxoid fibroma
Ossifying fibroma
Osteosarcoma
Giant cell tumour
Mucocele of paranasal sinuses

Table 18.3 Tumours and tumour-like lesions of the middle ear which may extend into the cranial cavity

Rhabdomyosarcoma
Cholesteatoma
Paragangloma
Ceruminoma
Squamous cell carcinoma
Papillary adenocarcinoma

Squamous cell carcinomas of the middle ear are uncommon lesions that can spread into the temporal bone and mastoid, sometimes invading the middle cranial fossa.[136–138]

Papillary adenocarcinoma of the middle ear, termed low grade adenocarcinoma of the endolymphatic sac, may grow into the intracranial cavity.[139–142] This lesion has been associated with von Hippel–Lindau disease (Chapter 19).

Tumours of the orbit

Tumours of the CNS may extend into the orbit and, on occasion, orbital tumours may extend back to involve the anterior skull base. The range of orbital tumours that are likely to extend back to involve the nervous system include meningiomas, malignant fibrous histiocytomas, rhabdomyosarcoma, malignant melanoma, lymphoma, and malignant tumours of lacrimal gland – especially adenoid cystic carcinoma[143,144] (Table 18.4).

Tumours of the nose and paranasal sinuses (Table 18.5)

Olfactory neuroblastoma (aesthesioneuroblastoma)

This is a relatively rare but well recognised tumour that develops high in the nasopharynx, commonly involving the cribriform plate with a potential for intracranial extension.[145] The tumours can occur across a wide age range, with bimodal peaks in the second and fifth

Table 18.4 Orbital tumours that may extend into the cranial cavity

Optic nerve astrocytoma/anaplastic astrocytoma/glioblastoma
Meningioma
Lymphoma
Rhabdomyosarcoma
Malignant melanoma
Malignant fibrous histiocytoma
Lacrimal gland carcinoma (adenoid cystic)
Haemangioma

Table 18.5 Tumours and tmour-like lesions of the nose and paranasal sinuses which may involve the cranial cavity

Olfactory neuroblastoma
Olfactory neuroepithelioma
Neuroendocrine carcinoma
Sinonasal teratocarcinoma
Nasopharyngeal carcinoma
Sinonasal undifferentiated carcinoma
Juvenile angiofibroma
Mucocele of paranasal sinuses

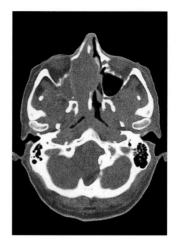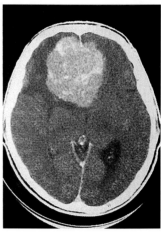

Fig. 18.31 **Olfactory neuroblastoma.** A large contrast enhancing tumour is shownin this CT scan, which fills the nasal cavity and invades the adjacent sinuses and skull base to involve the inferior frontal lobe. H & E.

decades. Most patients present with nasal obstruction or epistaxis, but some cases may present as intracranial lesions.[146] Imaging studies show bowing of the sinus walls, with the tumour in most cases invading the turbinates, septum, sinus walls and adjacent structures (Fig. 18.31). Variable signal and enhancement patterns have been described[145] but these are non-specific.

Histologically these tumours may show several patterns:

> Some tumours show a round cell almost neurocyte-like pattern with islands and cords of uniform cells having scant cytoplasm and forming well defined rosettes with a distinct neuropil. Mitoses are uncommon and the tumour appears bland (Figs 18.32–18.36). Ganglionic maturation may be seen. These cellular islands are typically surrounded by a population of cells staining for S-100 protein, resembling arrangements seen in paraganglioma.[147]

> Others show a pattern of malignant small blue cell tumour, resembling that seen in conventional neuroblastoma, including many mitoses and apoptotic bodies with rudimentary rosettes.

> In rare cases, a tubular or ribbon-like pattern of tumour cells with epithelioid features has been described, which may resemble a carcinoma of the nasopharynx. Immunocytochemical and ultrastructural studies will reveal its neuroectodermal nature, for which the term olfactory neuroepithelioma (aesthesioneuroepithelioma) has been employed.

Immunohistochemistry typically shows expression of markers of neuronal differentiation such as neuro-filament protein (NFP), neuron specific enolase (NSE), synaptophysin and chromogranin[147,148] (Fig. 18.37).

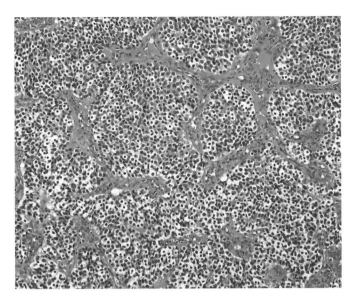

Fig. 18.32 **Olfactory neuroblastoma.** Most tumours are composed of well formed rounded nests of uniform small blue cells. In poorly fixed samples, an oligodendroglioma-like pattern of vacuolation can sometimes be seen. H & E.

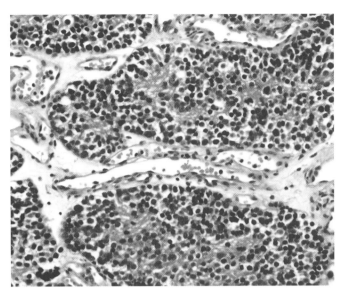

Fig. 18.33 **Olfactory neuroblastoma.** In a small proportion of tumours ill-defined rosettes can be seen. H & E.

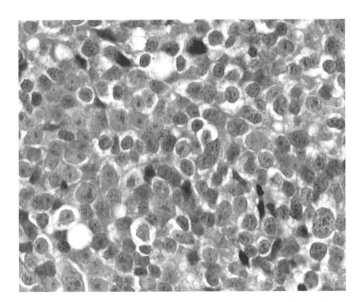

Fig. 18.34 **Olfactory neuroblastoma.** Nuclei are rounded with small nucleoli. Mitotic activity is variable, depending on tumour grade. H & E.

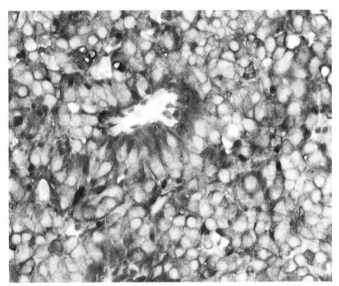

Fig. 18.35 **Olfactory neuroblastoma.** Chromogranin A immunoreactivity is high in this example. In others, this may be only focally present.

Epithelial markers are also expressed, but often in a patchy pattern.[149] Absence of *EWS/FLI1* gene fusion and *MIC2* expression in one study suggested that olfactory neuroblastoma is not related to the Ewing family of tumours,[150] but an opposite conclusion was obtained in another study.[151]

Olfactory neuroblastomas are radiosensitive and chemosensitive; localised tumours which are completely excised may carry a good prognosis. Invasion beyond the nasal cavity and paranasal sinuses is associated with an adverse prognosis, with a recurrence rate of around 50% of patients. Several staging and grading systems have been proposed for olfactory neuroblastomas, but these may not always allow accurate prediction of the clinical course in an individual patient.

The differential diagnosis includes *other types of peripheral primitive neuroectodermal tumours*, and the following rare lesions at this site.

Neuroendocrine carcinomas may arise in the nasopharynx and range from a small cell malignant

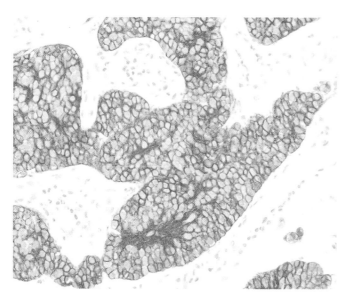

Fig. 18.36 **Olfactory neuroblastoma.** CD56 (Leu7) expression is strongly shown, including in rosettes.

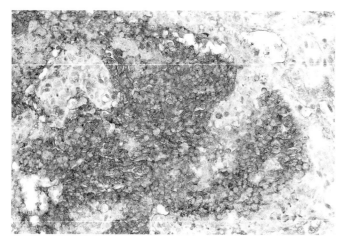

Fig. 18.37 **Olfactory neuroblastoma.** A strong positive reaction is shown in the cytoplasm of tumour cells within an infiltrating olfactory neuroblastoma. Immunocytochemistry for synaptophysin.

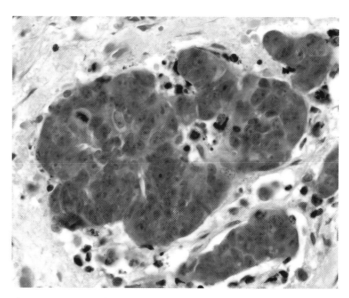

Fig. 18.38 **Neuroendocrine carcinoma.** Neuroendocrine carcinoma may resemble large cell undifferentiated carcinoma, as here, or may resemble small cell undifferentiated carcinoma. H & E.

neuroendocrine tumour, resembling oat cell carcinoma of the lung (termed small cell undifferentiated neuroendocrine carcinoma),[152] though to lesions that resemble atypical carcinoid tumours, and include forms with a recognisable epithelial pattern (Fig. 18.38). These lesions express neuroendocrine markers and also express epithelial markers such as cytokeratin.[153]

Sinonasal teratocarcinosarcomas are uncommon, aggressive, tumours of the paranasal sinuses or nasopharynx which can develop intracranial extension. Histologically they are composed of olfactory neuroblastoma-like areas associated with fetal-like squamous epithelium, glandular epithelium, immature mesenchyme and immature cartilage.[154]

Cases with areas resembling craniopharyngioma have been described.[155–157]

Nasopharyngeal carcinoma is a squamous pattern tumour which may be keratinising or non-keratinising. It may spread to involve the cavernous sinus and sometime invades into the anterior cranial fossa.[158]

Sinonasal undifferentiated carcinoma is an aggressive epithelial tumour which shows no evidence of squamous differentiation and may involve cranial nerves and brain with local spread. Histology shows sheets of large, pleomorphic hyperchromatic cells showing strong uniform cytokeratin expression (in contrast to olfactory neuroblastoma which shows patchy or weak expression).[159]

Some tumours of minor salivary glands may spread extensively, especially *adenoid cystic carcinoma*.[143,144,160] Tumours from nasal sinus are also well recognised as spreading to the nervous system by direct extension.[161]

Juvenile angiofibromas may be encountered in the cavernous sinus as well as the anterior cranial fossa (Figs 18.39 and 18.40).[162–164]

Soft tissue tumours

Soft tissue tumours and sarcomas may develop in a paraspinal distribution (Table 18.6) and may also occur around the skull base (Table 18.1). A detailed description of types and diagnostic interpretation is beyond the scope of this book but is well covered in standard texts. Increasingly a combination of cytogenetic, molecular, immunohistochemical and morphological assessments

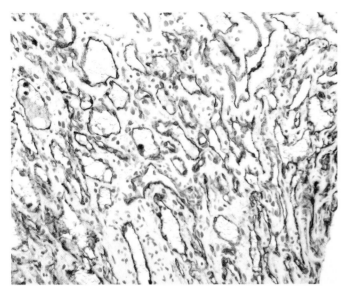

Fig. 18.39 **Juvenile angiofibroma.** Juvenile angiofibroma composed of vascular channels set in a fibrocollagenous stroma. In biopsy samples the extent of vascularity may be obscured as they collapse. H & E.

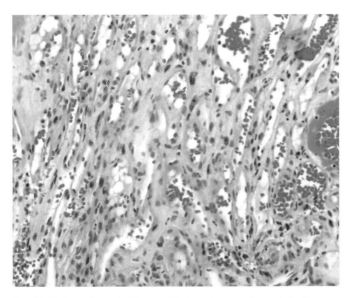

Fig. 18.40 **Juvenile angiofibroma.** Markers for vascular endothelium are a reliable way of highlighting vascular architecture.

Table 18.6 Paraspinal tumours and tumour-like masses presenting to neuropathologists for diagnosis

Chordoma
Chondroma/chondrosarcoma
Lipoma
Leukaemia/lymphoma
Plasmacytoma/myeloma
Neuroblastoma
Ewing's tumour/Askins' tumour
Malignant peripheral nerve sheath tumour
Sacrococcygeal teratoma
Tuberculosis
Bacterial abscess
Herniated nucleus pulposus

are becoming essential in making a correct diagnosis and guiding therapy in these types of tumour. Intraoperative consultation may allow diagnosis of a malignant spindle cell tumour and this should be followed by appropriate preservation and sampling of tumour to facilitate detailed investigation. Samples should be taken for cytogenetic analysis, frozen for later molecular genetic study if appropriate, and fixed for both light microscopic and ultrastructural assessment. Ewing's tumour, rhabdomyosarcoma and synovial sarcoma are amongst the commonest types encountered in personal neuropathological practice.

Ewing's tumour

Ewing's tumour is a form of malignant peripheral primitive neuroectodermal tumour that may present in childhood and adolescence in a paravertebral extradural location. Histologically they appear as uniform 'malignant small blue cell' tumours, usually without any distinctive histological pattern (Fig. 18.41), but variable PAS positivity is usually present in the tumour cell cytoplasm. As with all small cell tumours, the key to diagnosis rests in a combination of cytogenetic, molecular immunohistochemical and morphological assessment. Strong membrane immunoreactivity for CD99, a product of the *MIC2* gene, is characteristically present (Fig. 18.42). Many tumours also express beta-2 microglobulin, and there is variable expression of neuroendocrine markers such as NFP, synaptophysin, NSE and PGP9.5. Electron microscopy also shows evidence of neural differentiation, and many of the tumour cells contain aggregates of glycogen (Fig. 18.43). These tumours typically show a t(11;22)(q24;q12) translocation or other translocations involving the *EWS* gene on chromosome 22.[165–169]

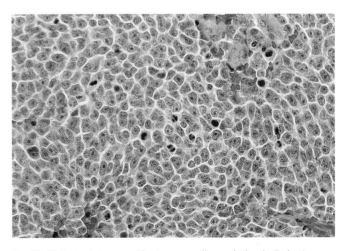

Fig. 18.41 **Ewing's tumour.** The tumour cell population in Ewing's tumour tends to form solid sheets of small primitive cells with slightly elongated or carrot-shaped nuclei. There is little evidence of rosette formation, but multiple mitotic figures are present in this case. H & E.

Fig. 18.42 **Ewing's tumour.** Immunocytochemistry for CD99 shows strong membranous and weaker cytoplasmic positivity in this case of Ewing's sarcoma.

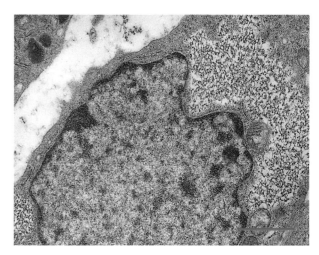

Fig. 18.43 **Ewing's tumour.** Electron microscopy shows a large paranuclear aggregate of glycogen in a tumour cell from a Ewing's sarcoma. Bar = 2 μm.

Germ cell tumours

Sacrococcygeal teratomas are uncommon lesions that typically present in early childhood or rarely in later life with neurological problems related to involvement of lower spinal nerve roots. These lesions are discussed more fully in Chapter 10. A distinction has been made between congenital spinal hamartomas and teratomas. In hamartomas histology has shown well formed elements related to the part affected such as bone, cartilage and tissue suggestive of urinary tract, cystic areas, adipose tissue and nerves. In the absence of neoplastic features it has been suggested that such lesions are better classsed as hamartoma rather than teratoma,[170] but the term 'mature teratoma' seems more appropriate.

REFERENCES

1. Jackson IT, Marsh WR. Anterior cranial fossa tumors. Ann Plast Surg, 1983; 11:479–489

Ecchordosis physaliphora

2. Rengachary SS, Grotte DA, Swanson PE. Extradural ecchordosis physaliphora of the thoracic spine: case report. Neurosurgery, 1997; 41:1198–1201
3. Ng SH, Ko SF, Wan YL et al. Cervical ecchordosis physaliphora: CT and MR features. Br J Radiol, 1998; 71:329–331
4. Macdonald RL, Cusimano MD, Deck JH et al. Cerebrospinal fluid fistula secondary to ecchordosis physaliphora. Neurosurgery, 1990; 26:515–518
5. Wolfe JTD, Scheithauer BW. 'Intradural chordoma' or 'giant ecchordosis physaliphora'? Report of two cases. Clin Neuropathol, 1987; 6:98–103
6. Stam FC, Kamphorst W. Ecchordosis physaliphora as a cause of fatal pontine hemorrhage. Eur Neurol, 1982; 21:90–93
7. Macdonald RL, Deck JH. Immunohistochemistry of ecchordosis physaliphora and chordoma. Can J Neurol Sci, 1990; 17:420–423
8. Sarasa JL, Fortes J. Ecchordosis physaliphora: an immunohistochemical study of two cases. Histopathology, 1991; 18:273–275

9. Ho KL. Ecchordosis physaliphora and chorodoma: a comparative ultrastructural study. Clin Neuropathol, 1985; 4:77–86

Chordoma

10. Salisbury JR. The pathology of the human notochord. J Pathol, 1993; 171:253–255
11. Dorfman HD, Czerniak B. Bone cancers. Cancer, 1995; 75:203–210
12. Thodou E, Kontogeorgos G, Scheithauer BW et al. Intrasellar chordomas mimicking pituitary adenoma. J Neurosurg, 2000; 92:976–982
13. Cable DG, Moir C. Pediatric sacrococcygeal chordomas: a rare tumor to be differentiated from sacrococcygeal teratoma. J Pediatr Surg, 1997; 32:759–761
14. Coffin CM, Swanson PE, Wick MR et al. Chordoma in childhood and adolescence. A clinicopathologic analysis of 12 cases. Arch Pathol Lab Med, 1993; 117:927–933
15. Forsyth PA, Cascino TL, Shaw EG et al. Intracranial chordomas: a clinicopathological and prognostic study of 51 cases. J Neurosurg, 1993; 78:741–747
16. Doucet V, Peretti-Viton P, Figarella-Branger D et al. MRI of intracranial chordomas. Extent of tumour and contrast enhancement: criteria for differential diagnosis. Neuroradiology, 1997; 39:571–576
17. Meyers SP, Hirsch WLJ, Curtin HD et al. Chordomas of the skull base: MR features. AJNR. Am J Neuroradiol, 1992; 13:1627–1636
18. Boriani S, Weinstein JN, Biagini R. Primary bone tumors of the spine. Terminology and surgical staging. Spine, 1997; 22:1036–1044
19. Fleming GF, Heimann PS, Stephens JK et al. Dedifferentiated chordoma. Response to aggressive chemotherapy in two cases. Cancer, 1993; 72:714–718
20. Hruban RH, Traganos F, Reuter VE et al. Chordomas with malignant spindle cell components. A DNA flow cytometric and immunohistochemical study with histogenetic implications. Am J Pathol, 1990; 137:435–447
21. Meis JM, Raymond AK, Evans HL et al. Dedifferentiated chordoma. A clinicopathologic and immunohistochemical study of three cases. Am J Surg Pathol, 1987; 11:516–525
22. Tomlinson FH, Scheithauer BW, Forsythe PA et al. Sarcomatous transformation in cranial chordoma. Neurosurgery, 1992; 31:13–18
23. Brooks JJ, LiVolsi VA, Trojanowski JQ. Does chondroid chordoma exist? Acta Neuropathol, 1987; 72:229–235
24. Brooks JJ, Trojanowski JQ, LiVolsi VA. Chondroid chordoma: a low-grade chondrosarcoma and its differential diagnosis. Curr Top Pathol, 1989; 80:165–181
25. Walker WP, Landas SK, Bromley CM et al. Immunohistochemical distinction of classic and chondroid chordomas. Mod Pathol, 1991; 4:661–666
26. Jeffrey PB, Biava CG, Davis RL. Chondroid chordoma. A hyalinized

chordoma without cartilaginous differentiation. Am J Clin Pathol, 1995; 103:271–279

27. Bouropoulou V, Bosse V, Roessner A et al. Immunohistochemical investigation of chordomas: histogenetic and differential diagnostic aspects. Curr Top Pathol, 1989; 80:183–203

28. Abenoza P, Sibley RK Chordoma: an immunohistologic study. Hum Pathol, 1986; 17:744–747

29. Heikinheimo K, Persson S, Kindblom LG et al. Expression of different cytokeratin subclasses in human chordoma. J Pathol, 1991; 164:145–150

30. Folpe AL, Agoff SN, Willis J et al. Parachordoma is immunohistochemically and cytogenetically distinct from axial chordoma and extraskeletal myxoid chondrosarcoma. Am J Surg Pathol, 1999; 23:1059–1067

31. Naka T, Iwamoto Y, Shinohara N et al. Cytokeratin subtyping in chordomas and the fetal notochord: an immunohistochemical analysis of aberrant expression. Mod Pathol, 1997; 10:545–551

32. O'Hara BJ, Paetau A, Miettinen M. Keratin subsets and monoclonal antibody HBME-1 in chordoma: immunohistochemical differential diagnosis between tumors simulating chordoma. Hum Pathol, 1998; 29:119–126

33. Holton J, Steel T, Luxsuwong M et al. Skull base chordomas: correlation of tumour doubling time with age, mitosis and Ki67 proliferation index. Neuropathol Appl Neurobiol, 2000; 26:497–503

34. Gibas Z, Miettinen M, Sandberg AA. Chromosomal abnormalities in two chordomas. Cancer Genet Cytogenet, 1992; 58:169–173

35. Stepanek J, Cataldo SA, Ebersold MJ et al. Familial chordoma with probable autosomal dominant inheritance. Am J Med Genet, 1998; 75:335–336

36. Bridge JA, Pickering D, Neff JR. Cytogenetic and molecular cytogenetic analysis of sacral chordoma. Cancer Genet Cytogenet, 1994; 75:23–25

37. Buonamici L, Roncaroli F, Fioravanti A et al. Cytogenetic investigation of chordomas of the skull. Cancer Genet Cytogenet, 1999; 112:49–52

38. Dalpra L, Malgara R, Miozzo M et al. First cytogenetic study of a recurrent familial chordoma of the clivus. Int J Cancer, 1999; 81:24–30

39. DeBoer JM, Neff JR, Bridge JA. Cytogenetics of sacral chordoma. Cancer Genet Cytogenet, 1992; 64:95–96

40. Miozzo M, Dalpra L, Riva P et al. A tumor suppressor locus in familial and sporadic chordoma maps to 1p36. Int J Cancer, 2000; 87(1):68–72

41. Scheil S, Bruderlein S, Lieher T et al. Genome-wide analysis of sixteen chordomas by comparative genomic hybridization and cytogenetics of the first human chordoma cell line, U-CHI. Genes Chromosomes Cancer, 2001; 32:203–211

42. Klingler L, Shooks J, Fiedler PN et al. Microsatellite instability in sacral chordoma. J Surg Oncol, 2000; 73:100–103

43. Coffin CM, Swanson PE, Wick MR et al. An immunohistochemical comparison of chordoma with renal cell carcinoma, colorectal adenocarcinoma, and myxopapillary ependymoma: a potential diagnostic dilemma in the diminutive biopsy. Mod Pathol, 1993; 6:531–538

44. Byers PD. A study of histological features distinguishing chordoma from chondrosarcoma. Br J Cancer, 1981; 43:229–242

45. Keel SB, Bhan AK, Liebsch NJ et al. Chondromyxoid fibroma of the skull base: a tumor which may be confused with chordoma and chondrosarcoma. A report of three cases and review of the literature. Am J Surg Pathol, 1997; 21:577–582

46. Ricoy JR, Lobato RD, Baez B et al. Suprasellar chordoid glioma. Acta Neuropathol, 2000; 99:699–703

47. Couce ME, Aker FV, Scheithauer BW. Chordoid meningioma: a clinicopathologic study of 42 cases. Am J Surg Pathol, 2000; 24:899–905

48. Kepes JJ, Chen WY, Connors MH et al. Chordoid meningeal tumors in young individuals with peritumoral lymphoplasmacellular infiltrates causing systemic manifestations of the Castleman syndrome. A report of seven cases. Cancer, 1988; 62:391–406

49. Steilen-Gimbel H, Niedermayer I, Feiden W et al. Unbalanced translocation t(1;3)(p12–13;q11) in meningiomas as the unique feature of chordoid differentiation. Genes, Chromosomes Cancer, 1999; 26:270–272

50. Sangueza OP, White CRJ. Parachordoma. Am J Dermatopathol, 1994; 16(2):185–188

51. Carstens PH. Chordoid tumor: a light, electron microscopic, and immunohistochemical study. Ultrastruct Pathol, 1995; 19:291–295

52. Fisher C, Miettinen M. Parachordoma: a clinicopathologic and immunohistochemical study of four cases of an unusual soft tissue neoplasm. Ann Diagn Pathol, 1997; 1:3–10

53. Fisher C. Parachordoma exists – but what is it? Adv Anat Pathol, 2000; 7:141–148

54. Imlay SP, Argenyi ZB, Stone MS et al. Cutaneous parachordoma. A light microscopic and immunohistochemical report of two cases and review of the literature. J Cutan Pathol, 1998; 25:279–284

55. Party PTW. Proton therapy for base of skull chordoma: a report for the Royal College of Radiologists. The Proton Therapy Working Party, Clin Oncol (R Coll Radiol), 2000; 12:75–79

56. Cheng EY, Ozerdemoglu RA, Transfeldt EE et al. Lumbosacral chordoma. Prognostic factors and treatment. Spine, 1999; 24:1639–1645

57. al-Mefty O, Borba LA. Skull base chordomas: a management challenge. J Neurosurg, 1997; 86:182–189

58. O'Connell JX, Renard LG, Liebsch NJ et al. Base of skull chordoma. A correlative study of histologic and clinical features of 62 cases. Cancer, 1994; 74:2261–2267

59. Ashwood N, Hoskin PJ, Saunders MI. Metastatic chordoma: pattern of spread and response to chemotherapy. Clin Oncol (R Coll Radiol), 1994; 6:341–342

60. Bergh P, Kindblom LG, Gunterberg B et al. Prognostic factors in chordoma of the sacrum and mobile spine: a study of 39 patients. Cancer, 2000; 88:2122–2134

61. Chambers PW, Schwinn CP. Chordoma. A clinicopathologic study of metastasis. Am J Clin Pathol, 1979; 72:765–776

62. Fischbein NJ, Kaplan MJ, Holliday RA et al. Recurrence of clival chordoma along the surgical pathway. Am J Neuroradiol, 2000; 21:578–583

63. Mitchell A, Scheithauer BW, Unni KK et al. Chordoma and chondroid neoplasms of the spheno-occiput. An immunohistochemical study of 41 cases with prognostic and nosologic implications. Cancer, 1993; 72:2943–2949

Other bone lesions

64. Posnick JC. Fibrous dysplasia of the craniomaxillofacial region: current clinical perspectives. Br J Oral Maxillofac Surg, 1998; 36:264–273

65. Mohammadi-Araghi H, Haery C. Fibro-osseous lesions of craniofacial bones. The role of imaging. Radiol Clin North Am, 1993; 31:121–153

66. Haddad GF, Hambali F, Mufarrij A et al. Concomitant fibrous dysplasia and aneurysmal bone cyst of the skull base. Case report and review of the literature. Pediatr Neurosurg, 1998; 28:147–153

67. Slootweg PJ. Maxillofacial fibro-osseous lesions: classification and differential diagnosis. Semin Diagn Pathol, 1996; 13:104–112

68. O'Brien DP, Rashad EM, Toland JA et al. Aneurysmal cyst of the frontal bone: case report and review of the literature. Br J Neurosurg; 1994; 8:105–108

69. Wojno KJ, McCarthy EF. Fibro-osseous lesions of the face and skull with aneurysmal bone cyst formation. Skeletal Radio, 1994; 23:15–18

70. Clavier E, Thiebot J, Godlewski J et al. Intracranial aneurysmal bone cyst: a rare CT appearance. Neuroradiology; 1988; 30:269–271

71. Ameli NO, Abbassioun K, Azod A et al. Aneurysmal bone cyst of the skull. Can J Neurol Sci, 1984; 11:466–471

72. Capanna R, Albisinni U, Picci P et al. Aneurysmal bone cyst of the spine. J Bone Joint Surg Am, 1985; 67:527–531

73. de Kleuver M, van der Heul RO, Veraart BE. Aneurysmal bone cyst of the spine: 31 cases and the importance of the surgical approach. J Pediatr Orthop B, 1998; 7:286–292

74. Sanerkin NG, Mott MG, Roylance J. An unusal intraosseous lesion with fibroblastic, osteoclastic, osteoblastic, aneurysmal and fibromyxoid elements. Solid variant of aneurysmal bone cyst. Cancer, 1983; 51:2278–2286

75. Bertoni F, Unni KK, Beabout JW et al. Chondroblastoma of the skull and facial bones. Am J Clin Pathol, 1987; 88:1–9

76. Whitehead RE, Melhem ER, Kasznica J et al. Telangiectatic osteosarcoma of the skull base. Am J Neuroradiol, 1998; 19:754–757

77. Roodman GD. Paget's disease and osteoclast biology. Bone, 1996; 19:209–212

78. Mirra JM, Brien EW, Tehranzadeh J. Paget's disease of bone: review with emphasis on radiologic features. II. Skeletal Radiol, 1995; 24:173–184

79. Gallacher SJ. Paget's disease of bone. Curr Opin Rheumatol, 1993; 5:351–356

80. Jattiot F, Goupille P, Azais I et al. Fourteen cases of sarcomatous degeneration in Paget's disease. J Rheumatol, 1999; 26:150–155

81. Howarth DM, Gilchrist GS, Mullan BP et al. Langerhans cell histiocytosis: diagnosis, natural history, management, and outcome. Cancer, 1999; 85:2278–2290

82. Veyssier-Belot C, Cacoub P, Caparros-Lefebvre D et al. Erdheim–Chester disease. Clinical and radiologic characteristics of 59 cases. Medicine, 1996; 75:157–169

83. Kenn W, Eck M, Allolio B et al. Erdheim–Chester disease: evidence for a disease entity different from Langerhans cell histiocytosis? Three cases with detailed radiological and immunohistochemical analysis. Hum Pathol, 2000; 31:734–739

84. Wenger DC, Wold LC. Benign vascular lesions of bone: radiologic and pathologic features. Skeletal Radiol 2000; 29:63–74

85. Tucker WS, Nasser-Sharif FJ. Benign skull lesions. Can J Surg, 1997; 40:449–455

86. Noterman J, Massager N, Vloeberghs M et al. Monstrous skull osteomas in a probable Gardner's syndrome: case report. Surg Neurol, 1998; 49:302–304

87. Haddad FS, Haddad GF, Zaatari G. Cranial osteomas: their classification and management. Report on a giant osteoma and review of the literature. Surg Neurol, 1997; 48:143–147

Chondrosarcoma

88. Batsakis JG, Solomon AR, Rice DH. The pathology of head and neck tumors: neoplasms of cartilage, bone, and the notochord, part 7. Head Neck Surg, 1980; 3:43–57

89. Korten AG, ter Berg HJ, Spincemaille GH et al. Intracranial chondrosarcoma: review of the literature and report of 15 cases. J Neurol Neurosurg Psychiatry, 1998; 65:88–92

90. Inwards CY, Unni KK. Classification and grading of bone sarcomas. Hematol Oncol Clin North Am, 1995; 9:545–569

91. Rosenberg AE, Nielsen GP, Keel SB et al. Chondrosarcoma of the base of the skull: a clinicopathologic study of 200 cases with emphasis on its distinction from chordoma. Am J Surg Pathol, 1999; 23:1370–1378

92. Gadwal SR, Fanburg-Smith JC, Gannon FH et al. Primary chondrosarcoma of the head and neck in pediatric patients: a clinicopathologic study of 14 cases with a review of the literature. Cancer, 2000; 88:2181–2188

93. Meis JM. Dedifferentiation in bone and soft-tissue tumours. A histological indicator of tumor progression. Pathol Ann, 1991; 26 Part 1:37–62

94. Ramina R, Coelho Neto M, Meneses MS et al. Maffucci's syndrome associated with a cranial base chondrosarcoma: case report and literature review. Neurosurgery, 1997; 41:269–272

Uncommon bony lesions

95. Kaya S, Unal OF, Sarac S et al. Melanotic neuroectodermal tumour of infancy: report of two cases and review of literature. Int J Pediatr Otorhinolaryngol, 2000; 52:169–172

96. Caird J, McDermott M, Farrell M. 5 month old boy with occipital bone mass. Brain Pathol, 2000; 10:317–319

97. Rickert CH, Probst-Cousin S, Blasius S et al. Melanotic progonoma of the brain: a case report and review. Childs Nerv Syst, 1998; 14:389–393

98. el-Saggan A, Bang G, Olofsson J. Melanotic neuroectodermal tumour of infancy arising in the maxilla. J Laryngol Otol, 1998; 112:61–64

99. Nitta T, Endo T, Tsunoda A et al. Melanotic neuroectodermal tumor of infancy: a molecular approach to diagnosis. Case report. J Neurosurg, 1995; 83:145–148

100. Ghogawala Z, Moore M, Strand R et al. Clival chondroma in a child with Ollier's disease. Case report. Pediatr Neurosurg, 1991; 17:53–56

101. Terasaka S, Sawamura Y, Abe H. Surgical removal of a cavernous sinus chondroma. Surg Neurol, 1997; 48:153–159

102. Matz S, Israeli Y, Shalit MN et al. Computed tomography in intracranial supratentorial osteochondroma. J Comput Assist Tomogr, 1981; 5:109–115

103. Haddad GF, Haddad FS, Zaatari G. Dural osteochondroma: case report, review of the literature and proposal of a new classification. Br J Neurosurg, 1998; 12:380–384

104. Sato K, Kodera T, Kitai R et al. Osteochondroma of the skull base: MRI and histological correlation. Neuroradiology, 1996; 38:41–43

105. Beck DW, Dyste GN. Intracranial osteochondroma: MR and CT appearance. Am J Neuroradiol, 1989; 10:S7–8

106. Cervoni L, Innocenzi G, Raguso M et al. Osteoblastoma of the calvaria: report of two cases diagnosed with MRI and clinical review. Neurosurg Rev, 1997; 20:51–54

107. Slootweg PJ. Maxillofacial fibro-osseous lesions: classification and differential diagnosis. Semin Diagn Pathol, 1996; 13:104–112

108. Goel A, Bhayani R, Nagpal RD. Massive benign osteoblastoma of the clivus and atlas. Br J Neurosurg, 1994; 8:483–486

109. Aziz TZ, Neal JW, Cole G. Malignant osteoblastoma of the skull. Br J Neurosurg, 1993; 7:423–426

110. Figarella-Branger D, Perez-Castillo M, Garbe L et al. Malignant transformation of an osteoblastoma of the skull: an exceptional occurrence. Case report. Neurosurg, 1991; 75:138–142

111. Adler M, Hnatuk L, Mock D et al. Aggressive osteoblastoma of the temporal bone: a case report. J Otolaryngol, 1990; 19:307–310

112. Kroon HM, Schurmans J. Osteoblastoma: clinical and radiologic findings in 98 new cases. Radiology, 1990; 175:783–790

113. Brien EW, Mirra JM, Ippolito V. Chondroblastoma arising from a nonepiphyseal site. Skeletal Radiol, 1995; 24:220–222

114. Leong HK, Chong PY, Sinniah R. Temporal bone chondroblastoma: big and small. J Laryngol Otol, 1994; 108:1115–1119

115. Muntane A, Valls C, Angeles de Miquel MA et al. Chondroblastoma of the temporal bone: CT and MR appearance. AJNR Am J Neuroradiol, 1993; 14:70–71

116. Varvares MA, Cheney ML, Goodman ML et al. Chondroblastoma of the temporal bone. Case report and literature review. Ann Otol Rhinol Laryngol, 1992; 101:763–769

117. Horn KL, Hankinson H, Nagel B et al. Surgical management of chondroblastoma of the temporal bone. Otolaryngol Head Neck Surg, 1990; 102:264–269

118. Kurt AM, Unni KK, Sim FH et al. Chondroblastoma of bone. Hum Pathol, 1989; 20:965–976

119. Wolf DA, Chaljub G, Maggio W et al. Intracranial chondromyxoid fibroma. Report of a case and review of the literature. Arch Pathol Lab Med, 1997; 121:626–630

120. Commins DJ, Tolley NS, Milford CA. Fibrous dysplasia and ossifying fibroma of the paranasal sinuses. J Laryngol Otol, 1998; 112:964–968

121. Slootweg PJ. Maxillofacial fibro-osseous lesions: classification and differential diagnosis. Semin Diagn Pathol, 1996; 13:104–112

122. Marvel JB, Marsh MA, Catlin FI. Ossifying fibroma of the mid-face and paranasal sinuses: diagnostic and therapeutic considerations. Otolaryngol Head Neck Surg, 1991; 104:803–808

123. Zappia JJ, LaRouere MJ, Telian SA. Massive ossifying fibroma of the temporal bone. Otolaryngol Head Neck Surg, 1990; 103:480–483

124. Daw NC, Mahmoud HH, Meyer WH et al. Bone sarcomas of the head and neck in children: the St Jude Children's Research Hospital experience. Cancer, 2000; 88:2172–2180

125. Unni KK. Osteosarcoma of bone. J Orthop Sci, 1998; 3:287–294

126. Shinoda J, Kimura T, Funakoshi T et al. Primary osteosarcoma of the skull – a case report and review of the literature. J Neurooncol,1993; 17:81–88

127. Salvati M, Ciappetta P, Raco A. Osteosarcomas of the skull. Clinical remarks on 19 cases. Cancer, 1993; 71:2210–2216

128. Mark RJ, Sercarz JA, Tran L et al. Osteogenic sarcoma of the head and neck. The UCLA experience. Arch Otolaryngol Head Neck Surg, 1991; 117:761–766

129. Dreghorn CR, Newman RJ, Hardy GJ et al. Primary tumors of the axial skeleton. Experience of the Leeds Regional Bone Tumor Registry. Spine, 1990; 15:137–140

130. Rosenbloom JS, Storper IS, Aviv JE et al. Giant cell tumors of the jugular foramen. Am J Otolaryngol, 1999; 20:176–179

131. Bertoni F, Unni KK, Beabout JW et al. Giant cell tumor of the skull. Cancer, 1992; 70:1124–1132

132. Henderson BT, Whitwell H. Giant cell tumor of the skull: case report. Neurosurgery, 1988; 23:120–122

Ear, temporal bone and orbital tumours

133. MacArthur CJ, McGill TJ, Healy GB. Pediatric head and neck rhabdomyosarcoma. Clin Pediatr, 1992; 31:66–70

134. Said H, Phang KS, Razi A et al. Rhabdomyosarcoma of the middle ear and mastoid in children. J Laryngol Otol, 1998; 102:614–619

135. Wiatrak BJ, Pensak ML. Rhabdomyosarcoma of the ear and temporal bone. Laryngoscope, 1989; 99:1188–1192

136. Clark LJ, Narula AA, Morgan DA et al. Squamous carcinoma of the temporal bone: a revised staging. J Laryngol Otol, 1991; 105:346–348

137. Koriwchak M. Temporal bone cancer. Am J Otol, 1993; 14:623–626

138. Zhang B, Tu G, Xu G et al. Squamous cell carcinoma of temporal bone: reported on 33 patients. Head Neck, 1994; 21:461–466

139. Heffner DK. Low-grade adenocarcinoma of probable endolymphatic sac origin. A clinicopathologic study of 20 cases. Cancer, 1989; 64:2292–2302

140. Asano K, Sekiya T, Hatayama T et al. A case of endolymphatic sac tumor with long-term survival. Brain Tumor Pathol, 1999; 16:69–76

141. Poe DS, Tarlov EC, Thomas CB et al. Aggressive papillary tumors of temporal bone. Otolaryngol Head Neck Surg, 1993; 108:80–86

142. Reijneveld J, Hanlo P, Groenewoud G et al. Endolymphatic sac tumor: a case report and review of the literature. Surg Neurol, 1997; 48:368–373

143. Brunori A, Scarano P, Iannetti G et al. Dumbbell tumor of the anterior skull base. Meningioma? No, adenoid cystic carcinoma! Surg Neurol, 1998; 50:470–474

144. Gormley WB, Sekhar LN, Wright DC et al. Management and long-term outcome of adenoid cystic carcinoma with intracranial extension: a neurosurgical perspective. Neurosurgery, 1996; 38:1105–1112

Nose and paranasal sinus tumours

145. Meneses MS, Thurel C, Mikol J et al. Esthesioneuroblastoma with intracranial extension. Neurosurgery, 1990; 27:813–819; discussion 9–20

146. Ng HK, Poon WS, Poon CY et al. Intracranial olfactory neuroblastoma mimicking carcinoma: report of two cases. Histopathology, 1988; 12:393–403

147. Hirose T, Scheithauer BW, Lopes MB et al. Olfactory neuroblastoma. An immunohistochemical, ultrastructural, and flow cytometric study. Cancer, 1995; 76:4–19

148. Frierson HFJ, Ross GW, Mills SE et al. Olfactory neuroblastoma. Additional immunohistochemical characterization. Am J Clin Pathol, 1990; 94:547–553

149. Devaney K, Wenig BM, Abbondanzo SL. Olfactory neuroblastoma and other round cell lesions of the sinonasal region. Mod Pathol, 1996; 9:658–663

150. Argani P, Perez-Ordonez B, Xiao H et al. Olfactory neuroblastoma is not related to the Ewing family of tumors: absence of EWS/FLI1 gene fusion and MIC2 expression. Am J Surg Pathol, 1998; 22:391–398

151. Sorensen PH, Wu JK, Berean KW et al. Olfactory neuroblastoma is a peripheral primitive neuroectodermal tumor related to Ewing sarcoma. Proc Nat Acad Sci U S A, 1996; 93:1038–1043

152. Perez-Ordonez B, Caruana SM, Huvos AG et al. Small cell neuroendocrine carcinoma of the nasal cavity and paranasal sinuses. Hum Pathol, 1998; 29:826–832

153. Mills SE, Fechner RE. Undifferentiated neoplasms of the sinonasal region: differential diagnosis based on clinical, light microscopic, immunohistochemical, and ultrastructural features. Semin Diagn Pathol, 1989; 6:316–328

154. Pai SA, Naresh KN, Masih K et al. Teratocarcinosarcoma of the paranasal sinuses: a clinicopathologic and immunohistochemical study. Hum Pathol, 1998; 29:718–722

155. Kleinschmidt-DeMasters BK, Pflaumer SM, Mulgrew TD et al. Sinonasal teratocarcinosarcoma (mixed olfactory neuroblastoma-craniopharyngioma) presenting with syndrome of inappropriate secretion of antidiuretic hormone. Clin Neuropathol, 2000; 19):63–69

156. Naresh KN, Pai SA. Foci resembling olfactory neuroblastoma and craniopharyngioma are seen in sinonasal teratocarcinosarcomas. Histopathology, 1998; 32:84

157. Chang KC, Jin YT, Chen RM et al. Mixed olfactory neuroblastoma and craniopharyngioma: an unusual pathological finding. Histopathology, 1997; 30:378–382

158. Wenig BM. Nasopharyngeal carcinoma. Ann Diagn Pathol, 1999; 3:374–385

159. Houston GD, Gillies E. Sinonasal undifferentiated carcinoma: a distinctive clinicopathologic entity. Adv Anat Pathol, 1999; 6:317–323

160. Naficy S, Disher MJ, Esclamado RM. Adenoid cystic carcinoma of the paranasal sinuses. Am J Rhinol, 1999; 13:311–314

161. Cantu G, Solero CL, Mariani L et al. A new classification for malignant tumors involving the anterior skull base. Arch Otolaryngol Head Neck Surg, 1999; 125:1252–1257

162. Herman P, Lot G, Chapot R et al. Long-term follow-up of juvenile nasopharyngeal angiofibromas: analysis of recurrences. Laryngoscope, 1999; 109:140–147

163. Radkowski D, McGill T, Healy GB et al. Angiofibroma. Changes in staging and treatment. Arch Otolaryngol Head Neck Surg; 122:122–129

164. Tewfik TL, Tan AK, al Noury K et al. Juvenile nasopharyngeal angiofibroma. J Otolaryngol, 1999; 28:145–151

Ewing's tumour and hamartomas

165. Thorner PS, Squire JA. Molecular genetics in the diagnosis and prognosis of solid pediatric tumors. Pediatr Dev Pathol, 1998; 1:337–365

166. Kovar H. Ewing's sarcoma and peripheral primitive neuroectodermal tumors after their genetic union. Curr Opin Oncol, 1998; 10:334–342

167. Terrier P, Llombart-Bosch A, Contesso G. Small round blue cell tumors in bone: prognostic factors correlated to Ewing's sarcoma and neuroectodermal tumors. Semin Diagn Pathol, 1996; 13:250–257

168. Llombart-Bosch A, Contesso G, Peydro-Olaya A. Histology, immunohistochemistry, and electron microscopy of small round cell tumors of bone. Semin Diagn Pathol, 1996; 13:153–170

169. Dehner LP. Peripheral and central primitive neuroectodermal tumors. A nosologic concept seeking a consensus. Arch Pathol Lab Med, 1986; 110:997–1005

170. Morris GF, Murphy K, Rorke LB et al. Spinal hamartomas: a distinct clinical entity. J Neurosurg, 1998; 88:954–957

19 Dysgenetic syndromes

Dysgenetic syndromes may be defined as inherited malformative diseases which arise early in fetal life but show progression after postnatal body growth has ceased.[1] This definition embraces a wide variety of congenital multisystem disorders, not all necessarily affecting the nervous system, but those which are usually associated with neural manifestations are listed in Table 19.1. Some of the syndromes also involve the skin or neural crest-derived tissues, and this is reflected in the use of alternative terms such as phakomatosis and neurocristopathy in some of the older literature.[2,3]

The chromosomal abnormalities underlying individual dysgenetic syndromes have been the subject of intensive research activity in recent years, and in many instances there is now quite detailed understanding of the mechanisms involved in the development of their characteristic pathological lesions. In most of the tumour syndromes, for example, the affected gene normally acts as a tumour suppressor, its encoded protein down-regulating growth promotion. Examples include the genes responsible for tuberous sclerosis, both types of neurofibromatosis and von Hippel–Lindau (VHL) syndrome. In these conditions and possibly others, the continuing development of lesions into adult life can be explained by a 'two-hit' mechanism, in which inactivation of both copies of the gene is necessary for tumour formation: one allele is affected on an hereditary (i.e. germline) basis, whilst random 'second-hit' somatic mutations occurring postnatally at the same locus lead to the development of neoplasia.

Table 19.1 Dysgenetic syndromes with nervous system manifestations

	Synonyms	Chromosome locus	Gene name	Encoded protein
Tuberous sclerosis	Bourneville's disease	9q34	*TSC1*	Hamartin
		16p13	*TSC2*	Tuberin
Neurofibromatosis				
(i) Type 1	Von Recklinghausen's disease Peripheral neurofibromatosis	17q11	*NF1*	Neurofibromin
(ii) Type 2	Bilateral acoustic neurofibromatosis Central neurofibromatosis	22q12	*NF2*	Merlin (schwannomin)
von Hippel–Lindau disease	Lindau disease	3p25	*VHL*	VHL protein
Li–Fraumeni syndrome		17p13	*TP53*	p53 protein
		22q12	*hCKH2*	Checkpoint kinase 2
Turcot syndrome		5q21	*APC*	APC protein
Hereditary non-polyposis colorectal cancer syndrome		2p16, 2q31, 3p22, 7p22	DNA mismatch repair genes	DNA mismatch repair proteins
Gorlin syndrome	Naevoid basal cell carcinoma syndrome	9q31	*PTCH*	Patched transmembrane protein
Cowden syndrome	Multiple hamartoma and neoplasia syndrome	10q23	*PTEN*	Unknown
Neurocutaneous melanosis	Neurocutaneous melanomatosis	Unknown		Unknown
Angiomatous syndromes Sturge–Weber disease	Encephalotrigeminal angiomatosis	Unknown		Unknown
Hereditary haemorrhagic telangiectasia	Rendu–Osler–Weber disease	9q33	*HHT1*	Endoglin
		12q1	*HHT2*	Activin receptor-like kinase
Ataxia telangiectasia	Louis–Bar syndrome	11q22	*ATM*	ATM protein
Mesencephalo-oculo-facial angiomatosis	Wyburn-Mason syndrome Bonnet–Dechaume–Blanc syndrome Retinocephalic angiomatosis	Unknown		Unknown
Cutaneospinal angiomatosis Multiple cavernous angiomas	Cobb syndrome	Unknown 7q11 7p 3q	*CCM1*	Unknown KRIT 1 unknown unknown

An interesting paradox is raised by well documented accounts of individual patients with the combined clinical features of more than one syndrome.[4] Reported examples include patients with combined manifestations of Sturge–Weber syndrome and neurocutaneous melanosis,[5,6] and others with clinical features of both neurofibromatosis and either neurocutaneous melanosis[7] or VHL.[3,8] In some cases this may be explained by overlap in the spectrum of possible phenotypic manifestation resulting from a given gene defect. However, more than one entirely typical dysgenetic syndrome can also coexist in separate individuals of a single family,[8,9] suggesting that different gene mutations may occasionally segregate coincidentally within the same pedigree.[10]

Tuberous sclerosis

Tuberous sclerosis was initially characterised as a multisystem disorder by Bourneville in 1880,[11] although several years previously von Recklinghausen had described an affected patient with multiple cardiac rhabdomyomas.[12] The condition is sometimes referred to as Bourneville's disease and the term 'epiloia' has also been used in older literature.[13]

Incidence and genetics

The true prevalence of tuberous sclerosis is rather uncertain because mild and subclinical forms may often escape recognition,[14,15] but more recent surveys with the benefit of modern imaging techniques have indicated that the figure may exceed 1 in 30 000.[14,16] The condition is most often recognised in early life and the prevalence in children less than 10 years old has been estimated as 1 in 12 000.[16] It is also more often found in mentally retarded individuals, especially those suffering from epilepsy, and about 0.5% of patients in residential institutions for the intellectually subnormal are said to be affected.[17,18] There is no significant predilection for one or other sex.[19]

Tuberous sclerosis is inherited in an autosomal dominant pattern but with a high spontaneous mutation rate.[20,21] New gene mutations probably account for 60–70% of all cases, explaining why newly diagnosed cases often have no family history of the disease.[16,22] The high mutation rate also means that the risk of unaffected parents bearing a second affected child is much lower than might otherwise be expected.[15] There is a very high penetrance in inherited cases,[23,24] and examples where the disease has skipped a generation are rare.[25] The disorder is genetically heterogeneous, with two separate gene loci definitely identified so far.[26,27] In approximately one-third of affected pedigrees the mutant gene lies on chromosome 9q34 and is referred to as *TSC 1*.[27,28] Most of the remaining families examined have shown mutation of the *TSC 2* gene on chromosome 16p13,[29] but there are isolated reports of pedigrees linking to other chromosomes and the existence of a third locus has not been entirely excluded.[26,27]

Aetiology

Recent genetic studies have indicated that both *TSC 1* and *TSC 2* are growth suppressors.[30,31] The *TSC 2* gene on chromosome 16p13 encodes for the protein tuberin which is normally present in brain, cardiac and renal tissues.[30,32] Tuberin shows sequence homology with a guanosine triphosphate (GTP)-ase activating protein responsible for downregulating the *Rap 1* oncogene.[20] The *TSC 1* gene on chromosome 9q34 encodes a more recently identified protein called hamartin.[33] The function of hamartin is not yet fully defined, but it is also thought to be involved in the suppression of tissue growth.[31] Both proteins can be demonstrated immunocytochemically in the atypical giant cells of cortical tubers from tuberous sclerosis patients, regardless of which germline mutation is present, and are sometimes co-localised in the same cell.[34] Perhaps more predictably, loss of the appropriate allele has been found in several subependymal giant cell astrocytomas and a variety of hamartomas in individuals with each genetic type of the condition.[31,35] Development of the lesions is thought to follow a 'two-hit' mechanism, with isolated somatic mutations ('second-hit') occurring at the same loci as the inherited defect.[36]

In terms of development, the nervous system hamartomas are thought to result from a failure of cell migration and differentiation dating from an early stage of embryogenesis.[37,38] The disturbed neuronal architecture of cortical tubers is probably due to faulty migration of neuroblasts from the germinal matrix zone,[37,39] and this mechanism is also likely to account for the radially dispersed pattern of the white matter heterotopia.[13] An abnormal astrocytic component is found in all the different nervous system lesions and is perhaps caused by faulty transformation of the embryonic radial glia, or disturbances in the proliferation and differentiation of their progeny.[37] The origin of the giant cells present in most of the hamartomas is more controversial, but they appear to represent a heterogeneous population of abnormally developed cells which are pluripotential in terms of their neuronal and glial differentiating capacity.[40] Ultrastructural studies have mostly found evidence of astrocytic lineage in giant cells of both tubers and subependymal nodules,[41,42] but in some cases ganglionic features have also been reported.[43] Immunocytochemically, the giant cells may express glial fibrillary acidic protein (GFAP) or neuron specific enolase (NSE), but there are differences depending on their location. A majority of giant cells in subependymal nodules and white matter heterotopia express GFAP with only occasional examples immunostaining for NSE, whilst the opposite situation is found in cortical tubers.[44]

Clinical features

The classic triad of clinical features in severely affected cases of tuberous sclerosis consists of mental retardation, epilepsy and cutaneous manifestations.[13,19] Skin lesions are said to be present in up to 90% of cases and most often take the form of facial angiofibromas (adenoma sebaceum). Intellectual retardation is a less consistent feature than originally thought, but is the presenting clinical finding in 40–60% of cases and is usually progressive.[9,45] Epilepsy becomes more common with increasing age,[45] but in some individuals fits start in early infancy and are the earliest manifestation of the disease.[13] Depending on the age of the cohort, epilepsy has been found in 60–90% of cases[19,45] and more often occurs in individuals who are mentally retarded.[13,46] The electroencephalogram (EEG) is said to be abnormal in 85% of cases but there are no specific features and the changes are mostly of epileptiform type.[47] Focal neurological deficits are uncommon even in the presence of widespread central nervous system abnormalities, although in some cases obstruction of the foramen of Monro by subependymal nodules or giant cell astrocytomas leads to an acute clinical presentation with signs and symptoms of raised intracranial pressure.[13,48]

There is a considerable range of clinical and pathological expression in tuberous sclerosis and oligosymptomatic forms of the disease or 'formes frustes' are becoming increasingly well documented.[20,24] Phenotypic variation may occur both between and within affected families and the complete syndrome of retardation and epilepsy with nervous system, skin, eye and visceral lesions is rarely found in two consecutive generations.[20] Mildly affected cases with a known family history but normal intelligence may present with either skin changes, cardiac rhabdomyomas or pulmonary lesions as the sole manifestation of the disorder.[49,50] Modern imaging has also revealed central nervous system hamartomas in clinically normal patients,[15] and asymptomatic adult cases of tuberous sclerosis without fits or mental retardation may often pass entirely unnoticed.[51,52] In addition, phenotypic expression varies with the age of affected individuals, such that cardiac hamartomas usually manifest in early infancy, skin and central nervous system changes in childhood or adolescence, and renal or pulmonary lesions in adult life.[24] Currently accepted diagnostic criteria for tuberous sclerosis are summarised in Table 19.2, and are based on the pathological changes found in different tissues.[15,24]

Pathology

Systematic manifestations

Skin lesions[53,54] Facial angiofibromas, originally termed 'adenoma sebaceum', are the most common cutaneous manifestation of tuberous sclerosis. They are shiny, pinkish

Table 19.2 Tuberous sclerosis – clinical significance of pathological lesions

Definitive lesions (Diagnostic in isolation)	Presumptive lesions (Diagnostic if combined with a positive family history)	Suspicious lesions (Not diagnostic unless combined with other lesions)
Cortical tubers	Subependymal giant cell astrocytoma	Hypopigmented macules
Subependymal nodules	Solitary renal angiomyolipoma	Solitary cardiac rhabdomyoma
Facial angiofibromas	Solitary retinal hamartoma	Non-renal angiomyolipoma
Multiple renal angiomyolipomas	Multiple cardiac rhabdomyomas	
Multiple retinal hamartomas	Pulmonary myomatosis	
Ungual fibromas	Shagreen patch	

papules which progressively increase during childhood and are usually found in the nasolabial folds or over the chin, cheeks and forehead. Histologically they consist of hamartomatous masses of collagen fibres and dilated capillaries. Sebaceous glands are often entrapped in the abnormal tissue and in older lesions there may be a secondary sebaceous hyperplasia. Other typical skin changes include hypopigmented leaf-shaped macules, periungual fibromas (Koenen's tumours) and irregular areas of dermal sclerosis usually referred to as 'shagreen patches'. Skin lesions less specifically associated with tuberous sclerosis are fibrous nodules of the oral mucous membranes, multiple skin tags and café-au-lait spots.

Visceral lesions Renal hamartomas are the most frequently occurring visceral manifestation of tuberous sclerosis and are normally detected during adult life.[55,56] They typically consist of nodular masses of smooth muscle, fat and capillaries, and are sometimes termed 'angiomyolipomas'.[55] They are usually multiple and bilateral and occasionally cause serious haemorrhage or progressive renal failure.[55,56] Multicystic disease may also be present[55] but renal carcinoma and other malignancies are uncommon.[57] Cardiac rhabdomyomas are found in a quarter to half of all childhood cases but are much less commonly seen in patients surviving into adulthood.[54,58] They consist of hamartomatous masses of abnormal giant cells resembling the Purkinje cells of the cardiac conducting system.[49,55] The lesions are often multiple and may cause dysrhythmias or cardiac failure.[55] Diffuse pulmonary myomatosis occurs in less than 10% of cases and presents almost exclusively in adult females with progressive respiratory failure.[59,60] Other manifestations of tuberous sclerosis are often sparse in these patients and may be entirely absent.[59] The lungs undergo multicystic change with a diffuse overgrowth of connective tissue, smooth muscle and capillary vessels.[55,59] Other systemic lesions sometimes associated with tuberous sclerosis include myomatous hamartomas of the liver, bowel and ovary,[55,61] fibrous lytic lesions of small limb bones[13] and adenomas of the pancreas, thyroid and adrenal glands.[55]

Central nervous system manifestations

Hamartomas

Cortical tubers Tubers are focal hamartomas of cortical grey matter which represent one of the most characteristic and fundamental lesions of the tuberous sclerosis complex. Although varying greatly in number, they are usually multiple and bilateral, most typically involving frontal and parietal areas of cerebral cortex.[13] In some cases, the cerebellar cortex may also be affected.[62,63] Using computerised tomography (CT), tubers are rather poorly visualised as non-enhancing, hypodense areas, and are often not apparent at all unless calcified.[64,65] Magnetic resonance (MR) scans, however, are more sensitive at detecting tubers, which appear as high signal areas using T2-weighted sequences.[66,67] A high proportion of suspected or presumptive cases of tuberous sclerosis can be shown to have cortical tubers using MR scanning, and it has thus proved an effective screening procedure for the condition.[15,68]

At autopsy, affected brains are usually of normal size and weight, and with careful examination the tubers are visible externally as pale, firm areas of focally expanded gyrus (Fig. 19.1). They are slightly raised above the adjacent pial surface and sometimes show a central dimple-like depression. They usually involve the crowns of gyri and are separated by the lines of sulci from neighbouring, unaffected convolutions. On coronal slices, tubers appear as abnormally pale areas of widened gyrus which blend indistinctly with the surrounding cortex and white matter.

Histologically, affected areas of cortex show a disorganised architecture and loss of the normal laminar pattern. Remaining neurones are reduced in number and appear randomly orientated. They often show regressive changes, including vacuolation and increased lipofuscin. There is a generalised increase in astrocytic cells and the background neuropil shows diffuse gliosis with loss of intracortical myelinated fibres. The glial fibres are often condensed in the subpial region, especially in older patients, where they frequently form radially orientated, tuft-like bundles.[13] With increasing age, the lesions may also undergo focal calcification and cystic change. The most striking feature of tubers is the presence of atypical giant cells of varied and bizzare morphology (Fig.19.2). These vary greatly in number between lesions and may be isolated or grouped together in clusters. They typically have round, clear nuclei with prominent nucleoli, abundant cytoplasm and coarse cytoplasmic processes of variable

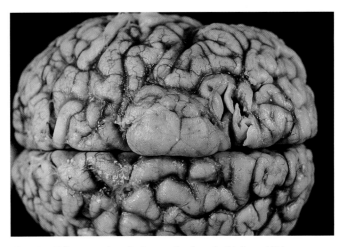

Fig. 19.1 **Tuberous sclerosis.** Parasagittal cortical tuber, visible as a circumscribed area of expanded gyrus, slightly raised above the surrounding convolutions.

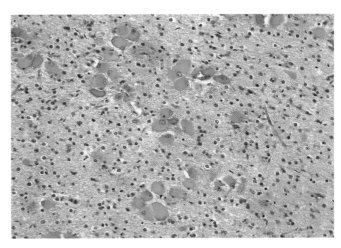

Fig. 19.2 **Tuberous sclerosis.** Cortical tuber. Atypical giant cells are set in a gliotic background containing numerous smaller astrocytic cells. H & E.

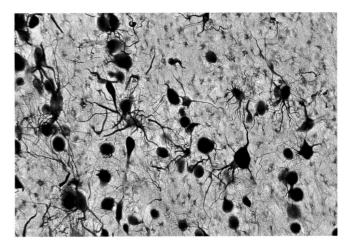

Fig. 19.3 **Tuberous sclerosis.** The giant cells of cortical tubers have an affinity for several different types of heavy metal impregnation. Cajal's gold sublimate stain.

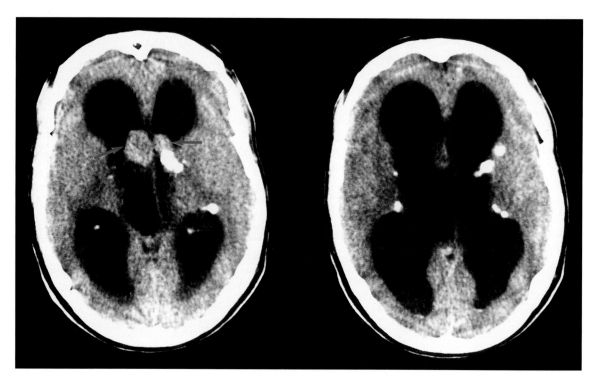

Fig. 19.4 **Tuberous sclerosis.** Non-enhanced computerised tomograms, showing multiple small subependymal nodules at both levels illustrated. Their bright signal is due to calcification. Subependymal giant cell astrocytomas are also visible in the left hand image (arrows), obstructing the foramina of Monro and causing hydrocephalus. These two tumours enhanced after administration of contrast medium.

configuration. Multinucleated examples are common, but mitoses do not occur. The giant cells in tubers have an affinity for heavy metal impregnations and frequently stain with both neuronal silver techniques such as Bielschowsky's stain and with Cajal's gold sublimate technique for astrocytes (Fig.19.3). Using immunocytochemistry, some stain intensely with antibodies to neuronal antigens, especially neuron specific enolase, whilst others appear to be unequivocally astrocytic in nature and express only GFAP.

In patients presenting purely with epilepsy, apparently solitary tubers are sometimes mistaken for tumours and surgically biopsied or excised before a diagnosis of tuberous sclerosis is suspected. For the pathologist, the differential diagnosis in this situation must include both focal cortical dysplasia and low grade ganglionic neoplasms. Areas of sporadic cortical dysplasia are not usually so well defined as tubers but may nevertheless show a similar disturbance of cortical architecture. In distinction, however, there is rarely such a prominent astrocytic gliosis and the bizzare atypical giant cells of tubers are not a feature. Similar cells may be seen in some gangliogliomas/ganglioneuromas, but the background stroma tends to be much more persuasive of an astrocytic neoplasm than gliotic cortical grey matter. In either case, it is obviously going to be important to make a careful check for other clinical stigmata of the syndrome or subtle radiological evidence of multiple lesions.

Radial white matter heterotopia Cortical tubers have ill-defined deep margins, and small groups of heterotopic neurons mixed with atypical, tuber-like giant cells are frequently present in the underlying white matter. These heterotopic foci are usually associated with focal loss of myelinated fibres and gliosis. They are typically distributed in a radial pattern between the ventricular surface and the overlying abnormal cortex, suggesting that they may lie along the migratory path of embryonic germinal matrix cells.[13,14]

Subependymal nodules These are said to be present in up to 80% of all tuberous sclerosis cases[65] and are usually clearly defined by CT due to calcification[69,70] (Fig.19.4). Unlike the subependymal giant cell astrocytomas occurring in similar locations, subependymal nodules do not enhance on CT scans after administration of contrast media.[64,71] They are less consistently detected by MR imaging and show a variable signal intensity depending on the extent of calcification.

Macroscopically, subependymal nodules are visible on coronally sliced autopsy brains as smooth white excrescences bulging from under the ventricular lining into the ventricular cavities. They typically have an elongated profile and have often been likened to congealed wax drippings on a candle, so-called 'candle-

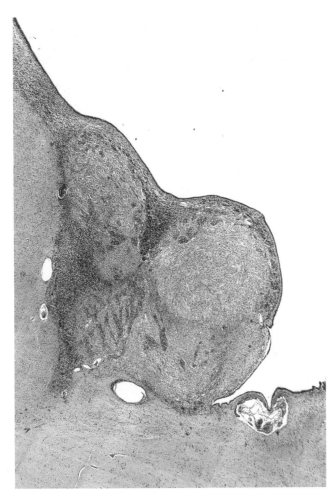

Fig. 19.5 **Tuberous sclerosis.** Subependymal nodules projecting into a lateral ventricle from the thalamostriate groove. This example comes from a neonate and darker areas of persisting germinal matrix are visible around the nodules. H & E.

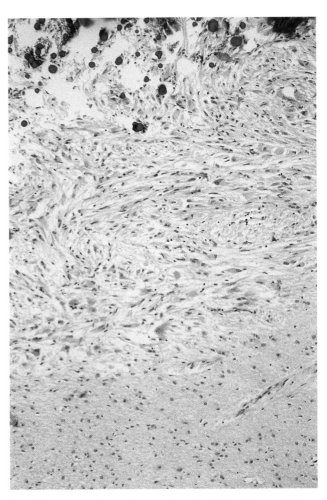

Fig. 19.6 **Tuberous sclerosis.** Subependymal nodule. At the periphery, the nodules consist of elongate, pilocytic-type astrocytes which merge with the adjacent brain (bottom). The central areas are often calcified (top). H & E.

gutterings'. They are often difficult to cut because of dense calcification. Subependymal nodules are nearly always multiple and vary in size from a few millimetres to several centimetres across. They may occur anywhere in the ventricular system but are most numerous in the lateral ventricles near the foramina of Monro, especially over the head of the caudate nucleus and in the thalamostriate groove[13] (Fig.19.5). Unlike cortical tubers, these subependymal hamartomas appear to have the capacity for slow enlargement during life, irrespective of the development of a subependymal giant cell astrocytoma.[13,63] Histologically, the central areas of the nodules are usually composed of closely-packed, atypical giant cells similar to those found in cortical tubers, although in older lesions these may be almost entirely effaced by areas of dense calcification. More peripherally, the lesions merge diffusely with adjacent brain and consist of masses of elongate, pilocytic-type astrocytes embedded in a dense meshwork of glial processes (Figs 19.6 and 19.7).

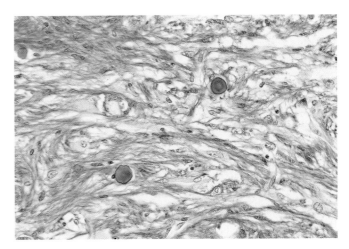

Fig. 19.7 **Tuberous sclerosis.** Subependymal nodule. There is widespread staining using immunocytochemistry for GFAP.

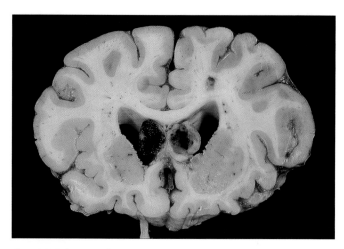

Fig. 19.8 Tuberous sclerosis. Bilateral subependymal giant cell astrocytomas obstructing the foramina of Monro. The patient had undergone surgery and the tumours are haemorrhagic.

Retinal hamartomas These are found in over half of all cases of tuberous sclerosis examined by fundoscopy, and are seen as multiple, small, flattened or lobulated masses projecting from the peripheral zones of the retina.[72,73] Histologically, they consist of gliotic masses within the ganglion cell or plexiform layers, and usually contain atypical giant cells similar to those seen in cortical tubers.[73,74]

Neoplasms

Subependymal giant cell astrocytoma These distinctive neoplasms, described in Chapter 4, have been estimated to occur in between 6% and 14% of all cases of tuberous sclerosis.[75,76] (Fig. 19.8) Although often considered pathognomonic of the condition, they are also found in otherwise normal individuals[70,77] and there is some debate as to whether this represents a 'formes fruste' of tuberous sclerosis, or whether the giant cell astrocytomas can occur as an unrelated phenomenon.[78] Where tuberous sclerosis is definitely present, the tumours are generally thought to arise from pre-existing subependymal nodules,[54,78] a view supported by sequential CT studies describing transformation of longstanding small nodules into large, histologically typical neoplasms obstructing the foramen of Monro.[79,80] Ultrastructural studies have suggested that the neoplastic cells derive from purely astrocytic elements within the subependymal nodules,[41,81] but the results of immunocytochemistry have been less clear-cut. Most studies have shown few or no GFAP staining cells in giant cell astrocytomas,[82,83] and strong expression of NSE.[70] This argues against a purely astrocytic origin, but is also in direct contrast to the staining pattern exhibited by the giant cells in subependymal hamartomas (Fig. 19.7). Even if subependymal giant cell astrocytomas are not directly related to the giant cells, however, it does seem likely that they arise from abnormally developed cells with a similar pluripotential capacity for neuronal and glial expression.[82,83]

Other neoplasms Other forms of nervous system neoplasm are very rare in tuberous sclerosis and may be incidental to the condition or simply reflect a generalised increase in potential for neoplastic change.[84] Subependymal nodules have been occasionally related to the development of typical ependymomas,[85] in some cases with intermingling of tumour and hamartomatous tissue.[86] Low grade astrocytomas,[75] glioblastomas[87] and gangliogliomas[84] have also been described in cases of tuberous sclerosis, but there is no evidence that these derive from cortical tubers, which are not thought to have the potential for significant growth or neoplastic change.[13,63]

Therapy and prognosis

Although some cases of tuberous sclerosis may survive into old age, survival rates are well below those of the normal population, with 30% of patients dying by 5 years of age and 75% by the end of the second decade of life.[13,15] Death is most commonly due to status epilepticus or intercurrent infection,[13,88] but renal, cardiac and pulmonary lesions also take their toll.[55,88] In about 3% of cases, death is related to the development of subependymal giant cell astrocytomas and obstruction of the foramina of Monro.[13] Ventricular shunting or surgical excision of the tumours is needed to relieve hydrocephalus in this situation,[89,90] but the success of surgical intervention is often hampered by the low tolerance of severely mentally retarded patients to such a procedure.[48,89] MR studies have indicated that whilst the absolute number of cortical tubers is poorly correlated with the final degree of intellectual defect in retarded patients, their size and location are good indicators of mental prognosis.[15,66] Surgery has little part to play where tubers are concerned, but in occasional individuals epilepsy can be related to a fixed EEG focus correlating with a focal abnormality on MR scans, and removal of the abnormal tissue in these patients can dramatically reduce the incidence of fits.[91,92]

Neurofibromatosis types 1 and 2

The first detailed account of neurofibromatosis is usually attributed to von Recklinghausen,[93] and the two cases he described in 1882 would now be regarded as typical of neurofibromatosis type 1 (NF1), the peripheral form of the disease also sometimes referred to as 'von Recklinghausen's neurofibromatosis'.[94] It has since become clear that there is a clinically and genetically distinct form of neurofibromatosis with predominantly central neuraxial manifestations, neurofibromatosis type 2 (NF2), which has been variously called 'bilateral acoustic neurofibromatosis' (BANF) or 'central neurofibromatosis'.[95,96] Several other, less common clinical variants have also been proposed, although it is not clear whether these are genetically distinct from the classic, peripheral form of the condition.[96,97] The designation of the peripheral and central forms of the disease as distinct entities (NF1 and NF2 respectively) has been substantially reinforced by the results of molecular genetic studies in these conditions.[96,98]

Neurofibromatosis type 1

Incidence and genetics

Neurofibromatosis type 1 (NF1) is said to have a prevalence of between 1 in 2000 and 1 in 3000,[99] although the true frequency of the aberrant gene is uncertain because of the unknown proportion of clinically unrecognised 'formes frustes' of the condition.[97] There is a predominance of males in most series.[94] The inheritance is autosomal dominant, with a variable but high penetrance rate.[97,99] However, over half of all cases represent new mutations and will not have a family history.[97] The *NF1* gene is located on chromosome 17q11 and normally encodes for neurofibromin, a ubiquitous protein involved in the control of cell proliferation and differentiation.[100] Although the gene is very large and may exhibit a variety of differing germline mutations,[101] the widely varying clinical expression found in individuals with NF1 may be partly determined by their genotype at other modifying loci, which alter the *NF1* gene product at post-translational level.[102,103]

The *NF1* gene product, neurofibromin, contains sequence homology with a family of proteins known as GTPase activating proteins.[100,104] These normally act to downregulate the p21 *ras* oncogene, which is important in the control of cell proliferation and differentiation.[105,106] The *NF1* gene may thus be classed as a tumour suppressor gene.[107] In addition to the germline mutations seen in individuals with NF1, somatic mutations have been found in a variety of systemic and neuroectodermal neoplasms, including neurofibromas.[104,108,109] This has led to the suggestion that a 'two-hit' mechanism may operate in NF1, with one allele inactivated on a hereditary (germline) basis and a second, somatic mutation leading to the development of tumours in postnatal life.[109]

Clinical features

NF1 is characterised by a great variability of clinical expression, and even within the same family affected individuals can exhibit a wide range of severity and differing patterns of disease involvement.[96,110] Only about one-third of known cases have severe systemic or neurological manifestations, and many appear to be mildly affected 'formes frustes', often only with cutaneous lesions.[97] In contrast to some other dysgenetic syndromes, NF1 has an obviously progressive clinical course and its manifestations become increasingly apparent throughout the lifespan of any one individual.[96] Cutaneous lesions, described below, are usually noticed prior to the development of any neurological symptoms, and in some cases are present at birth.[94] Short stature is a common feature of NF1, and about 8% of patients show a variable degree of mental retardation or learning difficulty.[94,96] Fits develop in 5–12% of affected individuals, often with no demonstrable neoplasm or other focal abnormality on CT or MR brain scans.[94,96] Focal neurological manifestations due to peripheral or central nervous system tumours in NF1 may appear any time up to late middle age.[94] Common symptoms include pain and weakness in limbs severely affected by large plexiform neurofibromas and radicular pain or other focal symptoms caused by a spinal root tumour.[94,110] NF1 patients may also present with a myriad of other signs and symptoms relating to the visceral or skeletal manifestations of the condition, as outlined below. Currently acceptable minimum diagnostic criteria for NF1 are shown in Table 19.3.[110,111]

Systemic and cutaneous manifestations

Cutaneous and deep soft tissue lesions

The characteristic skin lesions In NFI comprise axillary or inguinal freckling, café-au-lait spots and cutaneous

Table 19.3 Minimum clinical criteria for neurofibromatosis types 1 and 2

NF1		NF2	
Two or more of:		*One of:*	
1. Café-au lait spots	Prepubertal > 6 spots > 5 mm diameter Postpubertal > 6 spots > 15 mm diameter	1. Radiological or surgical evidence of bilateral acoustic Schwannomas	
2. Neurofibromas	> 2 of any type > 1 of plexiform type	2. Affected first degree relative and: (i) evidence of a unilateral acoustic Schwannoma; or	
3. Axillary or inguinal freckling			
4. Optic nerve glioma		(ii) evidence of ≥ 2 meningiomas, gliomas or Schwannomas at any site.	
5. Lisch iris nodules	> 2 nodules		
6. Typical skeletal anomaly	Sphenoid wing dysplasia Tibial bowing/pseudarthrosis		
7. Affected first degree relative			

neurofibromas.[96,112] *Café-au-lait spots* are usually present at birth but rapidly increase in size and number during puberty. In adults they may be very numerous and up to several centimetres across. Pigmentation is due to an increase both in the number of melanocytes in the basal layer of epidermis and in their melanin content. *Cutaneous neurofibromas* lie in the dermis or immediate subcutis and relate to small dermal nerve branches. They are visible as sessile or pedunculated skin nodules, usually appearing during childhood and again increasing in size and number during puberty. Histologically typical cutaneous neurofibromas are usually covered by smooth ('molluscoid') skin, but the large, pendulous lesions covered by wrinkled ('elephantiasic') skin are usually of plexiform type. *Plexiform neurofibromas* only occur almost exclusively in NF1 and are characteristic of the condition even in isolation.[113,114] Although usually superficial in location, they may become very extensive and diffusely infiltrate deeper tissues, engulfing major subcutaneous nerve trunks or plexuses.[110,112] Histologically, the plexiform lesions are not encapsulated by perineurial sheaths but show proliferation of spindle cell tumour elements outside the expanded fascicles of affected nerves (Fig. 19.9). Where subcutaneous fat becomes incorporated, the appearances are sometimes referred to as 'neurofibrolipomatosis'.[114] In addition to this lack of circumscription, plexiform neurofibromas also differ from ordinary neurofibromas in showing a bizzare, distorted architecture of intertwining tumour cell fascicles, a significant degree of nuclear pleomorphism and a tendency to lose their myxoid stroma and become increasingly hyalinised with age. They also carry a much greater risk of malignant transformation (see below).

Visceral lesions

Visceral neurofibromas and the other abnormalities described below are found only in NF1 or variants such as intestinal NF, and are not a feature of NF2. Systemic neurofibromas may occur in any part of the body in NF1 but are most commonly found in the upper gastro-intestinal tract, nasopharyngeal structures, the lungs and thoracic cavity and the genitourinary system.[96,115] The gastrointestinal tract may also be affected by leiomyomas and a diffuse hyperplasia of the colonic submucosal autonomic plexus, sometimes referred to as 'colonic ganglioneuromatosis'.[116,117] Other less commonly described types of visceral tumour are legion, but include thyroid adenomas, renal cortical adenomas and pancreatic carcinomas.[15] An association of NF1 with both phaeo-chromocytoma and duodenal carcinoid tumours has been repeatedly observed.[118,119] Vascular anomalies are not uncommon in NF1, and are typified by cervical vertebral artery aneurysms or arteriovenous fistulae.[120] In addition, either renal artery stenosis or aortic coarctation may be a cause of systemic hypertension.[96,121]

Eye lesions

Small iris hamartomas known as Lisch nodules are found in over 95% of all NF1 cases[122,123] and appear to be unique to the condition and are not present in NF2.[96] The nodules are typically multiple and bilateral, only a few millimetres in diameter and pigmented[124] (Fig. 19.10). They are thought to be of melanocytic origin, and consist histologically of a condensation of spindle cells on the anterior surface of the iris, sometimes with an associated underlying pigmented stromal naevus[125] (Fig. 19.11). The

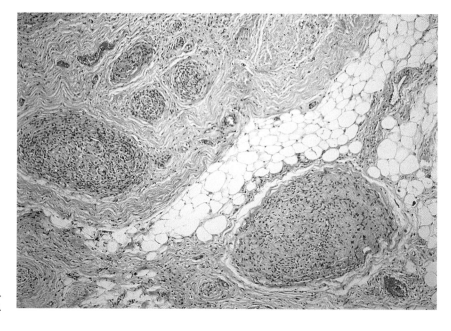

Fig. 19.9 **Neurofibromatosis type 1.** Subcutaneous plexiform neurofibroma. There is proliferation of spindle-cell tumour elements outside the expanded fascicles of nerve and the lesion is infiltrating adipose tissue. H & E.

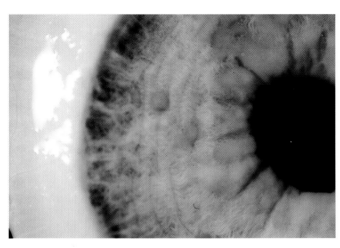

Fig. 19.10 **Neurofibromatosis type I.** Lisch nodules. These hamartomas are visible macroscopically as multiple, flattened, pigmented papules on the anterior surface of the iris.

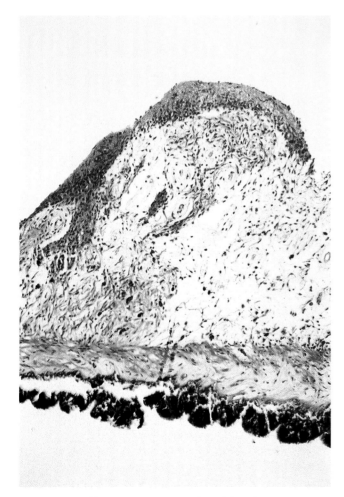

Fig. 19.11 **Neurofibromatosis type 1.** Lisch nodules. There is a condensation of spindle cells on the anterior aspect of the iris (top) and an underlying pigmented stromal naevus. H & E.

eye may also be affected by plexiform neurofibromas of the lids in NF1, but retinal manifestations are unusual.[124]

Skeletal lesions

Bony abnormalities are common in NF1.[126,127] Angular spinal scoliosis is the most frequent anomaly, and is sometimes associated with dysplastic changes in the vertebral bodies or arches.[114,127] Other characteristic skeletal manifestations of NF1 include congenital bowing of the tibia, sometimes with a tibial pseudoarthrosis,[114,127] and dysplasia of the sphenoid bone with partial absence of the bony walls of the orbit.[124,126]

Nervous system manifestations

Hamartomatous lesions

Nervous system hamartomas are relatively uncommon in NF1 and most often take the form of subependymal gliofibrillary nodules.[128] These are small, often multiple, polypoid masses of astrocytic tissue which project into the ventricular cavity, usually with focal loss of the overlying ependyma. They may occur anywhere in the ventricular system but typically involve the aqueduct, where they may cause obstructive hydrocephalus.[128,129] A diffuse, hyperplastic gliosis of the brainstem or cerebellum has also been reported in NF1.[128,130] This process appears to represent some sort of proliferative response rather than true neoplasia, but may extend into the overlying meninges in a similar manner to the diffuse astrocytomas in NF1 patients. Other dysplastic abnormalities of the brain reported in NF1 include focal disorder of cerebral cortex laminar architecture, glial nodules and glomeruloid vascular proliferations in cortical grey matter and heterotopic neurons in deep white matter.[128,131] Some of these abnormalities may be related to the intellectual retardation found in some NF1 patients.[131]

Neoplastic lesions

The neoplasms occurring in NF1 and NF2 are summarised in Table 19.4.

Neurofibroma and Schwannoma Non-cutaneous tumours of peripheral nerves are neurofibromas rather than Schwannomas and are almost exclusively a feature of NF1.[94,96] They may affect any major nerves or nerve trunks and are frequently found at multiple sites along the course of a given nerve.[94,112] With the exception of dermal plexiform neurofibromas which have engulfed adjacent large nerve trunks, the neurofibromas affecting major peripheral nerves in NF1 are histologically identical to their solitary counterparts.[112,114] As mentioned above, plexiform neurofibromas are virtually pathognomonic of NF1. These may extensively involve major nerve trunks or plexuses.[110,112] Spinal root tumours

Table 19.4 Nervous system tumours in neurofibromatosis types 1 and 2

	NF1	NF2
Typical cutaneous neurofibroma	+	Very rare
Plexiform neurofibroma	+	−
Peripheral nerve neurofibroma	+	−
Spinal root neurofibroma	+	−
Spinal root Schwannoma	−	+
Cranial nerve Schwannoma	−	VIII nerve
Plexiform Schwannoma	−	+
Malignant PNST	+	−
Optic nerve glioma	+	−
Diffuse astrocytoma	+	Rare
Spinal cord ependymoma	−	+
Meningioma	−	+

are much less common in NF1 and are almost always neurofibromas, although possible solitary dorsal root Schwannomas have been reported in the early literature.[94,96] Very rarely, Schwannomas have also been reported in intracerebral or spinal intramedullary sites, but these cases must also be viewed with some caution given the rarity of true Schwannomas in NF1.[132,133]

Optic nerve glioma This lesion, also described in Chapter 4, is said to occur in 15–20% of NF1 patients,[96,134] although the true frequency is uncertain because a significant proportion of cases is asymptomatic and only comes to attention after radiological screening.[135,136] The tumour is not found in NF2,[96] but taken in isolation it cannot be considered diagnostic of NF1 as up to three-quarters of patients show no other evidence of neurofibromatosis.[137] Whether these represent 'formes frustes' of NF1 or truly sporadic tumours is uncertain.[94,132] In patients with proven NF1, optic nerve gliomas tend to present at an earlier age than in the apparently sporadic cases,[138] often becoming symptomatic in childhood.[136,139] The lesions in NF1 are bilateral in 30% of cases[136] and are more likely to be located anteriorly in the optic nerves, sparing the chiasm.[135,138] Optic nerve gliomas are also more likely to have a benign, relatively static growth pattern in NF1 patients, sometimes exhibiting long periods of dormancy or even spontaneous clinical regression.[115,140] In view of this, it has been suggested that some of the lesions in NF1 are hamartomatous rather than neoplastic,[96] a theory supported by reports of NF1 patients showing diffuse hyperplasia of both glial and mesenchymal optic nerve elements.[128,141] Histologically, even the more typical lesions in NF1 differ from isolated optic nerve gliomas in showing a circumferential, perineural pattern of growth rather than a simple expansion of the endoneural compartment.[141] The residual nerve is still diffusely involved by tumour, but it becomes ensheathed in a thick mantle of intermingled tumour and arachnoidal elements, which occupy the expanded subarachnoid space outside the boundary of the old pial sheath. In some cases, the arachnoidal hyperplasia may predominate to such an extent that the lesion is mistaken for an 'en plaque' meningioma ensheathing the optic nerve.[142]

Glioma In addition to optic nerve gliomas, a variety of histologically typical glial tumours may occur in NF1, although some of these types, such as ependymomas, are regarded as being more characteristic of NF2 (see below).[134,143] Any grade of astrocytic tumour from pilocytic lesions to glioblastomas may occur,[94] but in NF1 the most common gliomas are very diffuse, low grade astrocytomas, frequently cerebellar in location, which have a pronounced tendency to infiltrate the overlying meninges.[132,139] These tumours often show 'glial bridging' between the parenchymal tumour and that within the leptomeninges, a phenomenon regarded as typical of NF1.[139] Although many of these cerebellar tumours have been described as fibrillary astrocytomas,[132,139] it is also generally accepted that pilocytic astrocytomas can also occur in the cerebellum in NF1. Pilocytic astrocytomas of the third ventricle region are also sometimes associated with NF1.[94,139]

Malignancy in NF1

Patients with NF1 have an increased overall lifetime risk of developing malignancy compared with the general population,[96] and this constitutes their commonest single cause of death.[144] Malignant tumours of the nervous system taken in isolation are also more common than expected and occur at younger ages than in patients without NF1.[144] Some of these are central nervous system gliomas such as glioblastomas,[139,143] but malignancy is most often encountered in peripheral nerve sheath tumours (PNSTs).[145,146] Malignant PNSTs (see also Chapter 15) are said to develop in anything between 2.4% and 4.6% of all NF1 cases,[145,147] and the majority present some time in the second and third decades of life.[96,147] They typically manifest as a painful, enlarging mass[145,146] and are most common in central locations relating to the trunk, pelvic and shoulder girdles.[145,146] The retroperitoneal compartment is a particularly frequent site.[145] A majority of examples result from malignant change occurring within a pre-existing neurofibroma,[145,146] although some appear to arise de novo from nerve trunks.[113,146] Malignant transformation is most likely to occur in deep-sited[96] or plexiform neurofibromas[113] and rarely affects typical cutaneous neurofibromas.[112,114] Most malignant PNSTs developing in NF1 display Schwannian differentiation[146,148] and are likely to be of higher grade malignancy than similar lesions occurring in patients without neurofibromatosis.[145] Mesenchymal differentiation is found in a significant proportion of NF1 malignant PNSTs, usually in the form of focal chondrosarcomatous or osteosarcomatous change.[145,146] Malignant 'Triton' tumours with rhabdomyoblastic differentiation may also occur and are almost pathognomonic of NF1.[145,146] Malignant transformation of neurofibromas in NF1 is associated with CDKN2A/p16 inactivation; immunocytochemistry shows that, although all neurofibromas express p16 protein, malignant PNSTs are essentially immuno-negative.[149] The prognosis in NF1 patients developing peripheral nerve malignancy is poor, with a high recurrence and metastasis rate, despite radical surgery and radiotherapy,[150] and a 5-year survival rate of only about 15%.[145,146] Non-nervous system malignancy is rather less common in NF1, but leiomyosarcomas,[151] angiosarcomas,[96] malignant fibrous histiocytomas[152,153] and non-lymphoid leukaemias[111,154] have all been reported as showing an increased incidence in the condition. In particular, childhood chronic myeloid leukaemia is highly suggestive of NF1.

Neurofibromatosis type 2

Incidence and genetics

Neurofibromatosis type 2 (NF2) is much less common than NF1, with an estimated incidence of only 0.1 in 100 000.[95] Published series have not reported a pre-dilection for either sex.[143] The condition is again inherited in an autosomal dominant fashion with very high penetrance,[96,155] but the spontaneous mutation rate is lower than that found in NF1.[95] The gene associated with NF2 lies on chromosome 22q12 and encodes a highly conserved cytoskeletal protein which has been named merlin or schwannomin.[156] Differing types of germline mutation have been correlated with the severity and age of onset of the clinical syndrome, but the same mutation may lead to differing degrees of severity in different families.[156,157]

The *NF2* gene functions as a tumour suppressor gene, with its encoded product merlin (schwannomin) exerting a growth inhibitory effect.[156,158,159] Merlin is one of a family of similar proteins that link the outer membrane of cells to their internal cytoskeleton.[156] Somatic mutations in the *NF2* gene are found in sporadic Schwannomas and meningiomas as well as those occurring in the context of the dysgenetic syndrome,[106,160] but gene alterations have not been found in other tumour types, including gliomas.[161,162] In patients with NF2, tumour genesis is again thought to follow the two-hit sequence, with a somatic mutation occurring against a background germ-line abnormality.[162] Western blotting and immunohisto-chemical studies have shown that merlin is not expressed in Schwannomas (including those lacking evidence of biallelic *NF2* gene inactivation); loss of the *NF2* gene and merlin expression have been demonstrated in the early 'tumourlet' stage of Schwannoma development in patients with NF2.[163,164]

Clinical features

NF2 is more relatively constant in its clinical expression and lacks the systemic features of NF1, including retardation, skeletal anomalies and visceral lesions. The clinical presentation is nearly always related to the development of nervous system tumours, in most cases with onset of symptoms some time during the second and third decades of life.[155,165] The majority of patients present with deafness and vestibular dysfunction caused by eighth nerve Schwannomas.[155,166] Although the tumours are usually bilateral, initial symptoms may relate purely to the worst affected side, the contralateral lesion being manifest only after radiological examination.[155] Up to half of NF2 patients will develop gliomas, meningiomas or nerve sheath tumours of the spine, and in some cases these are the earliest manifestation of the disease.[165] Spinal meningiomas and Schwannomas are often multiple, but lesions at cervical levels usually produce the earliest neurological symptoms, with brachial radiculopathy and evidence of high cord compression.[94] Signs and symptoms in NF2 may also relate to intracranial gliomas and meningiomas, which are again frequently multiple.[143] Malignant tumours are very rare in NF2. Minimum diagnostic criteria for NF2 are shown in Table 19.3 (p. 593). It should be emphasised there are undoubted 'formes frustes' which fall short of these guidelines, particularly unilateral eighth nerve Schwannomas in young age groups and patients with multiple spinal or cranial meningiomas but no family history.[110,111]

Systemic and cutaneous manifestations

Cutaneous manifestations in NF2 are often entirely absent, but a proportion of otherwise typical cases have small numbers of café au lait spots or typical cutaneous neurofibromas which fall short of the minimum criteria for the diagnosis of NF1.[95,155] Plexiform Schwannomas may occur in NF2, but plexiform neurofibromas have not been reported.[113] A variety of cataracts commonly occur in NF2, including juvenile posterior subcapsular opacities and cortical wedge lesions.[167] Skeletal and visceral abnor-malities are not a feature of NF2.[96]

Nervous system manifestations

Hamartomatous lesions

Dysplastic and hamartomatous lesions are more fre-quently encountered in the brains and cords of NF2 patients, but they are nearly always incidental autopsy findings and are of unknown clinical significance.[128] *Meningioangiomatosis* (see Chapter 13) consists of circum-scribed, often multiple foci of arachnoidal proliferation around parenchymal blood vessels.[128,168] The lesions can resemble miniature, very vascular meningiomas and are

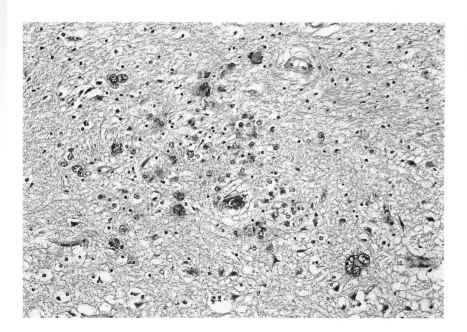

Fig. 19.12 **Neurofibromatosis type 2.** Hamartomatous focus of bizarre atypical glial cells at the margin of the amygdala. Incidental autopsy finding. H & E.

most common in cerebral cortex, although the basal ganglia and brainstem may also be affected. *Atypical nests of glial cells,* sometimes with an immature cytological appearance, may also be found in the cerebral cortex (Fig. 19.12), often in association with foci of meningio-angiomatosis.[128,169] In the spinal cord, parenchymal Schwann cell proliferation ('Schwannosis') is not uncommonly found in the posterior grey horn regions and has been variously interpreted as reactive[170] or dysplastic in nature.[128] *Ependymal ectopias* can also occur in the spinal cord, and may be the origin of the multiple cord ependymomas which are characteristic of NF2.[128]

Neoplastic lesions

The neoplasms occurring in NF2 and NF1 are summarised in Table 19.4.

Schwannoma Spinal nerve root tumours are almost exclusively Schwannomas in NF2 and are usually found at multiple levels[96,166] (Fig. 19.13). Some examples may be centred on a vertebral root foramen and have a 'dumbbell' distribution, with intra- and extraspinal components.[132] *Cranial nerve root* tumours are almost always a manifestation of NF2 and have been described as typical Schwannomas.[94] They are most commonly sited on the vestibular (VIII) nerves, which are affected in over 90% of all patients with NF2.[96,171] The involvement is bilateral in over 80% of affected individuals[143] (Fig. 19.14). Less commonly, NF2 Schwannomas have been reported on other cranial nerves, especially at lower anatomical levels, including IX, X and XI.[94]

Meningioma Meningiomas are a hallmark of NF2, being the next most frequent tumour after eighth nerve Schwannomas.[94,95] They are often multiple and may be intracranial, intraspinal or in both locations.[155,166] Intra-

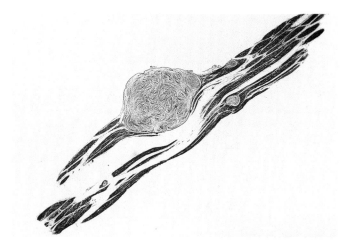

Fig. 19.13 **Neurofibromatosis type 2.** A spinal root Schwannoma with several smaller satellite lesions. Similar tumours were present at nearly every spinal level in this autopsy case. Solochrome cyanin.

cranial examples occur in the same sites as sporadic meningiomas,[94] and there are no specific histological differences between sporadic examples and those found in NF2 patients.[132] Multiple meningiomas may also occur in the absence of any other features of NF2, sometimes as an inherited syndrome,[172] but the germline mutation involved is at a separate locus on chromosome 22 from that of the NF2 gene.[173]

Glioma A wide range of glial tumours have been described in NF2. These are often multiple ependymomas and have a particular predilection for the upper spinal cord.[143] Multiple spinal cord ependymomas are especially common in NF2 and are said to occur in up to half of all cases.[132,143]

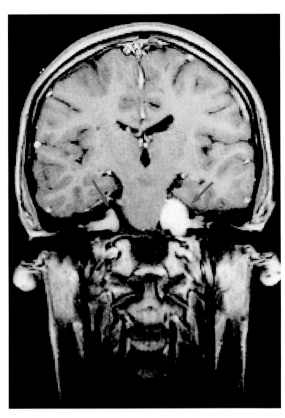

Fig. 19.14 **Neurofibromatosis type 2.** Coronal T1-weighted magnetic resonance scan, showing bilateral accoustic Schwannomas, brightly enhancing after administration of contrast medium (arrows). Both lesions have a narrow neck, representing intracanalicular tumour.

Other variants of neurofibromatosis

A number of other variants of neurofibromatosis have been defined on the basis of differing patterns of pathological and clinical expression, but it is not yet clear whether any of these are genetically distinct conditions, or whether they are all simply extreme manifestations of the NF1 gene.[96,97] Patients with *mixed NF* have bilateral acoustic Schwannomas, together with a combination of iris Lisch nodules, multiple café au lait spots or cutaneous neurofibromas, which meets the minimum clinical criteria for NF1.[174] In some of these cases there may be both typical NF1 and NF2 in different first degree relatives.[175] In *segmental NF* patients have cutaneous manifestations of NF1 which are confined to one or more dermal segments, commonly a unilateral body quadrant and the adjacent limb.[176,177] Most of these cases appear to be spontaneous somatic mutations, as both a family history and evidence of transmission are uncommon.[177,178] *Schwannomatosis* is a rare condition associated with multiple non-vestibular Schwannomas, which occurs without meningiomas, spinal cord ependymomas or any of the other characteristic lesions of NF2.[179] Studies of the *NF2* gene in this condition have revealed that, although the tumours frequently contain typical truncating

mutations, no heterozygous changes are identified in normal cells,[180] a finding which requires further investigation. Other variants of neurofibromatosis with restricted clinical and pathological manifestations include *familial café au lait spots, late onset cutaneous neurofibromas* and *intestinal NF*.[96,181]

von Hippel–Lindau disease

This syndrome was first fully characterised by Lindau in 1926,[182] some years after von Hippel's description of patients with multiple retinal haemangioblastomas.[183] Manifestations of the most complete form of the disorder include haemangioblastomas of the craniospinal axis and retina, together with a variety of cystic, vascular and neoplastic lesions affecting systemic organs.[184] In current terminology, retinal haemangioblastomas occurring in isolation are usually referred to as von Hippel's disease or retinal angiomatosis.[185] Where there are other nervous system and/or visceral abnormalities, the term von Hippel–Lindau disease (VHL) is now normally favoured, regardless of whether retinal lesions are also present.[184,186] Some authors have used 'Lindau's disease' specifically to denote cases lacking retinal haemangioblastomas, but this distinction is generally felt to be of little practical value.[184] The term 'Lindau's tumour' is simply an eponym for cerebellar haemangioblastoma and does not necessarily imply the presence of VHL.

Incidence and genetics

The true incidence of VHL is rather uncertain because of the unknown proportion of asymptomatic and undiagnosed cases, but the prevalence of heterozygotes has been estimated as being between 1 in 40 000 and 1 in 50 000 live persons,[187,188] and the incidence of the condition at birth is likely to be higher than this.[188,189] The sexes are equally affected.[190,191]

The gene responsible for VHL lies near the tip of the short arm of chromosome 3 at 3p25[192] and a wide variety of germline mutations have been found at this locus in over three-quarters of pedigrees tested.[193] Variations in phenotypic expression are thought to relate to differing types of mutation occurring at this single locus.[193] In particular, pedigrees where phaeochromocytomas occur appear to be genetically distinct from those which lack this manifestation of the syndrome.[193,196] The mutant gene is inherited in an autosomal dominant fashion[194,195] and the new mutation rate probably lies somewhere between 2 and 4×10^{-6} per gene per generation.[188] Although only a minority of the members of affected kindreds manifest the condition,[196] the gene is thought to exhibit almost complete penetrance, and the apparent lack of clinical expression associated with skipped generations is felt to be due to undiagnosed 'formes frustes'.[184,188]

Aetiology

The *VHL* gene on chromosome 3 normally encodes for a ubiquitous protein of 284 amino acids and is thought to act as a tumour suppressor gene.[193] It is expressed in all three germ cell layers and their derivatives, with enhancement in the normal epithelial components of lung, kidney and eye.[197] Somatic mutations or loss of heterozygosity have been found in most sporadically occurring renal cell carcinomas[198,199] and in at least 20% of sporadic central nervous system haemangioblastomas,[200,201] suggesting a critical role in the origin of these tumours in otherwise normal individuals. In patients with VHL, inactivation of both copies of the gene appears to be necessary for tumorigenesis, with 'second-hit' somatic defects adding to the existing germline mutation.[199,201]

Clinical features

Although the possible visceral and nervous system manifestations of VHL are varied and numerous, relatively few of the lesions regularly cause clinical symptoms.[190] Family screening and autopsy studies have revealed that the condition is clinically silent in up to a quarter of all cases.[184,190] In symptomatic patients, the commonest clinical manifestation is visual deterioration due to retinal haemangioblastomas, which occurs in over half of all cases.[185] The retinal lesions are initially symptomless, but if untreated they cause progressive loss of acuity, eye pain and eventual blindness due to secondary glaucoma or retinal detachment.[197,203] Clinical evidence of raised intracranial pressure or cerebellar dysfunction caused by cerebellar haemangioblastomas occurs in about a third of cases,[190,203] and a much smaller proportion of patients present with symptoms due to haemangioblastomas in the brain stem or spinal cord.[184,190] Renal cell carcinoma and phaeochromocytoma present symptomatically in a significant minority of patients,[190] but it is unusual for the other visceral lesions associated with VHL to cause signs or symptoms.[184] Polycythaemia is present in about one-fifth of cases[204] and may be associated with haemangioblastomas, renal cell carcinomas or phaeochromocytomas.[184,205] The initial clinical presentation most often occurs sometime in the third or fourth decade of life, with no documented cases manifesting before puberty and less than 5% after the age of 60.[206,207] There appears to be a distinct temporal sequence in the evolution of the lesions associated with VHL, the retinal and cerebellar haemangioblastomas being the most common cause of first presentation.[190,201] When retinal lesions occur, they often present symptomatically before the cerebellar ones,[202,203] but despite this, cerebellar haemangioblastomas in VHL are usually diagnosed earlier in life than in patients without other evidence of the syndrome.[191] Visceral lesions tend to become symptomatic later than the nervous system ones,[184] with renal carcinomas first presenting clinically at a mean age of 44 years in one series.[207] Patient survival in VHL is significantly below that of the general population, and the mean age at death is just under 50 years.[207] A majority of cases die from the complications of renal carcinomas or cerebellar haemangioblastomas.[204]

Pathology

Systemic manifestations

The visceral manifestations associated with VHL are extremely diverse (Table 19.5) and will only be briefly outlined here (for review see Ref. 209). *Renal lesions* are present in about two-thirds of cases coming to autopsy[183,190] and about one-third of all patients will eventually develop renal carcinomas.[190,207] The carcinomas are frequently bilateral[210] and become increasingly common with advancing age.[211] Other renal lesions include simple cysts[196,203] and cortical adenomas.[190,209] *Pancreatic lesions* are usually asymptomatic but have been found in over 70% of autopsied cases.[190] They are most often cysts or cystadenomas[209,212] but islet cell tumours may also occur (see below). Cysts and adenomas may be present in the liver[203,209] and cysts have also been found in the *spleen, lungs and bones*.[203,209] Lesions histologically resembling nervous system haemangioblastomas have been described in the liver, kidney and pancreas, although some of these may be simple angiomas.[190,203] *Papillary cystadenomas* of the epididymis are particularly associated with VHL[213,214] and similar lesions may occur in females in the mesosalpinx.[215] Locally aggressive *papillary tumours arising the middle ear and temporal bone* are again characteristic of VHL and can be bilateral.[216,217] They are thought to be of endolymphatic sac origin, but sometimes invade the cranial cavity in the cerebellopontine angle region and have been mistaken for choroid plexus tumours.

Table 19.5 Visceral manifestations associated with von Hippel–Lindau syndrome

Kidney	Carcinoma
	Cyst
	Cortical adenoma
	Angioma
Pancreas	Cyst
	Cystadenoma
	Islet cell tumour
Liver	Cyst
	Adenoma
	Angioma
Adrenal	Phaeochroromocytoma
Epididymis	Papillary cystadenoma
Lung	Cyst
Temporal bone	Aggressive papillary middle ear tumour

Endocrine tumours are also found in some patients with VHL and may be multiple, although there is a clear genetic distinction from the multiple endocrine neoplasia syndromes. Phaeochromocytomas,[190,207] and pancreatic islet cell tumours[218] are the most commonly reported types of endocrine tumour and occasionally occur together.[219] Carcinoid tumours have also been reported.[220] *Cutaneous lesions* are not normally found in VHL but very occasional cases have been reported to show vascular or pigmented naevi.[203,221]

Nervous system manifestations

Retinal haemangioblastoma Only about a quarter of patients with retinal haemangioblastomas are known to exhibit other manifestations of VHL,[202,222] but the lesions are present in almost two-thirds of patients known to have the syndrome.[204,207] The tumours tend to involve the periphery of the retina and are frequently multiple and bilateral.[202,223] They are typically only a few millimetres in size[221,222] and project into the posterior chamber of the globe from the plexiform layer.[202,224] The nodules are usually associated with tortuous and dilated retinal vessels, which can be detected by fundoscopy before the lesions themselves are visible.[202,203] Histologically, retinal haemangioblastomas are identical to those occurring elsewhere in the nervous system[184,202] and are associated with a pronounced marginal gliosis. Other secondary changes often present in the adjacent retina include cystic degeneration, haemorrhage and proliferation of the pigment layer.[202,224] The lesions may also undergo calcification or even ossification, a feature not found in haemangioblastomas of the brain or spinal cord.[202,226] If diagnosed early enough, before the onset of retinal detachment, haemorrhage and glaucoma, retinal haemangioblastomas can be successfully treated by photocoagulation.[223]

Brain and spinal cord haemangioblastomas Brain and cord haemangioblastomas have been found in half to three-quarters of patients with VHL, depending on the method of screening used.[191,227] The lesions are multiple in at least half of affected cases[191,227] and occur at similar sites to solitary, sporadic examples of the tumour.[184,191] Over two-thirds of haemangioblastomas in VHL arise in the cerebellum,[191,204] most often in the posterior and lateral parts of the hemispheres[184] (Fig. 19.15). The spinal cord is rather less frequently involved, although it accounted for over 40% of tumours in one published series.[227] The medulla is the third most common site and is affected in less than 20% of cases.[190,227] Supratentorial haemangioblastomas in VHL are extremely rare but well documented, and may be multiple.[191,228] Regardless of site, the haemangioblastomas occurring in VHL may be either solid or cystic[184,191] and cystic examples sited in the spinal cord are often associated with an elongate, syrinx-

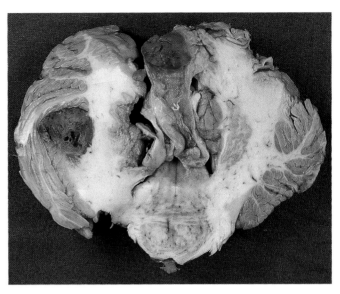

Fig. 19.15 **von Hippel–Lindau disease.** Two small, non-cystic haemangioblastomas are present in the cerebellum, one in the posterior vermis, the other in the lateral part of one hemisphere. This patient had undergone resection of another cerebellar haemangioblastoma several years prior to death, and old surgical scarring is visible in the vermis and one adjacent dentate nucleus.

like cavity.[190,229] Histologically, the tumours are again identical to the isolated lesions occurring in patients without other manifestations of VHL (see Chapter 14).[191,230]

Other nervous system tumours *Metastatic carcinoma* is an important diagnosis to consider in cases of VHL, both because of the increased incidence of visceral cancer and also because of the potential for confusion between a renal carcinoma metastasis and a neuraxial haemangioblastoma.[191,231] The difficulty here may be compounded if the two lesions occur simultaneously, or a renal metastasis arises in the site of a previously excised haemangioblastoma.[232] Histological distinction between the two lesions may be impossible using routine stains, especially if the metastasis is of the clear cell type, but immunocytochemical stains for both epithelial membrane antigen and cytokeratins can be used to positively identify the lesion as a carcinoma.[191,231] Nervous system tumours other than metastases and haemangioblastomas are exceedingly rare in VHL, and may possibly be purely coincidental when they do occur.[191] Anecdotal examples reported in patients with the syndrome have included ependymomas,[190,233] astrocytomas[191] and neuroblastomas.[234] An exception to this appears to be paragangliomas of the paravertebral sympathetic chain, which have been found often enough to suggest a definite association with VHL.[190,203]

Diagnosis

Patients with VHL exhibit a wide spectrum of clinical and pathological features, and it is relatively unusual to encounter the 'complete' syndrome of multiple nervous system haemangioblastomas and visceral cysts or neoplasms occurring in the context of a positive family history.[186,190] A majority of patients with solitary haemangioblastomas in the retina or cerebellum lack other evidence of VHL at the time of presentation and cannot be regarded as suffering from the syndrome.[202,230] It should be noted, however, that about a fifth of such cases will later develop other manifestations of VHL.[191] In addition, there are a wide variety of 'formes frustes' which still fall short of the full-blown clinical syndrome, some of which may be genetically distinct (Fig. 19.16). These include familial solitary cerebellar haemangioblastomas,[235] familial renal carcinomas,[236] phaeochromocytoma occurring in combination with renal carcinoma,[237] and patients with more than one nervous system haemangioblastoma in differing sites.[184,186] Bearing these comments in mind, the minimum clinical criteria normally quoted for the diagnosis of VHL are as follows:[184,186]

Either

1. At least two haemangioblastomas or typical visceral lesions in the absence of a positive family history.
   or
2. A single haemangioblastoma or typical visceral lesion with an affected first degree relative.

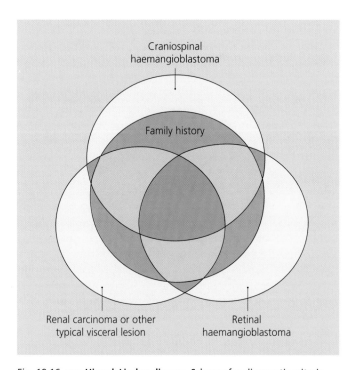

Fig. 19.16 von Hippel–Lindau disease. Schema for diagnostic criteria. The darker central area represents the most complete form of the syndrome, with the shaded areas outside this indicating the spectrum of acceptable 'formes frustes'. The diagramatic zones outside the shaded areas are not definitely diagnostic of VHL, except where visceral lesions or craniospinal haemangioblastomas are multiple.

Finally, genetic screening of at-risk individuals is now becoming more widely available, and although not providing complete certainty of prediction, confidence limits of above 0.98 have been claimed in nearly 90% of asymptomatic relatives.[238]

Miscellaneous familial tumour syndromes

Li–Fraumeni syndrome

First described in 1969, this condition manifests as multiple primary neoplasms in children and young adults.[239] There is a predominance of soft tissue sarcomas, osteosarcomas and breast malignancies, but brain tumours, leukaemias and adrenocortical carcinomas also occur more frequently than expected in the general population.[240] The minimum clinical criteria for diagnosis of the syndrome require a sarcoma before the age of 45 years and either a first degree relative with any tumour before the age of 45, or any relative with a malignancy before the same age.[241,242] Approximately half of the Li–Fraumeni pedigrees investigated have been found to carry germline mutations of the *TP53* tumour suppressor gene on chromosome 17p13[243] and the syndrome may also arise from germline *hCHK2* mutations.[244,245] Only half of all families with germline *TP53* mutations satisfy the clinical criteria for diagnosis. Of families carrying *TP53* gene defects 84% have point mutations, with only a small incidence of deletions, splice mutations and insertions. This corresponds closely to the spectrum of somatic *TP53* anomalies found in sporadic human tumours.[246] An investigation of 475 tumours from 91 pedigrees with germline *TP53* defects showed that breast carcinoma was the most frequently occurring neoplasm (24%), followed by bone sarcomas, brain tumours and soft tissue sarcomas, all with an incidence of about 12%.[245] There are marked tumour-specific differences in the mean age of presentation, with most adrenocortical carcinomas arising in the first decade of life, sarcomas in the second and breast tumours towards the end of the fourth.[245] Adrenocortical carcinoma is virtually diagnostic of a germline *TP53* mutation when occurring in childhood.[247] Of nervous system tumours, about two-thirds are astrocytic and just under a fifth are primitive neuroectodermal tumours, including medulloblastomas.[248] There is a bimodal age of presentation, with a first peak in childhood and second one in the third and fourth decades of life.[249] The astrocytic tumours can be of any malignant grade and tend to present at much younger ages than their sporadic counterparts, especially the glioblastomas.[248] A single report has suggested that germline *TP53* mutations are preferentially associated with gliomas which are multifocal.[250] There is current uncertainty over the relationship between typical Li–Fraumeni families and those which suffer hereditary occurrence of gliomas without full features of the syndrome. Some of these lack germline *TP53* mutations, but familial glioma pedigrees that do have *TP53* defects often display other, non-glial malignancies and may represent 'formes frustes' of the Li–Fraumeni phenotype.[251]

Turcot syndrome

The association between malignant tumours of the central nervous system and familial polyposis coli was initially recognised in 1959 and is now usually referred to as Turcot syndrome.[252,253] Affected pedigrees have a high incidence of multiple colorectal adenomas and primary brain tumours, which may occur either separately or in the same individual.[253] The brain tumours are most often medulloblastomas, which have a 100-fold increased incidence, but glioblastomas may also form part of the syndrome.[254] Most, but not all, affected families have germline mutations in the adenomatous polyposis coli (*APC*) gene on chromosome 5q21.[254,255] This is thought to act as a tumour suppressor gene in the nervous system but somatic *APC* mutations are rarely found in sporadic glioblastomas and medulloblastomas.[255] It therefore seems possible that genes distinct from the *APC* locus may be responsible both for the brain tumours occurring in families with *APC*-associated Turcot syndrome and also for those pedigrees that do not show germline *APC* mutations.[251] Some kindreds with familial glioblastomas carry germline mutations in DNA mismatch-repair genes and several of these genes are also associated with hereditary non-polyposis colorectal cancer.[254] It currently seems likely that kindreds with *APC* mutations and typical Turcot syndrome are most likely to develop medulloblastomas whilst families with inherited DNA repair defects and non-polyposis cancers are most at risk from glioblastomas.[254]

Gorlin syndrome

This syndrome was first described in 1987 and is also referred to as naevoid basal-cell carcinoma syndrome (NBCCS).[256] Affected individuals have a predisposition for developing cutaneous basal cell carcinomas and show an increased incidence of medulloblastomas.[251,256] They may also display a wide variety of developmental anomalies, including jaw cysts, bifid ribs, spina bifida occulta, dysgenesis of the corpus callosum, bridging of the sella turcica and calcification of the falx.[256] The *PTCH* gene is a homologue of the *Drosophila* patched gene and is located on chromosome 9q31.[257,258] It encodes a putative transmembrane protein and a wide variety of different

mutations are found in both affected family members and sporadically occurring basal cell carcinomas.[259] Patients often develop basal cell carcinomas in fields of therapeutic irradiation and their fibroblasts have been shown to be hypersensitive to ionising radiation in tissue culture.[260] Between 3% and 5% of affected individuals will develop medulloblastomas, usually before the age of 5 years, and it has been estimated that as many as 2% of all medulloblastomas may arise in the context of Gorlin syndrome.[258] They are frequently of the desmoplastic variant.[262] There have also been occasional reports of meningiomas[263] and astrocytomas[264] occurring in patients with Gorlin syndrome, but it is not clear whether these were genetically related events.

Cowden syndrome

Patients with Cowden syndrome have a predisposition for the development of mucocutaneous hamartomas and a variety of tumours in systemic organs.[251] There is also a consistent association with Lhermitte–Duclos syndrome of the cerebellum (see Chapter 8).[265] The condition is inherited in an autosomal dominant fashion, arising from germline mutations of the PTEN gene on chromosome 10q23.[266] Affected pedigrees may show increasingly severe clinical manifestations over successive generations, and different phenotypes resulting from maternal and paternal transmission may suggest imprinting.[267] The most common mucocutaneous lesions are tricholemmomas, hyalinising mucous fibromas, acral keratosis, oral papillomas and colorectal polyps.[268–276] Lesions in systemic organs include ovarian cysts and polyps, fibrocystic breast disease and tumours of uterus and thyroid gland.[251,269] As many as one-third of all cases of Lhermitte–Duclos disease occur in the context of Cowden syndrome and although the genetics are not yet fully understood, it has been suggested that the two conditions are part of the same dysgenetic syndrome.[271,272] When Lhermitte–Duclos disease presents during adolescence there is a particularly high likelihood of Cowden syndrome, since the mucocutaneous and systemic lesions do not usually manifest until the second or third decade of life.[273] In addition to Lhermitte–Duclos disease, megalencephaly is a common feature of Cowden syndrome, seen in up to 70% of affected individuals.[274] Less consistently, associations have also been claimed with both meningiomas[275] and medulloblastomas.[276]

Neurocutaneous melanosis

Incidence

This condition was first described by Rokitansky in 1861,[277] the term neurocutaneous melanosis being introduced over 80 years later by van Bogaert.[278] It is characterised by large or multiple pigmented skin naevi together with an increase in leptomeningeal melanocytic cells or a primary meningeal melanoma.[279,280] Neurocutaneous melanosis is normally classified alongside the other dysgenetic syndromes, despite its lack of inheritance and uncertain aetiology.[279,281] The condition is extremely uncommon, with less than 40 definite cases documented in the literature by 1991.[280] It probably accounts for about one-quarter of all cases of primary meningeal melanoma.[282] There is no racial bias, and the sexes are equally affected.[279,282]

Aetiology

Neurocutaneous melanosis is congenital in origin, and both the cutaneous and leptomeningeal changes can be demonstrated in stillbirths and neonates.[279] The abnormally increased pial melanocytic cells are presumed to take origin from normal leptomeningeal melanocytes or their precursors.[280,283] Differentiated melanocytic cells are found in the leptomeninges from quite early during normal fetal development, increasing up to the age of puberty.[279,284] They may be visible as dusky pigmentation of the meninges in brains from healthy individuals, and are mostly concentrated over the base of the cerebral hemispheres, the anterior aspect of the brain stem and the cervical cord.[279,285] Both pial and cutaneous melanocytes are thought to have a common origin in the developing neural crest,[280,286] leading to suggestions that neurocutaneous melanosis is a form of congenital dysplasia of the neural crest.[280,286]

The syndrome appears to be entirely sporadic in occurrence, and no cases with affected family members have been reported.[280,287] Even where they are not associated with leptomeningeal changes, the congenital giant hairy naevi typical of neurocutaneous melanosis are not associated with a family history of similar naevi[288] and can be discordantly expressed in identical twins.[289] Very occasionally, patients with the complete syndrome have had family members with multiple pigmented skin naevi, but these have not been giant hairy naevi and there have been no associated neurological abnormalities in the affected relatives.[287,290] The genetic basis for neurocutaneous melanosis is therefore uncertain, although it has been suggested that there may be a dominant, lethal gene which survives by mosaicism.[280,291]

Clinical features

The typical skin lesions of neurocutaneous melanosis, described in more detail below, consist of congenital giant hairy naevi or sometimes just multiple naevi of normal type, and are present from birth.[279,280] The syndrome characteristically manifests itself when neurological disturbances supervene in individuals already known to have these cutaneous abnormalities.[279,280] In over half of all cases, the neurological presentation occurs in the first 2 years of life, the remainder presenting before the end of the third decade.[279,280] In about two-thirds of cases, the neurological decline is due to hydrocephalus,[280,292] and this is almost always the case in infants, who typically present with head enlargement and signs and symptoms of raised intracranial pressure.[280,293] The hydrocephalus is of communicating type in a majority of instances, and is probably due to the increased pial melanocytic cells causing obstruction of the cerebrospinal fluid (CSF) spaces at the base of the brain or interfering with CSF absorption in the arachnoid villi.[280,292] In some cases the hydrocephalus may be non-communicating in nature, and this is usually the result of abnormal melanocytic cells obstructing the aqueduct or fourth ventricle exit foramina.[280] In older children and adults, the acute presentation may include focal signs and symptoms relating to a discrete intracranial mass lesion, particularly if the pial melanocytic cells have undergone malignant change.[279,280] The spinal cord can also be affected, with clinical evidence of a myelopathy.[286] A rapid clinical deterioration with focal neurological involvement in older patients can either occur in the absence of any previous neurological symptoms, or follow a longer history of epilepsy or mild meningism.[279]

Examination of the CSF in neurocutaneous melanosis may often reveal increased protein levels and xanthochromia, but atypical or pigmented cells are an inconstant finding in cytospin preparations unless there has been overt malignant change in the pial infiltrate.[279,280] Radiologically, thickening and enhancement of the meninges around the basal cisterns and brain stem are characteristic findings, most likely to be visible using contrast-enhanced CT or T1-weighted MR imaging after administration of gadolinium.[280,294]

Pathology

Cutaneous manifestations

Congenital giant naevi are found in about two-thirds of cases of neurocutaneous melanosis.[280] They most characteristically involve the pelvic area ('bathing trunk' type) or upper back ('cape' type) and may extend over the adjacent limb[280,288] (Fig. 19.17). They are often hairy, and may have a smooth or verrucous surface.[279,288] Giant naevi are present at birth and grow in proportion to general body growth.[288] Histologically, they are benign compound or intradermal naevi, indistinguishable from the giant naevi found in patients without other manifestations of neurocutaneous melanosis.[279,280] The dermal component not infrequently shows spindle cell or 'neuroid' differentiation and occasionally there may also be a blue naevus component.[288,295] Smaller naevi may

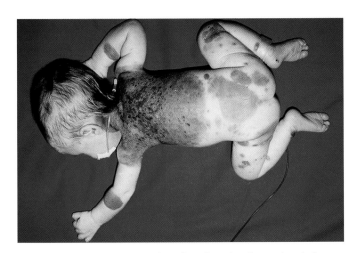

Fig. 19.17 **Neurocutaneous melanosis.** Infant showing a giant hairy naevus of 'cape' distribution over the upper back. Multiple smaller naevi are also present.

occur as satellites to a giant naevus or have a random distribution.[279,288] They are present at birth but may continue to appear up to the age of puberty.[285] Histologically, they are typical junctional or compound naevi.[288]

Nervous system manifestations

Meningeal melanosis The craniospinal changes of neurocutaneous melanosis are typified by a diffuse proliferation of melanocytic cells in the leptomeninges, sometimes referred to simply as 'melanosis'. As with physiological pigmentation of the meninges, melanosis most commonly affects the base of the cerebral hemispheres, cerebellum, brain stem and cervical spinal cord.[279,280] In some cases, the cerebral convexities and lower parts of the spinal cord may also be involved.[279,286] Externally, melanosis is apparent on naked eye examination in nearly all cases, and is seen as a diffuse thickening and brownish-black discolouration of the leptomeninges. A similar pigmentation is often visible on sectioning through the underlying neural parenchyma, especially in the cerebellum and brain stem, and this sometimes gives a mottled appearance to the cut surface of the tissue (Fig. 19.18). Occasionally, the ventricular lining and choroid plexus may also appear pigmented.[279]

Histologically, the leptomeninges and subarachnoid space are occupied by an infiltrate of melanocytic cells which are often markedly pleomorphic and can be spindle shaped, rounded, polygonal or stellate in outline. They may either be arranged in discrete cell nests like those found in cutaneous naevi (Fig. 19.19), or lie in diffuse sheets over the pial surfaces of the brain and spinal cord. There is frequently quite widespread infiltration of the underlying neural tissue along perivascular sheaths, visible in sections as discrete cuffs of melanocytic cells around parenchymal vessels. Mitoses

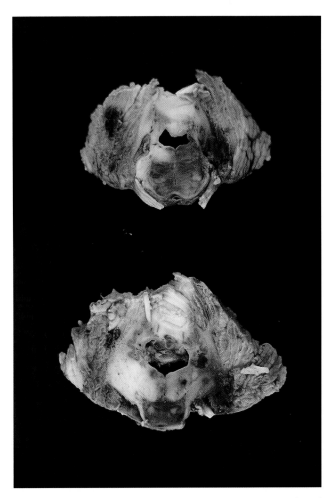

Fig. 19.18 **Neurocutaneous melanosis.** There is extensive parenchymal melanin pigmentation involving the cerebellum and brain stem.

may be found in some otherwise typical cases, suggesting a spectrum with diffuse melanomatosis (see below). The amount of pigment visible in the melanocytic cells is also very variable, but melanin granules are usually readily demonstrated in associated phagocytic cells, particularly in association with perivascular invasion of the parenchyma (Fig. 19.20).

Meningeal melanoma and diffuse melanomatosis Malignant transformation of the meningeal component of neurocutaneous melanosis is thought to occur in over 50% of cases,[279,283] although the true incidence is uncertain and may well have been overestimated in some earlier reported series.[279,280] About one-third of patients develop clear evidence of malignancy in the form of a discrete melanoma tumour mass, arising in a background of diffuse melanosis.[279,296] Such focal lesions are macroscopically and histologically identical to primary meningeal melanomas occurring in patients lacking any other features of the syndrome (see Chapter 14) and are most commonly located in the cerebellum, pons or temporal lobes.[296] They may present at any time from birth

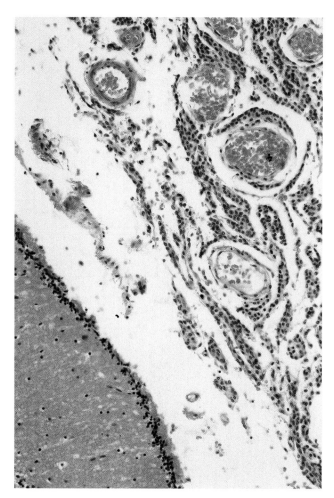

Fig. 19.19 **Neurocutaneous melanosis.** The leptomeninges over the cerebellum are infiltrated by nests of small, rounded naevus cells (top right). H & E.

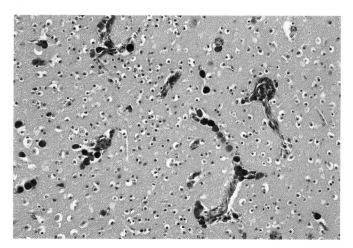

Fig. 19.20 **Neurocutaneous melanosis.** Capillaries in the cerebral cortex are cuffed by melanin-laden macrophages occupying the Virchow–Robin spaces. H & E.

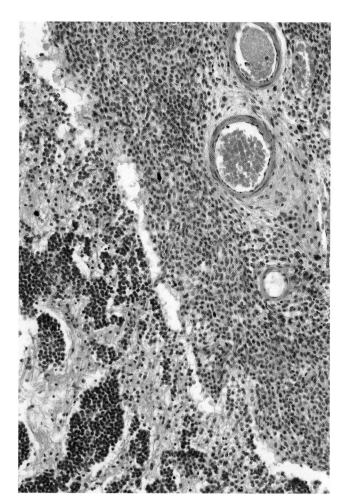

Fig. 19.21 **Neurocutaneous melanosis with diffuse malignant transformation.** The naevus cells in the meninges show a dense, sheet-like growth pattern (top right, compare Fig. 19.19). There is diffuse subpial parenchymal infiltration in addition to perivascular cuffing of cells (bottom left). H & E.

onwards, but tend to manifest at much younger ages than primary cutaneous melanomas.[296]

In patients without a discrete meningeal tumour mass, the biological potential of the diffuse melanocytic cells remains controversial, and probably varies between different cases.[280,295] In some instances, the infiltrate has an indolent appearance similar to that of benign cutaneous naevi, but in many cases there are histological features suggesting active growth, and some authors have suggested that the cells are always neoplastic rather than hamartomatous in nature.[281] However, the diagnosis of true diffuse malignancy needs to be made with caution, since features such as cellular pleomorphism, a sheet-like growth pattern and infiltration of parenchymal perivascular spaces mays all be associated with relatively benign clinical behaviour.[279,280] To be certain of diffuse malignant change, there ideally needs to be evidence of parenchymal invasion outside the perivascular sheaths, involving melanocytic cells and not just pigment laden macrophages[279] (Fig. 19.21). Other less definitive features which suggest diffuse malignancy include cell necrosis, focal haemorrhages and a high mitotic rate.[279,280]

Associated nervous system abnormalities Other nervous system lesions are uncommon in neurocutaneous melanosis, and may often be purely incidental to the syndrome. A possible exception to this is the Dandy–Walker syndrome,[297,298] where it has been postulated that the disrupted development of the cerebellum and fourth ventricle may very occasionally have been caused by an underlying hindbrain melanosis.[297] Other abnormalities described anecdotally in patients with neurocutaneous melanosis include spina bifida,[299] pial telangiectasis,[300] arachnoid cysts[301] and intraspinal lipomas.[301,302] Meningeal- related lesions such as arachnoid cysts and spinal lipomas may themselves be melanotic in some cases.[300]

Diagnosis

The mildest definite examples of neurocutaneous melanosis are usually felt to be cases of giant pigmented cutaneous naevi which are shown to have non-specifically increased pial pigmentation as an incidental autopsy finding.[279,293] However, patients with no skin lesions but a diffuse proliferation of benign melanocytic naevus cells in the meninges may also represent 'formes frustes' of the syndrome.[279,283] This has led to speculation that a spectrum exists between the classical manifestations of neurocutaneous melanosis and isolated primary malignant melanoma of the leptomeninges.[281] Giant or multiple cutaneous naevi are only present in about one-quarter of patients with primary intracranial melanoma,[282] but in some two-thirds of these cases the melanoma is a diffuse meningeal lesion.[283,303] Even where skin lesions are absent, it has been suggested that such diffuse primary malignancies may arise from a pre-existing benign melanosis of the meninges, and thus be distantly related to typical cases of the full neurocutaneous syndrome.[279,281]

The definition of neurocutaneous melanosis is also complicated by the need to be certain that the leptomeningeal component is not simply the result of metastasis, either from an undisclosed primary systemic melanoma or from a cutaneous naevus which has undergone malignant change.[279,280] To this end, earlier definitions of the syndrome have rejected patients with evidence of either a systemic melanoma deposit or malignant cutaneous naevi.[279,286] Unfortunately, this practice undoubtedly excludes some genuine cases of the syndrome, since giant naevi can become malignant and metastasise systemically or to the cranial cavity, and primary leptomeningeal melanomas can be a source of metastasis to systemic sites, including the skin.[280,288] More recently it has been proposed that genuinely simultaneous melanocytic lesions of the skin and meninges can

be more selectively distinguished from metastatic disease if the lesions at either site are known to be histologically benign.[280] The following minimum diagnostic criteria have thus evolved:

1. Large or multiple congenital cutaneous naevi associated with leptomeningeal melanosis or melanoma.
2. No evidence of cutaneous melanoma unless the meningeal lesions examined histologically are benign.
3. No evidence of meningeal melanoma unless the cutaneous lesions examined histologically are benign.

Based on the experience of definite cases of the syndrome, it has further been proposed that cutaneous naevi should be considered large enough if they exceed 20 cm diameter in adults or 6 cm in infants (9 cm if the lesion is cephalic), and that there should be at least three separate lesions if they are smaller than this.[280]

Therapy and prognosis

A small number of patients with neurocutaneous melanosis have a benign clinical course without significant neurological symptoms, and in some the meningeal changes may be a purely incidental autopsy finding.[279,280] In the majority of symptomatic cases, however, there is a rapid and progressive clinical decline, with early death from the complications of malignant change or hydrocephalus.[279,280] The interval from onset of neurological symptoms to death is usually little more than 6 months, with almost two-thirds of all patients dying before 2 years of age and few cases surviving into the third decade of life.[292,295] CSF shunting may produce transient clinical improvement where hydrocephalus is a prominent feature at presentation, but there is a high risk of patients developing systemic metastases via the shunt tube, especially where ventriculoperitoneal drainage systems are used.[280] Although the reported experience is very limited, radiotherapy and chemotherapy have not been found to alter significantly the clinical course.[280,299]

Angiomatous conditions involving the nervous system

Sturge–Weber syndrome

In its classic form, Sturge–Weber syndrome is characterised by the triad of an upper facial angiomatous naevus, a choroidal angioma and an ipsilateral meningeal angioma associated with adjacent cerebral calcification[304,305] (Table 19.6). The earliest clinical account of the disorder was by Sturge in 1879,[306] but it was not until

Table 19.6 Nature and distribution of vascular angiomatous syndromes involving the nervous system

	Cutaneous	Nervous system	Ocular	Visceral
Sturge–Weber disease	Upper facial capillary angioma	Meningeal capillary angioma	Choroidal angioma	Variable visceral capillary angiomas
Hereditary haemorrhagic telangiectasia	Multiple telangiectasia	Arteriovenous malformations or capillary telangiectases (some cases only)	–	Multiple mucosal telangiectases Pulmonary arteriovenous fistula Hepatic telangiectases
Ataxia-telangiectasia	Telangiectasia of face and extremities	Venous ectasia or capillary telangiectases (some cases only)	Scleral telangiectases	Oral telangiectases
Mesencephalo-oculo-facial angiomatosis	Facial capillary angioma or arteriovenous malformation	Arteriovenous malformation of mid brain, thalamus and optic nerve	Retinal arteriovenous malformation	–
Cutaneospinal angiomatosis	Capillary angioma of back	Spinal arteriovenous malformation or cord venous angioma (at same segmental level)	–	–
Multiple cavernous angiomas	Cavernous angiomas	Multiple cavernous angiomas	–	Variable visceral cavernous angiomas

1901 that the predicted intracranial angioma was demonstrated at autopsy examination.[307] Sturge–Weber syndrome is also occasionally referred to as 'encephalo-trigeminal angiomatosis'.[308,309] There are no reliable prevalence statistics for the condition in the general population, but it has been found in about 1 in 1000 admissions to institutions for patients with chronic epilepsy and mental subnormality.[310,311] It has been described in all ethnic groups and occurs with equal frequency in both sexes.[304,309]

Aetiology

Sturge–Weber syndrome appears to be sporadic when typically expressed, and a genetic basis for the condition remains uncertain.[311] In some cases there may be a family history of facial angiomatous naevi, mental retardation, epilepsy, or intracranial calcification, each occurring as isolated phenomenon, but relatives with definite evidence of the syndrome have not been reported.[311,312] It has been suggested that there may be a lethal gene mutation which only allows embryonic cells to survive in the mosaic state, but evidence to support this hypothesis is lacking at present.[313]

The pathogenesis of the condition is thought to involve abnormal development or persistence of the anterior segment of the embryonic vascular plexus.[304,308] Before its differentiation into mature vasculature, this part of the vascular plexus is closely related to embryonic face tissues, the optic vesicle and that part of the developing neural tube destined to become the occipital lobe.[308] These structures are all intimately juxtaposed during early embryogenesis, but with subsequent growth of the embryo the facial tissues and occipital cerebrum become widely distanced, thus explaining the anatomical separation of the facial and occipital meningeal components of the angiomatous malformation.[304,305] Although the facial naevi typically affect areas supplied by the upper divisions of the trigeminal nerve, a neurogenic origin is usually discounted because the vascular changes frequently transgress the boundaries of trigeminal innervation.[304,305]

Clinical features

The angiomatous facial naevi of Sturge–Weber syndrome are present at birth (see below), but affected infants are otherwise often normal in the immediate perinatal period.[304] Epilepsy is nearly always the earliest neurological manifestation of the syndrome, and is present in three-quarters of patients by the age of 15, often commencing the first few years of life.[304,309] The seizures are typically focal, affecting the opposite side of the body from the facial naevus, and initially the attacks may be separated by quite long periods of remission.[304] Even with appropriate medical treatment, however, the epilepsy usually becomes progressively severe, and in at least half of all cases it is accompanied by gradually increasing mental retardation.[304] As body growth progresses, a significant proportion of patients develop hemiparesis and sometimes hemiatrophy on the contralateral side to the facial naevus.[304,309] There may also be a homonymous hemianopia, which relates to the brain on the same side as the facial lesion.[304] Ocular signs and symptoms are found in over one-third of cases, and are usually due either to infantile buphthalmus or to the later-onset complications of choroidal angiomas, including haemorrhage, retinal detachment and glaucoma.[314]

Intracerebral calcification is visible on plain skull X-rays in about two-thirds of children with Sturge–Weber syndrome at the time of first presentation.[309] It has a characteristic gyriform pattern, with double contours representing the opposing surfaces of calcified cerebral cortical convolutions.[304] The calcification is also clearly seen using CT, which may in addition demonstrate convolutional atrophy and cortical enhancement in the same area.[315,316] MR scans are very sensitive at detecting the focal cerebral atrophy and accompanying parenchymal degenerative changes, but do not show the typical calcification as clearly.[319,317] The meningeal angioma may be visualised either by traditional angiography[318] or by using gadolinium-enhanced MR scans.[316,319]

Pathology

Extracranial manifestations

Cutaneous lesions The congenital facial naevus of Sturge–Weber syndrome, sometimes described as a 'naevus flammeus' or 'port wine stain', is a capillary angioma of the face and scalp[304,320] (Fig. 19.22). The naevus may affect either side of the face, and in rare instances can be bilateral.[314,317] Its precise distribution varies, but it is usually confined to the upper half of the face and always involves the ocular region.[304] Although there is overlap with the area innervated by the ocular division of the trigeminal nerve, the naevus often extends outside this territory.[304,305] It has a purplish-red colour and is flat in infancy, but may become verrucous with increasing age.[320] Histologically, it consists of numerous dilated, intradermal, capillary vessels, each formed from a single layer of flattened endothelium with variable surrounding collagen.[320]

Visceral lesions In fully-expressed cases of the syndrome, capillary or cavernous angiomas may occur in a variety of systemic organs including kidney, liver, spleen, pancreas, thyroid gland, adrenal glands, ovaries, anterior pituitary gland and gastrointestinal mucosa.[322,323] Such visceral angiomas are usually asymptomatic, and therefore unsuspected except in cases subjected to a detailed autopsy examination.[323]

Ocular lesions *Congenital choroidal angiomas* occur ipsilaterally in at least a third of all cases of Sturge–Weber syndrome, in many instances remaining occult and clinically undiagnosed.[314] On fundoscopy, they are usually visible as red or grey areas of retinal elevation, ranging in size from a few millimetres to over a centimetre in diameter, and are usually associated with engorged retinal vessels. Histologically, the retinal and pigment layers are unaffected and the cluster of dilated, thin-walled vascular channels is confined to the choroid

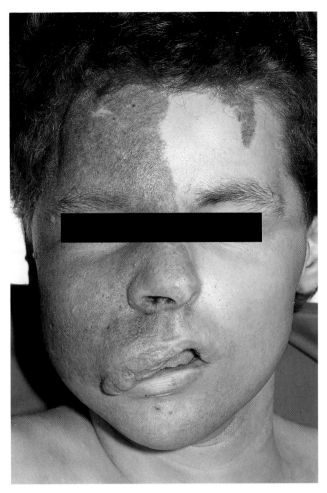

Fig. 19.22 **Sturge–Weber syndrome.** The hemifacial angiomatous naevus, or 'naevus flammeus' is an intradermal capillary angioma.

tissue.[308] In some cases there may be haemorrhage and secondary retinal detachment.[314] *Buphthalmus*, or globe enlargement due to congenitally raised intraocular pressure, is found in about 70% of affected infants.[314] Like the choroidal angiomas, it usually occurs on the same side as the facial and meningeal naevi.[304,314] Simple *glaucoma* of open-angle type develops in about one-third of older patients[314] and is thought to be due to raised episcleral venous pressure caused by the adjacent facial angioma.[324,325]

Intracranial manifestations

Macroscopic appearance The meningeal and parenchymal changes have the same distribution and are practically always unilateral. They most often involve the occipital lobe with variable encroachment of the adjacent temporal and parietal regions, but in severe cases the entire hemisphere can be involved.[304] Externally, the pial surface is obscured by a dense meshwork of tortuous, engorged blood vessels, which give the affected area of

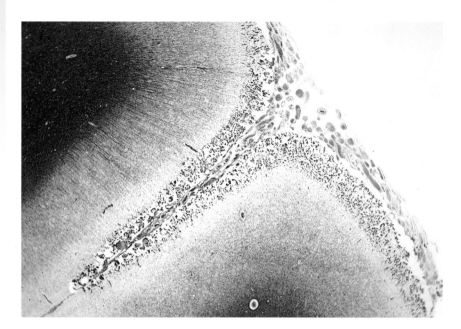

Fig. 19.23 **Sturge–Weber syndrome.** The subarachnoid space contains numerous small vascular channels, and there is a subpial zone of stippled mineralisation in the underlying cortex. Luxol fast blue-cresyl violet.

meninges a purplish colour. The meningeal angioma is usually well circumscribed at its margins but can be patchy, with underlying brain visible in focally unaffected areas. Beneath the angioma there is nearly always marked convolutional atrophy of the brain, which is more obvious on cut section. The affected cerebral tissue is gritty on slicing due to calcification and may be very difficult to cut cleanly when there are large calcified masses.

Histological features The subarachnoid space is filled by a myriad of closely-packed, thin-walled vascular channels (Figs 19.23 and 19.24). These follow the pial surface into the sulci, but are rarely seen to penetrate the underlying brain tissue. They are usually composed of a single endothelial layer with no elastic or muscular tissue and only sparse collagen, but some may show hyaline thickening of their walls. The calibre varies widely, but a majority range from capillary to small venule in size (Fig. 19.24). These vessels are not mineralised, but scattered arteries are also present and these frequently show intramural calcification. Arterialised veins are never seen and there are no features to suggest arteriovenous shunting. In some cases, a similar angiomatous malformation may be found in the choroid plexus of the affected hemisphere, and radiological studies have indicated that choroid plexus involvement may be more common than initially recognised.[322,326] The underlying cortex does not show true angiomatous change, but the capillaries and small veins are prominently outlined by stippled encrustations of calcified material (Figs 19.23 and 19.25). In larger parenchymal veins there may be a denser, concentric, intramural calcification associated with hyaline collagenous thickening. The parenchymal vascular mineralisation tends to be most severe in outer layers of

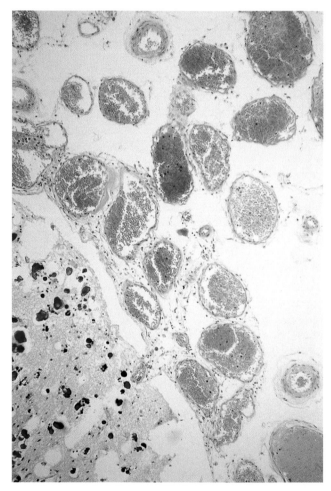

Fig. 19.24 **Sturge–Weber syndrome.** The angiomatous vessels in the subarachnoid space are mostly thin-walled and of quite small calibre. H & E.

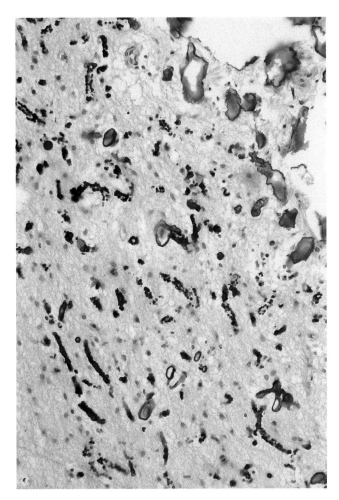

Fig. 19.25 **Sturge–Weber syndrome.** Intracortical capillaries are encrusted by finely stippled calcification. Larger calcospherites are present near to the pial surface (top right). H & E.

cortex but may also involve deeper cortical lamina and adjacent gyral stalk white matter. In addition to the vascular changes, there are usually numerous calcified concretions lying free within the cortical neuropil (Fig. 19.25). These vary in size from tiny calcospherites to huge, confluent masses, the larger examples tending to lie more superficially. All the calcified material stains strongly with Prussian blue, and appears to consist of a mixture of iron and calcium salts. The cortical mineralisation is associated with variable gliosis and neuronal loss, and in some cases there may be areas of frank infarction or cavitation. Immediately underlying white matter may also show gliosis and myelin loss, especially when affected by mineralisation.

Pathogenesis of the parenchymal changes Whilst the meningeal angioma is a static, congenital lesion, the underlying parenchymal changes are progressive, and appear to represent a secondary degeneration, consequent on the overlying angioma.[327,328] Parenchymal mineralisation

may be occasionally found in neonates,[329] but it more usually appears in infancy and increases with the age of the patient.[328] Calcified material is first detected in the pericytes of vessel walls,[328] and the extravascular mineralisation, gliosis and degeneration appear to follow as a result of the intramural vascular changes.[308] In the absence of overt malformation of the parenchymal vessels, however, it is not clear whether the initial intramural mineralisation is simply the result of stasis and ischaemia caused by the meningeal angioma, or whether there is some underlying functional abnormality of the vessels affecting their permeability.[328]

Diagnosis

Like many other neurocutaneous disorders, Sturge–Weber syndrome is quite variable in its pathological expression, and many cases do not exhibit all three of the major cutaneous, ocular and intracranial manifestations.[304] Such 'formes frustes' include patients with typical facial and ocular lesions but no intracranial abnormality, and cases of combined facial and meningeal angioma which lack ocular changes.[304] In some instances there may be typical facial naevi and meningeal lesions, but without calcification or focal degeneration of the cerebrum adjacent to the affected meninges.[330,331] The minimum diagnostic criteria usually quoted require the presence of at least two of the main characteristic features of the syndrome[305,312] and can be summarised as follows:

1. Congenital facial angiomatous naevus, which must always involve the ocular region.
2. At least one of: (i) Choroidal angioma;
                     (ii) Meningeal angioma.

Patients with isolated meningeal angiomas or facial naevi combined with idiopathic epilepsy are thus excluded by this definition, although their relationship to the typical syndrome must remain a matter of speculation.[305,327]

Therapy and prognosis

Without surgical intervention, up to one-third of children with Sturge–Weber syndrome can be expected to have a poor quality of life due to mental retardation, hemiparesis, blindness or progressively uncontrollable epilepsy.[309] Rare cases with bilateral intracranial involvement are associated with earlier onset seizures and a worse prognosis for mental development.[332] Intractable focal epilepsy has been successfully treated by lobectomy of the affected area of cerebral hemisphere, which can result in cessation of fits or at least greatly improved medical control.[309,333] In view of the risk of permanent mental impairment due to severe chronic epilepsy, some authors have advocated early surgical intervention in infants before seizures have become chronic and poorly controlled.[304]

Hereditary haemorrhagic telangiectasia

Hereditary haemorrhagic telangiectasia (HHT), also known as Rendu–Osler–Weber disease, is a form of systemic fibrovascular dysplasia associated with telangectases and arteriovenous fistulae widely distributed throughout the body vasculature[334,335] (Table 19.6). The condition is inherited in an autosomal dominant fashion with high penetrance,[335,336] and has an estimated prevalence of about 1 in 5000 of the general population.[337] At least three separate gene loci are involved, and at two of these the mutant genes have been identified. *HHT 1* on chromosome 9q33 encodes for endoglin and *HHT 2* on chromosome 12q1 for activin receptor-like kinase 1.[338] Both these proteins are members of the transforming growth factor-beta (TGF-beta) receptor family and are heavily expressed in vascular endothelial cells, leading to the hypothesis that the vascular lesions of HHT are caused by a dysregulated TGF-beta response.[338] Patients typically present in adolescence or young adulthood with bleeding from multiple mucocutaneous telangiectatic lesions.[336,337] The lesions are commonest over the face, upper limbs and the lining of the mouth and nasopharynx[338,339] The most frequent site of haemorrhage is the nasopharynx, with significant epistaxis occurring in over 90% of all cases.[335] In about one-quarter of patients, the mucosal lesions are more widespread, and in these cases there can be haemorrhage from almost anywhere in the respiratory, gastrointestinal or genitourinary tracts.[335,339] Between a third and half of all cases also develop clinically significant pulmonary arteriovenous fistulae[337,340] and in some patients the liver parenchyma is involved by telangiectatic lesions, which can ultimately result in cirrhosis.[336,341] Detailed study of the mucocutaneous lesions has shown that they initially consist of simple telangiectatic dilation of capillaries and post-capillary venules, but as they increase in size haemodynamic alterations lead to the loss of the intervening capillary element and the formation of a direct arteriovenous communication.[342]

Pathology

Nervous system manifestations

Neurological involvement occurs in only about 10% of cases of HHT, and may relate either to the complications of pulmonary arteriovenous fistulae or to the presence of primary intracranial vascular malformations.[336,337] Intracranial complications of the pulmonary fistulae include cerebral abscesses caused by septic emboli,[340,343] sterile embolic infarcts or transient ischaemic attacks[333,334] and more generalised hypoxic damage resulting from the associated polycythaemia.[336] Intracranial vascular mal-

formations are rather less common and account for around one-third of cases with neurological symptomatology.[336,337] The most frequent primary vascular lesions are arteriovenous malformations and venous angiomas, which may be sited anywhere in the brain or spinal cord.[336,344] The arteriovenous malformations usually present clinically with acute haemorrhage[337,345] and on rare occasions they have been identified antenatally.[346] Capillary telangiectases similar to those found elsewhere in the body may also occur in the brain or leptomeninges and are usually multiple.[336,344] They are often asymptomatic and are detected only at autopsy examination, but there have been occasional reports of progressive neurological deterioration, coma and death in cases with multiple parenchymal telangiectases and no evidence of haemorrhage.[344,347]

Ataxia telangiectasia

Ataxia telangiectasia, also known as Louis–Bar syndrome, is an autosomal recessively inherited condition characterised by immune deficiency, cerebellar degeneration and multiple vascular telangiectases[348,349] (Table 19.6). The disorder is rare, with an estimated incidence of three per million live births.[350] The *ATM* gene is located on chromosome 11q22 and encodes a protein which is largely confined to the nuclei of fibroblasts and lymphoid cells.[351,352] The precise function of this protein is not entirely clear, but it appears to be important both in ensuring the fidelity of DNA repair and in the activation of cellular defence mechanisms against oxidative stress.[352] Affected individuals show deficiencies of both the cellular and humoral immune mechanisms, including selective depletion of immunoglobulin A (IgA) and a poor delayed hypersensitivity response.[348,349] This is associated with a significantly increased risk of malignancies, especially of lymphoid type,[353,354] and also a greatly increased susceptibility to respiratory tract infections.[348,349] In addition, there is a generalised defect in the normal ability of DNA to respond to radiation damage.[355] This is presumed to be the origin of the bizarre, presumably aneuploid, nucleocytomegalic cells which are scattered throughout body organs and tissues, including the nervous system.[349,356] Patients typically present in infancy with progressive ataxia, eye movement disorders, choreoathetosis, mental retardation and recurrent respiratory tract infections.[349,357] Capillary telangiectases first appear on the sclera and later spread to the face, extremities and oral mucus membranes.[348,349] Visceral manifestations include thymic atrophy or aplasia, generalised lymphoid hypoplasia and gonadal hypoplasia.[349,356] Vascular lesions are not usually found in systemic organs, but multiple telangiectasias have occasionally been found in the liver.[358]

Pathology

Nervous system manisfestations

The typical degenerative changes found in the central nervous system include selective cerebellar cortical atrophy with loss of Purkinje and granule layer neurons, secondary degeneration of the olivary and dentate nuclei, axonal spheroids in the gracile and cuneate nuclei, ghost cells in the spinal anterior horns and posterior column degeneration of the cord.[358,359] In addition, there are usually bizarre cytomegalic endothelial cells scattered throughout the central nervous system. In the peripheral nervous system, there are often similar bizarre cytomegalic changes in dorsal root ganglion satellite cells and peripheral nerve Schwann cells[356,359] and there may also be evidence of peripheral neuropathy and skeletal muscle denervation.[349,360] Some individuals develop central nervous system tumours, including medulloblastomas and gliomas, and this may reflect their generalised susceptibility to malignancy.[361,362] Vascular malformations of the brain and cord are most uncommon in ataxia telangiectasia, and many of the changes described are of rather questionable significance.[349] In most cases, the abnormalities have consisted only of isolated ectatic veins in the meninges, cerebral white matter or brain stem.[363,364] Very occasionally, however, there have been reports of multiple capillary telangiectases in the brain and cord, and these have sometimes been associated with bizarre astrocytic cytomegaly, suggesting they are an integral part of the systemic disorder.[361,368]

Mesencephalo-oculo-facial angiomatosis

This is a rare form of neurocutaneous angiomatosis which has been variously referred to in the literature as retinocephalic angiomatosis, Wyburn-Mason syndrome or Bonnet–Dechaune–Blanc syndrome.[366,367] It is characterised by arteriovenous malformations involving the retina and upper brain stem, usually with an ipsilateral congenital vascular naevus of the face (Table 19.6). The facial lesion may be a dermal capillary angioma like that seen in Sturge–Weber syndrome, or a subcutaneous extension of the arteriovenous malformation.[366] The condition can be distinguished from non-calcified 'formes frustes' of Sturge–Weber syndrome angiographically, since the intracranial lesion is a true arteriovenous fistula rather than a simple meningeal angioma.[368,369] The genetic basis of this syndrome remains unknown. Patients typically present in childhood with exophthalmos, which may be pulsatile.[367,368] Neurological manifestations relate to the intracranial vascular malformation and include varied features of brain stem dysfunction, oculomotor cranial nerve palsies, homonymous hemianopia and epilepsy.[366] Occasionally there may be an acute clinical episode precipitated by brain stem haemorrhage.[370] Although the retinal and intracranial arteriovenous malformations may appear to be separate lesions in some cases, autopsy and radiological studies have shown that they are often connected by a variable meshwork of arterialised veins extending through the thalamic region and along the optic nerve.[369,370] The lesions are usually fed by multiple branches of both the carotid and vertebral vascular trees, and venous drainage is mostly via the vein of Galen and skull base venous sinuses.[366,368]

Cutaneospinal angiomatosis

Cutaneospinal angiomatosis and Cobb syndrome are terms used to describe cases of intraspinal vascular malformation with a coexisting cutaneous vascular lesion of the back at the same segmental level[371] (Table 19.6). There is no known genetic basis for the condition. The spinal lesion is nearly always a typical transdural arteriovenous fistula (see Chapter 17), although venous angiomas of the cord may also form part of the syndrome. The cutaneous naevus is usually a dermal capillary angioma, and its occurrence at the same anatomical level as the intraspinal lesion is thought to indicate a common embryonic pathogenesis.[371] A distinction needs to be made with Klippel–Trenaunay– Weber syndrome, where cutaneous angiomas are associated with limb hypertrophy in the absence of any underlying spinal or nervous system involvement.[372]

Familial cavernous angiomas

Multiple cavernous angiomas confined to intracranial sites are not an uncommon phenomenon (see Chapter 17), but in a significant proportion of patients the condition is inherited in an autosomal dominant fashion with similar angiomas affecting the skin and other systemic tissues.[373,374] (Table 19.6). Linkage studies have identified gene loci on chromosomes 7q,7p and 3q, and the *CCM1* gene on 7q11 is now known to produce a protein, KRIT1, which interacts with the ras family of GTPases.[375] The precise mechanism of angiogenesis is not yet known. The lesions are all typical cavernous angiomas and in addition to the brain and skin, affected individuals may show involvement of a variety of internal organs, including heart, liver and kidneys.[374]

REFERENCES

1. Musgar A. Dermatological aspects of the phakomatoses. In: Vinken PJ, Bruyn GW, eds. Handbook of clinical neurology, vol. 14. The phakomatoses. Amsterdam: North Holland, 1972: pp 562–618
2. Van der Hoeve J. Les phakomatoses de Bourneville, de Recklinghausen et de von Hippel–Lindau. J Belge Neurol Psychiat, 1933; 33:752–762

3. Bolande RP. The neurocristopathies. A unifying concept of disease arising in neural crest maldevelopment. Human Pathol, 1974; 5:409–429

4. Grossman M, Melmon KL. Von Hippel–Lindau disease. In: Vinken PJ, Bruyn GW, eds. Handbook of clinical neurology, vol. 14. The phakomatoses. Amsterdam; North Holland, 1972: pp 241–259

5. Bentz MS, Towfighi J, Greenwood S et al. Sturge–Weber syndrome. A case with thyroid and choroid plexus haemangiomas and leptomeningeal melanosis. Arch Pathol Lab Med, 1982; 106:75–78

6. Novotny EJ Jr, Urich H. The coincidence of neurocutaneous melanosis and encephalofacial angiomatosis. Clin Neuropathol, 1986; 5:246–251

7. Fox H. Neurocutaneous melanosis. In: Vinken PJ, Bruyn GW, eds. Handbook of clinical neurology, vol.14. The phakomatoses. Amsterdam: North Holland, 1972: pp 414–428

8. Chapman RC, Kemp VE, Teleaferro 1. Phaeochromocytoma associated with multiple neurofibromatosis and intracranial hemangioma. Am J Med, 1959; 26:883–890

9. Moller PM. Another family with von Hippel–Lindau's disease. Acta Ophthalmol, 1952; 30:154–165

10. Tishler PV. A family with coexistent von Recklinghausen's neurofibromatosis and von Hippel–Lindau's disease. Diseases possibly derived from a common gene. Neurology, 1975; 25:840–844

Tuberous sclerosis

11. Bourneville DM. Sclérose tubérose des circonvolutions cérébrales: idiotie et épilepsie hémiplégique. Arch de Neurol, 1880; 1:81–91

12. Von Recklinghausen F. Ein Herz van einem Neugebovenen, welches mehrere, theils nach aussen, thiels nach der Höhlen prominierende Tumoren (Myome) trug. Monatsschr Geburts Gynäkol, 1862; 20:1–2

13. Donegani G, Grattarola FR, Wildi E. Tuberous sclerosis. In: Vinken PJ, Bruyn GW, eds. Handbook of clinical neurology, vol 14. The phakomatoses. Amsterdam: North Holland, 1972: pp 340–389

14. Shepherd CW, Beard CM, Gomez MR et al. Tuberous sclerosis complex in Omsted County, Minnesota, 1950–1989. Arch Neurol, 1991; 48:400–401

15. Webb DW, Osborne JP. New research in tuberous sclerosis. Br Med J, 1991; 304:1647–1648

16. Sampson JR, Scahill SJ, Stephenson JB et al. Genetic aspects of tuberous sclerosis in the west of Scotland. J Med Genet, 1989; 26:28–31

17. Ross AT, Dickerson WW. Tuberous sclerosis. Arch Neurol Psychiatry (Chic) 1943; 50:233–257

18. Wilson GC, Lo D: Tuberous sclerosis: a case with pulmonary and lymph node involvement. Med J Aust, 1964; 2:795–796

19. Gomez MR. Clinical experience at Mayo clinic. In: Gomez MR, ed. Tuberous sclerosis. New York: Raven Press, 1979: pp 11–26

20. Koch G. Genetic aspects of the phakomatoses. In: Vinken PJ, Bruyn GW, eds. Handbook of clinical neurology, vol. 14. The phakomatoses. Amsterdam: North Holland, 1972: pp 488–561

21. Nevin NC, Pearce WG. Diagnostic and genetical aspects of tuberous sclerosis. J Med Genet, 1968; 5:273–280

22. Osborne JP, Fryer AE, Webb DW. Epidemiology of tuberous sclerosis. Ann NY Acad Sci, 1991; 615:125–127

23. Kandt RS, Pericak-Vance MA, Hung WY et al. Linkage studies in tuberous sclerosis. Chromosome 9?, 11?, or maybe 14! Ann NY Acad Sci, 1991; 615:284–297

24. Gomez MR. Phenotypes of the tuberous sclerosis complex with a revision of diagnostic criteria. Ann NY Acad Sci, 1991; 615:1–7

25. Webb DW, Osborne JP. Non-penetrance in tuberous sclerosis. J Med Genet, 1991; 28:417–419

26. Povey S, Burley MW, Attwood J et al. Two loci for tuberous sclerosis: One on 9q34 and one on 16p13. Ann Hum Genet, 1994; 58:107–127

27. Short MP, Richardson, EP Jr, Haines JL et al. Clinical, neuropathological and genetic aspects of the tuberous sclerosis complex. Brain Pathol, 1995; 5:173–179

28. Haines LJ, Short MP, Kwiatkowski DJ et al. Localization of one gene for tuberous sclerosis within 9q32-9q34, and further evidence for heterogeneity. Am J Hum Genet, 1991; 49:764–772

29. The European chromosome 16 tuberous sclerosis consortium. Identification and characterisation of the tuberous sclerosis gene on chromosome 16. Cell, 1993; 75:1305–1315

30. Wienecke R, Konig A, DeClue JE. Identification of tuberin, the tuberous sclerosis-2 product. Tuberin possesses specific Rap 1 GAP activity. J Biol Chem, 1995; 270:16409–16414

31. Green AJ, Johnson PH, Yates JR. The tuberous sclerosis gene on chromosome 9q34 acts as a growth suppressor. Hum Mol Genet, 1994; 3:1833–1834

32. Geist RT, Gutmann DH. The tuberous sclerosis gene is expressed at high levels in the cerebellum and developing spinal cord. Cell Growth Differ, 1995; 6:1477–1483

33. van Slegtenhorst M, de Hoogt R, Hermans C et al. Identification of the tuberous sclerosis gene TSC 1 on chromosome 9q34. Science, 1997; 27:805–808

34. Johnson M W, Emelin J K, Park S-H et al. Co-localisation of TSC 1 and TSC 2 gene products in tubers of patients with tuberous sclerosis. Brain Pathol, 1999; 9:45–54

35. Green AJ, Smith M, Yates JR. Loss of heterozygosity on chromosome 16p13.3 in hamartomas from tuberous sclerosis patients. Nature Genet, 1994; 6:193–196

36. Sampson JR, Harris PC. The molecular genetics of tuberous sclerosis. Hum Mol Genet, 1994; 3:1477–1480

37. Caviness VS Jr, Takahashi T. Cerebral lesions of tuberous sclerosis in relation to normal histogenesis. Ann NY Acad Sci, 1991; 615:187–195

38. Huttenlocher PR, Wollman RL. Cellular neuropathology of tuberous sclerosis. Ann NY Acad Sci, 1991; 615:140–148

39. Huttenlocher PR, Heydemann PT. Fine structure of cortical tubers in tuberous sclerosis. A Golgi study. Ann Neurol, 1984; 16:595–602

40. Chou TM, Chou SM. Tuberous sclerosis in the premature infant: a report of a case with immunohistochemistry on the CNS. Clin Neuropathol, 1989; 8:45–52

41. Trombley IK, Mirra SS. Ultrastructure of tuberous sclerosis: cortical tuber and subependymal tumor. Ann Neurol, 1981; 9:174–181

42. Ribadeau-Dumas JL, Poirier J, Escourolle R. Etude ultrastructurale des lesions cérébrales de la sclérose tubérose de Bourneville. Acta Neuropathol (Berl), 1973; 25:259–270

43. Arseni C, Alexianu M, Horvat L et al. Fine structure of atypical cells in tuberous sclerosis. Acta Neuropathol (Berl), 1972; 21:185–193

44. Stefansson K, Wolman RL. Distribution of glial fibrillary acidic protein in central nervous system lesions of tuberous sclerosis. Acta Neuropathol (Berl), 1980; 52:135–140

45. Webb DW, Fryer AE, Osborne JP. On the incidence of fits and mental retardation in tuberous sclerosis. J Med Genet, 1991; 28:395–397

46. Lagos JC, Gomez MR. Tuberous sclerosis: re-appraisal of a clinical entity. Mayo Clin Proc, 1967; 42:26–49

47. Westmoreland BF. Electroencephalographic experience at the Mayo Clinic. In: Gomez MR, ed. Tuberous sclerosis. New York: Raven Press, 1979: pp 55–68

48. Kapp JP, Paulson. GW, Odom GL. Brain tumours with tuberous sclerosis. J Neurosurg, 1967; 26:191–202

49. Elliott GB, MacGeachy WG. The monster Purkinje-cell nature of so-called 'congenital rhabdomyoma of heart'. A forme fruste of tuberous sclerosis. Am Heart J, 1962; 63:636–643

50. Kofman O, Hyland HH. Tuberous sclerosis in adults with normal intelligence. Arch Neurol (Chic), 1959; 81:43–48

51. Duvoisin RC, Vinson VM. Tuberous sclerosis: report of three cases without mental defect. J Am Med Asoc, 1961; 175:869–873

52. Fryer AE, Osborne JP, Tan R et al. Tuberous sclerosis: a large family with no history of seizures or mental retardation. J Med Genet, 1987; 24:547–548

53. Musgar A. Dermatological aspects of the phakomatoses. In: Vinken PJ, Bruyn GW, eds. Handbook of clinical neurology, vol. 14. The phakomatoses. Amsterdam: North Holland, 1972: pp 572–580

54. Reznik M. Cutaneous neuropathology: neurofibromas, Schwannomas and other neural neoplasms with cutaneous and extracutaneous expressions. Clin Neuropathol, 1991; 10:225–231

55. Schmitt J. Visceral aspects of the phakomatoses. In: Vinken PJ, Bruyn GW, eds. Handbook of clinical neurology, vol. 14. The phakomatoses. Amsterdam: North Holland, 1972: pp 682–691

56. Stillwell TJ, Gomez MR, Kelalis PP. Renal lesions in tuberous sclerosis. J Urol, 1987; 138:477–481

57. Bernstein J, Robbins TO. Renal involvement in tuberous sclerosis. Ann NY Acad Sci, 1991; 615:36–49

58. Smith HC, Watson GH, Patel RG et al. Cardiac rhabdomyomata in tuberous sclerosis: their course and diagnostic value. Arch Dis Child, 1989; 64:196–200

59. Dawson J. Pulmonary tuberous sclerosis and its relationship to other forms of the disease. Q J Med, 1954; 23:113–145

60. Schaper J, Konig T. Tuberous sclerosis: rare pulmonary manifestations. Monatsschr Kinderheilhd, 1990; 138:451–453
61. Fleury P, Smits N, van Ball S. The incidence of hepatic hamartomas in tuberous sclerosis. Evaluation by ultrasonography. ROFO Fortschr Geb Rontgenstr Nuklearmed, 1987; 146:694–696
62. Schafer JA, Berg BO, Norman D. Cerebellar calcification in tuberous sclerosis. Arch Neurol, 1975; 32:642–643
63. Richardson EP Jr. Pathology of tuberous sclerosis. Neuropathologic aspects. Ann NY Acad Sci, 1991; 615:128–139
64. Gerard G, Weisberg L. Tuberous sclerosis; CT findings and differential diagnosis. Comput Radiol, 1987; 11:189–192
65. Houser OW, McLeod RA. Roentgenographic experience at the Mayo Clinic. In: Gomex MR, ed. Tuberous sclerosis. New York: Raven Press, 1979: pp 27–53
66. Roach ES, Williams DP, Laster DW. Magnetic resonance imaging in tuberous sclerosis. Arch Neural, 1987; 44:302–303
67. Wippold FJ 2d, Baber WW, Gado M et al. Pre-and postcontrast MR studies in tuberous sclerosis. J Comput Assist Tomogr, 1992; 16:69–72
68. Nixon JR, Houser OW, Gomez MR et al. Cerebral tuberous sclerosis: MR imaging. Radiology. 1989; 170:869–873
69. Altman NR, Purser RK, Post MJ. Tuberous sclerosis: characteristics at CT and MR imaging. Radiology, 1988; 167:527–532
70. Bonnin JM, Rubinstein LJ, Papasozomenos S Ch et al. Subependymal giant cell astrocytoma. Significance and possible cytogenetic implications of an immunohistochemical study. Acta Neuropathol (Berl) 1984; 62:185–193
71. Moran V, O'Keeffe F. Giant cell astrocytoma in tuberous sclerosis: computed tomographic findings. Clin Radiol, 1986; 37:543–545
72. Robertson DM. Ophthalmic manifestations of tuberous sclerosis. Ann NY Acad Sci, 1991; 615:17–25
73. François J. Ocular aspects of phakomatoses. In: Vinken PJ, Bruyn GW, eds. Handbook of clinical-neurology, vol.14. The phakomatoses. Amsterdam: North Holland, 1972: pp 619–624
74. Ulbright TM, Fulling KH, Helveston EM. Astrocytic tumours of the retina. Differentiation of sporadic tumours from phakomatosis-associated tumours. Arch Pathol Lab Med, 1984; 108:160–163
75. Shepherd CW, Scheithauer B, Gomez MR. Brain tumours in tuberous sclerosis. A clinicopathological study of the Mayo Clinic experience. Ann NY Acad Sci, 1991; 615:378–379
76. Kingsley DP, Kendalal BE, Fitz CR. Tuberous sclerosis: a clinicoradiological evaluation of 110 cases with particular reference to atypical presentation. Neuroradiology, 1986; 28:38–46.
77. Chow CW, Klug GL, Lewis EA. Subependymal giant-cell astrocytoma in children: an unusual discrepancy between histology and clinical features. J Neurosurg, 1988; 68:880–883
78. Russell DS, Rubinstein LJ. Pathology of tumours of the nervous system. London: Edward Arnold, 1989: pp 766–769
79. Fujiwara S, Takaki T, Hikita T et al. Subependymal giant-cell astrocytoma associated with tuberous sclerosis. Do subependymal nodules grow? Childs Nery Syst, 1989; 5:43–44
80. Morimoto K, Mogami M. Sequential CT study of subependymal giant-cell astrocytoma associated with tuberous sclerosis. J Neurosurg, 1986; 65:874–877
81. De Chadarevian JP, Hollenberg RD. Subependymal giant cell tumour of tuberous sclerosis: a light and ultrastructural study. J Neuropathol Exp Neurol, 1979; 38:419–433
82. Iwasaki Y, Yoshikawa H, Sasaki M et al. Clinical and immunohistochemical studies of subependymal giant cell astrocytomas associated with tuberous sclerosis. Brain Dev, 1990; 12:478–481
83. Tanaka J, Kawakami S, Hashimoto K. Immunocytochemistry of subependymal giant cell astrocytoma associated with tuberous sclerosis. No To Hattatsu, 1989; 21:222–226
84. Davis RL, Nelson E. Unilateral ganglioglioma in a tuberosclerotic brain. J Neuropathol Exp Neurol, 1961; 20:571–581
85. Norman RM, Taylor AL. Congenital diverticulum of the left ventricle of the heart in a case of epiloia. J Pathol Bact, 1940; 50:61–68
86. MacCarty WC, Russell DG. Tuberous sclerosis: report of a case with ependymoma. Radiology, 1958; 71:833–839
87. Paomalatha C, Harruff RC, Ganick D et al. Glioblastoma multiforme with tuberous sclerosis. Arch Pathol Lab Med, 1980; 649–650
88. Shepherd CW, Gomez MR, Lie JT et al. Causes of death in patients with tuberous sclerosis. Mayo Clin Proc, 1991; 66:792–796
89. Bret P, Remond J, Pialat J et al. Tuberous sclerosis and trigonoseptal tumors. Neurochirurgie, 1988; 34:235–241
90. Ruberti R, Zotti G. Sclerosi tuberosa e tumore cerebrale (considerazioni sul trattamenta chirurgico). G Psichiatr Neuropat, 1961; 89:113–1160
91. Bye AM, Matheson JM, Tobias VH et al. Selective epilepsy surgery in tuberous sclerosis. Aust Paediatr J, 1989; 25:243–245
92. Perot P, Weir B, Rasmussen T. Tuberous sclerosis. Surgical therapy for seizures. Arch Neurol (Chic), 1966; 15:498–506

Neurofibromatosis types 1 and 2

93. Recklinghausen F von. Uber die multiplen Fibrome der Haut und ihre Beziehung zu der multiplen Neuromen. Berlin: Hirschwald, 1882
94. Canale DJ, Bebin J. Von Recklinghausen disease of the nervous system. In: Vinken PJ, Bruyn GW, eds. Handbook of clinical neurology, vol.14. The phakomatoses. Amsterdam: North Holland, 1972: pp 132–162
95. Huson SM, Thrush DC. Central neurofibromatosis. Q J Med, 1985; 55:213–224
96. Riccardi VM, Eichner JE. Neurofibromatosis. Phenotype, natural history and pathogenesis. Baltimore: John Hopkins Univ Press, 1986
97. Carey JC, Baty BJ, Johnson JP et al. The genetic aspects of neurofibromatosis. Ann NY Acad Sci, 1986; 486:45–56
98. Baldwin RL, LeMaster K. Neurofibromatois-2 and bilateral acoustic neuromas: distinctions from neurofibromatosis-1 (von Recklinghausen's disease). Am J Otol, 1989; 10:439–442
99. Koch G. Genetic aspects of the phakomatoses. In: Vinken PJ, Bruyn GW, eds. Handbook of clinical neurology, vol.14. The phakomatoses. Amsterdam: North Holland, 1972: pp 488–493
100. von Deimling A, Krone W, Menon AG Neurofibromatosis type 1: Pathology, clinical features and molecular genetics. Brain Pathol, 1995; 5:153–162
101. Upadhyaya M, Maynard J, Osborn M et al. Characterisation of germline mutations in the neurofibromatosis type gene (NF1) gene. J Med Genet, 1995; 32:706–710
102. Easton DF, Ponder MA, Huson SM et al. An analysis of variation in expression of neurofibromatosis (NF) type 1 (NF1). Evidence for modifying genes. Am J Hum Genet, 1993; 53:305–313
103. Metheny LJ, Cappione MS, Skuse GR. Genetic and epigenetic mechanisms in the pathogenesis of neurofibromatosis type 1. J Neuropathol Exp Neurol, 1995; 54:753–760
104. Li Y, Bollag G, Clark R et al. Somatic mutations in the neurofibromatosis 1 gene in human tumours. Cell, 1992; 69:275–281
105. Hattori S, Ohmi N, Maekawa M et al. Antibody against neurofibromatosis type 1 gene product reacts with a triton-insoluble GTPase activating protein towards ras p21. Biochem Biophys Res Commun, 1991; 177:83–89
106. Johnson MR, DeClue JE, Felzmann S et al. Neurofibromin can inhibit Ras-dependant growth by a mechanism independant of its GTPase-accelarating function. Mol Cell Biol, 1994; 14:641–645
107. DeClue JE, Papageorge AG, Fletcher JA et al. Abnormal regulation of mammalian p21ras contributes to malignant tumor growth in von Recklinghausen (type 1) neurofibromatosis. Cell, 1992; 69:265–273
108. Theil G, Marczinek K, Neumann R et al. Somatic mutations in the neurofibromatosis 1 gene in gliomas and primitive neuroectodermal tumours. Anticancer Res, 1995; 15:2495–2499
109. Colman SD, Williams CA, Wallace MR. Benign neurofibromas in type 1 neurofibromatosis (NF1) show somatic deteions of the NF12 gene. Nat Genet, 1995; 11:90–92
110. Martuza RL, Rouleau G. Genetic aspects of neurosurgical problems. In: Youmens JR, ed. Neurological surgery, 3rd edn, vol.2. Philadelphia: Saunders, 1990: Ch 38, pp 1061–1080
111. Rubenstein AE. Neurofibromatosis. A review of the clinical problem. Ann NY Acad Sci, 1986; 486:1–13
112. Musger A. Dermatological aspects of the phakomatoses. In: Vinken PJ, Bruyn GW, eds. Handbook of clinical neurology, vol. 14. The phakomatoses. Amsterdam: North Holland, 1972: pp 562–618
113. Harkin JC. Pathology of nerve sheath tumours. Ann NY Acad Sci, 1986; 486:147–154
114. Scheithauer BW, Waadruff JM, Erlandsen RA. Tumors of the Peripheral Nervous System. Atlas of Tumor Pathology, 3rd series, Fascicle 24. Washington: Armed Forces Institute of Pathology, 1999

115. Schmitt J. Visceral aspects of the phakomatoses. In: Vinken PJ, Bruyn GW, eds. Handbook of clinical neurology, vol. 14. The phakomatoses. Amsterdam: North Holland, 1972: pp 668–730

116. Snover DC, Weigent CE, Sumner HW. Diffuse muscosal ganglioneuromatosis of the colon associated with adenocarcinoma. Am J Clin Pathol, 1981; 75:225–229

117. Urschel JD, Berendt RC, Anselmo JE. Surgical treatment of colonic ganglioneuromatosis in neurofibromatosis. Can J Surg, 1991; 34:271–276

118. Wheeler MH, Curley IR, Williams ED. The association of neurofibromatosis, pheochromocytoma, and somatostatin-rich duodenal carcinoid tumor. Surgery, 1986; 100:1163–1169

119. Ohtsuki Y, Sonobe H, Mizobuchi T et al. Duodenal carcinoid (somatostatinoma) combined with von Recklinghausen's disease. A case report and review of the literature. Acta Pathol Jpn, 1989; 39:141–146

120. Schievink WI, Piepgras DG. Cervical vertebral artery aneurysms and arteriovenous fistulae in neurofibromatosis type 1: case reports. Neurosurgery, 1991; 19:760–765

121. Mallmann R, Roth FJ. Treatment of neurofibromatosis associated renal artery stenosis with hypertension by percutaneous transluminal angioplasty. Clin Exp Hypertens (A), 1986; 8:893–899

122. Flueler U, Boltshauser E, Kilchhofer A. Iris hamartomata as diagnostic criterion in neurofibromatosis. Neuropediatrics, 1986; 17:183–185

123. Huson S, Jones D, Beck L. Ophthalmic manifestations of neurofibromatosis. Br J Ophthalmol, 1987; 71:235–238

124. Francois J. Ocular aspects of the phakomatoses. In: Vinken PJ, Bruyn GW, eds. Handbook of clinical neurology, vol. 14. The phakomatoses. Amsterdam: North Holland, 1972: pp 624–639

125. Williamson TH, Garner A, Moore AT. Structure of Lisch nodules in neurofibromatosis type 1. Ophthalmic Paediatr Genet, 1991; 12:11–17

126. Hunt JC, Pugh DG. Skeletal lesions in neurofibromatosis. Radiology, 1961; 76:1–20

127. Crawford AH. Neurofibromatoses in children. Acta Orthop Scand, 1986; 57:Suppl 218:1–60

128. Rubinstein LJ. The malformative central nervous system lesions in the central and peripheral forms of neurofibromatosis. A clinicopathological study of 22 cases. Ann NY Acad Sci, 1986; 486:14–29

129. Balestrazzi P, de Gressi S, Donadio A et al. Periaqueductal gliosis causing hydrocephalus in a patient with neurofibromatosis type 1. Neurofibromatosis, 1989; 2:322–325

130. Walker AE. Astrocytosis arachnoideae cerebelli: A rare manifestation of von Recklinghausen's neurofibromatosis. Arch Neurol Psychiatry, 1941; 45:520–532

131. Rosman NP, Pearce J. The brain in multiple neurofibromatosis (von Recklinghausen's disease): a suggested neuropathological basis for the associated mental defect. Brain, 1967; 90:829–838

132. Russell DS, Rubinstein LJ. Pathology of tumours of the nervous system, 5th edn. London: Arnold, 1989: pp 769–784

133. Cruz Sanchez F, Cervos-Navarro J, Kashihara M et al. Intracerebral neurinomas in a case of von Recklinghausen's disease (neurofibromatosis) Clin Neuropathol, 1987; 6:174–178

134. Lund AM, Skovby F. Optic gliomas in children with neurofibromatosis type 1. Eur J Pediatr, 1991; 150:835–838

135. Lewis RA, Gerson LP, Axelson KA et al. Von Recklinghausen neurofibromatosis II. Incidence of optic gliomata. Ophthalmology, 1984; 91:929–935

136. Listernick R, Charrow J, Greenwald MJ et al. Optic gliomas in children with neurofibromatosis type 1. J Pediatr, 1989; 114:788–792

137. Borit A, Richardson EP Jr. The biological and clinical behaviour of pilocytic astrocytomas of the optic pathways. Brain, 1982; 105:161–187

138. Stern J, Jakobiec FA, Housepian EM. The architecture of optic nerve gliomas with and without neurofibromatosis. Arch Ophthalmol Ann, 1980; 98:505–511

139. Ilgren EB, Kinneir-Wilson LM, Stiller CA. Gliomas in neurofibromatosis: a series of 89 cases with evidence of enhanced malignancy in associated cerebellar astrocytomas. Pathol Ann (Part I), 1985; 20:331–358

140. Easley JD, Scharf L, Chou JL et al. Controversy in the management of optic pathway gliomas. 29 patients treated with radiation therapy at Baylor College of Medicine from 1967 through 1987. Neurofibromatosis, 1988; 1:248–251

141. Spencer WH, Borit A. Diffuse hyperplasia of the optic nerve in von Recklinghausen's disease. Am J Ophthalmol, 1967; 64:638–642

142. Cooling RJ, Wright JE. Arachnoid hyperplasia in optic nerve glioma: confusion with orbital meningioma. Br J Ophthalmol, 1979; 63:596–599

143. Rodriguez HA, Berthrong M. Multiple primary intracranial tumours in von Recklinghausen's neurofibromatosis. Arch Neurol, 1966; 14:467–475

144. Sorensen SA, Mulvihill JJ, Nielsen A. On the natural history of von Recklinghausen neurofibromatosis. Ann NY Acad Sci, 1986; 486:30–37

145. Ducatman BS, Schiethauer BW, Piepgras DG et al. Malignant peripheral nerve sheath tumours. A clinicopathological study of 120 cases. Cancer, 1986; 57:2006–2021

146. Guccion JG, Enzinger FM. Malignant Schwannoma associated with von Recklinghausen's neurofibromatosis. Virchows Arch (A), 1979; 383:43–57

147. Riccardi VM, Powell PP. Neurofibrosarcoma as a complication of von Recklinghausen neurofibromatosis. Neurofibromatosis, 1989; 2:152–165

148. D'Agostino AN, Soule EH, Miller RH. Sarcomas of the peripheral nerves and somatic soft tissues associated with multiple neurofibromatosis (von Recklinghausen's disease). Cancer, 1963; 16:1015–1027

149. Neilsen GP, Stemmer-Rachamimov AO, Ino Y et al. Malignant transformation of neurofibromas in neurofibromatosis 1 is associated with CDKN2A/p16 inactivation. Am J Pathol, 1999; 155:1879–1884

150. Storm IK, Eilber FR, Mirra J et al. Neurofibrosarcoma. Cancer, 1980; 45:126–129

151. Ishizaki Y, Tada Y, Ishida T et al. Leiomyosarcoma of the small intestine associated with von Recklinghausen's disease: report of a case. Surgery, 1992; 111:706–710

152. Ducatman BS, Scheithauer BW, Dahlin DC. Malignant bone tumors associated with neurofibromatosis. Mayo Clin Proc, 1983; 58:578–582

153. Katz RN, Waye JD, Batzel EL et al. Malignant fibrous histiocytoma of the gastrointestinal tract in a patient with neurofibromatosis. Am J Gastroenterol, 1990; 85:1527–1530

154. Goerg C, Goerg K, Pflueger KH et al. Neurofibromatosis and acute monocytic leukemia in adults. Cancer, 1989; 64:1717–1719

155. Kanter WR, Eldridge R, Fabricant R et al. Central neurofibromatosis with bilateral accoustic neuroma: genetic, clinical and biochemical distinctions from peripheral neurofibromatosis. Neurology, 1980; 30:851–859

156. Louis DN, Ramesh V, Gusella JF. Neuropathology and molecular genetics of neurofibromatosis 2 and related tumours. Brain Pathol, 1995; 5:163–172

157. Ruttledge MH, Anedrmann AA, Phelan CM et al. Type of mutation in the neurofibromatosis type 2 gene (NF2) frequently determines severity of disease. Am J Hum Genet, 1996; 59:331–342

158. Tikoo A, Varga M, Ramesh et al. An anti-Ras function of neurofibromatosis type 2 gene product (NF2/Merlin). J Biol Chem, 1994; 269:23387–23390

159. Lekanne Deprez RH, Bianchi AB, Groen NA et al. Frequent NF2 gene transcript mutations in sporadic meningiomas and vestibular Schwannomas. Am J Hum Genet, 1994; 54:1022–1029

160. Sanson M. A new tumour suppressor gene responsible for type 2 neurofibromatosis is inactivted in neurinoma and meningioma. Rev Neurol, 1996; 152:1–10

161. De Vitis LR, Tedde A, Vitelli F et al. Analysis of the neirofibromatosis type 2 gene in different human tumours of neuroectodermal origin. Hum Genet, 1996; 97:638–641

162. Merel P, Haong-Xuan K, Sanson M et al. Predominant occurrence of somatic mutations of the NF2 gene in meningiomas and Schwannomas. Genes Chromosomes Cancer, 1995; 13:211–216

163. Stemmer-Rachamimov AO, Xu L, Gonzalez-Agosti C et al. Universal absence of merlin, but not other ERM family members, in Schwannomas. Am J Pathol, 1997; 151:1649–1654.

164. Stemmer-Rachamimov AO, Ino Y, Lim ZY et al. Loss of the NF2 gene and merlin occur by the tumorlet stage of Schwannoma development in neurofibromatosis 2. J Neuropathol Exp Neurol, 1998 57:1164–1167

165. Yalcinkaya C, Sarioglu A, Boltshauser E. Neurofibromatosis 2 (bilateral acoustic neurofibromatosis). Schweiz Med Wochenschr, 1989; 14:1416–1420

166. Martuza RL, Ojeman RG. Bilateral acoustic neuromas: Clinical aspects, pathogenesis and treatment. Neurosurgery, 1982; 10:1–12

167. Gutmann DH, Aylsworth A, Carey JC et al. The diagnostic evaluation and multidisciplinary management of neurofibromatosis 1 and neurofibromatosis 2. JAMA, 1997; 278:51–57

168. Halper J, Scheithauer BW, Okazaki H et al. Meningo-angiomatosis: a report of six cases with special reference to the occurrence of neurofibrillary tangles. J Neuropathol Exp Neurol, 1986; 45:426–446

169. Wiestler OD, von Siebenthal K, Schmitt HP et al. Distribution and immunoreactivity of cerebral micro-hamartomas in bilateral acoustic neurofibrillary (neurofibromatosis 2). Acta Neuropathol (Berl), 1989; 79:137–143

170. Hori A. Über intraspinale Schwannosen der Zona terminalis (Lissauer) Formes frustes der Neurofibromatose Recklinghausen oder 'reaktiv'? Acta Neuropathol (Berl), 1973; 25:89–94

171. Constantino PD, Friedman CD, Pelzer HJ. Neurofibromatosis type II of the head and neck. Arch Otolaryngol Head Neck Surg, 1989; 115:380–383

172. Eljamel MS, Foy PM. Multiple meningiomas and their relation to neurofibromatosis. Review of the literature and report of seven cases. Surg Neurol, 1989; 32:131–136

173. Pulst S-M, Rouleau GA, Marineau C et al. Familial meningioma is not allelic to neurofibromatosis 2. Neurology, 1993; 43:2096–2098

174. Michels VV, Whisnant JP, Garrity JA et al. Neurofibromatosis type 1 with bilateral acoustic neuromas. Neurofibromatosis, 1989; 2:213–217

175. Sadeh M, Martinovits G, Goldhammer Y. Occurrence of both neurofibromatoses 1 and 2 in the same individual with a rapidly progressive course. Neurology, 1989; 39:282–283

176. Calzavara PG, Carlino A, Anzola GP et al. Segmental neurofibromatosis. Case report and review of the literature. Neurofibromatosis, 1988; 1:318–322

177. Rawlings CE III, Wilkins RH, Cook WA et al. Segmental neurofibromatosis. Neurosurgery, 1987; 20:946–949

178. Sloan JB, Fretzin DF, Bovenmyer DA. Genetic counselling in segmental neurofibromatosis. J Am Acad Dermatol, 1990; 22:461–467

179. MacCollin M, Woodfin W, Kronn D, Short MP. Schwannomatosis: a clinical and pathological study. Neurology 1996; 46:1072–1059

180. Jacoby LB, Jones D, Davis K et al. Molecular analysis of the NF2 tumor-suppressor gene in schwannomatosis. Am J Hum Genet 1997: 61:1293–1302

181. Theiler R, Stocker H, Boltshauser E. The classification of atypical forms of neurofibromatosis. Schweiz Med Wochenschr, 1991; 121:446–455

von Hippel–Lindau disease

182. Lindau A. Studien über Kleinhirncysten. Bau, Pathogenese und Beziehungen zur Angiomatosis retinae. Acta Pathol Microbiol Scand, 1926; Suppl 1, 1–128

183. von Hippel E. Die anatomische Grundelage der von mir beschreienen sehr seltenen Erkrangung der Netzhaut'. Albrecht v Graefes Arch Ophthalmol, 1911; 79:350

184. Grossman M, Melmon KL. Von Hippel–Lindau disease. In: Vinken PJ, Bruyn GW, eds. Handbook of clinical neurology, vol. 14. The phakomatoses. Amsterdam: North Holland, 1972: pp 241–259

185. Manschot WA. Juxtapapillary retinal angiomatosis. Arch Ophthalmol, 1968; 80:775–776

186. Russell DS, Rubinstein LJ. Pathology of tumours of the nervous system, 5th edn. London: Arnold, 1989; Ch 11, pp 784–787

187. Neumann HP, Wiestler OD. Clustering of features of von Hippel–Lindau syndrome: evidence for a complex genetic locus. Lancet, 1991; 337:1052–1054

188. Maher ER, Iselius L, Yates JR et al. Von Hippel–Lindau disease: a genetic study. J Med Genet, 1991; 28:443–447

189. Koch G. Genetic aspects of the phakomatoses. In: Vinken PJ, Bruyn GW, eds. Handbook of clinical neurology, vol. 14. The phakomatoses. Amsterdam: North Holland, 1972; pp 502–505.

190. Horton WA, Wong V, Eldridge R. Von Hippel–Lindau disease. Clinical and pathological manifestations in nine families with 50 affected members. Arch Int Med, 1976; 136:769–777

191. Neumann HPM, Eggert HR, Scheremet R et al. Central nervous system lesions in von Hippel–Lindau syndrome. J Neurol Neurosurg Psychiatry, 1992; 55:898–901

192. Latif F, Tory K, Gnarra J et al. Identification of the Hippel–Lindau disease tumour suppressor gene. Science, 1993; 260:1317–1320

193. Neumann HP, Lips CJ, Hsia YE et al. Von Hippel–Lindau syndrome. Brain Pathol, 1995; 5:181–193

194. Chen F, Kisheda T, Yao M et al. Germline mutations in the von Hippel–Lindau disease tumour suppressor gene: correlations with phenotype. Hum Mutat, 1995; 5:66–75

195. Glavac D, Neumann HP, Wittke C et al. Mutations in the VHL tumour suppressor gene and associated lesions in families with von Hippel–Lindau disease from central Europe. Hum Genet, 1996; 98:271–280

196. Christoferson LA, Gustafson MB, Petersen AG. Von Hippel–Lindau's disease. J Am Med Assoc, 1961; 178:280–282

197. Kessler PM, Vasavada SP, Rackley RR et al. Expression of the von Hippel–Lindau tumour suppressor gene, VHL, in human fetal kidney and during mouse embryogenesis. Mol Med, 1995; 1:457–466

198. Gnarra JR, Tory K, Weng Y et al. Mutations of the VHL tumour suppressor gene in renal carcinoma. Nat Genet, 1994; 7:85–90

199. Decker HJ, Neuhaus C, Jauch A et al. Detection of a germline mutation and somatic homozygous loss of the von Hippel–Lindau tumor-suppressor gene in a family with a de novo mutation. A combined genetic study, including cytogenetics, PCR/SSCP, FISH and CGH. Hum Genet, 1996; 97:770–776

200. Kanno H, Kondo K, Ito S et al. Somatic mutations of the von Hippel–Lindau tumour suppressor gene in sporadic central nervous system haemangioblastomas. Cancer Res, 1994; 54:4845–4847

201. Oberstrass J, Reifenberger G, Reifenberger J et al. Mutation of the von Hippel–Lindau tumour suppressor gene in capillary haemangioblastomas of the central nervous system. J Pathol, 1996; 179:151–156

202. Francois J. Ocular aspects of the phakomatoses. In: Vinken PJ, Bruyn GW, eds. Handbook of clinical neurology, vol. 14. The phakomatoses. Amsterdam: North-Holland, 1972: Ch 22, pp 644–649

203. Melmon KL, Rosen SW. Lindau's disease. Review of the literature and study of a large kindred. Am J Med, 1964; 36:595–617

204. Hardwig P, Robertson DM. Von Hippel–Lindau disease: a familial, often lethal multi-system phakomatosis. Ophthalmology, 1984; 91:263–270

205. Bradley TE, Young JD, Lentz G. Polycythaemia secondary to phaeochromocytoma. J Urol (Baltimore), 1961; 86:1–6

206. Huson SM, Harper PS, Hourihan MD et al. Cerebellar haemangioblastoma and von Hippel–Lindau disease. Brain, 1986; 109:1297–1310

207. Maher ER, Yates JR, Harries R et al. Clinical features and natural history of von Hippel–Lindau disease. Q J Med, 1990; 77:1151–1163

208. Lamiell JM, Balazar FG, Hsia YE. Von Hippel–Lindau disease affecting 43 members of a single kindred. Medicine (Baltimore), 1989; 68:1–29

209. Schmitt J. Visceral aspects of the phakomatoses. In: Vinken PJ, Bruyn GW, eds. Handbook of clinical neurology, vol. 14. The phakomatoses. Amsterdam: North Holland, 1972: pp 691–696

210. Malek RS, Omess PJ, Benson RC Jr et al. Renal cell carcinoma in von Hippel–Lindau syndrome. Am J Med, 1987; 82:236–238

211. Maher ER. Genetic mechanisms in von Hippel–Lindau disease. Lancet, 1991; 337:1478–1479

212. Le Borgne J. Pancreatic cystadenoma. Ann Chir, 1989; 43:451–457

213. Kragel PJ, Pestaner J, Travis WD et al. Papillary cystadenoma of the epididymis. A report of three cases with lectin histochemistry. Arch Pathol Lab Med, 1990; 114:672–675

214. de Souza Andrade J, Bambirra EA, Bicalho OJ et al. Bilateral papillary cystadenoma of the epididymis as a component of von Hippel–Lindau's syndrome: report of a case presenting as infertility. J Urol, 1985; 133:288–289

215. Gersell DJ, King TC. Papillary cystadenoma of the mesosalpinx in von Hippel–Lindau disease. Am J Surg Pathol, 1988; 12:145–149

216. Poe DS, Tarlov EC, Thomas CB et al. Aggressive papillary tumours of temporal bone. Otolaryngol Head Neck Surg, 1993; 108:80–86

217. Gaffey MJ, Mills SE, Boyd JC. Aggressive papillary tumor of middle ear/temporal bone and adnexal papillary cystadenoma. Manifestations of von Hippel–Lindau disease. Am J Surg Pathol, 1994; 18:1254–1260

218. Hull MT, Warcfel KA, Muller J et al. Familial islet cell tumours in von Hippel–Lindau's disease. Cancer, 1979; 44:1523–1526

219. Griffiths DF, Williams GT, Williams ED. Duodenal carcinoid tumours, phaeochromocytoma and neurofibromatosis: islet cell tumour, phaeochromocytoma and the von Hippel–Lindau complex: two distinctive neuroendocrine syndromes. Q J Med, 1987; 64:769–782

220. Fellows IW, Leach IH, Smith PG et al. Carcinoid tumour of the common bile duct: a novel complication of von Hippel–Lindau syndrome. Gut, 1990; 31:728–729

221. Hall GS. Blood vessel tumours of the brain with particular reference to the Lindau syndrome. J Neurol Psychopathol, 1935; 15:305–312

222. Jakobiec FA, Fond RL, Johnson FB. Angiomatous retinae: An ulstrastructural study and lipid analysis. Cancer, 1976; 38:2042–2056

223. Ridley M, Green J, Johnson G. Retinal angiomatosis: the ocular manifestations of von Hippel–Lindau disease. Can J Ophthalmol, 1986; 21:276–283

224. Goldberg MF, Duke JR. Von Hippel–Lindau disease. Histopathologic findings in a treated and untreated eye. Am J Ophthalmol, 1968; 66:693–705

225. Nicholson DH, Green WR, Kenyon KR. Light and electron microscopic study of early lesions in angiomatosis retinae. Am J Ophthalmol, 1976; 82:193–204

226. Carr TA, Stuard BH. A case of angio-gliomatosis retinae with pathological report. Brit J Ophthalmol, 1933; 17:525–528

227. Filling-Katz MR, Choyke PL, Oldfield E et al. Central nervous system involvement in von Hippel–Lindau disease. Neurology, 1991; 41:41–46

228. Miller MH, Tucker WS, Bilbao JM. Supratentorial hemangioblastoma associated with von Hippel–Lindau disease: case report and review of the literature. Can Assoc Radiol J, 1986; 37:35–37

229. Pou-Serradell A, Mares-Segura R, Lamarca-Ciuro JL. Combined medullary hemangioblastoma and syringomyelia in a patient with von Hippel–Lindau disease: pathological study. Rev Neurol (Paris), 1988; 144:456–458

230. Boughey Am, Fletcher NA, Harding AE. Central nervous system haemangioblastoma: a clinical and genetic study of 52 cases. J Neurol Neurosurg Psychiatry, 1990; 53:644–648

231. Clelland CA, Treip CS. Histological differentiation of metastatic renal carcinoma in the cerebellum from cerebellar haemangioblastoma in von Hippel–Lindau's disease. J Neurol Neurosurg Psychiatry, 1989; 52:162–166

232. Goodbody RA, Gamlen TR. Cerebellar haemangioblastoma and genitourinary tumours. J Neurol Neurosurg Psychiatry, 1974; 37:606–609

233. Craig W McK, Wagener HP, Kernohan JW. Lindau von–Hippel disease: a report of four cases. Arch Neurol Psychiatry, 1941; 46:36–54

234. Pearl GS, Takei Y, Stefanis GS et al. Intraventricular neuroblastoma in a patient with von Hippel–Lindau's disease. Light and electron microscopic study. Acta Neuropathol (Berl), 1981; 53:253–256

235. Bonebrake RA, Siquera EB. The familial occurrence of solitary haemangioblastoma of the cerebellum. Neurology, 1964; 14:743

236. Brinton LF. Hypernephroma – familial occurrence in one family. J Am Med Assoc, 1960; 173:888–890

237. Horbach JM, Brenninkmeyer SJ, van de Velde CJ et al. A forme fruste of von Hippel–Lindau disease: a combination of adrenal phenochromocytoma and ipsilateral renal cell carcinoma: a case report. Surgery, 1989; 105:436–441

238. Olschwang S, Boisson C, Richard S et al. DNA-based presymptomatic diagnosis for the von Hippel–Lindau disease by linkage analysis. Eur J Hum Genet, 1995; 3:108–115

Miscellaneous familial tumour syndromes

239. Li FP, Fraumeni JF Jr. Soft-tissue sarcomas, breast cancer, and other neoplasms. A familial syndrome? Ann Int Med, 1969; 71:747–752

240. Li FP, Fraumeni JF Jr, Hulvihill et al. A cancer family syndrome in twenty-four kindreds. Cancer Res, 1988; 48:5358–5362

241. Birch JM, Hartley AL, Blair V et al. Cancer in the families of children with soft tissue sarcoma. Cancer, 1990; 66:2239–2248

242. Garber JE, Goldstein AM, Kantor AF et al. Follow up study of twenty-four families with Li–Fraumeni syndrome. Cancer Res, 1991; 51:6049–6097

243. Malkin D, Li FP, Strong LC et al. Germ line p53 mutations in a familial syndrome of breast cancer, sarcomas and other neoplasms. Science, 1990; 250:1233–1238

244. Bell DW, Varley JM, Szydlo TE et al. Heterozygous germ line hCHK2 mutations in Li-Fraumeni syndrome. Science, 1999; 286:2528–2531

245. Kleihues P, zurHausen A, Schaube B et al. Tumours associated with p53 germline mutations. A synopsis of 91 families. Am J Pathol, 1997; 150:1–13

246. Greenblatt MS, Bennett, WP, Holstein M et al. Mutations in the p53 tumour suppressor gene: Clues to cancer aetiology and molecular pathogenesis. Cancer Res, 1994; 54:4855–4878

247. Sameshima Y, Tsunematsu Y, Watanabe S et al. Detection of novel germ-line p53 mutations in diverse cancer-prone families identified by selecting patients with childhood adrenocortical carcinoma. J Natl Cancer Inst, 1992; 84:703–707

248. Ohgaki H, Eibl RH, Schwab M et al. Mutations of the p53 tumour suppressor gene in neoplasms of the human nervous system. Mol Carcinogen, 1993; 8:74–80

249. Watanabe K, Tachibana O, Sato K et al. Over expression of the EGF receptor and TP53 mutations are mutually exclusive in the evolution of primary and secondary glioblastomas. Brain Pathol, 1996; 6:217–224

250. Kyritsis AP, Bondy ML, Xiao M et al. Germline p53 gene mutations in subsets of glioma patients. J Natl Cancer Inst, 1994; 86:344–349

251. Louis DN, von Deimling A. Hereditary tumour syndromes of the nervous system: Overview and rare syndromes. Brain Pathol, 1995; 5:145–151

252. Turcot J, Despres JP, St Pierre F. Malignant tumours of the central nervous system associated with familial polyposis of the colon. Dis Colon Rectum, 1959; 2:465–468

253. Itou H, Hirat K, Ohsato K. Turcot's syndrome and familial adenomatuos polyposis associated with brain tumour: Review of related literature. Int J Colorectal Dis, 1993; 8:87–94

254. Hamilton SR, Lui B, Parsons RE et al. The molecular basis of Turcot's syndrome. New Engl J Med, 1995; 332:839–847

255. Mori T, Nagase H, Horii A et al. Germline and somatic mutations of the APC gene in patients with Turcot syndrome and analysis of APC mutations in brain tumours. Genes Chromosomes Cancer, 1994; 9:168–172

256. Gorlin RJ. Nevoid basal-cell carcinoma syndrome. Medicine, 1987; 66:98–113

257. Gailani MR, Bale SJ, Leffell DJ et al. Developmental defects in Gorlin syndrome related to a putative tumour suppressor gene on chromosome 9, Cell, 1992; 69:111–117

258. Johnson RL, Rothman AL, Yie J et al. Human homologue of patched, a candidate gene for the basal cell nevus syndrome. Science, 1996; 272:1668–1771

259. Unden AB, Holmberg E, Lundh-Rozell B et al. Mutations in human homologue of Drosophila patched (PCTH) in basal cell carcinomas and the Gorlin syndrome – different in vivo mechanisms of PCTH inactivation. Cancer Res, 1996; 56:4562–4565

260. Chan GL, Little JB. Cultured diploid fibroblasts from patients with the nevoid basal cell carcinoma syndrome are hypersenitive to ionising radiation. Am J Pathol, 1983; 111:50–55

261. Evans DG, Farndon PA, Burnell LD et al. The incidence of Gorlin syndrome in 173 consecutive cases of medulloblastoma. Br J Cancer, 1991; 64:959–961

262. Schofield D, West DC, Anthony DC et al. Correlation of loss of heterozygosity at chromosome 9q with histological subtype in medulloblastomas. Am J Pathol, 1995; 146:472–480

263. Albrecht S, Goodman JC, Rajagopolan S et al. Malignant meningioma in Gorlin's syndrome: Cytogenetic and p53 gene analysis. Case report. J Neurosurg, 1994; 81:466–471

264. Evans DG, Birch JM, Orton CI. Brain tumours and the occurrence of severe invasive basal cell carcinoma in first degree relatives with Gorlin syndrome. Br J Neurosurg, 1991; 5:643–646

265. Albrecht S, Haber RM, Goodman JC et al. Cowden syndrome and Lhermitte–Duclos disease. Cancer, 1992; 70:869–876

266. Liaw D, Marsh DJ, Li J et al. Germline mutations of the PTEN gene in Cowden disease, an inherited breast and thyroid cancer syndrome. Nature Genet, 1997; 16:64–67

267. Hanssen AM, Werquin H, Suys E et al. Cowden syndrome; Report of a large family with macrocephaly and increased severity of signs in subsequent generations. Clin Genet, 1993; 44:281–286

268. Starink TM, Meijer CJ, Brownstein MH. The cutaneous pathology of Cowden's disease: New findings. J Cutan Pathol, 1985; 12:83–93

269. Starink TM. Cowden's disease: Analysis of fourteen new cases. J Am Acad Dermatol, 1984; 11:1127–1141

270. Carlson GJ, Nivatvongs S, Snover DC. Colorectal polyps in Cowden's disease. Am J Surg Pathol, 1984; 8:763–770

271. Vinchon M, Blond S, Ljeung JP et al. Association of Lhermitte–Duclos disease and Cowden disease; report of a new case and review of the

literature. J Neurol Neurosurg Psychiatry, 1994; 57:699–704

272. Padberg GW, Schot JD, Vielvoye GJ et al. Lhermitte–Duclos disease and Cowden disease: A single phakomatosis. Ann Neurol, 1991; 29:517–523

273. Wells GB, Lasner TM, Yousem DM et al. Lhermitte–Duclos disease and Cowden's syndrome in an adolescent patient. J Neurosurg, 1994; 81:133–136

274. Starink TM et al. The Cowden syndrome: a clinical and genetic study in 21 patients. Clin Genet, 1986; 29:222–223

275. Lyons CJ, Wilson CB, Horton JC. Association between meningioma and Cowden's disease. Neurology, 1993; 43:1436–1437

276. Bagan JV, Penarrocha M, Vera-Sempere F. Cowden syndrome: clinical and pathological considerations in two new cases. J Oral Maxillofacial Surg, 1989; 47:291–294

Neurocutaneous melanosis

277. Rokitansky J. Ein ausgezeichneter Fall von Pigment-Mal mit ausgebreiteter Pigmentierung der inneren Him-und Ruckenmarkshäute. Allg Wein Med Ztg, 1861; 6:113–116

278. Van Bogtaert L. La mélanose neurocutanée diffuse héréadofamiliale. Bull Acad Roy Med (Belg), 1948; 13:397–427

279. Fox H Neurocutaneous melanosis. In: Vinken PJ, Bruyn GW, eds. Handbook of clinical neurology, vol. 14. The phakomatoses. Amsterdam: North Holland, 1972: pp 414–428

280. Kadonaga JN, Frieden IJ. Neurocutaneous melanosis: definition and review of the literature. J Am Acad Dermatol, 1991; 24:747–755

281. Russell DS, Rubinstein LJ. Pathology of tumours of the nervous system, 5th edn. London: Arnold, 1989; pp 792–797

282. Banborschke S, Ebhardt G, Szehes-Stock B et al. Review and case report: primary melanoblastosis of the leptomeninges. Clin Neuropathol, 1985; 4:47–49

283. Fox H, Emery JL, Goodbody RA et al. Neurocutaneous melanosis. Arch Dis Child, 1964; 39:508–516

284. Farnell FJ, Globus JM. Primary melanoblastosis of the leptomeninges and brain. Arch Neurol Psychiatry, 1931; 25:803–823

285. Taft AE. Pigmented cells of pia and of meningeal tumours. Arch Pathol, 1940; 30:1073–1078

286. Faillace WJ, Okawara SH, McDonald JY. Neurocutaneous melanosis with extensive intracerebral and spinal cord involvement. Report of two cases. J Neurosurg, 1984; 61:782–785

287. Koch G. Genetic aspects of the phakomatoses. In: Vinken PJ, Bruyn GW, eds. Handbook of clinical neurology, vol. 14. The phakomatoses. Amsterdam: North Holland, 1972; pp 524–526

288. Musgar A. Dermatological aspects of the phakomatoses. In: Vinken PJ, Bruyn GW, eds. Handbook of clinical neurology, vol. 14. The phakomatoses. Amsterdam: North Holland, 1972; pp 593–601

289. Amir J, Metzker A, Nitzan M. Giant pigmented nevus occurring in one identical twin. Arch Dermatol, 1982; 118:188–189

290. Fischer S. Primary perivascular cerebral cerebellar and leptomeningeal melanoma (congenital aphasia and familial predispostion to naevi verrucosi). Acta Psychiatr Scand, 1956; 31:21–34

291 Happle R. Lethal genes surviving by mocaicism: a possible explanation for sporadic birth defects involving the skir. J Am Acad Dermatol, 1987; 16:899–906

292. Hoffman HJ, Freman A. Primary malignant leptomeningeal melanoma in association with giant hairy naevi. Report of two cases. J Neurosurg, 1967; 26:62–71

293. Humes RA, Roskamp J Eisenbrey AB. Melanosis and hydrocephalus: Report of four cases. J Neurosurg, 1984; 61:365–368

294. Rhodes RE, Friedman HS, Hatten HP Jr et al. Contrast-enhanced MR imaging of neurocutaneous melanosis. Am J Neuroradiol, 1991; 12:380–382

295. Reed WB, Becker SW Sr, Becker SW Jr et al. Giant pigmented nevi, melanoma and leptomeningeal melanocytosis. Arch Dermatol, 1965; 91:100–119

296. Morris U, Danta G. Malignant cerebral melanoma complicating giant pigmented naevus: a case report. J Neurol Neuro surg Psychiatry, 1968; 31:628–632

297. Kadonaga JN, Barkovich AJ, Edwards MB et al. Neurocutaneous melanosis in association with the Dandy-Walker complex. Pediatr Dermatol, 1992; 9:37–43

298. Narayanan HS, Gandhi DH, Girimaji SR. Neurocutaneous melanosis associated with Dandy-Walker syndrome. Clin Neurol Neurosurg, 1987; 89:197–200

299. Sawamura Y, Abe H, Murai H et al. An autopsy case of neurocutaneous melanosis associated with intracerebral malignant melanoma. No To Shinkei, 1987; 39:789–795

300. Wilcox JC. Melanomatosis of the skin and central nervous system in infants. Am J Dis Child, 1939; 57:391–400

301. Kasantikul V, Shuangshoti S, Pattanaruenglia A et al. Intraspinal melanotic arachnoid cyst and lipoma in neurocutaneous melanosis. Surg Neurol, 1989; 31:138–141

302. Van Heuzen EP, Kaiser MC, de Slegte RG. Neurocutaneous melanosis associated with intraspinal lipoma. Neuroradiology, 1989; 31:349–351

303. Slaughter JC, Hardman JM, Kempe LC et al. Neurocutaneous melanosis and leptomeningeal melanomatosis in children. Arch Pathol, 1969; 88:298–304

Sturge–Weber syndrome

304. Alexandre GL. Sturge–Weber Syndrome. In: Vinken PJ, Bruyn GW, eds. Handbook of clinical neurology, vol. 14. The phakomatoses. Amsterdam: North Holland, 1972; pp 223–240

305. Urich H. Malformations of the nervous system, perinatal damage and related conditions in early life. In: Blackwood W, Corsellis JAN, eds. Greenfield's neuropathology, 3rd edn. London: Arnold, 1976; pp 417–419

306. Sturge WA. A case of partial epilepsy, apparently due to a lesion of one of the vasomotor centres of the brain. Trans Clin Soc London, 1879; 12:162–167

307. Kalischer S. Ein Fall von Teleangiectasie (Angiom) des Gesichts und der weichen Himhaut. Arch Psych Nervenkrank, 1901; 34:171–180

308. Craig JM Encephalo-trigeminal angiomatosis (Sturge–Weber's disease). J Neuropathol Exp Neurol, 1949; 8:305–318

309. Peterman AF, Hayles AB, Dockerty MB. Encephalotrigeminal angiomatosis (Sturge–Weber disease). Clinical study of thirty-five cases. J Am Med Assoc, 1958; 167:2169–2176

310. Berg JM, Crome I. Les phakomatoses dans la deficience mentale. In: Michaux L, Feld M, eds. Les phacomatoses cérébrales. Paris: SPEI, 1963: pp 297–304

311. Koch G. Genetic aspects of the phakomatoses. In: Vinken PJ, Bruyn GW, eds. Handbook of clinical neurology, vol. 14. The phakomatoses. Amsterdam: North Holland, 1972; pp 507–514

312. Russell DS, Rubinstein LJ. Pathology of tumours of the nervous system, 5th edn. London: Arnold, 1989; pp 787–792

313. Happle R. Lethal genes surviving by mosaicism: a possible explanation for sporadic birth defects involving the skin. J Am Acad Dermatol, 1987; 16:899–906

314. Francois J. Ocular aspects of the phakomatoses. In: Vinken PJ, Bruyn GW, eds. Handbook of clinical neurology, vol. 14. The phakomatoses. Amsterdam: North Holland, 1972; pp 639–644

315. Wasenko JJ, Rosenbloom SA, Duchesneau PM et al. The Sturge–Weber syndrome: comparison of MR and CT characteristics. Am J Neuroradiol, 1990; 11:131–134

316. Marti-Bonmati L, Menor F, Poyatos C et al. Diagnosis of Sturge–Weber syndrome: comparison of the efficacy of CT and MR imaging in 14 cases. Am J Roentgenol, 1992; 158:867–871

317. Chamberlain MC, Press GA, Hesselink JR. MR imaging and CT in three cases of Sturge–Weber syndrome: prospective comparison. Am J Neuroradiol, 1989; 10:491–496

318. Poser CM, Tavernas JM. Cerebral angiography in encephalotrigeminal angiomatosis. Radiology, 1957; 68:327–336

319. Sperner J, Schmauser I, Bittner R et al. MR imaging findings in children with Sturge–Weber syndrome. Neuropediatrics, 1990; 21:146–152

320. Arnold PG, Meland NB. Tumours of the scalp. In: Youmans JR, ed. Neurological surgery, 3rd edn, vol. 5. Philadelphia: Saunders, 1990: p 3691

321. Fritsch G, Sacher M, Nissen T. Clinical aspects and course of Sturge–Weber syndrome in childhood. Monatsschr Kinderheilkd, 1986; 134:242–245

322. Roizin L, Gold G, Berman HH et al. Congenital vascular anomalies and their histopathology in Sturge–Weber–Dimitri syndrome (naevus flammeus with angiomatosis and encephalosis calcificans). J Neuropathol Exp Neurol, 1959; 18:75–97

323. Schmitt J. Visceral aspects of the phakomatoses. In: Vinken PJ, Bruyn GW, eds. Handbook of clinical neurology, vol. 14. The phakomatoses. Amsterdam: North Holland, 1972; pp 696–699

324. Jorgensen JS, Guthoff R. Sturge–Weber syndrome: glaucoma with elevated episcleral venous pressure. Klin Monatsbl Augenheilkd, 1987; 191:275–278

325. Wagner RS, Caputo AR, Del Negro RG et al. Trabeculectomy with cyclocryotherapy for infantile glaucoma in the Sturge–Weber syndrome. Ann Ophthalmol, 1988; 20:289–291

326. Stimac GK, Solomon MA, Newton TH. CT and MR of angiomatous malformations of the choroid plexus in patients with Sturge–Weber disease. Am J Neuroradiol, 1986; 7:623–627

327. Lichtenstein BW, Rosenberg C. Sturge–Weber–Dimitri's disease. A report of an abortive case with observations of the form, chemical nature and pathogenesis of cerebral cortical concretions. J Neuropathol Exp Neurol, 1947; 6:369–382

328. Norman MG, Schoene WC. The ultrastructure of Sturge–Weber disease. Acta Neuropathol (Berl), 1977; 37:199–205

329. Nellhaus G, Haberland C, Hill BJ. Sturge–Weber disease with bilateral intracranial calcifications at birth and unusual pathologic findings. Acta Neurol Scand, 1967; 43:314–317

330. Divry P, van Bogaert L. Une maladie familiale caractérisee par une angiomatose diffuse corticoméningée non calcifiante at une démyélinisation progressive de la substance blanche. J Neurol Neurosurg Psychiatry, 1946; 9:41–54

331. Haemerlinck C, Myle G, von Bogaert L. Angiomatose encéphalo-trigéminée (Sturge–Weber) sans calcifications radiologiquement decelables. Observation anatano-clinique. J Neurol Neurosurg Psychiatry, 1947; 10:93–100

332. Bebin EM, Gomez MR. Prognosis in Sturge–Weber disease: comparison of unihemispheric and bihemispheric involvement. J Child Neurol, 1988; 3:181–184

333. Ito M, Sato K, Ohnuki A et al. Sturge–Weber disease: operative indications and surgical results. Brain Dev, 1990; 12:473–477

Hereditary haemorrhagic telangiectasia

334. Peery WH. Clinical spectrum of hereditary hemorrhagic telangiectasia. Am J Med 1987; 82:989–997

335. Plauchu H, de Chadarevian JP, Bideau A et al. Age-related clinical profile of hereditary hemorrhagic telangiectasia in an epidemiologically recruited population. Am J Med Genet, 1989; 32:291–297

336. Roman G, Fisher M, Perl DP et al. Neurological manifestations of hereditary hemorrhagic telangiectasia (Rendu-Osler-Weber disease): report of 2 cases and a review of the literature. Ann Neurol, 1978; 4:130–144

337. Jessurun GA, Nossent JC. Cerebrovascular accidents at a young age in Rendu–Osler–Weber disease: a survey in the Netherlands Antilles. Ned Tijdschr Geneeskd, 1992; 136:428–431

338. Shovlin CL. Molecular defects in rare bleeding disorders: hereditary haemorrhagic telangiectasia. Thromb Haemostasis, 1997; 78:145–150

339. Kissel P, Dureux JB. Ullman syndrome Systemic angiomatosis. In: Vinken PJ, Bruyn GW, eds. Handbook of clinical neurology, vol. 14. The phakomatoses. Amsterdam: North Holland, 1972; pp 446–454

340. Piepgras U, Sielecki S. Lung involvement in Osler's disease and its cerebral complications. Radiologe, 1986; 26:27–30

341. Zelman S. Liver fibrosis in hereditary haemorrhagic telangiectasia. Fibrosis of diffuse insular character. Arch Pathol, 1962; 74:66–72

342. Braverman IM, Keh A, Jacobson BS. Ultrastructure and three-dimensional organization of the telangiectases of hereditary hemorrhagic telangiectasia. J Invest Dermatol, 1990; 95:422–427

343. Peruzzi P, Scherpereel B, Rouger C et al. Cerebral abscess and Osler–Rendu disease. Apropos of 4 cases. Neurochirurgie, 1988; 34:179–187

344. Heffner RR Jr, Solitaire GB. Hereditary haemorrhagic telangiectasia: neuropathological observations. J Neurol Neurosurg Psychiatry, 1969; 32:604–608

345. Aesch B, Lioret E, de Toffol B et al. Multiple cerebral angiomas and Rendu–Osler–Weber disease: case report. Neurosurgery, 1991; 29:599–602

346. Lesser BA, Wendt D, Miks VM et al. Identical twins with hereditary hemorrhagic telangiectasia concordant for cerebrovascular arteriovenous malformations. Am J Med, 1986; 81:931–934

347. Snyder LH, Doan CA. Studies in human inheritance: is homozygous form of multiple telangiectasia lethal? J Lab Clin Med, 1944; 29:1211–1216

348. McFarlin DE, Strober W, Waldmann TA. Ataxia telangiectasia. Medicine, 1972; 51:281–314

349. Sedgwick RP, Boder E. Ataxia telangiectasia. In: Vinken PJ, Bruyn GW, eds. Handbook of clinical neurology, vol. 14. The phakomatoses. Amsterdam: North Holland, 1972; pp 267–339

350. Swift M, Morrell D, Cromartie E et al. The incidence and gene frequency of ataxia-telangiectasia in the United States. Am J Hum Genet, 1986; 39:573–583

351. Lange E, Borresen AL, Chen X et al. Localisation of an ataxia-telangiectasia gene to an approximately 500-kb interval on chromosome l1 q23.1: linkage analysis of 176 families by an international consortium. Am J Hum Genet, 1995; 57:112–119

352. Rotman G, Shiloh Y. The ATM gene and protein: possible roles in genome surveillance, checkpoint controls and cellular defence against oxidative stress. Cancer Surv, 1997; 29:285–304

353. Hayakawa H, Kobayashi N, Yata J. Primary immunodeficiency diseases and malignancy in Japan. Jpn J Cancer Res, 1986; 77:74–79

354. Morrell D, Cromartie E, Swift M. Mortality and cancer incidence in 263 patients with ataxia-telangiectasia. J Natl Cancer Inst, 1986; 77:89–92

355. McKinnon PJ. Ataxia-telangiectasia: an inherited disorder of ionizing-radiation sensitivity in man. Progress in the elucidation of the underlying biochemical defect. Hum Genet, 1987; 75:197–208

356. Aguilar MJ, Kamoshita S, Landing BH et al. Pathological observations in ataxia-telangiectasia. A report on five cases. J Neuropathol Exp Neurol, 1968; 27:659–676

357. Woods CG, Taylor AM. Ataxia telangiectasia in the British Isles: the clinical and laboratory features of 70 affected individuals. Q J Med, 1992; 82:169–179

358. Amromin GD, Boder E, Teplitz R. Ataxia-telangiectasia with a 32-year survival. A clinico-pathological report. J Neuropathol Exp Neurol, 1979; 38:621–643

359. Strich SJ. Pathological findings in three cases of ataxia-telangectasia. J Neurol Neurosurg Psychiatry, 1966; 29:489–499

360. Barbieri F, Santoro L, Crisci C et al. Is the sensory neuropathy in ataxia-telangiectasia distinguishable from that in Friedreich's ataxia? Morphometric and ultrastructural study of the sural nerve in a case of Louis–Bar syndrome. Acta Neuropathol (Berl), 1986; 69:213–219

361. Hart RM, Kimler BF, Evans RG et al. Radiotherapeutic management of medulloblastoma in a pediatric patient with ataxia telangiectasia. Int J Radiat Oncol Biol Phys, 1987; 13:1237–1240

362. Young RR, Austen KF, Moser HW. Abnormalities of serum gamma 1A globulin and ataxia telangiectasia. Medicine (Baltimore), 1964; 43:423–433

363. Boder E, Sedgwick RP. Ataxia telangiectasia. A familial syndrome of progressive cerebellar ataxia, oculocutaneous telangectasia and frequent pulmonary infection. Pediatrics, 1958; 21:526–554

364. Solitaire GB, Lopez VF. Louis–Bar's syndrome (ataxia telangiectasia). Neuropathological observations. Neurology, 1963; 17:23–31

365. Sourander P, Bonnevier JO, Olsson Y. A case of ataxia-telangiectasia with lesions in the spinal cord. Acta Neurol Scand, 1966; 42:354–366

366. Lecuire J, Dechaume JP, Bret P. Bonnet–Dechaume–Blanc syndrome. In: Vinken PJ, Bruyn GW, eds. Handbook of clinical neurology, vol. 14. The phakomatoses. Amsterdam: North Holland, 1972; pp 260–266

Mesencephalo-oculo-facial angiomatosis

367. Kikuchi K, Kowada M, Sakamoto T et al. Wyburn–Mason syndrome: report of a rare case with computerised tomography and angiographic evaluations. J Comput Tomogr, 1988; 12:111–115

368. Fujita H, Nakano K, Kumon Y et al. A case of Wyburn–Mason syndrome. Rinsho Skinkeigaku, 1989; 29:1039–1044

369. Maeda H, Fujieda M, Morita H et al. Wyburn–Mason syndrome: a case report. No To Hattatsu, 1992; 24:65–69

370. Wyburn-Mason R. Arteriovenous aneurysm of mid-brain and retina, facial naevi and mental changes. Brain, 1943; 66:163–203

Cutaneous angiomatosis

371. Kissel P, Xureux JB. Cobb syndrome. Cutaneomeningo-spinal angiomatosis. In: Vinken PJ, Bruyn GW, eds. Handbook of clinical

neurology, vol. 14. The phakomatoses. Amsterdam: North Holland, 1972; pp 429–445

372. Lie JT. Pathology of angiodysplasia in Klippel–Trenaunay syndrome. Pathol Res Pract, 1988; 183:747–755

Familial cavernous angiomas

373. Smit LME, Barth PG, Stam FC et al. Congenital multiple angiomatosis with brain involvement. Childs Brain, 1981; 8:461–467

374. Wood MW, White RJ, Kernohan JW. Cavernous hemangiomatosis involving the brain, spinal cord, heart, skin and kidney. Mayo Clin Proc, 1957; 32:249–254

375. Couteulx SL, Jung HH, Labauge P et al. Truncating mutations in CCM1, encoding KRIT1, cause hereditary cavernous angiomas. Nature Genet, 1999; 23:189–193

20 Complications of tumours and effects of treatment

The complications of nervous system tumours can be divided into three main categories: their mass effect on surrounding structures, the problems resulting from surgical intervention and the adverse results of adjuvant therapy. For intracranial lesions, mass effect is perhaps the most significant clinical problem because of the resulting increase in intracranial pressure and its life threatening sequelae. However, the effects of surgery and adjuvant antineoplastic therapy are also recognised as causing serious problems in both the brain and spinal cord. Such treatment related complications are common and relate to both radiotherapy and chemotherapy. Importantly, some of the changes cause by radiotherapy may be clinically confused with disease recurrence and the distinction between radiation necrosis and tumour growth can be a diagnostic challenge.

Mass effect and raised intracranial pressure

The rigid confines of the intracranial compartment mean that any mass lesion at this site has the potential to cause an increase in intracranial pressure. This is especially true of neoplasms because of their capacity for continuing growth, and the clinical results of increased pressure are clearly most threatening in malignant, rapidly growing tumours. Raised intracranial pressure is not just caused by intrinsic tumour bulk, however, and the most important causes of tumour related mass effect are as follows:

- Tumour growth
- Cerebral oedema
- Intratumoral haemorrhage
- Hydrocephalus.

Additionally, biopsy or treatment related events may cause swelling either within tumour or surrounding brain, thereby contributing to mass effects. In one large published series the most common findings on computerised tomography (CT) scanning in patients with elevated intracranial pressure after elective neurosurgery were cerebral oedema and bleeding into the tumour bed.[1]

Cerebral oedema

Cerebral oedema associated with tumours is believed to be vasogenic in origin and is seen in relation to intrinsic glial, metastatic and some extrinsic tumours, especially meningiomas. Ultrastructural studies of vessels in tumour and adjacent brain support this. Tumour blood vessels show an increase in pinocytotic vesicles, with vacuolation in endothelial cells. Peritumoral blood vessels also show increased pinocytotic vesicles.[2,3] In severe oedema, transendothelial channels can be seen formed by chains of fused pinocytic vacuoles.[4] In experimentally induced brain tumours in rats protein extravasation across tumour vessels occurs via pinocytotic vesicles. Serum proteins then spread through the extracellular space.[5]

Estimates of the rate of production of oedema fluid have been made in vivo in patients with gliomas and metastatic tumours, suggesting ranges between 0.09 and 1.63 ml/h in metastases and between 0.42 and 3.49 ml/h in gliomas. The speed of oedema propagation has also been estimated, ranging from 0.2 to 2.2 mm/h. Such studies suggest that in large tumours most oedema fluid is draining into the ventricular and/or subarachnoid cerebrospinal fluid (CSF).[6] Positive correlations have been found between water content and both serum protein levels and sodium content in tumours and peritumoral oedema, suggesting that both these components are important in driving the extravasation of plasma derived oedema fluid.[7]

Vascular endothelial growth factor (VEGF) (formerly known as vascular permeability factor, (VPF) has been suggested as a likely mediator of disrupted blood–brain barrier (BBB) function in tumour capillaries.[8–11] Other mediators have been proposed. Intracarotid infusion of leukotrienes, bradykinin and other vasoactive agents can cause disruption of the BBB leading to oedema and this has been proposed as a way of increasing drug delivery to the brain.[12] Tumour prostaglandin levels have been suggested to correlate with oedema around supratentorial meningiomas.[13] The possible contribution of peritumoral inflammation has also been suggested.[14] In a case of malignant brain oedema after stereotactic radiosurgery, tissue showed very high levels of gelatinase B (92 kDa type IV collagenase) and urokinase type plasminogen activator suggesting a role in pathogenesis.[15] Corticosteroids have been shown to be effective in the clinical management of vasogenic oedema associated with cerebral tumours by decreasing the increased capillary permeability of the BBB. It has been suggested that dexamethasone may decrease brain tumour associated vascular permeability by two glucocorticoid receptor dependent mechanisms: reduction of the response of the vasculature to tumour derived permeability factors (including VEGF), and reduction of VEGF expression by tumour cells.[9]

Oedema related specifically to meningiomas has been investigated in several studies, implicating both tumour derived and vascular factors. Peritumoral oedema has been found to be least in meningiomas lacking a cerebral-pial supply[16] and in those with little VEGF expression. It has been suggested that VEGF expression may only contribute to oedema formation in meningiomas which have a cerebral-pial blood supply.[17] The growth fraction of meningiomas, as determined by Ki-67/MIB-1 immunostaining, shows a relationship between tumour proliferation and oedema development.[18] Lastly, the idea that tumour related venous obstruction plays a role in the development of oedema has not been substantiated for the majority of meningiomas.[19] However, compression and obstruction of normal perivascular fluid drainage

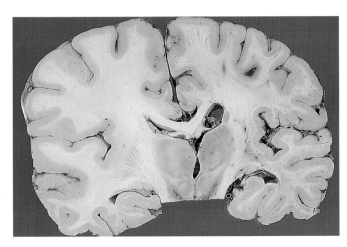

Fig. 20.1 **Cerebral oedema.** There is marked oedema of the left cerebral hemisphere with flattening of surface convolutions and midline shift.

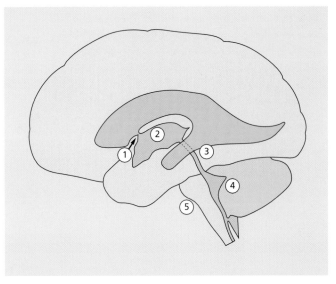

Fig. 20.2 **Hydrocephalus.** Diagram of the brain and the ventricular system showing common sites at which the CSF flow may be obstructed by tumour. **(1)** Foramen of Monro between the lateral ventricles and the third ventricle; **(2)** third ventricle; **(3)** aqueduct of Sylvius; **(4)** fourth ventricle; **(5)** subarachnoid space on the surface of the brain.

pathways has been proposed as a mechanism of oedema development.[20] Peritumoral vasogenic oedema has been implicated in the development of tumour related cysts.[21,22]

Macroscopically, brain affected by oedema shows expansion of the white matter with flattening of overlying cortex (Fig. 20.1). Oedema may be seen to spread along fibre tracts including the visual pathways or the corpus callosum. The mass effect of oedematous brain may distort adjacent structures. Histologically oedematous brain shows microvacuolation in white matter. Swollen astrocytes may be seen, especially in cases of long standing oedema.

Hydrocephalus

CSF is produced by the choroid plexuses of the lateral ventricles, third ventricle and fourth ventricle. Fluid produced in the lateral ventricles flows into the third ventricle through the relatively narrow foramina of Monro, and through the third ventricle into the narrow aqueduct between the third and fourth ventricles. Leaving the fourth ventricle through the paired foramina of Luschka and the median foramen of Magendi, CSF enters the subarachnoid space from which it flows either into the spinal canal, into the cisterns over the front of the pons and between the cerebral peduncles or over the surface of the brain to drain into the blood via the arachnoid granulations and villi in the major venous sinuses such as the superior sagittal sinus and cavernous sinus.

Obstruction to the flow of CSF by a tumour may occur at various points along the outflow pathway (Fig. 20.2), but is especially seen with tumours adjacent to the cerebral aqueduct or the exit foramina at the base of the brain.[23] If such an obstruction occurs, dilatation of the ventricular system occurs with the onset of obstructive hydrocephalus. The major effects of hydrocephalus on the brain are seen

initially in the periventricular white matter of the cerebral hemispheres. As the pressure in the ventricles rises, CSF is forced into the periventricular white matter, resulting in interstitial oedema which may be identified as low density areas on CT or magnetic resonance imaging (MRI). If the high pressure persists, there is progressive destruction of nerve fibres in the white matter and gliosis. The acute onset of hydrocephalus in adults in whom the sutures of the skull have fused leads to a rapid rise in intracranial pressure which, if not relieved, may result in death of the patient. In infants with unfused sutures, expansion of the skull occurs with separation of the skull bones and widening of the sutures, but with little rise in intracranial pressure. Nevertheless, distruction of brain tissue occurs with hydrocephalus in the infant brain, with axonal degeneration and gliosis in the periventricular white matter and relative sparing of the periventricular grey matter and the cortex. If the hydrocephalus becomes stablised, the periventricular oedema may disappear but the ventricles remain enlarged with thinning and gliosis of the periventricular white matter.

There are a number of different sites at which different tumours may grow and cause hydrocephalus. These sites are depicted in Fig. 20.2 and in Table 20.1.

Raised intracranial pressure and cerebral herniation

Clinical effects of raised intracranial pressure are a common complication of a tumour either in presentation or following therapy. In one series the most important risk

Table 20.1 Brain tumour as a cause of hydrocephalus
(tumours commonly causing obstruction at sites depicted in
Figure 20.2)

1. *Foramen of Monro*
   Choroid plexus papilloma
   Colloid cyst
   Central neurocytoma
   Thalamic astrocytoma compressing the foramen
   Subependymal giant cell astrocytoma
   Metastatic carcinoma

2. *Third ventricle*
   Pituitary adenoma
   Craniopharyngioma
   Neurocytoma
   Thalamic astrocytoma
   Choroid plexus papilloma
   Pineal tumours

3. *Aqueduct of Sylvius*
   Pineal tumours
   Astrocytoma of the midbrain

4. *Fourth ventricle*
   Ependymoma
   Choroid plexus papilloma
   Cerebellar primitive neuroectodermal tumour
      (medulloblastoma)
   Cerebellar pilocytic astrocytoma
   Cerebellar metastasis
   Pontine astrocytoma
   Schwannoma
   Meningioma
   Glomus jugulare tumour
   Metastatic carcinoma in the cerebellum

5. *Subarachnoid space*
   Carcinomatous meningitis

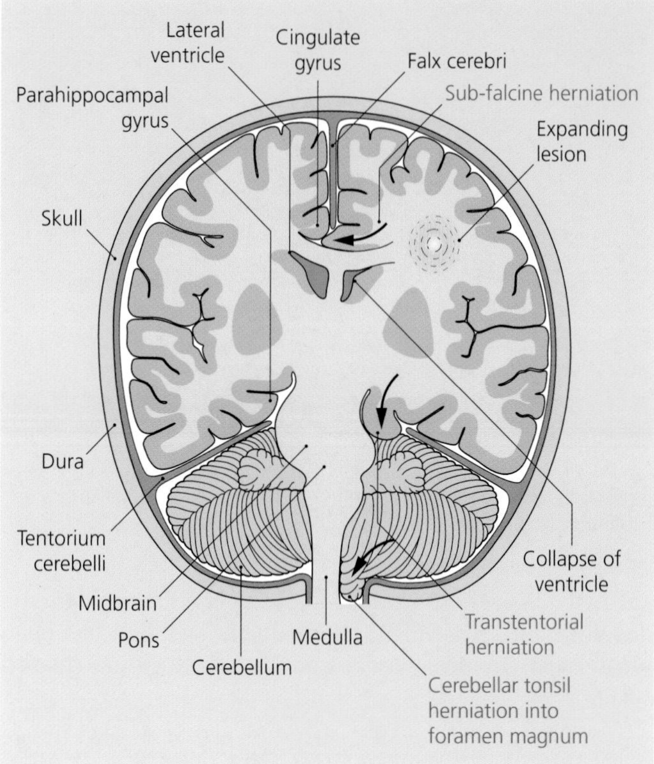

Fig. 20.3 **Types of internal herniation resulting from an intracranial mass lesion.** Pressure gradients resulting from a tumour sited in one cerebral hemisphere may result in sideways midline shift with subfalcine herniation of the cingulated gyrus and/or downward displacement through the tentorial orifice with herniation of the parahippocampal gyrus. Further downward pressure gradients across the posterior fossa lead to herniation of cerebellar tonsils through the foramen magnum.

factors for postoperative intracranial pressure elevation were: resection of glioblastoma, repeat surgery cases, and protracted surgery (greater than 6 h). About 50% of patients who develop postoperative raised intracranial pressure have an associated clinical deterioration.[1]

Intracranial pressure When pressure begins to exceed the upper range of normal for minutes at a time brain damage may occur:

- Mild rises to 15–22 mmHg are reasonably well tolerated.
- Moderate rises to 30 mmHg require intervention.
- Severe rises above 37.5 mmHg are associated with ischaemic brain damage.
- Pressures above 60 mmHg often indicate a terminal state.
- When intracranial pressure reaches the level of arterial pressure then cerebral blood flow ceases and all neurological functions fail.

When intracranial pressure cannot be controlled there may be development of internal cerebral herniations (Fig. 20.3).

Reduced volume of intracranial CSF is an important mechanism in spatial compensation. However, when CSF volumes are reduced in a particular region the localised reductions in pressure cause brain substance to flow into the space (away from the increased pressure produced by the lesion). This can result in the movement of brain tissue from one cranial compartment into another – herniation (Figs 20.4–20.6). There are three sites at which this often occurs to give supracallosal, tentorial and tonsillar herniation.

With severe, persisting herniation there is descent of diencephalic structures and descent of the pons. The brain stem becomes kinked in an anterior – posterior direction and penetrating vessels leading into the upper pons come under traction. This leads to bleeding into the upper pons. This is termed a Duret haemorrhage and is a late secondary consequence of raised intracranial pressure (Figs 20.7–20.13). Early lesions are seen as linear areas of haemorrhage in the midline, while later lesions show extensive haemorrhagic necrosis of the pons. In coronal section the pattern of lesions and relation to

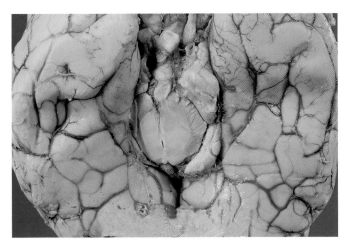

Fig. 20.4 **Cerebral herniation.** Parahippocampal gyral hernia. There has been herniation of the parahippocampal gyrus through the tentorial hiatus leading to a groove produced by the free edge of the tentorium cerebelli. Histological examination of the herniated region reveals small haemorrhages and necrosis.

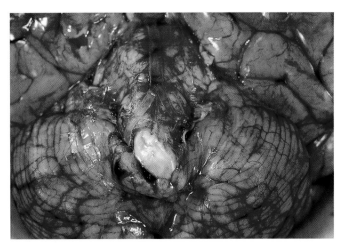

Fig. 20.6 **Tonsillar hernia.** There has been herniation of the cerebellar tonsils and medulla. Prominent cerebellar tonsils are often mistaken for herniated cerebellar tonsils. Histological examination, showing necrosis of herniated tissue, will usually resolve any diagnostic uncertainty.

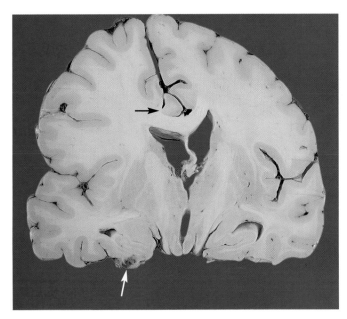

Fig. 20.5 **Cerebral herniation.** Herniation contusions (arrow) may be visible where the uncus or parahippocampal gyrus has been pressed against the free edge of the tentorium. Histological examination would reveal small haemorrhages and necrosis. There has also been displacement of midline structures causing subfalcine herniation of the cingulated gyrus (arrowhead).

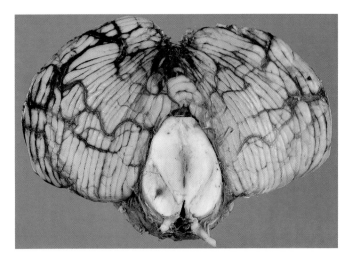

Fig. 20.7 **Effects of internal herniation.** With severe persisting herniation there is downwards displacement of diencephalic structures and descent of the pons, resulting in anteroposterior kinking of the brain stem with traction on the extramedullary segments of penetrating arteries and compression of their intramedullary segments. This results in foci of necrosis, and haemorrhages termed Duret haemorrhages, in the midbrain and upper pons. Small Duret haemorrhages appear as a linear area of midline haemorrhage.

kinking of the upper brain stem can be seen (Figs 12.11–12.12). It is important to recognise the secondary nature of this lesion and not attribute the bleeding to primary pontine haemorrhage.

A further complication of downward transtentorial herniation is caused by kinking and compression of the posteror cerebral arteries as they pass over the free edge of the tentorial membrane. In severe cases this compression leads to infarction of the inferior and medial parts of the occipital lobe, which may be uniateral or bilateral depending on whether the herniation is symmetric or one-sided (Figs 20.14–20.16). The calcarine branches are particularly susceptible, and in some surviving patients selective calcarine cortex infarction may lead to cortical blindness.

Effects of biopsy and surgery

Complications of surgical intervention in brain tumours can be divided into three groups (Table 20.2).[24–33]

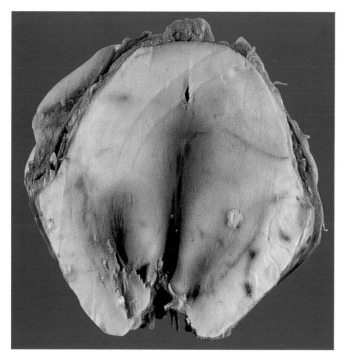

Fig. 20.8 **Effects of internal herniation.** A more severe lesion associated with haemorrhage in the midline and substantia nigra.

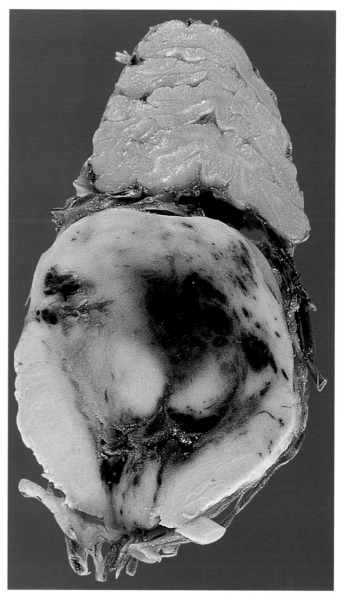

Fig. 20.9 **Effects of internal herniation.** Duret haemorrhages appearing as extensive foci of haemorrhagic necrosis.

The mechanical effects of the surgical procedures themselves constitute an iatrogenic form of trauma and can be associated with a wide range of complications and secondary effects. The risks of surgery will obviously depend on the skill of the surgeon, the site and accessibility of the tumour and the precise nature of the procedure – in particular whether a biopsy or larger scale craniotomy debulking is being performed. Modern microsurgical techniques and the advent of image guidance have greatly diminished complications directly related to surgery in tumour patients, and the trauma to the brain caused by stereotactic biopsy is usually remarkably small, despite the invasive nature of many such procedures (Figs 20.17–20.20). Haemorrhage and acute brain swelling are the most important adverse events that can arise at the time of surgery, but there are a number of delayed effects which may complicate the postoperative period and are directly related to the operative procedure. Prominent among these are delayed brain swelling or haemorrhage, CSF leaks, infection and epileptic seizures (Table 20.2).

Effects of adjuvant antineoplastic therapy

Radiotherapy

Effects of radiotherapy on tumours The histology of tumours may be altered by previous radiotherapy which may lead to problems in diagnosis. Radiotherapy may cause the following effects:

Table 20.2 Complications of surgical intervention in brain tumours

Intraoperative	Immediate postoperative	Late postoperative
Haemorrhage	Brain swelling	Meningitis
Acute brain swelling	Haemorrhage	Ventriculitis
	CSF leak	Cerebritis
	Diabetes insipidus	Aneurysm
	(especially seen in	CSF leak
	postsurgical excision	Epilepsy
	of craniopharyngioma	
	or pituitary adenoma)	

CSF, cerebrospinal fluid

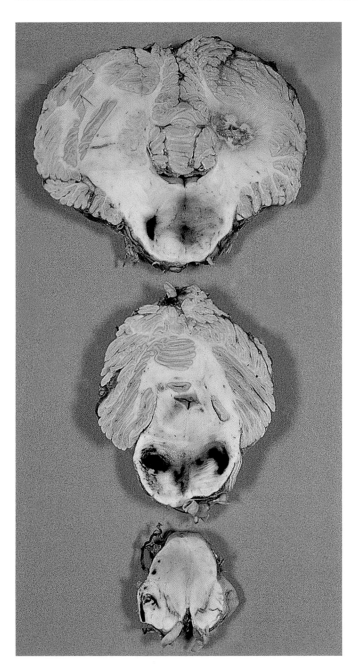

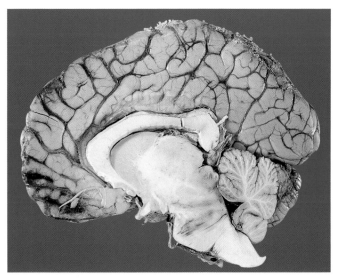

Fig. 20.11 **Effects of internal herniation.** Sagittal section demonstrating buckling of the upper brain stem and the distribution of early Duret haemorrhages.

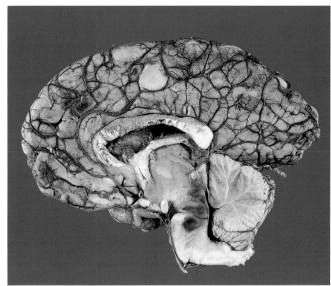

Fig. 20.12 **Effects of internal herniation.** Sagittal section demonstrating buckling of the upper brain stem and the distribution of later, more extensive Duret haemorrhages.

Fig. 20.10 **Effects of internal herniation.** Marked haemorrhage and necrosis in the pons.

Necrosis Following therapeutic irradiation, tumours commonly develop large areas of necrosis. Later, areas of necrosis are replaced by cystic areas lined by astroglial cells associated with hyalinised blood vessels.

Fibrinoid necrosis in vessels is seen in vessels in both tumour and adjacent brain. This may be seen in the early as well as late stages of radiotherapy.

Nuclear pleomorphism and hyperchromasia are seen as cytological features in both neoplastic and reactive cells in the radiotherapy field. In some cases the interpretation of repeat biopsies following radiotherapy may be confused by the presence of such pleomorphic cells. The main problem is in distinguishing between residual tumour and delayed radionecrosis (see below).

In the interpretation of any repeat biopsy sample, awareness that there has been previous radiotherapy is vital if the changes listed above are to be properly interpreted.

Effects of radiotherapy on normal brain Post-irradiation reactions in the brain can be divided into acute/subacute and late reactions.[34] While most cases have been associated with irradiation of intracranial lesions, some have

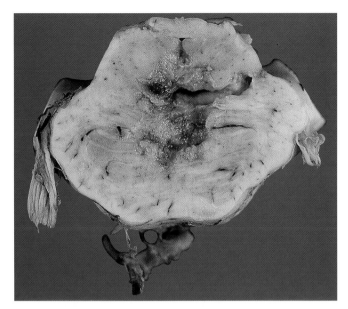

Fig. 20.13 **Effects of internal herniation.** Although internal herniation and brain stem haemorrhage are usually terminal events, rarely survival is long term, in which case the lesions in the midbrain and pons undergo organisation and appear as soft cystic areas of cavitation.

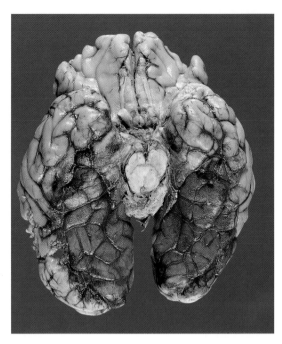

Fig. 20.15 **Infarction of occipital lobes secondary to transtentorial herniation.** In this case, the infarction is extensive and symmetrical (in contrast to Fig. 20.14).

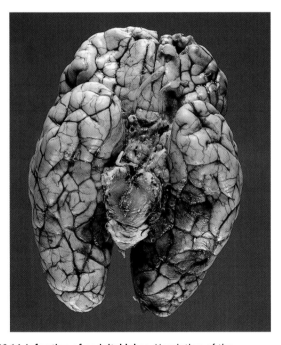

Fig. 20.14 **Infarction of occipital lobes.** Herniation of the parahippocampal gyrus causes branches of the posterior cerebral vessels supplying the occipital lobe to be compressed.

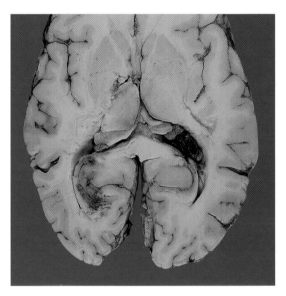

Fig. 20.16 **Infarction of occipital lobes secondary to transtentorial herniation.** It is important to recognise the secondary nature of the infarction and not mistake this for a primary pathology.

been described associated with extracranial lesions.[35] Brain necrosis in adults is rarely seen below 6000 cGy using conventional fractionation, and imaging and clinically symptomatic effects are generally observed only above 5000 cGy.[36] Radiation encephalopathy is a clinical diagnostic term that refers to the presence of significant cognitive or emotional dysfunction following radiation therapy to the brain. Studies suggest that about 30% of patients who receive cranial irradiation develop this syndrome, although the morphological basis in all cases remains uncertain.[37]

Acute complications of radiotherapy are mainly related to development of oedema and are commonly associated with symptoms which are treatable with steroids, and are

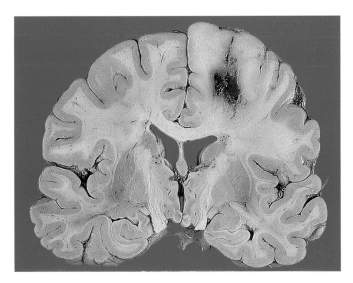

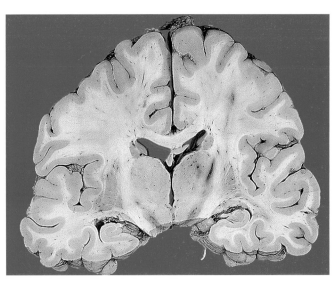

Fig. 20.17 Stereotactic biopsy track. This patient with a low grade oligodendroglioma underwent stereotactic biopsy approximately 2 days before sudden death from pulmonary thromboembolism. Note the area of haematoma at the site of biopsy. Mass effect is attributed to the tumour rather than the biopsy procedure. The ventricular system is not distorted.

Fig. 20.18 Stereotactic biopsy track. This patient died of a pulmonary thromboembolism 1 week after a stereotactic biopsy of a lesion in the pons. The track can be seen running down from the cortex, past the internal capsule.

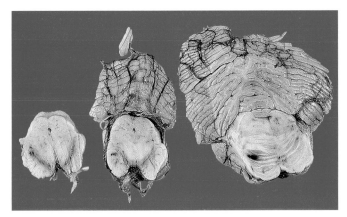

Fig. 20.19 Stereotactic biopsy track. Same patient as in Fig. 20.18. The track passses down adjacent to the cerebral peduncle in the midbrain.

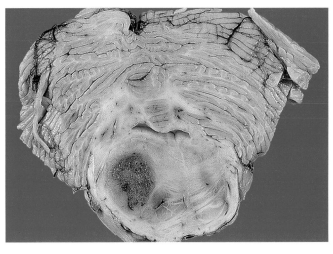

Fig. 20.20 Stereotactic biopsy track. Same patient as in Figs 20.18 and 20.19. The lesion in the pons was determined to be a high grade astroglial neoplasm.

transient in the majority of cases.[38–40] In one series the incidence of symptomatic oedema after radiosurgery for meningioma was 16%, being more common with larger tumours.[41] The main risk factors for the development of panhemispheric oedema are therapy for large tumours, administration of single fraction stereotactic radiosurgery, or the use of more than 600 cGy per fraction.[42]

Late radiation injury is an important complication of brain irradiation and occurs in two forms, focal and diffuse, related to dose.[43] In experimental studies, vascular damage is thought to be the main pathogenic mechanism[44] and is

believed to be dose dependent.[45] Late development of focal oedema is commonly noted on imaging following focal or large volume irradiation and is usually asymptomatic.[43]

Focal radionecrosis may occur as either a subacute or late effect of radiotherapy. CT and MRI show features of a heterogeneous mass lesion, and this is usually associated with clinical evidence of neurological deterioration and, when extensive, features of raised intracranial pressure. Macroscopically, affected areas appear as geographic areas of necrosis, often surrounded by firm,

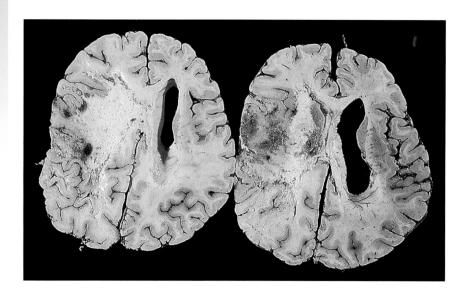

Fig. 20.21 **Focal radiation necrosis.** Extensive necrosis in cerebral hemisphere with mass effect as a result of irradiation necrosis.

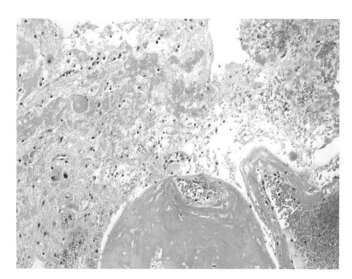

Fig. 20.22 **Radiation necrosis histology.** Necrotic lesion showing hyalinisation of vessels.

yellow rubbery tissue (Fig. 20.21). Multifocal lesions have been described.[46] Histologically, necrotic lesions show hyalinisation and fibrinoid necrosis of vessels (Fig. 20.22). White matter at the margin of lesions may show myelin loss and astrocytic gliosis while in the central regions there is overt coagulative necrosis. Foam cells may be prominent in some lesions.[47,48] Cytokine expression in macrophagic cells has been shown in one study.[49] In addition to external radiotherapy, brachytherapy of tumours is also associated with focal damage and may produce space occupying radionecrosis.[50,51]

The discrimination between late development of radionecrosis and recurrent tumour may be problematic. Functional imaging by positron emission tomography is an important tool that is capable of discriminating between recurrent tumour and focal radiation necrosis

with positive and negative predictive values for tumour of 80–90%.[43] In some cases, the use of magnetic resonance spectroscopy can reduce the need for biopsy in difficult cases.[52] Surgical intervention is such cases may be required to debulk a lesion to control raised intracranial pressure. Alternatively, biopsy may be indicated in cases of diagnostic uncertainty to ascertain whether recurrent tumour is present. An intraoperative opinion may be sought by a surgeon. It is reasonable to rely on smear preparations when the finding is of high cellularity tumour, of a similar pattern to that encountered in previous biopsies. However, the finding of necrotic tissue associated with sparse, pleomorphic cells poses difficult interpretive problems and in these circumstances resorting to frozen sections is often helpful.

- Radionecrosis is suggested by the presence of hyaline vessels and strongly reinforced by finding fibrinoid necrosis in vessel walls (Fig. 20.22). Pleomorphic, hyperchromatic cells are seen in low density and there is no evidence of mitotic activity (Fig. 20.23).
- Necrotic, high grade tumour is suggested by an absence of the vascular changes seen in radionecrosis and the presence of pleomorphic, hyperchromatic cells in focal clusters around surviving vessels (Fig. 20.24). The finding of mitotic figures in atypical cells is a feature that suggests tumour rather than radionecrosis.

Diffuse late radiation injury to the brain is seen as low attenuation regions seen in periventricular white matter on CT imaging or high signal on T2-weighted MRIs. Many patients with these features are asymptomatic but some show progressive cognitive decline. Cerebral atrophy, shown as dilatation of the temporal horns, neighbouring cisterns and Sylvian fissures may be seen on imaging but this is of uncertain clinical significance.[43,53,54] Histology

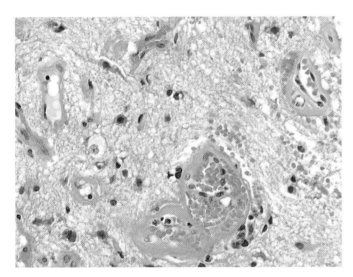

Fig. 20.23 **Radiation necrosis histology.** Vascular changes with plump 'activated' endothelial cells associated with vascular hyalinisation and fibrinoid change. H & E.

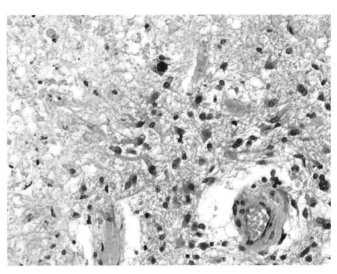

Fig. 20.24 **Residual glioblastoma.** This biopsy shows residual nectrotic high grade astroglial tumour, with no changes suggestive of radiation necrosis. H & E.

shows local spongy demyelination with loss of the oligodendroglia and astrocytic gliosis together with hyalinisation of vessels.[48,55] In one series, affected patients developed progressive dementia, ataxia and urinary incontinence causing severe disability within a median of 14 months after treatment, leading to death in 7 cases. Cortical atrophy and low attenuation lesions in white matter were seen with contrast enhancing lesions in a small proportion of patients, correlating with areas of radionecrosis on biopsy. Post-mortem examination in two patients showed diffuse oedema of hemispheric white matter with no evidence of tumour recurrence.[54] In other pathological descriptions histology has suggested two main patterns of reaction:

1. Diffuse loss of axons and myelin from white matter, associated with multiple small foci of necrosis disseminated in white matter;
2. Diffuse spongiform vacuolation of white matter.[56]

Irradiation of the brain in early childhood is associated with progressive cognitive deficits. Additionally, growth hormone impairment is a common form of neuro-endocrinologic dysfunction.[57]

Radiation induced telangiectatic lesions may develop in the irradiated brain. These may be seen as focal or multifocal hypointense lesions on T2-weighted MRIs. Histological correlation with imaging has shown that these lesions consist of ectatic thin walled vessels surrounded by hemosiderin and gliosis.[58] Lacunes may also be caused by radiotherapy induced vasculopathy in children with brain tumours, with the most significant predictor being age less than 5 years at the time of radiotherapy.[59] Late radiation injury of large arteries may cause an obliterative angiopathy, leading to cerebral

ischaemic changes and is an occasional cause of post-radiation cerebral injury that may have a latency of up to 20 years. Histology of these lesions mimics accelerated focal arteriosclerosis.[60-67] Aneurysmal lesions are also described as a late complication of radiation therapy.[68-70]

Radiation myelopathy Radiation myelopathy is a serious potential complication associated with radiation therapy either directly to the spinal cord or sustained by the spinal cord when adjacent lesions are irradiated.[36] Clinically the most common syndromes are acute transient radiation myelopathy and chronic progressive radiation myelitis.[71,72] Cord damage is related to a number of factors including radiation fraction size, total dose, treatment time, co-administration of chemotherapy, and the area of cord irradiated.[71,73-77] Several cases have been attributed to accidental administration of high radiation doses. It has been suggested that the 5% documented incidence of radiation myelopathy probably lies between 5700 and 6100 cGy to the spinal cord in the absence of dose modifying chemotherapy.[36]

Cell biological aspects that may relate to pathogenesis of myelopathy include effects on vessels, effects on glial cells and involvement of local growth factors.[78] Damage to white matter and vascular damage appear to be separate phenomena that may independently contribute to the development of radiation myelopathy in animal models.[79] Myelopathy of the lumbar cord has been found to have a shorter latent period compared to the cervical cord. The latent period from irradiation to clinical features of myelopathy is short in re-treated patients and paediatric or adolescent age groups.[75]

Findings on imaging vary according to the duration from onset of clinical signs. In one series, when imaging was performed within 8 months following the onset of the myelopathy, cord enlargement was usually encountered, but when patients were evaluated more than 8 months after clinical onset, cord atrophy was always seen. The main focus of cord damage was nearly always included within the irradiated cord segment.[80–82] Aseptic vertebral necrosis due to irradiation has been noted in association with a spinal cord lesion.[83]

Macroscopically, affected cord is generally atrophic but may be swollen in cases where death has taken place within about 8 months of clinical features becoming evident. In the irradiated area mineralisation, foamy macrophages and swollen astrocytes are commonly seen in the white matter associated with variable myelin loss. Hyalinisation of the walls of intramedullary vessels may also be present. Less commonly, fibrinoid necrosis of vessels and necrosis of the cord may be seen, often correlating with cord swelling. In some longstanding cases the affected region of cord is reduced to a soft, partly cystic gliotic ribbon devoid of myelin, axons and neurons.[84–88] Wallerian degeneration of relevant tracts is seen above and below areas of focal damage. Radiation lesions in the spinal cord have been classified into three groups:[89]

- type 1 – primarily white matter parenchymal lesions;
- type 2 – primarily vascular lesions;
- type 3 – combination of vascular and white matter lesions.

Factors affecting survival following irradiation myelopathy are the level of the lesion, the age of the patient and the latent period of the injury.[90]

Radiation optic neuropathy and other cranial nerve palsies Radiation optic neuropathy is a cause of visual loss following radiotherapy. Diagnostic criteria include acute visual loss (monocular or binocular), visual field defects indicating optic nerve or chiasmal dysfunction, absence of optic disc oedema, onset usually within 3 years of therapy (peak: 1–$1\frac{1}{2}$ years), and no CT evidence of visual pathway compression.[91]

Of the other cranial nerves that may develop radiation induced palsy following treatment of head and neck tumours, the twelfth nerve is commonest, involved alone or in combination with multiple nerves.[92,93]

Post-irradiation tumours Therapeutic irradiation is known to confer an increased risk of subsequent development of neoplasia.[94] Cranial irradiation is associated with a variety of secondary tumours, discussed in other specific sections of this book. The commonest tumours that arise following cranial radiotherapy are meningiomas and sarcomas but other tumours including gliomas and primary neuroectodermal tumours are described.[94–104] Spinal cord gliomas have also been reported following irradiation, many of which have an aggressive clinical course.[105] In a study on meningiomas arising after radiotherapy, the average time from therapy to diagnosis was

24 years (range 5 to 40 years). The latency of meningioma formation appeared to be influenced by both the radiation dose and the age of the patient at irradiation.[95] Following radiotherapy for pituitary lesions, one study has shown gliomas arising with a latency of 8–15 years after therapy. The cumulative actuarial risk of secondary glioma after radiation therapy was 1.7% at 10 years and 2.7% at 15 years.[106] Homozygous *TP53* gene mutation in a radiation induced glioblastoma has been documented 10 years after treatment for an intracranial germ cell tumour.[107]

Chemotherapy

Chemotherapy, either for treatment of brain tumours or tumours elsewhere, is recognised to cause complications in the nervous system.[108–111]

Complicated migraine-like episodes characterised by severe intermittent unilateral headaches, nausea, episodic visual loss, hemiparesis, aphasia, or hemisensory loss have been described in children following cranial irradiation and chemotherapy as a complication of therapy, but the pathological basis for this is unknown.[112]

Clinical or subclinical necrotising leucoencephalopathy has been described in patients after treatment for malignancy with cranial radiation therapy and parenteral or intrathecal chemotherapy, especially involving methotrexate (Figs 20.25–20.28).[113–118] Brain stem necrosis has also been described.[119] Chemotherapy in combination with radiotherapy has been implicated in a dementia syndrome in adults following treatment of CNS tumours.[56] It has been suggested that radiation opens the BBB, allowing high concentrations of parenteral drug to reach the nervous system.[120] In experimental models, radiation followed by chemotherapy has been shown to be associated with a higher risk of toxic effects.[121]

Leucoencephalopathy, characterised by white matter necrosis, also develops following chemotherapy alone with a variety of agents including BCNU, cisplatin, cytarabine, 5-fluorouracil, ifosfamide, L-asparaginase, methotrexate, procarbazine, corticosteroids, tegafur, interferon, interleukin-2.[122–126] Pathology of biopsy samples in cases following administration of 5-fluorouracil and levamisole has been investigated. Histology showed active demyelinating disease with sparing of axons associated with perivascular lymphocytic inflammation. Numerous macrophages were present both around vessels as well as in white matter.[127] MRI is a sensitive tool for detection of white matter changes in this condition.[128] Reversible posterior leucoencephalopathy has been described with several agents.[129–131]

Post-mortem examination of the brain has been described in six patients who had received chemo/radiotherapy and in whom a decrease in white matter density was seen on CT scan. Two of these cases were histologically normal, two cases showed some white

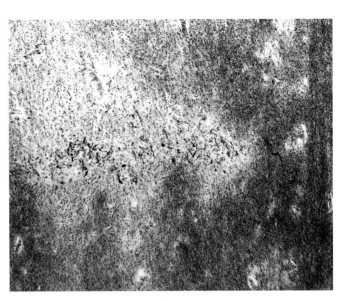

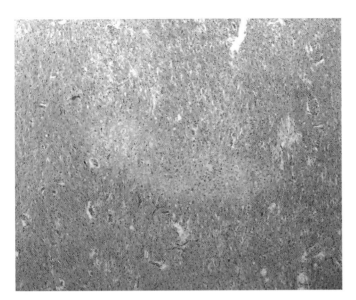

Fig. 20.25 **Necrotising leucoencephalopathy.** At low magnification white matter pallor can be seen in which the basophilic stippling of mineralisation can just be seen. H & E.

Fig. 20.26 **Necrotising leucoencephalopathy.** The same area stained with Luxol fast blue shows myelin loss and highlights the focal mineralisation.

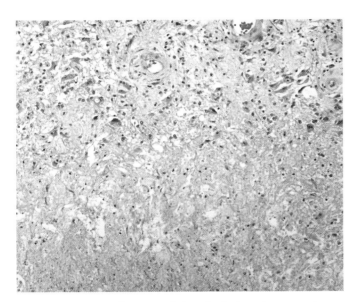

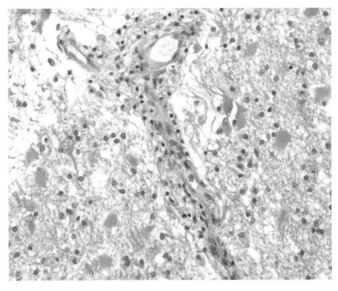

Fig. 20.27 **Necrotising leucoencephalopathy.** Lesions show necrosis (bottom) bounded by a zone containing reactive astrocytic cells and foamy macrophages. H & E.

Fig. 20.28 **Necrotising leucoencephalopathy.** Other areas show lymphocytic aggregates around vessels with both myelin and axonal loss, associated with florid reactive astrocytic gliosis. H & E.

matter rarefaction, one case contained multiple foci of white matter and vessel wall necrosis.[132]

Intra-arterial chemotherapy for brain tumour treatment has been advocated as a therapeutic option.[133] Intracarotid BCNU can result in a severe leucoencephalopathy similar to that seen with methotrexate or delayed radionecrosis.[117,134–136] However, recent series have reported few complications.[133,137–139]

In children with central nervous system neoplasia who have undergone cranial irradiation, or radiation combined with chemotherapy, delayed intracranial haemorrhage may develop.[140]

Complications have been described following intraventricular chemotherapy using an Ommaya reservoir and intraventricular catheter system used to treat patients with leptomeningeal metastases combined with radiotherapy. In this series the most common problem was catheter infection, and serious complications requiring surgery were infrequent (6%). Aseptic meningitis affected 43% of patients.[141] Ommaya devices may be associated with development of pericatheter white matter lesions, seen on CT scan as focal areas of lucency sometimes with contrast enhancement and/or mass effect. These changes, which may be associated with clinical signs in some cases, appear to be related to back flow of CSF into peri-ventricular white matter and resolve with removal of the catheter.[142] Malfunctioning devices can also be associated with leucoencephalopathy.[143]

Myelopathy may complicate intrathecal treatment with a variety of chemotherapeutic agents. It is also potentiated by radiotherapy.[77,118,144] Anterior lumbosacral radiculopathy has been described as a complication associated with intrathecal methotrexate treatment.[145] A severe myelopathy is seen following inadvertent intrathecal administration of vincristine.[146] At present, CSF lavage is the only treatment for intrathecal vincristine injection.[147] Inadvertent intrathecal injection of daunorubicin with a fatal outcome has also been described.[148]

Steroid complications Corticosteroids are commonly used in neurosurgical practice, especially in the management of cerebral oedema in relation to tumours and post-radiation effects. With the dosages and duration of therpy required in clinical management, side-effects of therapy are common. Steroid myopathy is the most frequently occurring serious complication seen in neuro-oncology patients, others include gastrointestinal haemorrhage, opportunistic infections, secondary diabetes, and the emotional distress caused by cushingoid skin and facial changes induced by steroids.[149]

REFERENCES

Raised intracranial pressure and oedema

1. Constantini S, Cotev S, Rappaport ZH et al. Intracranial pressure monitoring after elective intracraniani surgery. A retrospective study of 514 consecutive patients. J Neurosurg, 1988; 69(4):540–544
2. Roy S, Sarkar C. Ultrastructural study of micro-blood vessels in human brain tumours and peritumoral tissue. J Neurooncol, 1989; 7(3):283–292
3. Shibata S, Jinnouchi T, Mori K. Brain edema in delayed radiation necrosis: study of capillary ultrastructure – case report. Neurol Med Chir, 1989; 29(1):44–47
4. Castejon OJ. Electron microscopic study of capillary wall in human cerebral edema. J Neuropath Exp Neurol, 1980; 39(3):296–328
5. Hurter T. Experimental brain tumours and edema in rats. II. Tumor edema. Exp Pathol, 1984; 26(1):41–48
6. Groger U, Huber P, Reulen HJ. Formation and resolution of human peritumoral brain edema. Acta Neurochir, (Suppl), 1994; 60:373–374
7. Bodsch W, Rommel T, Ophoff BG et al. Factors responsible for the retention of fluid in human tumour edema and the effect of dexamethasone. J Neurosurg, 1987; 67(2):250–257
8. Strugar J, Rothbart D, Harrington W et al. Vascular permeability factor in brain metastases: correlation with vasogenic brain edema and tumor angiogenesis. J Neurosurg, 1994; 81(4):560–566
9. Heiss JD, Papavassiliou E, Merrill MJ et al. Mechanism of dexamethasone suppression of brain tumor-associated vascular permeability in rats. Involvement of the glucocorticoid receptor and vascular permeability factor. J Clin Invest, 1996; 98(6):1400–1408
10. Goldman CK, Bharara S, Palmer CA et al. Brain edema in meningiomas is associated with increased vascular endothelial growth factor expression. Neurosurgery, 1997; 40(6):1269–1277
11. Provias J, Claffey K, delAguila L et al. Meningiomas: role of vascular endothelial growth factor/vascular permeability factor in angiogenesis and peritumoral edema. Neurosurgery, 1997; 40(5):1016–1026
12. Cloughesy TF, Black KL. Pharmacological blood-brain barrier modification for selective drug delivery, [Review] [39 refs]. J Neurooncol, 1995; 26(2):125–132
13. Constantini S, Tamir J, Gomori MJ et al. Tumor prostaglandin levels correlate with edema around supratentorial meningiomas. Neurosurgery, 1993; 33(2):204–210; discussion 211
14. Lee ST, Hsueh S. Cerebral edema associated with meningioma. Can J Neuro Sci, 1989; 16(2):211–213
15. Adair JC, Baldwin N, Kornfeld M et al. Radiation-included blood-brain barrier damage in astrocytoma: relation to elevated gelatinase B and urokinase. J Neurooncol, 1999; 44(3):283–289
16. Bitzer M, Wockel L, Luft AR et al. The importance of pial blood supply to the development of peritumoral brain edema in meningiomas. J Neurosurg, 1997; 87(3):368–373
17. Yoshioka H, Hama S, Taniguchi E et al. Peritumoral brain edema associated with meningioma: influence of vascular endothelial growth factor expression and vascular blood supply. Cancer, 1999; 85(4):936–944
18. Ide M, Jimbo M, Yamamoto M et al. MIB-1 staining index and peritumoral brain edema of meningiomas. Cancer, 1996; 78(1):133–143
19. Bitzer M, Topka H, Morgalla M et al. Tumor-related venous obstruction and development of peritumoral of brain edema in meningiomas. Neurosurgery, 1998; 42(4):730–737
20. Kida S, Ellison DW, Steart PV et al. Perivascular edema fluid pathway in astrocytic tumors. Acta Neurochir (Suppl), 1994; 60:384–386
21. Lohle PN, Verhagen IT, Teelken AW et al. The pathogenesis of cerebral gliomatous cysts. Neurosurgery, 1992; 30(2):180–185
22. Lohle PN, Wurzer HA, Seelen PJ et al. The pathogenesis of cysts accompanying intra-axial primary and metastatic tumors of the central nervous system. J Neurooncol, 1998; 40(3):277–285
23. Raimondi AJ, Tomita T. Hydrocephalus and infratentorial tumors. Incidence, clinical picture, and treatment. J Neurosurg, 1981; 55(2):174–182

Effects of biopsy and surgery

24. Bernstein M, Parrent AG. Complications of CT-guided stereotactic biopsy of intra-axial brain lesions. J Neurosurg, 1994; 81(2):165–168
25. Sawin PD. Hitchon PW, Follett KA et al. Computed imaging-assisted stereotactic brain biopsy: a risk analysis of 225 consecutive cases. Surg Neurol, 1998; 49(6):640–649
26. Whittle IR, Viswanathan R. Acute intraoperative brain herniation during elective neurosurgery: pathophysiology and management considerations. J Neurol Neurosurg Psychiatry, 1996; 61(6):584–590
27. Hall WA. The safety and efficacy of stereotactic biopsy for intracranial lesions. Cancer, 1998; 82(9):1749–1755
28. Levy RM, Wilson CB. Contralateral intracerebral hemorrhage as a complication of tumor biopsy. Surg Neurol, 1987; 27(4):386–390
29. Fritsch MJ, Leber MJ, Gossett L et al. Stereotactic biopsy of intracranial brain lesions. High diagnostic yield without increased complications: 65 consecutive biopsies with early postoperative CT scans. Stereotact Funct Neurosurg, 1998; 71(1):36–42
30. Sahrakar K, Boggan JE, Salamat MS. Traumatic aneurysm: a complication of stereotactic brain biopsy: case report. Neurosurgery, 1995; 36(4):842–846
31. Voges J, Schroder R, Treuer H et al. CT-guided and computer assisted stereotactic biopsy. Technique, results, indications. Acta Neurochir, 1993; 125(1–4):142–149
32. Pattisapu JV, Walker ML, Heilbrun MP. Stereotactic surgery in children. Pediatr Neurosci, 1989; 15(2):62–65
33. Auer LM, Holzer P, Ascher PW et al. Endoscopic neurosurgery. Acta Neurochir, 1988; 90(1–2):1–14

Effects of radiotherapy

34. Plowman PN. Stereotactic radiosurgery. VIII. The classification of postirradiation reactions. Br J Neurosurg, 1999; 13(3):256–264
35. Vallee B, Malhaire JP, Person H et al. Delayed cerebral pseudo-tumoral radionecrosis following scalp-tumour irradiation. Case report and review of literature. J Neurol, 1984; 231(3):135–140

36. Schultheiss TE, Kun LE, Ang KK et al. Radiation response of the central nervous system [published erratum appears in Int. J Radiat Oncol Biol Phys, 1995 Jul 15; 32(4):1269]. Int J Radiat Oncol Biol Phys, 1995; 31(5):1093–1112

37. Crossen JR, Garwood D. Glatstein E et al. Neurobehavioral sequelae of cranial irradiation in adults: a review of radiation-induced encephalopathy. J Clin Oncol, 1994; 12(3):627–642

38. Alexander E 3rd, Loeffler JS. Radiosurgery for primary malignant brain tumors. [Review] [49 refs]. Semin Surg Oncol, 1998; 14(1):43–52

39. Young RF. Radiosurgery for the treatment of brain metastases. Semin Surg Oncol, 1998; 14(1):70–78

40. Grabb PA, Lunsford LD, Albright AL et al. Stereotactic radiosurgery for glial neoplasms of childhood. Neurosurgery, 1996; 38(4):696–701; discussion 701–702

41. Kondziolka D, Flickinger JC. Perez B. Judicions resection and/or radiosurgery for parasagittal meningiomas: outcomes from a multicenter review. Gamma Knife Meningioma Study Group. Neurosurgery, 1998; 43(3):405–413; discussion 413–414

42. Kalapurakal JA, Silverman CL, Akhtar N et al. Intracranial meningiomas: factors that influence the development of cerebral edema after stereotactic radiosurgery and radiation therapy. Radiology, 1997; 204(2):461–465

43. Valk PE, Dillon WP. Radiation injury of the brain. [Review] [90 refs]. AJNR Am J Neuroradiol, 1991; 12(1):45–62

44. Martins AN, Severance RE; Henry JM et al. Experimental delayed radiation necrosis of the brain. Part 1: Effect of early dexamethasone treatment. J Neurosurg, 1979; 51(5):587–596

45. Yoshii Y, Phillips TL. Late vascular effect of whole brain X-irradiation in the mouse. Acta Neurochir, 1982; 64(1–2):87–102

46. Safdari H, Boluix B, Gros C. Multifocal brain radionecrosis masquerading as tumor dissemination. Surg Neurol, 1984; 21(1):35–41

47. Husain MM, Garcia JH. Cerebral 'radiation necrosis': vascular and glial features. Acta Neuropathol, 1976; 36(4):381–385

48. Jellinger K. Human central nervous system lesions following radiation therapy. Zentralbl Neurochir, 1977; 38(2):199–200

49. Kureshi SA, Hofman FM, Schneider JH et al. Cytokine expression in radiation-induced delayed cerebral injury. Neurosurgery, 1994; 35(5):822–829; discussion 829–830

50. Moringlane JR, Voges M, Huber G et al. Short-term CT and MR changes in brain tumours following 125I interstitial irradiation. J Comput Assist Tomogr, 1997; 21(1):15–21

51. Oppenheimer JH, Levy ML, Sinha U et al. Radionecrosis secondary to interstitial brachytherapy: correlation of magnetic resonance imaging and histopatholgy. Neurosurgery, 1992; 31(2):336–343

52. Lin A, Bluml S, Mamelak, AN. Efficacy of proton magnetic resonance spectroscopy in clinical decision making for patients with suspected malignant brain tumors. J Neurooncol, 1999; 45(1):69–81

53. Hu JQ, Guan YH, Zhao LZ et al. Delayed radiation encephalopathy after radiotherapy for nasopharyngeal cancer: a CT study of 45 cases. J Comput Assist Tomogr, 1991; 15(2):181–187

54. DeAngelis LM, Delattre JY, Posner JB. Radiation-induced dementia in patients cured of brain metastases. Neurology, 1989; 39(6):789–796

55. Schiffer D, Soffietti R, Giordana MT et al. Tissue alterations induced by radio- and chemotherapy in brain with malignant gliomas. Acta Neuropathol (Supp); 1981; 7:109–110

56. Vigliani MC, Duyckaerts C, Hauw JJ et al. Dementia following treatment of brain tumors with radiotherapy administered alone or in combination with nitrosourea-based chemotherapy: a clinical and pathological study. J Neurooncol, 1999; 41(2):137–149

57. Packer RJ. Meadows AT, Rorke LB et al. Long-term sequelae of cancer treatment on the central nervous system in childhood. Med Pediatr Oncol, 1987; 15(5):241–253

58. Gaensler EH, Dillon WP, Edwards MS et al. Radiation-induced telangiectasia in the brain simulates cryptic vascular malformations at MR imaging. Radiology, 1994; 193(3):629–636

59. Fouladi M, Langston J, Mulhern R et al. Silent lacunar lesions detected by magnetic resonance imaging of children with brain tumors: a late sequela of therapy. J Clin Oncol, 2000; 18(4):824–831

60. Murros KE, Toole JF. The effect of radiation on carotid arteries. A review article. Arch Neurol, 1989; 46(4):449–455

61. Mitchell WG, Fishman LS, Miller JH et al. Stroke as a late sequela of cranial irradiation for childhood brain tumors. J Child Neurol, 1991; 6(2):128–133

62. Brant-Zawadzki M, Anderson M, DeArmond SJ et al. Radiation-induced large intracranial vessel occlusive vasculopathy. AJR Am J Roentgenol, 1980; 134(1):51–55

63. Montanera W, Chui M, Hudson A. Meningioma and occlusive vasculopathy: coexisting complications of past extracranial radiation. Surg Neurol, 1985; 24(1):35–39

64. Grenier Y, Tomita T, Marymont MH et al. Late postirradiation occlusive vasculopathy in childhood medulloblastoma. Report of two cases. J Neurosurg, 1998; 89(3):460–464

65. Hirata Y, Matsukado Y, Mihara Y et al. Occlusion of the internal carotid artery after radiation therapy for the chiasmal lesion. Acta Neurochir, 1985; 74(3–4):141–147

66. Hayashida K, Nishimura T, Imakita S et al. Embolic stroke following carotid radiation angiopathy demonstrated with I-123 IMP brain SPECT. Clin Nucl Med, 1991; 16(8):580–582

67. Horimoto M, Kodama N, Takamatsu H. Bilateral internal carotid artery disease secondary to cervical radiation. A case report. Angiology, 1996; 47(6):609–613

68. Benson PJ, Sung JH. Cerebral aneurysms following radiotherapy for medulloblastoma. J Neurosurg, 1989; 70(4):545–550

69. Girishkumar HT, Sivakumar M, Andaz S et al. Pseudo-aneurysm of the carotid bifurcation secondary to radiation. J Cardiovasc Surg, 1999; 40(6):877–888

70. Casey AT, Marsh HT, Uttley D. Intracranial aneurysm formation following radiotherapy. Br J Neurosurg, 1993; 7(5):575–579

71. Rampling R, Symonds P. Radiation myelopathy. Curr Opin Neurol, 1998; 11(6):627–632

72. Schultheiss TE, Stephens LC. Invited review: permanent radiation myelopathy. Br J Radiol, 1992; 65(777):737–753

73. Lavey RS, Taylor JM, Tward JD et al. The extent, time course, and fraction size dependence of mouse spinal cord recovery from radiation injury. Int J Radiat Oncol Biol Phys, 1994; 30(3):609–617

74. Macbeth FR, Wheldon TE, Girling DJ et al. Radiation myelopathy: estimates of risk in 1048 patients in three randomized trials of palliative radiotherapy for non-small cell lung cancer. The Medical Research Council Lung Cancer Working Party. Clin Oncol, (Royal College of Radiologists) 1996; 8(3):176–181

75. Schultheiss TE, Higgins EM, El-Mahdi AM. The latent period in clinical radiation myelopathy. [Review] [87 refs]. Int J Radiat Oncol Biol Phys, 1984; 10(7):1109–1115

76. Goldwein JW. Radiation myelopathy: a review. Med Pediatr Oncol, 1987; 15(2):89–95

77. Watterson J, Toogood I, Nieder M et al. Excessive spinal cord toxicity from intensive central nervous system-directed therapies. Cancer, 1994; 74(11):3034–3041

78. Nieder C, Ataman F, Price RE et al. Radiation myelopathy: new perspective on an old problem. Radiat Oncol Invest, 1999; 7(4):193–203

79. Ruifrok AC, Stephens LC, van der Kogel AJ. Radiation response of the rat cervical spinal cord after irradiation at different ages: tolerance, latency and pathology. Int J Radiat Oncol Biol, Phys, 1994; 29(1):73–79

80. Melki PS, Halimi P, Wibault P et al. MRI in chronic progressive radiation myelopathy. J Comput Assist Tomogr, 1994; 18(1):1–6

81. Wang PY, Shen WC, Jan JS. MR imaging in radiation myelopathy. AJNR Am J Neuroradiol, 1992; 13(4):1049–1055; discussion 1056–1058

82. Wang PY, Shen WC, Jan JS. Serial MRI changes in radiation myelopathy. Neuroradiology, 1995; 37(5):374–377

83. Martin D, Delacollette M, Collignon J et al. Radiation-induced myelopathy and vertebral necrosis. Neuroradiology, 1994; 36(5):405–407

84. Koehler PJ, Verbiest H, Jager J et al. Delayed radiation myelopathy: serial MR-imaging and pathology. Clin Neurol Neurosurg, 1996; 98(2):197–201

85. Jellinger K, Sturm KW. Delayed radiation myelopathy in man. Report of twelve necropsy cases. J Neurol Sci, 1971; 14(4):389–408

86. Howel DA. Radiation myelopathy. Dev Med Child Neurol, 1979; 21(5):653–656

87. Godwin-Austen RB, Howell DA, Worthington B. Observations on radiation myelopathy. Brain, 1975; 98(4):557–568

88. Godwin-Austen RB, Howell DA, Worthington BS. Proceedings: A combined clinico-pathological and radiological study of radiation myelopathy. Br J Radiol, 1975; 48(571):608–609

89. Schultheiss TE, Stephens LC, Maor MH. Analysis of the histopathology of radiation myelopathy. Int J Radiat Oncol Biol Phys 1988; 14(1):27–32

90. Schultheiss TE, Stephens LC, Peters LJ. Survival in radiation myelopathy. Int J Radiat Oncol Biol Phys, 1986; 12(10):1765–1769

91. Kline LB, Kim JY, Ceballos R. Radiation optic neuropathy. Ophthalmology, 1985; 92(8):1118–1126

92. Berger PS, Bataini JP. Radiation-induced cranial nerve palsy. Cancer, 1977; 40(1):152–155

93. Amato AA, Collins MP. Neuropathies associated with malignancy. Semin Neurol, 1998; 18(1):125–144

94. Cavin LW, Dalrymple GV, McGuire EL et al. CNS tumor induction by radiotherapy: a report of four new cases and estimate of dose required. Int J Radiat Oncol Biol Phys, 1990; 18(2):399–406

95. Mack EE, Wilson CB. Meningiomas induced by high-dose cranial irradiation. J Neurosurg, 1993; 79(1):28–31

96. Aydin F, Ghatak NR, Leshner RT. Possible radiation-induced dural fibrosarcoma with an unusually short latent period: case report. Neurosurgery, 1995; 36(3):591–594; discussion 594–595

97. Slavik T, Bentley RC, Gray L et al. Solitary fibrous tumor of the meninges occurring after irradiation of a mixed germ cell tumor of the pineal gland. Clin Neuropathol, 1998; 17(1):55–60

98. Shapiro S, Mealey JJ, Sartorius C. Radiation-induced intracranial malignant gliomas. J Neurosurg, 1989; 71(1):77–82

99. Brustle O, Ohgaki H, Schmitt HP et al. Primitive neuroectodermal tumors after prophylactic central nervous system irradiation in children. Association with an activated K-ras gene. Cancer, 1992; 69(9):2385–2392

100. Lee YY, Van Tassel P, Nauert C et al. Craniofacial osteosarcomas: Plain film, CT, and MR findings in 46 cases. AJR Am J Roentgenol, 1988; 150(6):1397–1402

101. Sznajder L, Abrahams C. Parry DM et al. Multiple schwannomas and meningiomas associated with irradiation in childhood. Arch Int Med, 1996; 156(16):1873–1878

102. Barasch ES, Altieri D, Decker RE et al. Primitive neuroectodermal tumor presenting as a delayed sequela to cranial irradiation and intrathecal methotrexate. Pediatr Neurol, 1988; 4(6):375–378

103. Perry JR, Ang LC, Bilbao JM et al. Clinicopathologic features of primary and postirradiation cerebral gliosarcoma. Cancer, 1995; 75(12):2910–2918

104. Tiberin P, Maor E, Zaizov R et al. Brain sarcoma of meningeal origin after cranial irradiation in childhood acute lymphocytic leukemia. Case report. J Neurosurg, 1984; 61(4):772–776

105. Grabb PA, Kelly DR, Fulmer BB et al. Radiation-induced glioma of the spinal cord. Pediatr Neurosurg, 1996; 25(4):214–219

106. Tsang RW, Laperriere NJ, Simpson WJ et al. Glioma arising after radiation therapy for pituitary adenoma. A report of four patients and estimation of risk [published erratum appears in Cancer 1994 Jan 15; 73(2):492]. Cancer, 1993; 72(7):2227–2232

107. Tada M, Sawamura Y, Abe H et al. Homozygous p53 gene mutation in a radiation-induced glioblastoma 10 years after treatment for an intracranial germ cell tumor: case report. Neurosurgery, 1997; 40(2):393–396

Effects of chemotherapy

108. Allen JC. Complications of chemotherapy in patients with brain and spinal cord tumors. Pediatr Neurosurg, 1991; 17(4):218–224

109. Duffner PK, Cohen ME. The long-term effects of central nervous system therapy on children with brain tumors. Neurol Clin, 1991; 9(2):479–495

110. Keime-Guibert F, Napolitano M, Delattre JY. Neurological complications of radiotherapy and chemotherapy. J Neurol, 1998; 245(11):695–708

111. Shapiro WR, Young DF. Neurological complications of antineoplastic therapy. Acta Neurol Scand, 1984 (Suppl 100):125–132

112. Shuper A, Packer RJ, Vezina LG et al. 'Complicated migraine-like episodes' in children following cranial irradiation and chemotherapy. Neurology, 1995; 45(10):1837–1840

113. Allen JC, Thaler HT, Deck MD et al. Leukoencephalopathy following high-dose intravenous methotrexate chemotherapy: quantitative assessment of white matter attenuation using computed tomography. Neuroradiology, 1978; 16:44–47

114. Devivo DC, Malas D, Nelson JS et al. Leukoencephalopathy in childhood leukemia. Neurology, 1977; 27(7):609–613

115. Boogerd W, Sande JJ, Moffie D. Acute fever and delayed leukoencephalopathy following low dose intraventricular methotrexate. J Neurol Neurosurg Psychiatry, 1988; 51(10):1277–1283

116. Glass JP, Lee YY, Bruner J et al. Treatment-related leukoencephalopathy. A study of three cases and literature review. Medicine, 1986; 65(3):154–162

117. Lee YY, Nauert C, Glass JP. Treatment-related white matter changes in cancer patients. Cancer, 1986; 57(8):1473–1482

118. Macdonald DR. Neurologic complications of chemotherapy. Neurol Clin, 1991; 9(4):955–967

119. Watterson J, Simonton SC, Rorke LB et al. Fatal brain stem necrosis after standard posterior fossa radiation and aggressive chemotherapy for metastatic medulloblastoma. Cancer, 1993; 71(12):4111–4117

120. Qin D, Ma J, Xiao J et al. Effect of brain irradiation on blood-CSF barrier permeability of chemotherapeutic agents. Am J Clin Oncol, 1997; 20(3):263–265

121. Remsen LG, McCormick CI, Sexton G et al. Long-term toxicity and neuropathology associated with the sequencing of cranial irradiation and enhanced chemotherapy delivery. Neurosurgery, 1997; 40(5):1034–1040; discussion 1040–1042

122. Freilich RJ, Delattre JY, Monjour A et al. Chemotherapy without radiation therapy as initial treatment for primary CNS lymphoma in older patients [see comments]. Neurology, 1996; 46(2):435–439

123. Gay CT, Bodensteiner JB, Nitschke R et al. Reversible treatment-related leukoencephalopathy. J Child Neurol, 1989; 4(3):208–213

124. Critchley P, Abbott R, Madden FJ. Multifocal inflammatory leukoencephalopathy developing in a patient receiving 5-fluorouracil and levamisole. Clin Oncol (Royal College of Radiologists), 1994; 6(6):406

125. Kimmel DW, Schutt AJ. Multifocal leukoencephalopathy: occurrence during 5-fluorouracil and levamisole therapy and resolution after discontinuation of chemotherapy. Mayo Clin Proc, 1993; 68(4):363–365

126. Lovblad K, Kelkar P, Ozdoba C et al. Pure methotrexate encephalopathy presenting with seizures: CT and MRI features. Pediatr Radiol, 1998; 28(2):86–91

127. Hook CC, Kimmel DW, Kvols LK et al. Multifocal inflammatory leukoencephalopathy with 5-fluorouracil and levamisole. Ann Neurol, 1992; 31(3):262–267

128. Atlas SW, Grossman RI, Packer RJ et al. Magnetic resonance imaging diagnosis of disseminated necrotizing leukoencephalopathy. J Comput Assist Tomogr, 1987; 11(1):39–43

129. Ito Y, Arahata Y, Goto Y et al. Cisplatin neurotoxicity presenting as reversible posterior leukoencephalopathy syndrome. AJNR Am J Neuroradiol, 1998; 19(3):415–417

130. Lewis MB, Cyclosporin neurotoxicity after chemotherapy. Cyclosporin causes reversible posterior leukoencephalopathy syndrome. Br Med J, 1999; 319(7201):54–55

131. Pavlakis SG, Frank Y, Chusid R. Hypertensive encephalopathy, reversible occipitoparietal encephalopathy, or reversible posterior leukoencephalopathy: three names for an old syndrome. J Child Neurol, 1999; 14(5):277–281

132. Wang AM, Skias DD, Rumbaugh CL et al. Central nervous system changes after radiation therapy and/or chemotherapy: correlation of CT and autopsy findings. AJNR Am J Neuroradiol, 1983; 4(3):466–471

133. Gelman M, Chakeres DW, Newton HB. Brain tumors: complications of cerebral angiography accompanied by intraarterial chemotherapy. Radiology, 1999; 213(1):135–140

134. Kleinschmidt-DeMasters BK. Intracarotid BCNU leukoencephalopathy. Cancer, 1986; 57(7):1276–1280

135. Kleinschmidt-DeMasters BK, Geier JM. Pathology of high-dose intraarterial BCNU. Surg Neurol, 1989; 31(6):435–443

136. Cohen ME, Duffner PK, Terplan KL. Myelopathy with severe structural derangement associated with combined modality therapy. Cancer, 1983; 52(9):1590–1596

137. Watne K, Nome O, Hager B et al. Combined intra-arterial chemotherapy and irradiation of malignant gliomas. Acta Oncol, 1991; 30(7):835–841

138. Watne K, Hannisdal E, Nome O et al. Combined intra-arterial chemotherapy followed by radiation in astrocytomas. J Neurooncol, 1992; 14(1):73–80

139. Watne K, Hannisdal E, Nome O et al. Prognostic factors in malignant gliomas with special reference to intra-arterial chemotherapy. Acta Oncol, 1993; 32(3):307–310

140. Poussaint TY, Siffert J, Barnes PD et al. Hemorrhagic vasculopathy after treatment of central nervous system neoplasia in childhood: diagnosis and follow-up. AJNR Am J Neuroradiol, 1995; 16(4):693–699

141. Chamberlain MC, Kormanik PA, Barba D. Complications associated with intraventricular chemotherapy in patients with leptomeningeal metastases. J Neurosurg, 1997; 87(5):694–699

142. Lemann W, Wiley RG, Posner JB. Leukoencephalopathy complicating intraventricular catheters: clinical, radiographic and pathologic study of 10 cases. J Neurooncol, 1988; 6(1):67–74

143. Stone JA, Castillo M, Mukherji SK. Leukoencephalopathy complicating an Ommaya reservoir and chemotherapy. Neuroradiology, 1999; 41(2):134–136

144. Lopez-Andreu JA, Ferris J, Verdeguer A et al. Myelopathy after intrathecal chemotherapy: a case report with unique magnetic resonance imaging changes. Cancer, 1995; 75(5):1216–1217

145. Koh S, Nelson MD, Jr, Kovanlikaya A et al. Anterior lumbosacral radiculopathy after intrathecal methotrexate treatment. Pediatr Neurol, 1999; 21(2):576–578

146. Williams ME, Walker AN, Bracikowski JP et al. Ascending myeloencephalopathy due to intrathecal vincristine sulfate. A fatal chemotherapeutic error. Cancer, 1983; 51(11):2041–2047

147. Al Ferayan A, Russell NA, Al Wohaibi M et al. Cerebrospinal fluid lavage in the treatment of inadvertent intrathecal vincristine injection. Childs Nerv Syst, 1999; 15(2–3):87–89

148. Mortensen ME, Cecalupo AJ, Lo WD et al. Inadvertent intrathecal injection of Daunorubicin with fatal outcome. Med Pediatr Oncol, 1992; 20(3):249–253

149. Koehler PJ. Use of corticosteroids in neuro-oncology. Anticancer Drugs 1995; 6(1):19–33

Index

W

Waldenstrom's macroglobulinaemia, 307
Western blot, 8, 9
WHO grading system, 75–6
Wyburn–Mason syndrome *see* mesencephalo-
oculo-facial angiomatosis

X

xanthoastrocytoma, 12, 30
see also pleomorphic xanthoastrocytoma

Y

yolk sac tumour, 285–6